# Key Features

## Teaching TIPS

## healthy people 2010

## A view from the field

# CONGRATULATIONS
## You now have access to Mosby's "Get Connected" Bonus Package!

### Here's what's included to help you "Get Connected":

**sign on at:**

http://www.mosby.com/MERLIN/Clemen-Stone/

A website just for you as you learn community health nursing with the new 6th edition of **Comprehensive Community Health Nursing: Family, Aggregate, and Community Practice**

**what you will receive:**

Whether you're a student, an instructor, or a clinician, you'll find information just for you, such as:
- Content Updates
- Links to Related Products
- Author Information...and More

**plus:**

 **WebLinks**

An exciting new program that allows you to directly access hundreds of active websites keyed specifically to the content of this book. The WebLinks are continually updated and new ones are added as they develop.

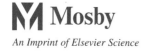 **Mosby**

*An Imprint of Elsevier Science*

www.mosby.com

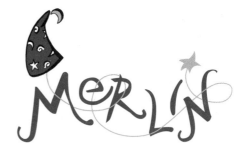

**M**osby's **E**lectronic **R**esource **L**inks & **I**nformation **N**etwork

COMPREHENSIVE
# COMMUNITY
## HEALTH NURSING

*Family, Aggregate, & Community Practice*

The logo for the book, interconnecting systems and subsystems, highlights a major focus in community health nursing practice—helping clients bring together in a meaningful way all the forces in their environment that influence their health and quality of life. Clients served by community health nurses, including individuals, families, populations at risk, and communities, frequently encounter forces that impede or facilitate growth. Community health nurses are uniquely positioned to help clients understand these forces and to mobilize community partnerships for the purpose of developing healthy, nurturing environments.

# COMPREHENSIVE
# COMMUNITY
# HEALTH NURSING

## *Family, Aggregate, & Community Practice*

**Susan Clemen-Stone, RN, MPH**

Associate Professor
University of Michigan
Community Health Nursing
Division of Health Promotion and Risk Reduction Programs
School of Nursing
Ann Arbor, Michigan

**Sandra L. McGuire, RN, EdD**

Associate Professor
University of Tennessee
College of Nursing
Knoxville, Tennessee

**Diane Gerber Eigsti, RN, MS**

Food Net Coordinator/Surveillance Officer
Tennessee Department of Health
Communicable and Environmental Disease Services
Nashville, Tennessee

**SIXTH EDITION**

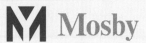

*An Imprint of Elsevier Science*

St. Louis   London   Philadelphia   Sydney   Toronto

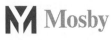

*An Imprint of Elsevier Science*

*Vice President and Publishing Director, Nursing:* Sally Schrefer
*Executive Editor:* Darlene Como
*Managing Editor:* Brian Dennison
*Publishing Services Manager:* Catherine Jackson
*Project Manager:* Marc P. Syp
*Design Manager:* Amy Buxton

Mosby, Inc.
*An Imprint of Elsevier Science*
11830 Westline Industrial Drive
St. Louis, Missouri 63146

Printed in the United States of America

**ISBN 0-323-01345-7**

02 03 04 05 06 GW/RRDW 9 8 7 6 5 4 3 2 1

# Contributors

**Ella M. Brooks, RN, PhD**
Vice President for Academic Affairs
Huron University
Huron, South Dakota

**Kathy Jo Ellison, RN, DSN**
Associate Professor
Auburn University
School of Nursing
Montgomery, Alabama

**Timothy Jones, MD**
Deputy State Epidemiologist
Tennessee Department of Health
Nashville, Tennessee

**Mary Ann Modrcin-Talbott, RN PhD**
Professor and Chair
Lincoln Memorial University
Department of Nursing
Horrogate, Tennessee

**Maureen Nalle, RN, PhD**
Assistant Professor
University of Tennessee
College of Nursing
Knoxville, Tennessee

**Joan Uhl Pierce, RN, PhD, FAAN**
Professor
University of Tennessee
College of Nursing
Knoxville, Tennessee

**Debra C. Wallace, RN, PhD**
Professor
University of North Carolina, Greensboro
School of Nursing
Greensboro, North Carolina

# To Our Significant Others

**Denver Stone,** for his love, unfailing support, and knowing just the right time to assist.

**Verna and Al J. Clemen,** for their special love that promoted growth, family cohesiveness, and independent thinking.

**John and Sharon Clemen** and **Sara and Henry Parks,** for their caring, friendship, and encouragement.

**Teresa and Rick Stone,** for their patience and understanding.

**Holly Marie and Tyler Huling,** for bringing the joys of childhood into our life and for their loving ways.

To the memory of **Ike.**

**Heiki-Lara Eigsti Nyce** and **Inge-Marie Eigsti,** along with **Jim, Mark, James** and **Conrad,** for their patience and loving.

**John E. Gerber,** for the joy he has brought.

**Joseph, Kelly, and Kerry McGuire** and **Matthew Currin,** for their love, support, and encouragement.

**Donald and Mary Lue Johnson,** for their pride in this publication, their continued encouragement, and their love and interest.

**Arthur and Sally Johnson,** for the belief they instilled in the value of education, the role modeling they provided, and their constant love.

**Judy Simpson,** for her continued faith in and support of the nursing profession.

**Alma Weale,** for recognizing the importance of this publication and for her unfailing encouragement.

# Preface

The first edition of *Comprehensive Community Health Nursing: Family, Aggregate, and Community Practice* was published in 1981 to generate excitement about population- and community-focused nursing practice as well as individual- and family-oriented care. It was obvious at that time that multiple societal and health care trends would significantly increase the opportunities and challenges for nurses in the community setting. The 1980s and 1990s were indeed characterized by major changes that have reshaped and expanded community health nursing practice. Clearly, health care delivery is shifting from the acute care setting to the community setting. Unprecedented need in the community—including demands such as the increasing bioterrorism, continuing and emerging biopsychosocial and spiritual issues, and environmental concerns—is calling for new and innovative interventions for promoting health and preventing disease. Community health nursing's rich heritage in the community places this nursing specialty at a competitive advantage for stimulating innovation in practice.

Community health nurses are uniquely poised to provide dynamic leadership in a health care system characterized by continuous and overlapping change. The emphasis in health care during the 1990s has moved from a national, holistic focus on health care reform to an era of rapidly evolving integrated managed care systems competing for public and private monies. These systems are designed to provide cost-effective, quality care for individuals and families. The challenge for community health professionals in the future will be to mobilize the resources necessary to meet the needs of populations at risk, as well as individuals and families, and to maintain a safety net for disadvantaged populations. Community health nurses have a strong background for mobilizing community resources and using them to help diverse client groups move effectively across the health care continuum. The expanding ethnic diversification in our nation will increase the demand for culturally appropriate services in all health care settings.

The future community health mission will be to build healthy, healing communities that provide access to health care for all. To assist practitioners to achieve this vision, the sixth edition of this text continues to provide a comprehensive foundation for community health nursing practice, including evolving approaches for addressing contemporary health issues. The educational preparation that makes community health nursing unique is its emphasis on community-oriented, population-focused practice from an interdisciplinary, partnership perspective.

## THE SIXTH EDITION

Following trends in the field, the sixth edition helps students and practitioners understand the importance of using a preventive approach, in partnership with clients and other stakeholders, to address community needs. The reader is provided the concepts essential for identifying the distinguishing features of community health nursing practice and the challenging nature of a specialty field committed to meeting the needs of vulnerable populations. The sixth edition speaks to the increasing challenges community health professionals will face as they strive to achieve health for all in the twenty-first century. It addresses the need to maintain a strong public health infrastructure to ensure access to care during a time of dwindling health care resources. Expanded discussion of the core public health functions of assessment, assurance, and policy development, as well as community health nursing interventions in relation to these functions has been included. The value of building broad-based coalitions that work in partnership with communities to promote health is highlighted throughout this text.

Extensive revision of the book enhances its usefulness for students and practitioners. The role managed care plays in promoting the public's health is carefully explored. Opportunities as well as challenges for the community health nurse in a managed care environment are identified. Expanded discussion on care management will help strengthen students' understanding of the pivotal role of community health nurses in helping populations in need access essential, culturally appropriate health care. Strategies for addressing the needs of populations at risk and health care access disparities have also been identified. Discussion on how the *Healthy People 2010* initiative guides the analysis of community needs and health planning efforts has been strengthened.

The profession is faced with unprecedented societal and health care changes that are significantly influencing client need and community health nursing practice. Two new chapters, Chapter 12, "Theoretical Models for Health Education and Health Promotion," and Chapter 20, "School

Health Nursing," have been added to present a more thoroughly developed discussion of population-focused, contemporary community health issues. Chapter 12 expands on the concepts essential for understanding health behavior change and health education interventions. Chapter 20 highlights the health promotion role of the community health nurse in the school setting. Expanded content on the new technologies and contemporary challenges in epidemiology (Chapter 11) helps the reader to understand the importance of public health surveillance activities and how technology can be used to mobilize disease control and prevention efforts worldwide.

Nurses share with all health care professionals the need to examine carefully the delivery of their services in light of changing societal demands. Health care providers will face several critical challenges during the twenty-first century as they strive to maintain quality in health care delivery. They will need to become more accountable to those who purchase and use health services and more focused on demonstrating that they can provide cost-effective care that is measurable. Expanded content on nursing interventions and an increased focus on outcome assessment throughout the text helps students to identify and evaluate appropriate community health nursing outcomes. It is envisioned that a much stronger emphasis will be placed on providing preventive health services in the coming century. This emphasis has been highlighted throughout the text. Other trends are also well documented.

## Organization

The overall acceptance of the past five editions of this book have challenged us to preserve the basic framework of the original text while extensively revising the content to reflect the dynamic changes in health care service delivery. The framework for this text stems from the philosophy of community and public health nursing practice delineated by the definitions of the American Nurses Association, the American Public Health Association, and the Quad Council of Public Health Nursing Organizations. These philosophies articulate the need for community health nurses to understand the environment in which they are functioning. They also address the unique orientation that community health nurses bring to any health care team: a holistic approach to promoting and protecting the health of individuals, families, and populations at risk from a community perspective. The two major parts of this book explore the unique role of the community health nurse from this perspective.

Part One presents a philosophical foundation for nursing practice in the community. It analyzes the origin, scope, and changing nature of community health nursing practice and examines community dynamics and societal and health care trends that influence the delivery of health, welfare, and environmental services. The emphasis is on the direct service functions of the community health nurse within the context of change and diversity. In Part One the reader is helped to analyze the concept of client from four perspectives—individual, family, populations at risk, and community—with a focus on providing culturally competent care. Special attention is placed on analyzing how the community health nurse uses the family-focused nursing process in collaboration with clients to implement and evaluate client-centered interventions.

Part Two stresses the value of working with populations at risk in the community. The needs of populations across the life span are examined, and interventions for addressing these needs are presented. The importance of using the *Healthy People 2010* objectives to guide community assessment processes is articulated. The epidemiological process is presented as a tool for studying the determinants of health and disease frequencies in populations and for analyzing contemporary health issues. Models for health behavior change and health education are also presented. The emphasis is on using a partnership approach to health planning to build healthy, nurturing communities. In Part Two the reader is also helped to gain an understanding of the role of the community health nurse in a variety of community settings such as schools, nursing centers, parishes, clinics, and work sites and how these settings provide important vehicles for reaching specific population groups. An increasing number of driving forces, including altered demographics, an emerging global and knowledge economy, technological innovation, growing consumer expectations, and emerging threats to the health of our society, are influencing the competencies needed by practitioners to provide population-based care in the twenty-first century. The implications of these driving forces for nursing, as well as skills needed by future health care providers, are highlighted in Part Two. There is no question about the need for future practitioners to have strong critical thinking skills, effective communication capabilities, cultural skills, political competencies, business management and leadership skills, and lifelong learning skills. There is also no question about the increasing need to consider the ethical dimensions of practice and the importance of documenting the effectiveness of nursing interventions. Part Two reflects a strong futurist perspective.

## Pedagogical Features

*Comprehensive Community Health Nursing: Family, Aggregate, and Community Practice* provides a foundation for discussion, dialogue, debate, and action both in the classroom and clinical setting. It was built on the belief that learning is a dynamic, collaborative process where students, faculty, and practitioners learn together. This book is designed to serve as a stimulus for bringing together the resources needed to address current and future health issues. It is envisioned that the classroom setting will serve as an environment where students can critically think about real client situations and clinical practice issues in the community setting.

Several teaching/learning features of this text will prepare students for this type of classroom experience. *Objectives* and *key terms* are included at the beginning of each chapter to focus students' attention on the critical concepts needed to formulate guidelines for effective family- and population-based nursing interventions. Illustrations and boxes throughout the text help students to identify quickly significant concepts, content, and nursing interventions. Careful attention was given to defining key terms in the text to facilitate students' understanding of them. Extensive *References* and a *Selected Bibliography* of historic and current information relevant to each chapter aid students in gaining a practical view of community health nursing practice. Several of these references encourage the student to challenge "what is" and dream about "what can be." These references can be used to promote lively debate in the classroom setting. The teaching/learning features of this text were designed to foster an *interactive approach* between faculty and students.

Other features of the book will help students obtain a realistic perspective of nursing care in the community setting. A *View from the Field* boxes enable the reader to understand community health nursing practice from the perspective of an experienced practitioner or client. These boxes help the student to examine the scope and exciting nature of nursing practice in the community setting, including workload management issues and client perceptions of health care delivery. Numerous *Case Scenarios* developed from clinical situations assist students in examining client needs and applying theoretical concepts. *Critical Thinking Exercises* at the end of each chapter and *Stop and Think About It* boxes throughout the chapters help students to think critically about client situations and the relevant concepts covered in the chapter. These critical thinking experiences reflect current issues encountered in the practice setting and encourage discussion and debate. The *Teaching Tips* boxes in Part Two help students to identify client learning needs and provide resources for facilitating the teaching process. The *Appendixes* provide valuable assessment tools and data that enhance students' abilities to use the nursing process with diverse client groups.

*Course Resources to Accompany Comprehensive Community Health Nursing: Family, Aggregate, and Community Practice,* an online supplement for instructors, is accessible at *http://www.mosby.com/MERLIN/Clemen-Stone.* Instructors who adopt the textbook for course use may obtain a passcode from their Mosby sales representative or by calling Faculty Support at 1-800-222-9570. Revisions to the *Course Resources* will assist educators in promoting an interactive style of learning. The *Instructor's Manual* portion highlights key concepts covered in each chapter and provides learning activities that promote critical thinking. Teaching aids for faculty are shared in the manual, including *Class Preparation Resources* and *Learning Activities. Course Resources* also offers an *Electronic Image Collection*, which contains important illustrations from the textbook, and a *Test Bank* of approximately 800 questions.

## ACKNOWLEDGMENTS

The authors are greatly indebted to family, friends, colleagues, students, and former faculty and associates for their support, guidance, and assistance as we revised this book. Special appreciation is extended to the following individuals:

- Beverly Smith, our administrative secretary and a special friend, whose painstaking efforts, patience, and dedication to our project made it a reality. This book could never have been published without her help.
- Bill Smith, whose "it only takes a little more to do it right" encouragement, as we began this process over 20 years ago, provided the impetus to move forward. His willingness to share his wife's time will never be forgotten.
- Our contributors who freely shared their time to bring to the reader relevant content in their area of expertise.
- Shu-Chen Chang, Marilyn Franecki, and Mo Qu, for their invaluable assistance with research of the literature.
- Henry Parks and Edward Richardson for helping us with our artwork and photography.
- Denver Stone, who willingly devoted considerable time to the tedious aspects of the manuscript preparation process. His commitment to quality was an inspiration to all of us.
- The reviewers of the book, who provided significant direction for the sixth edition revision.
- Colleagues from the service setting who have shared with us materials their staffs developed to facilitate the delivery of quality client services.
- Publishers and authors who graciously granted us permission to use information from their writings.
- The Mosby staff, especially Darlene Como, Brian Dennison, Catherine Jackson, Marc Syp, and Renee Duenow for their support, understanding, and concrete assistance.
- All our friends and family members who "understood" and allowed us to postpone events and activities.

*Susan Clemen-Stone*
*Sandra L. McGuire*
*Diane Gerber Eigsti*

# Contents

# COMPREHENSIVE COMMUNITY HEALTH NURSING

*Family, Aggregate, & Community Practice*

# PART ONE

# A Foundation for Community Health Nursing Practice

Public health nurses have been leaders in improving the quality of health care for people since the late 1800s. They have been the vanguard of change for both the nursing profession and society as a whole, stressing the importance of establishing standards for nursing education and practice and promoting social reform to improve quality of life for all individuals. Key concepts that delineate community health specialty practice emphasize the importance of culturally sensitive, population-based practice, with a focus on primary prevention and the community. Individual, family, and system interventions occur within the context of population-based, community-oriented practice.

Our early leaders were role models for effective change. They dealt with community dynamics and worked to influence legislative processes that shape the direction of health, welfare, and environmental systems and policies at all levels of government. Using multiple intervention strategies, they worked in partnership with communities to promote health and prevent disease.

Our heritage involves over a century of caring—for communities, populations, families, and individuals. To continue the progress made by their early leaders, community health nurses must understand where and how their specialty began, the nature of current community health nursing practice, and how community forces contribute to or distract from the health of families and populations at risk. Part One presents the theoretical concepts essential for understanding community health nursing practice and discusses the *Healthy People 2010* initiative. This initiative addresses current health issues in the United States and its objectives guide community health nursing efforts. The organization of our evolving health, welfare, and environmental systems is discussed within the context of needed health care reform. The challenges are great. The opportunities to promote the health of communities are endless.

# 1

# Historical Perspectives on Community Health Nursing

*Sandra L. McGuire*

## OBJECTIVES

*Upon completion of this chapter, the reader should be able to:*

1. Understand the historical development of public and community health nursing.
2. Understand the contributions of William Rathbone, Florence Nightingale, Lillian Wald, Mary Breckinridge, and other public health leaders to community health nursing.

3. Discuss the development of public and community health nursing in the United States.
4. Discuss the differences in visiting, public health, and community health nursing.
5. Summarize the evolution of educational preparation for public and community health nursing practice.

## KEY TERMS

Mary Breckinridge
Community health nursing
District nursing
Ruth B. Freeman
Frontier Nursing Service (FNS)
Mary Sewall Gardner
*Goldmark Report*
Healthy People Initiative
Henry Street Settlement (HSS)

*The House on Henry Street*
Mademoiselle Le Gras
Pearl McIver
Metropolitan Life Insurance Company
National League for Nursing (NLN)
National Organization for Public
  Health Nursing (NOPHN)
Florence Nightingale
Marie Phelar

Queen's Nurse
William Rathbone
St. Vincent de Paul
Sisters of Charity
Standards of practice
Town and Country Nursing Service
Visiting nursing
Lillian Wald

---

*Histories make [wo]men wise.*

FRANCIS BACON

In 1993 public health nurses across the United States celebrated "A Century of Caring" (Division of Nursing, 1992). That year, nurses and the American public celebrated public health nursing's first century of service and recognized the accomplishments of early public health nurses and their leaders, among them Lillian Wald, a brilliant political and social activist and the founder of public health nursing; Mary Breckinridge, a staunch advocate for children's health and founder of the Frontier Nursing Service; Mary Sewall Gardner, author of the first public health nursing textbook; and Lavinia Lloyd Dock, a nurse who devoted herself to women's rights and wrote extensively on

the history of nursing. Today's nurses should be proud of such early public health nursing leaders. They are heroines and role models for persons committed to nursing, health care, and humanity. Public health nursing in the United States has a strong and proud history. From the origins of public health nursing with Lillian Wald in 1893 to today, its practice represents a strong tradition of caring for communities, aggregates, and families (Box 1-1).

Historically, nurses have believed in human dignity and the need to alleviate human suffering. Early visiting and public health nurses cared for the sick in their homes, used health teaching as a means of preventing illness, and realized that family and community greatly contributed to a patient's illness and recovery. Examining history helps us understand how the concepts critical to today's specialty field

**BOX 1-1**

## A Century of Caring (1893-1993) and Beyond: Select Community Health Nursing Events in the United States

| | |
|---|---|
| 1893 | Lillian Wald and Mary Brewster found what becomes the Henry Street Settlement in New York City. |
| 1895 | Ada Mayo Stewart becomes the first industrial nurse. |
| 1898 | Nurses' Settlement is established in San Francisco. |
| 1900 | Nurses' Settlement is established in Richmond, Virginia. |
| 1902 | Lina Rogers, a Henry Street Settlement nurse, becomes the first school nurse. |
| 1909 | Metropolitan Life Insurance Company employs public health nurses. |
| 1910 | A public health nursing course is taught at Teacher's College, Columbia University. |
| 1912 | National Organization for Public Health Nursing (NOPHN) is established. American Red Cross Rural Nursing Service is established, and changes its name to Town and Country Nursing Service the next year. It later will be known as the Bureau of Public Health Nursing. Children's Bureau is established. *Public Health Nurse* is first published (formerly *The Visiting Nurses Quarterly* and later to become *Public Health Nursing* and then *Nursing Outlook*). |
| 1916 | Mary Sewall Gardner writes *Public Health Nursing.* |
| 1921 | Sheppard-Towner Act provides funding to improve the health of women, infants, and children, stimulates the formation of state health departments and increases the demand for public health nursing services. |
| 1925 | Mary Breckinridge founds the Frontier Nursing Service in Kentucky. |
| 1933 | Pearl McIver, a public health nurse, is appointed to U.S. Public Health Service (USPHS) and becomes the first public health nursing consultant for state health departments. |
| 1942 | American Association of Industrial Nurses is established (later becomes American Association of Occupational Health Nurses). |
| 1946 | Division of Nursing (DN) is formed in the USPHS, and public health nursing is one of the three DN offices. Lucille Petry Leone is the first Director of the DN and Pearl McIver heads up the Office of Public Health Nursing. |

| | |
|---|---|
| 1952 | NOPHN and other professional nursing organizations merge to become the National League for Nursing (NLN). |
| 1963 | Public health nursing content is required as part of baccalaureate nursing programs. |
| 1973 | American Nurses Association (ANA) publishes *Standards of Community Health Nursing Practice.* |
| 1980 | ANA and American Public Health Association (APHA) develop definitions for practice in community and public health nursing. |
| 1984 | National Consensus Conference on the Essentials of Public Health Nursing Practice and Education is held. |
| 1986 | National Center for Nursing Research is established. ANA revises *Standards of Community Health Nursing Practice* and develops *Standards for Home Health Nursing Practice.* |
| 1988 | Institute of Medicine publishes *The Future of Public Health.* |
| 1989 | National Consensus Conference on the Educational Preparation of Home Care Administrators is held. |
| 1990 | Association of Community Health Nursing Educators (ACHNE) publishes *Essentials of Baccalaureate Nursing Education for Entry Level Community Health Nursing Practice.* |
| 1991 | ACHNE publishes *Essentials of Master's Level Nursing Education for Advanced Community Health Nursing Practice.* |
| 1992 | ACHNE publishes *Essentials of Research Priorities for Community Health Nursing.* |
| 1993 | National Center for Nursing Research becomes the National Institute for Nursing Research, and community-based practice is part of the nursing research agenda. ACHNE publishes *Essentials of Differentiated Practice in Community Health.* |
| 1995 | ACHNE publishes *Essentials of Community/Public Health Advanced Practice Nurse (C/PHAPN) Position Statement.* |
| 1996 | APHA Public Health Nursing Section adopts a revised position statement on the *Definition and Role of Public Health Nursing.* |
| 1999 | ANA publishes *Scope and Standards of Public Health Nursing Practice.* |

of community health nursing evolved. Community health nursing today is a culmination of the work that extraordinary women and men accomplished over a great many years.

## IN THE BEGINNING

Nursing began when humanity began.

The word *nurse* is a reduced form of the Middle English *nurice*, which was derived through the old French *norrice*,

from the Latin *nutricius* (nourishing). In Roman mythology, the Goddess Fortuna, in addition to her usual function as goddess of fate, also was worshipped as Jupiter's nurse (Fortuna Praeneste) and prayed to for hygiene in the public baths (Fortuna Balnearis). Early history shows that people provided care for the sick, acquired knowledge of pain-relieving remedies, and sought to discover means of preventing disease. The true ancestors of the modern nurse were noble deaconesses, nuns, and early Christian women who were trying to do for their day what the nurse of today is doing for hers (Gardner, 1916, p. 3). Nursing roles developed in the desire to alleviate human suffering (Kalisch, Kalisch, 1995, p. 1).

Visiting nursing, or the care of ill people at home, has existed throughout the ages. Before the Christian era, rabbis declared it the responsibility of every Jew to visit the sick, in order to show them sympathy and to cheer, aid, and relieve them in their suffering (Gardner, 1916, p. 4). The New Testament is replete with stories of how the sick were visited. The Apostle Paul wrote of Phoebe in Romans 16:1-2, "I commend to you our sister Phoebe, a deaconess of the church at Cenchreae . . . help her in whatever she may require from you, for she has been a helper of many and of myself as well." Phoebe is probably the first visiting nurse we know by name.

During the Middle Ages (500-1500 AD) there was practically no organized care of the sick in their homes (Brainard, 1922, p. 18), and superstition and folk medicine dominated health practices. During this time epidemics of infectious diseases such as smallpox, plague, typhoid, yellow fever, and cholera were common. The bubonic plague, or "Black Death," epidemic of 540 AD had an estimated death toll of 100 million, and some 800 years later it would claim a death toll of more than 60 million people (Kalisch, Kalisch, 1995, p. 12). At this time, numerous factors added to the problem of infectious disease. Refuse was allowed to accumulate in streets and dwellings, human waste was dumped into public water supplies, and foods were often improperly stored and prepared. Personal hygiene was often neglected, and "to take a bath was to confess oneself ill" (Brainard, 1922, p. 29).

Throughout the Middle Ages monasteries and convents were erected in all parts of the world, and hospitals often were connected with them (Brainard, 1922, p. 16). Some religious orders existed primarily to provide nursing care to the sick. These early nurses included men who were drawn into military nursing orders, such as the Knights Hospitallers, Teutonic Knights, and Knights of St. Lazarus (Dock, 1938, p. 59). In such religious orders "the high born and rich and those of lowly birth alike gave their services to the care of the sick" (Gardner, 1916, p. 5).

The Renaissance (approximately 1500-1700 AD) brought about great political, social, and economic expansion and a revival of learning. Two important names from this period are St. Vincent de Paul and Mademoiselle Le Gras. Mary Sewall Gardner says of de Paul that "there is perhaps no more prominent figure in the history of public health nursing" (Gardner, 1916, p. 6).

In 1633 de Paul organized the Sisters of Charity (Kalisch, Kalisch, 1995, p. 28). The Sisters went from home to home, visiting the sick. As the movement spread and its numbers increased, problems with supervision arose. St. Vincent reorganized the group and appointed Mademoiselle Le Gras as supervisor. Together they made great contributions to the development of visiting and public health nursing, including providing education for those helping the poor and the sick, recognizing the need for professional supervision of caregivers, and helping people to help themselves. De Paul and Le Gras believed that one must determine the needs of the poor and disadvantaged, investigate the causes, and help supply solutions. Taken for granted by people today, these were entirely new concepts of charity for this time (Maynard, 1939). For centuries monasteries and convents stood for all that was best in nursing and made great efforts to care for the sick (Gardner, 1916, p. 4). Toward the end of the Renaissance, religious organizations began to withdraw from the provision of nursing care. When this happened nursing practice deteriorated, and a dark period for nursing emerged.

## A Dark Period for Nursing

Nursing, like so many other things the history of which may be studied from century to century, has had its bright periods of inspired effort, and its black periods of temporary degradation. It is difficult to imagine how nursing could have sunk to the low levels it did between the end of the seventeenth century to the middle of the nineteenth century. The change from nursing care given by devoted deaconesses to nursing care given by drunks and prostitutes is baffling. In *Martin Chuzzlewit*, published in 1844, Charles Dickens immortalized the prototype of the nurse of this era by describing a drunken, untrained servant, Sairy Gamp, as a nurse. It is not to the Sairy Gamps that the ancestry of the modern nurse is to be traced. Sairy was but an unhappy incident in the history of nursing (Gardner, 1916, p. 3).

Nursing care in the Western world had degenerated from care being given by deaconesses, sisters, and Christian women to care being given by beggars and vagrants. This change in the way nursing care was provided began during the time of the Reformation (around 1500-1600 AD), when many church organizations were overthrown. After the Reformation the lack of nursing sisterhoods was deeply felt (Brainard, 1922, p. 70). Without the protection and acceptance lent it by the church, nursing lost much of its social standing. "Even during this dark period good and devoted women were giving their lives to the relief of suffering, but it was only individual effort, and as a rule in every country the great body of the sick poor were being cared for by overworked, ignorant, and unprincipled women, while the sick rich fared but little better" (Gardner, 1916, p. 8).

Nursing now existed in a low and dismal state, without organization or social standing. No one who could possibly earn a living in some other way performed this service (Deloughery, 1977, p. 24). Those who sought nursing as a profession "lost caste thereby, for as one is judged partly by the company one keeps, a woman who began to practice nursing was almost certain to become corrupted if she were not so already" (Deloughery, 1977, p. 24).

At the middle of the nineteenth century, assistance programs for the poor and disadvantaged did not exist as we know them today, and social classes were rigidly stratified. Many people were starving, child labor was practiced routinely, housing frequently was overcrowded and inadequate, and personal hygiene and matters of public health often were ignored. The huge slums of the city bred disease. Life expectancy was short and mortality rates were high. The scientific basis for medicine was unknown, and health care was based on folklore and superstition. With this background in mind, the contributions of Florence Nightingale to nursing, to public health, and to women are inestimable. Indeed, when Florence Nightingale began her career, nursing was not thought of as a respectable career for a "proper" young woman.

## FLORENCE NIGHTINGALE'S LEGACY

Florence Nightingale was the second child of William and Frances Nightingale. She was born on May 12, 1820 in Florence, Italy; her older sister Parthenope had been born the previous year in Naples. Her family was well traveled, wealthy, and influential. Unlike other English girls of the day, Florence and her sister were well educated. As a young girl, Florence mastered the fundamentals of Greek and Latin; studied history, mathematics, and philosophy; and wrote essays (Kalisch, Kalisch, 1995, p. 30). To her family's chagrin, Florence remained unmarried and expressed a longing to be a nurse. Her numerous requests to train as a nurse were rejected by her parents. Finally, at age 31 she obtained her family's reluctant permission to train as a nurse at Kaiserswerth, Germany (Dock, 1938, p. 119).

### Kaiserswerth

Theodor Fliedner was pastor in the town of Kaiserswerth. He and his young wife, Frederika, had started a Woman's Society for visiting and nursing the sick poor in their homes (Brainard, 1922, p. 74). In 1836 he started a hospital and a training school for deaconesses that is considered to be the first modern order of nursing deaconesses (Kalisch, Kalisch, 1995, p. 28). It was the Kaiserswerth training school that young Florence became determined to attend.

In the winter of 1849 Florence was touring Egypt with family and friends and spent time in Alexandria with the Sisters of Charity of St. Vincent de Paul (Kalisch, Kalisch, 1995, p. 31). The next spring she set out unaccompanied for Kaiserswerth, stayed there for 2 weeks, and left determined to return to train as a nurse (Kalisch, Kalisch, 1995, p. 31). The following year, with her ailing sister about to journey to the mineral springs of Carlsbad, Nightingale went to Kaiserswerth for nurses' training. Permission was granted on the condition that no one outside the family learn of her destination. Her training at Kaiserswerth lasted for 3 months (Dock, 1938, p. 119), and upon returning home, she entered the profession of nursing.

### The Crimea

Shortly after her return to England, the Crimean War would offer Nightingale a great opportunity and challenge as "Superintendent of the Female Nursing Establishment of the English General Hospitals in Turkey" (Kalisch, Kalisch, 1995, p. 32). The story of Miss Nightingale in the Crimea is legendary. Her work at Scutari has been chronicled by many, among them Longfellow, in his "Santa Filomena." It was there that she demonstrated that thousands of lives could be saved by nursing care and that capable nurses were needed in hospitals. She accomplished this in the face of overwhelming obstacles. Although the hospital at Scutari was designed to accommodate 1700 patients, when Nightingale arrived in 1854 there were 3000 to 4000 wounded men in it (Kalisch, Kalisch, 1995, p. 32). Many of these men lay naked, with no bed or blanket and no eating or laundry facilities. Within days of her appearance at Scutari, she had a food kitchen and laundry operating and was working diligently to improve the unsanitary environmental conditions present. Factors Nightingale considered important in optimizing the physical environment of the ill person included pure air, pure water, efficient drainage, cleanliness, and light (Nightingale, 1859). She organized all of the hospitals throughout the Crimea and supervised the work of some 200 nurses (Dock, 1938, p. 122). When Nightingale arrived at the Barrack Hospital, its mortality rate was almost 60%; when she left, it was less than 1% (Dock, 1938, pp. 121-122). Statistics she had kept on her work in the Crimea would later be used for hospital reform in England. When the war ended in 1856, she returned to England determined to establish a training school for nurses.

### The First Modern Training School for Nurses

Upon returning to London, Nightingale established the first modern training school for nurses at St. Thomas Hospital in 1860. Interestingly, when the training school began, most London physicians opposed the project; of the 100 physicians asked, only 4 favored the school (Kalisch, Kalisch, 1995, p. 36).

The opening of the St. Thomas Training School for Nurses offered a new beginning for nursing. Nightingale visualized nursing as a profession; in earlier times it had been seen as religious dedication and a form of religious life. Nursing was envisioned as a "calling" to a high duty and demanded the age-old characteristics of love, kindness, patience, and self-sacrifice, but now added to that was training (Brainard, 1922, p. 84). Nightingale saw training as crucial to nursing and refined women were admitted to the program to become trained nurses.

The principle that training was necessary to make a competent professional nurse was accepted. However, the knowledge of what training was needed was vague, and it was left to Florence Nightingale to show the way (Brainard, 1922, p. 84). Nightingale's training school incorporated assessment, intervention, and evaluation into the role of the professional nurse, which began the professional focus on the nursing process. In her *Notes on Nursing,* she envisioned nursing as that care that puts a person in the best possible condition for nature to either restore or preserve health, to prevent or cure disease or injury (Nightingale, 1859). From the very beginning of her career, Nightingale focused on the use of a scientific process to guide nursing practice. "Nightingale (1885) encouraged nurses to be clear thinkers and independent in their judgments" (Reed, Zurakowski, 1996, p. 47). Nightingale intended that the school's graduates would teach and train other nurses, and as such would be "health missioners" (Dock, 1938, p. 126). Nightingale's training school set an example for other schools, including the one at Bellevue Hospital in New York City in 1873. It eventually lead to the establishment of university schools of nursing in the United States at Case Western Reserve and Yale (Winslow, 1946, p. 331).

Nightingale visualized the nurse as not merely an attendant for the sick but also as a teacher of hygiene and health. This was an early affirmation of the principle that individuals are responsible for their own health and the role of the nurse is to promote the client's self-care capabilities. These early beliefs fit well into what was to become a system of visiting nursing in England.

## The Establishment of Visiting Nursing in England

The modern concept of a nurse who visits and provides care to families in the home was visualized and established in 1859 by **William Rathbone** of Liverpool, England. "It is to Mr. Rathbone that we owe the first definitely formulated district nursing association and in that sense he may be called the father of the present movement" (Gardner, 1916, p. 10). Rathbone was a wealthy businessman and philanthropist. His wife died after a long illness, and he had been impressed and comforted by the skilled home nursing care given to her in the months before she died. Rathbone had long been interested in helping the poor people of Liverpool. If nursing care could help his wife, who had everything that money could buy, how much more might it do for people whose physical illnesses were made increasingly burdensome by their poverty. To test his idea, he employed Mary Robinson, the nurse who had cared for his wife, to visit the "sick poor" in their homes. She was to instruct both the patient and the family in the care of the sick, give care, and teach hygienic practices. The experiment was so successful that Rathbone decided to establish a permanent system of visiting nursing in Liverpool (McNeil, 1967, p. 1). A major problem in advancing visiting nursing was the lack of nurses prepared to do such work.

## Standardized Training for Visiting Nurses

In 1859, with the assistance of Florence Nightingale, Rathbone founded a school for the training of visiting nurses on the grounds of the Liverpool Royal Infirmary. In her paper, *Sick Nursing and Health Nursing,* Nightingale discussed the visiting nurse as a "health visitor," a guide and teacher of positive health in the home. Within 4 years, 18 visiting nurses had graduated and were providing care for the sick poor in their homes. They all were trained in the profession, were not to dispense material relief, and were not to interfere with the religious beliefs of their patients (Gardner, 1916, p. 12). Because they were frequently assigned to work in specific districts or villages, the term **district nursing** was soon synonymous with visiting nursing. In 1890 Rathbone wrote *Sketch of the History and Progress of District Nursing.* This book presented a clear idea of the profession and is considered to be the most important book of the nineteenth century on the subject (Carr, 1988, p. 82)

The visiting nurse movement in England spread rapidly. In 1887 the Queen lent her support by establishing the Queen Victoria's Jubilee Institute for Nurses with money received from the Women's Jubilee offering. This royal patronage conferred upon each graduate the title of **"Queen's Nurse."** The objective of the Institute was to promote the education and maintenance of nurses for the sick poor in their own houses (Cohen, 1997, p. 86). Selection of trainees and training were rigorous. A Queen's Nurse had to be intelligent and spiritually inspired to serve mankind without fear, fatigue, greed, or pain (Cohen, 1997, p. 86). The Institute set standards for both the preparation of visiting nurses and the care given by them. Nightingale was a firm believer in the need for visiting nurses to receive training in addition to their hospital training (Carr, 1988, p. 81). "A Queen's nurse was in every instance a graduate of a hospital giving a three years' course, and in addition she receives a six months post-graduate training in one of the homes of the Institute" (Gardner, 1916, p. 15). In 1890 Darce Craven wrote *A Guide to District Nurses and Home Nursing* as a training manual for the Institute. It was the first book written by a trained visiting nurse for visiting nurses (Carr, 1988, p. 82).

Nightingale wrote numerous papers on the topic of district nursing, including "Notes on Nursing for the Labouring Classes," "Improving the Nursing Service for the Sick Poor," "On Trained Nursing for the Sick Poor," and "Health Teaching in Towns and Villages: Rural Hygiene" (Cohen, 1997, p. 98). She supported and maintained involvement in the development and expansion of visiting nursing in both England and the United States.

## VISITING NURSING IN THE UNITED STATES

The Old World had been making rapid progress in the care of the sick poor in their homes, but little was happening in the New World. In early America there were few hospitals, few trained physicians, and only occasionally a trained midwife. Churches frequently provided some form of care to the sick in their homes. The poor usually chose to stay at home during illnesses, and they often depended on the women of the household, close friends, or neighbors. The quality of the nursing care given was dependent on the skill and experience of these caretakers, whether good or bad. Home care for middle and upper class Americans was more likely to be supervised by visits from the family physician or in a hospital's pay or private rooms (Buhler-Wilkerson, 1983).

In 1798 Dr. Valentine Seaman organized the first formal training course for nurses at New York Hospital (Dock, 1907, p. 339; Smillie, 1955, p. 405). This training consisted of 24 hours of basic lectures and instruction (Smillie, 1955, p. 405). Formal nursing education was slow to evolve in the United States. In 1861 the Philadelphia Hospital opened a training school, but the first modern training school in the United States is considered to be the New England Hospital for Women and Children established in 1872 and graduated Miss Linda Richards, the first American trained nurse (Gardner, 1916, p. 20). The following year Bellevue Hospital in New York City; New Haven Hospital in New Haven, Connecticut; and Massachusetts General Hospital in Boston all established nursing training programs. However, none of these programs offered training in visiting nursing.

In the early 1800s women philanthropists began to hire "nurses" to care for the sick poor in their homes (Brainard, 1922; Buhler-Wilkerson, 1983). In 1813 the Ladies' Benevolent Society of Charleston, South Carolina established what is considered to be the first visiting nursing service in America (Smillie, 1955, p. 406). This service was started following a yellow fever epidemic that devastated the city. Home nursing care was provided by members of the Society and nurses employed by them. This method of caring for the sick of Charleston lasted until the time of the Civil War (Gardner, 1916, p. 20). However, these early visiting nurses had no formal nursing or visiting nursing training.

In 1849 Theodor Fliedner of Kaiserswerth had accompanied four of his deaconesses to Pittsburgh in an endeavor to start visiting nursing in that city, but the undertaking did not prosper (Gardner, 1916, p. 20; Smillie, 1955, p. 406). A few other efforts were made to establish nursing sisterhoods and to introduce the Sisters of Charity into the homes of America's sick poor, but these efforts did not arouse the support of the public and were unsuccessful (Brainard, 1922, p. 194).

Other than the Ladies' Benevolent Society of Charleston, few notations of organized efforts for home care for the sick poor in America existed before 1877. In 1877 the Woman's Board of the New York City Mission, a voluntary philanthropic organization, hired a nurse, Miss Frances Root, to visit the sick poor (Brainard, 1922, p. 194). Miss Root was a graduate of the Bellevue Training School for nurses in New York City. She was hired as a "missionary nurse" and was expected to use every opportunity to introduce religious counsel and words of Christian comfort (Brainard, 1922, p. 196). Her work was successful, and other such nurses were hired.

The following year the New York Society for Ethical Culture hired missionary nurses. In 1898 the city health department in Los Angeles employed a nurse to provide home nursing care to welfare recipients and to visit the public schools, the first recorded hiring of a nurse by an official, tax-supported agency (Rosen, 1958, p. 380; Smillie, 1955, p. 411).

By the late 1800s large numbers of Americans were becoming increasingly concerned with the poverty and misery experienced by so many people. Poverty was beginning to be seen as the result of social problems and conditions. People rallied around causes such as working to improve maternal and child health, abolish child labor, provide decent housing, and procure women's right to vote. American cities were growing fast and had large immigrant populations, large slum areas, and high rates of disease. Dismal tenement houses were built for this huge influx of people, and living conditions were horrible. Even young children were expected to work 12 to 14 hours a day in dark, airless factories, and many slept on the streets at night. America's overcrowded cities posed many serious health problems. Such conditions saw a rise in social consciousness for the conditions of the poor, the formation of visiting nurse associations, and the birth of public health nursing.

## Associations for Visiting Nursing

Organized visiting nursing in the United States, just as in England, was begun by people who were greatly distressed by the conditions in which many poor people lived. As in England, visiting nursing involved both direct patient care and health teaching. Unlike England, in the United States there was a lack of standardized, formalized training for visiting nurses.

The first group of nurses organized in America for the sole purpose of providing skilled care for the sick poor in their homes was the District Nursing Association in Boston in 1886. The association was heavily involved in teaching, as well as care of the sick, and soon changed its name to the Instructive District Nursing Association. Its original purposes and some nursing rules are given in Box 1-2. The Visiting Nurse Society of Philadelphia was founded later that same year. The Philadelphia society had as its stated purpose "to furnish visiting nurses to those otherwise unable to secure skilled attendance in time of sickness, to teach cleanliness and the proper care of the sick" (Brainard, 1922, p. 219). Service also was given to people of moderate means who could afford to pay some for the care given, and this became one of the earliest known fee-for-service programs. It is noteworthy that both of these organizations had health instruction as part of the visiting nursing visit; this would become an integral part of public health nursing later in the century.

More visiting nurse associations were founded in Chicago (1889), Buffalo (1891), Kansas City (1892), Detroit (1894), and Baltimore (1896). Visiting nursing was now well established in the United States. By 1905 there were 171 separate associations engaged in visiting nursing in the United States (Fitzpatrick, 1975, p. 7).

As these organizations evolved, there was discussion as to what to call them. In England the term *district nursing* was often used. In the United States the terms *district nursing*, *visiting nursing*, and *instructive visiting nursing* were used. Harriet Fulmer in her 1902 article states, "In adopting a name for any new society doing this work we would advise the use of the term 'Visiting Nursing' as being more comprehensive than 'District Nursing,' and less cumbersome than "Instructive Visiting Nursing" (Fulmer, 1902, p. 413). In 1909 Yssabella Waters published *Visiting Nursing in the United States.* This book compiled statistical information on all visiting nursing organizations in the United States (Carr, 1988, p. 83). Cities and towns often established their own visiting nurse services, and there was great diversity in the scope and quality of care given.

In 1896 the Nurses' Associated Alumni (now the American Nurses Association [ANA]) was formed and helped organize all the nurses of the country into a professional group. However, there was no specialty nursing organization, standardized training, or standards of practice for visiting nursing. Additionally, public health nursing had only recently been established.

### BOX 1-2

## *Instructive District Nursing Association of Boston: 1886*

### Original Purposes

1. To provide and support thoroughly trained nurses, who, acting under the immediate direction of the outpatient physicians of the Boston Dispensary, shall care for the sick poor in their own homes instead of in hospitals.
2. By precept and example to give such instruction to the families which they are called upon to visit as shall enable them henceforth to take better care of themselves and their neighbors by observing the rules of wholesome living and by practicing the simple arts of domestic nursing.

### Some Nursing Rules

1. Each nurse shall work for eight hours daily, employment on Sunday and holidays shall be exceptional, also night duty.
2. Nurses must be examples of neatness, cleanliness, and sobriety.
3. Nurses attending to contagious diseases shall be subject to special limitation in their attendance on other patients.
4. Nurses shall not interfere with the religious or political opinion of the patient.
5. Nurses shall not receive presents from patients, nor give money nor its equivalent.

From Brainard AM: *The evolution of public health nursing,* Philadelphia, 1922, WB Saunders, pp. 207, 210-211.

## A LOOK AT THE DIFFERENCE: VISITING NURSING AND PUBLIC HEALTH NURSING IN THE UNITED STATES

Early agencies providing nursing care for the sick poor in the United States were located primarily in northeastern cities where there were high rates of immigration, poverty, and disease (Buhler-Wilkerson, 1983, p. 90). Early visiting nurses and public health nurses both provided nursing care for the sick poor in their homes. However, as public health nursing evolved in the United States, nursing services focused more on the preventive aspects of care—health education, for instance, rather than illness care (Schulte, 2000, p. 4). While visiting nurses continued to visit the sick poor in their homes, public health nurses diligently worked to improve social conditions and improve the health of communities (see "A View from the Field").

Visiting nurses often worked for associations that were voluntary and nonprofit in nature (see Chapter 5), and funding was largely derived from charitable contributions and fee-for-service. Public health nurses often worked for state and local health departments, official governmental agencies supported by tax dollars. Visiting nursing associations usually were administered by nurses and existed solely to provide home nursing care of the sick. The administration of health departments often was under the direction of a physician, and health departments offered numerous services in addition to public health nursing. Agencies and settings in which visiting and public health nurses worked in 1912 are given in Table 1-1. These nurses could be found in both urban and rural settings. Definitions of public health nursing and the more contemporary term, community health nursing, are provided in Chapter 2. Public health nursing in the United States was founded by a great American, Lillian Wald.

### TABLE 1-1

## *Distribution of Public Health Nurses in 1912*

| | |
|---|---|
| Visiting nurse associations | 205 |
| City and state boards of health and education | 156 |
| Private clubs and societies | 108 |
| Tuberculosis leagues | 107 |
| Hospitals and dispensaries | 87 |
| Business concerns | 38 |
| Settlements and day nurses | 35 |
| Churches | 28 |
| Charity organizations | 27 |
| Other organizations | 19 |

From Gardner MS: *Public health nursing,* ed 3, New York, 1936, Macmillan, p. 40.
NOTE: This list gives a reasonably true picture of the general distribution of nursing work among the different types of agencies.

$A$ *view*
*from the field*

**ABSTRACT Historical Reprint**

In 1923 when this article first appeared in the February issue of *The Public Health Nurse,* it was fairly common for board members to go with a public health nurse on her rounds for a day. Many agencies today would welcome the same opportunity, but unfortunately the volunteer board member has less time available for this inside look into an agency. We may smile at the datedness of some of the descriptions but we will be quickly reminded that much of what was practiced then is practiced today. Read and enjoy!

The author of this piece was a member of the nursing committee, Public Health Nursing Department, The United Workers of Norwich, Connecticut.

Ruth N. Knollmueller
Historical Editor

A uniform of sober gray, relieved only by collar and cuffs of immaculate white linen, an armband bearing the letters P.H.N.—all of us know this uniform, most of us know the meaning of the letters, but how many stop to think of the deeper significance of the Public Health Nurse in terms of her community-wide service? Perhaps if the nurse tells us a bit about her daily travels it may help us to understand.

"How many calls have I made today? Twelve, no— thirteen in all. First I went to see a dear little girl, two years old, who has been so ill with empyema that for days we feared that we might lose her. A month ago she was operated on, and then a week later the doctor said that a second operation must be performed or the child would die. The Polish parents, almost frantic with anxiety, at first objected strongly, but finally consented to the second operation, and now the little girl is well on the road to recovery. Today I found her temperature normal for the first time in many weeks.

"My next patient was a young Greek woman who has a very interesting history. She had been an olive picker in her own country, but her eyes were turned toward the golden promise of America. The weary journey took three months, she tells me, and at the end was Ellis Island, with all that means of filth and disease. Small wonder that she caught an infectious skin trouble! I've been dressing the eruption every day for two weeks, but this is my last call, for the places are practically healed.

"In the near neighborhood there lives another Greek family. The children have been brought to our clinic and

so I ran in for a friendly visit, before I went on to my case. We call in the homes of all our clinic babies, you know, to see if we can give help or advice or instruction.

"From babyhood to old age, from the cradle to the grave, indeed! My next patient was an old lady, and she died in my arms. But at least I had made her last days comfortable and she did so enjoy the attention. In all her long lifetime she had never known ill-health, had never had a nurse, and so my coming was a great event for her.

"The last call this morning I made on the three weeks' old baby of a young Russian woman. The mother had no doctor when her child was born, and her condition afterwards became so serious that a doctor had to be called. The doctor sent for me to assist in giving the necessary treatment, but all too soon it became evident that an operation must be performed. So the young mother was taken to the hospital and the wee baby was left in the care of a kind neighbor. I've been making friendly calls on the mother in the hospital, as well as keeping an eye on the new baby.

"After lunch I went to dress a bad case of leg-ulcers. My patient is a dear old lady, who has been suffering for forty years, hobbling about as best she could on crutches. At last the sores became so troublesome that she sent for a doctor, and he, realizing the necessity for constant attention, asked our department to send in a nurse. For five months I've been going there to do the dressings, and you simply can't imagine what improvement my patient has made. Already the crutches are discarded, and I have hopes that before long the ulcers will have disappeared. Think what that will mean to her, after all these long years of suffering. Do you wonder that I find a warm welcome in that home?

"Next I called on a young woman who had just come home from the hospital after an operation. The wound is not yet entirely healed, and so I have to dress it, but more than all that I try to cheer her up, because the period of convalescence seems endless to her and she gets so discouraged.

"After I left that little woman I stopped to see a young tuberculosis patient who has insisted upon coming home from the sanatorium, much against all advice. I do hope he is using the knowledge he gained in the sanatorium for his own progress and the protection of his family. I called upon him because he came to the tuberculosis clinic, and we try to keep in touch with all our clinic cases through friendly calling.

"The next case was an hourly nursing call—a case of grippe, needing baths to reduce temperature, and after I

*Continued*

*A view
    from the field*

had finished making the patient more comfortable I made several short visits in the homes of clinic babies nearby.

"My last patient for the day was an old colored woman, who was once a slave. She's ninety-five and bedridden, needing daily care, but the house is spotlessly clean and she's such a cheerful old soul that it is a pleasure to do for her.

"It hasn't been a very exciting day, you see; there was nothing new or unusual, just a quiet day."

A quiet day! The work she does is as quiet and inconspicuous as the gray gown she wears, and yet it's so inclusive that today or tomorrow, directly or indirectly, it finds us all within the limits of its service.

From Young EE: A quiet day: a peep at some of the varied homes visited by a district nurse in the course of one "quiet day," *Public Health Nurs* 6:43-44, 1989.

## PUBLIC HEALTH NURSING IN THE UNITED STATES: ENTER LILLIAN WALD

**Lillian Wald** coined the expression public health nursing and founded public health nursing in this country (Figure 1-1). Although Nightingale had originated the idea of "health nursing," it was Wald who added the word *public* so that all people would know that this type of service was available to them (Haupt, 1953, p. 81). "Wald claimed she chose the title 'public health nurse' to place emphasis on the 'community value of the nurse' whose work was built upon an understanding of the social and economic problems invariably accompanying patients' ills" (Buhler-Wilkerson, 1993, p. 1780). *The House on Henry Street* (Wald, 1915) is her story of the work she did as director of the Henry Street Settlement.

Lillian Wald was born in 1867 and grew up in Rochester, New York. Her father, an optical goods dealer, provided a comfortable living for her family. She considered her childhood a spoiled, joyous one surrounded by love (Yost, 1965, p. 23). She studied at a private school and was an excellent student. Wald chanced to meet a graduate of the Bellevue Hospital Training School for Nurses who had assisted her sister during pregnancy. It was in this manner that she became interested in nursing. She graduated from training at New York Hospital in 1891 and supplemented her nursing instruction with a period of study at Women's Medical College. During this medical college experience, she was asked to give home nursing classes to a group of immigrant women living in the Lower East Side tenement district. The classes were held in a school on Henry Street. What she found amazed her—there was filth, squalor and smells, an unhealthy pallor to the children, and sickness and disease surrounding her (Yost, 1965, p. 26). One day when she was teaching a child approached her and asked her to go with her to attend her sick mother. This would become a turning point in Wald's career, and the point at which public health nursing was born:

From the schoolroom where I had been giving a lesson in bed-making, a little girl led me one drizzling March morning. She had told me of her sick mother, and gathering from her incoherent account that a child had been born, I caught up the paraphernalia of the bed-making lesson and carried it with me.

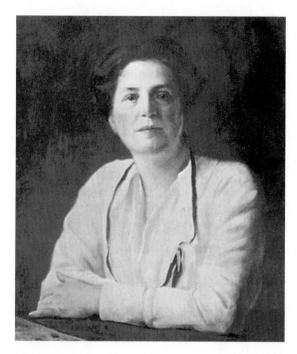

**FIGURE 1-1** Lillian Wald, the nurse leader who was the "predecessor of modern public health nursing," was far ahead of her time. She promoted health and social reform at a time when it was not the norm for women to engage in such activity. Her accomplishments truly reflect the mark of a professional nurse. (Courtesy of the Visiting Nurse Service of New York City.)

The child led me over broken roadways—there was no asphalt, although its use was well established in other parts of the city—over dirty mattresses and heaps of refuse—it was before Colonel Waring had shown the possibility of clean streets even in that quarter—between tall, reeking houses whose laden fire escapes, useless for their appointed purpose, bulged with household goods of every description. The rain added to the dismal appearance of the streets and to the discomfort of the crowds which thronged them, intensifying the odors which assailed me from every side. Through Hester and Division Streets we went to the end of Ludlow; past odorous fish-stands, for the streets were a marketplace, unregulated, unsupervised, unclean; past evil-smelling, uncovered garbage-cans; and—perhaps worst of all, where so many little children played—past the trucks brought down from more fastidious quarters and stalled on these already over-crowded streets, lending themselves inevitably to many forms of indecency.

The child led me on through a tenement hallway, across a court where open and unscreened closets were promiscuously used by men and women, up into a rear tenement, by slimy steps whose accumulated dirt was augmented that day by the mud of the streets, and finally into the sickroom.

All of the maladjustments of our social and economic relations seemed epitomized in this brief journey and what was found at the end of it. The family to which the child led me was neither criminal nor vicious. Although the husband was a cripple, one of those who stand on street corners exhibiting deformities to enlist compassion, and masking the begging of alms by a pretense at selling; although the family of seven shared their two rooms with boarders—who were literally boarders, since a piece of timber was placed over the floor for them to sleep on—and although the sick woman lay on a wretched, unclean bed, soiled with a hemorrhage two days old, they were not degraded human beings, judged by any measure of moral values.

In fact, it was very plain that they were sensitive to their condition, and when, at the end of my ministrations, they kissed my hands (those who have undergone similar experiences will, I am sure, understand), it would have been some solace if by any conviction of the moral unworthiness of the family I could have defended myself as a part of a society which permitted such conditions to exist. Indeed, my subsequent acquaintance with them revealed the fact that, miserable as their state was, they were not without ideals for the family life, and for society, of which they were so unloved and unlovely a part.

That morning's experience was a baptism of fire. Deserted were the laboratory and the academic work of the college—I never returned to them. On my way from the sickroom to my comfortable student quarters my mind was intent on my own responsibility. To my inexperience, it seemed certain that conditions such as these were allowed because people did not know, and for me there was a challenge to know and to tell. When early morning found me still awake, my naive conviction remained that, if people knew things—and "things" meant everything implied in the condition of this family—such horrors would cease to exist, and I rejoiced that I had a training in the care of the sick that in itself would give me an organic relationship to the neighborhood in which this awakening had come. (Wald, 1915, pp. 4-8)

This "baptism by fire" changed the life of Lillian Wald. She was finished with the thought of becoming a doctor; she would provide nursing care to the sick poor.

## The Henry Street Settlement

Wald had an exceptional ability to inform and convince people about the need for health care and social change (Backer, 1993, p. 122). She and her family had many wealthy friends and Wald eagerly approached them to help provide funding for nursing services to the sick poor. These friends did not disappoint her. In 1893 she and Mary Brewster, her friend and classmate, were able to obtain funds to establish a nurses' Settlement House on Jefferson Street in a slum section of the Lower East Side of New York. From the settlement house nurses would serve the sick poor and live among them (Box 1-3). Wald and Brewster became acquainted with their neighbors, let them know that they were trained nurses who would give

### BOX 1-3
### *Nursing Settlements*

The idea of the settlement house began in London in the late nineteenth century. The settlement movement was based on the belief that educated professionals could make a unique contribution to the lives of those less fortunate. Students and professionals established settlement houses in poor areas, lived as part of the community, and worked toward the betterment of the community. Settlement houses emerged in Europe and the United States. Two well-known settlement houses in the United States were Hull House in Chicago and the College Settlement in New York.

Lillian Wald and Mary Brewster founded what is considered the first nursing settlement in the United States, the Henry Street Settlement. However, it was not the only nursing settlement. It is uncertain just how many nursing settlements were established, but they are known to have existed in San Francisco, California, and Richmond, Virginia. Little is known of the settlement in San Francisco. The nurse's settlement at Richmond is considered the most comparable to Henry Street (Brainard, 1922, p. 254). This settlement was started in 1900 by the entire graduating class of Richmond's Old Dominion Hospital. Unlike the Henry Street Settlement, no fees were charged. Other differences included the requirement that the Richmond nurses have other jobs, "volunteer" at the settlement in their off-duty hours, and agree to pay $5 every month for rent plus board for the days actually spent there (Erickson, 1987, pp. 17, 20). Within a short time the Richmond settlement reorganized, and three paid nurses were employed. The concept of nursing settlements was short lived in the United States.

their services to the sick, and were busy immediately (Yost, 1965, p. 28). "By the end of the first month, Wald had begun to mobilize a vast array of the city's disjointed private relief and medical establishments to remedy her neighbors' ills" (Buhler-Wilkerson, 1991, p. 316).

The settlement was nonsectarian because Wald believed that a nurse could be most effective if she were independent of any religious agency. She thought that nurses should live in the neighborhood where they practiced so that they could better identify with the needs of the families served. Wald and her nurses lived at the settlement house and became an integral part of the community in which they lived.

Wald insisted that nurses should be available to anyone who needed them, without the intervention of a doctor, establishing early in the history of nursing that the profession should be an independent one. Families could refer themselves to the settlement's service without a physician referral. "Wald and Brewster quickly established the concept of the nurse ready to give her services in the home to all who needed them, making no distinction between those who could pay and those who could not, allied with no religious group, seeking to educate as well as to heal" (Kalisch,

### BOX 1-4

*Some Accomplishments of Lillian Wald*

Lillian Wald's accomplishments are legendary and involve numerous "firsts" in nursing. She devoted her life to nursing, was the founder of public health nursing, and transformed nursing care into health and social policy. She is a truly amazing woman whose ideas were far ahead of her time. Her accomplishments are even more remarkable considering that she achieved them in a time when women did not even have the right to vote. Some of her Henry Street Settlement nurses, including Lavinia Dock, were active in the suffragette movement. Inspired by Wald and her work, many of her settlement nurses went on to leadership positions in nursing. The following list notes some of Wald's accomplishments:

- Originated the term "public health nursing"
- Founded the Henry Street Settlement
- Established school nursing in the United States
- Was instrumental in establishing the American Red Cross Town and Country Nursing Service to provide rural visiting nursing
- Originated the idea of and helped establish the U.S. Children's Bureau
- Was instrumental in securing changes in national child labor laws
- Established and taught courses in public health nursing
- Founder and first president of the National Organization for Public Health Nursing
- Originated the idea of family-focused nursing
- Stressed the importance of health teaching in preventing disease and promoting health
- Established "milk stations" in New York City, where safe milk for infants and children could be obtained
- Was instrumental in securing better housing conditions in tenement districts in New York City
- Was instrumental in the development of city recreation centers, parks, and playgrounds for children in New York City (she put playgrounds in the backyards of the nursing settlement houses)
- Provided camp and recreational experiences for poor inner city children
- Helped establish graded public school classes for mentally disabled children
- Provided culturally sensitive, humanistic care for immigrants to the United States
- Elected to the Hall of Fame for Great Americans

Kalisch, 1995, p. 175). Wald insisted that the nurse must help in ways other than just caring for the sick and called upon them to keep aware of the conditions under which people lived and worked. She firmly believed in the dignity and independence of the people she served and in helping them to help themselves. Her vision was to provide comprehensive health care from the client's point of view and encourage personal and public responsibility for health—a vision that is still appropriate today.

In 1895 the settlement house moved to 265 Henry Street and became the **Henry Street Settlement (HSS)**. Her friend, Miss Brewster, was no longer with her because of poor health, but Lillian Wald continued on as the head resident—the nursing director. Soon branches of the settlement existed throughout the city. By 1910 the settlement staff of 54 nurses was making more than 143,000 home visits a year (Buhler-Wilkerson, 1993, p. 1780), and nursing service from the settlement was available 24 hours a day (Fitzpatrick, 1990, p. 94). Those who could pay were charged 10¢ to 25¢ a visit to detach the stigma of charity or missionary work (Coss, 1989). The HSS became known as an innovative force for health and human betterment in New York City and a model for other nursing agencies (Erickson, 1987, p. 18). "The Settlement House became not only the place where anyone could come for nursing aid when there was illness in the home . . . but also a center of community life and activity" (Yost, 1965, pp. 36-37). Wald was a true humanist, committed to helping people improve the quality of their lives. She and her settlement nurses advocated for improved housing, child labor laws, clean streets, better schools and parks, and garbage disposal and established playgrounds, libraries, clubs, and organizations for the members of the community. Some of her numerous achievements are highlighted in Box 1-4.

Chapters in Wald's book, *The House on Henry Street*, include information on the nurse and the community, education and the child, the handicapped child, children who work, the nation's children, social forces, and "new Americans." The HSS sponsored welfare, civic and social work, and visiting nursing and raised the level of social consciousness of the nurses working there. Many nurses who worked at the HSS made significant contributions to nursing, public health, and social reform. These nurses included Yssabella Waters, Annie Goodrich, Lavinia Dock, and Ruth B. Freeman (Table 1-2). Lavinia Dock worked at the HSS for almost 20 years and stated, "I never began to think until I went to Henry Street and worked with Miss Wald" (Estabrook, 1995, p. 143). Dock would later be a founder of the International Council of Nurses, write *The History of Nursing* (volumes 1-4) and *Short History of Nursing*, and become famous as a women's rights activist and suffragette. She became one of Lillian Wald's closest friends, and they worked together on many social causes. Mary Sewall Gardner, author of the first text on public health nursing, visited the settlement to learn about the work there. She and Lillian Wald became lifelong friends and inspired each other in their work (Nelson, 1953, p. 669).

Toward the end of Wald's life as she was thinking "of the vast fields that are as yet unexplored in the relationships between public health nursing and public health in its social entirety. I am envious of the younger leaders, who can transmit into programs and action the things that are within a nurse's responsibility" (Yost, 1965, p. 40). She remains an inspiration and role model for public health nurses today.

**TABLE 1-2**

*Selected Early Community and Public Health Nurse Leaders*

| LEADER | CONTRIBUTIONS |
|---|---|
| Mary Breckinridge (1877-1965) | Founder of the Frontier Nursing Service, pioneer in nurse-midwifery and in bringing modern nursing to rural America |
| Charity Collins (1882-*) | First African-American public health school nurse in the country |
| Lavinia Lloyd Dock (1858-1956) | Prolific nurse author and historian, an advocate for social reform, leader in the women's rights and labor movement, and a suffragette; helped to develop the American Nurses Association, one of the founders of the National Organization of Public Health Nurses |
| Ruth B. Freeman (1906-1982) | Prolific nurse author on public and community health nursing; worked as a Henry Street Settlement nurse, went on to achieve a doctorate, taught nursing and public health at John Hopkins and New York Universities, was the director of nursing of the American Red Cross, assumed leadership roles in the American Public Health Association, and was president of the National League for Nursing |
| Mary Sewall Gardner (1871-1961) | Wrote the first text on public health nursing; was a prolific author, one of the founders of the National Organization of Public Health Nurses and its second president, director of the Providence District Nursing Association for 25 years, director of the Town and Country Nursing Service of the American Red Cross, active abroad in World War I public health nursing services, and chaired the public health nursing section of the International Council of Nurses |
| Annie Goodrich (1866-1954) | Served as director of the Henry Street Settlement; was an outstanding nurse educator and crusader for professional nursing, first dean of the Army School of Nursing, first dean of the Yale University School of Nursing; received numerous national and international awards, including the Distinguished Service Medal of the USPHS; was President of the International Council of Nurses |
| Pearl McIver (1893-1976) | First nurse on the staff of the U.S. Public Health Service, director of the Office of Public Health Nursing in the USPHS and director of the Division of Nursing USPHS; expanded public health nursing services on the state and national level; served as Executive Director of the *American Journal of Nursing* |
| Margaret Sanger (1879-1966) | Provided the leadership for the birth control movement in the United States; launched the American Birth Control League, which became the Planned Parenthood Federation of America |
| Ada Mayo Stewart (1870-1945) | First occupational health nurse in the United States |
| Lina Rogers Struthers (1870-1946) | First school nurse in the United States, a Henry Street Settlement nurse |
| Lillian Wald (1867-1940) | Originator of the term "public health nursing"; started the public health nursing movement in the United States, founded the Henry Street Settlement in 1893 in New York City, staunch social rights advocate, instrumental in the formation of the Children's Bureau in 1912 (see Box 1-4) |

Modified from Kaufman M, Hawkins JW, Higgins LP, et al.: *Dictionary of American nursing biography*, Westport, Conn, 1988, Greenwood Press; Kalisch P, Kalisch BJ: *The advance of American nursing*, ed 3, Boston, 1995, Little, Brown; Yost E: *American women of nursing*, Philadelphia, 1965, JB Lippincott.

You can still visit the original HSS. The Visiting Nurse Service of New York City evolved from the original settlement and provides an extensive range of nursing and home care services.

*Stop and Think About It*

Many early nursing leaders lived and worked at the Henry Street Settlement. These nursing leaders made great strides in public health, nursing, and social reform and were role models for other nurses. Who are some of the local, state, and national nursing leaders today you see making a difference in health care delivery and society? What will your future leadership role be in nursing?

## School Nursing

School nursing has historically been a public health nursing role and was begun in the United States by Lillian Wald (see Chapter 20). In 1902 health conditions of school children in New York City were appalling. Large numbers of students were being sent home from school with diseases such as trachoma (an infectious eye disease), pediculosis, ringworm, scabies, and impetigo. They then played outside with the children from whom they had previously been excluded in the classroom (Wald, 1915, p. 51). Wald believed that with the assistance of a well-prepared nurse, fewer children would lose valuable school time and that it would be possible to treat those who needed it.

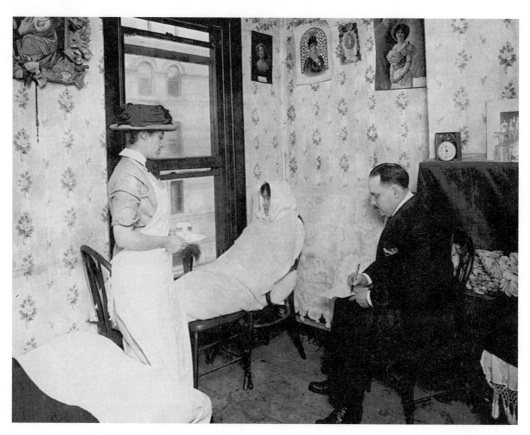

**FIGURE 1-2**  Convalescing from typhoid fever, New York City, 1912. (Courtesy of the Metropolitan Life Insurance Company of New York.)

Wald loaned Lina Rogers, an HSS nurse, to the New York City Health Department for a 1-month trial period as a school nurse. Miss Roger's stated, "I selected four schools in the most crowded part of the city, which I visited daily, spending about one hour in each, after which visits were made to the homes. First of all, crude dispensaries were improvised in each school, and these were equipped each day with supplies donated by the Settlement" (Brainard, 1922, p. 269). The experiment was so successful that the New York Board of Health appointed 12 other nurses to assist in carrying on the work (Brainard, 1922, p. 270). The sum of $30,000 was approved for the employment of these nurses—the first municipalized school nurses in the world (Wald, 1915, p. 53). By 1911, New York City was employing 150 nurses for school work, and school nursing had become an important part of public health nursing across the country (Fitzpatrick, 1975, p. 11). Under her married name of Struthers, Lina Rogers published the first book on school nursing, *The School Nurse*, in 1917. When Mary Sewall Gardner first wrote *Public Health Nursing* (1916), a chapter was dedicated to school nursing. School nursing remains an integral part of community health nursing today.

Wald was a great advocate for children. When she determined it was often a problem for neighborhood children to study in their homes, she assigned settlement rooms as study rooms and provided tutors. When she determined that some children in the neighborhood were not receiving adequate lunches for school, lunches were provided. Through her efforts, classes were established for children with disabilities. She started camp and recreational programs and built children's playgrounds behind the settlement houses. Many city children had no place to play, and these playgrounds were a new concept for the time. The first playground was referred to as "Bunker Hill" after the first battle of the American Revolution (Wald, 1915, p. 83). It became so popular that times had to be assigned for the children to visit, with toddlers and mothers coming in the morning and school children in the afternoons. Wald started the Outdoor Recreational League to develop neighborhood parks and convinced wealthy supporters to open their country homes to neighborhood children for outdoor recreational experiences; some of these homes were later bequeathed to the settlement. Wald said, "If I appear to lay too much stress upon the importance of play and recreation, it may be well to point out that it is one way of recognizing the dignity of the child" (Wald, 1915, p. 95). Wald's efforts resulted in city parks, playgrounds, and recreation areas, and police began to sponsor recreation and play activities for children. The governor of New York advocated that public schools should be surrounded by playgrounds and provided the impetus to a national play and recreation movement for children.

*Stop and Think About It*
Think about school nursing in your community. How are nursing services provided in the schools? Are the school nurses provided through the local health department, hired by the schools, or nonexistent? What services do these nurses provide? What is their level of education?

## Tuberculosis Nursing

Surveillance for infectious disease control was a major function of early public health nurses and continues to be a function of public health nurses today (Figure 1-2). Throughout the nineteenth century tuberculosis was a leading killer among infectious diseases in the United States. The isolation of the tuberculosis bacillus in 1882 by Robert Koch showed the dreaded disease was transmissible. By 1915 there were more than 1500 antituberculosis associations in the United States, including 35 state organizations (Gardner, 1916, p. 222). Tuberculosis patients were generally bedridden, and nursing care was often provided for them at home.

Lillian Wald was an originator of the concept of the tuberculosis nurse. HSS nurses regularly instructed patients and families about preventing and treating the disease (Wald, 1915, p. 54). In 1900, Jessie Sleet, an African-American nurse, was hired by New York City's Charitable Organization Society to try to reduce the spiraling incidence of the disease among the city's African-American population (Mosley, 1995, p. 65). In 1903, spearheaded by Lillian Wald, the New York City Health Department appointed three nurses (annual salary $900 each) to visit tuberculosis patients at home and teach the patients about sputum disposal and other aspects of care (Smillie, 1955, p. 412). The program was successful, and in 1905 the number of nurses was increased to 14. Across the country, agencies began to hire tuberculosis nurses. Ella LaMotte, a pioneer in tuberculosis nursing, wrote *The Tuberculosis Nurse* in 1915. When Mary Sewall Gardner first wrote *Public Health Nursing* (1916), an entire chapter was dedicated to tuberculosis nursing. Tuberculosis, once thought to be a dreaded disease of the past, has made a resurgence today.

## Occupational Health Nursing

Nurses from the HSS were keenly aware of the problems of child labor and unhealthy working conditions. Lillian Wald fought for the passage of child labor laws. Some HSS nurses provided nursing service in industrial settings. Settlement members Lavinia Dock and Lenora O'Reilly worked for labor reform (Estabrook, 1995, pp. 152-153). Occupational health nursing historically has been considered a public health nursing role. Ada Mayo Stewart, considered the first occupational health nurse in the United States, was hired by the Vermont Marble Company in 1897 to provide occupational health nursing services to workers in their homes and in the industry. She is considered the first occupational health nurse in the United States. When Mary Sewall Gardner first wrote *Public Health Nursing* (1916), an entire chapter was dedicated to industrial nursing. In this text, Chapter 21 discusses occupational health nursing.

## A Vision for National Coverage for Home-Based Care

In the early 1900s a unique partnership between a private enterprise and a public health nursing organization greatly expanded public health nursing services and provided nationwide insurance coverage for home-based nursing care. Lillian Wald was convinced that home nursing care was a cost-effective investment for insurance companies (Buhler-Wilkerson, 1993, p. 1781). She and Dr. Lee Frankel, of the **Metropolitan Life Insurance Company,** convinced the board of directors at Metropolitan that visiting nurses could care for policyholders during illness and that healthy policyholders would live longer, healthier lives and ultimately save the company money. In 1909 Metropolitan initiated the first public health nursing program for insurance policyholders (Haupt, 1953, p. 81). Rather than employing their own nurses, the company primarily contracted for services from existing visiting nursing associations. Three years after the program started, Metropolitan had contracts with more than 400 associations across the United States (Roberts, 1954, pp. 86-87). These associations made 1 million nursing visits a year nationwide (Buhler-Wilkerson, 1993, p. 1781). Partnering with Metropolitan Life generated important funding for visiting nursing associations and in many cases amounted to almost one third of the association's budget revenues (Buhler-Wilkerson, 1993, p. 1782). Because policyholder responses were positive, other insurance companies such as John Hancock funded similar services.

The Metropolitan project remained in place for 44 years. Numerous contributions to public health nursing occurred as a result of the project, including the provision of a national system of home nursing, the establishment of a cost-accounting system for visiting nurses, the achievement of outcomes linking nursing visits to a reduction in mortality rates, and the benefits of nurses and business working together to promote health. Over the lifetime of the program more than 1 billion home visits were made! Today, rather than life insurance policies covering home-based care, many health insurance policies offer such coverage on a limited basis.

## A Vision to Create a National Program of Public Health Nursing

While public health nursing in cities and towns was developing at a rapid rate at the beginning of the century, nursing service in rural areas was progressing slowly. Lillian Wald was acutely aware of this problem and looked to create a national program of public health nursing service in the United States (Buhler-Wilkerson, 1993, p. 1782). Wald was a member of the American Red Cross and expressed strong dissatisfaction at seeing this national organization limited to service only in war or disaster. She believed that the Red Cross was a logical facility to promote public health nursing on a national scale (Dock, Pickett, Noyes, et al., 1922, p. 1212). She proposed that the Red Cross standardize public health nursing in rural areas and coordinate the work of isolated nurses and nursing organizations under a central agency (Buhler-Wilkerson, 1993, p. 1782).

Wald asked her wealthy friend, Jacob Shiff, to donate money to the Red Cross so that a national system of public health nursing could be developed. As a result, in 1912 the Red Cross began the Rural Nursing Service, soon to be called the **Town and Country Nursing Service,** and Mary Sewall Gardner was its first director. The purpose of the department was to supply rural areas and small towns with trained public health nurses and to supervise their work. (Rural nursing services are discussed further in Chapter 3.) However, the Red Cross did not assume the financial responsibility for this work. Local voluntary and charitable organizations, as well as fee-for-service, financed the nursing care given.

Services initially sprang up all over the country and at one time there were nearly 3000 programs. However, by 1947, because of problems with funding, support, and administration, the number of programs had decreased to less than 100 and the service was discontinued (Buhler-Wilkerson, 1993, p. 1784). The administration of such programs moved away from the national leadership provided by the Red Cross back to local leadership.

### A Great American

Lillian Wald's work was widely recognized both in this country and abroad. On September 12, 1971, Wald became the first nurse and only the tenth woman elected to the Hall of Fame for Great Americans (Griffin, Griffin, 1973, p. 103). A bronze bust of Wald was placed in the Hall of Fame for Great Americans. An editorial about this event stated the following:

The kind of health care Lillian Wald began preaching and practicing in 1893 is the kind the people of this country are still crying for. She demonstrated with no need to rest on formal research that nursing could serve as the entry point—not only for health care, but for dealing with many other social ills of which sickness is only a part. She felt that nurses should go to the sick, instead of expecting the sick to come to them (and waiting for physicians to refer them); that care of persons in the home, especially of children, was far more effective and much less expensive except perhaps for those needing, to use her own word, "intensive" care (A Prophet Honored, 1971, p. 53).

The words of a noted nursing historian, Karen Buhler-Wilkerson, pay tribute to Wald and give us a vision to strive for:

We can be reinvigorated by Wald's vision of the public health nurse: providing care from the patient's point of view; encouraging personal and public responsibility; and providing a unifying structure for the delivery of comprehensive, equally available health care. To reinvent that vision for the 21st century would be a fitting and lasting tribute to Wald (Buhler-Wilkerson, 1993, p. 1785).

## MARY BRECKINRIDGE

**Mary Breckinridge** was a contemporary of Lillian Wald. In 1925 she founded the Frontier Nursing Service to provide public health nursing services to families in rural Kentucky. Like Wald, this remarkable woman dedicated her life to improving the health of the poor and underserved.

Almost from birth, Breckinridge held a fondness and affinity for the people of Kentucky. Her father had been born and raised in Lexington, Kentucky. Her Grandmother Lees, a Kentuckian by birth, was a wealthy and charitable woman who spent a large part of her fortune on the education of Kentucky children. Mary said of her grandmother, "I doubt if she ever refused to help any Kentucky mountain child whose need she knew" (Breckinridge, 1952, p. 4). Young Mary would sit at her grandmother's feet and listen as she read letters from the children she was helping. Later in life Mary would state, "Nearly a lifetime later, when I was living on money that came from my Grandmother Lees, it seemed altogether right to use this money to start the Frontier Nursing Service in the Kentucky mountains" (Breckinridge, 1952, p. 4).

Mary's family was well-to-do and traveled extensively. Although it was not deemed "proper" for her to receive a college education, Mary and her sister were educated by governesses and learned to speak both German and French. Mary loved her family and enjoyed her life but said, "I chafed at the complete lack of purpose in the things I was allowed to do. Several times I suggested to my mother that it would be nice to do something useful, but I never got anywhere with such an idea" (Breckinridge, 1952, p. 45). Later in life Mary would remedy that situation.

As a girl Mary frequently visited her uncle's plantation, and it was there that she learned to ride a horse—a skill that was a great asset to her in the Frontier Nursing Service. She would say of these times, "The happiest hours of my girlhood were spent on Oasis plantation in Mississippi and I loved it more than any place in the world. . . . We rode constantly when I was young, not only for fun but often because it was the easiest way to get about" (Breckinridge, 1952, p. 36). Figure 1-3 is a photograph of Mary Breckinridge, possibly on her beloved horse Teddy Bear.

Following the early death of her first husband, she enrolled in nursing school at St. Luke's Hospital in New York City (Wilkie, Moseley, 1969, p. 27). She remarried after graduation, but this marriage ended after the death of her two children—Polly, an infant daughter, and Breckie, her 4-year-old son. Her children gone and her marriage over, she began to devote herself to the work that would consume the rest of her life. She cherished the memories of her lost children and devoted her life to promoting the health of disadvantaged women and children (Browne, 1966, p. 54). Breckinridge (1952) stated, "My life was dedicated to the service of children" (p. 111).

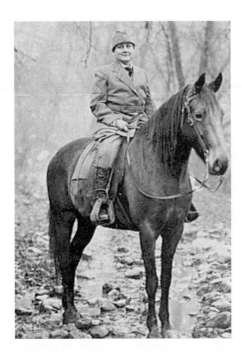

**FIGURE 1-3** Mary Breckinridge founded the Frontier Nursing Service in Kentucky. Her nurses used horses to provide service to families in the hills of Kentucky. (Courtesy of the Frontier Nursing Service of Wendover, Kentucky.)

At the end of World War I she volunteered for the American Committee for Devastated France. In postwar France and England she developed programs for war-devastated children and pregnant women and became interested in midwifery. A unique program she developed in France was the "goat crusade" through which Americans donated goats to provide milk for hungry infants (Browne, 1966, p. 54). When she returned to the United States, she wanted to continue her work with women and children and her idea for the Frontier Nursing Service was born.

### The Frontier Nursing Service

In 1925 Mary Breckinridge founded the Kentucky Committee for Mothers and Babies, and in 1928 the name was changed to the **Frontier Nursing Service (FNS)**. The service was based in rural Hyden, Kentucky. The area surrounding Hyden was mountainous, isolated, and with little access to health care. In December 1925 the Wendover outpost, just south of Hyden, was completed. Mary Breckinridge's 79-year-old father and his fox terrier, Patch, the dog that had belonged to her son, came to live with her at Wendover. There was a housewarming that Christmas and a bronze plaque placed on the chimney in the Wendover living room commemorating the day that stated: "To the glory of God and in memory of Breckie and Polly. Dedicated Christmas 1925" (Breckinridge, 1952, p. 180). Each year Christmas festivities with gifts for the local children and families were held at all the FNS outposts. Dolls were a favorite gift of the young girls.

Through the FNS, the Hyden Hospital was built in Hyden, Kentucky in 1928. The hospital was the first in the area and provided desperately needed services. Eventually, the area serviced by the FNS was divided into 8 districts of about 78 square miles each (Kalisch, Kalisch, 1995, p. 278). An outpost nursing center consisting of a log cabin was erected in the middle of each district. Two nurses lived at the outpost and provided care to the people of the district, usually about 200 families (Kalisch, Kalisch, 1995, p. 278). Because there were few highways in the area, much of the nurses' travel was done by horse. A fee of $1 a year was charged for general nursing and care and $5 was charged for maternity care (Breckinridge, 1952, p. 202). In relation to these fees Breckinridge (1952) states:

There was so little 'cash money' in the mountains for years after we started our work that our five-dollar midwifery fee...was rarely paid in money. In lieu of this fee we accepted quilted 'kivers' from the women, homemade split bottom chairs from the husbands, food from those who had a small surplus and the husband's labor in mending fences and whitewashing barns. The one dollar a year that we asked each cabin to pay for general nursing care was more often paid in cash if it could be paid at all (p. 202).

The FNS nursing service offered numerous services, including general nursing, midwifery, children's health, and public health. Services for children were extensive, according to Kalisch and Kalisch (1995):

The Frontier Nursing Service offered care for infants and children. Babies under one year of age were examined twice a month, preschool children from one to six were seen every month, and schoolchildren were examined once every three months. During these visits mothers were taught about diet, cleanliness, health habits, general sanitation, and preventive care. Inoculations against typhoid and diphtheria and vaccinations for smallpox were also given (p. 280).

The FNS was an effort of love and caring and a great success. By 1930 the outpost nursing centers served nearly 10,000 people in southeastern Kentucky (Browne, 1966, p. 55). The FNS is still in operation today, and many agencies have modeled their programs after the work of Mary Breckinridge and the FNS.

**NURSE-MIDWIFE SERVICES.** All the nurses in the FNS were required to have nurse-midwifery education in addition to their nursing and public health training. This was rather difficult at the time because such training was not offered in the United States. The nurses traveled abroad to Scotland or England to receive such training. The first nurse-midwife to the Wendover outpost, Ellen Halsall, came in 1926 and was soon joined by Gladys Peacock and Mary Willeford (Breckinridge, 1952, p. 189). The midwives were very successful and greatly reduced maternal and infant mortality. In looking at the first 1000 midwifery cases of the FNS, it was noted that there were one third fewer stillbirths and one third fewer deaths among infants in the first year of life than among the general population of Kentucky, and that if such a service were available to all U.S. women there would be a savings of 10,000 mothers' lives a year, 30,000 fewer stillbirths, and

30,000 more infants alive at the end of the first month of life (Dublin, 1932, pp. 1-2; Kalisch, Kalisch, 1995, pp. 279-280).

## ORGANIZING PUBLIC HEALTH NURSES

Professional nursing organizations were beginning to form during the later part of the nineteenth century. In 1893 the Society of Superintendents of Schools of Nursing was formed with Elizabeth Hampton as president. In 1896 she became president of the newly formed Nurses Associated Alumnae (later to become the ANA) under her married name of Elizabeth Hampton Robb (Griffin, Griffin, 1973, p. 101). Robb's early death at the age of 50 was a loss to nursing of an influential and dynamic leader. Public health nursing leaders including Lillian Wald, Mary Sewall Gardner, Lavinia Dock, and Ella Crandall also recognized the need to develop a professional organization and professional standards of practice for public health nursing. They felt that only a new organization "whose sole object should be public health nursing would adequately meet the need" (Gardner, 1919, p. 41).

### National Organization for Public Health Nursing

A momentous day in the history of American public health nursing was June 7, 1912. On that day, at the annual meeting of the ANA and the National League of Nursing Education (formerly the Society of Superintendents of Training Schools for Nurses), the National Organization for Public Health Nursing (NOPHN) was voted into existence. Lillian Wald was the organization's first president and Mary Sewall Gardner its second. The organization was devoted to public health nursing and its stated purposes included the expansion of public health nursing, the development of professional standards of practice and ethics, and the furthering of relationships among all people interested in the public's health (Fitzpatrick, 1975, p. 27). It was the first national nursing organization to have a headquarters and paid staff. For a long period in the development of nursing, it grew in power, set standards for practice, and influenced education by requiring certain curriculum content as a basis for employment (Fagin, 1978, p. 752). The organization achieved standardization for public health nursing practice through accreditation of programs and certification of practitioners (Olson, Wood, 1999, p. 27). Collaborative relationships among health and social agencies have always been a strength of public health nursing. A unique feature of the NOPHN was that its membership was open to people and agencies outside of nursing.

In 1952 the NOPHN merged with the National League for Nursing Education and the Association of Collegiate Schools for Nursing to become the National League for Nursing (NLN). When this happened, there was no longer a separate nursing organization dedicated solely to public health nursing. The lack of a separate organization dedicated to public health nursing significantly weakened the leadership of the profession.

However, other organizations had public health nursing constituencies and activities. When the American Public Health Association (APHA) was founded in 1872, its establishment spearheaded the development of state and local health departments and public health services in the United States. It is the nation's longest standing public health organization and continues to have a strong public health nursing section. The association's public health nursing section continues to organize public health nurses nationwide and has recently worked in conjunction with ANA to write standards of public health nursing practice. A more contemporary nursing organization, the Association for Community Health Nursing Educators (ACHNE), is a strong group of community health professionals who continuously look at community health nursing education and scope of practice.

## EDUCATION FOR PUBLIC HEALTH NURSES

In the early days of public health nursing, all nurses were prepared in hospital-based programs. Frequently, curriculum content was determined by the needs of the hospital and was controlled by physicians. Nursing education was illness- and individual-oriented and did not adequately prepare nurses to promote wellness and work in the community. Public health nursing demanded that nurses receive training beyond the basic hospital program. It was believed that public health nurses needed to be knowledgeable in subjects such as economics, politics, culture, hygiene and sanitation, food safety and preparation, bacteriology, social services, sociology, psychology, and principles and practice of district nursing (Fitzpatrick, 1975, pp. 13-14).

The first formal course in public health nursing was offered by the Boston Instructive Nursing Association in 1906 (McNeil, 1967, p. 4). This course was offered to graduate nurses wishing to practice in public health. Public health nursing leaders were at the forefront of the effort in establishing university affiliation for nursing education (Olson, Wood, 1999, p. 29). An early nursing leader, Elizabeth Hampton Robb, was instrumental in having the first university course for graduate nurses in public health offered at Teachers College in New York in 1910 (Griffin, Griffin, 1973, p. 101). The course at Teacher's College was taught in affiliation with the HSS.

In 1919, under the auspices of the Rockefeller Foundation and at the urging of concerned nursing leaders, the Committee for the Study of Public Health Nursing Education was founded. Josephine Goldmark was secretary of the committee, and the study was later to bear her name the *Goldmark Report*. The purposes of the committee were to study public health nursing education; to look at typical examples of public health nursing education and service; and to study the education afforded by hospital training schools, graduate courses for public health nurses, and special schools of a non-nursing type (Committee for the Study of Nursing Education, 1923, p. 2). The study was expanded the following year to look at the entire field of nursing education. The conclusions reached profoundly affected the course of nursing and public health nursing. The study recommended state legislation in regard to nursing licensure and standards, higher quality nursing education, additional training for nursing faculty, and increased funding for nursing education. A major recommendation of the study was that, following basic hospital training, nurses practicing in public health needed postgraduate education that included class and field work in public health nursing. Agencies sought to hire nurses with this training in public health, but training was scarce and the demand for such nurses increasing. At this time, fewer than 7% of the nurses working in public health had adequate public health training (Roberts, Heinrich, 1985, p. 1164).

By 1921, 15 colleges and universities in the United States offered postgraduate public health nursing courses that met NOPHN standards. These courses taught preventive medicine, covering topics such as how to examine a class of children, how to find those who were developing measles, and how to visit in a home and evaluate tuberculosis contacts (Jensen, 1959, p. 236). In 1944 the first baccalaureate program in nursing became accredited as including adequate preparation for public health nursing so that graduates did not need postgraduate study to practice (NOPHN, 1944, p. 371). National nursing organizations began considering making public health nursing coursework a required part of baccalaureate nursing education. Today, such preparation is a part of all baccalaureate nursing programs.

## Public Health Nursing Becomes Part of the Baccalaureate Nursing Program

In 1963 the NLN, an accrediting body for schools of nursing education, required that a baccalaureate nursing program have coursework in public health nursing in order for the program to be accredited. Since that time, public health coursework has continued to be a major difference between the educational programs of baccalaureate nurses and diploma and associate degree programs.

The educational preparation necessary for community health nursing has continued to be a topic of discussion. During the 1980s a national consensus conference was held (U.S. Department of Health and Human Services [USDHHS], 1985) and national studies were conducted (Blank, McElmurry, 1988; Jones, Davis, Davis, 1987) to examine the educational preparation needed to practice as a generalist (baccalaureate prepared) and specialist (master's prepared) in public health nursing. A national consensus conference also was held to address education preparation for a specialist in home care (Cary, 1989). During this conference participants believed that a home care specialist needed strong preparation in public health nursing. Currently several documents address the essential concepts needed to function effectively in public and community health nursing (ACHNE, 1990, 1991, 1993; ANA, 1986, 1999; APHA, 1996; ASTDN, 2000; Blank, McElmurry, 1988; Jones, Davis, Davis, 1987; USDHHS, 1985). The ANA also has standards on a variety of community health nursing specialties such as home health

care nursing, hospice nursing, and prison health. Professional books and journals assist nurses in keeping up-to-date.

## Specialty Books and Journals

Books and journals are an important part of nursing education. It is through books and journals that the nurse learns, stays current, and finds out about progress in research and clinical practice.

In 1916 **Mary Sewall Gardner,** an HSS nurse and nursing leader, wrote the first public health nursing text, titled *Public Health Nursing.* This text went into three editions (1916, 1924, 1936) and was translated into French, Chinese, Spanish, Japanese, and Korean (Griffin, Griffin, 1973, p. 104; Nelson, 1954, p. 38). It is considered a classic in the field and had worldwide influence (Nelson, 1954, p. 39). Gardner wrote numerous articles on public health nursing and, after her retirement, wrote books on public health nursing for lay readers. These later books were *So Build We* (1942) that detailed public health nursing administration, principles, and policies and *Mary Kent* (1946), which is considered somewhat autobiographic (Nelson, 1954, p. 38).

When Gardner retired from professional writing with the last edition of *Public Health Nursing,* there was a great need for someone to continue the tradition. **Ruth B. Freeman,** a new, and soon to be prolific, writer in the field of public health nursing would fill this need. Freeman graduated from nursing school in 1927 and would later obtain both masters and doctoral education. She worked as an HSS nurse, taught nursing and public health at New York University and John Hopkins University, was the director of nursing at the American Red Cross, was active in leadership roles in the APHA, and served as president of the NLN. She received the NLN Mary Adelaide Nutting Award and the Pearl McIver Public Health Nurse Award (Griffin, Griffin, 1973, p. 106; Safier, 1977, p. 77). Freeman wrote books on public health nursing including *Public Health Nursing Practice* (1950), *Techniques of Supervision in Public Health Nursing* (1944, 1950), and *Community Health Nursing Practice* (1970, 1981). Her writings in the field are considered classic, have gone into numerous editions, and were used by many schools of nursing as texts into the 1980s. Students often find it interesting to look at some of these early public health nursing texts and compare them to contemporary readings. Today numerous texts address the practice of community health nursing.

The first nursing journal in the United States, the *American Journal of Nursing,* began publication in 1900. Nurses were the founders and original stockholders of this journal (Dolan, 1969, p. 314). The journals early issues contained numerous articles on visiting and public health nursing. On the very day that the NOPHN was formed in 1912, the Cleveland Visiting Nurses' Association presented its magazine, *The Visiting Nurses' Quarterly,* to the organization as a gift. *The Quarterly* later became *Public Health Nurse,* then *Public Health Nursing,* and finally *Nursing Outlook.* Contemporary nursing journals such as the

*Journal of Community Health Nursing, Public Health Nursing,* and *Home Healthcare Nurse* help disseminate information on public and community health nursing. Other public health and health behavior journals such as the *American Journal of Public Health, Public Health Reports,* and the *Journal of Health Education* are valuable resources. Although there were many early publications in the field of public health nursing, a specific set of professional standards of practice did not exist.

## STANDARDS OF PRACTICE

Standards of practice are a hallmark of a profession, provide guidance in achieving excellence of care, and reflect current knowledge in the field. It was long recognized that standards of practice needed to be developed for public health nursing but they were slow to evolve. The first comprehensive statement of public health nursing objectives and functions was prepared by the NOPHN in 1931 (McIver, 1949, p. 65). *Standards of Community Health Nursing Practice* were first written by the ANA in 1973. In 1999 the Quad Council of the ANA published *Scope and Standards of Public Health Nursing Practice.* These standards are discussed in Chapter 2. The Quad Council is a group of specialty organizations that focuses on public health nursing.

## 1900-1919: PUBLIC HEALTH NURSING

At the turn of the century the future of public health nursing appeared bright. Public health nurses were an economical and effective way to help the poor and combat the spread of communicable disease. Buhler-Wilkerson (1983) states:

Within a decade the public health nurse's role had expanded to include a variety of preventive services, not only for those suffering from infectious diseases like tuberculosis, but also for mothers, babies, school children, and industrial workers. Since public health nurses fit neatly into the system of social and medical care that was evolving at the time, it was not surprising that the number and variety of agencies seeking their services increased steadily (p. 89).

The number of agencies employing public health nurses increased from 58 in 1901 to almost 2000 by 1914, and 60 different organizations employed public health nurses in New York City alone (Buhler-Wilkerson, 1983, p. 91). The formation of the NOPHN in 1912 gave public health nurses a strong professional organization.

By the time of World War I in 1917, the role of the public health nurse was well established and respected. The U.S. Armed Forces saw a need to develop public health nursing programs for military outposts, and a nurse was loaned to the U.S. Public Health Service (USPHS) from the NOPHN for program development. This was the first public health nursing service to be established within the federal government (Gardner, 1919). The war resulted in the involvement of thousands of nurses in military service, and general and public health nursing services in the United States were threatened by this wartime nursing demand.

The nation looked for ways to address this nursing shortage. The American Red Cross established a roster of available nurses to facilitate providing health care services and placed emphasis on providing health education and communicable disease services to American communities (Roberts, 1954, p. 131). In an effort to ease the nursing shortage, the American Red Cross helped establish the Vassar Training Camp for Nurses, where the typical 3-year nursing course was shortened to 2 years for students who had graduated from college majoring in other subjects. Annie Goodrich, an early public health nursing leader and prominent nurse educator, and Isabel Maitland Stewart, another prominent nurse educator, were instrumental in the development and leadership of the training camp program (Griffin, Griffin, 1973, pp. 104-105). Graduates of this program numbered 435; the program ended with the Armistice.

## AFTER WORLD WAR I

Rapid changes came with peace. Economic prosperity, reaction to Prohibition, and the increasing use of the automobile created radical changes in the way people lived. These trends brought subsequent changes in public health nursing. For instance, the use of the automobile permitted nurses to have easy access to rural areas and made once-closed areas accessible. The previous use of walking, bicycles, and horse and buggies made it difficult to reach many underserved populations and public health nursing services rapidly expanded (Figure 1-4).

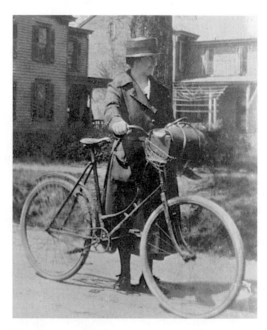

**FIGURE 1-4** Public health nurse using a bicycle before the advent of the automobile. (Courtesy of the Metropolitan Life Insurance Company of New York.)

In 1920 only 28 states had a statewide public health nursing program, and only 5 had divisions of public health nursing within state health departments (Roberts, 1954, p. 168). After the war, public health became a subject of nationwide interest and concern (Smillie, 1952, p. 10). The poor physical condition of the nation's men, made evident in wartime, shocked the nation. About 29% of those called for service were unfit for military duty because of problems that in many cases were preventable (Roberts, 1954, p. 164). Health programs to address these concerns grew as a result.

During this time voluntary (non–tax-supported) agencies were very active in public health nursing activities. Some of these organizations were the American Red Cross, the National Tuberculosis Association (forerunner of today's American Lung Association), the Metropolitan Life Insurance Company, and the John Hancock Life Insurance Company. Insurance companies paid public health nurses to visit their subscribers. The Red Cross often supplemented the work of health agencies, and Red Cross supervisors served as public health nursing supervisors in some state health departments. The National Tuberculosis Association provided public health nursing services to tuberculosis patients in many states (Fox, 1920, p. 180).

Postwar studies by the Children's Bureau showed that the United States had a higher maternal death rate than most other developed countries. The passage of the Shepherd-Towner Act of 1921 became a historic milestone in the evolution of public health nursing and helped address our nation's appalling maternal-child health statistics. This act, administered by the Children's Bureau, gave grants to states to develop programs that provided nursing care to mothers, infants, and children.

**Marie Phelan** was appointed in 1923 as the first nurse consultant to the federal government in peacetime. At the request of state health departments, she helped develop programs that promoted the health of mothers and children (Figures 1-5 and 1-6). Her work created a demand for public health nurses, and the work of these nurses was instrumental in lowering the national maternal and infant death rate. In 1933 **Pearl McIver** was appointed to the USPHS as a public health nursing consultant. She would later head the Office of Public Health Nursing and the Division of Nursing within the USPHS.

By the 1930s and 1940s more Americans were moving from a system of health care at home to the acceptance and provision of health care in hospitals and long-term care settings. As hospitals gained in number and popularity, the need for visiting nurse services subsided. It was also during this period that psychiatric hospitals and institutional settings for people who were mentally retarded and mentally ill gained in number and popularity.

At this time, national research studies showed that, although communicable diseases remained important causes of morbidity and mortality, the United States was having to address the rising incidence of chronic disease. Americans were living longer than ever before and chronic diseases had become a national health problem. Chronic diseases continue to be a contemporary health problem, and we are far from having reached resolution on their prevention or treatment.

## The Great Depression and the Social Security Act

Possibly no single event took as great a toll on the nation's health as the Great Depression. The Depression of 1929 forced many hospitals and schools of nursing to close, and the supply of nurses far exceeded the demand. Unemployment was high, and people could not afford even basic food, shelter, and clothing. Unrest among the general population

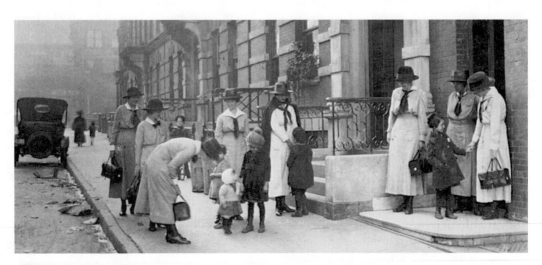

**FIGURE 1-5** To these nurses of the 1930s, the city's streets were hospital corridors and family bedrooms their wards. Each carried cakes of soap to protect herself from germs and a whistle to guard herself from danger. (Courtesy of the Visiting Nurse Service of New York City.)

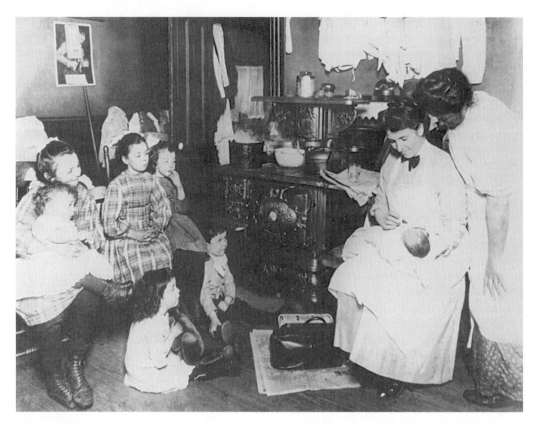

**FIGURE 1-6** Involving the family in infant care, Boston, 1912. (Courtesy of the Metropolitan Life Insurance Company of New York.)

was high, and a cry from the people for more governmental intervention in matters of health and welfare was heard across the country. Promoting the general welfare of the people was outlined in the U.S. Constitution, and now was a time when governmental agencies were called on to assume more responsibility in this area. In an effort to deal with many of the problems brought on by the Depression, the Social Security Act of 1935 introduced government health and welfare programs and provided monies that aided in the expansion of public health nursing services (see Chapter 5).

### The Social Security Act and Public Health

Title VI of the Social Security Act focused on public health programs; its overall purpose was to elicit a public health program that would protect and promote the nation's health. Title VI was directly responsible for expanding and developing state and local public health nursing programs and provided money for nurses to study public health. As a result of this legislation, the public health nurse became an integral part of local health departments.

Before 1935 only one third of the states had a public health nursing section within the state health department. At the same time only 7% of the public health nurses employed had adequate preparation in public health nursing (Fitzpatrick, 1975; Roberts, Heinrich, 1985, p. 1164). The

Social Security provided funding for training of public health nurses. During 1936, the first year that training money became available, over 1000 nurses received money to study public health nursing and by 1940, 3000 nurses had received public health training (Williams, 1951, p. 156). This funding for public health nursing provided an impetus for states to implement public health nursing services. By 1938 every state had established public health nursing programs (Roberts, Heinrich, 1985, p. 1164).

Historically, maternal-child health has been a major focus of community health nursing. As already mentioned, Lillian Wald and Mary Breckinridge were staunch advocates for children's rights and maternal-child health. Funds from Title V of the act were designed to improve the health of mothers and children who did not have access to adequate health care, particularly those from low-income families, and significantly expanded the scope of public health nursing services. It is under the Social Security Act that today's Medicaid program providing health care services to young families exists.

### WORLD WAR II AND INTO THE 1950s

After World War II began in 1941, an acute nurse shortage existed in the United States. The National Nursing Council, composed of six national nursing organizations, along with the aid of the U.S. Department of Education, requested funding to enlarge facilities for nursing education. Funding programs for nurses' training included Training for Nurses for National Defense, the GI bill, the Nurse Training Act of 1943, and Public Health and Professional Nurse traineeships.

Under the leadership of Surgeon General Thomas Parran, the Public Health Service Act of 1944 was passed. Long overdue, this act consolidated existing federal public health legislation under one piece of legislation and provided for numerous public health programs (see Chapter 5). Today this act incorporates our National Institutes of Health and funding for training of health professionals and other national public health measures.

During World War II the country had to take a close look at use of health care resources and services; maximum use of personnel was essential. To better use personnel, official public health agencies often combined with voluntary agencies to avoid service duplication. However, combination agencies would prove difficult to fund and administer, and many of them returned to their separate structures. Public health nursing services usually were housed in state and local health departments, while visiting nursing "home health care" services were provided by voluntary agencies in the community.

During the war years the establishment of priorities for health care became a topic for discussion, but it would be decades before the country would form national health objectives (see Chapter 4). The importance of public health nursing service was clearly recognized, and public health nurses were declared essential for civilian work and promoting the nation's health. The war helped the nation recognize its serious undersupply of nurses. The war also forced the country to look at health care delivery in the United States.

## Considering A National Health Program

At many times during our country's history, a national health program has been considered, but not implemented. With the end of World War II in 1945, President Harry Truman presented to Congress a recommendation for a comprehensive, national health program in which nursing would have played an important role (Kalisch, Kalisch, 1995, p. 364). Truman recommended the following:

1. Federal grants for construction of hospitals and related facilities
2. Expansion of public health, maternity, and child health services
3. Federal grants for medical education, nursing education, and research
4. Establishment of a national social insurance program for the prepayment of medical costs
5. Expansion of present social insurance systems to furnish protection against loss of wages from sickness and disability

Charges of socialism from the American Medical Association ended the quest for a national health insurance program (Kalisch, Kalisch, 1995, p. 366). Today the United States still has not realized Truman's goal.

## Public Health Nursing Expands

In 1946 the Division of Nursing was organized in the USPHS with Lucile Petry as its first director (USPHS, 1997, p. 4). The Division had three offices: Public Health Nursing, Nurse Education, and Resources and Hospital Nursing. The first director of the Office of Public Health Nursing was Pearl McIver.

To better define public health nursing roles and avoid duplication of services, a committee of representatives from numerous agencies published guidelines in 1946 on how public health nursing should be organized (Desirable Organization, 1946, p. 387). The guidelines adopted by the committee agreed that a population of 50,000 was needed to support a comprehensive public health program and that there should be one public health nurse for every 2000 people. Other principles included the following:

- That each public health nurse should combine the functions of health teaching, control of disease, and care of the sick
- That the community should adopt one of three patterns of organization that would best serve that community:
  1. All public health nursing service, including care of the sick at home, is administered by the local health department.
  2. Preventive services are carried on by the health department with one voluntary agency, in close coordination with the health department, carrying responsibility for bedside nursing care—a combined agency.
  3. A combination service is jointly administered and financed by official and voluntary agencies, with all service given by a single group of public health nurses.

In 1948 Esther Lucile Brown's study of nursing education, *Nursing for the Future*, recommended that nurses should be educated in colleges and universities. This would become increasingly important to public health nursing as public health content began to emerge as part of the curricula of these programs.

## Other Happenings

The Hospital Survey and Construction Act of 1946, often called the Hill Burton Act, provided funding for the building and remodeling of nonprofit hospitals throughout the country. Priority was given to the construction of hospitals and public health centers in rural and underserved areas (Kalisch, Kalisch, 1995, p. 591). The availability of more hospitals had an impact on the need for public health nursing services. At the same time, amendments to the Social Security Act lead to the closing of many public homes for the aging and a rise in proprietary nursing homes (Kalisch, Kalisch, 1995, p. 591).

A great success of the 1950s was the development of the polio vaccine and its use on a national scale. State and local health departments were instrumental in the success of the vaccination campaign. Immunization services became an important part of local health department service provision and remain so today. Public health nurses staffed child health and immunization clinics.

As previously mentioned, a major blow to visiting nursing occurred in the 1950s when the Metropolitan and John Hancock Life Insurance companies stopped funding visiting nursing services for their policyholders. At the same time the American Red Cross discontinued its national program of visiting nursing in rural areas. With the closing of such programs, visiting nursing agencies lost a valuable source of funding in the United States, and some of these agencies were forced to reorganize or ceased to exist.

### Stop and Think About It

If a client you were visiting asked you about visiting nurse services in your community what would you tell them? In your community how are visiting nursing services provided? Who pays for these services? What types of service are covered? Does coverage vary from one insurance provider to another?

### Changes in Public Health Service Delivery

Changes also occurred in the delivery of public health services during the 1950s. By the mid-1950s more than 70% of all counties in the United States had local health departments in which public health nurses played a major role in service provision. However, at the same time, expenditures of public health departments were experiencing a sharp decline. Federal grants-in-aid to the states for public health programs declined from $45 million in 1950 to $33 million in 1959 (Fee, 1997, p. 23). Nationally, there was an increased emphasis on hospital-based services and a decline in home health services. Health departments quickly were becoming underbudgeted and understaffed and losing their visibility in our nation's communities. Public health funding continues to be in jeopardy today.

## THE DECADES OF THE 1960s AND 1970s

Dating from the 1960s the federal government more aggressively took on the role of guardian of the nation's health. President Kennedy's inaugural address in 1961 is remembered for the words, "Ask not what your country can do for you—ask what you can do for your country." "Great Society" programs emerged, a new social consciousness swept the nation, and a war on poverty began. At the same time, the Constitution of the World Health Organization holistically defined health as "complete physical, mental, and social well-being and not just the absence of disease." Additionally, many changes were occurring in nursing education and research.

In 1962 the ANA established nursing research priorities and published "Blueprint for Research in Nursing" in the *American Journal of Nursing*. In 1965 the ANA held the first nursing research conference funded by a grant from the Division of Nursing of the U.S. Public Health Service. In 1969 the first Center for Nursing Research in a college of nursing was established at Wayne State University College of Nursing in Detroit, Michigan with H. Harriet Werley as the director (Werley, Shea, 1973, p. 217). Many early studies from the Center focused on community health nursing issues.

In 1963 the NLN required that content in public health nursing be included in all baccalaureate nursing programs as a requirement for accreditation of the school. From 1963 on, every nurse graduating from an accredited baccalaureate program has received education in public health nursing. This is very different from the postgraduate education required of such nurses during Lillian Wald's time.

Similar to reports in the 1940s and 1950s, the Surgeon General's Consultant Group on Nursing reported that there were too few nursing schools and not enough nurses (USPHS, 1963). Based on these conclusions, the Nurse Training Act of 1964 was passed and provided money for nursing school construction, student nursing loans, and nursing scholarships. Many nurses still use Nurse Training Act monies today to obtain their education. USPHS Fellowships became available for nurses to study public health nursing at leading universities throughout the country. Nurses nationwide have a valuable funding resource made available to them through such legislation.

The establishment of the advanced practice nursing movement was a significant event in the 1960s. This movement began in 1965 with Loretta Ford and Dr. Silver starting the first nurse practitioner program in the country at the University of Colorado. Loretta Ford's public health nursing background gave the program a strong public health component from the onset. The program prepared nurses to provide comprehensive well-child primary care in home and ambulatory settings. This led the way for such programs to be developed nationwide, and today there are numerous educational programs for advanced practice nursing. The acceptance of advanced practice nurses (APNs) by the general public has been extremely positive, and today's APNs provide valuable primary care services in various community settings. Some consider early public health nurses to have been the first nurse practitioners, providing primary care in American homes and communities.

During the 1960s and 1970s more nonhealth and allied health professionals, including social workers, physical therapists, occupational therapists, physicians' assistants, and home health aides, began to work in the community. Health maintenance organizations, neighborhood health centers, free clinics, and numerous home health care programs sprang up in local communities. By the 1970s all areas of nursing, including parent and child nursing, psychiatric nursing, and medical and surgical nursing, began discovering the community. Subspecialities in public health nursing, including school nursing, occupational health nursing, home health care nursing, and nurse midwifery, flourished. An array of nurses and other health care professionals were practicing in the community. The line of distinction for public health nursing practice was beginning to blur.

This provided an impetus for community health nurses and public health leaders to define the scope of practice. In 1973 the ANA published *Standards of Practice for Community Health Nursing*. This led to the more common usage of the "umbrella" term community health nurse. The term **community health nursing** was seen as better reflecting the holistic scope of practice and the care given to the community. The term *public health nurse* continued to be used by most nurses working in official public health agencies such as state and local health departments.

### 1965: A Turning Point in Public Health Legislation

The year 1965 is considered by many to be a very significant year in public health legislation in the United States (see Chapter 4). In 1965 the passage of Medicaid and Medicare under the *Social Security Act* greatly affected the provision of nursing services and public health nursing. Medicare reimbursement to service providers helped many visiting nursing organizations expand their services. Medicaid had many maternal-child health provisions and public health nurses became very involved in services such as early, periodic, screening, diagnosis, and treatment (EPSDT) provided for under that legislation. However, the administration of the Medicaid and Medicare programs was through social welfare agencies and not state and local health departments. The *Economic Opportunity Act* provided funding for many community health programs, including neighborhood health centers and Head Start. The *Older Americans Act* resulted in health resources and services for older Americans. Legislation created the Environmental Protection Agency and the environmental health movement became a national health issue. State and local health departments provided environmental health services.

### The 1970s

In the 1970s public health departments often became the providers of care for people who were uninsured or underinsured and for Medicaid clients who could not receive care through private practitioners (Fee, 1997, p. 25). This engulfed a large part of the budgets of state and local health departments. At the same time, the need for a strong public health infrastructure was becoming lost in the minds of legislators and the general public (Fee, 1997).

The desire to reexamine the education necessary for public health nursing practice lead to a 1973 U.S. Department of Health, Education and Welfare (USDHEW) conference.

The conference publication, *Redesigning Nursing Education for Public Health* (USDHEW, 1973), suggested that basic generalist preparation for public health nursing require knowledge of epidemiology, biostatistics, principles of health education, community health models, and approaches to aggregate-based nursing (Schulte, 2000, p. 4).

## COMMUNITY HEALTH NURSING IN THE 1980S AND 1990S

In the 1980s our nation's health status data reflected a dismal state of affairs. "Every key measure of maternal and child health in the United States worsened, failed to improve, or improved at a slower rate than in previous years. As a result, the United States has fallen behind other countries with fewer resources on important health indicators such as infant mortality and low birth weight" (Children's Defense Fund, 1992, p. 1). The Institute of Medicine, in its classic report, *The Future of Public Health*, addressed the fact that health care professionals and consumers were having to deal with immediate, enduring, and growing health care challenges (e.g., AIDS, chronic disease, an aging population, poverty, and homelessness) with increasingly fewer resources (Institute of Medicine, 1988). During the Reagan administration of the 1980s federal funding for public health programs was cut (Fee, 1997, p. 25).

The 1980s were a time for reflection for consumer groups, health care professionals, and political leaders. Recognizing the serious state of affairs, all of these groups pushed for health care reform. Health care delivery issues such as quality, accountability, and access came to the forefront, as did an increasingly well-educated and sophisticated consumer of health care. There was intense interest about skyrocketing health care costs and cost-containment measures were enacted at the federal and state levels. Recognition grew that nurses are valuable resources in the health care system and can provide cost-effective preventive services. Renewed interest in home care services emerged, as did a greater focus on health promotion and disease prevention. The nation began to look at health promotion and disease prevention as important public health mandates. National health objectives were established with the Healthy People Initiative (see Chapter 4).

Nursing was able to strengthen its focus on health promotion and disease prevention through the establishment of the National Center for Nursing Research (NCNR). The NCNR was authorized under the Health Research Extension Act of 1985 (Public Law 99-158) and was established on April 18, 1986, as part of the National Institutes of Health (NIH) in the USPHS. Its major purpose was to conduct a program of grants and funding to support nursing research and research training, expand the knowledge base in nursing, and promote health across the life span. The NCNR was the first national center for nursing research in the world. With its establishment, nursing research funding and studies increased; however, little research was occurring in public health nursing.

## The Healthy People Initiative

Probably one of the most significant occurrences in the 1980s was the beginning of the **Healthy People Initiative** with the publication of *Healthy People* in 1979 by the federal government. This document outlined health care problems in America. The following year, *Promoting Health, Preventing Disease: Objectives for the Nation* (USDHEW, 1980) outlined specific health priority areas and objectives that would guide the nation in its quest for health in the decade of 1980 to 1990. This was the first time that the federal government had set national health priority areas and objectives and attempted to chart a course for the public health of the nation. With the publication of *Healthy People 2000* in 1990 (USDHHS, 1990), the Healthy People Initiative was continued for the decade of 1990 to 2000, and the publication of *Healthy People 2010* (USDHHS, 2000) in the year 2000 continues the initiative into the twenty-first century. Nursing organizations were instrumental in the writing of the Healthy People documents, and nurses are playing a major role in accomplishing its objectives. These objectives are presented throughout the text.

## Happenings in the 1990s

As the decade of the 1990s came to an end, it was evident that the acute-care model of care delivery and disease-focused care and payment systems did not promote health; many Americans remained uninsured and underinsured; as America aged, many of the health care needs of the elderly went unmet; managed care was not the answer to everyone's health care needs; and vulnerable groups such as minorities and people who were disabled or elderly often had difficulty accessing appropriate health care. During the 1990s the nation continued to work toward achieving the national health objectives of the Healthy People Initiative but was not always successful. Drugs, tobacco, violence, mental health, and environmental health continued as national health problems. As health insurance paid for shorter and shorter hospital stays, more care moved into the community and there was a proliferation of home care agencies.

The growing role of the APN saw a rise in the use of such nurses in public health settings. Many health departments had clinics that used the services of a variety of APNs such as family nurse practitioners, women's health nurse practitioners, adult health nurse practitioners, psychiatric clinical nurse specialists, and community health nurse practitioners. School districts and health departments also hired school nurse practitioners.

Although "health care for all" was a goal being promoted worldwide, it is not a reality for many Americans. However, APNs are increasingly addressing many primary health care needs for Americans, and the need for a sound public health infrastructure is increasingly being recognized. Unfortu-

nately, many local health departments continue to struggle to maintain an adequate funding base.

## A LOOK TO THE FUTURE

There is a cyclic nature to community health nursing problems. Many of the problems that have faced community health nurses before continue to exist. In fact, many of the issues that face community health nurses today are amazingly like those faced by Lillian Wald and her contemporaries. Impoverished families, lack of elder care, malnutrition, lack of health care for the disadvantaged, infants born to destitute parents, violence, mental health issues, and sexually transmitted diseases are problems that cross centuries. New communicable diseases such as AIDS, a resurgence in communicable disease, and a host of drug-resistant organisms also are pressing community health problems. Human needs do not change or diminish—only our methods of dealing with them do.

A key issue that will continue to challenge the profession is the spiraling cost of health care and lack of national health insurance. Medical costs are the fastest growing item in the federal government's budget. Yearly spending for health care is now in the trillions of dollars. If current rates of health care spending are maintained, problems with growing poverty, drug and alcohol abuse, unintended pregnancies, family violence, and the AIDS epidemic will have limited attention. Managed health care seems destined to expand, but with it come many questions, including health care rationing and access to necessary health care services. A significant challenge for nurses is to ensure quality care while delivering cost-effective care. Use of APNs in the community can help control health care costs.

State and local health departments have been the mainstay of public health activities in the United States and major employers of public health nurses. These departments will need to examine their programs and look beyond traditional health department activities to provide for the health needs of the community. They need to work in partnership with communities to promote community health. Health departments need to become more visible in their communities. Media campaigns to promote local health department services and to enlist community support for these departments can aid in this visibility and help communities to see the need for increased funding.

Methods to link health care management decisions to systematic information about outcomes of practice are necessary to improve the effectiveness of care and provide a firm basis for economic decision making. Often programs lack adequate documentation of the effectiveness of community health nursing interventions. Preventive efforts and those that are long term in nature are often difficult to evaluate. However, nurses need to research the outcomes of such interventions and make such research a priority.

Alternatives to the health care system that we now have in place need to be explored. Nurses need to support their professional organizations in their efforts to provide quality, affordable, accessible health care for all Americans. Professional organizations work diligently to promote comprehensive health care to all, protect the rights of high-risk groups, and support the nursing profession. Nurses need to be members of their professional organizations.

"Helping families to help themselves" was a creed of the earliest nurses who visited families in their homes, and it remains important for the contemporary community health nurse. This creed can be expanded to "helping communities to help themselves." Nurses will need to become increasingly involved and visible in community partnership activities to promote health.

Nursing research needs to become more community focused. Nursing's national research agenda should emphasize knowledge development in providing care to aggregates at risk in the community and testing models of community-based care (Naylor, Buhler-Wilkerson, 1999, pp. 126-127). Nursing research also needs to expand and aggressively address outcome and quality issues. Nurse researchers need to make valiant efforts to have nursing research findings disseminated in the literature and translated into clinical practice.

Public health nurses must position themselves in leadership roles on all levels of government—local, state, and national. They need to be active in the development of public health legislation and social welfare programs. Nurses need to create alliances to create socially responsible care systems (Naylor, Buhler-Wilkerson, 1999, p. 127).

The challenges that need to be addressed in the twenty-first century are not insurmountable. Early public health nurse pioneers set the standards for the development of the nursing profession and for reform in health care delivery. They were on the cutting edge of the suffragette movement, the birth control movement, and the social reform movement that brought health care and civil rights to women, children, immigrants, prisoners, and the mentally ill. Their names are seen in the books that tell the story of our nation's history. Table 1-2 presents an overview of early nurse leaders whose lives we can celebrate today. They are models for our own professional and personal growth. Nursing leaders need to continue to have a strong voice in the public health of our nation.

## SUMMARY

The beginnings of nursing can be traced to the beginnings of humankind, for there has always been a need for reducing pain with comfort measures. The early Christian church's contributions to nursing were significant, as were the organizational contributions of St. Vincent de Paul and Mademoiselle Le Gras to public health nursing. Florence Nightingale's legacy to professional nursing and to public health, along with the contributions of William Rathbone,

the founder of public health nursing in England, provided the basis for public health nursing in the United States. Events in society at large have shaped nursing as a whole and the development of public health nursing. Public health nursing can be proud of its strong early leaders, such as Lillian Wald, Mary Breckinridge, Mary Sewall Gardner, and Lavinia Dock. We need to look to such leaders for inspiration, motivation, and encouragement.

Public health nurses used advances in the public health sciences to deal with the problems they encountered. The title of community health nurse came into being to emphasize that this field was for the community, not just people who were poor enough to use public assistance programs. How community health nurses organized themselves, along with methods of education for this area of nursing, shaped not only the development of this specialty area but also the entire field of nursing. Emphases in community health nursing, as well as nursing in general, are changing; the health scene is chaotic because there is no overall health plan. Community health nursing, with its focus on the health of aggregates, can involve nurses in health planning and in the necessary task of bringing order out of chaos.

## CRITICAL THINKING
*exercise*

Nursing recognizes the importance of using its history. Nursing can better evaluate its values and goals and chart its course to fulfill them if nurses have a fuller understanding of who they are and what they do, wish to be, and need to know.

If nursing is to continue to grow as a profession, knowledge of what has been done in the past and what factors influenced its growth are vitally important. It is in looking at nursing's history that safeguards can be established to ensure that the profession profits by its errors and recognizes its successes. If nursing does not study its history, its educational advances, its research, and its publications, it is doomed to repeat the same mistakes" (Hezel, Linebach, 1991, p. 272).

After reading this chapter and considering the state of our current health care system, complete one of the following exercises:

1. Select a current societal issue (e.g., provision of home care to the uninsured) and examine the progress or lack of progress made in addressing the problem.

2. Examine the characteristics of the current immigrants to the United States and consider how they are similar to and different from the immigrants in the early part of the twentieth century. How can community health nurses assist recent immigrants with their health needs?

3. Think about some of the achievements of early nursing leaders such as Lillian Wald and Mary Breckinridge and identify factors that facilitated and hindered their ability to accomplish goals. How would you personally deal with these inhibiting factors today?

## REFERENCES

American Nurses Association (ANA): *Standards of community health nursing practice*, Kansas City, Mo, 1986, ANA.

American Nurses Association (ANA) Quad Council of Public Health Nursing Organizations: *Scope and standards of public health nursing practice*, Washington, DC, 1999, ANA.

American Public Health Association, Division of Nursing: *A century of caring: a celebration of public health nursing in the United States: 1893-1993*, Washington, DC, 1992, APHA.

American Public Health Association (APHA): *The definition and role of public health nursing: a statement of APHA public health nursing section*, Washington, DC, 1996, APHA.

Association of Community Health Nursing Educators (ACHNE): *Essentials for entry level community health nursing practice*, Louisville, Ky, 1990, ACHNE.

Association of Community Health Nursing Educators (ACHNE): *Essentials of master's level nursing education for advanced community health nursing practice*, Lexington, Ky, 1991, ACHNE.

Association of Community Health Nursing Educators (ACHNE): *Differentiated nursing practice in community health*, Lexington, Ky, 1993, ACHNE.

Association of State and Territorial Directors of Nursing (ASTDN): *Public health nursing: a partner for healthy populations*, Washington, DC, 2000, American Nurses Publishing.

Backer BA: Lillian Wald: connecting caring with action, *Nurs Health Care* 14(3):122-129, 1993.

Blank JJ, McElmurry BJ: A paradigm for baccalaureate public health nursing education, *Public Health Nurs* 5:183-189, 1988.

Brainard AM: *The evolution of public health nursing*, Philadelphia, 1922, Saunders.

Breckinridge M: *Wide neighborhoods: a story of the Frontier Nursing Service*, New York, 1952, Harper & Brothers.

Browne HE: A tribute to Mary Breckinridge, *Nurs Outlook* 14(5):54-55, 1966.

Buhler-Wilkerson K: False dawn: the rise and fall of public health nursing in America 1900-1930. In Lagemann EC, editor: *Nursing history. New perspectives, new possibilities*, New York, 1983, Teachers College Press.

Buhler-Wilkerson K: Lillian Wald: public health pioneer, *Nurs Res* 40(5):316-317, 1991.

Buhler-Wilkerson K: Public health then and now. Bringing care to the people: Lillian Wald's legacy to public health nursing, *Am J Public Health* 83(12):1778-1786, 1993.

Carr A: Development of public health nursing literature, *Public Health Nurs* 5(2):81-85, 1988. Edited reprint from *Public Health Nurse* 18(2):83-90, 1926.

Cary A: *Strategies for a collaborative future: the consensus report for the National Consensus Conference on the Educational Preparation of Home Care Administrators*, Washington, DC, 1989, Catholic University of America School of Nursing.

Children's Defense Fund: *The state of America's children 1992*, Washington, DC, 1992, The Fund.

Cohen S: Miss Loane, Florence Nightingale, and district nursing in late Victorian Britain, *Nurs Hist Rev* 5:83-103, 1997.

Committee for the Study of Nursing Education: *Nursing and nursing education in the United States*, New York, 1923, Macmillan.

Coss C: Lillian D. Wald: progressive activist, *Public Health Nurs* 10(2):134-138, 1989.

Craven D: *A guide to district nurses and home nursing*, London, 1890, Macmillan.

Deloughery GL: *History and trends of professional nursing*, ed 8, St Louis, 1977, Mosby.

Desirable organization of public health nursing for family service, *Public Health Nurs* 38:387-389, 1946.

Dock L: *A history of nursing*, vol 2, New York, 1907, Putnam and Sons.

Dock L: *A short history of nursing*, ed 4, New York, 1938, Putnam and Sons.

Dock L, Pickett SE, Noyes CD, et al: *History of American Red Cross nursing*, New York, 1922, Macmillan.

Dolan JA: *History of nursing*, ed 2, vol 12, Philadelphia, 1969, WB Saunders.

Dublin LI: *The first one thousand midwifery cases of the Frontier Nursing Service*, New York, 1932, Metropolitan Life Insurance Company.

Erickson G: Southern initiative in public health nursing: the founding of the Nurses' Settlement and Instructive Visiting Nurse Association of Richmond, Virginia, 1900-1910, *J Nurs History* 3(1):17-22, 1987.

Estabrook CA: Lavinia Lloyd Dock. The Henry Street years, *Nurs Hist Rev* 3:143-172, 1995.

Fagin CM: Primary care as an academic discipline, *Nurs Outlook* 26:750-753, 1978.

Fee E: History and development of public health. In Scutchfield DF, Keck CW, editors: *Principles of public health practice*, Albany, 1997, Delmar Publishers.

Fitzpatrick ML: *The National Organization for Public Health Nursing 1912-1952: Development of a field of practice*, New York, 1975, National League for Nursing.

Fitzpatrick ML: Lillian Wald: prototype of an involved nurse, *Imprint* (April/May):92-95, 1990.

Fox EG, editor: Red Cross public health nursing, *Public Health Nurs* 12:175-181, 1920.

Freeman RB: *Techniques of supervision in public health nursing*, Philadelphia, 1944, WB Saunders.

Freeman RB: *Techniques of supervision in public health nursing*, ed 2, Philadelphia, 1950, WB Saunders.

Freeman RB: *Public health nursing practice*, Philadelphia, 1950, WB Saunders.

Freeman RB: *Community health nursing practice*, Philadelphia, 1970, WB Saunders.

Freeman RB, Heinrich, J: *Community health nursing practice*, ed 2, Philadelphia, 1981, WB Saunders.

Fulmer H: A history of visiting nurse work in America, *Am J Nurs* 2(3):411-425, 1902.

Gardner MS: *Public health nursing*, New York, 1916, Macmillan.

Gardner MS: *Public health nursing*, ed 1, revised, New York, 1919, Macmillan.

Gardner MS: *Public health nursing*, ed 2, New York, 1924, Macmillan.

Gardner MS: *Public health nursing*, ed 3, New York, 1936, Macmillan.

Gardner MS: *So build we*, New York, 1942, Macmillan.

Gardner MS: *Mary Kent*, New York, 1946, Macmillan.

Griffin GJ, Griffin JK: *Historical trends of professional nursing*, St Louis, 1973, Mosby.

Haupt AC: Forty years of teamwork in public health nursing, *Am J Nurs* 53:81-84, 1953.

Hezel LF, Linebach LM: The development of a regional nursing history collection: its relevance to practice, education, and research, *Nurs Outlook* 39(5):268-272, 1991.

Institute of Medicine, Committee for the Study of the Future of Public Health: *The future of public health*, Washington, DC, 1988, National Academy Press.

Jensen DM: *History and trends of professional nursing*, ed 4, St Louis, 1959, Mosby.

Jones DC, Davis JA, Davis MC: *Public health nursing education and practice*, Rockville, Md, 1987, Division of Nursing, USDHHS.

Kalisch P, Kalisch BJ: *The advance of American nursing*, ed 3, Boston, 1995, Little, Brown.

Kaufman M, Hawkins JW, Higgins LP, et al., editors: *Dictionary of American nursing biography*, Westport, Conn, 1988, Greenwood Press.

LaMotte E: *The tuberculosis nurse*, New York, 1915, Putnam.

Maynard T: *The apostle of charity: the life of St. Vincent de Paul*, New York, 1939, Dial Books.

McIver P: Public health nursing responsibilities, *Public Health Nurs* 41:65-66, 1949.

McNeil EE: *Transition in public health nursing*, John Sundwall Lecture, Ann Arbor, 1967, University of Michigan.

Mosley MOP: Satisfied to carry the bag. Three black community health nurses' contributions to health care reform, 1900-1937, *Nurs Hist Rev* 4:65-82, 1995.

National Organization for Public Health Nursing: Approval of Skidmore College of Nursing as preparing students for public health nursing, *Public Health Nurs* 36:371, 1944.

Naylor, MD, Buhler-Wilkerson K: Creating community-based care for the new millennium, *Nurs Outlook* 47(3):120-127, 1999.

Nelson SC: Mary Sewall Gardner (Part 1), *Nurs Outlook* 1(12):668-670, 1953.

Nelson SC: Mary Sewall Gardner (Part 2), *Nurs Outlook* 2(1):37-39, 1954.

Nightingale F: *Notes on nursing*, London, England 1859, Harris and Sons.

Nightingale F: Nurses, training of. In Quain R, editor: *A dictionary of medicine*, ed 9, New York, 1885, Appleton.

Olson V, Wood J: Public health and community health nursing. In Schoor TM, Kennedy MS, editors: *100 years of American nursing*, Philadelphia, 1999, Lippincott.

A prophet honored, *Am J Nurs* 17:53, 1971 (editorial).

Rathbone W: *Sketch of the history and progress of district nursing*, London, 1890, Macmillan.

Reed PG, Zurakowski TL: Nightingale: foundations of nursing. In Fitzpatrick JJ, Whall AL, editors: *Conceptual models of nursing: analysis and application*, ed 3, Stamford, Conn, 1996, Appleton & Lange.

Roberts DE, Heinrich J: Public health nursing comes of age, *Am J Public Health* 75:1162-1172, 1985.

Roberts MM: *American nursing—history and interpretation*, New York, 1954, Macmillan.

Rosen G: *A history of public health*, New York, 1958, MD Publications.

Safier G: *Contemporary American leaders in nursing. An oral history*, New York, 1977, McGraw-Hill.

Schulte J: Finding ways to create connections among communities: partial results of an ethnography of urban public health nurses, *Public Health Nurs* 17(1):3-10, 2000.

Smillie WG: *Preventive medicine and public health*, ed 2, New York, 1952, Macmillan.

Smillie WG: *Public health. Its promise for the future*, New York, 1955, Macmillan.

Struthers L: *The school nurse*, New York, 1917, Putnam.

US Department of Health, Education, and Welfare (USDHEW): *Redesigning nursing education for public health: report of the conference, May 23-25, 1973*, Pub No HRA75-75, Bethesda, Md, 1973, USDHEW.

US Department of Health, Education, and Welfare (USDHEW): *Healthy people*, Washington, DC, 1980, US Government Printing Office.

US Department of Health and Human Services (USDHHS): *Promoting health, preventing disease: objectives for the nation*, Washington, DC, 1980, US Government Printing Office.

US Department of Health and Human Services (USDHHS): *Consensus conference on the essentials of public health nursing practice and education*, Rockville, Md, 1985, Division of Nursing, USDHHS.

US Department of Health and Human Services (USDHHS): *Healthy people 2000: objectives for the nation*, Washington, DC, 1990, US Government Printing Office.

US Department of Health and Human Services (USDHHS): *Healthy people 2010: conference edition*, Washington, DC, 2000, US Government Printing Office.

US Public Health Service (USPHS): *Toward quality in nursing: needs and goals. Report of the Surgeon General's consultant group on nursing*, Washington DC, 1963, US Government Printing Office.

US Public Health Service (USPHS): *50 years at the Division of Nursing*, Washington, DC, 1997, US Government Printing Office.

Wald L: *The house on Henry Street*, New York, 1915, Holt.

Werley HH, Shea FP: The first center for research in nursing: its development, accomplishments, and problems, *Nurs Res* 22(3):217-231, 1973.

Wilkie KE, Moseley ER: *Frontier nurse: Mary Breckinridge*, New York, 1969, Julian Messner.

Williams R: *The United States public health service*, Bethesda, Md, 1951, Commissioned Officers Association of the US Public Health Service.

Winslow C-EA: Florence Nightingale and public health nursing, *Public Health Nurs* 2:330-332, 1946.

Yost E: *American women of nursing*, Philadelphia, 1965, JB Lippincott.

Young EE: A quiet day: a peep at some of the varied homes visited by a district nurse in the course of one "quiet day," *Public Health Nurs* 6:43-44, 1989.

## SELECTED BIBLIOGRAPHY

Bigbee JL, Crowder ELM: The Red Cross Rural Nursing Service: an innovative model of public health nursing delivery, *Public Health Nurs* 2:109-121, 1985.

Buhler-Wilkerson K: Bringing care to the people: Lillian Wald's legacy to public health nursing, *Am J Public Health* 83(12):1778-1786, 1993.

Carr AM: Development of public health nursing literature, *Public Health Nurs* 5(2):81-85, 1988.

Christy TE: Portrait of a leader: Lavinia Lloyd Dock, *Nurs Outlook* 17:72-75, 1969.

Christy TE: Portrait of a leader: Lillian Wald, *Nurs Outlook* 18:50-54, 1970.

Daniels DG: *Always a sister: the feminism of Lillian D. Wald*, New York, 1995, Feminist Press.

Dock L: School-nurse experiment in New York, *Am J Nurs* 2(11):108-109, 1902.

Dossey BM: *Florence Nightingale: mystic, visionary healer*, Springhouse, Pa, 2000, Springhouse.

Fee E: The origins and development of public health in the United States. In Holland WW, Detels R, Knox G, editors: *Oxford textbook of public health*, ed 2, Oxford, 1991, Oxford University Press.

Frachel RR: A new profession: the evolution of public health nursing, *Public Health Nurs* 5:86-90, 1988.

Gardner MS: The National Organization for Public Health Nursing, *Visiting Nurse Q* 4:13-18, 1912.

Hamilton D: Clinical excellence, but too high a cost: the Metropolitan Life Insurance Company Visiting Nurse Service (1909-1953), *Public Health Nurs* 5:235-240, 1988.

Rathbone W: *History and progress of district nursing*, New York, 1890, Macmillan.

Wald L: The treatment of families in which there is sickness, *Am J Nurs* 17(6):427-431, 515-519, 602-606, 1917.

# 2

# Defining Community Health Nursing

*Susan Clemen-Stone*

## OBJECTIVES

*Upon completion of this chapter, the reader should be able to:*

1. Articulate the distinguishing characteristics of community health nursing practice.
2. Formulate a personal definition of community health nursing practice, incorporating key concepts delineated by professional organizations.
3. Discuss the key concepts inherent in community health nursing practice.
4. Describe the mission of public health and how the concept of "Health for All" relates to this mission.
5. Understand the concept of client from the community health nursing perspective.
6. Identify the roles community health nurses assume in practice and in settings in which these nurses work.

## KEY TERMS

Access to health care
Community-based nursing
Community health nursing
Community partnership
Core public health functions
Determinants of health
Educative nursing interventions
Enforcement nursing interventions

Engineering nursing interventions
Environmental health
Health for All mandate
*Healthy People 2010* initiative
Partnership process
Personal health
Population-based individual services
Populations at risk

Primary health care (PHC)
Public health nursing
Quad Council of Public Health
    Nursing Organizations
White's Construct for Public Health
    Nursing Model

---

*The dogmas of the quiet past are inadequate for the stormy present and future. As our circumstances are new, we must think anew, and act anew.*

ABRAHAM LINCOLN

Daunting challenges and exciting opportunities have emerged for community health nurses in the twenty-first century. With the community becoming the focal point for health care, community health nurses are in a unique position to provide leadership in evolving managed care and integrated health systems. Their past heritage has provided them with the knowledge and skill to assist clients in moving across the health care continuum. However, with the health system changing so rapidly, the past cannot be the only indicator for providing direction in practice. Circumstances are new and, accordingly, community health nurses must think anew and act anew!

The managed care movement has provided a stimulus for developing innovative approaches for addressing client needs in a more efficient manner. As these new approaches evolve, it is essential for community health nurses to establish mechanisms for monitoring client outcomes and for ensuring that the needs of all clients, regardless of their socioeconomic status, are met. "Despite the nation's vast riches and enormous resources certain (vulnerable) populations continue to fall outside the medical and economic mainstream and have little or no access to stable health care coverage" (Institute of Medicine [IOM], 2000, p. 1).

Although change is occurring in every aspect of the nursing profession, the basic values of community health nursing have remained viable over time and have become increasingly important. The emphasis in community health nursing on using population-based, community-oriented interventions to build healthy communities is making a major contribution in health care delivery. Community health nurses are playing a key role in helping to identify community health strengths and problems using these type of interventions.

## PERSPECTIVES ON COMMUNITY HEALTH NURSING AND COMMUNITY-BASED NURSING PRACTICE

When public health nursing began in the early 1900s, it was a simple matter to define it as a specialty area within nursing. **Public health nursing** took place outside the hospital setting. It was "nursing without walls," nursing that was community focused and family and population oriented. Early public health nurses functioned relatively independently and worked to maintain and improve the health of the entire community. Public health nursing was *"nursing for the public health"* (Brainard, 1921, p. 5).

Today, as the focus of health care continues to move outside the hospital setting and as more and more nurses assume expanded roles, defining community health nursing as a specialty area is less easily done. The definition becomes sharper and clearer, however, when one understands that the *nature of the practice*, not the *setting*, defines community health nursing as a specialty area. Nursing outside the walls is not necessarily community health nursing. It may be **community-based nursing** or nursing in a variety of community settings focused on the care of individuals and families with acute and chronic conditions and self-care needs (Table 2-1). For example, pediatric nurses who do assessments of newborns in physicians' offices and nurses who counsel clients in mental health centers are probably functioning as specialty-focused nurse *practitioners*. These nurses have advanced physical assessment skills and preparation to exercise independent and collaborative judgment in the management of clients' health care needs. The holistic *community* focus characteristic of community health nursing practice is not a major emphasis of nurse practitioners in many ambulatory care and other community-based health care settings. These practitioners place emphasis on managing acute or chronic conditions from an individual and family perspective. They may not be oriented to the community (Goeppinger, 1984; Hemstrom, Ambrose, Donahue, et al., 2000; Zotti, Brown, Stotts, 1996).

Several distinguishing characteristics differentiate community health nursing from community-based practice focused at the individual and family level of care (see Table 2-1). **Community health nursing** is "nursing for the community's health." Its uniqueness lies in its emphasis on the health of the population as a whole. Because their focus is on the community, community health nurses provide care to individuals, families, and groups within the context and framework of the community (ACHNE, 1993). This implies that community health nurses use information obtained from assessment and evaluation at individual and family levels to identify health needs and concerns at the community level (Conley, 1995; Keller, Strohschein, Lia-Hoagberg, et al., 1998; Minnesota Department of Health [MDH], 1997). In other words, community health nurses compile data from their contacts with individuals and families and use these data to raise community awareness about major community health problems affecting large numbers of people, such as domestic violence or lack of access to primary health care services.

"Interventions at the individual and family levels are critical to the population-based role of public (community) health nursing, because they provide the linkage necessary to effectively interact with the community" (Conley, 1995, p. 4). However, community health nurses address both the

**TABLE 2-1**

*Practice Models of Community-Based Nursing and Community Health Nursing Compared*

| MODEL COMPONENT | COMMUNITY-BASED NURSING | COMMUNITY HEALTH NURSING |
|---|---|---|
| Goals | Manage acute or chronic conditions<br>Promote self-care | Preserve/protect health<br>Promote self-care |
| Client | Individual and family | Community |
| Underlying philosophy | Human ecologic model | Primary health care |
| Autonomy | Individual and family autonomy | Community autonomy<br>Individual rights may be sacrificed for good of community |
| Client character | Across the life span | Across the life span with emphasis on high-risk aggregates |
| Cultural diversity | Culturally appropriate care of individual and families | Collaboration with and mobilization of diverse groups and communities |
| Type of service | Direct | Direct and indirect |
| Home visiting | Home visitor | Home visitor |
| Service focus | Local community | Local, state, federal, and international |

Modified from Zotti ME, Brown P, Stotts RC: Community-based nursing versus community health nursing: what does it all mean? *Nurs Outlook* 44:211-217, 1996, p. 212.

personal and the environmental aspects of health and deal with community factors that either inhibit or facilitate healthy living when providing individual-focused, population-based services.

**Personal health** involves the biopsychosocial and spiritual aspects of individual, family, and group functioning, whereas **environmental health** deals with people's surroundings—settings such as homes, schools, workplaces, or recreational facilities—and factors within these settings that influence health behavior. Community health nurses enter the environment in which people live and practice within that environment, in sharp contrast to the situation where the client enters the nurse's environment in a hospital or ambulatory care setting. In addition to the one-to-one or single-family approach to health care, the community health nurse thinks in terms of populations within caseloads, districts, census tracts, cities, and group settings. Aggregates at risk within these populations, including families at risk, are identified so that preventive measures and resources can be targeted for them. This kind of community focus involves educating individuals and groups and changing the social and physical environments that cue and reinforce the choices people make. Environmental factors that generate patterns of disease and social problems in populations must be addressed to resolve many of our contemporary health concerns, such as AIDS, teenage pregnancy, and toxic waste contamination (Koopman, 1996; U.S. Department of Health and Human Services [USDHHS], 2000).

The emphasis in community health nursing practice is on promoting health and preventing disease. Community health nursing interventions focus on providing health promotion services in family environments as well as group settings such as neighborhood centers or churches. Community health nursing interventions also include activities like screening programs that are community based; environmental and organizational changes through persuasion, as illustrated by the public's use of seat belts; and regulation and the use of mass media to promote healthy life styles (Association of State and Territorial Directors of Nursing [ASTDN], 1998; National Institutes of Health [NIH], 1995). The fact that smoking is now considered a health hazard and is no longer chic is a superb illustration of education at the community level through the mass media.

Examples can best illustrate how the community health nurse expands community-based nursing by focusing on populations at risk and the community.

**CASE** *Scenario* Kathy Barnes, a community health nurse working for an official health department, was assigned a census tract as her population to be served. This census tract was located in a decaying area of town with substandard housing and no transportation, playgrounds, or parks. A large industrial complex lay in the census tract, and consequently large numbers of young laborers and their families lived there. No hospital was lo-

cated in the area and only one physician practiced there. The community health nurse received numerous referrals from the physician and outlying hospitals to visit young mothers who needed support with parenting their newborn children. The nurse assessed the need for a parenting group by talking with the families whom she served as well as with her supervisors. She and the families she visited planned a weekly sharing and support group that met in a neighborhood church. The group was well attended and generated community interest in developing a coalition designed to address the needs of young families with children. In addition to maintaining the support group, this coalition helped families in the neighborhood address other areas of concern. For example, churches in the community obtained volunteers to transport families in need to medical appointments and established recreational activities for school-age children.

The nurse in this case scenario demonstrated critical elements of community health nursing: providing care to the basic unit of service—the family—and concurrently planning preventive health measures for a population at risk—young families needing parenting and other family support services. This is a step beyond providing primary health care to families who need that level of nursing intervention and is different from the one-to-one focus of care to a sick person in the hospital or ambulatory care setting. Another case scenario helps clarify how community nursing concepts are applied in the practice setting when nurses work with families that have an ill family member.

**CASE** *Scenario* John Stone is a community health nurse employed by a hospital-based home health agency. His caseload typically has a large percentage of people over 65 years of age with diagnoses such as congestive heart failure, diabetes, pneumonia, and hypertension. A common concern that John encounters with his clients is their inability to shop for food because they often are unable to drive or walk. Relying on neighbors is difficult, and families frequently live long distances away from the inner-city neighborhood served by John. John worked with a local church to develop an organized cadre of volunteers who shop for groceries for those clients who need this service. These volunteers also provide respite services that help prevent caregiver role strain. Many primary caregivers in John's caseload are elderly and have major health concerns. Caregiving responsibilities are often very stressful for these elderly caregivers.

As was the situation with Kathy Barnes, John Stone demonstrated how delivering one-on-one care to ill clients provided a window of opportunity for identifying population-focused needs (grocery shopping; respite services) within the community. John also worked collaboratively with a significant community system to meet crucial client needs and to provide a long-term solution to a community health problem.

As mentioned previously, the unique aspects of community health nursing practice do not negate direct individual client service or community-based nursing. Many services provided in the pursuit of protecting the general health of the public are the same as those needed to address the specific health concerns of individuals (Gebbe, 1995). These types of services are labeled population-based individual services. Population-based individual services are person-to-person interventions that focus on creating changes in knowledge, attitude, belief, skill, practice, and behavior, either singly or in families, classes, or groups. Persons are receiving these services because they are identified as belonging to a targeted group, such as high-risk mothers or children (MDH, 1997).

Although community-based practice and managed care are clearly emerging as major health care delivery strategies, community health nurses will continue to play a significant role in providing population-based services and ensuring that the needs of vulnerable populations and communities are met. They will work in partnership with clients and other health care providers in monitoring access to care and in identifying unmet needs among underserved groups. Financing a managed care program for low-income populations does not by itself resolve problems created by diverse barriers to care. Nor does it necessarily provide a safety net for those near poor populations that are uninsured and have other health problems (Gold, Sparer, Chu, 1996). Public health agencies and managed care organizations have already recognized the need to establish mutually beneficial collaborative models for maintaining and improving the health of populations and communities (Beery, Greenwald, Nudelman, 1996). The partnership model is increasingly being used to guide family and population-focused practice in the community setting (Courtney, Ballard, Fauver et al., 1996). This model is presented later in this chapter.

### Stop and Think About It

You are interested in working in a community health nursing setting that addresses the needs of high-risk children and their parents. What organizations in your local community serve this population? What type of services are these organizations providing? Are they providing community health nursing services or community-based services?

## EVOLUTION OF TITLE OVER TIME

Historically, varying titles have been used to describe the type of nursing provided in the community setting, including district nursing, home health nursing, visiting nursing, public health nursing, and community health nursing (McNeil, 1967). *District nursing*, which was the origin of our present concept of public health–community health nursing, was the title used by Rathbone when he hired nurses in England to care for the sick poor in their homes (see Chapter 1).

When home nursing services were started in the United States, the term *visiting nursing* was used to identify the specialty area of practice that emphasized home-based nursing care of the ill. *Home health nursing* and *home care* were other titles that emerged with the development of the home health care industry. Government policy changes beginning in the 1970s, including Medicare's prospective payment system and the progressive use of third-party payments for noninstitutionalized care, fostered a rapid growth in home health care.

The title, *public health nursing*, has its historical roots in Florence Nightingale's *health nurse* and Lillian Wald's *public health nurse*. Wald thought the word *public* denoted a service that was available to *all* people and, thus, coined the term *public health nursing* when she was director of the Henry Street Settlement in New York City. She hoped that by doing so the public would realize that the nursing services provided by the Henry Street Settlement were available to all individuals in the community. However, as federal, state, and local governments increased their involvement in the delivery of health services, the term *public health nursing* became associated with "public," or official, agencies and in turn with the care of poor people.

The phrase *community health nursing* emerged out of an interest in reaffirming the original thrust of public health nursing practice: nursing for the health of the entire public/community rather than nursing only for the public who are poor. Some people use the terms *community health nursing* and *public health nursing* interchangeably. It must be remembered, however, that not every nurse who works in the community setting is a public health nurse or a community health nurse who addresses the needs of the community as a whole. Public, or community, health nurses have a definitive philosophy of practice that is described in a later section of this chapter.

In this text, the terms *community health nurse* and *community health nursing* are used to emphasize the major focus of the nurse's work—the *community*—as well as the underlying philosophy of *population-focused practice*. Community health nursing is viewed as a specialty area in nursing, oriented to promoting and protecting the health of populations. The reader will find that a variety of titles (e.g., home health nursing, visiting nursing, community health nursing, and public health nursing) are used in practice settings to identify nurses who work with populations as well as individuals and families.

It is common for official agencies such as public health departments or departments of health and human services to use the term *public health nursing* to describe the population-focused practice of nurses employed by these agencies. Nurses in official agencies have traditionally placed emphasis on population-based, community-oriented practice, which focuses on creating changes in community norms, attitudes, awareness, standards, or practices (MDH, 1997). Recently there has been a renewed interest in focusing on using the term *public health nursing* to describe this type of practice (Quad Council of Public Health Nursing Organizations, 1999). This is occurring to highlight the need to maintain a strong emphasis on the role of public health departments in building healthy communities and the importance of adequately funding health improvement community activities.

## DEFINING COMMUNITY HEALTH NURSING: STANDARDS FOR PRACTICE

Community health nurses have consistently examined the nature of their practice within the context of societal needs and have focused attention on developing standards for practice to guide quality improvement efforts. The National Organization for Public Health Nursing (NOPHN), founded in 1912, grew out of a concern for the rights and safety of clients. At that time, community health nursing professionals were finding that as their specialty-based practice was rapidly expanding to meet the needs of vulnerable populations nationwide, "there were no generally accepted standards for anything" (Gardner, 1975, p. 17). They "realized a body of poorly prepared and unsupervised nurses, some of whom might be without an ethical background for this work, were a dangerous element to let loose in the homes of the people and might easily jeopardize, in a short time, all the confidence we had been building throughout the country" (Gardner, 1975, p. 17).

One of the major purposes of the NOPHN was to promote standardization of community health nursing practice. "It was believed that the general public, as well as those involved in public health nursing affairs, had to be made aware of the importance of nursing standards" (Fitzpatrick, 1975, p. 38). Ella Crandall, the executive secretary of NOPHN, traveled over 32,000 miles in 1915 to carry out this mission (Fitzpatrick, 1975). She spoke to countless lay and professional groups to inform the public about community health nursing and to promote a standard setting within the profession.

In recent times, the Quad Council of Public Health Nursing Organizations has carried on the tradition of the NOPHN. This council is comprised of four professional organizations that represent community health nurses on the national level (Box 2-1). Documents that delineate the essence of community–public health nursing practice and that clarify the role of specialty prepared community health nurses in the delivery of health care have been published by the Quad Council, ANA, and APHA. The latest definitions written by these organizations are presented in Boxes 2-2, 2-3, and 2-4. Professional standards for practice are presented in selected chapters throughout the text to illustrate the scope of services community health nurses provide when they work with a variety of at-risk populations (e.g., school-age children, the elderly, home health care clients, and clients needing rehabilitation services).

## UNIQUENESS OF COMMUNITY HEALTH NURSING PRACTICE

The emphasis in community health nursing, promoting the health of the community, has not changed over time. In 1912 the NOPHN stated in its constitution that "the object of this organization shall be to stimulate responsibility for the health of the community" (NOPHN, 1975, p. 27). The ANA, APHA, and the Quad Council reaffirm this goal, the importance of which is recognized worldwide. For example, the Canadian Public Health Association's definition for community–public health nursing (Box 2-5) articulates this

**BOX 2-1**

*Quad Council of Public Health Nursing Organizations: Membership*

- American Nurses Association (ANA), Council for Community, Primary, and Long-term Care Nursing Practice
- American Public Health Association (APHA), Public Health Nursing Section
- Association of Community Health Nursing Educators (ACHNE)
- Association of State and Territorial Directors of Nursing (ASTDN)

**BOX 2-2**

*The American Nurses Association's Definition of Community Health Nursing*

Community health nursing practice promotes and preserves the health of populations by integrating the skills and knowledge relevant to both nursing and public health. The practice is comprehensive and general, and is not limited to a particular age or diagnostic group; it is continual, and is not limited to episodic care. . . .

Community health nursing practice promotes the public's health. The programs, services, and institutions involved in public health emphasize promotion and maintenance of the population's health, and the prevention and limitation of disease. . . . While community health nursing practice includes nursing directed to individuals, families, and groups, the dominant responsibility is to the population as a whole.

From American Nurses Association, Council of Community Health Nurses: *Standards of community health nursing practice,* Pub No CH-10 Kansas City, Mo, 1986, ANA, pp. 1-2.

responsibility for nurses in Canada. The World Health Organization (WHO) also highlights this responsibility in documents describing community health nursing practice (WHO, 1974, 1978, 1985).

In 1997, the Quad Council of Public Health Nursing Organizations (1999) developed eight tenets of public health nursing to advance the goal of promoting and protecting the public's health. These tenets, delineated in Box 2-6, help nurses define the uniqueness of population-based, community-oriented practice carried out by public health and community health nurses. They reflect the belief that the uniqueness of community health nursing is related to its philosophy and scope of practice rather than the settings in which community health nurses function. They also highlight the dominant concern and obligation for the greater good of the population as a whole. This means that "what is in the best interest of the whole takes priority over the best interest of an individual or group" (Quad Council of Public Health Nursing Organizations, 1999, p. 4).

### BOX 2-3
### *The American Public Health Association's Definition of Public Health Nursing*

**Public health nursing is the practice of promoting and protecting the health of populations using knowledge from nursing, social, and public health sciences.**

Public health nursing practice is a systematic process by which:

- The health and health care needs of a population are assessed in order to identify subpopulations, families, and individuals who would benefit from health promotion or who are at risk of illness, injury, disability, or premature death;
- A plan for intervention is developed with the community to meet identified needs that takes into account available resources, the range of activities that contribute to health and the prevention of illness, injury, disability, and premature death;
- The plan is implemented effectively, efficiently, and equitably;
- Evaluations are conducted to determine the extent to which the interventions have an impact on the health status of individuals and the population;
- The results of the process are used to influence and direct the current delivery of care, deployment of health resources, and the development of local, regional, state, and national health policy and research to promote health and prevent disease.

From APHA, Public Health Nursing Section: *The definition and role of public health nursing, a statement of APHA public health nursing section*, Washington, DC, 1996, APHA, pp. 1-2.

### BOX 2-4
### *Scope of Public Health Nursing*

Public health nursing is the practice of promoting and protecting the health of populations using knowledge from nursing, social, and public health sciences (American Public Health Association, Public Health Nursing Section, 1996). Public health nursing is population-focused, community-oriented nursing practice. The goal of public health nursing is the prevention of disease and disability for all people through the creation of conditions in which people can be healthy.

Public health nurses most often partner with nations, states, communities, organizations, and groups, as well as individuals, in completing health assessment, policy development, and assurance activities. Public health nurses practice in both public and private agencies. Some public health nurses may have responsibility for the health of a geographic or enrolled population, such as those covered by a health department or capitated health system, whereas others may promote the health of a specific population, for example, those with HIV/AIDS.

Public health nurses assess the needs and strengths of the population, design interventions to mobilize resources for action, and promote equal opportunity for health. Strong, effective organizational and political skills must compliment their nursing and public health expertise.

Quad Council of Public Health Nursing Organizations: *Scope and standards* of *public health nursing practice*, Washington, DC, 1999, American Nurses Publishing, p. 2.

### BOX 2-5
### *The Canadian Public Health Association's Definition of Community Health/Public Health Nursing*

Community health/public health nursing is an art and a science that synthesizes knowledge from the public health sciences and professional nursing theories. Its goal is to promote and preserve the health of populations and is directed to communities, groups, families and individuals across their life span, in a continuous rather than episodic process.

Community health/public health nurses play a pivotal role in identifying, assessing, and responding to the health needs of given populations. They work in collaboration with, among others, communities, families, individuals, other professionals, voluntary organizations, self-help groups, informal health care providers, governments, and the private sector.

From Canadian Public Health Association (CPHA): *Community health/ public health nursing in Canada: preparation and practice*, Ottawa, Ontario, 1990, CPHA, p. 3.

### BOX 2-6

## *Tenets of Public Health Nursing*

- Population-based assessment, policy development, and assurance processes are systematic and comprehensive.
- All processes must include partnering with representatives of the people.
- Primary prevention is given priority.
- Intervention strategies are selected to create healthy environmental, social, and economic conditions in which people can thrive.
- Public health nursing practice includes an obligation to actively reach out to all who might benefit from an intervention or service.
- The dominant concern and obligation is for the greater good of all of the people or the population as a whole.
- Stewardship and allocation of available resources supports the maximum population health benefit gain.
- The health of the people is most effectively promoted and protected through collaboration with members of other professions and organizations.

Quad Council of Public Health Nursing Organizations: *Scope and standards* of *public health nursing practice*, Washington, DC, 1999, American Nurses Publishing, pp. 2-5.

The scope of community health nursing practice is very broad and involves the delivery of a continuum of preventive health services aimed at enhancing the health of individuals, families, groups, and communities. Community health nurses place priority on delivery of *primary* prevention services, believing that the most effective way to address community health problems is to prevent them from occurring. When providing preventive services to individuals, community health nurses view these services within the context of the family and the community. Community health nurses recognize that the health of individuals can affect the health of families and communities. They also recognize that families and communities provide an environment that influences the health of individuals. The family is seen as a significant entry point from which to identify community strengths, needs, and resources, related to the delivery of health care services (Figure 2-1).

Community health nursing practice is comprehensive and general, not limited to a particular age group or diagnostic group (ANA, 1986, p. 2). Community health nurses work with clients across the life span. They are committed to improving *the health of the community* by identifying subpopulations, families, and individuals who would benefit from health promotion or who are at risk of illness, injury, disability, and premature death (APHA, 1996, p. 1). Deter-

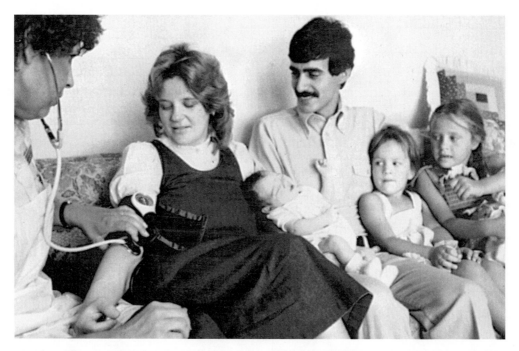

**FIGURE 2-1** The family is seen as a basic unit of service in community health nursing practice. Families provide a significant entry point from which to identify community assets and needs. (Courtesy of Genesee Region Home Care Association, Rochester, New York.)

mining specific populations at risk facilitates the identification of individuals and families at risk.

WHO defined the following three necessary components of community health nursing that continue to delineate the uniqueness of this nursing specialty (WHO, 1974):

- Community health nurses are responsible for ensuring that needed health services are provided in the community. This does not imply that community health nurses provide all of these services. Rather, it focuses attention on the need for nurses to participate in community assessment efforts that identify community health concerns and health planning activities that address community health problems.
- The care of vulnerable groups in a community is a priority. A major reason for involvement in the health care of populations at risk is their vulnerability. The long involvement of community health nursing in the care of mothers, children, and disadvantaged groups is based on this belief.
- The client (individual, family, group, or community) must be a partner in planning and evaluating health care.

The Quad Council's tenets of public health nursing (see Box 2-6) reinforce the value of WHO's elements of community health nursing as well as the partnership approach to health care service delivery.

Community health nurses must have a broad knowledge base to accomplish their goals and to apply basic principles (see Box 2-6) of practice. Because community health nursing is a *synthesis of nursing and public health* practice, community health nurses use the knowledge and skills of professional nursing and the philosophy, content, and methods of public health when delivering services in the community. Essential features of contemporary nursing practice are identified in Box 2-7. "The nursing profession remains committed to the care and nurturing of both healthy and ill people individually or in groups and communities" (ANA, 1995, p. 6). However, "the extent to which individual nurses engage in the total scope of nursing practice is dependent on their educational preparation, experience, roles, and the nature of the patient populations they serve" (ANA, 1995, p. 12). Public health preparation helps community health nurses extend their scope of practice to populations and communities. This preparation includes the philosophy, content, and methods of epidemiology, biostatistics, social policy, health planning, public health organization and administration, and public health law.

The classic definition of public health is presented in Box 2-8. The values reflected in this definition have guided public health and community health nursing practice over time and are reflected in the current, essential public health services (Figure 2-2). These services were articulated and adopted in the 1990s to help focus public health efforts. The Association of State and Territorial Directors of Nursing (ASTDN) developed a practice model in the late 1990s to illustrate the link between nursing practice, these essential public health services, and the core public health functions. This model (see Figure 2-2) illustrates that the knowledge and skills of professional nursing influence how nurses implement the functions of assessment, policy development, and assurance and the ten essential public health services. Chapters 4 and 5 significantly expand on public health practice, including the core public health functions and essential services. The core public health functions are summarized briefly later in this chapter.

**BOX 2-7**
*Essential Features of Contemporary Nursing Practice*

Definitions of nursing frequently acknowledge four essential features of contemporary nursing practice:
- Attention to the full range of human experiences and responses to health and illness without restriction to a problem-focused orientation;
- Integration of objective data with knowledge gained from an understanding of the patient or group's subjective experience;
- Application of scientific knowledge to the processes of diagnosis and treatment; and
- Provision of a caring relationship that facilitates health and healing.

American Nurses Association (ANA): *Nursing's social policy statement,* Washington, DC, 1995, American Nurses Publishing, p. 6.

**BOX 2-8**
*Classic Definition of Public Health*

Public health is the science and art of preventing disease, prolonging life, and promoting physical and mental health and efficiency through organized community efforts focused toward:
- Maintaining a sanitary environment;
- Controlling communicable diseases;
- Providing education regarding principles of personal hygiene;
- Organizing medical and nursing services for early diagnosis and treatment of disease; and
- Developing social machinery to ensure everyone a standard of living adequate for health maintenance, so organizing these benefits as to enable every citizen to realize his birthright of health and longevity.

From Winslow C-EA: *Man and epidemics,* Princeton, NJ, 1952, Princeton University Press, p. 60.

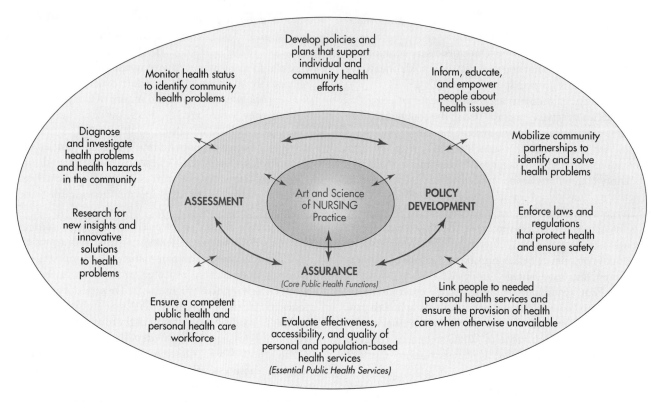

**FIGURE 2-2** ASTDN's public health nursing practice model: essential public health services and public health nursing. (From Association of State and Territorial Directors of Nursing (ASTDN): *Public health nursing: a partner for progress: a document which links nursing, public health core functions and essential services*, Washington, DC, 1998, ASTDN.)

## Partnership Approach to Service Delivery

Over the decades it has been learned that "community partnerships, particularly when they reach out to nontraditional partners (e.g., businesses and civic and religious organizations) can be among the most effective tools for improving health in communities" (USDHHS, 2000, p. 4). A **community partnership** is a union of people that is focused on collective action for a common endeavor or goal (Bracht, Kingsbury, Rissel, 1999).

Courtney, Ballard, Fauver, et al. (1996) and other professionals in the field (ASTDN, 1998, 2000; Berkowitz, 2000; Flynn, 1998) believe that strengthening a community's health competencies requires a partnership approach that focuses on community strengths and active client participation in all aspects of the health planning process. In contrast, the professional clinical model uses a client problem or deficiency approach and often places the client in a passive role. Further differences between the professional model and the partnership model are presented in Table 2-2. The **partnership process** is an exciting approach for helping clients address their health needs. This process is highlighted throughout the text.

## A MODEL FOR COMMUNITY HEALTH NURSING PRACTICE

Community health nurses are practicing in a health care environment that is presenting emerging opportunities for creating healthy communities as well as challenges that impede individuals and populations from receiving quality health care. As they navigate in this environment, it is important for these nurses to use a conceptual framework that clearly focuses their sites on the basic concepts of their specialty. **White's Construct for Public Health Nursing Model** (Figure 2-3) provides a framework for systematically addressing the population-based, community-oriented processes that distinguish community health–public health nursing from other nursing specialties. Developed in the early 1980s, this model has stood the test of time and remains particularly relevant as communities focus their efforts on achieving Healthy People goals and objectives. The determinants of the health framework in White's model were adapted from those presented in the first Healthy People document. The determinants of health presented in this first report remain viable and are providing a systematic approach to community health improvement (USDHHS,

**TABLE 2-2**

*Comparison of Professional Model with Partnership Model*

| PROFESSIONAL MODEL | PARTNERSHIP MODEL |
|---|---|
| *Focus* | |
| The problem or the diagnosis | Fostering the skills and capacity of the partner as a primary focus in the process of improving health and well-being (the initial stimulus may be a problem, but the primary focus will be strengthening/facilitating empowerment of the partner) |
| *Health Professional's Role* | |
| Expert who does "to" or "for," not "with"; the professional serves as decision maker and problem solver | Professional working "with," not "doing to"; facilitator, enabler, resource person who shares leadership and power with partner; services are provided in nonjudgmental, noncontrolling manner |
| *Partner's Role* | |
| Often passive recipient of "service" that is defined by professional | Active and willing participant in self-determination of strengths, problems, and solutions |
| *Nature of Relationship* | |
| Professional is director of the process, instructing or "telling" others what to do; interventions tend to be standardized and are seldom tailored to individual or cultural needs; interventions tend to focus on the problem, not the person | Professional actively facilitates the partner's participation in the relationship; requires ongoing negotiation of goals, roles, and responsibilities; respects individual and cultural differences |
| *Goal/Plan* | |
| Determined by the professional; focused totally on the problem | Mutual goal setting; plan of action developed with partner who is involved as active participant |
| *Activity/Service* | |
| Unilateral action by the professional to diagnose problem, establish intervention, assess progress, and revise intervention as needed | Joint action and assessment of progress that includes ongoing negotiation of roles and responsibilities; implements the partnership process; emphasizes involving natural helpers; families, groups, and/or coalitions as resources |
| *Expected Outcome* | |
| The problem is solved or corrected or the patient is considered noncompliant | The partner's capacity to act more effectively on his or her own behalf is strengthened (i.e., more empowered); the "problem" may or may not be solved, but the partner's capacity is enhanced to prevent future problems or to address them more effectively |

From Courtney R, Ballard E, Fauver S, et al.: The partnership model: working with individuals, families, and communities toward a new vision of health, *Public Health Nurs* 13:177-186, 1996, p. 179.

2000). The national determinants of health framework is presented in Chapter 4.

White's conceptual model for public health nursing practice (see Figure 2-3) visualizes the interrelationships between the determinants of health and public health nursing practice priorities, dynamics, interventions, and values. White (1982) conceptualizes the scope of practice as being very broad, extending from "one-to-one nursing to a global perspective of world health" (p. 528). Her global perspective on practice is especially valuable as the profession addresses the impact of the globalization movement. This movement, discussed further in Chapter 26, has highlighted the significant link between environmental conditions; socioeconomic development; and other determinants of disease, mortality, and health disparities (Olshansky, Carnes, Rogers, et al., 1998). It is clear that globalization will have both a positive and negative impact on health outcomes worldwide.

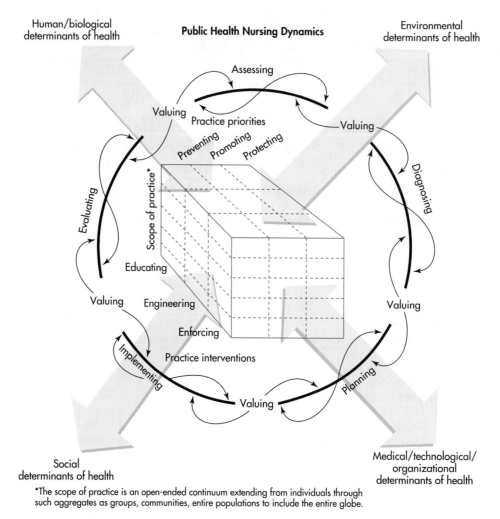

**FIGURE 2-3** A public health nursing conceptual model. The determinants of the health framework presented are modified from those in *Healthy People: the Surgeon General's Report on Health Promotion and Disease Prevention,* 1979. (From White MS: Construct for public health nursing, *Nurs Outlook* 30:529, 1982.)

## Determinants of Health

White argues that health or illness results from the interplay of multiple factors. She identifies four categories of determinants of health—*human/biologic; social; environmental;* and *health care system* or medical, technologic, and organizational factors—that influence the level of wellness among individuals, families, populations, and communities. Implicit in White's model is the belief that having an understanding of the multidimensional nature of health assists the community health nurse in planning health-promoting interventions (White, 1982). During the community health nursing assessment process, it is important for nurses to gather data that help them identify the consequences of the determinants of health. When this information is known, community health nurses are more effective in tailoring nursing interventions to address these determinants. Chap-

ters 6 and 11 examine the determinants of health in greater detail.

## Practice Priorities

"The overall focus of public health nursing is achieving and maintaining the public's health—at all times" (White, 1982, p. 528). Community health nursing services are grounded in the belief that changing communities or populations as a whole changes the lives of individuals within the community. In other words, a focus on the public's health that strengthens the health capabilities of the community can strengthen a community's ability to address the health of individuals within the community.

White's model places emphasis on keeping populations well and preventing disease occurrence to minimize the consequences of disease and poor health. In keeping with this emphasis, White highlights three practice priorities—prevention, promotion, and protection. These practice priorities focus on preventive interventions that are designed to address the adverse determinants of health. Providing immunizations for populations across the life span is an example of a disease preventing or specific protection nursing intervention. Teaching caregivers of ill clients stress management techniques or providing "Healthy Heart" meals in employee cafeterias are examples of health promotion interventions. An elaboration on the continuum of preventive interventions can be found in Chapter 11.

White envisions the need for preventive public health nursing interventions that promote healthy public policy as well as healthy lifestyles. In the pursuit of health, community health nurses develop health policies that support health action and use the nursing process to tailor preventive interventions for targeted individuals, populations, and communities. Community health nurses play a vital role in helping build healthy communities through the delivery of health promotion and other preventive services.

## Practice Dynamics

White proposed that two key processes help nurses identify health promoting and disease prevention needs among client populations and establish priorities for community health nursing intervention. These are the *nursing process* and the *valuing process*. The nursing process is used to assess and diagnose client needs and to plan, implement, and evaluate effective nursing interventions. This process is used in community health nursing to assess community and individual needs as well as to deliver and evaluate nursing services from a population-based perspective (see Chapters 9 and 14).

*Valuing,* the second dynamic process in White's model, guides nursing interventions and decision making and influences the development of goals and priorities for care. *Valuing* is "the process of assigning or determining the worth or merit of something" (White, 1982, p. 529). The influence that valuing has on decision making becomes particularly evident during times of scarce resources. When resources are limited, professionals must critically examine their beliefs about practice and target resources so that they are used effectively and efficiently.

Community health professionals place a high priority on targeting resources for at-risk populations in the community (APHA, 1996). Identifying service priorities for populations at risk and planning services to achieve these priorities benefits the population as a whole. Populations at risk *are those populations that engage in certain activities or have certain characteristics that increase their potential for contracting an illness, injury, or health problem.* Individuals who smoke, for example, constitute a population at high risk for developing cancer. The at-risk concept is basic to public health practice. It guides epidemiologic study of health and disease occurrence. It also provides a framework for assessing the

health status of clients across the continuum of practice and for developing health promoting intervention. This concept is addressed extensively in Chapter 11.

## Nursing Interventions

White classifies community health nursing interventions into three major categories: education, engineering, and enforcement. Educative nursing interventions help clients voluntarily acquire knowledge essential for understanding healthy functioning, develop attitudes that foster preventive health behaviors, and establish practices conducive to effective living. Educative strategies are commonly used in community health nursing practice in a variety of situations. Community health nurses help families learn about normal growth and development and childcare; conduct discussions related to sexuality issues in the school setting; and distribute health education materials in clinics, industrial plants, and other community health settings. Nurses visiting clients whose care is being reimbursed by Medicare also help clients learn about their health concerns. They may, for example, teach clients about their many medications, including why, when, and how to take them, or ways clients and families can deal with their health care needs.

Because the community health nurse believes that clients and families are in charge of their own lives and will ultimately make the decisions that influence their own health, education is considered a strategic intervention. Community health nurses work on the principle that people need to be active participants in the health care process and that knowledge helps empower people to make informed health care decisions.

Engineering nursing interventions focus on environmental modification for the purpose of eliminating or managing environmental risk factors that affect healthy living. Campaigning against television advertisements that promote alcohol and cigarette use, conducting clinics for the treatment of sexually transmitted diseases, promoting actions to eliminate safety hazards in a schoolyard, and creating a system to help elderly clients safely take their many medications, are all examples of engineering nursing interventions.

Enforcement nursing interventions are actions that impose regulatory controls and are designed to prevent disease, promote health, and protect society from harmful substances and conditions. Enforcement actions encourage the passage of regulations and legislation, such as seat belt, helmet, and drug abuse laws, that mandate health-promoting behaviors. Laws also may mandate that high-risk clients with infectious diseases such as tuberculosis (TB) (e.g., the drug-addicted, those with failed TB treatment, the homeless, and those who have problems understanding the disease) take their pills under a direct observation therapy program. This type of intervention focuses attention on the value "for the public good."

The Construct for Public Health Nursing Model provides a futuristic organizing framework for expanding the scope of practice to "nursing for the public's health." It is a dynamic model that integrates public health and nursing concepts to facilitate the analysis of health issues and to plan appropriate population-based, community-oriented interventions. The circular nature of the nursing process reflects the importance of ongoing assessment and intervention to assure the public's health.

### Stop and Think About It

You identify in your local community that the homeless have limited access to health care services. Describe how you would use White's Construct for Public Health Nursing Model to implement care for this at-risk population. Specifically, identify how you would go about obtaining information about the determinants of health in your local community that decrease access to health care. Searching the web for information on community health needs and resources and the demographic characteristics of your local community (census data) could be helpful here. Additionally, identify potential health promoting interventions that could impact access to care issues.

### *HEALTHY PEOPLE 2010* INITIATIVE GUIDES PRACTICE

The **Healthy People 2010 initiative,** the nation's vision for improving the health of the nation, provides a framework for identifying populations at risk and for developing prevention strategies that address population-based needs. This initiative builds on Healthy People activities pursued over the past two decades (USDHHS, 2000). The history addressing this initiative is shared in Chapter 4.

*Healthy People 2010* identifies a national strategy for increasing the span of *healthy* life among Americans, reducing health disparities, achieving universal access to quality health care, strengthening public health services, and improving the availability of health-related information (USDHHS, 2000). It also establishes directives for addressing the prevention of major chronic illnesses, injuries, and infectious diseases. These directives target population groups that are at highest risk of premature death, disease, and disability and promote a comprehensive strategy for achieving improvements in health that are possible through prevention and access to quality health care. The vision is to provide "every community member the *right services*, at the *right time*, in the *right way*" (Health Resources and Service Administration, Bureau of Primary Health Care [HRSA, BPHC], 2000).

*Healthy People 2010* challenges professionals and the American public to establish specific goals and objectives for improving health in local communities. This initiative emphasizes building healthy communities that provide a nurturing environment for its citizens. It also articulates the importance of developing preventive interventions that address the needs of at-risk populations across the life span and provides a framework for helping communities target

scarce resources and develop public policies that promote health and prevent disease.

*Healthy People 2010* objectives are used throughout this text to assist the reader in identifying major health needs among population groups across the life span and in formulating strategies for addressing these needs. Community health nurses nationwide are using the *Healthy People 2010* document (USDHHS, 2000) to develop a community health profile and health programs that effectively and efficiently address community health needs. Innovative initiatives are being developed at the local level to address health concerns identified by community residents. These initiatives provide exciting opportunities for an interdisciplinary cadre of health care professionals. "One of the most compelling and encouraging lessons learned from the *Healthy People 2000* initiatives is that we, as a nation, can make dramatic progress in improving the Nation's health in a relatively short period of time" (USDHHS, 2000, p. 3).

### HEALTH FOR ALL MANDATE

"What unites people around public (community) health is the focus on society as a whole, the community, and the aim of optimal health status" (IOM, 1988, p. 39). This is the theme that guides community health action at all levels of national and international government. In 1978, 158 countries attending the International Conference on Primary Health Care, held in Alma-Ata, USSR, set for themselves a common goal, "Health for All (HFA) by the Year 2000" (WHO, 2001). The **Health for All mandate** is a process founded on the fundamental belief of *social justice*. This process focuses on helping all people in all countries obtain access to health services that permit them to lead economically and socially productive lives (WHO, 1998). **Access to health care** is a complex concept that involves examining system, personal, and socioeconomic issues that facilitate or hinder an individual, a population, or a community in obtaining *essential health care services*, including public health services (see Figure 2-2).

Several key values guide the Health for all Process: "providing the *highest attainable standard of health as a fundamental right*; strengthening application of *ethics* to health policy, research, and service provision; implementing *equity-oriented* policies and strategies that emphasize *solidarity*; and incorporating a *gender* perspective into health policies and strategies" (WHO, 1998, p. V). These values are strongly linked and are aimed at improving quality of life and increased life expectancy for all people. However, despite unprecedented prosperity worldwide, the absolute number of people living in poverty is steadily increasing (WHO, 1998). *Poverty is strongly linked with poor health outcomes.*

The Declaration of Alma-Ata specifies that primary health care is the key vehicle for attaining the Health for All goal. The new global health policy, "Health for All in the Twenty-First Century," reinforces the importance of primary health care in combating health care access issues (WHO, 1998). **Primary health care (PHC)** is a blend of essential health services, personal responsibility for one's own health, and health promoting action taken by the community. The original elements of PHC addressed during the Alma-Ata conference were as follows (WHO, 1988, p. 23):

- Education concerning prevailing health problems and the methods of preventing and controlling them
- Promotion of food supply and proper nutrition
- Provision of an adequate supply of safe water and basic sanitation
- Provision of maternal and child health care, including family planning
- Immunization against the major infectious diseases
- Prevention and control of locally endemic diseases
- Appropriate treatment of common diseases and injuries
- Provision of essential drugs

The current Health for All mandate extended these original eight PHC elements to include expanded options for immunization, reproductive health needs, provision of essential technologies for health, health promotion services, prevention and control of noncommunicable disease, and food safety and provision of selected food supplements (WHO, 1998).

PHC facilitates client entry into a comprehensive health care system and promotes coordinated health care services and active client participation in health care delivery. Community health nurses carry out multiple functions to promote equitable access to the elements of primary care. For example, they advocate for services when they are lacking; deliver PHC services in a variety of settings such as homes, schools, clinics, and worksites; and help people gain the information needed to make knowledgeable health care decisions.

The "Health for All in the Twenty-First Century" mandate challenges all nations to ensure access to PHC for all people and to place greater emphasis on providing comprehensive quality health care throughout the life span (WHO, 1998). In response to this challenge, the USDHHS Bureau of Primary Health Care has proposed the use of a comprehensive, community-based health service delivery model for attaining the future vision in primary care: *100% access and 0 health disparities*. This proposal recognizes the importance of a community-wide responsibility for providing health care to all and incorporates the partnership approach previously discussed (HRSA, BPHC, 2000).

Community health nurses worldwide will play an instrumental role in helping their country create new models to reach the "100% access and 0 health disparities" vision. Because no one discipline alone can address all of the health needs in a community, an increasing emphasis will be placed on an interdisciplinary, community partnership approach to health care delivery. This approach will involve clients as well as health care professionals, ancillary services, and a range of staff from community agencies. "Government cannot single-handedly solve the health care crisis in the United States, and neither can corporate America or community leaders. But by pooling our resources—and that includes our creativity, not just our money—we can reach people, who, without us, probably won't ever get any health care" (HRSA, BPHC, 2001, p. 29).

## SETTINGS, WORK FORCE, AND ROLES

Community health nurses implement a variety of roles in multiple practice settings and provide a broad range of health promoting services. They work in diverse health and health-related organizations. Changing health care delivery trends have resulted in a need for increased numbers of nurses who can function in the community setting. It is anticipated that community-based and community-oriented service delivery will expand significantly in the future (American Association of Colleges of Nursing [AACN], 2001).

### Settings in Which Community Health Nurses Function

An exciting aspect of community health nursing is the existence of varied settings and modalities for practice. Community health nurses were first employed by visiting nurse associations, where they responded to the needs of people at greatest risk by nursing the sick in their homes and in neighborhood health centers and by providing instruction to both manage illness and remain well (Figure 2-4). With the increase demand for home care, this remains an important avenue for reaching individuals and targeted populations. Community health nurses also are employed by official health departments and other tax-supported agencies, such as schools and protective social services agencies. Additionally they work in a range of non–tax-supported agencies, including occupational health programs, churches, health maintenance organizations, and volunteer organizations focused on addressing specific populations such as clients with diabetes or developmental disabilities.

The type of community health services provided by nurses in these setting varies, based on the mission of the organization. For example, state and local health departments are mandated to protect the health of the community and, therefore, to provide a broad range of services that addresses the needs of groups across the life span. Visiting nurse associations, on the other hand, primarily emphasize the delivery of home health services, or direct hands-on nursing care.

Some community health settings mainly serve a specific segment of the community. Illustrative of this are health programs in schools and occupational settings. School-age children are the focus in school health programs, whereas the well adult is the target of service in the occupational health setting. Migrant health clinics, prisons, rural and urban nursing centers, homeless shelters, senior citizen centers, neighborhood health centers, and churches are other

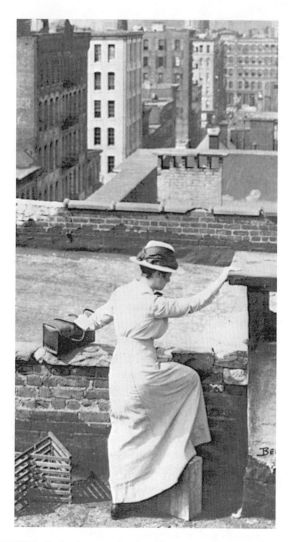

**FIGURE 2-4** Community health nurses traditionally have gone into a variety of community settings to serve individuals, families, and groups. In this picture, a Henry Street Settlement nurse is climbing over a tenement roof on New York's Lower East Side to visit her clients in the home. Today, community health nurses usually do not climb over rooftops. They do, however, reach out to clients in all types of settings (e.g., homes, schools, rural clinics, neighborhood health centers, and sheltered workshops). (Courtesy of Visiting Nurse Service of New York City.)

settings in which community health nurses work and where services are often targeted for specific populations. In the evolving health care system, community health nurses also are working in a variety of care management agencies established to assist specific client groups in accessing needed health care services.

In these settings the following elements are common: (1) an emphasis on independent practice by the practitioner, (2) an understanding that the physical and social environment is critical to the state of health, and (3) a focus on the concept that clients need to be active participants in the health care delivery process. As discussed previously, it is also important for community health nursing

organizations to focus on population-based, community-oriented practice. Some agencies find it difficult to address community-focused interventions from a comprehensive perspective, but they do value that problems are caused and solved at the community level. Usually health departments and other local health planning agencies are more likely than home health and private organizations to focus on comprehensive community intervention.

The Public Health Nursing Section of the American Public Health Association (APHA) (1996) has provided guidelines to assist nurses in expanding their community-focused efforts when they are working in private, voluntary, or nonofficial agencies. Often these types of agencies only serve a specific segment of the community, such as clients who need home health care services or individuals and families in a specific church or school district. In these settings, APHA recommends that nurses first analyze the needs of clients served by the organization and then extend their scope of service to individuals and families within the community who are eligible for service but have not availed themselves of the care offered (APHA, 1996, p. 9). This "targeted outreach" helps "the nurse to move away from solely meeting the needs of consumers as individually presented and toward practicing public (community) health nursing for all individuals or families within the population group or program focus" (APHA, 1996, p. 9).

## Size of the Work Force in Community Health Nursing

The earliest known count of public health nurses in the United States was reported in 1901 by Harriett Fulmer at the International Congress of Nurses in Buffalo, New York. At that time, 58 public health nursing organizations employed about 130 nurses. By 1912 Mary Gardner found that approximately 3000 nurses were engaged in delivering community health nursing services (Gardner, 1975). By the year 2000 approximately 403,000 registered nurses were working in public/community health settings, representing 18.3% of the registered nurse work force in the United States (USDHHS, 2001). Between 1992 and 1996, the number of registered nurses working in community health settings climbed by 42% (AACN, 2001). Public and community health settings continued to show the largest increase in the employment of registered nurses when the Seventh National Survey of Nurses was conducted in the year 2000 (USDHHS, 2001). These settings include state and local health departments, all types of home health care agencies, schools, community health centers, and occupational health programs. It is forecasted that 1 of every 10 nurses will be employed in homecare by 2005 (Shindul-Rothschild, Berry, Long-Middleton, 1996).

## Roles and Functions of Community Health Nurses in a Managed Care Environment

We are mobilizing public and private resources to make sure that the question of how healthy we are is determined

**BOX 2-9**

## *Selected Roles Assumed by Community Health Nurses*

### Advocate

Community health nurses facilitate clients' efforts in obtaining needed health services and in negotiating an appropriate care management plan. They also promote community awareness of significant health problems, lobby for beneficial public policy, and stimulate supportive community action for health.

### Caregiver

Community health nurses provide care to individuals, families, and vulnerable populations in a variety of settings (e.g., churches, safe houses for domestic violence victims, homes, homeless shelters, migrant health camps, and worksites). This care includes a range of activities such as hands-on physical care, educating a client about his or her health problems, and screening for undiagnosed health conditions.

### Care Manager

Community health nurses help clients make decisions about appropriate health care services and achieve service delivery integration and coordination. They advocate for services when needed and make referrals as necessary.

### Casefinder

Community health nurses conduct targeted outreach to identify clients in need of service and to assist clients in accessing appropriate care. They also observe for clients who may have potential or actual service needs during their daily course of activities.

### Counselor

Community health nurses are often in a unique position to help clients cope with normative and nonnormative stressors that could lead to crises and to adapt to changes in the environment. When assuming this role, they help clients express emotions and feelings, clarify facts in the situation, confront the stress in manageable doses, and accept assistance if needed.

### Educator

Community health nurses apply the principles of teaching and learning to promote positive health action and to facilitate behavioral change. They use these principles to help clients across the age continuum learn about new events and healthy functioning and apply acquired knowledge.

### Epidemiologist

Community health nurses use the epidemiologic method to analyze health problems among population groups and to develop population-focused interventions.

### Group Leader

Community health nurses use the group process to provide targeted preventive services and to manage caseload responsibilities. Through group process, community health nurses are able to assist small client or community groups to learn new knowledge and skills, to support group members during stressful times, or to problem-solve around issues important to the community.

### Health Planner

Community health nurses use the health planning process to develop, implement, and evaluate health services for populations at risk. This process is used to provide community-wide or population-specific health services.

### Manager

Community health nurses are responsible for managing caseload demands in an effective and efficient manner. They are also often responsible for managing problems and activities of other members of the health care team.

---

by disease and science, not by race or gender, income or address, or any other characteristic (e.g., health care financing) (HRSA, BPHC, 2001). A major Institute of Medicine (1988) report on the Future of Public Health identified three core public health functions—assessment, policy development, and assurance—that need to be implemented to achieve this goal. These functions are currently guiding community health nursing and public health practice. Briefly summarized, the core public health functions involve assessing the health status of the community; promoting the development of comprehensive health policies; and assuring constituents that services necessary to achieve agreed-upon goals are provided, by encouraging actions by other entities, requiring such action through regulation, or providing services directly (IOM, 1988). Assurance also involves determining "a set of high-priority personal and community-wide health ser-

vices that governments will guarantee to every member of the community" (IOM, 1988, p. 8). In partnership with the community and other health care providers, community health nurses are implementing the core public health functions to address the needs of clients across the continuum of practice and to build healthy communities (ASTDN, 1998, 2000; Conley, 1995).

Community health nurses assume a variety of roles and plan, implement, and evaluate a range of interventions when addressing the needs of clients in the community (ASTDN, 2000; Keller, Strohschein, Lia-Hoagberg, et al., 1998; Kosidlak, 1999; MDH, 1997; Smart, 1999). Select community health nursing interventions were addressed in an earlier section of this chapter. A partial listing of the types of roles commonly implemented by community health nurses across settings is displayed in Box 2-9. These roles and interventions are discussed throughout the text.

In the rapidly changing managed health care environment there is clearly a call for innovation in service delivery and a reformulation of health care provider roles. New opportunities for improving and expanding health care delivery are emerging. "We are building a system whereby communities can implement solutions that respond to their unique needs, a system that empowers individuals to participate in their own health care" (HRSA, BPHC, 2001). Community health nurses are assuming vital roles in helping communities meet their unique needs.

## SERVICES PROVIDED BY COMMUNITY HEALTH NURSES

To achieve their goals, community health nurses provide multiple and diverse direct and indirect client services. Direct client services usually involve a personal relationship between the nurse and client (who can be a person, a family, a targeted population, or the community). Teaching, hands-on bedside care, health risk appraisal, counseling, health planning with consumers, and the delivery of clinic services are examples of direct client services. Indirect client services include such things as record keeping, talking to a community agency about available resources to meet client needs, and supervising the care provided by a home health aide.

Provided are two "A View from the Field" discussions that chronicle a day in the life of two community health nurses: Charlene is employed by a county health department, and John is employed by a large voluntary visiting nurses' association. The stories illustrate the range of services commonly provided by nurses in various community settings.

The community health nurses in these two stories illustrate several important community health nursing concepts. The community health nurse is a generalist and serves all population groups. She or he works in the client's setting, using principles of prevention. The community health nurse also serves vulnerable populations such as those in clinics and schools. Concepts from the public health sciences of biostatistics, epidemiology, and administration help the nurse identify the needs of these populations.

The range of services provided by community health nurses is extensive. Although some community health nurses focus on addressing the needs of a specific segment of the population, such as John Roethke, who is working with clients who need home health care services, all community health nurses extend themselves to promote the development of a system of care that addresses population-focused needs. Additionally, community health nurses in all settings collaborate with other community agencies to ensure that needs of clients across the age continuum are addressed. Community health nursing is "nursing for the community's health."

## SUMMARY

Community health nursing is a synthesis of nursing and public health practice applied to promoting and preserving the health of populations (ANA, 1986). The community health nurse's philosophy and scope of practice distinguishes him or her from other nurses in the practice setting. Community health nurses serve individuals and targeted populations (groups of people) across the life span on a continuing basis. Their major goal is to protect and promote the health of the community. Primary prevention is their major focus. Identifying at-risk populations within the community assists community health nurses to effectively and efficiently provide preventive health care services. Nursing and public health concepts provide the foundation for population-based community-oriented practice.

Community health nurses work in a variety of settings and implement multiple roles such as casefinder, educator, group worker, and health planner. Changing health care delivery trends have increased the demand for community-based services and, in turn, the number of qualified community health nurses. The excitement of this specialty area lies in its diversity.

## CRITICAL THINKING
*exercise*

The definition of community health nursing states that it is a synthesis of nursing and public health practice. Discuss examples from the "A View from the Field" stories about a day in the life of a community health nurse and a day in the life of a visiting nurse (pp. 47-50) where concepts of public health and nursing are applied.

*A view from the field*

## A DAY IN THE LIFE OF A COMMUNITY HEALTH NURSE

Charlene's first stop by 8 am each day is at her desk in the health department to pick up messages from the day before, make phone calls, and plan her day's schedule.

After morning coffee with the other nurses, which offers time for comparisons, she starts her calls.

"Sometimes you've had a dark day and you need input, you need to talk to someone," she explains. "I could get depressed if I allowed myself, but I realize whose problem it is. It's not my problem. It's only my place to help when I'm accepted."

Many calls start with a request from a school or another public health nurse, or Charlene's own casefinding.

Her first stop on a gray, cheerless day recently was a happy one, to visit a new baby. Paul Daniel Conner had spent 2 months in a hospital nursery after being born prematurely, weighing only 3 lbs, 7 oz. Now 2 1/2 months old, he has adjusted easily to his mother's style in the 2 weeks he has been home.

"He's a perfect baby," says his mother, Julie. "He doesn't ever cry." But she does have a few questions, written on a scrap of paper.

"I was surprised how easy it has been. I've been just really relaxed with him," she tells Charlene.

The routine on a visit to a new baby includes leaving a sheaf of pamphlets for the mother's spare-time reading. Topics include first aid, exercises for the mother, feeding, birth control, and descriptions of the free services offered by the health department.

Charlene advises Mrs. Conner not to put Paul Daniel to bed with a bottle.

"A baby will get a pool of milk, juice, or Kool-Aid in its mouth that causes tooth decay. I see children with nothing but little brown stubs left of their teeth," she explains.

"You can use your blender to make baby food from table food, then freeze it in an ice cube tray and put it in a bag. But be sure to freeze it."

The telephone number for the Western Michigan Poison Center and instructions on taking a baby's temperature are all part of the routine, which ends with a full examination of the baby and measurement of his height and weight.

Charlene tells Mrs. Conner she can take her baby to the health department's well-baby clinic, in the Belmont area, for children from birth to school age.

"It's one of your benefits as a taxpayer. You can take the baby in for his shots, but continue to see the doctor."

The idea appeals to Mrs. Conner. She takes the information, the telephone number she would use for an appointment.

"You can call me anytime," Charlene says as she leaves. "I'm usually in early in the morning."

Few newborns in Kent County are seen by a public health nurse. Many don't need it; more probably do. All it would take is a call—from the hospital, from the mother, or even from a relative.

"There are many out there I'm not getting, mothers who are having problems adjusting to a new baby, who didn't like children or babies before and now overcompensate," Charlene explains.

A stop at West Oakview School is squeezed in before the students' lunch break to check a girl with bites on her arms and legs (probably flea bites from a cat, Charlene thinks) and to make a progress report from a class for emotionally impaired youngsters.

At North Oakview School, after lunch, Charlene calls in to her office for messages. Then she visits a "readiness room" for 5- to 7-year-olds taught by Ann Westerhof.

"If Charlene didn't come in once a week, I don't know what I'd do," Mrs. Westerhof exclaims. "She's the go-between for me and the families. She helps me know what I can and can't do."

The "star" of this visit is Jim Fragale, 6, who is sporting a new brace, an unusual contraption with a tripod base and straps that keep his legs bent to aid healing of the hip joints.

The cause of Jim's hip problem is unknown, Charlene explains. "The ball joint of the hip softens, then starts coming back. But the regeneration is dependent on rest and nutrition."

Jim had a little trouble balancing when he was first fitted with the brace, and even fell backwards, Mrs. Westerhof explains. "And he was a little embarrassed by it at first. But now he can show the other students tricks they can't do."

Charlene's link was knowing what agency to contact to make the brace a reality. "So many times, parents can't afford the treatment needed, and Char knows how to get it," Mrs. Westerhof adds.

From the young to the old—that switch in thinking is typical for public health nurses.

Twice a month, Charlene is in charge of the well-baby clinic in Belmont. She sees humanity at its beginnings there, in the tots brought in for free care—routine physical

Modified from Haradine J: Public health nurse makes a difference, *Grand Rapids Press,* December 3, 1978, pp. 29-33.

*Continued*

*A view from the field*

## A DAY IN THE LIFE OF A COMMUNITY HEALTH NURSE—cont'd

examinations by a doctor, immunizations, and advice for parents.

Although the wait can be long, the time can be used to ask a public health nurse about the little doubts, those questions that seem too insignificant for the doctor.

"I thought he'd outgrow it by this time. I guess he won't," one mother was overheard commenting to one of the three nurses staffing the clinic.

These chats, informal and friendly, offer help on parenting to start the young out right.

When the young, at 14 or 15, stumble along the way, Charlene and the other public health nurses are there, just a telephone call away.

Sometimes it's the child's problem, and sometimes it's the parent's, spreading over to the child. "Rare is the teenager who will say, 'Hey, I've got a problem,'" Charlene notes. "Some social workers do refer kids to me.

"We see some child abuse cases and we see neglect, which is so hard to prove. It's insidious and camouflaged. Sometimes the parents are too wrapped up in themselves, or it might be a lack of resources, of money.

"We have to know what help is available from the different agencies."

The old pose a different problem, when loneliness and loss have taken their toll. Charlene pulls into a driveway along the Grand River, next to a small house with a tidy yard. It's a call to the other end of life.

"They say I'll live to be 90, but I don't care to," says Josephine Robbins as Charlene takes her blood pressure.

"I know that," Charlene replies, acceptingly, as she removes the blood pressure cuff from the arm of the woman, who is 80.

The youngest of seven, Josephine says, "The others, they're all gone. My sister was 92."

Her husband, Lloyd, died in March. "What do I have to live for?" she asks.

In answer to Charlene's questions on her health, she reports only "a catch in my side" now and then. But she takes "just a little Lydia Pinkham's and it goes away."

An active woman now very lonely and anxious, Josephine looks forward to the weekly nurse visit. "You're not taking any of those pills, are you?" Charlene asks in a warning tone.

"No, I threw them out." A neighbor had given Josephine two drugs, Librium (a tranquilizer) and nitroglycerine (a heart drug), saying, "They always helped me. Maybe they'll help you."

Charlene had become aware of them on her last visit when she had asked what medications Josephine was taking.

Josephine worries about getting her things in order, her will, her records and being able to pledge her eyes and kidneys before she dies. "They said I had to come down and sign in front of two witnesses, but I can't get down there," she tells the nurse. Charlene explains, "Not necessary; just witnesses, here in your home."

Besides the decisions for her will, on the who and what of all she owns, Josephine must finish the mural she is painting on one wall, then paint a scene in a window and refinish some furniture. And then. . . .

"There's just an awful lot of red tape," the gray-haired woman comments sadly. "I'm never going to be through."

The public health nurse visits often when the need is great, then as the crisis eases, the visits taper off, to make time and room for someone else with other pressing needs.

Days are filled with joy and sadness. Charlene believes she gets as much as she gives in her 8-to-5 job. "I need people. I see myself as a helping person and they are fulfilling to me."

But in public health the rewards are seldom quick in coming. "You see something grow. You see a person who has never had any self-confidence make strides.

"I'm really in preventive medicine," Charlene says. "By educating others and by my intervention, I believe I'll make a difference."

From Haradine J: Public health nurse makes a difference, *Grand Rapids Press,* December 3, 1978, pp. 29-33.

*A view from the field*

## A DAY IN THE LIFE OF A VISITING NURSE

Shortly before noon on yet another 90-plus-degree September day, John Roethke is praising automobile air-conditioning as he navigates the streets of West Philadelphia in search of a particular shopping center.

A few minutes later he finds it and, more importantly, the pay phone he uses to inform his next patient that he's just around the corner.

When Roethke pulls up to Derrick Smith's building in Yeadon, a family member already has a third-floor window open. Smith and his aunt have trouble climbing the three flights of stairs, so they have devised a ritual: Roethke calls when he gets close, honks his horn when he arrives, and they toss him the front-door key from the third floor.

Just another day for a home health care nurse.

Before joining the Visiting Nurse Association of Greater Philadelphia, Roethke worked in the trauma center at Albert Einstein Medical Center and as an emergency room nurse manager at Parkview Hospital.

"I thought I'd be bored silly working in home care after being in emergency rooms for so long." the 34-year-old Bethlehem native says. "But that hasn't happened. I'm working with a lot of high-tech equipment and teaching patients how to use it. It really astounds me that I'm teaching a 78-year-old woman how to work a CADD pump."

The computer-assisted delivery device, the size of a transistor radio, pumps medication into a patient's veins at a preset rate.

"It sounds kind of corny, but patients really do better at home where they are in familiar surroundings," Roethke says. "Hospitals in the 21st century won't be anything like they are today. They'll have an emergency room, a huge outpatient department and intensive-care units for surgery and that's it. Everything else will be home care."

Roethke's work day begins around 8 AM, when he contacts patients to let them know when he will be coming by.

His first stop on this oppressively hot day is in South Philadelphia, a few blocks from where Connie Mack Stadium once stood. The patient, 72-year-old Early Yearwood, suffers from cardiomyopathy—his heart is having a difficult time pumping fluid to his kidneys.

Roethke, who at 6-foot-6 is not the prototype nurse, attracts a few curious stares as he lifts his bag from the car's trunk.

Inside, Early and his wife, Mary, are watching a television game show. The lights are off and two fans are oscillating in the heat.

"How do you feel today, Earl?" Roethke asks, as he checks Yearwood's blood pressure.

"Bad," he responds.

For a half-hour Roethke examines Yearwood and administers 50 mg of Lasix, a treatment for cardiomyopathy. At the same time he quizzes Yearwood's wife on how and when she should change Yearwood's bandages. Home health aides are available to help patients get out of bed and dressed, but the idea, Roethke explains, is to have the family do as much as it can. If a nurse thinks the family can't handle the responsibility, a recommendation will be made to return the patient to the hospital.

Though Yearwood is stoic for most of the visit, Roethke gets him to smile occasionally.

"Now, no jogging around the block," Roethke says, as he packs up his equipment.

"I don't think I could do that," Yearwood answers with a grin.

On the way to his next patient, Derrick Smith, Roethke tells of two events that lead him to home health care.

He is going through a divorce and has joint custody of his children. Working as a home health care nurse allows him to set his own schedule so he can spend more time with his three daughters.

He also had the experience of becoming a patient after getting stuck with a needle and contracting hepatitis B.

"When you become a patient they just don't strip away your clothes, they strip away your dignity," Roethke says. "I'm not trying to come down hard on the hospitals because they have a tremendous job to do."

But it made him an advocate for home care.

Roethke says he is unconcerned about visiting patients in high-crime areas, but he agrees maybe he should be.

"Some of the other nurses told me, in the drug-infested areas the drug dealers know you're there to care for the elderly in the neighborhood and they leave you alone," he says. "I don't bank on that, but I never had any problems."

Smith, the 44-year-old Yeadon patient, also suffers from cardiomyopathy.

"This is great," Smith says of being treated at home. "I've been in the hospital so much for so long. I don't want to go back."

"I've seen so much improvement." Roethke spent 40 minutes with Smith, checking his vital signs and administering about 200 mg of Lasix, seemingly oblivious to Smith's niece and nephew playing and yelling just a few feet away.

Modified from George J: For John Roethke, the job of visiting nurse is anything but dull, *Philadelphia Business Journal*, October 7, 1991, pp. 1, 3-4.

*Continued*

*A view from the field*

## A DAY IN THE LIFE OF A VISITING NURSE—cont'd

Before he leaves, the children hug Roethke, wrapping their arms around his knees.

"People are always giving you food or little gifts. It's amazing," Roethke says. "They're welcoming you into their home. When I worked in the emergency room it was often on patients who didn't want to be there. They'd fight you. If I didn't get called a MF at least once a shift I didn't feel loved."

Roethke's third visit on this day is a marked departure from the first two. His patient, Shirley Channick, lives in King of Prussia.

The key isn't tossed out the window. The maid lets him in after a security guard buzzes him through the lobby.

Channick has rheumatoid arthritis and an infection stemming from a hip replacement. Her arthritis keeps Channick from administering medication to herself, so she is being treated with antibiotics delivered by a CADD pump.

Roethke's next stop is the office, where he will spend hours tackling the Medicare and Medicaid forms the job generates.

"I thought I'd find it difficult to work in long-term care where you don't always see improvement," he says. "I haven't found that to be the case. Maybe I should stop looking."

Modified from George J: For John Roethke, the job of visiting nurse is anything but dull, *Philadelphia Business Journal*, October 7, 1991, pp. 1, 3-4.

## REFERENCES

American Association of Colleges of Nursing (AACN): *Your nursing career: a look at the facts*, Washington, DC, 2001, AACN.

American Nurses Association (ANA): Council of Community Health Nurses: *Standards of community health nursing practice*, Pub No CH-10, Kansas City, Mo, 1986, ANA.

American Nurses Association (ANA): *Nursing's social policy statement*, Washington, DC, 1995, American Nurses Publishing.

American Public Health Association (APHA), Public Health Nursing Section: *The definition and role of public health nursing, a statement of APHA public health nursing section*, Washington, DC, 1996, APHA.

Association of Community Health Nursing Educators (ACHNE): *Differentiated nursing practice in community health*, Skokie, Ill, 1993, ACHNE.

Association of State and Territorial Directors of Nursing (ASTDN): *Public health nursing: a partner for progress: a document which links nursing, public health core functions and essential services*, Washington, DC, 1998, ASTDN.

Association of State and Territorial Directors of Nursing (ASTDN): *Public health nursing: a partner for healthy populations*, Washington, DC, 2000, American Nurses Publishing.

Beery WL, Greenwald HP, Nudelman PM: Managed care and public health: building a partnership, *Public Health Nurs* 13:305-310, 1996.

Berkowitz B: Collaboration for health improvement models for state, community, and academic partnerships, *J Public Management and Practice* 6(1):67-72, 2000.

Bracht N, Kingsbury L, Rissel C: A five-stage community organization model for health promotion: empowerment and partnership strategies. In Bracht N, editor: *Health promotion at the community level: new advances*, ed 2, Thousand Oaks, Calif, 1999, Sage.

Brainard A: *Organization of public health nursing*, New York, 1921, Macmillan.

Canadian Public Health Association (CPHA): *Community health/public health nursing in Canada: preparation and practice*, Ottawa, Ontario, 1990, CPHA.

Conley E: Public health nursing within core public health functions: "back to the future," *J Public Health Management Practice* 1(3):1-8, 1995.

Courtney R, Ballard E, Fauver S, et al.: The partnership model: working with individuals, families, and communities toward a new vision of health, *Public Health Nurs* 13:177-186, 1996.

Fitzpatrick ML: *The National Organization for Public Health Nursing, 1912-1952: development of a practice field*, New York, 1975, National League for Nursing.

Flynn BC: Communicating with the public in community-based nursing practice, *Public Health Nurs* 15(3):165-170, 1998.

Gardner MS: Typewritten Reminiscences, Feb. 5, 1948, NOPHN Archive Microfilm H25. In Fitzpatrick ML, editor: *The National Organization for Public Health Nursing, 1912-1952: development of a practice field*, New York, 1975, National League for Nursing.

Gebbe K: Follow the money: funding streams and public health nursing, *J Public Health Management and Practice* 1(3):23-28, 1995.

George J: For John Roethke, the job of visiting nurse is anything but dull, *Philadelphia Business Journal*, pp. 1, 3-4, October 7, 1991.

Goeppinger J: Primary health care: an answer to the dilemmas of community nursing, *Public Health Nurs* 1:129-140, 1984.

Gold M, Sparer M, Chu K: Medicaid managed care: lessons from five states, *Health Affairs* 15:153-166, 1996.

Haradine J: Public health nurse makes a difference, *Grand Rapids Press*, pp. 29-33, December 3, 1978.

Health Resources and Service Administration, Bureau of Primary Health Care (HRSA, BPHC): *Visioning the future in primary care: creating a new model to research 100% access and 0 health disparities: comprehensive, community-based health service delivery*, Rockville, Md, 2000, HRSA, BPHC.

Health Resources and Service Administration, Bureau of Primary Health Care (HRSA, BPHC): *Changing lives, changing communities through primary health care*, Rockville, Md, 2001, HRSA, BPHC.

Hemstrom M, Ambrose M, Donahue G, et al.: The clinical specialist in community health nursing: a solution for the 21st century, *Public Health Nurs* 17(5):386-391, 2000.

Institute of Medicine (IOM), Committee for the Study of the Future of Public Health: *The future of public health*, Washington, DC, 1988, National Academy Press.

Institute of Medicine (IOM): *America's health care safety net: intact but endangered*, Washington, DC, 2000, National Academy Press.

Keller L, Strohschein S, Lia-Hoagberg B, et al.: Population-based public health nursing interventions: a model from practice, *Public Health Nurs* 15(3):207-215, 1998.

Koopman JS: Comment: emerging objectives and methods in epidemiology, *Am J Public Health* 86:630-632, 1996.

Kosidlak J: The development and implementation of a population based intervention model for public health nursing practice, *Public Health Nurs* 16(5):311-320, 1999.

McNeil E: Transition in public health nursing, *U Michigan Medical Center J* 33:286-291, 1967.

Minnesota Department of Health (MDH), Section of Public Health Nursing: *Public health interventions: examples from public health nursing*, Minneapolis, 1997, MDH.

National Institutes of Health (NIH): *Making health communication programs work: a planner's guide*, Atlanta, 1995, US Department of Health and Human Services.

National Organization for Public Health Nursing (NOPHN): Constitution of the National Organization for Public Health Nursing, Article 2, 1912, Wald: New York Public Library folder: NOPHN No. 1. In Fitzpatrick ML, editor: *The National Organization for Public Health Nursing, 1912-1952: development of a practice field*, New York, 1975, National League for Nursing.

Olshansky S, Carnes B, Rogers R, et al.: The challenge of prediction: the fifth stage of epidemiological transition, *World Health Stat Q* 51(2/3/4):99-119, 1998.

Quad Council of Public Health Nursing Organizations: *Scope and standards of public health nursing practice*, Washington, DC, 1999, American Nurses Publishing.

Shindul-Rothschild J, Berry D, Long-Middleton E: Where have all the nurses gone? Final results of AJN's patient care survey, *Am J Nurs* 96:25-37, 1996.

Smart J: Public health nursing in children's protective services, *Public Health Nurs* 16(6):390-396, 1999.

US Department of Health and Human Services (USDHHS): *Healthy People 2010: understanding and improving health*, vol I and II, ed 2, Washington, DC, 2000, US Government Printing Office.

US Department of Health and Human Services (USDHHS): *The registered nurse population: National Sample Survey of Registered Nurses—March 2000: preliminary findings*, Washington, DC, 2001, Division of Nursing, Health Resources and Services Administration.

White MS: Construct for public health nursing, *Nurs Outlook* 30:527-530, 1982.

Winslow C-EA: *Man and epidemics*, Princeton, NJ, 1952, Princeton University Press.

World Health Organization (WHO): *Community health nursing*, 1974 WHO Expert Committee Report 558, Geneva, 1974, WHO.

World Health Organization (WHO): *Alma-Ata 1978: primary health care: report of the International Conference on Primary Health Care*, Alma-Ata, USSR, Geneva, 1978, WHO.

World Health Organization (WHO): *A guide to curriculum review for basic nursing education: orientation to primary health care and community health*, Geneva, 1985, WHO.

World Health Organization (WHO): *Four decades of achievement: highlights of the work of WHO*, Geneva, 1988, WHO.

World Health Organization (WHO): *Health for all in the twenty-first century*, Geneva, 1998, WHO.

World Health Organization (WHO): *Health for all in the twenty-first century: history*, Geneva, 2001, WHO. Retrieved from the internet July 29, 2001. *http://www.who.int/archives/hfa/history.html*

Zotti ME, Brown P, Stotts RC: Community-based nursing versus community health nursing: what does it all mean? *Nurs Outlook* 44:211-217, 1996.

## SELECTED BIBLIOGRAPHY

Barnes D, Eribes C, Juarbe T, et al.: Primary health care: a confusion of philosophies, *Nurs Outlook* 43:7-16, 1995.

Eakin B, Brady J, Lusk S: Creating a tailored, multimedia, computer-based intervention, *Computers in Nursing* 19(4):152-163, 2001.

Glick D: Advanced practice community health nursing in community nursing centers, *Holistic Nurs Pract* 13(4):19-27, 1999.

Hanchett E: *Nursing frameworks and community as client: bridging the gap*, Norwalk, Conn, 1988, Appleton & Lange.

Heller B, Oros M, Durney-Crowley J: The future of nursing education: 10 trends to watch, *Nursing and Health Care Perspectives* 21(1):9-13, 2000.

Kenyon V, Smith E, Hefty LV, et al.: Clinical competencies for community health nursing, *Public Health Nurs* 7:33-39, 1990.

Kreuter M, Lezin N, Kreuter M, et al.: *Community health promotion ideas that work: a field-book for practitioners*, Boston, 1998, Jones and Bartlett.

Misener TR, Alexander JW, Blaha AJ, et al.: National delphi study to determine competencies for nursing leadership in public health, *Image J Nurs Sch* 29:47-51, 1997.

Nacion K, Fordham K, Burnett G, et al.: Validating the safety of nurse-health advocate services, *Public Health Nurs* 17(1):32-42, 2000.

SmithBattle L, Diekemper M, Drake M: Articulating the culture and tradition of community health nursing, *Public Health Nurs* 16(3):215-222, 1999.

Smith-Campbell B: A case study on expanding the concept of caring from individuals to communities, *Public Health Nurs* 16(6):405-411, 1999.

US Department of Health and Human Services, Public Health Service: *The public health workforce: an agenda for the 21st century, full report of the public health functions project*, Washington, DC, 1997, Public Health Services.

Wieck K: Health promotion for inner-city minority elders, *J Community Health* 17(3):131-139, 2000.

Williams A, Wold JL: Healthcare for the future: caring for populations in alternative settings, *Nurs Educ* 21:23-26, 1996.

Williams CA: Community health nursing: what is it? *Nurs Outlook* 24:250-254, 1977.

World Health Organization (WHO): *Health for all: origins and mandate, special publication: the world health report: life in the 21st century-vision for all*, Geneva, 1998, WHO.

World Health Organization (WHO): *The world health report 1998: life in the 21st century—a vision for all*, Geneva, 1998, WHO.

Zahner S: Public health nursing and immunization surveillance, *Public Health Nurs* 16(6):384-389, 1999.

Zerwekh J: A family caregiving model for public health nursing, *Nurs Outlook* 39:213-217, 1991.

Zerwekh J, Primomo J, Deal L, editors: *Opening doors: stories of public health nursing*, Olympia, Wash, 1992, Washington State Department of Health.

# 3

# Community as Partner

*Sandra L. McGuire*

## OBJECTIVES

*Upon completion of this chapter, the reader should be able to:*

1. Define the term *community*.
2. Discuss the concept of community as partner.
3. Discuss the meaning of community as client.
4. Describe the service systems of a community.
5. Discuss the functions of a community.
6. Discuss community dynamics.
7. Define the term *aggregate*.
8. Discuss Healthy Communities Initiatives.
9. Discuss health problems of rural communities.
10. Understand the importance of community assessment to community health nursing practice.

## KEY TERMS

Aggregates
Community
Community as client
Community as partner
Community assessment
Community autonomy
Community communication

Community components
Community dynamics
Community empowerment
Community functions
Community leadership
Community stressors
Flexible line of defense

Functional community
Healthy Community Initiatives
International communities
Neighborhoods
Normal line of defense
Rural communities
Service systems

*As discussed there can be no health without community: that sense of mutual values and goals held by people regardless of geographic boundaries and their collective responsibility for nurturing their biophysical environment.*

**DR. NANCY MILIO (1990)**

As discussed in Chapter 2, the uniqueness of community health nursing lies in the fact that nurses in this specialty area care for the "community." Community health nurses view the community as client, work in partnership with communities to promote health, and provide services to aggregates in the community. They work toward ensuring equal access to health services for everyone—health for all.

In its definition of community health nursing, the American Nurses Association (ANA) stated that nursing efforts to promote and maintain health in the community entail the understanding and application of (1) concepts of public health and community; (2) skills of community organization and development; and (3) nursing care of selected in-

dividuals, families, and groups for health promotion, health maintenance, health education, and coordination of care (ANA, 1986, p. 1). As health care moves from a treatment- and hospital-based system to a prevention- and community-based one, nurses need to be ready to provide interventions that lead to improved health outcomes for the entire population (Shoultz, Hatcher, 1997, p. 23). Nursing students need knowledge about communities and community-based problem solving (Feenstra, 2000, p. 156).

This chapter presents the concepts of community as partner and community as client, defines the terms community and aggregate, and discusses community dynamics. Chapters 2 and 15 build on this material and discuss how community assessment, diagnosis, and health planning processes assist public health professionals in working with communities.

## COMMUNITY AS PARTNER

Today, more than ever before, nurses are working in partnership with communities to promote health. The nurse assists communities to build on their strengths, works collaboratively with them in decision making, and facilitates community empowerment. "To be empowered means that one (community, family, individual) has the knowledge, skills and capacity for effective and self-determined action" (Courtney, 1995, p. 370; Courtney, Ballard, Fauver, et al., 1996, p. 180). Empowerment is a proactive, participatory change process that encourages people and organizations in communities to use their skills and resources in collective action to improve the quality of life within the community (Israel, Checkoway, Schulz, et al., 1994). As communities take action on their local health needs, they increase their capacity for health promotion (Flynn, 1998, p. 165).

A partnership is a union of people focused on collective action for a common endeavor or goal. Community as partner takes advantages of the increased opportunities for community partnerships to promote health (Flynn, 1998, p. 165). Partners share "in a common activity or interest that may include other members of interdisciplinary professionals groups, community members, policymakers, and community institutions and organizations" (ANA Quad Council, 1999, p. 24). Community partnerships require a high level of communication skills, and community health nurses are skilled in communication (Flynn, 1998, p. 166).

Community partners agree to be active participants in the process of mutually determining goals and actions that promote health and well-being (Courtney, Ballard, Fauver, et al., 1996, p. 180). "The ultimate goal of the partnership is to enhance the capacity of individual, family and community partners to act more effectively on their own behalf" (Courtney, Ballard, Fauver, et al., 1996, p. 180). Characteristics of a community partnership include negotiated power; mutual goal setting; active versus passive client participation; and mobilization of a client's capacity for effective, self-determined action. Such partnerships need to build on a community's strengths and assets and not merely focus on community needs and deficits (Kretzmann, McKnight, 1993; Kretzmann, McKnight, Sheehan, 1997).

Community partnerships recognize the value of community representatives and health care providers working together to create health care systems that are user friendly, accessible, culturally sensitive, and responsive to community needs (Pender, 1996, p. 296). They involve developing networks of people to take action for health, promoting broad-based community participation and equity in health, and focusing on what is best for the total community (Flynn, 1994, p. 55). The community's right to identify health problems and their solutions is recognized, and provider-community alliances are developed (Milio, 1992, p. 24). Public health nurses partner with the community to develop public policy and target health promotion and disease prevention activities (ANA Quad Council, 1999, p. 5).

Increasingly, the importance of developing partnerships to promote collective action for enhancing community health and quality of life is recognized. The tenets of public health nursing discussed in Chapter 2 stress the importance of partnering with the community. The healthy communities initiatives discussed later in this chapter illustrate examples of nurses working in partnership with communities to promote health and improve the quality of life. Nurses all over the country are working in partnership with communities. Examples of such nursing partnerships include CITYNET Healthy Cities at the University of Indiana School of Nursing (Flynn, 1996); the LIFE program at the University of Pennsylvania School of Nursing, designed to meet the needs of frail elders (Naylor, Buhler-Wilkerson, 1999); the de Madres a Madres program that addresses prenatal care issues of low income Hispanic women (McFarlane, Fehir, 1994); and a nurse-managed clinic in partnership with the Andrews University Department of Nursing and the Veteran's Administration Hospital in Battle Creek, Michigan (Box 3-1) (Allen, 2000). Community health nurses do not just work in the community, they work in partnership with communities to promote community health (McKnight, VanDover, 1994, p. 13).

 **BOX 3-1**

*Clinical Practice: A Community Partnership Initiative*

The Andrews University Department of Nursing, located in southwestern Michigan, is an example of a nurse-managed clinic that is providing a valuable community service. The clinic is funded by a third-party payor, the Veteran's Administration (VA). Before this nurse-managed clinic was opened, veterans from southwestern Michigan had to travel at least 1½ hours one way to receive primary care services. The Battle Creek VA saw the need to provide accessible primary care services to veterans in southwestern Michigan. In November 1999 the Department of Nursing at Andrews University approached the Battle Creek VA with a proposal to provide primary care for veterans in three southwestern Michigan counties through a nurse-managed clinic. Advanced practice nursing faculty provide primary care at the clinic and advanced practice nursing students participate through supervised practice. This partnership provides comprehensive primary care close to home. In the future, the nurse-managed clinic plans to expand services to offer health education classes and seminars at community Veterans of Foreign War (VFW) sites. Donald Olivia, director of the Veterans Services Office in one of the counties served by the clinic, stated, "I see this as something we've needed for a long time." By participating in these types of partnerships we all win. Clients get comprehensive, accessible care, nurses are visible in the community, students get practice sites, and important community health needs are addressed. Nurses are increasingly becoming involved in such innovative community partnerships.

Modified from Allen K: Nursing school, VA partnership benefits vets in rural Michigan, *The American Nurse* 32(3):31, 2000.

## COMMUNITY AS CLIENT

Conceptualizing **community as client** can be difficult for the nurse. In the acute care setting, nursing care is often provided to individuals and families, but not as often to aggregates or communities. Moving to a community focus requires an understanding of community dynamics and aggregate- and community-based care. Numerous services are provided in the community to aggregates at risk such as infants, school-age children, pregnant women, incarcerated juveniles and adults, elders, people who are disabled, and workers.

The importance of the concept of community as client has long been recognized in community health nursing practice. Lillian Wald, Mary Breckinridge, and other early community health nursing leaders realized that health problems, and their solutions, were deeply embedded in the structure of the community. These leaders promoted the idea that the dominant responsibility of the community health nurse was to the population as a whole, the community (ANA, 1980; National Organization for Public Health Nursing, 1975).

Today this responsibility has been integrated into the ANA's definitions of community health and public health nursing and the American Public Health Association's (APHA) definition of public health nursing (see Chapter 2). Public health nursing is "the practice of promoting and protecting the health of populations using knowledge from nursing, social, and public health sciences" (ANA Quad Council, 1999, p. 2; APHA, 1996, p. 1). The nurse works in partnership with the community to promote health and provide services to the community and its aggregates.

## DEFINING COMMUNITY

The concept of community is basic to public health practice and is a distinguishing feature of community health nursing. The word **community** has been in common use since its Latin origin as *communitas*, and there are no less than 100 definitions for the word *communis*, from which *community* was derived (Shamansky, Pesznecker, 1981, p. 182).

Health, social, urban, and political scientists have defined community from several different perspectives, and nursing literature reveals diverse usages and definitions of the term *community*. Characteristics that have emerged as being essential to a definition of community are (1) people, (2) social interaction, (3) area, and (4) common ties (Hillery, 1955, pp. 118-119; Wellman, Leighton, 1988, p. 58). Although communities have many similarities, each community is uniquely different.

People in a community share things in common such as land, history, culture, heritage, and even destiny (MacIver, Page, 1949, pp. 8-10; Moore, 2000). A community is where people live, maintain their homes, earn their living, become educated, rear their children, and carry on day-to-day activities (Poplin, 1979, p. 8). A community can be defined in a very broad sense as a group of people living in an environment that has the ability to meet their major life goals and needs such as food, shelter, and socialization.

The APHA (1991, p. 444) has said that the term *community* implies an entity from which the nature and scope of a public health problem, as well as the capacity to respond to that problem, can be defined and, depending on the problem area and response capacity, the definition of community may vary. According to the APHA, for most instances of public health, the community is defined as a geopolitical unit such as a town, city, or county. In the United States many public health services are provided by local health departments based on their geopolitical boundaries.

The definition of community used in this text is the World Health Organization (WHO) definition that is incorporated into the ANA's (1986) *Standards of Community Health Nursing Practice*. This definition states that a "community is a social group determined by geographic boundaries and/or common values and interests; community members know and interact with one another; the community functions within a particular social structure; and the community creates norms, values, and social institutions" (WHO, 1974).

### The American Community

The American community has been studied since the early 1900s. Early researchers of the American community were usually social scientists and included MacIver (1917), Hillery (1955), Sanders (1958), and Warren (1955, 1966). Many of these early studies have become classics in the field and are still cited in today's social science and nursing literature. These early researchers recognized that there was a relationship between the community and the health of its members. One of them, Irwin T. Sanders, published in the community health nursing literature. His article "The Community: Structure and Function" appeared in *Nursing Outlook* (Sanders, 1963). For interested readers, *The Community: An Introduction to a Social System* (Sanders, 1958, 1966, 1975), *The Community in America* (Warren, 1963, 1972, 1978, 1987), and *Studying Your Community* (Warren, 1955, 1965) are considered classic works on the American community.

Early research on the American community focused on the community as a natural area. This natural area is often a geopolitical area such as a city or town. Contemporary research on community has been broadened to reflect a natural network approach to defining and describing communities. The natural network approach is more relational in nature and takes into account the widening scope of resources and services necessary to maintain the health and well-being of a community in today's technologic, complex, and diverse society. This approach addresses some contemporary community health concerns such as health disparities, access to resources, resource distribution, and how communities network outside the community to obtain necessary resources and services.

### Communities as Social Units

Communities are social units and settings for social action. A community is the basic unit of social organization that transmits values, attitudes, and beliefs to its members (Arensburg, Kimball, 1972, p. 15). Community health nurses need to be aware of, and respect, the values, attitudes, and culture of the communities in which they work.

As a social unit, the community has a life within which individuals define their own lives (Moore, 2000). The community helps provide its members a sense of who they are and where they are going and perpetuates the culture and heritage of the community. A community can be differentiated from other social units, such as groups, in that one's life can basically be lived within its bounds (Arensburg, Kimball, 1972, p. 17; MacIver, Page, 1949, pp. 8-10; Warren, 1978, p. 6). This is possible because of the various services and functions that the community provides and offers its residents.

## Communities as Part of a Larger Society

A community is part of, and has ties to, the larger society, often on a county, state, national, or international level. In today's world such ties are necessary to maintain community function. A community's patterns of communication and leadership (discussed later in this chapter) link it to the larger society and its resources.

In many communities, health care resources are inadequate to meet the community's increasingly diverse, complex, and ever-changing health care needs. When a community's resources are inadequate, people have to go outside the community, to the larger society, to obtain necessary health care services. This results in a "community of solution" within which the problem can be solved and resources obtained. In American rural communities with shrinking health care resources, such networking is becoming increasingly necessary to meet health care needs.

## Community Autonomy

Some communities have a greater sense of **community autonomy** than others, and people have varying degrees of loyalty to their communities. In some places a sense of community exists, and in others it does not. Research has shown that a population base of 10,000 to 20,000 is preferred for maintaining a sense of community, that larger cities of up to 100,000 can still maintain this sense, and that cities or geographic areas larger than 100,000 often need to be broken down into target areas such as neighborhoods or districts to maintain a sense of community and provide effective health care delivery (Chamberlain, 1988, p. 302). Also, if a community has a relatively "mobile" or transient populace, it may be difficult for a sense of community to exist because people do not stay in the community long enough to develop ties to it and feel part of it.

## COMMUNITY DYNAMICS

Community dynamics occur as a result of interactions within the community and between the community and the larger society. These interactions are instrumental in determining what public health services are offered in the community and the level of community health, and for achieving healthy communities. Community dynamics involve interactions between the community's people; goals, needs, and assets; environment; service systems; patterns of communication and leadership; and community functions. Figure 3-1 is a flow chart that summarizes the information on community dynamics presented in this chapter and assists the reader in visualizing and conceptualizing the discussion that follows.

## Components of a Community

Community components include people; shared goals, needs and assets; environment; service systems; and boundaries. Communities also have patterns of communication and leadership and carry out various functions.

People are a community's most important resource: they are its essence and give the community its identity. They have responsibilities to the community, and the community has responsibilities to them.

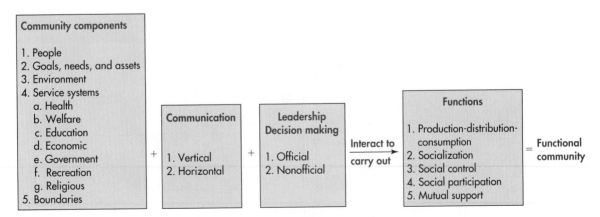

**FIGURE 3-1** Community dynamics. (Service systems data from Sanders IT: *The community: an introduction to a social system,* ed 2, New York, 1966, Ronald Press; communication and function data from Warren RL: *The community in America,* ed. 2, Chicago, 1972, Rand McNally.)

Knowledge of the values, attitudes, and beliefs of the people in the community and knowledge of basic community population characteristics, such as cultural and ethnic backgrounds, age, sex, and income and educational levels, is essential for effective community health planning and action. The community assessment section in Chapter 14 gives parameters to use in gathering data on the people of a community.

## Stop and Think About It

You are a public health nurse working at a local health department. In doing a community assessment, you become aware that the community in which you work has a large proportion of young families and school-age children. What resources and services would help meet the needs of this aggregate? You also have a significant number of senior citizens. What resources and services would commonly assist older people in a community?

Nurses work in partnership with communities to determine community health needs, establish health goals and action plans, and help them become healthier communities. Community health nurses' skills make them a valuable resource in assisting the community to assess, set, and achieve its health goals. The nurse also can serve as an advocate for the community in obtaining the health care resources and services necessary to achieve these goals. Community health goals and needs have been compared to Maslow's hierarchical order of basic needs (Higgs, Gustafson, 1985, p. 12; Meneshian, 1988, p. 116). Figure 3-2 shows a comparison of these needs. The healthy community initiatives discussed in this chapter are ways that nurses can help communities meet their goals and needs.

*Community environment* has physical, biologic, and sociocultural components. These components combine to make each community unique and have a major impact on the overall health of the community.

The *physical environment* of the community includes the geography, climate, terrain, natural resources, and structural entities (buildings such as schools, workplaces, and homes). The *biologic environment* of the community includes various flora, fauna, bacteria, viruses, molds, fungi, toxic substances, and food and water supplies. The *sociocultural environment* of the community reflects culture, values, attitudes, and demographic characteristics of the people of the community.

These environments play a significant role in community health. For example, in many rural communities well water is the only source of fresh water, and if this water is contaminated, health problems can develop. If a city's water supply is contaminated, community health also can be jeopardized. Environmental health concerns for the community health nurse are discussed in Chapter 6.

**Service systems** of a community help people meet basic needs of daily living as well as specific health and welfare needs. Sanders (1966, p. 170) viewed the major service systems of the community as (1) health, (2) social welfare, (3) educational, (4) economic, (5) governmental, (6) recreational, and (7) religious. These community service systems form a network of resources that deliver services to community members. All service systems are crucial and all have a role to play in maintaining and promoting community health. The nurse should assess a community's service systems, identify their resources and services, discover how each fits into the overall structure of the community, and use them to promote health.

Not all service systems have equal importance within the community, and sometimes they become out of balance with one another. An example of an imbalance in service systems is when the welfare system receives a disproportionate amount of the tax dollars and reduces the tax dol-

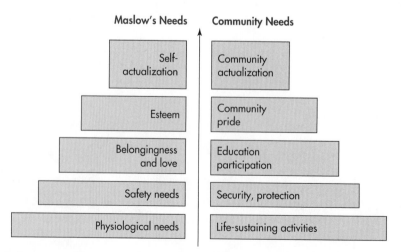

**FIGURE 3-2** A comparison of Maslow's identification of basic needs of the individual with those of the community as a client. (From Higgs ZR, Gustafson DD: *Community as client: assessment and diagnosis,* Philadelphia, 1985, FA Davis.)

lars available to other community systems such as education or health. Once this system equilibrium has been disturbed, it may never be restored, or it may take years to recover.

Also, service systems may have some form of authority over one another. For example, the religious system may influence the health practices of its members. The religious practices of fasting, eating or not eating certain foods, and prohibiting the use of certain health care services, such as general medical care, blood transfusions, and family planning methods, are examples of how religious beliefs make an impact on the health care system. The nurse must be aware of such religious and cultural beliefs and their effect on health (Box 3-2).

Although the health system is a central focus for the community health nurse, it is the economic system (economic sufficiency) that has long been recognized as the usual focus for the citizenry and leadership of the community (National Commission on Community Health Services, 1966, p. 7). Until a community's basic economic

 **BOX 3-2**
## *Clinical Practice: The Nurse, Religious Beliefs, and Health*

A recently graduated public health nurse was working in a city health department. The health department served a large Arab population, and many of these families were on the nurse's caseload. The nurse wanted to provide culturally sensitive care and thought it was important to learn more about the culture and beliefs of these families, most of whom had recently immigrated to the United States. She worked closely with the local university and community resources to learn more about Arab culture. The nurse noticed there were many young, married Arab women with infants in her caseload area. The children were not being immunized and the women refused to bring the children to the immunization clinic at the health department. Having learned about the culture, the nurse realized that these young women were not allowed to go outside their own neighborhoods unless escorted by a male relative, had limited transportation, and were unclear about the need for immunizations. The nurse suggested to her supervisor that an immunization clinic be opened in the neighborhood in which these young families lived. She also talked to local religious leaders about the lack of immunizations among the children and asked for their help with teaching the families about immunizations and making immunization services available. A demonstration clinic was opened near a neighborhood mosque, and information was provided through the health department and religious leaders about the benefits of immunizations. The young mothers started bringing children in for immunizations. The clinic became a regular part of health department services and other such clinic services were offered in other neighborhoods.

needs are met, it is not likely the populace will work diligently on other needs, such as health. The health system is discussed separately later in this chapter.

Service systems are made up of numerous agencies and organizations. If the service system cannot met the needs of the population's members, the community must find the necessary service elsewhere. When this happens a service area develops for the community within which the problem is defined and solved. A community of solution develops, and the service area for the community expands and networks outside its boundaries. An example of this is a rural county whose health service system does not offer open heart surgery and residents have to go to a metropolitan area 100 miles away.

*Community boundaries* serve to regulate the exchange of energies between the community and its external environment. In general, boundaries may be *concrete* or *conceptual/relational*. Concrete boundaries are more absolute and usually easier to see and define. They include geographic boundaries (mountains, valleys, and deserts), political boundaries (cities, towns, counties, states, and nations), situational boundaries (settings such as home, school, and work), and combinations of these such as geopolitical boundaries. In the United States, official public health services are often provided through the geopolitical units of state and local health departments. The service areas of these health departments are usually determined by their geopolitical boundaries (e.g., city or county). It is important that community health nurses working in these health departments remember that even their geopolitical service area may not reflect "the community" for the populace. Geopolitical boundaries may overlap for community members. For example, a person may live in one geopolitical community, work in another, and receive health care in yet another. Geopolitical boundaries fit with the definition of community used in this text.

A community's conceptual/relational boundaries are dynamic and less definite. These boundaries reflect how people group in the community, based on shared interests, age-related development, diagnostic groups, or socially defined roles and norms. Such boundaries often form aggregate groups in the community. Everyone belongs to multiple groups based on conceptual/relational boundaries.

### Community Communication Patterns

Community communication includes both horizontal and vertical patterns (Warren, 1978, pp. 163-164). Vertical patterns of communication link the community to the larger society (state, national, and international). Horizontal patterns of communication link the community to its people, environment, and systems. The strength and ease with which these patterns operate largely determines the extent to which the community is able to be self-sufficient and provide for the needs of its membership. Horizontal patterns of communication greatly influence the internal dynamics of the community. This communication within the community transmits community culture, tradition, values, and attitudes from generation to generation and helps preserve the community. It allows community members to know what is happening in the community and share information with each other.

## Community Leadership

**Community leadership** and decision making critically influence how well that community will function. A community usually has *official* (elected and appointed) leadership such as a mayor or city council, school board, and judges. This leadership is obvious to community members and other communities. However, much of a community's leadership is *nonofficial* (not elected or appointed).

Nonofficial community leadership is less obvious and may be more difficult to detect. However, this leadership often has more influence, power, and control over community action and decision making than the official leadership. The local community religious leader to whom people may go for advice and guidance, and the wealthy philanthropist who heavily subsidizes community health activities, are examples of nonofficial leaders.

Nonofficial leaders are often "heroes" of the community, those whom people in the community revere, trust, and respect. It is frequently these leaders that people turn to for advice and assistance. Nonofficial leaders can aid in the development, implementation, and utilization of community health activities.

The community health nurse will find it useful to identify and work with community leaders to promote health. Community leaders can encourage community residents to become active community workers (Moore, Puntenney, 1999, p. 1). They can assist in making health a community priority. An example of this is a research study by Wiist and Flack (1990) that showed how the support of religious leaders in a community made a large-scale cholesterol education program possible and successful.

Some aspects of community life are controlled by leadership decisions made outside the community. These decisions are commonly in the form of state, federal, and international laws and regulations. The community must adhere to such legal mandates even though they may be in conflict with its values, attitudes, and ideology. Examples include federal laws in relation to public health and state laws regarding child abuse and adult protective services. Health and welfare legislation that influences local communities is discussed throughout this text.

## Community Functions

To provide for the life goals and needs of its population, the community carries out several functions. Warren (1978, pp. 171-212) gives the following **community functions**:

PRODUCTION-DISTRIBUTION-CONSUMPTION.   The community produces, distributes, and uses goods and ser-

vices that are essential for meeting the health and welfare needs of its residents. This triad of activities involves extensive resource and service coordination.

SOCIALIZATION.  Socialization is the process by which prevailing knowledge, values, beliefs, customs, and behavior are transmitted to a community's members. It is a lifelong process that helps persons learn how to effectively relate in a social environment and to develop a philosophy of life.

SOCIAL CONTROL.  The community influences the behavior of its members through norms, regulations, and rules of social control. Social control has a legal component that is often enforced through law agencies, courts, and the government. It also has a social sanction component. Social control helps safeguard and protect the community by providing mechanisms for safety and order.

SOCIAL PARTICIPATION.  People have basic needs for self-expression and self-fulfillment. These needs are largely met through interaction with others. This function provides opportunity for members of the community to communicate, socially interact, and obtain support. It helps community members achieve psychosocial wellness. Social networks evolve though social participation.

MUTUAL SUPPORT.  Mutual support involves people lending assistance to one another. It is frequently offered through family, friends, neighbors, and religious groups as well as official and private health and social service organizations within the community.

These functions provide for the services and activities necessary to carry out everyday community life. The way a community carries out these functions affects how well it is able to meet the needs of the population. If there is a gap in production-distribution-consumption, the community may be unable to support the health resources needed to meet its needs. Or, if people have not been socialized to value preventive health care, the nurse's ability to implement preventive health care services can be hindered. If community health policy is inadequate or not enforced, the health of the community may be in jeopardy. If the members of the community do not value social interaction and participation, the community's response to clinics, classes, and group activities may not be maximized. If a community does not offer sufficient mutual support, there may be few health and welfare assistance programs for community members in need of them, and it may be difficult to engage the community in partnership activities.

## The Functional Community

The figure on community dynamics (see Figure 3-1) illustrated how components of the community interact to create a healthy, **functional community.** Functional communities can identify, prioritize, and address community assets and needs and are capable of problem solving and crisis resolution. Functional communities work in partnership with health care professionals to increase and maintain community competence.

According to Warren (1988, pp. 413-418), a functional community has the following characteristics: (1) people interact, participate, and have a degree of commitment to the community; (2) the community has some autonomy from the larger society; (3) people can confront their problems through concerted action (viability); (4) decision making is relatively equally distributed throughout the population and not concentrated (power distribution); (5) there is a balance of differences (degree of heterogeneity); and (6) the degree of conflict is manageable. Communities can become dysfunctional as a result of community stressors.

COMMUNITY STRESSORS. Community stressors are tension-producing stimuli that have the potential to cause disequilibrium and disruption in the community (Anderson, McFarlane, 1996, p. 172). They can arise from inside or outside the community and include natural and man-made disasters, social unrest, and economic crises. Stressors occur when service systems are unable to provide the necessary services for effective community functioning (e.g., the inability of a community to maintain a tax base sufficient to adequately operate the local health department). The reaction to these stressors may be reflected in community health statistics such as morbidity and mortality rates, crime statistics, and unemployment (Anderson, McFarlane, 1996). When community stressors arise, a functional community mobilizes resources to resolve them.

## AGGREGATES IN THE COMMUNITY

A community is made up of numerous aggregates, and community members belong to multiple aggregate groups. Aggregates are groups of persons who have one or more shared personal or environmental characteristics. "The care of communities requires valuing the aggregate good" (Flick, Reese, Harris, 1996, p. 36). Increasingly, community health activities are being provided to aggregates in clinics, classes, screening and health promotion activities. It is generally more cost-effective to provide aggregate-based services. "One certainty for nursing...is that nurses of the 21st century will be called upon to deliver aggregate-based care" (Doerr, Sheil, Baisch, et al., 1998, p. 214).

Historically, community health nurses have provided services to aggregates, based on developmental and at-risk characteristics. Community health nurses need to be able to identify aggregates of the population whose health is at highest risk and provide appropriate nursing interventions (ANA Quad Council, 1999). Students and nurses need to think in terms of assessing aggregates and providing services to them. By improving the health of aggregates, the health of individuals, families, and the community is improved (Feenstra, 2000, p. 156).

The *developmental approach* to aggregate-based services reflects developmental theory. Erikson's (1978) developmental stages of the life cycle (infancy, early childhood, play age, school age, adolescence, young adulthood, adult-hood, and senescence) have been used widely in nursing to guide both individual- and aggregate-based approaches to service delivery. Developmental theory postulates that individuals develop in their own way, yet conform to a common developmental pattern. It emphasizes that failure to accomplish developmental tasks at the appropriate time makes subsequent development more difficult. Using anticipatory guidance, health teaching, and health promotion activities, the nurse can facilitate achievement of developmental tasks and educate families and communities about developmental needs. Using the developmental approach, this text assists the reader in looking at nursing roles and services to aggregates such as preschool children, school-age children, adults, and the elderly.

Aggregates also can be looked at from an *at-risk approach.* Examples of aggregates at risk addressed in this text are adults who are disabled, children with developmental disabilities, persons with long-term care needs, persons with AIDS, teenage parents, homeless individuals and families, victims of domestic violence, individuals and families living in poverty, disadvantaged groups, and ethnic and racial minority groups. From an at-risk perspective, health care professionals can look at morbidity and mortality across the lifespan and implement primary prevention activities to reduce the incidence of these conditions.

Community health nurses work in partnership with communities to identify aggregate-based health promotion activities and interventions. It is envisioned that aggregate based services will expand in the future. Assessing and planning services for aggregates in the community are discussed in Chapters 14 and 15. Health education techniques that can be used with aggregates are discussed in Chapter 12, and working with groups in the community is discussed in Chapter 23.

## THE HEALTH SYSTEM AND THE COMMUNITY

As mentioned previously in this chapter, the health system is a community service system. The priority that the community places on health and the resources it has to promote health, will play a major role in the overall health of the community. There is growing emphasis on promoting health in communities, assisting communities to identify and solve their own health problems, and mobilizing community resources for health (McKnight, VanDover, 1994, p. 13). Initiatives to build healthy communities are discussed later in this chapter.

In the United States, health care is becoming increasingly complicated, costly, and diverse. Health resources in the community are found in both governmental and private sectors (see Chapter 5). The governmental (official) sector includes state and local health departments, Veteran's Administration hospitals, state mental health facilities, State Departments of Human or Social Services, and the Social

Security Administration. Private-sector provision of health care services includes resources such as hospitals, outpatient clinics, private practitioner's offices, community health volunteers, nursing homes, assisted-living facilities, pharmacies, laboratories, support groups (e.g., Alcoholics Anonymous, Associations for Retarded Citizens), and service agencies (e.g., American Red Cross, American Heart Association, American Lung Association, Arthritis Foundation, and the American Diabetes Association). Both sectors have various health care providers, including nurses, nurse practitioners, physicians, dentists, nutritionists, psychologists, social workers, environmental health workers, unlicensed health care personnel, and volunteers. Local health departments are an excellent source of information on community health resources and services.

A community has a level of health reached over time that is called its **normal line of defense** (Anderson, McFarlane, 1996, p. 169). This line of defense can include characteristics such as high immunity levels and low infant mortality and is contrasted with the community's **flexible line of defense**, which represents a state of health that is more dynamic or in flux owing to temporary stressors such as environmental disasters and epidemics (Anderson, McFarlane, 1996, p. 169). These lines of defense are considered in partnership with communities when engaging in health planning, implementation, and evaluation.

## Difficulties in the Community Health System

When analyzing the health care system in the United States, several issues are apparent. A major concern is that of access to health care services. Many Americans do not have access to appropriate health care services for reasons such as cost, transportation, and lack of an appropriate resource. Millions of Americans are uninsured or underinsured for health. You may be one of those underinsured Americans.

### Stop and Think About It

Many Americans with health insurance are underinsured. They have insurance policies that do not cover long-term care, physical examinations, preventive health services, dental care, outpatient physical therapy, prescriptions, and optical or durable medical products, and/or they have "caps" on the amount of money that can be spent for a specific medical occurrence. How will you help your clients in the clinical setting obtain the health care services they need but cannot afford? What resources are available in your community to provide services to those individuals?

Funding for public health in the community has historically been low and has continued to decrease in recent years. Local health departments usually receive a large part of their funding from local tax dollars and have historically been underfunded. Many community residents are not aware of the services offered by their local health department and do not realize how important this agency is to maintaining community health.

Communication between the health care system and the other community systems has historically been weak. In many communities official local health departments have little contact with private health care resources and community welfare resources. The health system of the community may have little communication with the people of the community, and partnerships for community health may not exist. However, as the health care system partners with community residents and other community resources, communication becomes strengthened.

No one agency has statutory (legal) responsibility for managing the health resources in the community, and responsibilities for who manages what resource are often vague and unclear even to health care professionals. The overall management of the health system is not coordinated, and the management skills of individual health providers may be weak. Health care professionals must understand the principles of management if the health care system is to carry out its functions effectively, work in partnership with communities, and promote community health. Unfortunately, health practitioners frequently do not have educational preparation in managing health care resources.

American communities have historically reacted better to disaster and catastrophic health events than to providing ongoing, preventive community health services. There is often indifference to a health problem if no obvious, serious, long-term, or personal effects are apparent. Traditionally, health insurance coverage pays for treatment of illness, but less often for preventive services. Healthy community initiatives can assist communities in taking responsibility for their own health and working to remove barriers to health action.

## HEALTHY COMMUNITIES

In Chapter 1 we discussed how nurses at the Henry Street Settlement, Frontier Nursing Service, visiting nurses, and public health nurses worked closely with communities to make them a healthier places to live. Historically, local health departments diligently worked with communities to promote health. Major public health achievements occurred in response to communities working in partnership with health professionals. A classic report by the National Commission on Community Health Services (1966) issued the following goals for achieving healthy communities:

Communities must take the actions necessary to provide comprehensive health services to all people in the community. These services should embrace health education and health promotion, application of established preventive measures, early detection and treatment of disease, prompt and rehabilitation activities and efforts to ameliorate environmental and social causes of diseases and conditions. This broad range of health services must be provided in a way to assure full and informed use by all members of the community (p. 132).

Today, many communities continue to work toward these goals.

The Healthy People Initiative in the United States (see Chapter 4) envisioned establishing healthy communities through the commitment of individuals, agencies, and organizations at the community level (U.S. Department of Health and Human Services [USDHHS], 1995a, p. 143). Healthy People 2000 established an objective for communities to take part in community health promotion programs and developed a set of public health indicators to assist communities in assessing their general health status and progress in achieving community health. The document supported states in formulating and promoting statewide disease prevention and health promotion objectives that could be the blueprint for local initiatives and encouraged involvement from both the public and private sectors in healthy communities programs (USDHHS, 1995a, pp. 143-145). Having healthy communities has become a national and international goal and public health nursing initiatives focus on improving the health of communities.

## HEALTHY COMMUNITY INITIATIVES

The idea for the contemporary healthy communities movement had its origins in the mid-1980s and was inspired by Drs. Len Duhl and Trevor Hancock (Norris, Pittman, 2000). It initially was endorsed by the Canadian Public Health Association. The World Health Organization (WHO) actively promotes such initiatives as part of its overall move toward the "health care for all" policy (Kenzer, 2000). Healthy community initiatives focus on the use of diverse community coalitions to assess their health priorities, develop effective community health promotion actions, and promote community health (Sasenick, 1994, p. 56). They use the previously discussed concept of "community as partner" to build on community assets and facilitate community empowerment for health action, making health a community priority.

Organized community effort to promote health and prevent disease is both valuable and effective (Institute of Medicine, 1988, p. 17). Such efforts encourage shared community-wide responsibility for health, involve local people, focus on hard-to-reach populations, and promote healthy public policies (Flynn, 1995, p. 6; Flynn, Rains, 1993, p. 24). They encourage communities to improve their physical and social environments and strengthen community resources (Flynn, 1996, p. 300; Hancock, Duhl, 1988). Helping communities develop initiatives that address social and health problems and consider the complex factors that contribute to wellness is an essential part of building healthy communities (Norris, Lampe, 1994, p. 2).

Healthy Community Initiatives put health on the agenda of local governments and create new structures and processes for achieving health (International Council of Nurses, 1991, p. 109). They challenge local communities to engage in collaborative problem solving to improve the quality of life, reduce disparities in health access and status, rethink approaches to health care delivery, and address factors that contribute to good health (National Civic League, 1995, p. 1; Norris, 1993, p. 6). Such initiatives facilitate community empowerment processes for health action, focus on the community, involve citizen participation and problem solving, and strive to improve the quality of life (Flynn, Ray, Rider, 1994, p. 395). There are several websites for information on healthy communities (e.g., *http://www.healthy.communities.org*).

Communities across the nation are involved in such initiatives, which are often coordinated through local health departments. These initiatives respond to the unique health needs of each community and focus on primary prevention. Chapter 15 discusses such initiatives in relation to health planning. Communities are becoming increasingly sophisticated in their efforts to address preventive health needs (Eisen, 1994, p. 236). Nationwide such initiatives are focusing on environmental health, community safety, immunizations, tobacco, teenage pregnancy, recreation for youth, and school-based services (Flynn, 1996, p. 301). A study of local health departments showed that the most frequently used models for healthy community activities were Model Standards (47%), Assessment Protocol for Excellence in Public Health (APEX/PH) (32%), Planned Approach to Community Health (PATCH) (12%), and Healthy Cities (6%) (Durch, Bailey, Stoto, 1997, p. 85). A brief discussion of these initiatives and selected others follows.

### Healthy Communities 2000: Model Standards

*Healthy Communities 2000: Model Standards* is a publication of the APHA (1991). It was developed in conjunction with the Centers for Disease Control and Prevention (CDC), the Association of State and Territorial Health Officials (ASTHO), the National Association of County and City Health Officials (NACCHO), and the Association of Schools of Public Health. The guidelines presented in the document assist communities in establishing achievable community health objectives in line with the national health objectives of the Healthy People Initiative (see Chapter 4). It provides detailed guidance and practical tools for constructing process and outcome objectives and implementation plans that address the community's public health problems (Scutchfield, Keck, 1997, pp. 149, 155). It has a readily usable "fill in the blank" format that assists communities in readily developing public health objectives. *Model Standards* provides a focus for health action efforts and is used in conjunction with a healthy communities process such as APEX/PH, PATCH, and Healthy Cities in developing healthy community initiatives (Scutchfield, Keck, 1997, p. 150). APHA also publishes the *Guide to Implementing Model Standards: Eleven Steps Toward a Healthy Community*. These steps are in Box 3-3 and are elaborated on throughout the text. For more information, contact the American Public Health Association, 800 I Street, Washington, D.C.,

### BOX 3-3

## *Model Standards: Eleven Steps Toward A Healthy Community*

1. Assess and determine the role of one's health agency.
2. Assess the lead agency's organizational capacity.
3. Develop an agency plan to build the necessary organizational capacity.
4. Assess the community's organizational and power structures.
5. Organize the community to build a stronger constituency for public health and establish a partnership for public health.
6. Assess health needs and available community resources.
7. Determine local priorities.
8. Select outcome and process objectives that are compatible with local priorities and national health objectives.
9. Develop community-wide intervention strategies.
10. Develop and implement a plan of action.
11. Monitor and evaluate the effort on a continuing basis.

American Public Health Association (APHA): *Guide to implementing model standards*, Washington, DC, 1993, APHA, pp 8-9.

20001-3710, (202) 777-APHA, or visit the association's website at *http://www.apha.org.*

## Assessment Protocol for Excellence in Public Health

The Assessment Protocol for Excellence in Public Health (APEX/PH) was jointly developed by NACCHO and the CDC to assist local health departments in meeting the needs of their communities through assessment, planning, and intervention strategies. It is a step-by-step process for local health departments to assess their capacity to build stronger partnerships with their community. It encompasses a three-part cycle: (1) organizational capacity assessment (a self-assessment process for local health departments), (2) the community process (a community health assessment process), and (3) completing the cycle (a discussion of how to monitor and evaluate the plans developed in parts 1 and 2) (NACCHO, 2000). It involves strong leadership from the local health department and involvement of community representatives and utilizes *APHA Model Standards.* For further information, contact NACCHO at 1100 17th Street, Second Floor, Washington, D.C. 20036, (202) 783-5550, or visit the organization's website at *http://www.naccho.org.*

## Planned Approach to Community Health

The CDC also sponsors the Planned Approach to Community Health (PATCH). PATCH is a community health planning model that has been operating since 1986. It was designed to strengthen state and local health department's

capacities to plan, implement, and evaluate community-based health promotion activities (Kreuter, 1992, p. 135).

PATCH assists a community to establish a health promotion team, collect and use local data, set health priorities, and design and evaluate interventions (National Center for Chronic Disease Prevention and Health Promotion [NCCDPHP], 1995, CG1-1). The goal of PATCH is to increase a community's capacity to plan, implement, and evaluate comprehensive, community-based health promotion and disease prevention programs targeted toward achieving the year 2010 national health objectives. The program expands community participation in setting health priorities and designing and implementing outcome-oriented intervention programs (Scutchfield, Keck, 1997, p. 149).

Five essential elements of PATCH are (1) community members actively participate in the process, (2) data guide the development of the programs, (3) participants develop a comprehensive health promotion strategy, (4) evaluation emphasizes feedback and program improvement, and (5) the community capacity for health promotion is increased. NCCDPHP (1995) states:

Community members analyze the factors that contribute to an identified health problem. They review community policies, services and resources and design an overall community health promotion strategy. Interventions, which may include educational programs, mass media campaigns, policy advocacy, and environmental measures, are conducted in various settings, such as schools, health care facilities, community sites, and the workplace. Participants are encouraged to relate intervention goals to the appropriate national health objective (p. CG1-3). CDC provides training and consultation to state and local health departments on the application of PATCH. Most state health departments play a major leadership role in the program and have a state coordinator for PATCH (p. CG1-2).

CDC helps network agencies that are using PATCH programs, which often target rural and underserved communities (Green, Kreuter, 1992, p. 140). The five phases of PATCH are given in Box 3-4. For more information, contact the National Center for Chronic Disease Prevention and Health Promotion, Centers for Disease Control and Prevention, Mailstop K-46, 4770 Buford Highway, N.E., Atlanta, GA 30341 or visit the NCCDPHP/CDC website at *http://www.cdc.gov.*

## Healthy Cities

Healthy Cities is a Healthy Communities Initiative in the United States. It began in Canada in 1984 and in 1986 the WHO European Healthy Cities Project was started. WHO continues to provide extensive technical and consulting support to Healthy Cities initiatives throughout the world. In the United States the WHO Collaborating Center on Healthy Cities is directed by a nurse, Dr. Beverly C. Flynn. This center conducts research and provides materials, consultation, leadership training, and technical support to communities interested in Healthy Cities (Flynn, 1996, p. 301). Dr. Flynn founded the Healthy Cities initiative in the

**BOX 3-4**

*The PATCH Process*

---

*Phase I: Mobilizing the Community*

Mobilizing the community is an ongoing process that starts in Phase I and continues throughout the process. In Phase I the community to be addressed is defined, participants are recruited from the community, partnerships are formed, and a demographic profile of the community is completed. The community group and steering committee are organized, and working groups are created. During this phase, the community is informed about PATCH so that support is gained, particularly from community leaders.

*Phase II: Collecting and Organizing Data*

Phase II begins when the community members form working groups to obtain and analyze data on mortality, morbidity, community opinion, and behaviors. These data, obtained from various sources, include quantitative data (e.g., vital statistics and survey) and qualitative data (e.g., opinions of community leaders). PATCH participants identify ways to share the results of data analysis with the community.

*Phase III: Choosing Health Priorities*

During this phase, behavioral and any additional data collected are presented to the community group. This group analyzes the behavioral, social, economic, political, and environmental factors that affect the behaviors that put people at risk for disease, death, disability, and injury. Health priorities are identified. Community objectives related to the health priorities are set and the health priorities to be addressed initially are selected.

*Phase IV: Developing a Comprehensive Intervention Plan*

Using information generated during Phases II and III, the community group chooses, designs, and conducts interventions during Phase IV. To prevent duplication and to build on existing services, the community group identifies and assesses resources, policies, environmental measures, and programs already focused on the risk behavior and to the target group. This group devises a comprehensive health promotion strategy, sets intervention objectives, and develops an intervention plan. This intervention plan includes strategies, a timetable, and a work plan for completing such tasks as recruiting and training volunteers, publicizing and conducting activities, evaluating the activities, and informing the community about results. Throughout Phase IV, members of the target groups are involved in the process of planning interventions.

*Phase V: Evaluating PATCH*

Evaluation is an integral part of the PATCH process. It is ongoing and serves two purposes: (1) to monitor and assess progress during the five phases of PATCH and (2) to evaluate interventions. The community sets criteria for determining success and identifies data to be collected. Feedback is provided to the community to encourage future participation and to planners for use in program improvement.

---

Source: U.S. Department of Health and Human Services (USDHHS): *Planned approach to community health: guide for the local coordinator*, Atlanta, 1995b, US Department of Health and Human Services, Centers for Disease Control and Prevention and National Center for Chronic Disease Prevention and Health Promotion, pp. CG1-4–CG1-5.

United States and directs the Institute of Action Research for Community Health at Indiana University School of Nursing. We can be proud that in the United States community health nurses have played an important role in the development of Healthy Cities. Healthy Cities began in the United States with two statewide initiatives, Healthy Cities Indiana and Healthy Cities California. Worldwide there are now more than 1000 such initiatives (Nakajima, 1996). Dr. Flynn (1996) states:

These Healthy Cities projects were built on the concepts of primary health care and health promotion, which included challenging communities to develop projects that reduce inequalities in health status and access to services, and to develop healthy public policies at the local level through a multisectoral approach and increased community participation in health decision making. The role of local government is central to the Healthy Cities concept....The Healthy Cities concept involves focusing on the whole community, with its strengths and problems, rather than being established under the rubric of categorical problems..." (p. 300).

Healthy Cities fosters collaborative working relationships with sectors of community life such as schools, universities, local health departments, local government, hospitals, arts and culture, business and industry, education, environmental groups, media, and religion (Flynn, 1994, p. 55). This approach energizes individuals to enact positive change and develop healthier communities through analysis, consensus, social action, and health policies (Flynn, 1993, p. 15). For additional information on Healthy Cities contact CITYNET Healthy Cities, Institute of Action Research for Community Health, Indiana University School of Nursing, 1111 Middle Drive, NU 236, Indianapolis, IN 46202-5107.

## Other Community Building Initiatives

In addition to the initiatives already mentioned other organized and grassroots initiatives exist. Selected initiatives are presented.

The National Healthy Communities Initiative was developed in 1989 by the National Civic League (NCL) in cooperation with the U.S. Public Health Service. It promotes a collaborative community-based approach to health promotion (NCL, 1995). The Colorado Healthy Communities Initiative was organized through the NCL. The NCL publishes the *Healthy Communities Handbook* and *A Guide to a Community-Oriented Approach to Core Public Health Functions* and sponsors the Healthy Community Program. For additional information, contact the National Civic League, 1445 Market, Suite 300, Denver, CO 80202-1717.

United Way also sponsors a community building initiative. It consists of training through courses on principles and practices of community building and publications such as *Community Input Through Neighborhood Partnerships*. It publishes COMPASS, a tool kit for community assessment that emphasizes community partnerships and offers community building awards. United Way is committed to improving the health of the nation's communities and incorporating healthy community concepts through collaborative community problem solving and provision of services. For additional information, contact United Way of America, 701 North Fairfax Street, Arlington, VA 22314-2045.

Community and Institutional Assessment Process (CIAP) was developed by the Public Health Resource Group. CIAP focuses on facilitating service development, based on the needs of individual communities. Planners utilize the epidemiologic process to develop a community profile that allows communities to generate rates of health-related behaviors/conditions and make comparisons with other communities. M-Power is a new tool developed by the group to deliver local health data for every zip code in the United States. For information, contact Public Health Resource Group, 120 Exchange Street, Portland, ME 04101.

Another initiative is through the Asset-Based Community Development Institute. It has developed numerous materials for local communities and neighborhoods to use their assets to promote community building. The institute publishes the guide *Building Communities from the Inside Out* (Kretzmann, McKnight, 1993), as well as workbooks on creating neighborhood information exchange, city-sponsored community building, strategies for achieving newspaper coverage of local community happenings, mobilizing the community skills of local residents, mapping and mobilizing association in local neighborhoods, and helping city officials build neighborhood capacity. For information, contact Asset-Based Community Development Institute at the Institute for Policy Research at Northwestern University, 2040 Sheridan Road, Evanston, IL 60208-4100.

The American Hospital Association Research and Education Trust's (AHARET) Healthcare Forum has initiated a Healthier Communities Fellows Program and presents annual Healthier Communities Awards. AHARET's Institute for Healthcare Improvement has initiated a community-wide health improvement learning collaborative (Flynn, 1996, pp. 301-302). All of the initiatives discussed demonstrate that health is not just the responsibility of individuals or health professionals but also is a mandate of the community as a whole (Flynn, 1993, p. 80).

Communities with such partnerships develop significantly more programs and policies than those communities without partnerships; partnerships produce community-wide results (Flynn, 1998, pp. 165-166). These initiatives are expanding and making an impact on public health across the United States and throughout the world. One important component of a community is neighborhoods. Many healthy community initiatives are using neighborhoods to promote health. To illustrate the significant influence of neighborhoods on the health of the community, a discussion of neighborhoods and health follows.

## NEIGHBORHOODS AND HEALTH

Nurses have long recognized the importance of neighborhoods in promoting health. Lillian Wald and the nurses of the Henry Street Settlement lived and worked in neighborhoods in New York City. Mary Breckinridge and the nurses of the Frontier Nursing Service lived and worked in rural neighborhoods in Kentucky. Her autobiography, *Wide Neighborhoods* (Breckinridge, 1952), addressed the work of the service in helping improve the health of rural neighborhoods.

**Neighborhoods** are small units in the community, and people often identify more closely with their neighborhood than with the community as a whole. Neighborhoods represent people with common ties, needs, concerns, and even history. There is often a high level of cohesiveness, cooperativeness, and comradery in neighborhoods. The smaller scale of neighborhood health initiatives often makes them more conducive to health action and reduces barriers to utilization of services such as transportation and promotes coordination among agencies and leadership. Neighborhood-based initiatives empower participants with a sense of ownership and involvement and offer a mechanism for directly targeting resources to at-risk populations.

Neighborhood health initiatives provide a level of social comfort that is conducive to health action (Eisen, 1994, p. 238). Many neighborhood health initiatives offer services such as child care, interpreters, and use of neighborhood community health volunteers. These volunteers are recruited from the community where the program is located, are trained to promote health, and are usually well received by the community (Sherer, 1994, p. 52). Such initiatives build on community strengths and assets to promote health. They give local residents and community leaders the chance to work together to make their neighborhood and community a better place to live.

Neighborhood health initiatives are increasingly being used to promote community health (Torres, 1998, p. 211). Environmental projects such as neighborhood beautification and clean-up programs have been a great sense of neighborhood pride. Neighborhood health initiatives such as immunization campaigns and neighborhood clinics have brought health care directly to the people. Savannah, Georgia, has a great success record with neighborhood initiatives, and for more than 25 years has successfully worked with neighborhoods to build stronger communities (Moore, Puntenney, 1999, p. 1). More and more neighborhoods are being looked to for community health planning and interventions. There are many types of neighborhoods. Some types are more likely than others to facilitate community-building efforts.

## Classifications of Neighborhoods

Warren (1977, pp. 224-229) classified neighborhoods to identify the differences between them. Descriptions of these classifications are given in Box 3-5 and are still meaningful today. Neighborhoods vary greatly in leadership, cohesiveness, and self-sufficiency. These variances have an impact on the health resources and services available.

Identifying the type of neighborhood in which nurses work can assist them to function in partnership with the community to meet health needs. For example, if a community health nurse is working in a parochial neighborhood, it would be important to work closely with neighborhood leaders in the delivery of health care services. The nurse may find that the parochial neighborhood readily becomes involved in providing services for its residents. However, there also may be more resistance in this type of neighborhood to health services proposed by the larger community, especially if these services do not coincide with neighborhood values and beliefs. On the other hand, in an anomic neighborhood the community health nurse may find little neighborhood leadership and may need to assist in developing this leadership to facilitate health action. In addition, the nurse may find that the anomic neighborhood offers few services to its residents and that services need to be sought from outside the neighborhood. Whatever the

**BOX 3-5**

*Classifications of Neighborhoods*

### Integral

The individuals in this setting have frequent face-to-face contacts. The norms, values, and attitudes of the neighborhood support those of the larger community. People are cohesive within the neighborhood but belong to other groups outside their area of residence. There is a form of power, authority, and leadership within this type of neighborhood, which aids its members to reach out to the larger society for assistance when a problem arises that cannot be handled internally.

### Parochial

People in this setting also have face-to-face contacts, but there is an absence of ties to the larger community. These neighborhoods tend to be protective of their status, to screen out values that do not conform to their own, and to enforce their own beliefs within the neighborhood. The power, authority, and leadership structure within this type of neighborhood encourages isolation from the larger community.

### Diffuse

Neighbors within this type of environment interact infrequently with each other and have few ties with the larger community. There is often a lack of shared norms, values, and attitudes. A primary tie between these neighbors is geographic proximity to one another. There may be little or no leadership in these areas. When leadership exists, it is often not representative of the entire neighborhood but is composed of an "elitist" leadership that ignores or subverts the values of most residents. Groups of residents, such as those living in a public housing unit, may be categorized and separated from the mainstream of the neighborhood.

### Stepping-stone

This type of neighborhood is characterized by a rapid membership turnover and families who have a weak sense of identity with the neighborhood. Members are willing to give up the ties established in the neighborhood if other commitments arise. They strive to attain a higher social status. Residents of these areas do, however, have close ties to the larger community and do interact regularly with neighbors. Leadership is usually not effective because of the high rate of mobility. Conflicts arise between the needs of the local neighborhood and the values of social mobility.

### Transitory

Members of this kind of neighborhood fail to participate in or identify with the local community. There is an emphasis on people keeping to themselves because links with others may interfere with the goals of the individual and the family. There may be a widespread feeling of mistrust in this type of neighborhood.

### Anomic

Such a neighborhood is completely disorganized. Its residents lack participation in and a common identification with the neighborhood or the larger community. This neighborhood reflects mass apathy and is not likely to influence or alter the values of its residents through any form of socialization. There is little interaction between people within the neighborhood or between the neighborhood and the larger community, and leadership activity is largely lacking.

Warren DI: Neighborhoods in urban areas. In Warren RL, editor: *New perspectives on the American community*, ed 3, Chicago, 1977, Rand McNally, pp. 224-237.

### BOX 3-6

## *Mantua: A Neighborhood-Based Nursing Model*

Mantua is a neighborhood in West Philadelphia with a population of approximately 10,000. The majority of Mantua residents (94%) are African Americans, 65% live in single-parent households, and more than 50% are in families at or below the poverty level. The infant mortality rate is among the highest in Philadelphia—28 per 1000 live births. Only 38% of Mantua residents have finished high school, and only 5% have completed college. Despite the presence of a renowned medical facility only blocks away and several other fine hospitals nearby, significant numbers of residents do not obtain health care. Of the children screened in West Philadelphia, 60% had elevated lead levels (it was estimated that only 10% had been screened), only 30% of 2-year-olds in Mantua were fully immunized, almost 25% of Mantua births were to adolescents, 32.7% of the women in Mantua delayed prenatal care or had none at all, 21% of the women had low-birth-weight infants, and rates of gonorrhea and syphilis were many times the national average. Based on these maternal-child health indicators, nurses and the community decided to develop a neighborhood-based health initiative in Mantua. The project's overall mission was to create a health care site that would minimize barriers to access, increase utilization of health services, and improve the health status of the community.

In the Mantua project, members of the community were the driving force in determining the appropriateness of services, and a "Neighborhood Advisory Council" was established. Services at the site included well-child care, focusing on immunizations and lead screenings; services for adolescents, focusing on sexually transmitted diseases screening and treatment; family planning; and walk-in pregnancy testing for women of all ages, with referrals to early prenatal care. Referral mechanisms and linkages between community agencies were developed, and community health improved.

The project is a success story for community health partnerships and neighborhood health initiatives. It received a U.S. Department of Health and Human Services "Secretary's Award for Innovations in Health Promotion and Disease Prevention." It is a model for others who are considering implementing neighborhood health initiatives.

Whelan E-M: The Health Corner: a community-based nursing model to maximize access to primary care, *Public Health Rep* 110(2):184-188, 1995.

### TABLE 3-1

## *States with More Than 40% of Their Population Residing in Rural Areas*

| STATE | PERCENTAGE OF POPULATION RESIDING IN RURAL AREAS |
|---|---|
| Vermont | 67.9% |
| West Virginia | 63.9% |
| Maine | 55.3% |
| Mississippi | 52.9% |
| South Dakota | 50.0% |
| North Carolina | 49.7% |
| New Hampshire | 49.0% |
| Kentucky | 48.2% |
| Montana | 47.4% |
| North Dakota | 46.7% |
| Arkansas | 46.5% |
| South Carolina | 45.3% |
| Idaho | 42.5% |

Sources: Ricketts TC, Johnson-Webb KD, Taylor PL: *Definitions of rural: a handbook for health policy makers and researchers*, Washington, DC, 1998, Federal Office of Rural Health Policy, p. 134; Census Bureau: *Urban and rural populations 1900-1990*. Retrieved from the internet July 6, 2000. *http://www.census.gov/*

Although neighborhoods in urban communities are frequently written about in the health literature, it is increasingly recognized that rural communities also have significant health issues. Rural health initiatives are being developed across the nation to address these issues and improve rural health.

### *Stop and Think About It*

Warren's classifications of neighborhoods are considered classic and have been used extensively. Are these classifications representative of the neighborhoods in which you have lived and worked? How would you classify the neighborhood you are currently residing in, and how might you mobilize residents in the neighborhood for health activities?

## RURAL COMMUNITIES

In the early 1800s approximately 90% of the U.S. population lived in **rural communities.** In 1900 that changed to about 60%, and today it is about 20% (Ricketts, Johnson-Webb, Randolph, 1999, p. 15). The population in rural communities continues to decline (Bushy, 1998, p. 66). The South has the highest proportion of its population living in rural areas and the Northeast the smallest. Interestingly, 77% of our nation's counties, 83% of the nation's land, and nearly 15,000 American towns are considered rural (Ricketts, Johnson-Webb, Randolph, 1999; Rural Information Center [RIC], 2000) (Figure 3-3). States in which 40% or more of the population is considered rural are listed in Table 3-1. Community

type of neighborhood, its structure has implications for the activities of the community health nurse. An enlightening example of a neighborhood health initiative is the neighborhood-based nursing model that addresses the specific health needs of the Mantua neighborhood in West Philadelphia (Box 3-6).

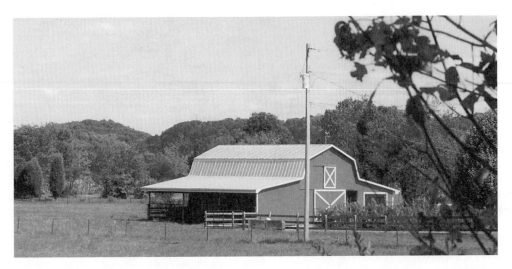

**FIGURE 3-3** Some 62 million Americans live in rural communities. Residents in rural settings are regularly exposed to environmental hazards such as pesticides, water and soil pollution, and toxic chemicals. Many rural Americans lack access to regular and emergency health care services. The shortage of health care in rural communities presents serious problems for many rural Americans, and public health efforts need to be strengthened in these communities. (Courtesy Ed Richardson.)

health nurses historically have provided services to rural communities.

## What Is a Rural Community?

A recent review of the *Journal of Rural Health* showed researchers used 26 different definitions of *rural* (Johnson-Webb, Leonard, Gesler, 1997, p. 254). Historically, communities have been defined as rural based on population. In the United States definitions of rural frequently used are those from the Census Bureau and the Office of Management and Budget (Box 3-7). In addition, the Administration on Aging and the Department of Agriculture have developed classifications of rural. This lack of consensus on a definition has consistently posed problems in rural resource provision and policy development.

All rural communities are not alike, just as all urban communities are not alike. A rural logging community in upper Michigan is different from a rural tourist community in South Carolina; a rural community of low-income minority or Native Americans is different from a rural community of affluent retirees. "Standard definitions of urban/rural...gloss over the richness of the multiple dimensions of rural life" (Weinert, Burman, 1999, p. 75). Weinert and Burman (1999) liken rural communities to a sampler quilt:

A sampler quilt contains a variety of colors, fabrics, and stitches. Each square is unique, yet when stitched together, the squares form a unified whole. The sampler quilt, through the images of bright prints, muted solid colors, and various textures and shapes, provides a metaphor of rural communities (p. 75).

Rural communities are often described in terms of their major economic activity or focus, which frequently includes farming, ranching, mining, logging, and fishing.

 **BOX 3-7**

## *Definitions of Rural*

There are many definitions of rural. In the United States the two principal definitions of rural used by the federal government in determining health care resources and policy are from the Census Bureau and the Office of Management and Budget (OMB).

The Census Bureau uses the terms rural and urban. Its definition of rural is based on a combination of factors, including population density, relationship to cities, and population size. The Census Bureau defines rural as territory, populations, and housing units having fewer than 2500 inhabitants. This population threshold of 2500 has been in use since 1910. The term "frontier" has been used to describe select rural communities with a population density of less than 6 people per square mile, as compared with between 6 to 99 per square mile for a rural community. Within rural communities, frontier communities have their own unique set of health needs and concerns.

The OMB uses the terms *nonmetropolitan* and *metropolitan* to classify counties on the basis of population and integration with large cities. Nonmetropolitan counties do not meet minimum population requirements, do not have a central city, and/or do not relate closely to larger urban places. Nonmetropolitan counties are outside the boundaries of metropolitan areas and have no cities with 50,000 or more residents. OMB classifies 2522 of 3139 American counties as nonmetropolitan.

Sources: Ricketts TC, Johnson-Webb KD, Taylor PL: *Definitions of rural: a handbook for health policy makers and researchers*, Washington, DC, 1998, Federal Office of Rural Health Policy, p. 134; Rural Information Center: Rural health services funding: a resource guide, Retrieved from the internet July 5, 2000. *http://www.nalusda.gov/ric/richs/*

More recently, rural communities have emerged primarily for retirees or for people wishing to escape urban life.

## Sociocultural Characteristics of Rural Communities

Researchers have consistently supported the existence of a unique rural culture (Bushy, 1991a; Bushy, 1991b; Bushy, 1991c). Rural communities differ from urban ones in several sociocultural characteristics. Many rural residents have lower incomes, poorer health, and less formal education than their urban counterparts. Rural communities have fewer minority residents and higher percentages of elderly.

Values prevalent in rural Americans are achievement, activity and work, traditional values and role orientation, group conformity, conservative political viewpoints, and a more religious nature (ANA, 1996b; Lee, 1991, p. 15). Rural residents are generally slower than urban dwellers to change values and attitudes (Bushy, 1991b, p.134). They are more likely to be familiar with local government and leadership. Rural residents may resist assistance from an outsider whom they may perceive as a stranger and prefer to interact with people they know and who are similar to themselves (Bushy, 1997, p. 28).

Rural communities are often closely knit and people tend to know one another. In contrast, urban communities are often known for the isolation that is evident when people living next to each other do not even know one another's names. In close-knit rural communities, friends, neighbors, church, and family traditionally assist those in need (Bushy, 1997, pp. 32-33).

Rural communities have higher rates of households of children living with both parents and have fewer households headed by women (Office of Technology Assessment [OTA], 1990, p. 40). Rural adults are more likely to have been married and more likely to be widowed than urban adults.

There is a higher incidence of poverty in rural populations. Nearly 5 million rural children live in poverty (Vulnerable populations, 1991, p. 128). The average rural family has a median income close to $10,000 less a year than the average urban family (Ricketts, Johnson-Webb, Randolph 1999, p.15). Forty percent of all rural families have incomes below the poverty level (Bushy, 1998, p. 66). Of the nation's 206 persistent poverty areas, almost all are located in rural areas (ANA, 1996b, p. 11).

Fewer minority Americans reside in rural areas than in urban areas. Exceptions to this minority status include communities with migrant farm workers and Native Americans. In general, rural minorities are poorer than the rest of the rural population and are at higher risk for health problems.

Rural America is "aging" faster than America in general. Although the elderly account for 12% of the U.S. population, they account for more than 15 % of the rural population (Ricketts, Johnson-Webb-Randolph, 1999, p. 13). Rural elderly have higher rates of poverty and report signif-

icantly poorer health than do their urban counterparts (Eggebeen, Lichter, 1993, p. 94). This elder population brings with it increased needs for health care resources and services. Rural communities have unique health care needs.

## Health and the Rural Community

Nurses can be proud that they have played a major role in providing primary health care to rural families and communities (Bushy, 1990, p. 34). Mary Breckinridge, a nurse and midwife, founded the Frontier Nursing Service in rural Kentucky, and it is still operating today. Lillian Wald was one of the first to advocate for rural health services. In 1915 Wald wrote:

In 1908 I began to urge that in a country dedicated to peace it would be fitting for the American Red Cross to consecrate its efforts to the upbuilding of life and the prevention of disaster . . . The concrete recommendation made was that the Red Cross should develop a system of visiting nursing in the vast, neglected country areas. This suggestion has been adopted and an excellent beginning made with a Department of Town and Country Nursing directed by a special Committee (p. 61).

The American Red Cross Rural Nursing Service was formally established in 1912, and the name was changed to Town and Country Nursing Service the following year (see Chapter 1). Wald's vision was that rural nursing services would become available across the nation. Although this vision was not actualized, the organized provision of rural nursing in the United States had been initiated. Today an awareness of populations at risk and the characteristics of rural communities assist the community health nurse in developing community partnerships for health and providing effective nursing services. The following discussion examines selected rural health statistics and needs.

PERCEIVED HEALTH STATUS AND PRACTICES. Research has shown that rural residents generally define health as the ability to work and to do what needs to be done (Long, 1993; Long, Weinert, 1989; Weinert, Burman, 1994; Weinert, Long, 1987). Such health beliefs are a determinant of health perception and health-seeking behaviors (Bushy, 1991b, p. 135). Rural residents consistently rate their physical health as poorer and are somewhat less happy than urban residents (Eggebeen, Lichter, 1993; Weinert, Burman, 1999, p. 77). However, they rate their social health as stronger (Weinert, Burman, 1994, p. 68).

Rural dwellers are more independent and self-reliant and resist accepting help or services, especially from those seen as "outsiders" or from agencies seen as national or regional "welfare" programs (Long, Weinert, 1989, p. 121). Rural residents often prefer an old and trusted health care resource rather than a newer "outsider" service. They will often prefer the "Old Doc," whom they know, to the new specialist, who is unfamiliar. They tend to wait longer to seek medical care or not seek it at all (Bushy, 1997, p. 28). When they finally obtain care, they tend to be sicker and may require more intensive services (Bushy, 1997, p. 28).

Research findings have indicated rural residents prefer to use informal resources (e.g., family, neighbors, friends) for help and support in dealing with health problems rather than formal resources (e.g., hospitals or clinics) (Long, Weinert, 1989, p. 121). Formal health care providers are often not trusted and are viewed as outsiders. Even when they live at a great distance, family, neighbors, and friends are frequently relied on to assist with health problems (Weinert, Long, 1993, p. 53; Weinert, Burman, 1994, p. 76). Rural residents respond favorably to the use of advanced practice nurses (APNs) for health care and a nurse run clinic may be the only clinic available in a rural area.

Rural residents are less likely to use seatbelts regularly (resulting in higher motor vehicle fatality rates); less likely to exercise regularly; more likely to be obese; and less likely to use preventive screening services such as Papanicolaou (PAP) smears, self-breast examination, and blood pressure checks (OTA, 1990, p. 43). Pregnant rural women tend to seek care later in pregnancy and make fewer prenatal visits (Weinert, Burman, 1999, p. 77). High death rates from motor vehicle accidents are attributed to high speed driving, hazardous road conditions, lack of use of seat belts, type and condition of vehicle, and limited access to emergency care (Weinert, Burman, 1999, p. 78).

There is a dramatic shortage of mental health professionals in rural areas, and rural residents are more likely than their urban counterparts to use their primary health care provider for mental health (Ricketts, 1999a, p. 159). Limited finances and work and distance constraints often mean that mental health therapy is only available as short-term treatment (Weinert, Long, 1990, p. 70). For rural residents needing long-term treatment for mental illness, the lack of specialty services in their community may mean that they have to move to where services are available (Hartley, Bird, Dempsey, 1999, p. 159).

HEALTH DISPARITIES. Rural residents have higher rates of chronic illness and higher incidence of diabetes, cancer, hypertension, heart disease, and lung disease (Summer, 1991; Weinert, Burman, 1999, p. 77). They have higher rates of disability, injury-related mortality, and maternal and infant mortality than their urban counterparts (Goeppinger, 1993, p. 1; OTA, 1990, pp. 5-6; Weinert, Burman, 1994, p. 72; Weinert, Burman, 1999, p. 77; Weinert, Long, 1993, p. 47). The rural setting predisposes residents to exposure to pesticides and other toxic agents, farm equipment injury, farm and motor vehicle accidents, and firearm injury (McGinnis, Foege, 1993; Weinert, Burman, 1999, p. 77). Rural communities have a higher rate of many communicable diseases than the general population (e.g., intestinal parasite diseases, tuberculosis, influenza, and pneumonia) but a lower rate of AIDS (Weinert, Burman, 1994, p. 72). However, AIDS cases are increasing in rural areas (Brooks, 1998, p. 1).

Maternal, infant, and child mortality rates are all higher in rural than urban areas (ANA, 1996b). Contributing to these rates is the limited availability of obstetric services, lack of use of prenatal care by rural residents, and lack of medical insurance. Little research has been done on the health of rural children and adolescents. Rural children are less likely to have a usual provider of ambulatory health care (ANA, 1996b, p. 10). School nurses can play an important role in the provision of health care services to rural children.

Agriculture is one of the few occupations in which children actively participate. Each year almost 100,000 children suffer a preventable injury associated with agricultural work (National Committee for Childhood Agricultural Injury Prevention, 1996, p. 5). It is estimated that each year more than 2 million farm children are at risk of accidental injury or trauma (Lee, Jenkins, Westaby, 1997, p. 207). Hundreds of children die each year in farm accidents (FORHP, 1993). Agricultural fatality rates are much higher in boys than girls, especially boys aged 15-19. As many as 29% of farm fatality victims are children younger than 16 (Lee, Jenkins, Westaby, 1997, p. 207; Purschwitz, 1990). Farm machinery and tractor rollovers account for one half of all the deaths of children living or working on farms (Weinert, Burman, 1999, p. 77). Other injuries and deaths are due to farm machinery, tools, livestock, and falls. Children in rural areas also are exposed to pesticides and other chemicals, noise, vibration, zoonoses, and stress.

Historically, farming is one of the most hazardous occupations in the United States and agricultural workers have some of the nation's highest rates of occupational illness, injury, disability, and death. Many farmers reported cutting back on safety measures to save money (Geller, Ludtke, Stratton, 1990; Weinert, Burman, 1999, p. 78). Hearing loss is common from the loud noise created by farm equipment and the infrequent use of hearing protection. The incidence of back problems is significantly higher in rural populations (Weinert, Burman, 1994, p. 72).

Public health problems such as smoking, smokeless tobacco, alcohol use, homelessness, mental illness, motor vehicle accidents, and family violence occur in rural communities. However, rural communities often have fewer resources available to work with such conditions, and the more traditional value systems of the community can affect service provision to these aggregates at risk.

The dynamics related to domestic violence are often intensified in rural communities because of traditional values and attitudes, isolation, lack of resources, and lack of privacy in seeking care (Goeckermann, Hamberger, Barber, 1994; Weinert, Burman, 1999, p. 78). Rural families are often hesitant to deal with mental health and substance abuse issues outside of a close network of family and friends and may hesitate to use such services in the community, especially if the practitioner involved is considered an outsider (Wagenfeld, Murray, Mohatt, et al., 1994).

Recent research has indicated that the prevalence of alcohol and other substance abuse among adults does not vary appreciably between rural and urban areas (Hartley, Bird, Dempsey, 1999, p. 160). However, research reflects that young adults in rural areas generally had lower rates of use of marijuana, stimulants, and cocaine than urban dwellers but had higher rates of smoking and smokeless tobacco use (Hartley, Bird, Dempsey, 1999). Rural counties have a considerably elevated rate of driving under the influence of alcohol (DUI) arrests when compared to urban areas, and al-

cohol use is a significant factor in rural motor vehicle accidents (Hartley, Bird, Dempsey, 1999, p. 161).

Suicide rates are a proxy measure for mental health problems and the rate of suicides among rural children and adolescents is higher than the urban rate (Hartley, Bird, Dempsey, 1999, pp. 161, 163). Rural elders have less access to services that support their independence such as homemaker and chore services, meal preparation, mobile meals, and home health (Hassinger, Hicks, Godino, 1993, p. 70). Boxes 3-8 and 3-9 give some interesting facts and figures on health in rural communities and resources for information on rural health.

BARRIERS TO HEALTH CARE. Access to services is a major problem for rural Americans. Poor roads, rough terrain, lack of transportation, lack of health insurance, lack of primary care resources, and work demands all contribute to this situation (Strategies, 1996, p. 101). Most rural counties in the United States do not have an adequate public transportation system. Rural residents travel almost twice the distance of urban residents to obtain health care services (Edelman, Menz, 1996, p. 200). Geography also can play a part in that in many rural area residents have mountains, rivers, and other geographic barriers between them and health care resources. Lack of access to appropriate health care has a negative effect on health status (Ramsbottom-Lucier, Emmett, Rich, et al., 1996, p. 386).

### BOX 3-8

### *Some Facts and Figures on Rural Communities*

1. Twenty percent of the U.S. population, approximately 62 million Americans, live in rural areas—a number larger than the population of the United Kingdom (58 million).
2. Thirteen states have 40% or more of their population residing in rural areas.
3. The South has the highest proportion of its population living in rural areas (29.1%) and the Northeast the least (11.8%).
4. Seventy-seven percent of U.S. counties are considered rural.
5. Ninety-eight percent of rural residents are native born Americans.
6. The average income of a rural American household is approximately $10,000 less than the average income of an urban American household.
7. One in five rural Americans lives in poverty (of these, nearly 5 million are children).
8. Forty percent of rural families have incomes below the poverty level.
9. Fewer minority Americans reside in rural areas, and minority residents have lower incomes than the rural population in general.
10. Rural America is aging faster than America in general.
11. Fewer rural residents (14.8%) have college educations than urban residents (25%).
12. In relation to health insurance coverage, more rural residents are uninsured than urban residents.
13. Although 25% of the nation's population lives in rural areas, only 9% of the nation's physicians practice there.
14. Almost 8 million rural Americans have no health insurance, and another 4.5 million are underinsured.
15. Millions of rural Americans live in federally designated "Health Professions Shortage Areas."
16. Many rural communities do not have a hospital.

Data from USDHHS: *Prevention resource guide: rural communities*, Rockville, Md, 1991, USDHHS; Ricketts TC, Johnson-Webb KD, Randolph RK: Populations and places in rural America. In Ricketts TC, editor: *Rural health in the United States*, New York, 1999, Oxford University Press, pp. 7-24; Bushy A: Rural nursing in the U.S.: where do we stand as we enter a new millennium? *Aust J Rural Health*, 6:65-71, 1998; Federal Office of Rural Health Policy: *On creating a composite statistical picture of rural America*, Washington, DC, 1993, US Government Printing Office.

### BOX 3-9

### *Rural Health Information Resources*

National Rural Health Association
One West Armour Boulevard, Suite 203
Kansas City, MO 64111
(816) 756-3140
*http://www.nrharural.org*

Rural Information Center (RIC)
U.S. Department of Agriculture
National Agricultural Library, Room 304
10301 Baltimore Boulevard
Beltsville, MD 20705-2351
(800) 633-7701
*http://www.nalusda.gov/ric/richs/*

Federal Office of Rural Health Policy (FORHP)
U.S. Department of Health and Human Services
5600 Fishers Lane, Room 9A-55
Rockville, MD 20857
(301) 443-0835
*http://www.ruralhealth.hrsa.gov/*

Rural Policy Research Institute
University of Missouri
200 Mumford Hall
Columbia, MO 65211-6200
(573) 882-0316
*http://www.rupri.org*

The rural characteristics of self-reliance, stoicism, and independence can contribute to lower utilization of available health care resources and prevent timely entry into the health care system (ANA, 1996b, p. 9; Bushy, 1991b, p. 137). Attitudes and beliefs that conditions are normal or natural, such as pregnancy, may prevent rural women from seeking prenatal care (ANA, 1996, p. 9). Rural families cite the fear of receiving insensitive treatment and fear that others may find out about the family's use of services as deterrents to using health services (Bushy, 1991b, pp. 136-137).

Economic barriers prevent many rural residents from receiving adequate health care. Almost 8 million rural Americans have no health insurance (FORHP, 1993). More than 50% of the nation's underinsured live in rural areas (Bosch, Bushy, 1997, p. 21). Many rural families cannot afford preventive care, and such care is usually not covered under health insurance. Many rural residents are uninsured or underinsured for health care. Hazardous or seasonal occupations in farming, ranching, mining, logging, and recreational operations such as ski resorts are often excluded entirely from health insurance coverage and Medicaid coverage has traditionally excluded more rural populations (ANA, 1996b, p. 9; Frenzen, 1993). Economic conditions such as low-income and lack of health insurance pose serious barriers to rural utilization of health care services. The high cost of health care often prohibits families from seeking it.

HEALTH CARE RESOURCES. The last few decades have witnessed rural economic decline and serious concerns about the viability of the rural health care system. A major problem in relation to rural health care resources is that of the closing of rural hospitals. Between 1980 and 1998 the number of rural hospitals declined almost 12% (Ricketts, Heaphy, 1999, p. 104), and many rural areas have no hospital at all.

Remaining rural hospitals must adapt and discover innovative ways to meet the challenges of the changing health care market. Innovative programs such as the Rural Hospital Flexibility Program have helped ease some of the financial problems of rural hospitals (Ricketts, 1999a, p. 168), and some alternative models for rural hospitals have been proposed (Avery, 1999, p. 171). The goal of such models is "to develop a hospital design that is feasible in isolated areas, with small populations and low utilization so that acute services can be maintained" (Avery, 1999, p. 171). California's Rural General Acute Care Hospital program and Montana's Medical Assistance Facility are state models that have tried to address the need of maintaining hospital services in rural areas (Avery, 1999).

When rural hospitals close, the loss of the surgical and emergency room services can be devastating on the community. In addition, without a hospital, it is often difficult for communities to recruit and retain physicians (Reiff, DesHarnais, Bernard, 1999, p. 207). Vulnerable populations such as the poor, medically fragile, children, and the elderly suffer more from rural hospital closures and have a

more difficult time accessing needed health care services (Reiff, DesHarnais, Bernard, 1999, pp. 208-209).

Rural America has a disproportionately higher proportion of Medicare beneficiaries, and rural hospitals rely heavily on Medicare reimbursement. Medicare pays for almost 50% of all rural hospital admissions (Ricketts, Heaphy, 1999, p. 102). Recent reductions in Medicare funding have great impact on rural hospitals (National Rural Health Association [NRHA], 2000). Because of funding mechanisms that take into consideration local wages and the average proportion of highly trained or educated employees, Medicare reimbursement to rural hospitals is lower than urban hospitals (NRHA, 2000). Many rural hospitals close because of a shortage of registered nurses. Rural hospitals have successfully utilized the services of APNs to maintain and expand acute and primary care services (Bergeron, Neuman, Kinsey, 1999).

Rural areas rely heavily on satellite clinics, often offered through hospitals or health departments, to provide primary health care to residents. Community and migrant health centers (see Chapter 21) are bringing primary care services to numerous underserved populations. Mobile clinics are delivering care to remote areas with significant success. Meals on Wheels programs are providing nutritious meals to homebound elders and others in the community. With scarce resources, some rural communities are networking with each other to provide health care services and health education programs (Hemman, McClendon, Lightfoot, 1995, p. 170).

Rural areas often have fewer health resources such as pharmacies, laboratory services, mental health, and physical and occupational therapy services. Twenty percent of rural counties have no mental health services, and 80% of rural hospitals offer no emergency psychiatric services (Hartley, Bird, Dempsey, 1999, p. 166, 171).

Emergency medical service (EMS) for rural areas is becoming an increasing problem. It is difficult to deliver EMS to widely dispersed populations quickly, efficiently, and cost effectively. There are often shortages of EMS personnel in rural areas. Rural ambulance services find they cannot support themselves financially.

Local health departments continue to provide a mainstay of public health services to rural areas. "Public/community health nurses play a critical role in rural health by providing traditional public health services, direct primary care services, and home care services" (ANA, 1996b, p. 19-20). Public health services commonly found in rural health departments include public health nursing, immunization clinics, maternal-child health services, school nursing, environmental and occupational health, communicable disease clinics, primary care clinics, Supplemental Food Program for Women Infants and Children (WIC), health education, community partnership initiatives, and mental health/substance abuse counseling.

States rely heavily on the federal government for assistance in maintaining and expanding rural health resources

(OTA, 1990, p. 9). Recent federal initiatives have facilitated rural health, rural nursing, and rural nursing research. The Agency for Health Care Policy and Research (AHCPR) has initiated a rural health research agenda, and AHCPR and the National Institute for Nursing Research

## BOX 3-10

### *Federal Programs to Enhance Rural Health*

*National Health Service Corps* provides placement services, scholarships, and educational loan repayment for physicians and other health professionals willing to serve in designated rural areas. It also provides grants to schools educating and training primary health care providers such as family practitioners and nurse practitioners.

*Area Health Education Centers (AHEC)* programs coordinate and support the training of health professionals with a focus on rural health. AHEC programs link medical centers and schools for health professionals with rural practice sites to provide students, faculty, and practitioners with rural clinical experience.

*Rural Outreach and Networks Grants Program* is administered by the Federal Office of Rural Health Policy and provides grants to nonprofit, public, or private health care facilities in rural areas to facilitate the provision of services to underserved rural populations; enhance the capacity or expand the service areas to increase access to rural health services; promote integration and coordination of services in or among rural communities; and enhance linkages, integration, and cooperation among the various entities eligible to receive grants.

*Rural Health Clinics* programs provide exceptions to normal reimbursement mechanisms for clinics and primary care delivery units to make use of advanced practice nurses and physician assistants in areas designated as underserved. The program was created to increase the number of primary care practitioners in rural, underserved communities by allowing for payment under Medicare and Medicaid for the services of these professionals. Today more than 35000 clinics are certified to provide service.

*Consolidated Rural Health Programs* are composed of four initiatives: Community Health Centers, Migrant Health Centers, the Health Care for the Homeless Program, and the Health Care for Residents of Public Housing Program. These programs are administered by the Bureau of Primary Health Care and guarantee the delivery of basic health care services, including prenatal care, immunizations, physical exams, and other preventive health care to families who lack access to health care, migrant and seasonal farm workers and their families, and children and adults who are homeless or are at risk for homelessness. There are over 630 centers operating at more than 1600 sites.

Source: Ricketts TC, Heaphy PE: Hospitals in rural America. In Ricketts TC, editor: *Rural health in the United States*, New York, 1999, Oxford University Press, pp. 101-112; Ricketts TC: Federal programs and rural health. In Ricketts TC, editor: *Rural health in the United States*, New York, 1999c, Oxford University Press, pp. 61-69; Ricketts TC: Rural communities and rural hospitals, *J Rural Health* 15:168-169, 1999a.

have jointly invited applications for research grants to study ways of improving the health and well-being of rural populations. Selected federal programs to enhance rural health resources are noted in Box 3-10.

HEALTH CARE PROVIDERS. Getting health care providers to practice in rural settings has been difficult. As mentioned previously, there are fewer health care providers in rural areas than urban. Almost one third of rural Americans live in federally designated "Health Professions Shortage Areas (HPSA)," or areas that have a primary care provider-to-patient ratio of 1 to 3500 or worse (FORHP, 1993). Only one tenth of urban Americans live in such areas (ANA, 1996b, p. 12).

Medical training in the United States has historically taken place in cities and only 70 of the nation's approximately 850 teaching hospitals are located in rural areas (Ricketts, 1999b, p. 7). Approximately 10% of the nation's physicians practice in rural areas (FORHP, 1997, p. 2; Rosenblatt, Hart, 1999, p. 38), and many rural doctors are expected to retire or leave their practices in the near future. More than 50% of rural physicians generally are in primary care specialties (FORHP, 1997, p. 1). Specialists are not available in many medical areas, and rural residents travel great distances to see them.

Additionally, shortages in public health professionals, psychologists, physical and occupational therapists, speech therapists, rehabilitation specialists, social workers, and other health care providers are drastically affecting the quality of health care available to rural communities. Recent research has looked at the problem of closure of rural pharmacies (Straub, Straub, 1999). There are estimated shortages of at least 45,000 registered nurses, 1200 psychiatrists, and nearly 1000 dentists in rural areas (FORHP, 1993). An adequate supply of primary health care profes-

## BOX 3-11

### *Nursing in Rural Communities: Selected Literature*

American Nurses Association: *Rural/Frontier nursing: the challenge to grow*, Washington, DC, 1996, ANA.

Bushy A: *Rural nursing*, vols 1 and 2, Newbury Park, Calif, 1991, Sage.

Long KA, Weinert C: Rural nursing: developing the theory base, *Scholar Inq Nurs Pract* 3(2):113-127, 1989.

Weinert C, Burman ME: Rural health and health-seeking behaviors. In Fitzpatrick JJ, Stevenson JS, editors: *Annual review of nursing research*, vol 12, New York, 1994, Springer, pp. 65-92.

Weinert C, Burman ME: Nursing of rural elders: myth and reality, *Adv Gerontol Nurs* 1:57-80, 1996.

Weinert C, Burman ME: The sampler quilt: a metaphor of rural communities. In Hinshaw, AS, Feetham S, Shaver JLF, editors: *Handbook of clinical nursing research*, Newbury Park, Calif, 1999, Sage, pp. 75-86.

sionals would resolve many of the problems of access to health care in rural areas. APNs are an excellent source of primary health care in rural communities.

## Nursing and the Rural Community

Nurses are highly respected in rural communities (ANA, 1996b, p. 15; Dunkin, Juhl, Stratton et al., 1992; Fuszard, Slocum, Wiggers, 1990). Rural residents show a high level of acceptance of nursing services and frequently utilize the services of APNs. Unfortunately, most rural areas have a shortage of nurses, and the number of registered nurses living in rural areas has declined (ANA, 1996b, p. 12). Until recently, little has been written to guide rural nursing practice, and students received little education on rural nursing. Bushy's (1991a) two-volume book, *Rural Nursing*, and some other selected readings on rural nursing are highlighted in Box 3-11. Rural nursing research and theory has been slow to develop. Weinert and Long (1987, 1990, 1991) laid a foundation for a theoretic framework for rural nursing (Box 3-12), but further research is necessary (Box 3-13). Nursing leaders in this field such as Mary Burman, Angeline

Bushy, Kathleen Long, and Clarann Weinert are helping the professional maintain a focus on rural health.

Rural nurses have high community visibility and close community ties and relationships and play a significant role in shaping health policy, developing programs, and initiating change in the community (ANA, 1996b, p. 16). Because of their visibility in the community, they are often sought out as caregivers outside of their jobs, as part of living in a rural community (Barger, 1996, p. 3).

Nurses practicing in rural areas often assume a generalist role, need to be a "jack of all trades," and have greater role diffusion (ANA 1996b, pp. 15-16; Barger, 1996; Long, Weinert, 1989, p. 123). Nurses in rural areas have the opportunity to assume a generalist role and to become involved with clients across the life span. Rural hospital nurses may find themselves working in the emergency department, labor and delivery, and a general medical floor all in the same day or week (Barger, 1996).

As a health care provider in a rural area, nurses often experience greater autonomy in practice. However, they tend to lack personal anonymity (ANA 1996b, pp. 15-16; Bushy, 1998, pp. 67-68), and rural communities may not be appropriate practice settings for nurses who prefer to maintain entirely separate professional and personal lives (Long, Weinert, 1989, p. 124).

---

### BOX 3-12
*Rural Health Nursing Theory:*
*Weinert and Long*

**Key Rural Concepts Identified**
Work and health beliefs
Isolation and distance
Independence and self-reliance
Lack of anonymity
Outsider/insider
Oldtimer/newcomers

**Initial Relational Statements**
Rural dwellers define health primarily as the ability to work, to be productive, and to do usual tasks.
Rural dwellers are self-reliant and resist accepting help from those viewed as outsiders. Help, including health care, is usually sought through an informal rather than a formal system.
Health care providers in rural areas must deal with a lack of anonymity and much greater role diffusion than providers in urban or suburban settings.

From Bushy A: Meeting the challenges of rural nursing research. In Bushy A, editor: *Rural nursing*, vol 2, Newbury Park, Calif, 1991b, Sage, pp. 304-318; Long KA, Weinert C: Rural nursing: developing the theory base, *Scholar Inq Nurs Pract* 3(2):113-127, 1989; Weinert C, Long KA: Understanding the health care needs of rural families, *Family Relations* 36:450-455, 1987; Weinert C, Long KA: Rural families and health care: refining the knowledge base, *J Marriage Fam Rev* 15(1): 57-75, 1990; Weinert C, Long KA: The theory and research base for rural nursing practice. In Bushy A, editor: *Rural nursing*, vol 1, Newbury Park, Calif, 1991, Sage; Weinert C, Burman ME: Rural health and health-seeking behaviors. In Fitzpatrick JJ, Stevenson JS, editors: *Annual review of nursing research*, vol 12, New York, 1994, Springer, p. 82.

---

### BOX 3-13
*Some Future Directions for*
*Rural Nursing Research*

1. Advancing the development and testing of rural nursing theory
2. Careful operationalization and measurement of rurality
3. Implementing studies to explore rural and urban differences
4. Developing a standard definition of rural while avoiding generalizations about rural dwellers
5. Evaluating, adapting, and developing measures that are valid, reliable, and sensitive to rural issues
6. Exploring innovative methods to capture the picture of rural life and rural health needs
7. Utilizing interdisciplinary research initiatives that focus on rural health delivery systems
8. Evaluating the clinical outcomes of rural nursing practice
9. Replication, multisite, and collaborative studies
10. Exploring what nursing education can do to prepare nurses to meet the needs of rural dwellers

Sources: Weinert C, Burman ME: Rural health and health-seeking behaviors. In Fitzpatrick JJ, Stevenson JS, editors: *Annual review of nursing research*, vol 12, New York, 1994, Springer, pp. 65-92; American Nurses Association: *Rural/frontier nursing: the challenge to grow*. Washington, DC, 1996, ANA; Weinert C, Burman ME: The sampler quilt: a metaphor of rural communities. In Hinshaw AS, Feetham SL, Shaver JLF, editors: *Handbook of clinical nursing research*, Newbury Park, Calif, 1999, Sage, p. 83.

Long and Weinert (1989) have noted that nurses who enter rural communities must allow for extended periods before being accepted and that involvement in diverse community activities such as civic organizations and recreational clubs may assist this endeavor. In rural communities acceptance as a health care professional is often tied to personal acceptance. According to Weinert and Long (1993), "The establishment of trust, based on consistency, longevity of relationship, and sincere effort to understand and appreciate the specific rural culture is an essential first step in implementing interventions with rural families" (p. 53). Rural nurses need to establish collaborative relationships with community leaders to promote health.

As care managers, nurses in rural areas face a unique challenge. The sparse population density, excessive distances to resources, scarce resources, and attitudes toward health care complicate this nursing role (Bushy, 1997, p. 27). Nurses need to be able to blend the formal health care system with the informal one that client's may prefer to use. The rural nurse must be skilled in accessing diverse information, networking clients with resources, and utilizing the referral process (see Chapter 10). The nurse needs to know how to obtain assistance from the informal support network of family, friends, neighbors, and church and civic organizations (Bushy, 1997, p. 32).

Challenges for the rural nurse are numerous, but not insurmountable. Rural nurses often see themselves as isolated from the professional mainstream and distanced from collegial support (ANA, 1996b; Davis, Droes, 1993, p. 160; Long, Weinert, 1989, p. 124). The nurse's social and professional roles tend to blur. Inadvertent breaches of confidentiality are a concern, as is the considerable demand to "be all things to all people" (ANA, 1996b, p. 16). The ANA (1996b, p. 16) has cited the following additional challenges: an inadequate supply of primary health care providers, lack of preparation for rural practice, few opportunities for advancement, reduced access to advanced and continuing education, and longer work hours.

In spite of the tremendous challenges and practice demands, rural nurses have exhibited less professional burn out and fatigue (ANA, 1996b, p. 16). Personal benefits of rural nursing practice include the beauty of rural areas, lower crime rates, close-knit relationships with the community, and professional autonomy (ANA, 1996b, p. 15). More nurses are needed to practice in rural areas, and the ANA has recommended increased use of APNs in rural communities.

APNS IN THE RURAL COMMUNITY. According to the ANA (1996b), APNs are more likely than the general registered nurse to practice in rural areas and their role in promoting rural health is becoming increasingly important. The National Advisory Committee on Rural Health (1989) recommended the use of APNs to meet primary health care needs in rural communities, and this recommendation has been repeated by other federal agencies (ANA, 1996b;

FORHP, 1990; National Advisory Committee on Rural Health, 1990; National Advisory Council of the National Health Service Corps, 1991).

A large number of U.S. counties without a physician are served by APNs, and certified nurse anesthetists are the sole providers of anesthesia services in the majority of rural hospitals (ANA, 1996b, p. 13). APNs have the potential to provide a large portion of the primary care needed in rural communities, and the use of APNs in rural communities needs to be expanded.

The ANA (1996b) has cited the need for APN training to be more accessible to nurses in rural communities and has issued a challenge to nursing education to help meet this need. In the future it is envisioned that more advanced practice distance learning opportunities will be made available to registered nurses in rural areas to pursue advanced practice education. Incentives for nurses to work in rural areas are educational loan repayment programs for health professionals practicing in rural areas and the direct reimbursement for advanced practice nursing services through programs such as Medicaid and Medicare.

## Future Directions for Rural Health

New and innovative ways need to be developed to bring health care to rural Americans and improve their access to health care. APNs have played a unique role in provision of rural health services, and this role is envisioned to expand. However, more health care professionals in all fields are needed to practice in rural communities.

As managed care moves more into rural areas, nurses will need to be assimilated into managed care systems. The generalist skills that have been useful in rural hospitals will be indispensable in managed care systems (Barger, 1996). Teaching skills, high level health assessment skills, and quality management will become important skills for the rural nurse of the future and development of prevention education programs will become an even more important nursing function (Barger, 1996, pp. 3-4). Rural communities have great need for preventive services such as health education and immunization services as well as screening clinics and mechanisms for early diagnosis and treatment of disease (Pickard, 1996).

A priority for nurse researchers is the development of rural nursing theory and a knowledge base relevant to the health care needs of rural populations (ANA, 1996b). Some have proposed that rural nursing become a specialty area within community health nursing. Innovative service delivery is being encouraged through federal grants to rural communities and has resulted in highly successful outreach programs. Nurses are bringing services to the home, schools, worksites, and other community-based settings in rural communities around the world (Randall, 1995).

Technology will play a major role in the provision of rural health services in the future. Computer-based technology will allow the nurse to link with other resources from the clients home, network with community agencies, input and retrieve data and explore health care databases. Such technology will help promote collaborative research and provide a means of nursing education in rural areas.

Nurses will take a much more visible and influential role in leading community partnership initiatives and developing community-based strategies for promoting rural health. Rural nurses need to be at the forefront of health care reform, and the impact it can have on facilitating rural health. They will help rural communities network and build coalitions to promote rural health.

## THE INTERNATIONAL COMMUNITY

International health is everyone's concern. As an outcome, international health is often viewed in terms of worldwide morbidity and mortality statistics. As a process, people, organizations, technology, and resources work together to promote international health. Morbidity and mortality are important indicators of world health and differ greatly among nations. Some diseases are endemic in one country and epidemic in another. Health statistics of **international communities** are presented throughout the book.

Worldwide the incidence of tuberculosis, AIDS, malaria, and waterborne diseases is increasing, and developing nations have much different health problems than developed nations. Examining international health statistics provides information about health status and trends in the world and the United States and assists in developing strategies to promote world health.

It is a small world after all, and we must preserve the environment and protect the world from threats to health. In terms of impact, diseases and conditions such as pollution and water shortages in one country can readily affect other countries. For example, ozone depletion and the polluting of the air and seas contribute to the destruction of the global environment (see Chapter 6). The impact of disease transmission, as exemplified with the worldwide AIDS epidemic, has helped people understand that one nation cannot afford to look at health conditions as other people's problems—they are our problems too.

Numerous agencies discussed in this text have an international health role. Examples include the CDC, the World Health Organization, the United Nations Children's Fund (UNICEF), and APHA, which are discussed in Chapter 5, and the American Red Cross, which is discussed in Chapter 6. The APHA publication, *Control of Communicable Diseases Manual* (Chin, 2000), now in its seventeenth edition, is the classic text on the world's communicable diseases and should be part of every community health nurse's library.

### Nursing and International Health

Lillian Wald and the Henry Street Settlement nurses worked with U.S. immigrants in New York City to promote health. Lillian Wald and her contemporaries, Lavinia Dock and Annie Goodrich, were instrumental in forming the In-

ternational Council of Nurses. They realized the importance of looking at culture in relation to health practices and beliefs and strove to provide culturally sensitive care.

Today, nurses are involved in numerous international health activities. Nursing organizations such as the International Council of Nurses (ICN), the Transcultural Nursing Society, Sigma Theta Tau, the ANA, and the National League for Nursing (NLN) all recognize the importance of international health. In its position statement on cultural diversity in nursing practice, the ANA (1996a) states, "Ethnocentric approaches to nursing practice are ineffective in meeting health and nursing needs of diverse cultural groups of clients. Knowledge about cultures and their impact on interactions with health care is essential for nurses in a clinical setting, education, research or administration" (p. 89).

Nurses need to be concerned about world health and involved in international health activities. The experience of one international nurse is given in *A View from the Field*. This nurse's story illustrates the contributions nurses can make worldwide. Nurses must understand and value diversity and promote world health. Nurses need to provide culturally sensitive care, and cultural aspects of nursing are integrated throughout this text. In today's world people are all inextricably linked.

## COMMUNITY ASSESSMENT

From the days of Lillian Wald, nurses have been assessing the health needs of the community. The community health nurse is in the unique position of working with the community on a day-to-day basis. Community health nurses provide services in community agencies, homes, schools, clinics and industry, and have multiple opportunities to comprehensively assess the community. Community assessment is identified as a critical public health skill (ANA, 1986; ANA Quad Council, 1999; Gerberich, Stearns, Dowd, 1995; Ruth, Eliason, Schultz, 1992).

**Community assessment** models include the collection of data, prioritization of problems and assets, intervention strategies, and ongoing evaluation (Stanley, Stein, 1998, p. 225). Chapter 14 addresses the community assessment process, and community assessment is briefly addressed here in relation to assisting the nurse in conceptualizing both the community as client and as partner.

The Committee for the Study of the Future of Public Health (Institute of Medicine, 1988, p. 7) recommended that every public health agency regularly and systematically collect, assemble, analyze, and make available information on the health of the community. In community health partnerships, assessment data are gathered as a collaborative effort. A community assessment provides a "window" through which to view the community. It provides the means for looking at community assets, problems, and potential problems. It can identify aggregates at risk

*A view from the field*

*Barbara Young*

With less than two years' experience of field public health nursing in the inner cities of Columbus and Dayton, Ohio, I was assigned the position of head nurse for a federal health post in the southern part of the state of Bahia in Brazil. The town where I would spend over two years, Ibicarai, had a population of 20,000 inhabitants, mostly poor. There was also a small upper class comprised of professionals and merchants. The middle class was almost nonexistent. The lower class were those who worked on the cacao plantations or did menial and domestic work. The major ethnic makeup of Ibicarai was a blend of the descendants of the original Tupi-Guandani Indian, Portuguese, and African. Lebanese and Syrians made up a small minority.

My home was of white stucco-type construction. Mud was packed between a lattice of upright sticks. White coating was painted over the dried mud. The floors were packed clay. My water source was a well in the back yard. The wood shack outhouse was "out back" and consisted of a raised platform with a hole in it. *Time* magazine was my favorite toilet paper because it was softer than the local variety. Cooking was done on my built-in charcoal stove. Refrigerators only existed at the local "vendas" where you could buy cold beer. Refrigerators were the status symbol. I had no such status. I learned that fresh meats should be purchased early in the morning and added to the daily black bean pot if you had fresh meat at all.

The federal public health post to which I was assigned stood in the center of town. Each weekday, the people would walk into town from the five surrounding *barrios* (neighborhoods), and I would assist with triage at the front door of the clinic. Those most in need were seen first. These were usually sick babies. Some less acute patients were told to return the next day. It was always difficult for me to see those patients who were turned away because I knew they had to walk miles to get to the clinic. My assignment included the supervision of four *visitadoras* (visiting nurses) and three attendants (aides to the clinic). I communicated in Portuguese, assisted with the triage, supervised the intravenous medications, supervised the local midwives and, generally, made this a healthier community!

The public health issues of this community were enormous. There were shoeless children with bloated abdomens. Although women enjoyed their social time together as they washed clothes against rocks in the river that ran through town, the river played a role in the life cycle of the schistosome, the parasite causing schistosomiasis.

Family planning existed only for the rich who could afford to purchase "the pill" at the local pharmacy. The local bishop, the fifteenth child in a large family, prohibited me from responding to requests for family planning. A woman in a distant barrio died of tetanus poisoning after childbirth. In another barrio, a woman died of placenta previa, partially because the nearest hospital was an hour away. My neighbor across the street swallowed her wedding band in a misguided attempt to abort an unwanted pregnancy.

The local daily diet consisted mainly of black beans, rice, and farina, a grainy substance of little nutritive value. Tropical fruits were abundant. Only wealthier families could add meat and vegetables to the bean pot.

How could one American public health nurse make a difference? It seemed overwhelming. Clearly, any change in this scene would take a great deal of time. It would take the commitment of many people. It would involve the education of the population. It would include the political leaders. Where would I begin?

The midwives came to the health post to receive free supplies. We scheduled their visit for supplies to coincide with a "refresher" class. I went with the visitadoras to walk to distant barrios to visit new mothers. We talked of nutrition. We encouraged the consumption of tropical fruits and vegetables rich in vitamins. Although I felt these visits were useful, I was obsessed with a concern about the contaminated river. The river, which ran behind the poorest homes, was used for washing family clothes and dishes. Women needed the social interaction with friends, but they did not need schistosomiasis and the resultant liver disease.

Luiz, a young man with a fifth-grade school education, came to our home one evening. He was an organizer. If we could help him and teach him what to do, he would help set up a literacy program. His participation provided the opportunity to use the rather radical teaching method of the exiled Brazilian Secretary of Education, Paulo Friere: "Train the Trainer." We began by teaching Luiz. He then taught ten young women who had graduated from high school. With the mayor's backing, we set up classes all over the city. The plantation workers came to class in their cleanly pressed clothes after a day in cacao groves. I remember one class including the following: "panela (pan). A utensil used to boil water to prevent disease." In this way, the teachers introduced health principles along with the literacy.

From Zerwekh J, Young B, Primono J, et al., editors: *Opening doors: stories of public health nursing*, Olympia, Wash, 1992, Washington State Department of Health, pp. 131-135. Used with permission.

*A view from the field*

Two days after Christmas, hard rains began. The river rose and topped the bridge from the camp. Water covered the roads and isolated the town. I was told that this was the "20-year flood waters." Twenty percent of the town's houses, particularly those belonging to the poor who lived along the river, were washed away or severely damaged. Families took refuge in church and school buildings. The three Italian Sisters of Charity and I collaborated to make visits to the homeless families. We obtained medical help when needed. We worked with city officials to avoid the possibility of a typhoid outbreak. Immunizations were given. Then we began to plan for the rebuilding.

Two and one-half years after I arrived in the town, it was time to prepare to leave. Peace Corp volunteers met in Rio de Janerio for a debriefing from the state department and we wanted to know, before we returned to the United States, how we would know if our presence had made a difference? The reply from the state depart-

ment official was this: "You may never know, but twenty years from now, someone may cast an important vote due to your work here. You must believe that your work here has made a difference."

It was almost twenty years later that I decided to return to Ibicarai. When I drove into town with Luiz as my guide, we first went to the barrio where Luiz had lived. The streets were paved. Street lighting was provided by a rural electrification project. His mother's home had running water from a city water system. A Coca-Cola bottling plant on the outskirts of the barrio provided jobs. Close to the town there was a beautiful new bus station with bright yellow Mercedes buses proudly moving in and out of stalls. An attractive woman in an orange attendant's dress saw me from across the lobby.

"Are you Dona Barbara?"

"Yes," I said, feeling a lump in my throat.

Tearfully hugging me, she said, "I prayed that you would return some day."

and gaps in community resources. It is the basis for community health planning and service provision.

It can be difficult for both neophytes and experienced professionals to collect all of the data that must be obtained when doing a community assessment. Community assessment tools can help students and professional nurses collect and organize community data. Stein and Eigsti (1982) have developed a tool to assist the practitioner in doing an initial, brief community assessment. This tool is based on a set of master categories that characterize community data. It provides observational information about a community's environment, mode of functioning, and social and health resources. Because community health nurses collect these data while driving through or walking around in a community, this form of community assessment has been termed a "windshield" survey of the community. A windshield assessment provides a beginning database about a community. Students are often required to do such assessments as part of class assignments.

Community assessment tools will vary in their comprehensiveness. An in-depth comprehensive assessment tool that assists health agencies to obtain a comprehensive profile of a community is presented in Appendix 14-1. Other community assessment tools and frameworks from which nurses can assess the community are found in Allor (1983), Anderson and McFarlane (1996), Caretto and McCormick (1991), Clark (1986), Edelman and Mandle (1990), Finnegan and Erwin (1989), Gikow and Kucharski (1987), Hanchett (1988), Martin (1988), Meneshian (1988),

Rauckhorst, Stokes, and Mezey (1980), Rodgers (1984), and Ruffing-Rahal (1987). White and Valentine (1993) developed an innovative computer-assisted video instructional program for community assessment, and Selby and Tuttle (1987) developed a community assessment learning module. The National Center for Chronic Disease Prevention and Health Promotion (NCCDPHP) developed a community profile as part of the PATCH program (NCCD-PHP, 1995). Through knowledge gained from a community assessment, the community health nurse has a database for community diagnosis and health planning.

Illustrative of how community assessment can assist in health planning was a project conducted by a local health department in a rural community. A group of community health nurses carried out a community assessment of their rural county. The nurses found that a major health problem was traffic deaths among males 16 to 24 years of age. The death rates for this age group were significantly higher than the expected death rates for the age group. After careful data analysis, factors contributing to this were determined to be narrow, winding, two-lane roads with no shoulders; an image among the young rural males that fast cars were "macho"; no recreational facilities except bars; unlighted roads; and the necessity of driving very long distances to employment sites. These data pointed out the urgent need for a traffic safety program, which was initiated in the local high school.

Community assessments can help communities determine community strengths and resources, and provide direction for the community in relation to health (Sasenick, 1994, p. 56). Community assessment assists in seeing the links among primary health care, health and social service programs, and the health and welfare needs of the community (White, Valentine, 1993, p. 349). Community assessment processes can help communities across our nation identify and address disparities in service delivery.

## SUMMARY

The community health nurse conceptualizes the community as a client and partner in health care delivery. As a client, each community is unique and has its own health care needs. Developing a conceptual understanding of the word community, community dynamics, and how health problems are assessed and solved within the community are crucial in caring for the community. Working with individuals, families, and aggregates at risk becomes far more exciting when the community health nurse understands community concepts. This knowledge, coupled with flexibility in meeting the changing and diverse health needs of the community, facilitates the achievement of healthy communities.

Nurses work in partnership with communities to promote health. Communities across the nation and the world are putting health on their agendas and working to build healthier communities. Nurses work in urban, rural, and international communities to promote health. Nurses gather information about the communities in which they work, they "assess" the community to identify health problems and needed resources, and they build on community strengths to promote health action. It is an exciting adventure to work as a community health nurse.

## CRITICAL THINKING
*exercise*

Review the beginning of the chapter where the term community was defined and discussed. Conceptualize in your mind the community you lived in during high school. Look at this community in terms of some of the major components of community dynamics, such as service systems, communication patterns, leadership, and community functions.

1. What were some of the major values held by this community?
2. What were some of the major strengths of this community?
3. What were some of the health needs of this community?
4. How could a nurse work collaboratively with this community to build on these strengths and facilitate community empowerment?

## REFERENCES

Allen K: Nursing school, VA partnership benefits vets in rural Michigan, *Am Nurse* 32(3):31, 2000.

Allor MT: The "community profile," *J Nurs Educ* 22:12-17, 1983.

American Nurses Association (ANA), Community Health Nursing Division: *Conceptual model of community health nursing*, Pub No CH-10, Kansas City, Mo, 1980, ANA.

American Nurses Association (ANA): *Standards of community health nursing practice*, St Louis, 1986, ANA.

American Nurses Association (ANA): *American Nurses Association position statement on cultural diversity in nursing practice*, Washington, DC, 1996a, ANA.

American Nurses Association (ANA): *Rural/frontier nursing. The challenge to grow*, Washington, DC, 1996b, ANA.

American Nurses Association, Quad Council (ANA Quad Council): *Scope and standards of public health nursing practice*, Washington, DC, 1999, ANA.

American Public Health Association (APHA): *Healthy communities 2000: model standards. Guidelines for implementing the year 2000 national health objectives*, Washington, DC, 1991, APHA.

American Public Health Association (APHA): *Guide to implementing model standards*, Washington, DC, 1993, APHA.

American Public Health Association, Public Health Nursing Section (APHA): *Definition and role of public health nursing*, Washington, DC, 1996, APHA.

Anderson ET, McFarlane JM: *Community-as-partner: theory and practice in nursing*, Philadelphia, 1996, Lippincott.

Arensburg CM, Kimball ST: *Culture and community*, Gloucester, Mass, 1972, Peter Smith.

Avery S: A limited-service rural hospital: the freestanding emergency department, *J Rural Health* 15:170-179, 1999.

Barger SE: Rural nurses: here today and gone tomorrow? *Rural Clinician Q* 6(3):3-4, 1996.

Bergeron J, Neuman K, Kinsey J: Do advanced practice nurses and physician assistants benefit small rural hospitals? *J Rural Health* 15:219-232, 1999.

Bosch D, Bushy A: The five A's of rural home care, *Caring* 16(1):20-25, 1997.

Breckinridge M: *Wide neighborhoods. A story of the Frontier Nursing Service*, New York, 1952, Harper & Brothers Publishers.

Brooks J: Increasing AIDS rates in rural Americans deserve more attention, *NRHA Rural Clin Q* 8(1):1, 1998.

Bushy A: Rural determinants in family health: considerations for community nurses, *Fam Comm Health* 12(4):29-38, 1990.

Bushy A, editor: *Rural nursing*, vols 1-2, Newbury Park, Calif, 1991a, Sage.

Bushy A: Rural determinants in family health: considerations for community nurses. In Bushy A, editor: *Rural nursing*, vol 1, Newbury Park, Calif, 1991b, Sage.

Bushy A: Meeting the challenges of rural nursing research. In Bushy A, editor: *Rural nursing*, vol 2, Newbury Park, Calif, 1991c, Sage.

Bushy A: Case management: considerations for coordinating quality service in rural communities, *J Nurs Care Qual* 12(1):26-35, 1997.

Bushy A: Rural nursing in the United States: where do we stand as we enter a new millennium? *Aust J Rural Health* 6:65-71, 1998.

Caretto VA, McCormick CS: Community as client: a "hands-on" experience for baccalaureate nursing students, *J Comm Health Nurs* 8(3):179-189, 1991.

Census Bureau: *Urban and rural populations 1900-1990*. Retrieved from the internet July 6, 2000. *http://www.census.gov/*

Chamberlain RW: *Beyond individual risk assessment: community-wide approaches to promoting the health and development of families and children—conference proceedings*, Washington, DC, 1988, National Center for Education in Maternal and Child Health.

Chin J, editor: *Control of communicable diseases manual*, 17th ed, Washington, DC, 2000, American Public Health Association.

Clark CC: *Wellness nursing: concepts, theory, research and practice*, New York, 1986, Springer.

Courtney R: Community partnership primary care: a new paradigm for primary care, *Public Health Nurs* 12:366-373, 1995.

Courtney R, Ballard F, Fauver S, et al.: The partnership model: working with individuals, families, and communities toward a new vision of health, *Public Health Nurs* 13:177-186, 1996.

Davis DJ, Droes NS: Community health nursing in rural and frontier counties, *Nurs Clin North Am* 28(1):159-169, 1993.

Doerr B, Sheil E, Baisch MJ, et al.: Beyond community assessment into the real world of learning aggregate practice, *Nurs Health Care* 19(5):214-219, 1998.

Dunkin J, Juhl N, Stratton T, et al.: Job satisfaction and retention of rural community health nurses in North Dakota, *J Rural Health* 8(4):268-275, 1992.

Durch JS, Bailey LA, Stoto MA, editors: *Improving health in the community*, Washington, DC, 1997, Institute of Medicine/National Academy Press.

Edelman CL, Mandle CL: *Health promotion throughout the lifespan*, ed 2, St Louis, 1990, Mosby.

Edelman MA, Menz BL: Selected comparisons and implications of a national rural and urban survey of health care access, demographics, and policy issues, *J Rural Health* 12(3):197-205, 1996.

Eggebeen DJ, Lichter DT: Health and well-being among rural Americans: variations across the lifecourse, *J Rural Health* 9(2):86-98, 1993.

Eisen A: A survey of neighborhood-based, comprehensive community empowerment initiatives, *Health Educ Q* 21(2):235-252, 1994.

Erikson EH: *Childhood and society*, ed 2, New York, 1978, Norton.

Federal Office of Rural Health Policy (FORHP): *White paper: national health service corps scholarship program*, Rockville, Md, 1990, FORHP.

Federal Office of Rural Health Policy (FORHP): *On creating a composite statistical picture of rural America*, Washington, DC, 1993, US Government Printing Office.

Federal Office of Rural Health Policy (FORHP): *Facts about...rural physicians*. Washington DC, 1997, US Government Printing Office.

Federal Office of Rural Health Policy (FORHP): *Facts about...rural physicians*. Retrieved from the internet on July 5, 2000. *http://www.ruralhealth.hrsa.gov/*

Feenstra C: Community based and community focused: nursing education in community health, *Public Health Nurs* 17:155-159, 2000.

Finnegan L, Erwin NE: An epidemiological approach to community assessment, *Public Health Nurs* 6:147-151, 1989.

Flick LH, Reese C, Harris A: Aggregate/community centered undergraduate community health nursing clinical experience, *Public Health Nurs* 13(1):36-41, 1996.

Flynn BC: Healthy cities: the future of public health. Restructuring how we live, *HealthC TrendsTransit* 4(3):12-18, 80, 1993.

Flynn BC: Partnerships for health, *HealthC Forum J* 37(3):55-56, 73, 1994.

Flynn BC: Healthy Cities: building partnerships for healthy public policy, *Nurs Policy Forum* 1(6):6-9, 20-25, 1995.

Flynn BC: Healthy Cities: toward worldwide health promotion, *Annu Rev of Public Health* 17:299-309, 1996.

Flynn BC: Communicating with the public: community based nursing research and practice, *Public Health Nurs* 15(3):165-170, 1998.

Flynn BC, Rains JW: Establishing community coalitions for prevention: healthy cities Indiana. In Knollmueller RN, editor: *Prevention across the lifespan: healthy people for the 21st century*. Washington DC, 1993, American Nurses Association.

Flynn BC, Ray DW, Rider MS: Empowering communities: action research through healthy cities, *Health Educ Q* 21(3):395-405, 1994.

Frenzen P: Health insurance coverage in U.S. urban and rural areas, *J Rural Health* 6(3):204-214, 1993.

Fuszard B, Slocum I, Wiggers D: Rural nurses, part I: surviving cost containment, *J Nurs Adm* 20(4):5-12, 1990.

Geller J, Ludtke R, Stratton T: Nonfatal farm injuries in North Dakota: a sociological analysis. *J Rural Health* 6:185-196, 1990.

Gerberich SS, Stearns SJ, Dowd T: A critical skill for the future: community health assessment, *J Comm Health Nurs* 12:239-250, 1995.

Gikow FF, Kucharski PM: A new look at the community: functional health pattern assessment, *J Comm Health Nurs* 4(1):21-27, 1987.

Goeckermann CR, Hamberger LK, Barber K: Issues of domestic violence unique to rural areas, *Wisc Med J* 93(4):473-479, 1994.

Goeppinger J: Health promotion for rural populations: partnership interventions, *Comm Health* 16(1):1-10, 1993.

Green LW, Kreuter MW: CDC's planned approach to community health as an application of PRECEDE and an inspiration for PROCEED, *J Health Educ* 23(3):140-147, 1992.

Hanchett ES: *Nursing frameworks and community as client*, Norwalk, Conn, 1988, Appleton & Lange.

Hancock T, Duhl L: *Promoting health in the urban context*, WHO Healthy Cities Paper No 1, Copenhagen, 1988, FADL.

Hartley D, Bird DC, Dempsey P: Rural mental health and substance abuse. In Ricketts TC, editor: *Rural health in the United States*, New York, 1999, Oxford University Press.

Hassinger EW, Hicks LL, Godino V: A literature review of health issues of the rural elderly, *J Rural Health* 9:68-75, 1993.

Hemman EA, McClendon BJ, Lightfoot SF: Networking for educational resources in a rural community, *J Contin Educ Nurs* 26(4):170-173, 1995.

Higgs ZR, Gustafson DD: *Community as client: assessment and diagnosis*, Philadelphia, 1985, FA Davis.

Hillery GA Jr: Definitions of community: areas of agreement, *Rural Sociol* 20(2):118-120, 1955.

Institute of Medicine: *The future of public health*, Washington, DC, 1988, National Academy Press.

International Council of Nurses: Cities in distress: a rescue strategy, *Int Nurs Rev* 38(4):105-117, 1991.

Israel BA, Checkoway B, Schulz A, et al.: Health education and community empowerment: conceptualizing and measuring perceptions of individual, organizational and community control, *Health Educ Q* 21(2):149-170, 1994.

Johnson-Webb KD, Leonard DB, Gesler WM: What is rural? Issues and considerations, *J Rural Health* 13(3):253-256, 1997.

Kenzer M: Healthy Cities: a guide to the literature, *Public Health Rep* 115:279-289, 2000.

Kretzmann J, McKnight J: *Building communities from the inside out*, Chicago, 1993, ACTA Publications.

Kretzmann J, McKnight J, Sheehan G: *A guide to capacity inventories: mobilizing the community skills of local residents*, Chicago, 1997, ACTA Publications.

Kreuter MW: PATCH: its origin, basic concepts, and links to contemporary health policy, *J Health Educ* 23(3):135-139, 1992.

Lee BC, Jenkins LS, Westaby JD: Factors influencing exposure of children to major hazards on family farms, *J Rural Health* 13(3):206-215, 1997.

Lee HJ: Definitions of rural: a review of the literature. In Bushy A, editor: *Rural nursing*, vol 1, Newbury Park, Calif, 1991, Sage.

Long KA: The concept of health: rural perspectives, *Nurs Clin North Am* 28:123-130, 1993.

Long KA, Weinert C: Rural nursing: developing the theory base, *Scholar Inq Nurs Pract* 3(2):113-127, 1989.

MacIver RM: *Community*, London, 1917, MacMillan.

MacIver RM, Page CH: *Society: an introductory analysis*, New York, 1949, Rinehart.

Martin A: Community assessment: the cornerstone of effective marketing, *Pediatr Nurs* 14:50-53, 1988.

McFarlane J, Fehir J: De madres a madres: a community, primary health care program based on empowerment, *Health Educ Q* 21(3):381-394, 1994.

McGinnis J, Foege W: Actual causes of death in the United States, *J Am Med Assoc* 270:2207-2212, 1993.

McKnight J, VanDover L: Community as client: a challenge for nursing education, *Public Health Nurs* 11(1):12-16, 1994.

Meneshian S: Nursing assessment of a community. In Caliandro G, Judkins B, editors: *Primary nursing practice*, Glenview, Ill, 1988, Scott, Foresman.

Milio N: Healthy cities: the new public health and supportive research, *Health Prom Int* 5(4):291-297, 1990.

Milio N: Stirring the social pot: community effects of program and policy research, *J Nurs Adm* 22(2):24-29, 1992.

Moore H, Puntenney D: *Leading by stepping back: a guide for city officials on building neighborhood capacity*, Chicago, 1999, ACTA Publications.

Moore T: *Conversation on the philosophy of community*, Knoxville, Tenn, Oct 2000, University of Tennessee, College of Nursing.

Nakajima H: World Health Day 1996: Healthy Cities for better life, *World Health* 49:300, 1996.

National Advisory Committee on Rural Health: *Second annual report to the Secretary of Health and Human Services*, Rockville, Md, 1989, Office of Rural Health Policy.

National Advisory Committee on Rural Health: *Third annual report to the Secretary of Health and Human Services*, Rockville, Md, 1990, Office of Rural Health Policy.

National Advisory Council of the National Health Service Corps: *Proposed strategies for fulfilling primary care professional needs, part II: nurse practitioners, physician assistants, and certified nurse-midwives*, Rockville, Md, 1991, Health Resources and Services Administration.

National Association for County and City Health Officials (NACCHO): APEX/PH. Retrieved from the internet July 5, 2000. *http://www.naccho.org*

National Center for Chronic Disease Prevention and Health Promotion (NCCDPHP): *Planned approach to community health: Guide for the local coordinator*, Atlanta, 1995, Centers for Disease Control and Prevention.

National Civic League: *National Civic League: a century of community building*, Denver, 1995, National Civic League.

National Commission on Community Health Services: *Health is a community affair*, Cambridge, Mass, 1966, Harvard University Press.

National Committee for Childhood Agricultural Injury Prevention: *Children and agriculture: opportunities for safety and health. A national action plan*, Marshfield, Wis, 1996, Marshfield Clinic.

National Organization for Public Health Nursing (NOPHN): Constitution of the National Organization for Public Health Nursing, Article 2, 1912, Wald: New York Public Library folder: NOPHN No 1. In Fitzpatrick ML, editor: *The National Organization for Public Health Nursing, 1912-1952: development of a practice field*, New York, 1975, National League for Nursing.

National Rural Health Association (NRHA): *Roadmap to a healthy rural America. Direction No. 4. Strengthen America's small, rural hospitals*. Retrieved from the internet July 5, 2000. *http://www.nrharural.org*

Naylor MD, Buhler-Wilkerson K: Creating community-based care for the new millennium, *Nurs Outlook* 47:120-127, 1999.

Norris T: *The healthy communities handbook*, Denver, 1993, National Civic League.

Norris T, Lampe D: Healthy communities, healthy people, *Natl Civ Rev* 83(3):2-11, 1994.

Norris T, Pittman M: The healthy communities movement and the coalition for healthier cities and communities, *Public Health Rep* 115:118-124, 2000.

Office of Technology Assessment (OTA), Congress of the United States: *Health care in rural America*, Washington DC, 1990, OTA.

Pender N: *Health promotion in nursing practice*, Stanford, Conn, 1996, Appleton & Lange.

Pickard MR: Rural nursing: a decade in review, *Rural Clinician Q* 6(3):1-2, 1996.

Poplin DC: *Communities: a survey of theories and methods of research*, ed 2, New York, 1979, Macmillan.

Purschwitz MA: *Fatal farm injuries to children*, Marshfield, Wis, 1990, Office of Rural Health Policy, Wisconsin Rural Health Research Center.

Ramsbottom-Lucier M, Emmett K, Rich EC, et al.: Hills, ridges, mountains, and roads: geographical factors and access to care in rural Kentucky, *J Rural Health* 12(5):386-394, 1996.

Randall T: *The outreach sourcebook: rural health demonstration projects 1991 to 1994*, Rockville, Md, 1995, Federal Office of Rural Health Policy.

Rauckhorst LM, Stokes SA, Mezey MD: Community and home assessment, *J Gerontol Nurs* 6:319-327, 1980.

Reiff S, DesHarnais S, Bernard S: Community perceptions of the effects of rural hospital closure on access to care, *J Rural Health* 15:202-209, 1999.

Ricketts TC: Rural communities and rural hospitals, *J Rural Health* 15:168-169, 1999a.

Ricketts TC: Policies for rural health care: they work...sometimes. *J Rural Health* 15:7-10, 1999b.

Ricketts TC: Federal programs and rural health, In Ricketts TC, editor: *Rural health in the United States*, New York, 1999c, Oxford University Press.

Ricketts TC, Heaphy PE: Hospitals in rural America. In Ricketts TC, editor: *Rural health in the United States*, New York, 1999, Oxford University Press.

Ricketts TC, Johnson-Webb KD, Randolph RK: Populations and places in rural America. In Ricketts TC, editor: *Rural health in the United States*, New York, 1999, Oxford University Press.

Ricketts TC, Johnson-Webb KD, Taylor PL: *Definitions of rural: a handbook for health policy makers and researchers*. Technical Issues Paper prepared for the Federal Office of Rural Health Policy (FORHP), Washington, DC, 1998, FORHP.

Rodgers SS: Community as client—a multivariate model for analysis of community and aggregate health risk, *Public Health Nurs* 1:210-222, 1984.

Rosenblatt RA, Hart LG: Physicians and rural America. In Ricketts TC, editor: *Rural health in the United States*, New York, 1999, Oxford University Press.

Ruffing-Rahal MA: Resident/provider contrasts in community health priorities, *Public Health Nurs* 4:242-246, 1987.

Rural Information Center: *Rural health services funding: a resource guide*. Retrieved from the internet July 5, 2000. *http://www.nalusda.gov/ric/richs/*

Ruth J, Eliason K, Schultz PR: Community assessment: a process of learning, *J Nurs Educ* 31(4):181-183, 1992.

Sanders IT: *The community: an introduction to a social system*, New York, 1958, Ronald Press.

Sanders IT: *The community: an introduction to a social system*, ed 2, New York, 1966, Ronald Press.

Sanders IT: *The community: an introduction to a social system*, ed 3, New York, 1975, Ronald Press.

Sanders IT: The community: structure and function, *Nurs Outlook* 11:642-645, 1963.

Sasenick SM: How healthy is your community? *Health Care Forum J* 37(3):56, 1994.

Scutchfield FD, Keck CW: *Principles of public health practice*, Albany, NY, 1997, Delmar.

Selby ML, Tuttle DM: Community health assessment and program planning in the nursing practitioner curriculum: evaluation of a guided design learning module, *Public Health Nurs* 4:160-165, 1987.

Shamansky SL, Pesznecker B: A community is . . . , *Nurs Outlook* 29:182-185, 1981.

Sherer JL: Neighbor to neighbor, *Hosp Health Netw* 68(20):52-56, 1994.

Shoultz J, Hatcher PA: Looking beyond primary care to primary health care: an approach to community-based action, *Nurs Outlook* 45(1):23-26, 1997.

Stanley SAR, Stein DS: Health Watch 2000: community health assessment in south central Ohio, *J Comm Health Nurs* 15(4):225-236, 1998.

Stein KZ, Eigsti DG: Utilizing a community database system with community health nursing students, *J Nurs Educ* 21:26-32, 1982.

Strategies to improve rural health, *Public Health Rep* 111(2):101, 1996.

Straub LA, Straub SA: Consumer and provider evaluation of rural pharmacy, *J Rural Health*, 15:403-412, 1999.

Summer L: *Limited access: health care for the rural poor*, Washington, DC, 1991, Center on Budget and Policy Priorities.

Torres MI: Assessing health in an urban neighborhood: community process, data results and implications for practice, *J Comm Health* 23(3):211-226, 1998.

US Department of Health and Human Services (USDHHS): *Prevention resource guide: rural communities*, Rockville, Md, 1991, USDHHS.

US Department of Health and Human Services (USDHHS): *Healthy People 2000 midcourse review and 1995 revisions*, Rockville, Md, 1995a, USDHHS.

US Department of Health and Human Services (USDHHS): *Planned approach to community health. Guide for the local coordinator.* Atlanta, Ga, 1995b, US Department of Health and Human Services, Centers for Disease Control and Prevention and National Center for Chronic Disease Prevention and Health Promotion.

Vulnerable populations. In Bushy A, editor: *Rural nursing*, vol 1, Newbury Park, Calif, 1991, Sage.

Wagenfeld M, Murray D, Mohatt D, et al.: *Mental health and rural America: 1980-1993*, NIH Pub No 94-3500, Washington, DC, 1994, US Government Printing Office.

Wald L: *The house on Henry Street*, New York, 1915, Henry Holt.

Warren DI: Neighborhoods in urban areas. In Warren RL, editor: *New perspectives on the American community*, ed 3, Chicago, 1977, Rand McNally.

Warren RL: *Studying your community*, Chicago, 1955, Rand McNally.

Warren RL: *The community in America*, Chicago, 1963, Rand McNally.

Warren RL: *Studying your community*, Chicago, 1965, Rand McNally.

Warren RL: *Perspectives on the American community*, Chicago, 1966, Rand McNally.

Warren RL: *The community in America*, ed 2, Chicago, 1972, Rand McNally.

Warren RL: *The community in America*, ed 3, Chicago, 1978, Rand McNally.

Warren RL: *The community in America*, ed 4, Chicago, 1987, Rand McNally.

Warren RL: The good community—what would it be? In Warren RL, Lyon L, editors: *New perspectives on the American community*, ed 5, Chicago, 1988, Rand McNally.

Weinert C, Burman ME: Rural health and health-seeking behaviors. In Fitzpatrick JJ, Stevenson JS, editors: *Annual review of nursing research*, vol 12, New York, 1994, Springer.

Weinert C, Burman ME: The sampler quilt: a metaphor of rural communities. In Hinshaw AS, Feetham SL, Shaver JLF, editors: *Handbook of clinical nursing research*, Newbury Park, Calif, 1999, Sage.

Weinert C, Long KA: Understanding the health care needs of rural families, *Fam Relations* 36:450-455, 1987.

Weinert C, Long KA: Rural families and health care: refining the knowledge base, *J Marr Fam Rev* 15(1):57-96, 1990.

Weinert C, Long KA: The theory and research base for rural nursing practice. In Bushy A, editor: *Rural nursing*, vol 1, Newbury Park, Calif, 1991, Sage.

Weinert C, Long KA: Support systems for the spouses of chronically ill persons in rural areas, *Fam Community Health* 16(1):46-54, 1993.

Wellman B, Leighton B: Networks, neighborhoods, and communities: approaches to the study of the community question. In Warren RL, Lyon L, editors: *New perspectives on the American community*, Chicago, 1988, Dorsey.

Whelan E-M: The Health Corner: a community-based nursing model to maximize access to primary care, *Public Health Rep* 110(2): 184-188, 1995.

White JE, Valentine VL: Computer assisted video instruction and community assessment, *Nurs Health Care* 14(7):349-353, 1993.

Wiist WH, Flack JM: A church-based cholesterol education program, *Public Health Rep* 105(4):381-388, 1990.

World Health Organization (WHO): *Community health nursing: report of a WHO expert committee*, Technical Report Series No 558, Geneva, 1974, WHO.

World Health Organization (WHO): *Building a healthy city: a practitioner's guide*, Geneva, 1995, WHO.

Zerwekh J, Young B, Primono J, et al., editors: *Opening doors: stories of public health nursing*, Olympia, Wash, 1992, Washington State Department of Health.

## SELECTED BIBLIOGRAPHY

Anderson ET, McFarlane JM, Helton A: Community-as-client: a model for practice, *Nurs Outlook* 34:220-224, 1986.

Chalmers K, Kristajanson L: The theoretical basis for nursing at the community level: a comparison of three models, *J Adv Nurs* 14:569-574, 1989.

Clark DK: The city government's role in community health improvement, *Public Health Rep* 115:216-221, 2000.

Goldstein G, Kickbusch I: A healthy city is a better city, *World Health* 49:4-6, 1996.

Hancock T: Healthy communities must also be sustainable communities, *Public Health Rep* 115:151-156, 2000.

Lee P: Healthy communities: a young movement that can revolutionize public health, *Public Health Rep* 115:114-115, 2000.

Norris T, Pittman M: The healthy communities movement and the coalition for healthier cities and communities, *Public Health Rep* 115:118-124, 2000.

Reif S, Ricketts TC: *The first year of the Medicare rural hospital flexibility program*, Chapel Hill, NC, 1999, University of North Carolina (Project of the North Carolina Rural Health Research Program and Cecil G. Sheps Center for Health Services Research with support from the Office of Rural Health Policy USDHHS CSURC0004-03).

Sharp PA, Greaney ML, Lee PR, et al.: Assets-oriented community assessment, *Public Health Rep* 115:205-211, 2000.

Sills GM, Goeppinger J: The community as a field of inquiry in nursing. In Werly HH, Fitzpatrick JJ, editors: *Annual review of nursing research*, vol 3, New York, 1985, Springer.

Smith N: The implementation and evaluation of a healthy communities process in central Alberta: some implications for public health practice, *J Public Health Management Practice* 6(2):11-20, 2000.

Wilcox R: Building communities that create health, *Public Health Rep* 115:139-143, 2000.

# 4

# Promoting Healthy People: Public Health Policies and Legislation

*Sandra L. McGuire*

## OBJECTIVES

*Upon completion of this chapter, the reader should be able to:*

1. Summarize the development of public health in the United States.
2. Discuss core public health functions and essential public health services.
3. Define public health.
4. Discuss the Healthy People Initiative.
5. List the central goals of *Healthy People 2010*.
6. Be familiar with the focus areas of *Healthy People 2010*.
7. Discuss the purpose and mandates of significant health and welfare legislation in the United States.
8. Explain how the Social Security Act and the Public Health Service Act have influenced health and welfare practices in the United States.
9. Discuss how health and welfare legislation affects community health nursing practice.

## KEY TERMS

Americans with Disabilities Act
*Chadwick Report*
Civil Rights Act of 1964
Core public health functions
Determinants of health
Economic Opportunity Act
Education for All Handicapped Children Act
Elizabethan Poor Law of 1601
Essential public health services

Family and Medical Leave Act
Healthy People Initiative
Individuals with Disabilities Education Act
Leading health indicators
Stewart B. McKinney Homeless Assistance Act
National Environmental Policy Act
Occupational Safety and Health Act
Older Americans Act

Preventive Health Amendments
Public health
Public Health Service Act
Rehabilitation Act
*Shattuck Report*
Social Security Act
State Workers' Compensation Acts
*The Future of Public Health*

---

*We have left undone those things which we ought to have done and we have done those things which we ought not to have done, and there is no health in us.*

BOOK OF COMMON PRAYER

Chapter 1 discussed the evolution of community health nursing in the United States. This chapter explores the evolution of public health, presents an overview of the Healthy People Initiative, discusses core public health functions, and looks at national health and welfare legislation. Chapter 5 expands on this chapter to examine U.S. health and welfare resources and services.

## PUBLIC HEALTH IN THE UNITED STATES

Public health has a proud history. Throughout the ages public health practices have prevented unnecessary illness, injury, disability, and death. These practices have been the mainstay of communicable disease prevention and control. They have provided the foundation for improvements in health, quality of life, and life expectancy. Unfortunately, the health care system and the public health system have often taken separate paths (Pearson, Spencer, Jenkins, 1995, p. 24). Historically, public health has been a stronghold for primary prevention, while the health care system has focused on a "treatment" model (U.S. Public Health Service [USPHS], 1994, p. 3).

## The Evolution of Public Health Practices

Across civilizations, early public health practices focused on controlling communicable disease. Early societies used communicable disease control measures such as isolation (often in the form of quarantine or banishment), burial of the dead, and protection and conservation of food and water supplies to promote health.

Egyptians of 1000 BC were possibly the healthiest of all ancient civilized people (Pickett, Hanlon, 1990, p. 21). They practiced rigorous personal hygiene measures; isolated lepers; had elaborate sewage, drainage, and water-supply systems; and used pharmaceutical preparations and surgical treatments. The Romans practiced public health measures that included provision of public sanitation services, including the removal of garbage and rubbish, protection of the public water supply, and supervision of public food and housing (Pickett, Hanlon, 1990, p. 22). As early as 1500 BC the Hebrews had a written hygienic code in Leviticus that dealt with personal and community hygiene (Pickett, Hanlon, 1990, p. 21).

Unfortunately, during the Middle Ages (500-1500 AD) many of the public health practices of previous times and cultures were not followed. In many European countries, refuse was allowed to accumulate in streets and dwellings, human waste was dumped into public water supplies, food was improperly stored and prepared, personal hygiene was often ignored, and child labor was common. Earlier public health practices were largely ignored.

During the Middle Ages epidemics of cholera, smallpox, typhoid, plague, and diphtheria raged. In the 1300s bubonic plague nearly exterminated the human race, reportedly killing up to half of the world's population (Pickett, Hanlon, 1990, p. 24). Epidemics of such magnitude have never been seen since, and public health practices evolved to control these communicable diseases. Over the centuries public health measures, technology, vaccines, and antibiotics have aided greatly in the control of communicable diseases. However, communicable diseases continue to be a public health problem with the worldwide epidemic of acquired immunodeficiency syndrome (AIDS), the resurgence of diseases such as tuberculosis, the continuing impact of influenza and pneumonia, and many bacteria becoming resistant to antibiotics.

Throughout the history of public health, two major factors have determined how problems were solved: the level of scientific and technical knowledge, and the content of public values and popular opinions (Institute of Medicine [IOM], 1988, p. 1). Two major indicators of a nation's health are morbidity and mortality statistics (see Chapter 11). Although the United States has an abundance of health care resources, it often lags behind other countries in relation to such statistics. The United States ranks twenty-sixth among industrial nations in the world in terms of infant mortality (Health Resources and Services Administration [HRSA], 2000, p. 22), nineteenth in female life expectancy, and twenty-fifth in male life expectancy (U.S.

**TABLE 4-1**

*Life Expectancy by Country*

| FEMALE | | MALE | |
|---|---|---|---|
| COUNTRY | YEARS OF LIFE EXPECTANCY | COUNTRY | YEARS OF LIFE EXPECTANCY |
| Japan | 82.9 | Japan | 76.4 |
| France | 82.6 | Sweden | 76.2 |
| Switzerland | 81.9 | Israel | 75.3 |
| Sweden | 81.6 | Canada | 75.2 |
| Spain | 81.5 | Switzerland | 75.1 |
| Canada | 81.2 | Greece | 75.1 |
| Australia | 80.9 | Australia | 75.0 |
| Italy | 80.8 | Norway | 74.9 |
| Norway | 80.7 | Netherlands | 74.6 |
| Netherlands | 80.4 | Italy | 74.4 |
| Greece | 80.3 | England and Wales | 74.3 |
| Finland | 80.3 | | |
| Austria | 80.1 | France | 74.2 |
| Germany | 79.8 | Spain | 74.2 |
| Belgium | 79.8 | Austria | 73.5 |
| England and Wales | 79.6 | Singapore | 73.4 |
| | | Germany | 73.3 |
| Israel | 79.3 | New Zealand | 73.3 |
| Singapore | 79.0 | | |
| **United States** | **78.9** | Northern Ireland | 73.1 |
| | | Belgium | 73.0 |
| | | Cuba | 73.0 |
| | | Costa Rica | 73.0 |
| | | Finland | 72.8 |
| | | Denmark | 72.8 |
| | | Ireland | 72.5 |
| | | **United States** | **72.5** |

From US Department of Health and Human Services: *Healthy People 2010, conference edition,* Washington, DC, 2000, U.S. Government Printing Office, p. 9.
Source: World Health Organization. United Nations. Centers for Disease Control and Prevention. National Center for Health Statistics. National Vital Statistics System. 1990-1995 and unpublished data.

Department of Health and Human Services [USDHHS], 2000, p. 9) (Table 4-1). Promoting the public's health is an important national concern.

## The Future of Public Health

*The Future of Public Health* is a landmark report on public health in the United States. Published in 1988 by the Institute of Medicine's (IOM) Committee for the Study of the Future of Public Health, this report examined the status of public health in the United States and provided a futuristic view for the public health system. The Committee broadly defined the mission of public health to be "the measures that we as a society take collectively to provide the conditions that ensure the people's health" (IOM, 1988, p. 17). The findings of this report continue to guide the development and revision of public health in the United States.

After careful study of the public health system, the Committee concluded that the nation had lost sight of its public health goals and that the public health system was in disarray and a threat to the health of the nation (IOM, 1988, p. 191). The Committee stated that decision making in public

### BOX 4-1
### *Ten Great Public Health Achievements in the United States, 1990-1999*

1. Vaccination
2. Motor vehicle safety
3. Safer workplaces
4. Control of infectious diseases
5. Decline in deaths from coronary heart disease and stroke
6. Safer and healthier foods
7. Healthier mothers and infants
8. Family planning
9. Fluoridation of drinking water
10. Recognition of tobacco as a health hazard

Source: Centers for Disease Control and Prevention (CDC): Ten great public health achievements—United States, 1900-1999. In Lee PR, Estes CL, editors: *The nation's health*, ed 6, Boston, 2001, Jones and Bartlett, pp. 225-227.

### BOX 4-2
### *Public Health: What It Does*

- Focuses on primary prevention
- Leads the development of sound health policy and planning
- Educates people about health risks and health promotion
- Prevents epidemics
- Protects the environment, workplaces, housing, food, and water
- Enforces laws and regulations that protect health and ensure safety
- Promotes healthy behaviors
- Links people to needed personal health services
- Monitors the health status of the population
- Mobilizes community action for health
- Responds to disasters
- Assures the quality, accessibility, and accountability of medical care
- Targets high-risk and hard-to-reach populations with clinical services
- Maintains diagnostic laboratory services
- Collects health statistics
- Researches to develop new insights and innovative solutions

Modified from US Public Health Service: *For a healthy nation: returns on investment in public health,* Washington, DC, 1994, USDHHS.

health is frequently driven by crises and the concerns of organized interest groups rather than by comprehensive analysis or the objective of enhancing the quality of life (IOM, 1988, p. 5). Some barriers cited to promoting public health included the lack of consensus on the mission of public health, inequities in public health services, problems in relationships among the several levels of government, the poor public image of public health, and fragmented decision making (IOM, 1988, p. 108). The Committee further noted that public health resources have become so fragmented and diverse that deliberate action is often difficult, if not impossible (IOM, 1988, p. 1).

The Committee contended that an impossible responsibility has been placed on America's public health resources "to serve the basic health needs of entire populations, while at the same time averting impending disasters, providing personal health care to those rejected by the rest of the health system, and taking on the new public health problems while confronting the old" (IOM, 1988, pp. 2, 138). According to the Committee, public health in the United States requires that threats to the public health be successfully countered, including: (1) *immediate crises* such as the AIDS epidemic and access to health and welfare services for the indigent; (2) *enduring problems* such as injuries, chronic illness, teen pregnancy, control of high blood pressure, smoking, and substance abuse; and (3) *growing challenges* such as the aging of the population, homelessness, and environmental health (IOM, 1988, pp. 19-30).

The Committee noted that many great public health achievements had been made (Box 4-1) but concluded that the American public has slackened its public health vigilance and has come to take for granted many of the successes of public health, such as control of communicable disease and provision of safe food and water. It is no wonder the American public health system is in trouble—"the wonder is that the system has done so much, for so long, with so little" (IOM, 1988, p. 2). In spite of lack of funding and a diluted public health workforce, some public health initiatives are making progress: more children than ever before are being immunized in the United States, and teen pregnancy rates are dropping (Gebbie, 2000). Boxes 4-2 and 4-3 outline what public health does and the public health ap-

### BOX 4-3
### *The Public Health Approach*

Defines the health problem
Identifies the risk factors associated with the problem
Develops community-level interventions to control or prevent the causes of the problem
Implements interventions to improve the health of the population
Monitors interventions to assess their effectiveness

From US Public Health Service: *For a healthy nation: returns on investment in public health,* Washington, DC, 1994, USDHHS, p. 5.

proach. The **core public health functions** developed by the Committee are discussed further.

## Core Public Health Functions

Core functions in ensuring public health in *The Future of Public Health* report were determined to be assessment, policy development, and assurance (IOM, 1988, pp. 7-8, 41-42, 141-142); these functions exist at all levels of government, and the government's role in ensuring them includes the following elements:

*Assessment.* Regularly and systematically collect, assemble, analyze, and make available information on the health of the community, including statistics on health status, community health needs, and epidemiologic and other studies of health problems (p. 7).

*Policy development.* Exercise responsibility to serve the public interest in the development of comprehensive public health policies by promoting use of the scientific knowledge base in decision making about public health and by leading in the development of public health policy. Agencies must take a strategic approach, developed on the basis of a positive appreciation for the democratic political process (p. 8).

*Assurance.* Ensure constituents that services necessary to achieve agreed-upon goals are provided, either by encouraging actions by other entities (private or public sector), by requiring such action through regulation, or by providing services directly. Public health leaders involve the general public and key policymakers in determining a set of high-priority personal and community-wide health services that governments will guarantee to every member of the community. This guarantee should include subsidization or direct provision of high-priority personal health services for those unable to afford them (p. 8).

In carrying out these core functions federal, state, and local agencies work to ensure a competent workforce, monitor health, diagnose and investigate health concerns, inform and educate, empower and mobilize community partnerships, develop health policies, enforce public health laws, and link consumers to care resources (Office of Disease Prevention and Health Promotion [ODPHP], 1999). Chapter 5 looks at these functions in relation to the service functions and activities of public health agencies such as state health authorities (SHAs) and local health departments (LHDs). As health care reform continues to take place in the United States, it will be interesting to note the collaborations and changes that occur in public health.

## Essential Public Health Services

In 1994, the Public Health Functions Steering Committee of the Public Health Service delineated ten **essential public health services** that build on the core public health functions (Association of State and Territorial Directors of Nursing, 2000; Novick, 2001; USDHHS, 1997). These services also build on the vision of public health to have healthy people in healthy communities and the mission of public health to promote physical and mental health and prevent disease, injury, and disability. Presently, national public health performance standards are being developed to

be able to measure our nation's progress toward providing essential public health services (Public Health Practice Program Office [PHPPO], 1999). Essential public health services are given in Box 4-4. Chapter 5 discusses service functions of state and local health departments and illustrates how these essential public health services are incorporated into practice.

## Public Health and Health Care Reform

Any proposals for health care reform need to incorporate public health provisions as part of a national health plan. Such proposals would include strengthening the nation's public health infrastructure, developing innovations in providing population-based community health services, outlining a public health research agenda, developing collaborative academic and practice research, establishing centers for public health practice, and increasing funding for prevention research (Mahan, 2000). Such research needs to be collaborative and include resources such as the Centers for Disease Control and Prevention (CDC); schools of public health; other health sciences schools; state and local health departments; community health centers; and representation from the private sector, including hospitals, long-term care institutions, managed care organizations, and practitioners (Mahan, 2000).

Unfortunately, "the American public has come to expect more from medicine than it can deliver and far less from public health than it can accomplish" (Robbins, Freeman,

**BOX 4-4**

*Essential Public Health Services*

- Monitor health status to identify community health problems
- Diagnose and investigate health problems and health hazards in the community
- Inform, educate, and empower people about health issues
- Mobilize community partnerships to identify and solve health problems
- Develop policies and plans that support individual and community health efforts
- Enforce laws and regulations that protect health and ensure safety
- Link people to needed personal health services and assure the provision of health care when otherwise unavailable
- Assure a competent public health and personal health care workforce
- Evaluate effectiveness, accessibility, and quality of personal and population-based health services
- Research for new insights and innovative solutions to health problems

From Public Health Functions Steering Committee Members: *Public Health in America Statement, July, 1995*. Retrieved from the internet August 19, 2001. *http://www.health.gov/phfunctions/public.htm*

1999, p. 120). We need to more fully use public health interventions to assist communities in promoting health and attacking sources of harm (Robbins, Freeman, 1999). Through a reformed public health system, we could be the first country to consciously link public health agencies with the medical care system (Robbins, Freeman, 1999, p. 122).

The integration of public health principles and services into managed care is crucial in public health reform and expanding public health practice (Association of State and Territorial Health Officials [ASTHO], 1999). Public health agencies can work cooperatively with managed care organizations (MCOs) to implement community health promotion interventions, perform community health assessments, develop MCO health promotion and health education guidelines, train managed care providers in health promotion and health education, implement school-based health programs, develop MCO public health performance standards, and influence legislation related to managed care as it affects the public's health (ASTHO, 1999).

Unfortunately, despite its centrality to the well-being of Americans, public health funding is jeopardized (USPHS, 1994, p. ii). Health care reform needs to ensure adequate funding and resources for public health. Historically, insufficient funds have been devoted to public health. In 1932 the United States spent $1 per person, 3.4% of the national health care expenditures, on public health (Committee on the Costs of Medical Care, 1932, p. 118). Recent research has shown about $36 per person, 1% of health care expenditures, is spent on public health (Public Health Foundation [PHF], 2000). Public health funding continues to decline at a time when serious public health problems such as AIDS, tuberculosis, and environmental health increase in scope. Public health remains grossly underfunded in the United States.

To strengthen public health in our nation, the public health infrastructure and public health workforce need to be strengthened. "An effective local public health system that serves all Americans is of vital importance to assuring a proficient national public health system" (Milne, 2000, p. 61). Health departments, in collaboration with schools of public health and other health science programs, can help enhance the public health workforce (Milne, 2000).

A performance measurement monitoring system for state and local public health agencies is being developed (Corso, Wiesner, Halverson, et al., 2000) and will assist local communities in measuring public health outcomes. Having this knowledge will help public health professionals know what works and what does not.

A strengthened public health system is vital as our nation confronts challenges to the health of the public (USPHS, 1994, p. ii). Public health must retain its leadership role in primary prevention and promoting healthy communities. The Healthy People Initiative is an attempt by our nation to strengthen and promote the public's health.

## THE HEALTHY PEOPLE INITIATIVE: PROVIDING FOR THE PUBLIC'S HEALTH

The word *health* was left out of the U.S. Constitution. The federal government bases its involvement in matters of health and welfare on the Preamble to the Constitution, which charges it with providing for the general welfare of the people. Public health has historically been the responsibility of the individual states and is provided for through state constitutions, legislation, and public health codes. Starting in the late 1970s the federal government took an enlightened role in helping provide for the public's health by establishing national health goals and objectives.

### Healthy People

In 1979, under the presidency of Jimmy Carter, the Surgeon General of the United States issued a landmark report. This report was *Healthy People: The Surgeon General's Report on Health Promotion and Disease Prevention*, often referred to as *Healthy People* (USDHEW, 1979). *Healthy People* set in motion a process, the **Healthy People Initiative,** to establish national health objectives and policy (Lee and Estes, 2001). This initiative made public health a national concern, changing the focus of care to health promotion and disease prevention, rather than treatment and cure (McGuire & Nalle, 2000). It is important that the nurse be familiar with the Healthy People Initiative because it will continue to shape health care policy decades into the future. Major documents in this initiative are presented in this chapter and are listed in Box 4-5.

*Healthy People* (USDHEW, 1979) analyzed the leading causes of death in the United States and suggested that many of these deaths were preventable. It was estimated that approximately half of all U.S. mortality was caused by unhealthful behavior, 20% by environmental hazards, 20% by human biological factors, and 10% by inadequacies in the health care system. Based on these findings, national health objectives were established to address behavioral and environmental aspects of illness as well as the biologic aspects of disease.

The *Healthy People* document shaped national health policy for the decade of 1980-1990. It established broad national health goals targeted for achievement by 1990 and challenged the nation to accomplish them. It launched an unprecedented initiative to promote healthful lifestyles and improve the health of Americans and called on the government and the public to work together to reduce preventable death and disability across the life span (USDHHS, 1986, p. v). This preventive, life span approach was revolutionary for a country that had previously focused on treatment of disease.

*Healthy People* established three target areas: (1) preventive health services (priority areas: family planning, pregnancy and infant care, immunizations, sexually transmitted diseases, and blood pressure control), (2) health protection

**BOX 4-5**

*Healthy People Initiative: Major Documents*

US Department of Health, Education, and Welfare (USDHEW): *Healthy People: the Surgeon General's report on health promotion and disease prevention*, Washington, DC, 1979, US Government Printing Office. (This document is commonly called *Healthy People*.)

US Department of Health and Human Services (USDHHS): *Promoting health/preventing disease: objectives for the nation*, Washington, DC, 1980, US Government Printing Office.

US Department of Health and Human Services (USDHHS): *The 1990 health objectives for the nation: a midcourse review*, Washington, DC, 1986, US Government Printing Office.

US Department of Health and Human Services (USDHHS): *Healthy People 2000: national health promotion and disease prevention objectives, full report, with commentary*, Washington, DC, 1991, US Government Printing Office. (This document is commonly called *Healthy People 2000*.)

US Department of Health and Human Services (USDHHS): *Healthy People 2000: midcourse review and 1995 revisions*, Washington, DC, 1995, US Government Printing Office.

US Department of Health and Human Services (USDHHS): *Healthy People 2010: conference edition*, Washington, DC, 2000, US Government Printing Office. (This document is commonly called *Healthy People 2010*.)

(priority areas: toxic agent control, occupational safety and health, accidental injury control, fluoridation of community water supplies, and infectious agents control), and (3) health promotion (priority areas: smoking cessation; reduction of the misuse of alcohol and drugs; stress control; and improvement of nutrition, exercise, and fitness). Specific objectives for each of these priority areas would be established in the subsequent document *Promoting Health/Preventing Disease: Objectives for the Nation*.

*Promoting Health/Preventing Disease: Objectives for the Nation* was published in 1980 and identified objectives to achieve the *Healthy People* national health goals (USDHHS, 1980). It established 226 national health objectives in 15 priority areas to be achieved over the following 10 years. Yearly reviews outlined the progress made toward achieving these objectives.

The *1990 Health Objectives for the Nation: A Midcourse Review* was published in 1986. It provided Americans with an assessment of how the nation was doing in its decade-long quest to improve the nation's health status. The midcourse review showed that the nation was on its way to achieving nearly half of the 226 objectives, that

about one fourth were unlikely to be achieved, and that in some cases the trend was away from reaching the 1990 targets (USDHHS, 1986, p. iii). Review data indicated reductions in both smoking and per-capita alcohol consumption; increased use of automobile seat belts; and reduced death rates from strokes, cirrhosis, and traffic accidents. However, it showed that Americans had regressed in the areas of weight control, illicit drug use, control of violent behavior, teenage pregnancy, infant health, family planning, physical fitness and exercise, provision of safe water, and control of sexually transmitted diseases. An interesting finding of the review was that states often had inadequate surveillance systems in place to report on progress toward *Healthy People* objectives. As a result, having adequate surveillance systems would become a priority area in *Healthy People 2000*.

## Healthy People 2000: The Initiative Continues

*Healthy People 2000: National Health Promotion and Disease Prevention Objectives*, often referred to as *Healthy People 2000*, "provided a vision for achieving improved health for all Americans" (USDHHS, 1995, p. 2). Published in 1991, it became the flagship of the initiative, building on the efforts of *Healthy People* and shaping U.S. health policy for the next decade (1990-2000). It was the product of a national effort involving almost 300 national organizations including SHAs, the American Nurses Association, the Institute of Medicine, the National Academy of Sciences, and the U.S. Public Health Service.

*Healthy People 2000* identified three broad national health goals: (1) to increase the span of healthy life for Americans, (2) to reduce health disparities among Americans, and (3) to achieve access to preventive services for all Americans. Under the broad approaches of health promotion, health protection, and preventive services, it outlined almost 300 national health objectives under 22 priority areas. Some priority areas were reorganized and new priority areas were added, including environmental health, food and drug safety, mental health and mental disorders, human immunodeficiency virus (HIV) infection, cancer, diabetes and chronic disabling conditions, clinical preventive services, educational and community-based programs, and surveillance and data systems. *Healthy People 2000* focused on working in partnership with communities to promote health, improving access to preventive health care and reducing health disparities. Yearly updates and a midcourse review outlined the progress made toward achieving objectives.

*HEALTHY PEOPLE 2000:* REVIEW AND REVISIONS. Yearly reviews outlined the progress made toward the year 2000 objectives and revised some objectives. *Healthy People 2000: Midcourse Review and 1995 Revisions* identified that progress had been made toward achieving 50% of the objectives, 18% were moving away from the target, 3% showed no change, and tracking data were not available for 29% (USDHHS, 1995, p. 12). Areas that were moving away from target included the number of overweight Americans, teen pregnancies, violent and abusive behavior, occupational work-related injuries, low-birth-weight infants, disability related to chronic conditions, pneumonia and influenza deaths, and financial barriers to preventive health services (USDHHS, 1995, pp. 15-17). The review stated that families, schools, worksites, and community programs all provide important preventive health opportunities and called for renewed commitment to improving the nation's health, stating:

*Healthy People 2000* cannot be accomplished by the Federal Government alone. Leadership must come from institutions and individuals throughout the Nation. Each person makes decisions about how fast to drive, whether to wear a safety belt, what to eat, and how much alcohol to drink. In families, parents have the opportunity to promote health and encourage healthy habits for their children. Community organizations—schools, religious institutions, and voluntary organizations—can become more actively engaged in promoting health. Employers can make worksites healthy. This midcourse review...outlines opportunities to renew the Nation's commitment to making a difference in the health of its citizens as the 21st century approaches. (USDHHS, 1995, p. 5)

Analysis of *Healthy People 2000* objectives showed that over the decade of 1990-2000 the nation ultimately achieved reductions in infant mortality, increased childhood vaccination rates, decreased incidence of teenage pregnancy, decreased death rates of coronary heart disease and stroke, reduced unintentional injuries, and made significant advances in the diagnosis and treatment of cancer (USDHHS, 2000, p. 3). During the same time period, there had been a leveling off of alcohol, tobacco, and illicit drug use (USDHHS, 2000). Unfortunately, it was noted that violence and abusive behavior continued to ravage homes and communities across the country, mental disorders continued to go undiagnosed and untreated, obesity in adults had increased 50% since 1980, almost 40% of adults engaged in no leisure time physical activity, smoking among adolescents had increased, the occurrence of diabetes and other chronic conditions continued to rise, and HIV remained a serious and untamed public health problem (USDHHS, 2000). A guide that communities used when working to meet national health objectives was *Healthy Communities 2000: Model Standards*.

*HEALTHY COMMUNITIES 2000:* MODEL STANDARDS. The Health Services Extension Act of 1977 (Public Law 95-83) mandated the development of model standards for community preventive health services in American communities. These model standards encompass all of the priority areas and national objectives in *Healthy People 2010* and assist communities in establishing community health objectives (American Public Health Association [APHA], 1991, p. ix). The publication, *Healthy Communities 2000: Model Standards* (APHA, 1991), was developed by APHA, the National Association of County Health Officials, the CDC, and the Association for State and Territorial Health Officials. The federal government encouraged SHAs and LHDs to use these model standards in developing public

health objectives. Chapter 3 discussed how these model standards are used across the nation to promote healthier communities.

## Healthy People 2010

*Healthy People 2010* represents the third time that the U.S. Department of Health and Human Services has developed a 10-year health plan for the nation. It builds on *Healthy People* and *Healthy People 2000*. The American public was given the opportunity to share its thoughts and ideas on development of the *Healthy People 2010* document through an interactive website, and more than 11,000 comments on draft materials were received by mail or via the internet from individuals in every state (USDHHS, 2000). The 1244-page document has 28 focus areas (previously called priority areas) and 467 objectives. Boxes 4-6 and 4-7 give an overview of the central goals and focus areas of *Healthy People 2010*. The first central goal addresses not just increasing longevity, but improving the quality of life and years of healthy life. The goal to eliminate health disparities is a great challenge for the nation. Historically, our nation has had great disparity between the health of minority groups and persons of poverty in comparison with the general population.

### *Stop and Think About It*

Box 4-7 presents the focus areas of *Healthy People 2010*. These focus areas are where our nation is placing its public health priorities for the next decade. Think of the community in which you live or work. Which focus areas would you select as the top three to work on? What community initiatives are happening in these areas in your community today? How could you be a part of these initiatives?

*Healthy People 2010* is built on a systematic approach to health improvement that is composed of four key elements: goals, objectives, determinants of health, and health status. It focuses on promoting healthy behaviors, promoting healthy and safe communities, and improving systems for personal and public health. This initiative stresses that "everyone can help achieve the *Healthy People 2010* objectives" (USDHHS, 2000, p. 4). It represents the best in public health planning and strives to achieve the vision of "Healthy People in Healthy Communities" (USDHHS, 2000, p. 3). The document notes that "community partner-

**BOX 4-6**
*Central Goals*

- Increase quality and years of healthy life
- Eliminate health disparities

From US Department of Health and Human Services (USDHHS): *Healthy People 2010, conference edition*, Washington, DC, 2000, US Government Printing Office, p. 2.

ships...can be among the most effective tools for improving the health in communities (USDHHS, 2000, p. 4). Such partnerships are discussed throughout the text.

For the first time, a set of **leading health indicators** (Box 4-8) assists individuals and communities in targeting the actions necessary to improve health (USDHHS, 2000). "The Leading Health Indicators illuminate individual behaviors, physical and social environmental factors, and important health system issues that greatly affect the health of individuals and communities. Underlying each of these indicators is the significant influence of income and education" (USDHHS, 2000, p. 11). The indicators are intended to assist people in understanding the importance of health promotion and disease prevention and to encourage wide participation in improving health in the next decade (USDHHS, 2000, p. 12). For each of the indicators, specific objectives will be used to track progress, highlight achievement, and identify the need for new strategies and actions (Davis, Fields, 2000).

The document looks extensively at **determinants of health,** or critical influences that determine the health of individuals and communities (Figure 4-1). Determinants of health include individual behavior, biology, and physical and social environmental influences on health. Policies and interventions and access to health care also greatly influence health. *Healthy People 2010* points out that about 70% of all premature deaths in the United States are due to individual behaviors and environmental factors.

"Developing and implementing policies and preventive interventions that effectively address these determinants of health can reduce the burden of illness, enhance quality of life, and increase longevity. Individual biology and behavior influence health through their interaction with each other and with the individual's social and physical environments. In addition, policies and interventions can improve health by targeting factors related to individuals and their environments, including access to quality health care" (USDHHS, 2000, p. 5).

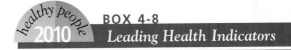

**BOX 4-8**
*Leading Health Indicators*

Physical activity
Overweight and obesity
Tobacco use
Substance abuse
Responsible sexual behavior
Mental health
Injury and violence
Environmental quality
Immunizations
Access to health care

From US Department of Health and Human Services (USDHHS): *Healthy People 2010, conference edition,* in two volumes, Washington, DC, 2000, US Government Printing Office, p. xx.

**BOX 4-7**
*Focus Areas*

1. Access to quality health services
2. Arthritis, osteoporosis, and chronic back conditions
3. Cancer
4. Chronic kidney disease
5. Diabetes
6. Disability and secondary conditions
7. Educational and community-based programs
8. Environmental health
9. Family planning
10. Food safety
11. Health communication
12. Heart disease and stroke
13. Human immunodeficiency virus (HIV)
14. Immunization and infectious diseases
15. Injury and violence prevention
16. Maternal, infant, and child health
17. Medical product safety
18. Mental health and mental disorders
19. Nutrition and overweight
20. Occupational safety and health
21. Oral health
22. Physical activity and fitness
23. Public health infrastructure
24. Respiratory disease
25. Sexually transmitted disease
26. Substance abuse
27. Tobacco use
28. Vision and hearing

From US Department of Health and Human Services (USDHHS): *Healthy People 2010, conference edition,* Washington, DC, 2000, US Government Printing Office, p. 17.

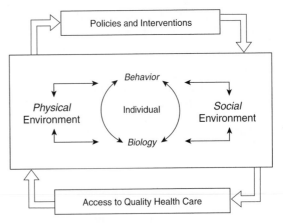

**FIGURE 4-1** Determinants of health. (From US Department of Health and Human Services [USDHHS]: *Healthy People 2010, conference edition,* Washington, DC, 2000, US Government Printing Office, p. 18.)

It is important for nurses to be familiar with *Healthy People 2010* and implement nursing interventions that assist in achieving national health objectives. This document is a valiant attempt by our nation to promote public health and improve the health of communities. Many organizations that the nurse works with will be involved in activities to meet these national objectives designed to facilitate healthy communities. *Healthy People 2010* is a national public health initiative. Many of its objectives are met through enabling health and welfare legislation.

## EVOLUTION OF U.S. HEALTH AND WELFARE LEGISLATION

Because the word *health* was left out of the U.S. Constitution, each state was responsible for legislating its own health laws and providing for the health of its citizens. Recognition of the need for control of communicable disease and the beliefs of divine causation, self-help, and minimal government intervention prevailed in the United States. Federal intervention in public health and welfare assistance was almost nonexistent in early America.

An examination of the historical evolution of health and welfare legislation in the United States demonstrates that it was often reactionary rather than preventive. Health

and welfare organization was decentralized and operated at all levels of government, as well as in the private sector. It would not be until 1980, as part of the Healthy People Initiative, that national health objectives were developed. Early U.S. health and welfare legislation was modeled after the Elizabethan Poor Law of 1601 and early public health practices were encouraged by the **Chadwick Report** and **Shattuck Report.**

### The Elizabethan Poor Law of 1601

A severe economic depression in England spurred the enactment of the Elizabethan Poor Law of 1601. Large-scale involuntary unemployment and the fear of insurrection stimulated the government to provide welfare aid (Coll, 1969, p. 5). This law granted the right to assistance through taxation and established three major categories of dependent people: the vagrant, the involuntarily unemployed, and the helpless (Coll, 1969, p. 5). The last two categories were deemed the "worthy" poor. The helpless included widows, the disabled, and dependent children. Poor law concepts are given in Box 4-9.

The Elizabethan Poor Law became a forerunner of U.S. welfare policy, and *all* of the original 13 colonies adopted it in some form. Following poor law tradition, the United States left administration of assistance programs largely under local control, implemented responsible relative clauses, administered means tests, provided minimal subsistence, generally mandated work or service, imposed restrictive residency, and derived welfare revenues through taxation. Restrictive residency laws are now unconstitutional in the United States. However, many original poor law concepts are part of contemporary health and welfare policy. A report written in England more than 200 years ago has provided the impetus for developing public health policy in the United States.

### The Chadwick Report

In 1832 the British Parliament appointed a royal commission to revise the poor law, and by 1834 the revisions were implemented. Edwin Chadwick was a member of this commission and in 1842, he published the *Report of the Labouring Population and on the Means of Its Improvement*, often referred to as the *Chadwick Report*. The report detailed the unsanitary conditions in which the laborers lived, the lack of proper refuse disposal, contaminated water supplies, high rates of morbidity and mortality, and generally poor living conditions of the laboring population.

At the time of Chadwick's report, one half of the children of working-class parents died before their fifth birthday, and in large English cities the average age of death for laborers was 16 years (Richardson, 1887, cited in Pickett, Hanlon, 1990, p. 26). Chadwick's report helped bring about the passage of the English Public Health Act of 1848, the establishment of a General Board of Health, and the writing of the *Shattuck Report* in the United States in 1850.

**BOX 4-9**

*Elizabethan Poor Law of 1601: Poor Law Concepts*

1. *Local administration.* It was the responsibility of local government to aid those in need. The locality decided who would receive aid and the amount and type of aid. Aid was frequently administered through the church.
2. *General aid.* General aid, usually in the form of food and shelter, was available to the worthy poor.
3. *Responsible relatives.* Relatives could be held responsible for the financial support of other family members.
4. *Restrictive residence.* The locality of the individual's origin was responsible for the financial support of the individual. An indigent who migrated from his or her locality of origin could be returned to it.
5. *Individual means test.* Aid was administered on an individual basis through tests that determined needs. Local jurisdictions exercised the right to use moral qualifications to determine who was worthy of assistance.
6. *Minimal subsistence.* A recipient was to receive no more assistance than necessary to exist.
7. *Compulsory work or service.* Work or service by the recipient was often compulsory to obtain assistance, and refusal to work could be a punishable crime. Workhouses for the indigent were commonplace.
8. *Funding through taxation.* Funds to administer the poor law were raised through local taxes.

## The Shattuck Report

The *Shattuck Report* was the forerunner of contemporary U.S. public health policy. It was written in 1850 by Lemuel Shattuck, a teacher, statistician, and legislator. The report recommended measures such as the creation of state and local boards of health; collection of vital statistics; supervision of housing, factories, sanitation, and foods; procurement of immunizations; community health control measures; and school health and health education. The majority of Shattuck's recommendations are still accepted today as sound public health practice.

Before the report, *local* boards of health had begun to emerge in the United States. Some of the earliest were in Baltimore, Maryland (1798); Charleston, South Carolina (1815); Philadelphia, Pennsylvania (1818); and Providence, Rhode Island (1832). Following the *Shattuck Report*, the number of local boards of health significantly expanded. In 1869 Massachusetts established the first *state* board of health in line with Shattuck's recommendations (Pickett, Hanlon, 1990, p. 32). These state and local boards of health were the forerunners of today's SHAs and LHDs. A National Board of Health existed briefly from 1879-1883. At the time of the *Shattuck Report* no major health and welfare legislation existed on a federal level. It would be more than 80 years before major federal health and welfare legislation would be enacted in the United States.

## THE SOCIAL SECURITY ACT: ESTABLISHING A FEDERAL PRESENCE IN HEALTH AND WELFARE

The *Great Depression* started with the stock market crash of 1929 and peaked in 1933 when 13 million persons, 25% of the work force, were unemployed, and 19 million persons were on state relief rolls. Neither private nor government-funded health or welfare programs could handle the demands created by this event. Possibly no other single event has had such an impact on U.S. health and welfare policy.

The Great Depression showed the general public that anyone could become poor. It dealt a mortal blow to the belief of divine causation because many people whom the general public believed were not deserving of poverty became impoverished. States and the general public put considerable pressure on the federal government to assist those in need. Economic times were desperate for millions of Americans.

A major concern that emerged out of the Depression was a large, young, and restless unemployed workforce. New jobs were hard to generate, and many jobs were held by older workers with seniority. Across the country demonstrations and protests took place to bring about government intervention to help ease unemployment and economic distress.

Retirement as we know it today was nonexistent. Without the benefit of retirement plans, most workers worked throughout their lives, not being able to afford to retire. In an attempt to move older workers out of the workplace and make room for younger unemployed workers, the idea of a federal retirement plan emerged. Retirement insurance became part of the Social Security Act of 1935, generated more jobs for young workers, and helped quiet the general unrest of the American people.

## The Social Security Act of 1935 (Public Law 74-721)

Out of the Depression, under the presidency of Franklin D. Roosevelt, came the Social Security Act. The passage of the act gave the United States the dubious distinction of being the last major industrial nation to develop a federal welfare program.

The Social Security Act included numerous health and welfare provisions. The Act established both *insurance programs* (contributory) and *assistance programs* (noncontributory). Contributory programs are financed through both taxation and individual contributions, whereas assistance programs are financed only through taxation. Box 4-10 outlines original and subsequent Social Security Act programs. Table 4-2 outlines these programs by type of benefit and type of program and gives information on where they are applied for. Chapter 5 expands on the type of services funded by this act.

The Social Security Act is a landmark piece of legislation. Since 1935 the Act has been amended numerous times to incorporate other health and welfare programs. It is one of many legislative acts that is important for the

**BOX 4-10**

*The Evolution of Social Security Act Programs*

*Original Programs*
Aid to the Blind (AB)
Old Age Assistance (OAA)
Aid to Dependent Children (ADC)
Old Age Insurance (OAI)
Unemployment Insurance

*Subsequent Programs*
1939: Old Age and Survivors Insurance (OASI)—*replaces* OAI
1950: Aid to the Permanently and Totally Disabled (APTD) Aid to Families of Dependent Children (AFDC)—*replaces* ADC
1956: Old Age, Survivors, and Disability Insurance (OASDI)—*replaces* OASI
1965: Medicaid and Medicare
1972: Supplemental Security Income (SSI)—*replaces* three programs: AB, OAA, APTD
1996: Temporary Assistance to Needy Families (TANF)*— *replaces* AFDC

*The name of this program varies from state to state.

**TABLE 4-2**

*Major Social Security Act Programs by Type of Benefit*

| TYPE OF BENEFIT | FEDERAL PROGRAMS* | PROGRAM ADMINISTRATION | |
| | | STATE-FEDERAL PROGRAMS† | FEDERAL-STATE PROGRAMS* |
| --- | --- | --- | --- |
| Welfare Insurance (Cash benefit) | Old Age, Survivors, and Disability Insurance (OASDI) | Unemployment Insurance [State Employment Security Commission] | None |
| Welfare Assistance (Cash benefit) | None | Temporary Assistance to Needy Families (TANF) [State Department of Human or Social Services] | Supplemental Security Income (SSI) |
| Health Insurance | 1. Medicare A—hospital insurance prepaid through social security contributions 2. Medicare B—medical insurance, individual premium required | None | None |
| Health Assistance | None | Medicaid [State Department of Human or Social Services] Various maternal and child health programs (e.g., services to children who are disabled, immunizations, EPSDT) [Local health departments, State Departments of Human or Social Services] | None |

*These programs are administered by the federal government and applied for at local branches of the Social Security Administration.
†These programs are administered by state government and applied for at various agencies (commonly used agencies appear in brackets).
Note: Programs such as Workers' Compensation, general assistance, and food stamps are not provided for under the Social Security Act (see Chapter 5).

community health nurse to understand and is discussed in depth later in this chapter.

The act provided for the general welfare by establishing a system of federal old-age insurance and assistance benefits and by enabling the states to make adequate provision for aged persons, blind persons, dependent and crippled children, maternal and child welfare, and the administration of state unemployment compensation laws. This act was a significant step toward safeguarding the health and welfare of Americans. Table 4-3 lists selected amendments to the act.

Today nearly every American family is involved with the Social Security Act in some form. Employers, employees, and the self-employed pay into the insurance programs of the act. Almost 95% of all U.S. workers contribute to these programs. The social security insurance protection, Old Age, Survivors, and Disability Insurance (OASDI), earned by workers stays with them even in a new job or residence. The contributions made by a worker determine the amount and type of benefits.

Numerous other acts have had a significant impact on provision of health and welfare services. A discussion of some of these acts follows.

## OTHER MAJOR U.S. HEALTH AND WELFARE LEGISLATION

Several acts of legislation had a major impact on the development of health and welfare policy and practices in the United States. The Social Security Act has already been discussed. Nurses need to be aware of this legislation because it has significant impact on the availability of health and welfare services. When nurses examine new legislation, they often find that it is an amendment to an existing law rather than an entirely new law and these amendments can significantly alter the original law. Federal laws are designated *public law* and are followed by the number of the congressional session and the sequential number of the law.

The Social Security Act of 1935 and the Public Health Service Act of 1944 are two of the most significant pieces of U.S. legislation ever enacted (Gerber, McGuire, 1995, p. 266). Many new laws are amendments to these two acts, and they provide numerous health and welfare services for clients.

The year 1965 has actually been called the turning point in U.S. public health law and federal involvement in matters

**TABLE 4-3**

## *Selected Amendments: Social Security Act of 1935*

1939    *Social Security Amendments* provided for the payment of insurance benefits to qualifying survivors of workers. The insurance program under the act now was Old Age and Survivors Insurance (OASI).

1950    *Social Security Amendments of 1950* provided for federal aid to states for financial assistance to people who were disabled under Aid to the Permanently and Totally Disabled. Under a new title, Title XIV, Aid to Dependent Children was broadened to include the relative with whom the child was living and became known as Aid to Families with Dependent Children.

1956    *Social Security Amendments of 1956* provided disability insurance benefits for qualifying disabled individuals and reduced to 62 the age at which benefits could be paid to women (The Social Security Amendments of 1961, Public Law 87-64, would make this the age for men also). The insurance portion of the act now was Old Age, Survivors, and Disability Insurance (OASDI).

1963    *Maternal and Child Health and Mental Retardation Planning Amendments* assisted states and communities in preventing mental retardation through expansion and improvement of maternal-child health and crippled children's programs.

1965    *Social Security Amendments of 1965* established Medicare (Title XVII) and Medicaid (Title XIX). These were landmark pieces of legislation and marked the advent of major federal government involvement in health care delivery. Medicare greatly influenced the expansion of home health care services.

1967    *Social Security Amendments of 1967* consolidated maternal and child health and crippled children programs under one authorization and provided for funding of family planning services. They established the Early, Periodic, Screening, and Development Testing (EPSDT) under Medicaid and allowed Medicaid recipients free choice in the selection of qualified medical facilities and practitioners.

1972    *Social Security Amendments of 1972* mandated the establishment of Professional Standard Review Organizations (PSROs) in health care. Established the assistance program of Supplemental Security Income (SSI) to replace the categorical assistance programs of Old Age Assistance, Aid to the Blind, and Aid to the Permanently and Totally Disabled. This change provided for more nationally uniform payment levels to qualifying individuals and set a minimum level of payment. Health insurance coverage for the disabled was made available under Medicare.

1977    *Social Security Act—Rural Health Clinic Amendments* provided payment for rural health clinic services and allowed for direct reimbursement for nursing services in these settings.

1982    *Tax Equity and Fiscal Responsibility Act of 1982* set forth a system of prospective payment for Medicare services called Diagnostic-Related Groups (DRGs).

1984    *Child Support Enforcement Amendments of 1984* amended the act to allow *mandatory* income withholding and other improvements in the child support enforcement program so that children in the United States who are in need of assistance in securing financial support from their parents will receive such assistance. Included provisions for increasing the availability of federal parent locator services to state agencies, collection of past-due support from federal tax refund, and the inclusion of medical support in child support orders.

1985    *Consolidated Omnibus Budget Reconciliation Act of 1985 (COBRA)* amended the act to extend Medicaid coverage for prenatal and postnatal care to low-income women in two-parent families where the primary breadwinner is unemployed, expanded Medicaid services available under home- and community-based services waivers, and permitted states to offer hospice services to the terminally ill as a Medicaid benefit.

1986    *Omnibus Budget Reconciliation Act of 1986 (OBRA)* amended the Social Security Act under Medicaid to allow states to have the option of expanding coverage for pregnant women, infants up to age 1, and children up to age 5 who had incomes below the federal poverty level; required states to continue Medicaid coverage to disabled individuals who lost their eligibility for SSI assistance as a result of work earnings; clarified Medicaid coverage policies with regard to aliens and homeless individuals; and gave states the option of expanding Medicaid coverage for respiratory care services in the home.

1988    *Family Support Act of 1988* reformed the federal welfare system and revised the AFDC program to emphasize work and child support. Established child support programs, job opportunities, and basic skills and training programs. Established a federal requirement that welfare recipients seek employment, and required that each state establish an education, training, and work (NETWork) program. Established rules regarding recipient rights.

1996    *Personal Responsibility and Work Opportunity Reconciliation Act of 1996* (commonly known as the "Welfare Reform Bill") amended the Social Security Act to reform the federal welfare system. It imposes a 5-year lifetime limit on welfare benefits and changes AFDC to temporary assistance to needy families (TANF). It also restricts benefits for legal immigrants.

**BOX 4-11**

*1965: The Turning Point in Health Law in the United States*

1. Drug Abuse Control Amendments of 1965 (PL 89-74).
2. Federal Cigarette Labeling and Advertising Act (PL 89-92).
3. Mental Retardation Facilities and Community Mental Health Centers Construction Act Amendments of 1965 (PL 89-105).
4. Community Health Services Extension Amendments of 1965 (PL 89-109).
5. Health Research Facilities Amendments of 1965 (PL 89-115).
6. Water Quality Act of 1965 (PL 89-234).
7. Heart Disease, Cancer, and Stroke Amendments of 1965 (PL 89-239).
8. The Clean Air Act Amendments and Solid Waste Disposal Act of 1965 (PL 89-272).
9. Health Professions Educational Assistance Amendments of 1965 (PL 89-290).
10. Medical Library Assistance Act of 1965 (PL 89-291).
11. The Appalachian Regional Development Act of 1965 (PL 89-4).
12. The Older Americans Act (PL 89-73).
13. The Social Security Amendments of 1965 (PL 89-97).
14. The Vocational Rehabilitation Act Amendments of 1965 (PL 89-333).
15. The Housing and Urban Development Act of 1965 (PL 89-117).

From Forgotson EH: 1965: the turning point in health law—1966 reflections, *Am J Public Health* 57(6):934-935, 1967.

of public health (Forgotson, 1967, p. 934). During 1965 numerous health-related laws were passed (Box 4-11).

Each year numerous laws with health and welfare implications are enacted, and many existing laws are amended (Figure 4-2). Health and welfare legislation should be examined in terms of its administration, funding, services offered, clients served, service delivery, and quality control. The responsibility to implement this legislation is often dispersed over several agencies at the federal, state, and local levels, with a resulting diffusion of responsibility and accountability (IOM, 1988, p. 115).

An in-depth perspective on laws can be obtained by reading materials specific to each piece of legislation in the *United States Code—Congressional and Administrative News* and the *United States Statutes at Large*. An understanding of this legislation is needed for the community health nurse to assist clients in obtaining services, identifying gaps in the delivery of health and welfare services, and working in partnership with communities to promote health. Discussion of some major U.S. health and welfare legislation follows.

## Public Health Service Act of 1944 (Public Law 78-410)

The Public Health Service Act consolidated and revised the laws relating to the Public Health Service and has since served to consolidate national public health legislation. It is the major piece of public health legislation in the country but inexplicably does not have administration over the Medicaid and Medicare programs of the Social Security Act.

This act incorporates legislation about health care personnel, health facility construction and modernization, and ser-

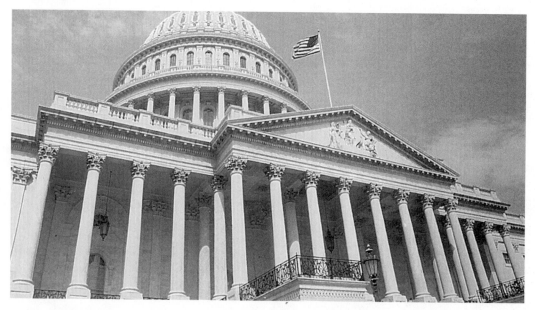

**FIGURE 4-2** The Capitol Building, Washington, D.C. Public health professionals need to monitor proposed laws to ensure that the health care needs of clients are met.

vices to specific population groups. Over the years, this law has been frequently amended to provide financing for traineeships for health care professionals (e.g., nurse training acts); grants-in-aid to schools of public health; construction of community mental health centers and facilities; national comprehensive health planning and resource development; the development of health maintenance organizations; health services for migratory workers; family planning services and communicable disease control; emergency medical services; and research and facilities for the prevention and control of conditions such as heart disease, cancer, stroke, kidney disease, sudden infant death syndrome, arthritis, Coo-

ley's anemia, sickle cell anemia, AIDS, and diabetes mellitus. Amendments such as the Heart Disease, Cancer, and Stroke Amendments gave research and service priority to some of the leading causes of death in this country. Table 4-4 lists some major amendments under this act.

## Civil Rights Act of 1964 (Public Law 88-352)

Most states and many municipalities have enacted civil rights laws that forbid discrimination and ensure constitutional rights. Federal civil rights legislation was enacted in the United States in 1866, 1870, and 1871. Contemporary civil rights acts were enacted in 1957, 1960, 1964, and

**TABLE 4-4**

## Selected Amendments: Public Health Service Act of 1944

| | |
|---|---|
| 1946 | *Hospital Survey and Construction Act,* often called the Hill-Burton Act, authorized grants to states for construction of health care facilities. |
| 1962 | *Migrant Health Act* authorized grants to family clinics for migratory workers. |
| 1964 | *Nurse Training Act* provided funding for nursing education and construction of nursing schools. |
| 1968 | *Health Manpower Act* extended and improved programs relating to the training of nursing, health professions, and allied health professions. |
| 1970 | *Communicable Disease Control Amendments* authorized grants for communicable disease control, vaccination assistance, and studies to determine community-based communicable disease programs designed to contribute to national protection against tuberculosis, venereal disease, rubella, measles, poliomyelitis, diphtheria, tetanus, pertussis, and other communicable diseases. |
| | *Family Planning Services and Population Research Act* established population research and voluntary family planning programs and improved coordination of family planning services and expanded research activities of the federal government. |
| 1971 | *Nurse Training Act* provided funding for nursing education through construction grants to schools of nursing and student loans, advanced practice traineeships, loan repayment and forgiveness, and capitation grants. Prohibited sex discrimination in student award selection. |
| | *Health Maintenance Organization Act* provided assistance for the establishment and expansion of HMOs. |
| 1974 | *National Health Planning and Resource Development Act* authorized the development of national health policy and state and area health planning resources development programs. Required the establishment of state health planning and development agencies. |

| | |
|---|---|
| 1977 | *Rural Health Clinics Act* established rural health clinics in underserved sections of the country. |
| 1981 | *Omnibus Budget Reconciliation Act* enacted many budget and program cuts under the Public Health Service Act. It revised health planning policy, eliminated Public Health Service Hospitals at the end of fiscal year 1981, consolidated many of the categorical programs into block grants to states, but left in place categorical funding for immunizations, tuberculosis, veneral disease, family planning, and migrant health. |
| 1988 | *Health Omnibus Programs Extension Act* created a new title to the act, Title XIV: Health services with respect to acquired immunodeficiency syndrome (AIDS). This new title provided comprehensive AIDS services. Extended nurse traineeships and health professions education. |
| 1990 | *Home Health Care and Alzheimer's Disease Amendments* authorized demonstration projects for home health care services on Alzheimer's disease, established the Task Force on Aging Research to implement research on the aging process and on diagnosis and treatment of disease, disorders, and disability related to aging to assist the aged individual in retaining independence. |
| | *Year 2000 Health Objectives Planning Act* established a program of grants to states for the development of state plans for meeting Healthy People 2000 objectives. |
| 1992 | *Preventive Health Amendments* placed major emphasis by the federal government on preventive health and primary prevention activities. Changed the name of the Centers for Disease Control to Centers for Disease Control and Prevention. Provided for more comprehensive services to Migrant Health Centers in the areas of maternal and child health and community education. Provided for international exchange programs for public health officials from the United States and abroad. |

1968. In 1980 the Civil Rights of Institutionalized Persons Act (Public Law 96-247) was enacted.

Of all the civil rights legislation, the **Civil Rights Act of 1964** is generally considered the most significant; it was designed to ensure fair and equal treatment for all. The act forbade discrimination on the basis of race or sex in public accommodations, public facilities, and public education. It also enforced the constitutional right to vote. It established the Commission on Equal Employment Opportunity and attempted to ensure fair employment practices. If a state or local government is found to be practicing discrimination, the federal Attorney General can sue to have that state's revenue-sharing funds cut off. The Civil Rights Restoration Act of 1987 (Public Law 100-259) clarified and enlarged the scope of the coverage of this act.

## Economic Opportunity Act of 1964 (Public Law 88-452)

The **Economic Opportunity Act** was designed to mobilize the human and financial resources of the nation to combat poverty. It included work training and study programs, established the Office of Economic Opportunity, authorized Volunteers in Service to America (VISTA), the Job Corps, Upward Bound, Neighborhood Youth Corps, Head Start, neighborhood health centers, and community action programs. An impetus to antipoverty programs, it also incorporated urban and rural community action programs and assistance to small businesses and work experience programs.

## Older Americans Act of 1965 (Public Law 89-73)

The **Older Americans Act** was passed to provide assistance in the development of programs to help older Americans. It provided grants to states for community planning and services and for training and research in the field of gerontology and aging. It established the Administration on Aging, which is now part of the Department of Health and Human Services. This act gave national attention to the needs of the elderly, established state and local agencies on aging, and facilitated the delivery of services to older Americans. It is discussed extensively in Chapter 19.

## National Environmental Policy Act of 1969 (Public Law 91-190)

The **National Environmental Policy Act** is one of the best known and most significant pieces of U.S. environmental health legislation. It established national environmental policy and authorized formation of the Environmental Protection Agency (EPA). Environmental health legislation is discussed in Chapter 6.

## Occupational Safety and Health Act of 1970 (Public Law 91-956)

The **Occupational Safety and Health Act** is the most comprehensive piece of legislation on occupational health and safety in the United States. Championed by organized labor, its intent is to protect the health of the worker, and it made worker health a public concern. The United States was the last major industrial nation to enact such a law. This act is discussed in depth in Chapter 21.

## Rehabilitation Act of 1973 (Public Law 93-112)

The Vocational Rehabilitation Act of 1920 (Public Law 66-236) was an outgrowth of the health care needs evidenced by veterans after World War I and was a forerunner of the 1973 act. The **Rehabilitation Act** replaced the 1920 act but retained its major components. This act extended and revised the authorization of grants to states for vocational rehabilitation services, emphasized services to persons with severe disabilities, expanded federal responsibilities and training programs, defined services necessary for rehabilitation programs, established the National Architectural and Transportation Barriers Board to enforce legislation designed to remove architectural barriers for persons who are severely disabled, and began affirmative action programs to facilitate employment for them. This act is discussed further in Chapter 18.

## Education for All Handicapped Children Act of 1975 (Public Law 94-142)

The **Education for All Handicapped Children Act** amended the Education of the Handicapped Act (Public Law 90-247). Through it the federal government took an active role in ensuring the educational rights of people who are disabled. The law helps provide free, public education for children who are disabled (see Chapters 16 and 20). Before its passage, many American children had been denied access to the public educational system because they were disabled.

## Stewart B. McKinney Homeless Assistance Act of 1994 (Public Law 100-77)

The **Stewart B. McKinney Homeless Assistance Act** dealt with the increasing problem of homelessness in America and provided urgently needed assistance to improve the lives of the homeless, with special emphasis on elderly persons, the disabled, and families with children. It established the Interagency Council on the Homeless, Emergency Food and Shelter Program National Board, Emergency Food and Shelter Grants, Supportive Housing Demonstration Program, Primary Health Services and Substance Abuse Services Grant Program, and Food Assistance for the Homeless Food Stamp Program. It authorized emergency food supplies for the homeless, HUD programs for emergency shelter, supportive housing, programs for primary health care, substance abuse services, community mental health care, adult education for the homeless, education for homeless children and youth, job training for the homeless, and studies of homelessness among youth and Native Americans.

## Individuals with Disabilities Education Act of 1990 (Public Law 101-476)

This act was formerly known as the Education for All Handicapped Children Act (just discussed). The **Individuals with Disabilities Education Act** mandates a free and appropriate public education for all children and youth with disabilities. Supreme Court decisions relating to this act have mandated that for certain services and benefits a noncategorical rather than a disease-specific approach be applied, which means that children with serious disabilities will not be denied services even when their specific disease or condition is not specified on an eligibility list.

## Americans with Disabilities Act of 1990 (Public Law 101-336)

The Americans with Disabilities Act was signed into law on July 26, 1990. The act is one of the most significant pieces of legislation in this country to help guarantee the rights of the nation's 43 million disabled citizens. It includes a new definition of disability and helped ensure equal access and opportunity in employment, transportation, education, public accommodations, and telecommunications. This landmark act increased the opportunity for people who are disabled to be integrated into the mainstream of society. It is further discussed in Chapter 18.

## Preventive Health Amendments of 1992 (Public Law 102-531)

The Preventive Health Amendments amended the Public Health Service Act of 1944. It mandated major federal involvement in preventive health and primary prevention activities. It changed the name of the Centers for Disease Control to Centers for Disease Control and Prevention (CDC). The act authorized prevention programs, including injury control; lead poisoning; preventable infertility from sexually transmitted diseases; vaccination services; screening and detection programs for breast, cervical, and prostate cancer; and international cooperation in preventive health measures. Further, the act provided additional services in Migrant Health Centers and established the National Foundation for the Centers for Disease Control and Prevention. The purpose of the foundation is to promote the public's health and support and implement prevention activities.

## Family and Medical Leave Act of 1993 (Public Law 103-5)

The Family and Medical Leave Act requires covered employers to provide up to 12 weeks (during a 1-year period) of unpaid, job-protected leave to "eligible" employees for family and medical reasons including the birth or adoption of a child; care of an ill child, spouse, or parent; or the employee's own illness. The employer must provide adequate protection of the employee's employment and health benefits during the leave. Upon return from family medical leave, most employees must be restored to their original or equivalent positions with equivalent pay and benefits; and the use of such leave cannot result in the loss of any employment benefit that accrued before the leave. The U.S. Department of Labor investigates Act violations, and employees may bring civil action against employers for violations of the law.

## State Workers' Compensation Acts

The State Workers' Compensation Acts are the oldest form of government health and welfare insurance in this country. The first state act was legislated in 1911, and by 1948 all states had such acts. The federal government provides workers' compensation benefits for federal employees. Workers' compensation programs vary greatly from state to state in the amount of cash and health care benefits provided. State workers' compensation laws are usually administered by the state labor department or an independent workers' compensation agency. Workers' compensation is discussed in Chapter 5.

## SUMMARY

The Healthy People Initiative and numerous pieces of legislation have worked toward promoting the public's health in the United States. The Healthy People Initiative is a dynamic, ongoing process that will be with us for decades to come. Its focus areas and objectives guide public health activities for the nation. Legislation enables many health and welfare programs. The federal government was slow to get involved in such legislation and the Social Security Act of 1935 signaled federal involvement in this arena. The Social Security Act and the Public Health Service Act remain two of the most important pieces of health and welfare legislation in the United States. Knowledge of health and welfare policy and legislation and the Healthy People Initiative is essential when nursing a community.

## CRITICAL THINKING
*exercise*

This chapter gives community health nurses an overview of the Healthy People Initiative and health and welfare legislation in the United States. Think in terms of one of the *Healthy People 2010* focus areas. Considering the needs in your community, what type of health legislation would assist your community in meeting its health needs in this focus area?

*We are indebted to Professor Dorothy Donabedian, colleague and friend, whose efforts stimulated both student and faculty awareness of the health and welfare systems as they apply to community health nursing practice. Her enthusiasm, encouragement, and suggestions will forever be greatly appreciated.*

## REFERENCES

American Public Health Association (APHA): *Healthy communities 2000: model standards. Guidelines for community attainment of the year 2000 national health objectives*, ed 3, Washington, DC, 1991, APHA.

Association of State and Territorial Directors of Nursing: *Public health nursing. A partner for healthy populations*, Washington, DC, 2000, American Nurses Publishing.

Association of State and Territorial Health Officials [ASTHO]: *Public health-managed care collaborations. ASTHO access brief*, Washington, DC, 1999, ASTHO.

Centers for Disease Control and Prevention (CDC): Ten great public health achievements—United States, 1900-1999. In Lee PR, Estes CL, editors: *The nation's health*, ed 6, Boston, 2001, Jones and Bartlett.

Coll BD: *Perspectives in public welfare: a history*, Washington, DC, 1969, US Government Printing Office.

Committee on the Costs of Medical Care: *Medical care for the American people*, Chicago, 1932, University of Chicago Press.

Corso LC, Wiesner PJ, Halverson PK, et al.: Using the essential services as a foundation for performance measurement and assessment of local public health systems, *J Public Health Management Practice* 6(5):1-18, 2000.

Davis M, Fields B: Healthy People 2010: a resource for health, *Tenn Nurse* 63(4):17-18, 2000.

Forgotson EH: 1965: the turning point in health law—1966 reflections, *Am J Public Health* 57(6):934-946, 1967.

Gebbie KM: Who's minding the public health store, *J Public Health Management Practice* 6(1):vii-viii, 2000.

Gerber DE, McGuire SL: Understanding contemporary health and welfare services: the Social Security Act of 1935 and the Public Health Service Act of 1944, *Nurs Outlook* 43:266-272, 1995.

Health Resources and Services Administration (HRSA): *Child health USA 2000*, Washington, DC, 2000, US Government Printing Office.

Institute of Medicine—Committee for the Study of the Future of Public Health: *The future of public health*, Washington, DC, 1988, National Academy Press.

Lee PR, Estes CL: *The nation's health*, Boston, 2001, Jones and Bartlett.

Mahan CS: A bold new future for public health or implementing the "Alexander Haig" idea, *J Public Health Management Practice* 6(1):73-77, 2000.

McGuire SL, Nalle M: Healthy People Initiative: an introduction, *Tenn Nurse* 63(4):11-12, 2000.

Milne TL: Strengthening local public health practice: a view to the new millennium, *J Public Health Management Practice* 6(1):61-66, 2000.

Novick LF: A framework for public health administration and practice. In Novick LF, Mays GP editors: *Public health administration: principles for population-based management*, Gaithersburg, Mass, 2001, Aspen.

Office of Disease Prevention and Health Promotion (ODPHP), *Core public health functions project: public health in America*, Washington, DC, 1999, US Government Printing Office.

Pearson TA, Spencer M, Jenkins P: Who will provide preventive services? The changing relationships between medical care systems and public health agencies in health care reform, *J Public Health Management Practice* 1(1):16-27, 1995.

Pickett G, Hanlon JJ: *Public health administration and practice*, ed 9, St Louis, 1990, Mosby.

Public Health Foundation (PHF): *Measuring expenditures for essential public health services. Executive summary*. Washington, DC, 2000, PHF. Retrieved from the internet October 20, 2000. *http://www.phf.org*

Public Health Functions Steering Committee Members: *Public Health in America Statement, July, 1995*. Retrieved from the internet August 19, 2001. *http://www.health.gov/phfunctions/public.htm*

Public Health Practice Program Office (PHPPO): *National public health performance standards*, Atlanta, 1999, Centers for Disease Control and Prevention.

Richardson BW: *The health of nations, a review of the works of Edwin Chadwick*, vol 2, London, 1887, Longmans, Green & Co.

Robbins A, Freeman P: How organized medical care can advance public health, *Public Health Rep* 114:120-125, 1999.

Shattuck L: *Report of the Sanitary Commission of Massachusetts*, Cambridge, Mass, 1948, Harvard University Press (originally published by Dutton & Wentworth in 1850).

US Department of Health, Education, and Welfare (USDHEW): *Healthy People: the Surgeon General's report on health promotion and disease prevention*, Washington, DC, 1979, US Government Printing Office.

US Department of Health and Human Services (USDHHS): *Promoting health/preventing disease: objectives for the nation*, Washington, DC, 1980, US Government Printing Office.

US Department of Health and Human Services (USDHHS): *The 1990 health objectives for the nation: a midcourse review*, Washington, DC, 1986, US Government Printing Office.

US Department of Health and Human Services (USDHHS): *Healthy people 2000: national health promotion and disease prevention objectives, full report, with commentary*, Washington, DC, 1991, US Government Printing Office.

US Department of Health and Human Services (USDHHS): *Healthy People 2000: midcourse review and 1995 revisions*, Washington, DC, 1995, US Government Printing Office.

US Department of Health and Human Services (USDHHS): *The public health workforce: an agenda for the 21st century. Full report of the Public Health Functions Project*, Washington DC, 1997, USDHHS.

US Department of Health and Human Services (USDHHS): *Healthy people 2010, conference edition*, in two volumes, Washington DC, 2000, US Government Printing Office.

US Public Health Service (USPHS): *For a healthy nation: returns on investment in public health*, Washington, DC, 1994, USDHHS.

## SELECTED BIBLIOGRAPHY

Aday LA, Quill BE: A framework for assessing practice-oriented scholarship in schools of public health, *J Public Health Management Practice* 6(1):38-46, 2000.

Barry MA: Can performance standards enhance accountability for public health, *J Public Health Management Practice* 6(5):78-84, 2000.

Berkowitz B: Collaboration for health improvement: models for state, community, and academic partnerships, *J Public Health Management Practice* 6(1):67-72, 2000.

Bialek R: Building the science base for public health practice, *J Public Health Management Practice* 6(5):51-58, 2000.

Dower C, Finocchio L: Strengthening the links between the public health community and health professions regulation, *Public Health Rep* 114:421-426, 1999.

Gebbie KM: State public health laws: an expression of constituency expectations, *J Public Health Management Practice* 6(2):46-54, 2000.

Hanlon JJ, Rogers F, Rosen G: A bookshelf on the history and philosophy of public health, *Am J Public Health* 50(4):445-458, 1960.

Health Resources Administration: *Health in America: 1776-1976*, Washington, DC, 1976, United States Public Health Service.

Keck CW: Lessons learned from an academic health department, *J Public Health Management Practice* 6(1):47-52, 2000.

Quill BE, Aday LA: Toward a new paradigm for public health practice and academic partnerships, *J Public Health Management Practice* 6(1):1-3, 2000.

Ravenel MP: A *half century of public health: jubilee historical volume of the American Public Health Association*, New York, 1921, American Public Health Association.

Rothstein WG: Trends in mortality in the twentieth century. In Lee PR, Estes CL, editors: *The nation's health*, Sudbury, Mass, 2001, Jones and Bartlett, pp. 9-29.

Smillie WG: The national board of health, 1879-1883, *Am J Public Health* 33(8):925-930, 1943.

Turnock BJ: Can public health performance standards improve the quality of public health practice? *J Public Health Management Practice* 6(5):19-25, 2000.

# 5

# Organization of Health and Welfare Resources and Services

*Sandra L. McGuire*

## OBJECTIVES

*Upon completion of this chapter, the reader should be able to:*

1. State the levels and sectors into which health care is organized and delivered in the United States.
2. Understand methods of health care financing in the United States.
3. Discuss the major agencies of the U.S. Department of Health and Human Services (USDHHS).
4. Discuss federal, state, and local governmental and private health care resources and services.

5. Discuss federal, state, and local governmental and private welfare resources and services.
6. Describe patterns of organizational structure between state health authorities (SHAs) and local health departments (LHDs).
7. Discuss service functions of SHAs and LHDs.

## KEY TERMS

Administration on Aging (AoA)
Administration on Children and Families
Centers for Medicare and Medicaid Services (CMS)
Corporation for National and Community Service
Health assistance
Health care reform
Health insurance
Health maintenance organization (HMO)

Individual payment
Local health department (LHD)
Managed care
Medically indigent
National Board of Health
*Nursing's Agenda for Health Care Reform*
Official agencies
Social Security Administration (SSA)
State health authority (SHA)

State public health code
United Nations (UN)
U.S. Department of Health and Human Services (USDHHS)
U.S. Public Health Service (USPHS)
Voluntary agencies
Welfare assistance
Welfare insurance
World Health Organization (WHO)

There are great disparities among Americans in regard to access to health care, and reducing this disparity has become a national health goal (see Chapter 4). Comprehensive health services exist in the United States, but they are unequally distributed, fragmented, and expensive. Amazingly, the average life expectancy of Americans continues to increase, the death rate is historically low, and the infant mortality rate continues to decline. However, compared to other developed nations, the United States lags behind on these and other important indicators of health. This chapter looks at strengths and needs in the U.S. health and welfare systems, the organization of health and welfare resources, and health and welfare services.

## THE U.S. HEALTH CARE SYSTEM

The United States is notable among countries of the world for its complicated policy relationships between levels of governments and its interweaving of private and public sector activity to maintain the public's health (Institute of Medicine [IOM], 1988, p. 37). Health and welfare resources and services are found at three levels of government and in

**BOX 5-1**

*Organization of U.S. Health and Welfare Resources*

> **Three Levels**
> Federal
> State
> Local
>
> **Two Sectors**
> Public (governmental)
> Private*

*Private-sector resources can be nonprofit or for-profit (proprietary) agencies.

**BOX 5-2**

*Some Interesting Facts About Health in the United States*

> • The United States spends more than $1 trillion a year on health care.
> • The United States spends more than any other industrial nation on health care.
> • Although the United States spends more on health care, it often has less to show for it. Worldwide, the United States ranks twenty-sixth in infant mortality, nineteenth in female life expectancy, and twenty-fifth in male life expectancy.
> • The United States and South Africa are the only industrialized countries without a form of national health insurance guaranteeing "health for all."
> • Forty-four million Americans do not have health insurance and millions of Americans who have health insurance are underinsured.
> • Medicare, a federal health program serving millions of older Americans, leaves them underinsured. (It does not cover the cost of things such as prescription drugs, eyeglasses, or hearing aids or long-term care).
> • Only 1% of the U.S. health care budget is spent on public health. The remainder is spent on secondary and tertiary care, making the United States a treatment rather than a prevention model of health care.
> • Failure to control rising health care spending will make it difficult, if not impossible, to bring the federal budget into balance. Americans can no longer afford their present health care.
> • Health expenditures are one of the leading causes of bankruptcy in the United States.

From Health Care Financing Administration: *1999 HCFA statistics*, Washington, DC, 2000, US Department of Health and Human Services; Health Resources and Services Administration: *Child Health USA 2000*, Washington, DC, 2000, US Government Printing Office; Leviss PS: Financing the public's health. In Novick LF, Mays GO, editors: *Public health administration. Principles for population-based management*, Gaithersburg, Md, 2001, Aspen, p. 413; Social Security Administration: *Annual statistical supplement to the Social Security Bulletin*, 1999, Washington, DC, 1999, SSA; US Department of Health and Human Services: *Healthy People 2010: conference edition*, Washington, DC, 2000, US Government Printing Office.

two sectors of the health care system in the United States (Box 5-1). Agencies in the governmental sector are often called official agencies.

Health care resources and services in the United States are often fragmented, unequally distributed, and increasingly expensive. There is little coordination between health care resources, and not all Americans have equal access to health care. The great complexity and diversity of the U.S. health care delivery system present problems for nurses when they attempt to educate clients about health care resources and coordinate services. Some interesting facts on this system are in Box 5-2.

In the government sector, public health activities are primarily carried out by the federal Department of Health and Human Services, state health authorities (SHAs), and local health departments (LHDs). These agencies are discussed later in this chapter. Under the Constitution individual states have primary responsibility for ensuring the public's health.

The Healthy People Initiative, discussed in Chapter 4, has made ensuring accessibility to preventive health care services a national health goal. However, health care is still sought and offered in this country primarily on a treatment rather than a preventive basis. Improving access to preventive care services requires addressing patient, provider, and system barriers (United States Department of Health and Human Services [USDHHS], 2000, pp. 1-4). According to *Healthy People 2010*, *patient barriers* include lack of knowledge, skepticism about the effectiveness of prevention, lack of a primary care source, and cost of services; *provider barriers* include limited time, lack of training in prevention, lack of perceived effectiveness of preventive services, and practice environments that fail to promote prevention; and *system barriers* include lack of resources, lack of coverage or inadequate reimbursement for services, and lack of systems to track quality and outcomes of care (USDHHS, 2000).

Preventable conditions such as heart disease, cancer, stroke, injuries, human immunodeficiency virus (HIV) in-

fection, alcoholism, drug abuse, low-birth-weight infants, and communicable diseases continue to occur in the United States at great personal and economic expense. The Centers for Disease Control and Prevention (CDC) estimates that nearly half the premature deaths among Americans could be avoided by changes in individual behaviors and another 17% by reducing environmental risk (USDHHS, 1995, pp. 3-4).

More than 44 million Americans, almost 16% of the population, do not have health insurance (Health Insurance Association of America [HIAA], 1999, p. 24; USDHHS,

**BOX 5-3**

*A Look at the Uninsured and Underinsured in the United States— Who Are They?*

- Sixteen percent of the U.S. population, 44 million people, are uninsured.
- Eleven million children are uninsured (30% are Hispanic, 20% African American, 17% Asian, and 11% Caucasian).
- The poor are more likely than other socioeconomic groups to be uninsured: 25% of families with incomes of less than $25,000 are uninsured, while only 8% of families with incomes greater than $75,000 are uninsured.
- The percentages of people who are uninsured vary greatly from state to state. Minnesota and Iowa have the lowest rate at 9.3% while Texas has the highest rate at 24.5%.
- The South is the region of the country with the highest rate of people who are uninsured.
- About 86% of uninsured persons are employed workers and their families.
- A disproportionate number of minorities are uninsured.
- Young adults (18 to 24) are the age group most likely to be uninsured.
- Millions of Americans who have health insurance are underinsured because their policies do not cover preventive health services (e.g., physical examinations, immunizations), prescriptions, eyeglasses, hearing aids, dental care, or long-term care. This includes many senior citizens on Medicare.
- Because of inadequate health insurance coverage, millions of Americans could become bankrupt or suffer severe financial distress in the event of a long-term or catastrophic illness.
- No legislators are uninsured.

From Health Resources and Services Administration: *Child Health USA 2000*, Washington, DC, 2000, US Government Printing Office; National Center for Health Statistics: *Health, United States, 2000*, Hyattsville, Md, 2000, US Public Health Service; Turner C, Campbell E: Counting the uninsured using state-level hospitalization data, *Public Health Rep* 114:149-156, 1999; 44.3 million in U.S. lack health insurance, *Public Health Rep* 114:491, 1999.

2000, pp. 1-6). Older Americans have access to health insurance through Medicare. The age group most likely to be uninsured is that composed of young adults aged 18 to 24.

Although the lack of health insurance is clearly an impediment to accessing health care, having health insurance does not guarantee that health care will be adequate, accessible, or affordable (USDHHS, 2000, pp. 1-6). Millions of Americans who have health insurance are underinsured. People who are underinsured may lack insurance coverage for things such as preventive services, prescriptions, dental care, assistive devices, eyeglasses and hearing aids, and long-term care.

The percentage of Americans who are uninsured varies greatly from state to state and within demographic groups (Turner, Campbell, 1999, p. 150). Box 5-3 gives information on the uninsured and underinsured in the United States. Figure 5-1 shows the percentage of people in the United States who are uninsured by age. The United States does not have national health insurance and this contributes to millions of Americans being uninsured.

*Stop and Think About It*

Do you have health insurance? Does your health insurance cover preventive health services, prescriptions, eyeglasses, dental care, and long-term care? If not, you could be one of America's underinsured. What can we do to provide "health care for all" in the United States?

**No National Health Insurance**

The United States is the only major industrial nation in the world not to have national health insurance. President Theodore Roosevelt proposed national health insurance in 1912, but his efforts were unsuccessful (Harrington, 1989, p. 214). The United States came close to enacting national health insurance in 1938 when President Franklin D. Roosevelt called a *National Health Conference* in Washington, D.C. At the conference a national health program was discussed and Annie Goodrich, former dean of the School of Nursing at Yale University, spoke in favor of a national program and stated that the strongest agent in such a program was the nurse (Kalisch, Kalisch, 1982, pp. 137-138). Following the conference, public interest in a national health program rose, but World War II shifted national priorities to the war effort (Kalisch, Kalisch, 1982, pp. 139-140). Following the war, President Harry Truman attempted to legislate a nationwide system of health insurance stating that "the real cost of medical services and the need for them cannot be measured merely by doctors' bills and medical bills. The real cost to society is in unnecessary human suffering and the yearly loss of hundred of millions of working days" (Kalisch, Kalisch, 1982, p. 142). However, national health legislation failed to be passed.

Numerous presidents since Truman have unsuccessfully attempted to enact national health insurance legislation. As recently as 1993 President Clinton proposed the *Health Security Act*, but the act did not pass. Health care reform legislation, including proposals for national health insurance, continues to be introduced in Congress. Proposed programs have varied as to whether they would be federally or privately administered, who would be covered, what would be covered, how they would be funded, and what quality control measures would be taken. The nation is presently looking at ways to reform the health care system to decrease costs, enhance access to services, improve service coordination, make services more equitable, enhance preventive services, and achieve better health outcomes.

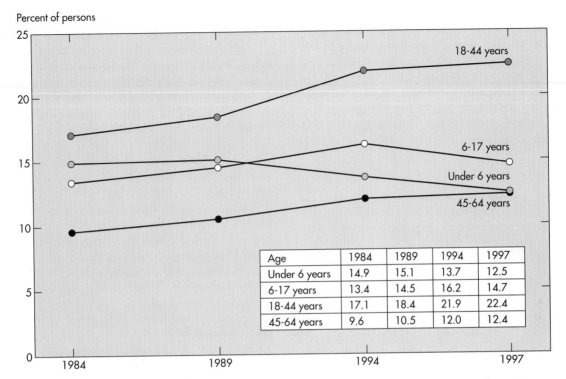

| Age | 1984 | 1989 | 1994 | 1997 |
|---|---|---|---|---|
| Under 6 years | 14.9 | 15.1 | 13.7 | 12.5 |
| 6-17 years | 13.4 | 14.5 | 16.2 | 14.7 |
| 18-44 years | 17.1 | 18.4 | 21.9 | 22.4 |
| 45-64 years | 9.6 | 10.5 | 12.0 | 12.4 |

**FIGURE 5-1** Percentage of persons under 65 years of age who are uninsured, by age. (From National Center for Health Statistics: *Health, United States, 2000,* Hyattsville, Md, 2000, US Public Health Service, p. 340).

## Health Care Facilities and the Health Care Workforce

The United States has a greater abundance of health care facilities than any other nation in the world. The first U.S. hospitals were private nonprofit institutions, primarily established for the care of the poor. The earliest of these hospitals were Pennsylvania Hospital in Philadelphia (established in 1752) and New York Hospital (established in 1771) (Needleman, 1999, p. 108). The first public hospitals, including the Marine Hospital Service, started about the same time in the late eighteenth and early nineteenth centuries (Needleman, 1999).

Today, there are 5,291 acute-care hospitals, 731 long-term hospitals, and 17,259 nursing homes in the United States (Social Security Administration [SSA], 1999, pp. 315, 319). Most acute-care hospitals in the private sector are organized as nonprofit. However, many nonprofit hospitals are converting to for-profit organizations (Needleman, 1999, p. 113). Government ownership of hospitals includes Veteran's Administration hospitals, federal and state prison hospitals, state long-term hospitals for people who are mentally ill and mentally retarded, and city and county hospitals. The U.S. government closed its Public Health Service hospitals at the end of fiscal year 1981.

The number of acute-care hospitals has been steadily declining over the last 20 years, especially in rural areas. As hospitals close, there has been a massive expansion in health care in ambulatory and community settings (Pew Health Professions Commission, 1995, p. i). This has great implications for community health nursing practice because the site of care is increasingly becoming the community.

Historically in the United States, rural and inner-city areas have had a significantly smaller health workforce than suburban areas, and affluent areas have had more health care resources than areas where there are high levels of poverty. The government offers educational and financial incentives to health-professions students and practitioners who agree to serve in areas with shortages of health care personnel.

Almost 12 million people are employed in health care occupations in the United States (National Center for Health Statistics [NCHS], 2000, p. 303). Health care is one of the nation's biggest businesses, and employment in the health care industry is growing more rapidly than civilian employment in general. For every 10,000 Americans there are approximately 27 physicians, 81 registered nurses, 6 dentists, 7 pharmacists, and 11 optometrists in practice today (NCHS, 2000, p. 308). There are almost 2.5 million registered nurses in the United States, but many areas are suffering nursing shortages. There is a great need for public health professionals (Pew Health Professions Commission, 1995).

## Health Care Cost

Health care in the United States is disproportionately inflationary. Despite decades of policy aimed at reducing health care costs, U.S. health care spending increases every year. The rise in national health expenditures from 1940 to 2000 is shown in Table 5-1. Health care spending has reached more than $1 trillion yearly in the United States. This spending includes approximately $585 billion in private spending and $507 billion in public spending (HIAA, 1999, p. 11). Public spending includes $367 billion of federal monies and $140 billion of state and local government funds (HIAA, 1999).

The United States spends more on health care than any other country in the world and frequently has fewer positive health outcomes. Life expectancy in the United States lags behind many industrial nations, and the United States ranks twenty-second in infant mortality (NCHS, 2000). Figure 5-2 compares health expenditures of the United States and selected countries related to gross domestic product (GDP). Most developed nations have been able to stabilize their health spending at less than 10% of their GDP and with a much lower per capita cost.

Rising health expenditures have placed an increased burden on federal, state, and local government budgets. Failure to control overall health care costs will make it difficult, if not impossible, to bring the federal budget into balance. Millions of Americans cannot afford even basic health care services. Health care reform measures need to be enacted to contain costs.

## Health Care Reform

Americans are taking a serious look at their health care system, and most Americans believe that health care reform is needed. In 1993 President Clinton's *Health Security Act* proposed a national health program. That legislation did not pass. Single-payor national health programs such as Canada's also have been proposed but have not been legislated.

### TABLE 5-1

*National Health Expenditures—United States*

| YEAR | (ROUNDED TO NEAREST BILLION) | PER CAPITA | PERCENT OF GNP |
|------|------------------------------|------------|----------------|
| 1940 | $4 | $29 | 4 |
| 1950 | $13 | $80 | 4.5 |
| 1960 | $27 | $141 | 5.1 |
| 1970 | $74 | $341 | 7.1 |
| 1980 | $251 | $1052 | 8.9 |
| 1990 | $697 | $2689 | 12.2 |
| 2000 (projected) | $1616 | $5712 | 16.4 |

From National Center for Health Statistics: *Health, United States, 2000,* Hyattsville, Md, 2000, US Public Health Service, p. 321.

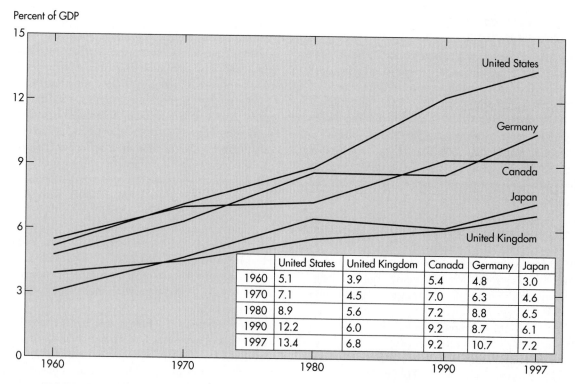

Percent of GDP

|  | United States | United Kingdom | Canada | Germany | Japan |
|------|------|------|------|------|------|
| 1960 | 5.1 | 3.9 | 5.4 | 4.8 | 3.0 |
| 1970 | 7.1 | 4.5 | 7.0 | 6.3 | 4.6 |
| 1980 | 8.9 | 5.6 | 7.2 | 8.8 | 6.5 |
| 1990 | 12.2 | 6.0 | 9.2 | 8.7 | 6.1 |
| 1997 | 13.4 | 6.8 | 9.2 | 10.7 | 7.2 |

**FIGURE 5-2** Health expenditures as a percentage of gross domestic product: selected countries. (From National Center for Health Statistics: *Health, United States, 2000,* Hyattsville, Md, 2000, US Public Health Service, p. 321).

State governments have felt the need to establish reforms because they play a major role in financing and providing health care. States are developing plans to reduce health care costs while at the same time providing more state residents with access to health care coverage.

The American Public Health Association (APHA) championed the platform of "health care for all" in the United States by the year 2000, but that year has come and gone. The American Nurses Association (ANA) has developed a national health care agenda, *Nursing's Agenda for Health Care Reform,* that advocates access, quality, and services at affordable costs (ANA, 1991). The agenda has been endorsed by more than 40 nursing organizations and calls for (1) a basic core of essential health care services available to everyone (universal coverage); (2) a restructured health care system focusing on consumers and their health, with services to be delivered in convenient sites by the most appropriate provider; (3) use of primary care providers, including nurse practitioners, clinical nurse specialists, and certified nurse midwives; and (4) a shift from the predominant focus on illness and cure to an orientation toward wellness and care (ANA, 1991). Nursing is promoting new models of health care delivery that emphasize wellness and care versus illness and cure. Nurses must carefully monitor all proposed national health programs to ensure that they actually provide the services.

The Pew Health Professions Commission (1995) examined characteristics that are needed to address the nation's health concerns. The characteristics of this health care system are given in Box 5-4. In addition the Commission predicted that this evolving system would be more accountable to consumers of health services; more responsive to the needs of enrolled populations; more reliant on outcomes data; less focused on treatment; and more concerned with education, prevention, and management.

To date, managed competition, or "managed care," has been a key feature of health care reform. However, managed care has not always met the expectations of what it proposes to provide. Serious concerns have arisen about the scope and quality of services, as well as ethical concerns about such issues as health care rationing. Managed care is both a structure and a process. From a structural perspective, managed care establishes organizational and financing mechanisms for delivery of services. Managed care as a case management process is discussed in Chapter 10.

## Managed Care

There is no universally accepted definition of **managed care,** and the term is used to refer to a variety of prepayment "capitation" plans. This differed from the traditional "fee-for-service" system in which health care services were paid for as billed and the provider of care set the fee schedule. *Capitation* is the acceptance of a prepaid, per-person payment for specified health services. Box 5-5 provides some information on managed care and Chapter 10 discusses the managed care process.

After failed efforts to enact national health insurance in the 1990s, managed care gained impetus as a method of controlling health care costs. It soon became a national strategy for ensuring comprehensive, quality care at affordable cost. An important part of the managed care mission was to keep people healthy, and most managed care plans offer extensive coverage for preventive health services.

Managed care actually began in the United States as early as the 1930s when prepaid group plans began to emerge. These plans provided a focus on prevention and covered many preventive services (e.g., physical examinations and

---

**BOX 5-4**

### *Characteristics of the Emerging Health Care System*

Orientation toward health
Population perspective
Intensive use of information
Focus on the consumer
Knowledge of treatment outcomes
Constrained resources
Coordination of services
Reconsideration of human values
Expectations of accountability
Growing interdependence

From Pew Health Professions Commission: *Critical challenges: revitalizing the health professions for the twenty-first century,* San Francisco, 1995, UCSF Center for the Health Professions, p. 2.

---

**BOX 5-5**

### *A Look at Managed Care*

**Theory**
Clients receive care through a single "seamless" system as they move from wellness to sickness back to wellness again. Continuity of care, prevention, and early diagnosis are stressed.

**What is Managed?**
Who: Provider network
What: Services covered
Where: Site of service
When: Duration of treatment

**How is Care Managed?**
Provider selection
Quality assurance
Care management/utilization management
Client and staff education and feedback
Financial arrangements

Modified from Gillis L, Thomas D: *Developing clinical systems for working in a managed care environment,* Washington, DC, June 7-9, 1996, Conference on Health Care for the Homeless.

immunizations) that were not usually covered under traditional, fee-for-service plans. Managed care plans historically have been characterized by the following components:

- Direct service provision to enrollees on a prepayment basis, with each enrollee paying a fixed amount regardless of the volume or expense of the services used
- Service provision through physicians, nurses, and other health care providers who are under contractual agreement with the managed care organization (Subscribers are limited to usage of the health workers employed by the plan, unless they choose a point-of-service plan [discussed later in this chapter] in which they have a different level of benefits based on their choice of a participating or nonparticipating provider.)
- Providers manage clients' care, referring them to additional services as necessary
- A defined package of benefits
- Comprehensive general practitioner services that include both inpatient and outpatient care and have an emphasis on preventive health practices
- Internal, self-regulatory mechanisms to ensure quality of care and cost control

Americans did not quickly embrace capitated health care, and managed care was initially slow in gaining momentum in this country. However, it gained great impetus after the failed health care reform efforts of the 1990s.

Almost 15% of Medicare enrollees are now in managed care plans (NCHS, 2000, p. 361). Almost 54% of the nation's Medicaid recipients are enrolled in managed care plans, and this percentage has rapidly increased in the last decade (NCHS, 2000, p. 344). States increasingly look to managed care to control rising health care costs. For example, Tennessee has 100% of its TennCare recipients in managed care plans (NCHS, 2000, p. 362).

**BOX 5-6**

*Major Methods of Health Care Financing in the United States*

---

*Individual Payment (Direct, Out-of-Pocket)*

*Health Insurance*
- Government: Medicare, Workers' Compensation
- Private: Blue Cross–Blue Shield, commercial insurance, self-insurance, health maintenance organizations (HMOs), preferred provider organizations (PPOs), and point-of-service organizations (POSs)

*Health Assistance*
- Government: Medicaid, Maternal-Child Health (MCH) Programs
- Private: Numerous services offered by voluntary, community, agencies, and individuals, such as the American Heart Association, the American Lung Association, local churches, and individual donations

---

Today more than 111 million Americans are enrolled in managed care organizations (NCHS, 2000, p. 362). Managed care is with us today and appears to be a trend in the future. However, it has not proved to be the "quick fix" to the nation's health care problems that it was hoped to be. It has continued to grow because of its popularity with insurance carriers, employers, and the government as an effective way to control health care costs. However, numerous concerns have arisen in relation to managed care (see Chapter 10).

Managed care enrollees have voiced concerns about access to services, quality of care, and whether the individual's health is given less importance than costs and profits. The following are some examples of recurrent questions: Do managed care organizations consistently act in the best interests of the client? How much will health care providers be restricted in telling clients about treatment options? Will health care providers be criticized for acting as client advocates? How ethical is it to offer bonuses to health care workers who save money for the managed care organization? Will expensive procedures be rationed? Managed care organizations have not routinely sought medically disadvantaged populations or provided services to people traditionally served by health assistance programs and public health (e.g., people who are uninsured, underinsured, and at risk groups such as people who are disabled).

There are many forms of managed care. Possibly the one most people are familiar with is the **health maintenance organization (HMO).** HMOs and other methods of health care financing are discussed later in this chapter.

## METHODS OF HEALTH CARE FINANCING IN THE UNITED STATES

The methods of health care financing in the United States are diverse and complicated. Methods of health care financing are found in both the government and private sectors. To help make this diverse system of financing clearer, a discussion of financing methods follows. Box 5-6 summarizes some major methods of health care financing in the United States. Keep in mind that future methods of financing health care in the United States may be significantly different.

### Individual Payment (Out-of-Pocket Spending)

**Individual payment** for health care services is exactly what it says—the individual pays for the health care directly out of his or her own pocket. The acronym for out-of-pocket spending, OOPS, is a fitting description. For the millions of Americans who are uninsured and underinsured, individual payment is a hard reality that often puts them at financial risk. When a person is paying for services directly, they tend to seek treatment and crisis health care rather than preventive care. Such health behaviors present serious consequences for individual, family, and community health.

Direct, out-of-pocket payment accounts for more than $20 billion each year (NCHS, 2000, p. 327). It is interesting to note that out-of-pocket payment for hospital expenses amounts to 3.4% of this amount, and almost 33% goes for nursing home care (NCHS, 2000, p. 230). Such expenditures put many families at financial risk, and many Americans file for bankruptcy each year as a result of health care costs. A form of health care financing that helps protect the individual and family from the financial risk of health care is health insurance.

## Health Insurance

Health insurance is a contractual agreement between an insurer and an insuree for the payment of specified health care costs. Most health insurance programs cover hospital, surgical costs, and major medical costs. Many insurance plans do not include preventive medical, dental, prescriptions, eyeglasses, hearing aids, health care equipment, or long-term care. Most Americans are extremely vulnerable to the cost of long-term health care and catastrophic illness. Chapter 22 examines this problem and the actions needed to correct it.

The rising costs of health insurance are prompting employers to limit the services covered. Even with health insurance, many people are involved in some form of individual payment because of insurance deductibles, premiums, co-payments/fixed payments, and uncovered expenses. A *de-*

*ductible* is a set expense that must be paid by the insuree before the insurer will reimburse for services (e.g., $500 deductible). A *premium* is the monthly amount that an insuree pays for an insurance plan. *Fixed payments* or *co-payments* are arrangements whereby only a specified amount for a health service is paid by the insurer, regardless of the cost to the client (e.g., $600 for antepartal care). *Uncovered services* are services that the insurer does not pay for, leaving payment to the insuree (e.g., prescription drugs under Medicare).

Health insurance is administered by both government and private agencies. Private health insurance programs serve the majority of the American people, whereas government programs are limited largely to serving people who are aged, disabled, and terminally ill. It has already been mentioned that we have no form of national health insurance.

GOVERNMENT HEALTH INSURANCE. Government health insurance did not exist in any significant form until 1965, when Medicare was passed as part of the Social Security Act. Two major forms of government health insurance: (1) Medicare and (2) Workers' Compensation are presented in Table 5-2. *Medicare* is a federal program created under the Social Security Act amendments of 1965, and Workers' Compensation is a state program. Publications describing Medicare include *Medicare and You*, an

---

**TABLE 5-2**

*Selected Government Health Insurance Programs*

| | |
|---|---|
| Medicare | Enacted in 1965, Medicare is a federal health insurance program for people 65 and over, and qualifying people who are disabled or terminally ill. It is the largest health insurance program in the United States, insuring almost 40 million people at a cost of almost $165 billion a year (Social Security Administration [SSA], 1999, pp. 313-314). It has two components: Medicare A and Medicare B. Medicare beneficiaries who have low-incomes and limited resources also may be eligible for Medicaid and are referred to as "dual eligibles." |
| | **MEDICARE A**<br>A mandatory, hospital insurance program, financed through Social Security contributions, Medicare A covers selected inpatient hospital care, inpatient care in a skilled nursing facility following a hospital stay, home health care, and hospice care. It sets limits on the number of hospital and extended care days covered and is subject to yearly changes in services and deductibles. |
| | **MEDICARE B**<br>Medicare B is a voluntary, supplemental medical insurance program with a monthly premium that changes regularly. In 2000 the monthly premium was $46.10. Covered services include physicians' services and selected services by other health professionals, including clinical psychologists, certified nurse anesthetists, nurse practitioners, clinical social workers, dentists, podiatrists, optometrists, and chiropractors; emergency treatment; outpatient physical therapy and speech therapy; specified equipment; and radiation therapy. It *excludes* coverage for prescription drugs, eyeglasses, dentures, hearing aids, yearly physical examinations, dental care, and routine foot care. Because of these exclusions, many persons 65 and older have obtained supplemental private health insurance, "Medigap" policies, discussed in this chapter under private health insurance.<br>**Apply at** local branches of the federal Social Security Administration. |
| Workers' Compensation | Established by state law and state administered, Workers' Compensation is funded primarily through employers. It provides medical care and cash benefits to qualifying workers who have an occupational illness or injury regardless of who is responsible for the occurrence.<br>**Apply at** State Employment Security Commission or other state office. |

**BOX 5-7**

## *Selected Types of Private Health Insurance*

### *Blue Cross–Blue Shield*

Every state has a tax-exempt, nonprofit, Blue Cross–Blue Shield (BCBS) organization that exists through specific state legislation. BCBS provides coverage to individuals and groups. Blue Cross is the hospital component, and Blue Shield is the major medical component. BCBS organizations insure almost 68 million Americans (HIAA, 1999, p. 39). The state insurance commissioner usually has powers of regulation over these programs, with rate increases being subject to public hearings and approval by the commissioner. They are allowed to contract with providers of service for agreed-upon fees, and payment is made directly to the service provider.

### *Commercial Insurance*

Commercial health insurance is provided by private, for-profit organizations. These organizations provide cover services similar to those offered under BCBS plans. Commercial insurers compete with BCBS. They contract with clients for prepaid premiums and benefits. Clients are expected to pay the service provider and are reimbursed by the insurer for the agreed-upon cost.

### *Health Maintenance Organizations*

Health maintenance organizations (HMOs) are a form of managed care and the most rapidly growing method of health insurance in the United States. The Health Maintenance Organization Act of 1973 (Public Law 93-222), an amendment to the Public Health Service Act of 1944, aided in HMO development. There are more than 650 HMOs in the United States insuring almost 67 million people (HIAA, 1999, p. 55). Figure 5-3 shows the steady increase in HMO enrollment since 1985. States with some of the highest rates of residents insured by HMOs are Oregon (47.2%), Massachusetts (44.6%), California (43.8%), Utah (40.7%), Delaware (38.8%), Maryland (38%), and New York (35.7%) (HIAA, 1999, p. 63). Medicaid and Medicare enrollees participating in HMOs are increasing. Historically, HMOs have operated on a prepayment (capitation) basis and focused on primary prevention, cost-containment, and case management. HMOs can be organized as nonprofit or for-profit but most are for-profit.

   HMOs provide a wide range of health care services for a specified group (enrolled, defined population) at a fixed, prepaid cost (capitation rate). In general, an HMO member is financially covered for health services only if the member receives them from providers participating in the plan (site-of-service restrictions) or if they are preauthorized to receive services from a provider outside the plan.

### *Preferred Provider Organizations*

Preferred provider organizations (PPOs) are a form of managed care. There are more than 2700 PPOs in the United States serving 117 million people (HIAA, 1999, p. 55). They offer the subscriber more flexibility in choosing service providers than do HMOs. These plans fall somewhere in between an HMO and traditional health insurance. In these plans a limited number of physicians (hospitals and other health care providers may be included) become "preferred providers" by contracting with an insurer who agrees to pay them to care for its subscribers on a fee-for-service basis, but at prenegotiated discount rates. Providers accept the negotiated PPO fee payment in full and do not bill clients for additional amounts. When the insuree strays from the PPO network of providers, he or she will pay more in out-of-pocket expenses.

### *Point-of-Service Plans*

Point-of-service (POS) plans are a form of managed care and sometimes referred to as HMO-PPO hybrids. They use a network of selected contracted, participating providers. Under this plan subscribers usually select a primary care physician who is responsible for managing health care and controls referrals to medical specialists (HIAA, 1999, p. 56). These plans are not as well established or used as the HMO and PPO options. For higher premiums, co-payments and/or deductibles, members can use non-POS health services.

### *Self-Insurance*

Self-insurance was stimulated by the passage of the Employee Retirement Income Security Act of 1974. Under this act, corporations and organizations can establish self-funded, nonprofit health plans and escape the taxes and regulations of state insurance laws. This is the method of insurance for more than 62 million Americans (HIAA, 1999, p. 40).

### *Medigap Insurance*

*Medigap* is voluntary, private insurance that supplements health care services not covered under Medicare A and B. It is purchased by 29 million Americans, almost 80% of those on Medicare (HIAA, 1999, pp. 19-20). The Omnibus Budget Reconciliation Act of 1990 (PL 101-508) required that Medigap policies include an open enrollment period for new Medicare beneficiaries aged 65 or older; forbade insurers to deny coverage or discriminate in the price of the policy; required that the policy could not be canceled or a renewal refused solely on the basis of the health of the policyholder; and mandated use of the same format, language, and definitions in all Medigap policies. Medigap is offered by BCBS and commercial insurance companies.

---

excellent handbook that is updated yearly and can be obtained free of charge by calling the SSA's toll-free number, 1-800-638-6833. The federal government also provides health services to veterans, federal employees, and Native Americans on reservations.

**PRIVATE HEALTH INSURANCE.** Private health insurance is provided through agencies not affiliated with the government. Employers often pay the premiums for this insurance. When premiums are not paid for by employers, the individual pays the premium, goes without insurance, or

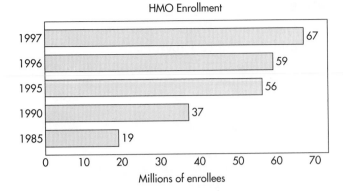

HMO Enrollment

FIGURE 5-3 Rise in HMO enrollment. (From Health Insurance Association of America (HIAA): *Source book of health insurance data, 1995,* Washington, DC, 1995, HIAA, p. 34; Health Insurance Association of America: *Source book of health insurance data, 1999,* Washington, DC, 1999, HIAA, p. 55).

may qualify for a government health insurance or assistance program.

The ancient Chinese had an interesting form of health insurance based on the custom of paying the doctor when in good health and discontinuing payment during periods of illness, and the Greeks and Romans offered some early forms of health insurance (HIAA, 1995, p. 1). In 1860 the Travelers Insurance Company of Hartford, Connecticut, offered health insurance, and by 1866 health insurance policies were being written by 60 companies in the United States (HIAA, 1999, p. 1).

In 1929 a group of teachers contracted with Baylor Hospital in Dallas, Texas, to provide specific health services at a predetermined cost (HIAA, 1999, p. 1). The monthly premium was 50¢, and the Baylor Plan offered 21 days of semiprivate care at Baylor Hospital in Dallas, Texas (Wilner, Walkley, O'Neill, 1978, pp. 138-139). Out of this plan emerged the Blue Cross–Blue Shield concept in 1939. When Blue Cross–Blue Shield started, less than 10% of the civilian population was covered by private health insurance (HIAA, 1983, p. 13). Today almost 70% of the population (almost 190 million Americans) are covered by private health insurance, and this insurance pays almost $300 billion a year in claims (HIAA, 1999, p. 11).

The most common forms of private health insurance in the United States are Blue Cross–Blue Shield, commercial insurance, self-insurance, various managed care insurance plans, and Medigap. The three major types of managed care plans are health maintenance organizations (HMOs), preferred provider organizations (PPOs), and point-of-service (POS) plans (HIAA, 1999, p. 14). These forms of private health insurance are presented in Box 5-7.

## Health Assistance

**Health assistance** programs provide services to qualifying individuals. Generally the individual does not participate in cost-sharing for the services (e.g., government programs such as Medicaid). Health assistance programs are found in

### BOX 5-8
## *Medicaid: A Health Assistance Program*

Medicaid is a health assistance program that provides health care services to America's poor. It is a state-federal cost-sharing program. The federal cost-sharing percentage for the program varies from 50% to 83%, depending on the state's economic status (SSA, 1999, p. 110). The federal government reimburses states for 100% of the cost of services provided through Indian Health Service facilities (SSA, 1999).

Almost 35 million people are enrolled in the program at a cost of more than $125 billion (SSA, 1999, p. 328). More than 15% of Medicaid recipients are enrolled in Medicaid HMOs (HIAA, 1999, p. 57).

Within broad federal guidelines each state (1) establishes its own eligibility standards; (2) determines the type, amount, duration, and scope of services; (3) sets the rate of payment for services; and (4) administers its own Medicaid program. Programs vary greatly from state to state in relation to covered services.

A state's Medicaid services must include inpatient and outpatient hospital services; prenatal care; vaccines for children; physician services; family planning services; rural health clinic services; home health care for eligible skilled nursing clients; laboratory and x-ray services; pediatric and family nurse practitioner services; nurse-midwife services; and early and periodic screening, diagnosis, and treatment (EPSDT) for children under 21 years old (SSA, 1999, p. 109). States have the option to provide other services. For the medically indigent, Medicaid pays for skilled nursing home care.

Individuals are generally eligible for Medicaid if they are on Temporary Assistance for Needy Families (TANF) or Supplemental Security Income (SSI). Other eligibles are pregnant women and children under age 6 whose family income is at or below 133% of the federal poverty level (FPL), recipients of adoption or foster care assistance under the Social Security Act, and children under age 19 in families with incomes at or below the FPL (SSA, 1999, p. 107). States have the option of providing services to other groups.

Some people are "dual eligibles" which means they qualify for both Medicaid and Medicare. The state's Medicaid program can pay the Medicare B premiums for such individuals. Medicaid supplements Medicare coverage with services such as prescriptions, hearing aids, eyeglasses, and long-term care. Unfortunately, many people eligible for this dual status are not participating because they are not aware that they are eligible.

**Apply at** local offices of the State Department of Human or Social Services.

the public and private sectors. The major governmental health assistance program is *Medicaid.* Medicaid is discussed in Box 5-8.

Medicaid was created by the same 1965 Social Security Act amendments that created Medicare. It is a federal-state entitlement program that provides health services for the **medically indigent** (i.e., people who are unable to meet their health care expenses and who fall within specified economic guidelines). Other government health assistance programs include maternal-child health and nutrition programs.

*Maternal-child health* (MCH) programs traditionally have been carried out by LHDs and voluntary agencies to meet the needs of high-risk mothers and children. Such programs include the *Supplemental Food Program for Women, Infants, and Children (WIC)*, health care services, and the *Children's Health Insurance Program (CHIP)*. CHIP is discussed in Chapter 16. The monies appropriated for these programs now are often available through federal block grants. Health assistance services of state and LHDs are discussed extensively later in the chapter.

Health assistance in the private sector is primarily of a voluntary, nonprofit nature. This volunteerism is prevalent, with many people donating time, money, and effort to help procure health services for others. Candy stripers in the local hospital, volunteer respite workers, and readers for the blind are examples of volunteers who are helping clients. The dedicated leadership, financial support, and personal service of volunteers and voluntary agencies have greatly aided the health care delivery system in this country. Service groups such as the American Cancer Society, American Diabetes Association, American Heart Association, Associations for Retarded Citizens, Lions' Clubs, Shriners, Rotarians, Knights of Columbus, and church groups often provide health assistance to those in need.

## THE U.S. WELFARE SYSTEM

The primary task of the welfare system is to alleviate the economic hardships of the most disadvantaged. Welfare programs reflect an effort to ensure a basic standard of living and to promote social well-being. Like the health care financing system, the welfare system is complex. In this text, programs are arbitrarily divided into welfare insurance and assistance programs. The benefits provided under insurance (contributory) programs have historically been better than those provided under assistance (noncontributory) programs. Box 5-9 outlines governmental welfare insurance and assistance programs. Private assistance programs generally are administered locally and vary greatly from community to community. Many people who use welfare assistance programs live in poverty.

### Poverty

Poverty is a serious health problem. Poor health status is strongly associated with low family income (Figure 5-4). Almost 36 million Americans, 14% of the population, have incomes below the poverty level (SSA, 1999, p. 151). Almost 14 million American children live in poverty (SSA, 1999). There is a great discrepancy in poverty among ethnic groups in the United States. Approximately 36% of African-American children, 34% of Hispanic children, and

### BOX 5-9

*Government Welfare Insurance and Assistance Programs*

**Welfare Insurance**
- Old Age, Survivors, and Disability Insurance (OASDI)
- Unemployment Insurance
- Workers' Compensation

**Welfare Assistance**
- Temporary Assistance to Needy Families (TANF)
- Supplemental Security Income (SSI)
- Food Stamps
- Supplemental Food Program for Women, Infants, and Children (WIC)
- General Assistance
- Subsidized Housing

17% of Asian children live in poverty, while only 10% of Caucasian children do (poverty statistics are further discussed in Chapter 13) (NCHS, 2000, p. 125).

In all states except Alaska and Hawaii, a family of one is considered living in poverty if annual family income is $8240 or less. This amount is added to in increments of $2820 for each additional household member. So, for a family of four, a yearly income of $16,700 or less would be considered living in poverty (Alaska: 1 person family = $10,320/increment of $3,520; Hawaii: 1 person family = $9,490/increment of $3,240) (SSA, 1999, p. 155).

### Welfare Insurance

Welfare insurance programs are contributory. The individual or someone on behalf of the individual, such as the employer or the government, pays a premium, and benefits are awarded by virtue of these past premium contributions. Welfare insurance programs are found in both the government and private sectors.

GOVERNMENT WELFARE INSURANCE. With the passage of the Social Security Act in 1935 (see Chapter 4), the federal government became extensively involved in providing government welfare insurance programs. This Social Security Act is the basis for many federal welfare insurance programs. State governments also legislate welfare insurance in the form of workers' compensation and unemployment insurance.

*Old Age, Survivors, and Disability Insurance (OASDI).* Old Age, Survivors, and Disability Insurance is a Social Security Act program and is the major form of federal welfare insurance. OASDI is commonly called "Social Security." A history of the term *Social Security* is given in Box 5-10.

OASDI provides cash benefits to a qualified worker and his or her family when the worker retires in old age, becomes severely disabled, or dies. It is the largest income maintenance program in the country. Presently more than

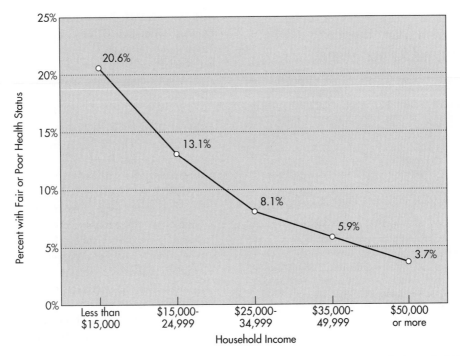

**FIGURE 5-4** Percentage of persons with fair or poor perceived health status by household income, United States. (From US Department of Health and Human Services: *Healthy People 2010: conference edition*, Washington, DC, 2000, US Government Printing Office, p. 11).

**BOX 5-10**

## *Origin of the Term "Social Security"*

Abraham Epstein is the person generally recognized as introducing the term "Social Security." He was a national leader in the social welfare movement in the first half of the twentieth century. Epstein authored three books. The most well known is *Insecurity, a Challenge to America* (1933).

From 1918 to 1927 Epstein served as the research director of the Pennsylvania Commission on Old Age Pensions and was instrumental in having the state adopt an old-age assistance law in 1923. When Epstein realized that the Pennsylvania Commission would not be continued, he decided to establish a national organization to boost public support for social legislation such as state old-age assistance and pension programs. In 1927 he founded the American Association for Old Age Security. In 1933 he changed the name of his organization to the American Association for Social Security.

When Epstein was asked by Wilbur Cohen, later Secretary of the Department of Health, Education, and Welfare,

why he chose the term "Social Security," he explained that at the time Germany was using the term "Social Insurance" and England was using the term "Economic Security," and he did not want to use either of these. Epstein responded that he wanted a term to convey a program that not only provided economic security for workers, but the type of security that would promote the welfare of society as a whole. In a letter to Cohen, Epstein stated, "I was convinced that no improvement in the conditions of labor can come except as the security of the people as a whole is advanced."

It was Epstein's term "Social Security" that became the title of one of our country's landmark pieces of legislation, the Social Security Act of 1935. It is a term that has become a household word and denotes economic security to millions of Americans.

From Origin of the term "Social Security," *Social Security Bulletin* 55(1)63-53, 1992. Original article based on letters:
1. Cohen to Abraham Epstein, March 3, 1941, Abraham Epstein Papers, Columbia University Library, New York.
2. Epstein to Wilbur J. Cohen, March 4, 1941, Abraham Epstein Papers, Columbia University Library, New York.
3. Frankel to Wilbur J. Cohen, October 1949, Abraham Epstein Papers, Columbia University Library, New York.

44 million Americans receive OASDI benefits. Eligibility is based on the amount of time worked and the amount of contributions made to the program. OASDI is applied for at local offices of the federal SSA.

Employers, employees, and the self-employed pay mandatory contributions into OASDI. The maximum amount of taxable earnings and worker contribution is updated each year. Employer and worker contributions to

**TABLE 5-3**

## Maximum Annual Worker Taxable OASDI Earnings and Annual Contributions

| YEAR | MAXIMUM ANNUAL WORKER TAXABLE EARNINGS | MAXIMUM WORKER ANNUAL CONTRIBUTIONS |
|------|------|------|
| 1939 | $3,000 | $30.00 |
| 1949 | $3,000 | $30.00 |
| 1959 | $4,800 | $120.00 |
| 1969 | $7,800 | $290.55 |
| 1979 | $22,900 | $991.59 |
| 1989 | $48,000 | $2,654.40 |
| 1999* | $72,600 | $3,884.10 |

From Social Security Administration: *Annual statistical supplement to the Social Security Bulletin, 1995,* Washington, DC, 1995, SSA, p. 51; Social Security Administration: *Annual statistical supplement to the Social Security Bulletin, 1999,* Washington, DC, 1999, SSA, pp. 36-37.
*Since 1999, the maximum annual worker taxable earnings are based on automatic adjustment in proportion to increases in the average wage level.

**TABLE 5-4**

## Projected Year of Retirement with Full OASDI Benefits:

| If you are an OASDI eligible worker who becomes 62 in: | | |
|------|------|------|
| 2000 | you can retire with | 65 and 2 months |
| 2001 | full benefits at | 65 and 4 months |
| 2002 | | 65 and 6 months |
| 2003 | | 65 and 8 months |
| 2004 | | 65 and 10 months |
| 2005-2016 | | 66 |
| 2017 | | 66 and 2 months |
| 2018 | | 66 and 4 months |
| 2019 | | 66 and 6 months |
| 2020 | | 66 and 8 months |
| 2021 | | 66 and 10 months |
| 2022 and later | | 67 |

From Social Security Administration: *Annual statistical supplement to the Social Security Bulletin, 1999,* Washington, DC, 1999, The Administration, p. 62.

OASDI have steadily increased over the years. Table 5-3 illustrates the maximum annual worker taxable earnings and contributions to OASDI for selected years. Table 5-4 indicates when a worker can retire with full old-age benefits.

The U.S. Social Security system is coordinated with the social security systems of various countries to help ensure benefits to people who have lived and worked in other nations. The United States presently has Social Security agreements with nations including: Austria, Belgium, Canada, Finland, France, Germany, Greece, Ireland, Italy, Luxembourg, Netherlands, Norway, Portugal, Spain, Sweden, Switzerland, and the United Kingdom.

OASDIs component parts—old age insurance, survivors insurance, and disability insurance—are presented in Table 5-5 along with the state welfare insurance programs of *Workers' Compensation* and *Unemployment Insurance.* Figure 5-5 gives the average monthly benefits for all OASDI programs. Figure 5-6 illustrates OASDI beneficiaries by type of benefit.

PRIVATE WELFARE INSURANCE. Private welfare insurance, often in the form of income replacement insurance, is available through a number of agencies. Major forms of private welfare insurance include retirement and disability insurance. Many of these programs are obtained through the workplace, whereas others are purchased individually by the consumer. Millions of American workers are covered by private retirement insurance through their place of employment. The Retirement Income Security Act of 1974 helped safeguard the financial integrity of these private retirement programs.

## Welfare Assistance Programs

**Welfare assistance** programs are noncontributory or minimally contributory programs for qualifying indigent individuals, and they provide cash and service benefits (e.g., food, shelter, and clothing). They exist largely as a result of state and federal legislation and are locally administered. Once a person's eligibility for a categorical government welfare assistance program has been determined, he or she usually receives cash benefits, social service benefits, and medical benefits through Medicare or Medicaid. Welfare assistance programs include both government and private programs.

GOVERNMENT WELFARE ASSISTANCE. Government welfare assistance programs provide subsistence benefits for those without other resources. Applicants often apply for these programs at local offices of the State Department of Human of Social Services or the federal Social Security Administration, depending on the program. Information that is often requested of applicants is given in Box 5-11. Some major categorical government welfare assistance programs include *Temporary Assistance to Needy Families (TANF); Supplemental Security Income (SSI);* food stamps; *Supplemental Food for Women, Infants, and Children (WIC);* and *General Assistance.* These programs are presented in Table 5-6.

The federal government is involved in numerous other assistance programs. Several of these are nutrition programs including school lunch programs, school breakfast programs, school milk programs, needy family commodity foods, and food programs for the elderly. These programs provide millions of meals each year and improve the nutritional status of Americans. In addition, state and local governments offer a number of other welfare services

**TABLE 5-5**

## *Government Welfare Insurance Programs*

| | |
|---|---|
| Old Age Insurance (OAI) | *Old Age Insurance (OAI)* is the retirement component of OASDI and commonly is called "Social Security." Almost 31 million people receive OAI and the average monthly benefit for a retired worker is $780 (SSA, 1999, p. 13). Social Security has kept millions of older Americans out of poverty, provides more than half the income for 60% of beneficiaries, and is a source of income for 90% of all older Americans (SSA, 1999, pp. 20-21). |
| | Full Social Security retirement benefits have historically begun at age 65. However, the age is gradually being raised to 67. People can start to receive benefits as early as age 62, but receiving benefits early permanently reduces the monthly cash benefits. Financial incentives accrue if a worker delays retirement past age 65. A recent change in Social Security legislation now allows a person to work after beginning retirement and still collect full Social Security retirement benefits. The Social Security Administration publishes a free booklet, *A Guide to Social Security Retirement Benefits,* which can be obtained free of charge by calling 1-800-772-1213. |
| | **Apply at** local offices of the federal Social Security Administration, or potential retirees can now apply online at *http://www.ssa.gov/applytoretire* or by phone at 1-800-772-1213. |
| Survivor's Insurance (SI) | The *Survivor's Insurance* component of OASDI provides benefits to qualifying families of deceased or disabled workers. Ninety-five percent of American children and their surviving parent are eligible for these benefits. The Social Security Administration publishes a booklet, *A Guide to Social Security Survivors Benefits,* which can be obtained free of charge by calling, 1-800-772-1213. |
| | **Apply at** local offices of the federal Social Security Administration. |
| Disability Insurance (DI) | The *Disability Insurance* component of OASDI provides benefits to qualifying persons under the age of 65 on the basis of medical evaluation of the person's continued ability to work. After age 65 the disabled worker can apply for OAI. More than 3 million disabled workers receive benefits with average monthly benefits of $661.70 (SSA, 1995, p. 173). The Social Security Administration publishes a free booklet, *A Guide to Social Security Disability Benefits* that can be obtained free of charge by calling, 1-800-772-1213. |
| | **Apply at** local offices of the federal Social Security Administration. |
| Unemployment Insurance | *Unemployment Insurance* was one of the original Social Security Act programs. It is not a part of OASDI. It is a state-federal program with state administration. It provides benefits to regularly employed members of the labor force who are involuntarily unemployed and actively seeking employment. States decide what agency administers the program, the amount and duration of benefits, and eligibility criteria. |
| | To be eligible for benefits, the worker must remain registered to work and actively seek employment while collecting benefits. Most states provide a maximum of 26 weeks of benefits each year and the average length of time on the program is 14 weeks (SSA, 1999, p. 332). For workers who have exhausted state benefits, a federal program of extended benefits may be available. Cash benefits vary greatly from state to state. More than 2 million workers collect unemployment benefits each year, with an average weekly benefit amount of $200 (SSA, 1999). |
| | **Apply at** local offices of the State Employment Security Commission or other state agency. |
| Workers' Compensation | *Workers' Compensation* is established by state law and is administered by the state but is funded primarily through employers. It was presented under government health insurance (see Table 5-2) because it has both an insurance and welfare component providing both health insurance and a cash benefit to qualifying workers. |
| | It provides survivors benefits to dependents of workers whose deaths resulted from occupational illness or injury. Benefits are awarded regardless of who is at fault for the occurrence. The amount of cash benefit is related to the degree and permanence of the injury, the worker's earnings, and the number of worker's dependents. Each state sets a minimum and maximum payment range. The maximum wage replacement averages about 67% of the worker's take-home earnings. |
| | Loss of ability to work is generally a criterion for awarding benefits. If the worker is injured on the job but suffers no loss of ability to work, such as with certain types of hearing loss, the injury may not be compensable. In some states, workers may receive benefits only for a specified period of time, and there may be waiting periods before the compensation can begin. However, if the condition appears to be permanent, most states provide for the payment of weekly benefits for life or the entire period of disability (SSA, 1995, p. 114). |
| | **Apply at** local offices of the State Employment Security Commission or other state agency. |

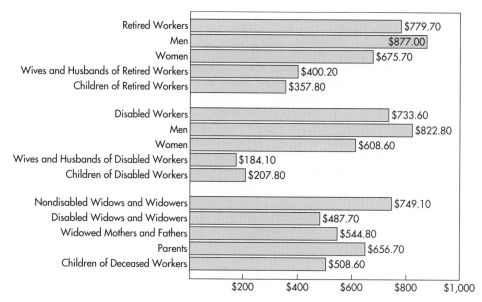

**FIGURE 5-5** Average monthly OASDI benefit amount. (From Social Security Administration: *Annual Statistical Supplement to the Social Security Bulletin, 1999,* Washington, DC, 1999, SSA, p. 18).

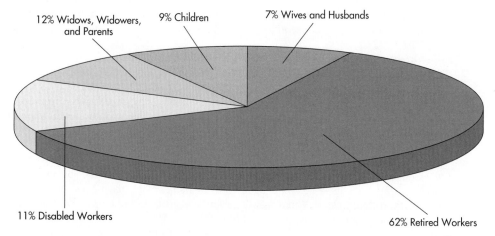

**FIGURE 5-6** OASDI beneficiaries by type of benefit. (From Social Security Administration: *Annual Statistical Supplement to the Social Security Bulletin, 1999,* Washington, DC, 1999, SSA, p. 16).

 **BOX 5-11**

*Applying for Government Welfare Assistance*

When applying for government welfare assistance an applicant is generally asked to provide some or all of the following information:
- Proof of residence
- Proof of gross income from all sources for all household members
- Record of all property, including savings accounts, checking accounts, bonds, and land owned
- Record of house payments or rent and also insurance and taxes

- Record of utility bills
- Record of current medical and dental expenses
- Birth dates and social security numbers of household members
- Records of child support and alimony
- Proof of tuition and other required educational expenses
- Records of child care payment for employment or training purposes

**TABLE 5-6**

*Selected Government Welfare Assistance Programs*

| | |
|---|---|
| Temporary Assistance to Needy Families (TANF) | TANF, formerly known as Aid to Families with Dependent Children (AFDC), is a state-federal program established by the Personal Responsibility and Work Opportunity Act of 1996 (PL 104-193), commonly known as the Welfare Reform Bill. It is state administered and provides financial assistance, funding for child care, and work opportunities for participants. Parents are helped to become self-sufficient through welfare-to-work programs and federal financial incentives are given to states that move families off their welfare roles. TANF cash benefits are provided on a *temporary* basis (5-year lifetime limit). An "employability" plan is developed for TANF families. |
| | Any U.S. citizen can apply for TANF. However, some restrictions apply regarding when legal immigrants are eligible to apply. Almost 4 million American families receive benefits from the program each year (SSA, 1999, pp. 15, 334). Monthly cash benefit amounts vary from state to state with an average benefit for a family of four of $490/month (SSA, 1999). TANF families are eligible for food stamps and Medicaid, but they must apply for them. The income of TANF families is below the poverty level and they frequently need other welfare assistance such as referrals for clothing, housing, and furniture. |
| | **Apply at** local offices of the State Department of Human or Social Services. |
| Supplemental Security Income (SSI) | SSI is federal-state assistance provided for under the Social Security Act and federally administered through the Social Security Administration. The objective for establishing this program was to develop a uniform national minimum cash income program to provide aid to the indigent aged, blind, and disabled. Almost 7 million people receive SSI each year (SSA, 1999, p. 25). |
| | The average federal SSI benefit is $500 per month for an individual and $751 per month for a couple (SSA, 1999, pp. 14, 25). The federal cash benefit is constant throughout the nation. State supplementation is available and averages about $125 (SSA, 1999, p. 14). State supplementary benefits vary and may be made directly to the beneficiary or paid through the federal Social Security Administration. |
| | Adults are usually the beneficiaries of SSI, but a child may be eligible if he or she suffers from an impairment that is expected to last a year or longer, such as mental retardation, terminal illness, or blindness. Qualifying United States citizens and legally admitted aliens are eligible. The Social Security Administration publishes a free booklet, *A Guide to the Supplemental Security Income Program*. |
| | **Apply at** local offices of the federal Social Security Administration. |
| Food Stamps | Food stamps were begun on a pilot basis in 1961 to improve the nutritional adequacy of low-income persons. The Food Stamp Act of 1964 formally established the program. It is a federal-state program under state administration; the federal sharing agency is the Department of Agriculture. The number of people participating in the program and program expenditures have decreased in recent years (SSA, 1999, p. 334). |
| | People on TANF and SSI are automatically eligible (SSA, 1999, p. 124). An eligible family of four persons receives approximately $419 per month in food stamps (SSA, 1999, p. 15). The average food stamp recipient has just a little more than $1 worth of food stamps to use for each meal ($102 per person per month). Almost 20 million Americans take part in this program at an annual cost to the government of almost $17 billion (SSA, 1999). |
| | Food stamp coupons are used like money at participating stores, and most grocery stores accept food stamps. Food stamps can be used only to purchase edible items; no imported foodstuffs, alcoholic beverages, or tobacco products can be bought with them. They must be used by the person to whom they were issued—they are not transferable. |
| | **Apply at** local offices of the State Department of Human or Social Services. |
| Supplemental Food Program for Women, Infants, and Children (WIC) | WIC is a federal nutrition and health assistance program authorized under the Child Nutrition Act of 1966 and administered at the federal level by the Food and Nutrition Service of the U.S. Department of Agriculture. Local nonprofit health and welfare agencies apply to their respective states to qualify for funds from this program, and there are almost 9000 approved local WIC sites. Most local health departments are WIC sites. |
| | WIC is designed to help pregnant and postpartum women, infants, and children up to 5 years of age who have been identified by health professionals as being at nutritional risk and who meet certain age and income requirements. The program includes food distribution, health assessment, and *mandatory* nutrition education. Participants receive vouchers that are redeemable at participating grocery stores for items such as infant formula, cereal, and juices; milk; cereals; and cheese. The WIC program has been very successful in promoting adequate nutrition and nutrition education. If a family is receiving food stamps, participation in WIC does not affect their food stamp eligibility. |

*Continued*

**TABLE 5-6—cont'd**

*Selected Government Welfare Assistance Programs*

| | |
|---|---|
| WIC—cont'd | **Apply at** local health departments, where the program is generally administered, but other community agencies can be designated WIC sites. |
| General Assistance | General assistance, or "direct assistance," is a state and locally funded and administered program offered in many states. No federal monies are involved. The program is often administered through the state Department of Human or Social Services. Assistance is usually in the form of cash benefits, vouchers, or payments to vendors. It is often the only form of government assistance available for individuals who are poor but who do not qualify for TANF, unemployment insurance, OASDI, or SSI. In many states, general assistance is limited to emergency relief (e.g., a catastrophic event such as a flood), short-term relief, and burial benefits. Any citizen can apply. Approximately 750,000 people receive general assistance in the United States each year (SSA, 1999, p. 335). **Apply at** local offices of the State Department of Human or Social Services. |

**BOX 5-12**

*Services Frequently Provided by Private Welfare Agencies*

*Individual and Family Services*
Counseling and referral services to families and children, family service agencies, adoption services, advocacy, emergency and disaster services, child day care services, and senior citizens services

*Residential Care*
Group foster homes, halfway homes, and shelters for the homeless

*Recreation and Group Work*
Such as YMCA, YWCA, Boy Scouts, and Girl Scouts

*Civic and Social Activities*
Provided by organizations such as Rotarians, Goodwill Industries, Lions Clubs, Jaycees, and churches

*Job Training and Vocational Rehabilitation*
Sheltered workshops, vocational rehabilitation agencies, and skill training centers

From Kerns WL, Glanz MP: Private social welfare expenditures, 1972-88, *Social Security Bulletin* 54(2):2-11, 1991, p. 6.

including foster care, adoption services, and facilities for people who are mentally ill and mentally retarded. The federal government also participates in housing and home assistance programs.

PRIVATE WELFARE ASSISTANCE. Following its volunteer tradition, the United States is one of the few countries in the world to offer such a magnitude of privately operated welfare resources and services. Historically, the private sector has played a significant role in the provision of welfare assistance services to local communities in the United States. Provision of such services costs private social welfare

agencies billions of dollars each year and countless volunteer hours.

A census survey involving a sample representing more than 100,000 social service agencies found that numerous services are frequently provided by private welfare agencies in the areas of individual and family services, residential care, recreation and group work, civic and social activities, and job training and rehabilitation. Examples of these services are given in Box 5-12. Most of these services involve short-term (acute) relief but do not provide long-term assistance for chronic problems.

GOVERNMENT HOUSING ASSISTANCE. Since the late 1930s the federal government has provided leadership and a commitment to providing decent, safe, sanitary, and affordable housing for all Americans in the form of public and assisted housing (SSA, 1993, p. 75). The Department of Housing and Urban Development (HUD) is the federal agency responsible for administering federal public housing programs for low-income families.

The *low-income home energy assistance program* provides eligible households with funds to meet heating and cooling costs and home energy crisis. On the federal level the program is administered by the Department of Health and Human Services. States make payments directly to eligible households or to home energy suppliers on behalf of eligible households. Payments may be provided in vouchers, cash, fuel, or prepaid utility bills. Each year Congress appropriates approximately $1 billion for the program (SSA, 1999, p. 129). This program has provided valuable assistance to many older and disabled Americans. The federal government also is involved in public and assisted housing.

*Public, low-rent housing units* are available to low-income families and people who are elderly or disabled. The units are owned, managed, and administered by a local Public Housing Agency. Rental charges are set by the federal government and are usually about 30% of the monthly adjusted income of the recipient's household.

*Rental assistance programs* are limited to very low-income families and designed to give them the opportunity to rent

**TABLE 5-7**

*Federal Government Health and Welfare Functions*

| FUNCTIONS | SELECTED ACTIVITIES |
|---|---|
| Assessment and planning | Includes a number of ongoing national assessments and collection planning of health and welfare statistics. Health planning activities include setting national health objectives and assisting states in their implementation. Stimulates debate on national health and welfare issues. |
| Assurance | Involves periodic evaluation of progress toward national health objectives and monitoring of the quality and effectiveness of national public health programs. Provides technical assistance and funds to states and localities to promote health and welfare. |
| Policy development | Includes enacting the necessary health and welfare legislation and making adequate appropriations for implementing legislative mandates. |
| Personal and community health | Carries out extensive personal and community health services, including services in the Healthy People 2010 priority areas, providing direct services to special population groups (e.g., Native Americans, Native Hawaiians, military personnel, rural Americans, and migrant workers). Supports programs such as VISTA, community mental health centers, rural health centers, and senior citizen centers. |
| International health and welfare | Is a member of and supports international health and welfare organizations including the United Nations, WHO, and the Peace Corps. Participates in foreign aid, international disaster relief, environmental health, and world peace and human rights activities. |
| Education and training | Supports knowledge development and dissemination. Subsidizes grants and loans for education and training of health and welfare professionals. Provides grants-in-aid to schools of public health and is involved in health education and public health programs. Offers numerous health and welfare publications at low or no cost to the general public. Maintains numerous national clearinghouses, which distribute educational materials, and the U.S. Government Printing Office. |
| Research | Subsidizes research for the advancement of health and welfare. The National Institutes of Health conduct rigorous research programs and collaborate on international research. The National Institute of Nursing Research is one of these national institutes. |

housing suitable to their needs. The family is free to locate a suitable dwelling unit that meets program housing quality standards. The family usually pays about 30% of their income toward the rent.

*Housing programs for the homeless* are administered by HUD. These programs cover emergency, transitional, and permanent housing. Safe Havens for battered women and their children may be part of such programs.

Supportive housing programs pay for the building of special housing units to be made available to low-income elderly and people who are disabled. This housing has been made handicap accessible and allows many people to remain living independently in their communities.

## ORGANIZATION OF U.S. HEALTH AND WELFARE RESOURCES

The United States has a wealth of health and welfare resources, the scope of which is not seen elsewhere in the world. However, the organization of these resources is diverse, fragmented, and complicated. Three levels of government providing varied and different services in both the public and private sectors create a system that is difficult to comprehend. Consumers are often confused about what services are offered

and where to go for services. Each level of government carries out significant public health responsibilities.

As mentioned in Chapter 4, a **National Board of Health** briefly existed in the United States from 1879-1883. Today there is no National Board of Health, however, many federal agencies are involved in matters of public health. Table 5-7 gives examples of some functions and activities of the federal government in relation to public health and welfare. The single most important agency in this area is the U.S. Department of Health and Human Services. Most of the health and welfare functions of the federal government are coordinated and administered through this department.

## U.S. DEPARTMENT OF HEALTH AND HUMAN SERVICES

This department assumed a cabinet-level position on April 11, 1953, as the Department of Health, Education, and Welfare (DHEW). In 1980 the DHEW split into the U.S. Department of Health and Human Services (USDHHS) and the Department of Education. Today, the USDHHS advises the President on federal income security programs and policies and on health and welfare issues. The department touches the lives of more Americans than any

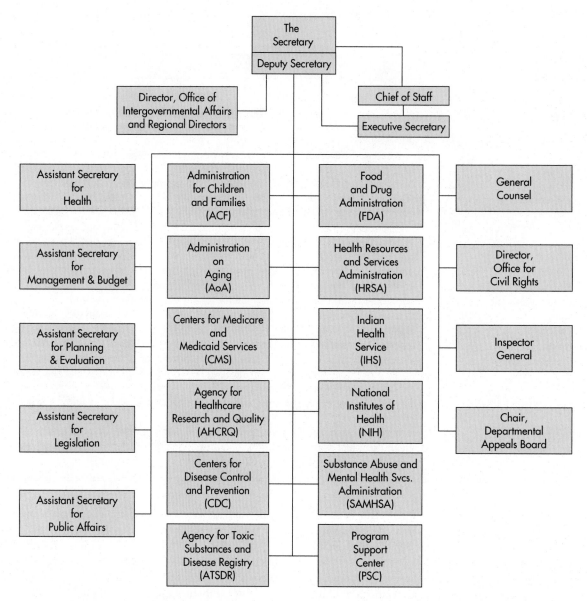

**FIGURE 5-7** U.S. Department of Health and Human Services. (From Office of the Federal Register, *United States government manual, 2000-2001,* Washington, DC, 2000, US Government Printing Office, p. 227)

other federal agency. It is charged with safeguarding the health and welfare of the nation. Major components of the USDHHS are discussed here, using information from the *United States Government Manual* (Office of the Federal Register [OFR], 2000). Figure 5-7 depicts the organization of the USDHHS.

## U.S. Public Health Service

The U.S. Public Health Service (USPHS) is the oldest and one of the best known services of the USDHHS. Its origins began in 1798 as the Marine Hospital Service, and it became the USPHS in 1912. Its early Hygienic Laboratory was the forerunner of the National Institutes of Health. Today the USPHS is under the Assistant Secretary for Health.

It carries out the mandates of the Public Health Act of 1944 and is charged with protecting and advancing the nation's physical and mental health. It is the nation's premier public health agency.

Through USPHS, broad-based public health assessments are conducted and preventive health services guidelines are developed. The USPHS provides leadership in research in disease prevention and health promotion, health promotion and disease prevention activities across the life span, women's health, minority health, mental health, food and drug safety, emergency preparedness, international and refugee health, HIV/AIDS policy, and public health research. The service has eight operating divisions within its structure.

**CENTERS FOR DISEASE CONTROL AND PREVENTION.** The Centers for Disease Control and Prevention (CDC) had its genesis in a World War II agency, Malaria Control in War Areas, which was converted to the Communicable Disease Center in 1946. The Centers for Disease Control was formally established in 1973, and in 1992 its name was changed to Centers for Disease Control and Prevention, but the acronym, CDC, remained the same. In 1995 it became an operating division of the USPHS. Some agencies that are part of the CDC are given in Box 5-13.

The CDC is the federal agency charged with protecting the public health of the nation by strengthening essential public health services and providing leadership and direction in prevention and control of diseases and conditions. The CDC's Public Health Practice Program Office coordinates the development of National Public Health Performance Standards with national, state, and local public health organizations (Public Health Practice Program Office, 1999). These standards are used to measure public health practice and outcomes as defined by the Essential Public Health Services (see Chapter 4).

The CDC works to develop prevention strategies and has Prevention Research Centers at major universities across the country. These centers serve as a national network and resource for effective prevention strategies and application of these strategies at the community level (CDC, 2000).

The CDC also works to strengthen our nation's response to public health emergencies, addresses chronic disease prevention and control, injury prevention and control, occupational safety and health, and international health. CDC coordinates the national immunization program, national quarantine measures, and the use of rare therapeutic and immunoprophylactic agents.

**FOOD AND DRUG ADMINISTRATION.** The Food and Drug Administration (FDA) was formally established in 1931 and touches the lives of virtually every American today. In 1995 it became an operating division of the USPHS. Its mission is to ensure that food, drugs, and biologic products are safe; medical devices are safe and effective; and electronic products that emit radiation (e.g., microwaves) are safe. Feed and drugs for pets and farm animals also come under FDA scrutiny. FDA ensures that products are labeled truthfully and with the information needed to use them properly. Major divisions of the administration include (1) Center for Drug Evaluation and Research, (2) Center for Biologics Evaluation and Research, (3) Center for Food Safety and Applied Nutrition, (4) Center for Veterinary Medicine, (5) Center for Devices and Radiological Health, and (6) National Center for Toxicological Research.

**AGENCY FOR TOXIC SUBSTANCES AND DISEASE REGISTRY.** The Agency for Toxic Substances and Disease Registry (ATSDR) was established in 1983 and became an operating division of the USPHS in 1995. The agency's mission is to prevent exposure to toxic and hazardous sub-

**BOX 5-13**

*Centers for Disease Control and Prevention: Network of Agencies*

- National Center for Chronic Disease Prevention and Health Promotion
- National Center for Environmental Health
- National Center for Health Statistics
- National Center for HIV, STD, and TB Prevention
- National Center for Infectious Diseases
- National Center for Injury Control and Prevention
- National Institute for Occupational Safety and Health
- Epidemiology Program Office
- International Health Program Office
- National Immunization Program
- Public Health Practice Program Office

stances and reduce sources of environmental pollution. It assists the Environmental Protection Agency (EPA) in identifying hazardous wastes that need to be regulated (see Chapter 6). ATSDR initiatives target populations at risk of exposure to hazardous substances and intervene to eliminate exposures and mitigate adverse health outcomes to hazardous substances. ATSDR compiles registries of human exposure to hazardous substances for long-term follow-up, maintains listings of areas restricted or closed to the public due to contamination, compiles data on the health effects of hazardous substances, sponsors research that evaluates relationships between hazardous substances in the environment and adverse health outcomes, and provides training and consultation to ensure adequate and safe response to public health emergencies. Through the Public Health Workforce Development Initiative, the agency is working to train public health workers in the skills necessary to respond to current and emerging public health threats (ATSDR, 2000).

**INDIAN HEALTH SERVICE.** The Indian Health Service (IHS) was established in 1924. It became an operating division of the USPHS in 1995. Its mission is to raise the physical, mental, social, and spiritual health of Native American and Alaska Natives to the highest level. Its goal is to ensure that comprehensive, culturally acceptable personal and public health services are available and accessible. It provides a comprehensive health services delivery system in cooperation with tribes and operates hospitals, health centers, and school health centers. The IHS assists tribes in developing health programs, coordinating health planning, and obtaining and utilizing health resources. It assists tribes in matters of public health and development of community sanitation facilities, and serves as a consultant and advocate for health care.

**NATIONAL INSTITUTES OF HEALTH.** The National Institutes of Health (NIH) was initially established in 1887 as the Hygienic Laboratory. It became an operating division of the USPHS in 1995. It is the world's premier medical research organization. Its mission is to uncover new knowledge that will lead to better health for everyone. It conducts research in its own laboratories and clinics and funds research and training in research institutions. NIH-conducted research helps determine medical treatment and disease prevention strategies. Among its many achievements, NIH research has played a major role in reducing mortality from heart disease and stroke, improving treatments for and detection of cancer, reducing paralysis from spinal cord injuries, increasing chances for survival of respiratory distress syndrome infants, increasing vaccinations for infectious disease, and advancing molecular genetics and genomics research. Institutes in the NIH are given in Box 5-14. The NIH also includes the National Library of Medicine, National Center for Research Resources, National Center for Human Genome Research, Clinical Center, Fogarty International Center, and the Division of Research Grants.

HEALTH RESOURCES AND SERVICES ADMINISTRATION. The Health Resources and Services Administration (HRSA) was established in 1982. It became an operating division of the USPHS in 1995. It houses the Division of Nursing (Division of Nursing, 1997) and is the principal primary health care service agency of the federal government. It directs national health programs, which improve the health of the nation by assuring quality health care to underserved,

vulnerable, and special-need populations and by promoting an appropriate health profession workforce, particularly in primary care and public health. HRSA operates a national network of community and migrant health centers and primary care programs. It maintains the National Health Service Corps, provides services to people with AIDS through the provisions of the Ryan White CARE Act, and administers the Maternal and Child Health Block Grant. It oversees the organ transplantation program, encourages organ donation, and ensures the equitable distribution of organs.

SUBSTANCE ABUSE AND MENTAL HEALTH SERVICES ADMINISTRATION. The Substance Abuse and Mental Health Services Administration (SAMHSA) was established in 1992. Its predecessor was the Alcohol, Drug Abuse, and Mental Health Administration. SAMHSA became an operating division of the USPHS in 1995. It provides national leadership in the prevention and treatment of addictive and mental disorders. SAMHSA works to improve the quality and availability of substance abuse prevention; addiction treatment; and mental health services for individuals, families, and communities. It houses three centers: the Center for Substance Abuse Prevention, the Center for Substance Abuse Treatment, and the Center for Mental Health Services.

AGENCY FOR HEALTHCARE RESEARCH AND QUALITY. The Agency for Healthcare Research and Quality (AHRQ) was established in 1999. Its forerunner was the Agency for Health Care Policy and Research. AHRQ provides evidence-based information on health care outcomes, quality, cost, use, and access. Its strategic goals include supporting improving health outcomes, strengthening quality measurement and improvement, identifying strategies that improve access, fostering appropriate health care use, reducing unnecessary health care expenditures, improving the quality of health care, promoting client safety and reducing medical errors, advancing the use of client care information technology, and conducting quality and outcomes research. The agency publishes many health care guidelines and protocols and single copies of most publications are available free of charge by calling 1-800-358-9295.

## Administration on Aging

The **Administration on Aging (AoA)**, created by the Older Americans Act of 1965, is the principal agency designated to carry out provisions of the act and is the lead USDHHS agency on all issues involving the elderly population. It develops policies, plans, and programs to promote the health and welfare of older Americans and administers grants to states to establish state and community programs for older persons. It strives to keep elders living independently in their communities and supports home-delivered meals, helps provide transportation and at-home services, and supports ombudsman services. The administration is discussed further in Chapter 19.

**BOX 5-14**
*National Institutes of Health*

- National Cancer Institute
- National Eye Institute
- National Heart, Lung, and Blood Institute
- National Institute of Alcohol Abuse and Alcoholism
- National Institute of Allergy and Infectious Diseases
- National Institute of Arthritis and Musculoskeletal and Skin Disorders
- National Institute of Child Health and Human Development
- National Institute of Dental and Craniofacial Research
- National Institute of Diabetes, Digestive, and Kidney Disease
- National Institute of Environmental Health Sciences
- National Institute of General Medical Sciences
- National Institute of Mental Health
- National Institute of Neurological Disorders and Stroke
- National Institute of Nursing Research*
- National Institute on Aging
- National Institute on Deafness and Other Communication Disorders
- National Institute on Drug Abuse

*The National Institute of Nursing Research (NINR) was founded in 1986 as the National Center for Nursing Research. In 1995 it became NINR. This institute is of special interest and importance to nurses.

## Administration on Children and Families

The Administration on Children and Families (ACF) was created April 15, 1991. It is responsible for federal programs that promote the economic and social well-being of families, children, individuals, and communities. ACF provides guidance to states in administering *Temporary Assistance for Needy Families* (TANF) discussed in this chapter and is active in assisting states in child support enforcement issues. Through its Administration on Developmental Disabilities (ADD) it administers State Developmental Disabilities Councils and Protection and Advocacy Grant Programs. Its Administration on Children, Youth, and Families (ACYF) administers many programs that enhance the lives of children and families. ACF provides federal matching funds to states for foster care and adoption assistance and child abuse prevention and treatment programs, provides funding for federally subsidized child care, administers Head Start, and administers runaway and homeless youth community programs.

## Centers for Medicare and Medicaid Services

The Centers for Medicare and Medicaid Services (CMS) was created in 2001. It was formerly called the Health Care Financing Administration (HCFA), created in 1977. The CMS administers the Medicare and Medicaid programs, which provide health care to about one in four Americans. The CMS also administers the Children's Health Insurance Program (CHIP) through approved state plans (see Chapter 16).

## SOCIAL SECURITY ADMINISTRATION

The Social Security Administration (SSA) was originally established on July 16, 1946, when its predecessor, the Social Security Board, was abolished. In 1995 the administration became an independent agency of the federal government. Before becoming an independent agency, it had been part of the USDHHS. Many American families are served by this agency.

The administration oversees the OASDI and SSI programs of the Social Security Act of 1935 discussed previously in this chapter. It is responsible for studying poverty and health care needs in the United States, assigning Social Security numbers, and maintaining individual records of Social Security earnings. It has 10 regional offices (Boston, New York, Philadelphia, Atlanta, Chicago, Dallas, Kansas City, Denver, San Francisco, and Seattle) and over 1300 local offices.

The administration is the major federal agency dealing with social welfare programs. Local offices of the administration have the responsibility to inform people about programs, assist in filing and processing claims, and help claimants file appeals. Requests can be made to local offices for information on Social Security. The administration can be contacted at 1-800-772-1213 for information on programs and publications.

## CABINET-LEVEL INVOLVEMENT

Cabinet-level departments are involved extensively in provision of health and welfare services to the American public. One cabinet-level department, the Department of Health and Human Services, has already been discussed. All cabinet-level departments sponsor research, education, and training opportunities. Box 5-15 looks at cabinet-level involvement in health and welfare activities.

Two important government agencies that do not have cabinet status are the Corporation for National and Community Service and the EPA (discussed in Chapter 6). The federal government also is involved in numerous international health activities.

---

**BOX 5-15**

*Cabinet-Level Involvement: United States*

The *Department of Agriculture* sets and enforces food and drug standards, offers farm assistance, and works to minimize hunger and malnutrition. Its national food programs serve one in six Americans and include Food Stamps; Supplemental Food for Women, Infants, and Children (WIC); Commodity Supplemental Food Program; National School Lunch Program; School Breakfast Program; Special Milk Program for Children; Child and Adult Care Food Program; Summer Food Service Program for Children; Emergency Food Assistance Program; Food Distribution Program; and Nutrition Program for the Elderly. Its Nutrition Education and Training Program grants funds to states for the development and dissemination of nutrition information. The Department of Agriculture works jointly with the U.S. Department of Health and Human Services in the review, revision, and dissemination of the publication, *Dietary Guidelines for Americans*. It maintains the National Agricultural Library, conducts agricultural research, operates cooperative extension services, and offers international food assistance programs. Its Forest Service oversees the national forest system.

The *Department of Commerce* promotes national economic development, encourages technologic advancements, and maintains a national measurement system. Its Bureau of the Census collects and disseminates national statistical data and census information and is discussed more thoroughly in Chapter 14.

The *Department of Defense* provides the military forces necessary to deter war and to protect the national security.

*Continued*

**BOX 5-15**

*Cabinet-Level Involvement: United States—cont'd*

It administers the health and medical care services for military forces as well as civilian dependents of service personnel. It also operates the National Civil Defense Program.

The *Department of Education* safeguards the nation's educational system. It oversees bilingual education, educational civil rights, education of people who are disabled, and vocational and adult education. It offers numerous services to the nation's schools and operates the Educational Resources and Information Clearinghouse (ERIC), a source of educational materials nationwide.

The *Department of Energy* provides the framework for a comprehensive national energy plan. It is responsible for energy conservation and regulations, radioactive waste management, environmental restoration, cleanup of inactive waste sites, and nuclear energy and weapons. It ensures that departmental programs are in compliance with environmental safety and health regulations.

The *Department of Health and Human Services* is discussed separately in this chapter. It is the lead federal agency in matters of health and welfare.

The *Department of Housing and Urban Development* is the principal agency concerned with national housing needs and fair housing opportunities. It provides public low-income housing and oversees the development and modernization of impoverished communities, the establishment of new communities, and emergency shelter grants. (Some of the housing programs under the department are discussed in this chapter.)

The *Department of the Interior* is the nation's major environmental conservation agency, responsible for protecting our natural resources. It implements policies for the protection of the environment pursuant to the National Environmental Protection Act of 1969, which is responsible for preserving historic places and national parks; assists communities in environmentally sound land use; and enforces laws concerning flood plains, wetlands, and endangered species. Its Bureau of Indian Affairs promotes improvement of health and welfare conditions for Native Americans.

The *Department of Justice* protects the American public by enforcing federal heath and welfare laws. It is instrumental in protecting civil rights; prosecuting high-level narcotic and drug offenders; and is involved in programs to help reduce homicide, violence, and drug addiction in the United States. It represents the United States in litigation involving environmental health and public lands and natural resources. Its Bureau of Prisons is responsible for all health, food, and sanitation services in federal prisons.

The *Department of Labor* promotes the health and welfare of workers, strives to improve working conditions of Americans, and helps protect the economic future and retirement security of working Americans. It administers provisions of various federal labor laws, including the Occupational Safety and Health Act of 1970, the Job Training and Partnership Act of 1982, and the Employment Retirement Income Security Act of 1974. The Department of Labor also coordinates federal compensation and unemployment programs and enforces safety standards and fair employment practices. Activities of the department's Occupational Safety and Health Administration (OSHA) and the Mine Safety and Health Administration focus on promoting worker health and safety. It oversees workers' compensation legislation and black lung benefits and compiles statistics about the American workforce.

The *Department of State* assists the President in formulating foreign policy, carries out foreign aid and trade agreements, assists in improving the quality of life in underdeveloped countries, is an advocate of international human rights, and is involved in international law enforcement. It is responsible for refugee programs, international travel, passports, and representing our country abroad. It develops, administers, and staffs a worldwide primary health care system for department employees and their eligible dependents residing abroad.

The *Department of Transportation* enforces certain air, land, and water standards in relation to interstate transport. Its U.S. Coast Guard is responsible for guarding the American coastline, promoting boating safety, and enforcing the federal Water Pollution Control Act and other laws relating to protection of the marine environment. Its National Highway Traffic Safety Administration is charged with reducing morbidity and mortality on U.S. highways, conducting programs aimed at reducing traffic accidents, and compiling transportation statistics. Its Federal Aviation Administration develops and implements programs and regulations to control aircraft noise, sonic booms, and other environmental effects of civil aviation. It sets and enforces regulations for the safe interstate transportation of hazardous materials and oversees transportation related to civil emergencies.

The *Department of the Treasury* assists other government agencies in preventing illegal drug traffic and illegal possession of firearms, alcoholic beverages, and tobacco products through the U.S. Customs Service and the Bureau of Alcohol, Tobacco, and Firearms.

Data from Office of the Federal Register [OFR]: *United States government manual 2000-2001,* Washington, DC, 2000, US Government Printing Office and websites of the various departments.

## CORPORATION FOR NATIONAL AND COMMUNITY SERVICE

The Corporation for National and Community Service was established by the National and Community Service Act of 1993. The goal of the corporation is to address the nation's critical problems in education, the environment, public safety, and other human needs, while fostering a service ethic and civic responsibility in participants and beneficiaries (Office of the Federal Register [OFR], 2000, p. 383). It mobilizes Americans of all backgrounds in volunteer, community-based service. In exchange for service, volunteers can receive education awards to repay college loans or help finance their college education. The corporation serves as a domestic Peace Corps and has three major divisions: (1) *AmeriCorps* (programs: AmeriCorps National Civilian Community Corps, AmeriCorps VISTA), (2) *Learn and Serve America* (programs: School-Based and Community-Based Programs, Higher Education Programs), and (3) *National Senior Service Corps* (programs: Retired and Senior Volunteer Program [RSVP], Foster Grandparent Program, Senior Companion Program). Its headquarters are in Washington, D.C.

## INTERNATIONAL INVOLVEMENT

The United States is involved with a number of agencies, groups, and governments on an international level to maintain and improve health, welfare, and environmental conditions throughout the world. Several intergovernmental agreements, especially in relation to disease control, trade, immigration, world peace, and respect for basic human rights, have been developed to enhance the well-being of all people.

### United Nations

The United States is extensively involved in international health and welfare issues through the **United Nations (UN).** This international assembly is dedicated to promoting welfare, peace, and health. Two major UN-sponsored groups with which the United States works are the World Health Organization and the United Nations' Children's Fund.

### World Health Organization

Efforts to organize international health activities took place between 1851 and 1909, when a series of meetings known as the International Sanitary Conferences occurred. These meetings were the precursor to the International Office of Public Health in 1909 (Pickett, Hanlon, 1990, p. 74). In 1948 the **World Health Organization (WHO)** was created as part of the United Nations. However, any nation can belong to WHO without being a UN member. A major goal of WHO is to achieve international cooperation for health throughout the world.

WHO focuses much of its international health activity on the control of communicable disease and maternal and child health. It sets international quarantine measures, collects epidemiologic data, is actively involved in coordinating international AIDS research and information, and is a clearinghouse for international health information. WHO also is concerned with establishing worldwide health standards and practices, standardizing international health regulations, providing statistical and health education services, promoting research, and training health workers. WHO publishes international health statistics and documents worldwide outbreaks of disease. The headquarters of WHO are located in Geneva, Switzerland.

### United Nations' Children's Fund

The United Nations' Children's Fund (UNICEF) attempts to meet the emergency and ongoing needs of children, particularly children in developing countries. It has improved maternal and child health by combating malnutrition (through food programs), preventing and controlling communicable diseases (through immunization and treatment programs), and providing food, shelter, and other basic welfare needs. UNICEF works closely with WHO to promote health and welfare services for at-risk mothers and children throughout the world.

### Peace Corps

The Peace Corps was established in 1961 and was made an independent agency by the International Security and Development Act of 1981. Americans of all ages and from all walks of life serve as volunteers in the Peace Corps. The Corps is charged with promoting a better understanding of the American people and promoting world peace and friendship by helping meet the needs of other countries.

Thousands of Peace Corps volunteers serve in Central and South America, the Caribbean, Africa, Asia, the Pacific, Europe, Russia, the Ukraine, and the Baltics. Volunteers work in areas of education, agriculture, health, environment, and small business and urban development. Community projects incorporate the skills of volunteers with the resources of the host country and international assistance programs. To increase international understanding, Corps volunteers make presentations in U.S. elementary, junior high, and senior high schools. Its main headquarters are in Washington, D.C.

## OTHER FEDERAL INVOLVEMENT IN HEALTH AND WELFARE

On the federal level numerous agencies have health and welfare functions. The Veterans' Administration provides hospital, nursing home, and outpatient medical and dental care to eligible veterans of military service; coordinates veteran compensation, pension, and assistance programs; and provides rehabilitation training for disabled veterans. Examples of agencies that are involved in health and welfare activities are the Endangered Species Committee, United States Information Agency, Architectural and Transportation Barriers Compliance Board, Commission on Civil Rights, the Tennessee Valley Authority, Disability Rights Council, President's Committee on Physical Fitness, and President's Committee on Employment of People with Disabilities. All U.S. cabinet-level departments provide services that relate to the improvement of national and international health and welfare conditions.

## PUBLIC HEALTH: STATE AND LOCAL GOVERNMENT

Each state is responsible for providing for the health of its residents and has a public health code and a state health authority (SHA) that deals with health. State public health codes establish what type of administrative relationship exists between SHAs and local health departments (LHDs). The SHAs and LHDs are official government agencies that are supported by taxes and provide health services to the general public.

### Administrative Relationships Between SHAs and LHDs

Historically four organizational patterns have characterized the administrative relationships between SHAs and LHDs: (1) *centralized administration* in which the SHA has direct administrative authority over the LHD, (2) *decentralized administration* in which the local government operates the LHD and has direct administrative authority over it, (3) *shared authority* between the SHA and LHD, and (4) *mixed jurisdiction* in which the SHA exercises centralized administration over some LHDs and decentralized administration over others (Mays, 2001, p. 83). SHAs usually share in the cost of LHD services, but the cost-sharing ratio varies greatly. LHDs provide many *direct services* to clients, whereas SHAs are more involved in *indirect service* provision. Services provided by SHAs and LHDs vary; some common service areas are discussed here.

## STATE HEALTH AUTHORITY

The U.S. Constitution empowers state governments to protect the health and welfare of their citizens. States are the central authorities in the nation's public health system and have the primary responsibility for public health (IOM, 1988, p. 8). The state health authority (SHA) is the agency or department dealing with health on the state level. The structure of SHAs differs from state to state. More than half of SHAs maintain regional or district offices that maintain close working relationships with LHDs

(Mays, 2001, p. 83). Figure 5-8 is an organizational chart depicting how an SHA might be organized.

There are 55 state and territorial health agencies. Two-thirds of states have an independent SHA, often a state Department of Health, and the remainder have a "superagency" approach (Mays, 2001, p. 80). A superagency combines public health, mental health, environmental and/or social service functions. The federal government's Department of Health and Human Services is a superagency.

The IOM's Committee for the Study of the Future of Public Health recommended that, in addition to the core functions of assessment, policy development, and assurance (see Chapter 4), the public health duties of states should include the following (IOM, 1988, p. 12):

- Assessment of health needs in the state based on statewide data collection
- Assurance of an adequate statutory base for health activities in the state
- Establishment of statewide health objectives, delegating power to LHDs (LHDs) as necessary and holding them accountable
- Assurance of statewide efforts to develop and maintain essential personal, educational, and environmental health services; provision of access to necessary services; and problem solving for public health
- Guarantee of a minimum set of essential health services
- Support of local service capacity, especially when disparities exist in local ability to raise revenue and/or administer programs

### State Public Health Code

Each state authorizes specific public health services through its legislated state public health code. These codes establish state public health law and designate what administrative relationship exists between SHAs and LHDs. The SHA can delegate responsibility for public health activities mandated

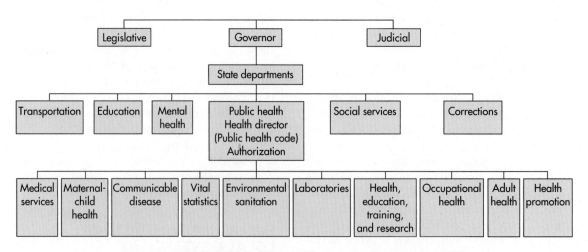

**FIGURE 5-8** Organizational chart of a state health authority (SHA).

in the code to LHDs, but ultimate responsibility for the activity rests with the state.

## Chief Executive

The chief executive of an SHA is often called the health officer. State health officers are frequently physicians who are political appointees. The average term of service is 2 years and greater continuity of leadership in such positions is needed (IOM, 1988, p. 148). Less than half of all SHA health officers have public health training or experience. Some states are now requiring their health officer to have graduate education in public health (IOM, 1988, p. 174).

## Spending

The total of all SHA funding is more than $11 billion each year (PHF, 1995, p. 2). SHA spending is financed primarily from state (41%) and federal funds (32%) (PHF, 1995). Recently states have not been a stable source of funding for SHAs (PHF, 1992, p. 2). Faced with deteriorating fiscal conditions and decreases in state funding, many SHAs are trimming their budgets and cutting back on services offered. Funding may be better in the future because strengthening the public health infrastructure has been added as a focus area in *Healthy People 2010* (see Chapter 4).

## Staff

The SHA is headed by a chief executive (health officer or other title) who is usually appointed by the governor. This person is traditionally a physician. Other staff members include administrators, clerical workers, and consultants in fields such as community health nursing, occupational health, mental health, epidemiology, statistics, maternal-child health, health education, and nutrition. SHAs have legal counsel available to them, often through the state attorney general's office. States may have regional directors who serve as intermediaries between their regions and the state department. Most SHA personnel, except for the chief executive, are civil service employees.

Community health nurses are a valuable part of SHA staffs. They are hired to provide consultant services and help establish state health policies, particularly in relation to maternal-child health and adult health services. They work closely with LHDs to improve the quality of care delivered to individuals, families, and aggregates at risk. Generally, community health nurses who work for state health departments are prepared at the master's or doctoral level and have community health nursing experience.

## Service Functions

An overall goal of state health authorities and LHDs is to enhance personal, public, and community health. SHAs and LHDs have a number of shared service functions, but play differing roles in provision of service. Table 5-8 presents these service functions and contrasts the service role of SHAs and LHDs.

## LOCAL HEALTH DEPARTMENT

The National Association of County and City Health Officials definition of a **local health department (LHD)** is displayed in Box 5-16. There are more than 2800 LHDs in the United States (Mays, 2001, p. 85). The LHD is the basic unit for the delivery of public health services and has primary responsibility for performing public health activities at the community level.

The IOM's Committee for the Study of the Future of Public Health recommends that, in addition to the core public health functions (see Chapter 4), LHDs also be responsible for the following activities (IOM, 1988, pp. 9-10):

- Assessment, monitoring, and surveillance of local health problems and needs and resources for dealing with them
- Policy development and leadership fostering local involvement and a sense of ownership, emphasizing local needs, and advocating equitable distribution of public resources and complementary private activities commensurate with community needs
- Assurance that high-quality services, including personal health services, needed for the protection of public health in the community are available and accessible to all persons; that the community receives proper consideration in the allocation of federal, state, and local resources for public health; and that the community is informed about how to obtain public health, including personal health, services, or how to comply with public health regulations

Almost two thirds of LHDs are county departments, 10% are combined city and county, 8% are multicounty, and 18% are operated by a city or a town (Mays, 2001, p. 85). LHDs have functions similar to those carried out by the state health department, but the services they provide are more direct (see Table 5-8).

Traditionally LHDs have offered personal health services focusing on maternal-child health and control of communicable disease. Almost all LHDs offer immunization services, 84% are actively involved in well-child care, two thirds offer sexually transmitted disease testing and treatment, and one third offer prenatal care (Mays, 2001, p. 86; National Association of County and City Health Officials, 1998). Other LHD services include school health, environmental health, laboratory services, chronic disease programs, family planning services, research, health education, and home care.

The delivery of primary care services by LHDs continues to be an issue of debate (Mays, 2001, p. 86). Although LHDs have historically provide primary care services such as immunizations and well-child care, expansion in this area of service remains controversial. The IOM has cautioned

**TABLE 5-8**

*Service Functions of State and Local Health Departments*

| | STATE HEALTH AUTHORITY (SHA) | LOCAL HEALTH DEPARTMENT (LHD) |
|---|---|---|
| Administrative | Assessment, policy development, and assurance are core functions of SHAs. They provide the legal, statutory basis for public health practice through their *Public Health Codes* and other legislation. SHAs may take action against an LHD that is not adhering to state health policies. Health planning activities are carried out to facilitate meeting *Healthy People 2010* objectives (see Chapter 4). Consultation services are provided to LHDs. SHAs administer federally aided health programs | Assessment, policy development, and assurance are core functions of LHDs. They conduct community assessments and community health profiles. LHDs promulgate and enforce local health standards, codes, and policies in relation to public health (e.g., food, water, and environmental safety). They inspect and license local health facilities such as hospitals, nursing homes, and restaurants and provide consulting services to community agencies and individuals. LHDs coordinate community initiatives to meet *Healthy People 2010* objectives, take part in healthy community initiatives, and mobilize community partnerships (see Chapter 3). |
| Communicable Disease (CD) | SHAs establish reporting guidelines for communicable disease, distribute vaccines, and develop quarantine measures. They determine what communicable diseases are to be routinely reported in accordance with national and international law and consult with LHDs on CD concerns. | LHDs are responsible for case finding, early diagnosis, and treatment of communicable disease. They offer immunization and communicable disease clinics (e.g., tuberculosis, sexually transmitted diseases) and conduct epidemiologic studies of individual cases of disease (e.g., hepatitis) and disease outbreaks. LHDs enforce disease reporting and local quarantine measures and maintain local CD statistics. They offer immunization and clinics on sexually transmitted and communicable diseases. LHDs must conform with state and federal regulations on reporting and follow-up of communicable disease. |
| Personal Health Services | SHAs administer federal block grant monies and consult with LHDs. They usually are not involved in direct provision of personal health services, with the exceptions of services to special populations at-risk such as people who are mentally ill or mentally retarded, migrants, occupational health clients, and children with disabilities. | Numerous services are provided through classes, clinics, schools, community agencies, and home visiting. Clinic services frequently include family planning, immunization, sexually transmitted diseases, and antepartal and well-baby care. Primary care clinics for the medically indigent, pharmacy services, and dental health may be provided. Health education offerings are extensive. School health historically has been an integral part of personal health services, and public health nurses provide numerous school nursing services (see Chapter 20). |
| Occupational Health | SHAs are the lead state agency for occupational health in only five states. Other states have freestanding Occupational Safety and Health Administrations (see Chapter 21). Several states require occupational health information on death certificates, and parental occupation on birth certificates to help pinpoint causes of death and congenital disorders. Some states have occupational disease registries. | These activities are largely conducted on the state level with little LHD involvement. Some industries are contracting with LHDs to provide diagnostic and screening programs and assist with recordkeeping. Some occupational health nurses (see Chapter 21) are consulting with LHDs in the development of health policies and procedures and the management of clinic facilities. |
| Environmental Health | SHAs are the lead state agency for environmental health in many states. Other states have freestanding agencies to deal with environmental health. | Frequently performed environmental health activities include food safety inspections, lead screening and abatement, sewage disposal monitoring, and drinking water monitoring. Other activities include air and water quality, land use, building codes and safety, noise pollution, waste management, vector and animal control, and toxic and hazardous substances. Environmental concerns dealing with terrorism and chemical warfare have recently emerged. |

**TABLE 5-8**

*Service Functions of State and Local Health Departments—cont'd*

| | STATE HEALTH AUTHORITY (SHA) | LOCAL HEALTH DEPARTMENT (LHD) |
|---|---|---|
| Vital Statistics | Vital statistics are an important responsibility of the SHA, and many states have Centers for Health Statistics. States develop standardized forms, including certificates of birth, death, fetal death, marriage, and epidemiologic reporting forms. SHAs disseminate statistical information to the general public, LHDs, and other agencies including the National Center for Health Statistics. | Vital statistics are collected by LHDs and used for local health planning as well as reporting to the state. LHDs keep statistics on births, deaths, and reportable communicable disease, maintain registers of individuals known to have specific communicable diseases for which carrier states exist (e.g., typhoid), conduct morbidity and mortality surveys as necessary, and maintain records on jurisdictional health facilities. An LHD may issue birth and death certificates to people within its jurisdiction. |
| Laboratory Services | Laboratories are operated by most SHAs and provided at free or low cost to LHDs. Laboratory services may be extended to hospitals, clinics, and private practitioners on a contractual, fee-for-service basis. The laboratory also certifies vaccines and other biologics. The diagnostic services are primarily in relation to CD control and environmental sanitation. | Many LHDs use state laboratory facilities or contract with local laboratory services to diagnose and investigate health problems and hazards in the community. Services include water analysis, serology, parasitology, identification of microorganisms, x-ray services for tuberculosis control, sanitation laboratory services, and metabolic and genetic screening for conditions such as phenylketonuria (PKU) and sickle cell anemia. Laboratory services are essential for communicable disease control and environmental sanitation and safety. |
| Health Education and Training | SHAs work in cooperation with community organizations and educational facilities to develop public health education, training, and in-service programs and often provide extensive public health education materials. Some states have expanded their health education activities to include advertising on radio, television, and the internet. Ad campaigns often address tobacco use, drug use, and sexually transmitted diseases. | LHDs provide extensive health education and serve as public health information centers. Public health nurses regularly take part in health education activities. Health education services are provided to individuals and groups, community health education programs are provided, health education materials are distributed, and staff in-service and continuing education programs are provided. LHDs utilize local media as health education resources. They may have health educators on staff and often offer tuition reimbursement for employees who take course work in public health or related fields. |
| Research | SHAs implement research studies to develop new insights and innovative solutions to public health problems. They also form links with academic institutions to conduct research. Research activities often look at leading causes of morbidity and mortality and Healthy People Initiative focus areas. | LHDs engage in research to promote public health in conjunction with local educational facilities and agencies. Studies related to local public health needs, service effectiveness and cost containment often are emphasized. |
| Emergency and Special Medical Services | Special medical services include the provision of hospital and institutional services for chronic or long-term conditions such as mental retardation, mental illness, and tuberculosis. In the event of epidemics, natural disasters, and man-made disasters, emergency services are made available to ensure that the necessary public health care is made available. | In the event of epidemics, natural disasters, and man-made disasters, such as terrorism and chemical warfare, emergency services are made available to ensure that the necessary public health care is made available. |

that provision of such services may drain vital resources away from population-wide services, that the U.S. public health system is inadequately equipped to address these needs, and that provision of primary care may pose a threat to the maintenance of important disease prevention and health promotion efforts (IOM, 1988, pp. 13, 152-153). The committee endorsed the idea that the ultimate responsibility for ensuring equitable access to health care for all

rests with the federal government. The privatization of certain public health functions has been mentioned as an option to this concern. However, many people in this country remain medically underserved, and until other health care resources are available, primary care services offered through LHDs provide valuable services to this at-risk aggregate.

LHDs are aware of the public health needs of their residents, and it is imperative that they assume leadership roles in the formulation of public health policy. Many people in the community are not aware of the services available at their LHD. A major role of the community health nurse is to familiarize the public with LHD programs and services. LHDs are one of our country's most valuable public health resources.

## Administration

LHDs usually have a board of health and a health officer. Each LHD will establish its own organizational pattern. An example of an organizational structure for a LHD is given in Figure 5-9.

**BOX 5-16**

*Definition of a Local Health Department*

An administrative or service unit of local or state government, concerned with health, and carrying some responsibility for the health of a jurisdiction smaller than a state.

Source National Association of County and City Health Officials (NACCHO): *National profile of local health departments*, Washington, DC, 1998, NACCHO, p. 2.

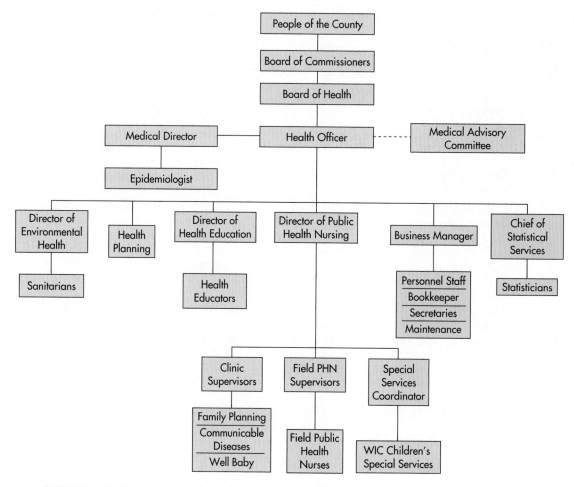

**FIGURE 5-9** Organizational chart of a local health department (LHD).

## Funding

LHDs receive the majority of their funding from the state and from local tax dollars (Mays, 2001, p. 87). Other funds come from fee-for-service, Medicaid and Medicare reimbursement, permits, and licensing fees. Fee-based revenue sources are becoming an increasingly important source of LHD funding (Mays, 2001; Wall, 1998). The average annual LHD budget is $5.5 million with a per capita expenditure of $41 per person (Mays, 2001). Recent years have seen cuts in LHD funding at a time when we need to be strengthening our public health infrastructure. Funding may be better in the future, with strengthening the public health infrastructure being added as a focus area in *Healthy People 2010* (see Chapter 4).

## Staff

Half of the nation's LHDs employ fewer than 20 full-time staff members (Mays, 2001, p. 87). LHD staffing varies, but the minimum staff usually includes (1) a health officer, (2) a community health nurse, (3) an environmental engineer (sanitarian), and (4) a clerk. Additional personnel often include an epidemiologist, health educator, nutritionist, dentist, dental hygienist, physical therapist, occupational safety and health specialist, statistician, mental health counselor, alcohol and substance abuse counselor, and/or a social worker. To provide comprehensive community health services, a basic multidisciplinary staff is necessary. Estimating the number of community health personnel needed in a local area is a complex task. Multiple factors, such as current health problems in the community, the supply of health professionals in an area, and the services offered by the LHD all influence workforce planning.

HEALTH OFFICER. Traditionally a health officer was a physician with public health training. Today many health officers are still physicians, but the field is opening up to other health professionals such as nurses and public health administrators. If the health officer is not a physician, a medical director is utilized to provide medical consultation for LHD programs. The health officer is responsible for seeing that all divisions and programs in the LHD operate efficiently, effectively implement public health services, coordinate service provision with other community agencies, and are cost effective.

### *Stop and Think About It*

Your health officer is interested in having a community-wide educational program focused on decreasing domestic violence. How would you work with the different disciplines in your LHD and community agencies to plan, implement, and evaluate this program?

PUBLIC HEALTH NURSE. Historically, the public health nurse has been the mainstay of LHD staffing. The history, scope, and standards of practice for public health nurses were presented in Chapters 1 and 2. Public health nurses use a synthesis of nursing and public health theory to promote community health.

The types of services offered by the nursing division in an LHD vary, depending on the workforce available and other community resources that have been developed to meet the health care needs of community citizens. Public health nurses work closely with community resources to assist in meeting client's health care needs and are extensively involved in health education activities.

Public health nurses staff health department clinics, implement health education programs, conduct screening clinics, and make home visits. Public health nurses implement nursing interventions in numerous settings discussed throughout this text. They work extensively in schools, providing health education, counseling, screening programs, and private direct nursing care (see Chapter 20).

Many LHDs use nurse practitioners to staff clinics such as antepartal, sexually transmitted diseases, family planning, and WIC. If the LHD offers home care, nurses will be used to provide skilled nursing care in the home.

Baccalaureate preparation is recommended for entry-level positions in community health (ANA, 1986; Anderson, Mejer, 1985; Jones, Davis, Davis, 1987). Baccalaureate-prepared nurses are required to have community health nursing content during their educational preparation and have a strong background in the human and social sciences.

ENVIRONMENTAL ENGINEER. The environmental engineer (sanitarian) applies engineering principles to control, eliminate, or prevent environmental health hazards (Public Health Functions Project, 1998, p. 23). Environmental engineers apply principles of public health, toxicology, health, education, law enforcement, and industrial health and use practical and technical measures to eliminate or control environmental health problems. They have historically been members of LHD staffs. Their efforts have facilitated communicable disease control, promoted environmental health, helped ensure food and water safety, and reduced environmental pollution.

SUPPORT STAFF. LHDs may employ many other people, including social workers, laboratory technicians, home health aides, and clerical staff. A clerk/secretary is usually responsible for maintaining the records and schedules of the health department. Clerical and support staff are very important to the day-to-day functioning of the LHD.

## STATE AND LOCAL GOVERNMENT WELFARE ORGANIZATION

The primary purpose of official governmental welfare agencies is to assist indigent individuals in meeting their basic needs of food, shelter, and clothing. Benefits provided by these agencies are usually in the form of cash, food, or shelter. Many of the programs discussed in this chapter provided for under the Social Security Act are administered by these agencies.

Each state has a state-level department, usually a state department of human or social services, that establishes rules and regulations, sets guidelines for service provision, and administers services. Local offices of this state department provide direct services to clients. These local offices administer state-subsidized programs such as TANF, food stamps, General Assistance, and Medicaid. Protective services for children and adults are also often administered through these local offices. Other programs such as OASDI and SSI are administered by the federal government through local SSA offices.

## PRIVATE HEALTH AND WELFARE ORGANIZATION

The United States abounds in private health and welfare resources. Private resources can be classified as either for-profit or nonprofit. Nonprofit agencies reflect our na-

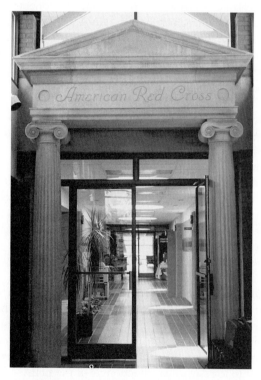

**FIGURE 5-10** For over 100 years the American Red Cross, a voluntary, nonprofit organization, has initiated the development and provision of health and welfare services. Established originally to assist and support military men and their families during times of war and to aid victims of disasters, this agency continues to make significant public health contributions. Some of its current efforts include the provision of selected health and welfare services based on community need. The American Red Cross continues to provide relief for disaster victims and to serve military families. Local chapters of this organization can be found in most major cities across the United States. (Courtesy Ed Richardson.)

tion's volunteer tradition. Historically, coordination between private and government resources has been limited, and private health and welfare resources are not centrally coordinated. As we move toward a partnership model in service delivery, an increasing number of cooperative ventures are being established between public and private resources in the community.

### The Volunteer Tradition

The United States has the strongest volunteer tradition of any country in the world. Tennessee is nicknamed the "Volunteer State." The American volunteer tradition has early roots. Early American settlers were often trying to break from the traditional and sometimes oppressive influences of church and state from which they came. In general, they were mistrustful of governmental intervention into matters of personal and public health and welfare. People helped each other, charities developed, and voluntary organizations emerged.

The United States went through what has been termed by some social and health researchers as the voluntaristic period. This was the time between the Civil War and 1935, and it was during this period that many voluntary agencies were founded. The passage of the Social Security Act of 1935 signaled governmental involvement in the provision of health and welfare services and eliminated some of the need for voluntary organizations. However, millions of Americans continue to "volunteer" their services each year. This voluntary tradition is to be applauded.

### Voluntary Agencies

When the term *voluntary* is used in relation to health and welfare services, it can be somewhat confusing. **Voluntary agencies** are private, nonprofit resources that are not under the auspices of federal, state, or local government. They are neither mandated by law nor tax supported and have no legal powers. Their services augment official (government) services. They frequently have paid staff, but extensively use volunteers to provide services.

Voluntary agencies are represented by professional societies, service organizations, agencies, and facilities. They are a unique part of American tradition and have a long and distinguished history. By the 1870s voluntary health and welfare organizations were emerging in the United States. In 1872 the American Public Health Association (APHA) was founded. Its first president was Dr. Stephen Smith. Today APHA remains one of our foremost public health organizations, helping to protect and promote the nation's health. In 1882 Clara Barton founded one of our country's best-known voluntary organizations, the American Red Cross (Figure 5-10). In 1892 the Anti-Tuberculosis Society of Philadelphia, a forerunner of today's American Lung Association, was established. Other voluntary organizations continued to develop.

Today there are thousands of voluntary health and welfare organizations in the United States, and nurses work extensively with these agencies. One voluntary service agency, the United Way, represents a large number of local voluntary resources with one central fund-raising campaign. Giving to the United Way campaign means giving to many voluntary resources with one donation.

Voluntary agencies rely heavily on donations, endowments, grants, and fee-for-service for funding. Voluntary agencies provide many services that would not otherwise be possible and are an important part of provision of health and welfare services. The federal government has encouraged private philanthropic giving to voluntary organizations by permitting contributions to be deducted from personal and corporate income tax. Box 5-17 briefly summarizes the characteristics of voluntary resources in the United States.

## Stop and Think About It

What are some of the voluntary agencies in your community? What health and welfare services do they provide? How are they funded?

## Private For-Profit Agencies

Private for-profit agencies are exactly as the term implies, agencies that make a profit out of providing services. This includes an increasing number of hospitals, a large percentage of nursing homes, health and welfare professionals in private practice, pharmacies, health business companies (e.g., medical equipment companies, hospital supplies), and proprietary social service agencies. These services are available on a fee-for-service basis and are organized primarily as companies and independent businesses.

## COORDINATION OF HEALTH AND WELFARE RESOURCES

The United States has great diversity in health and welfare resources. Lack of coordination among these resources presents a multitude of problems for both providers and recipients of service. Providers of service may become frustrated because they find it difficult to learn about the resources available and effect change in the system. Recipients of service are frustrated because they are not aware of resources, do not understand how to use them, and often receive fragmented care. A major role of the community health nurse is to explain and coordinate community services. Lack of resource coordination can adversely affect the quality of care delivered to clients, as demonstrated in the following case scenario.

**CASE** *Scenario*   John Falta, age 19, was in a motorcycle accident that necessitated an amputation below the right knee. He was hospitalized for 6 weeks and upon discharge was referred to a local home healthcare agency for skilled nursing services, the State Office of Vocational Rehabilitation for rehabilitation training, and the Department of Social Services for assistance with his medical expenses. In addition, a physical therapist from the hospital saw John on a weekly basis at home, and a volunteer from a local amputee self-help group visited and called him regularly to help him adapt to the changes that had occurred in his life. Each of these health and welfare resources provided a valuable service, but their services had not been coordinated and John became frustrated with working with so many "helping agencies" and the different goals that had been set for him. The nurse suggested that a conference be arranged between John, his family, and the involved resources, and John agreed that this was necessary. The conference helped coordinate John's care, enhanced John's involvement in the rehabilitation process, and allowed him to actively participate in establishing goals for his future. It is not uncommon to encounter clients like John. Coordination of service is an important issue for community health nurses.

Historically, there has been lack of coordination of health and welfare services in the United States. An early study by the National Commission on Community Health Services (1966, p. 132) identified lack of resource and service coordination between official (government) and private health care agencies. The National Health Planning and Resource Development Act of 1974 (Public Law 93-641) was passed to improve the delivery and coordination of government

**BOX 5-17**

*Voluntary Resources: Characteristics, Classifications, and Examples*

*Characteristics*
Voluntarily organized
Governed by a board of directors that includes lay and/or professional members
Have no legal powers
Receive support primarily from voluntary contributions, fees for service, third party payors, and grants
Usually provide services to a defined geographic location

*Classifications*
**PROFESSIONAL SOCIETIES**
American Nurses Association (ANA), American Public Health Association (APHA)

**SERVICE AGENCIES**
Visiting Nurse Association (VNA), American Cancer Society, American Red Cross, Alcoholics Anonymous, Rockefeller Foundation, United Community Services

**FACILITIES**
Universities, public museums, and libraries

**INDIVIDUALS**

health care services to all segments of the population. However, in 1981 the Omnibus Budget Reconciliation Act was passed and ended the federal mandate for Public Law 93-641 planning. A classic example of lack of coordination between health and welfare resources in the United States is the administration of the Medicare and Medicaid programs. These programs are locally administered by agencies that traditionally are not health agencies—the SSA and state departments of social service—without much input from public health agencies.

Lack of coordination between official and private health care agencies continues to be a contemporary problem. Nurses are in a unique position to influence coordination of care on both an individual and a community health planning level. On an individual level, community health nurses coordinate community resources for the families they visit. On a community level, community health nurses work with community agencies to coordinate care and prevent service duplication. As our nation moves towards cost containment in health care service delivery, we cannot afford to duplicate services, but instead must emphasize coordination of services.

Another issue closely linked to coordination is underutilization of services. For example, the nation's LHDs have been underutilized in American communities for decades. Such departments exist across the nation. The public health infrastructure could be strengthened by better utilizing these agencies, having SHAs and LHDs forming cooperative agreements with community agencies and practitioners for service provision, and making these agencies more visible to community residents. These agencies have the potential to play an even more important role in the public health of our nation.

## SUMMARY

The health and welfare system in the United States is complicated and diverse. Health and welfare services are found at the federal, state, and local levels and in the public and private sectors. Forty-four million Americans do not have health insurance and many Americans are underinsured. Frequently, Americans do not have access to necessary preventive health services or primary care. Such knowledge equips the nurse to more effectively deal with situations encountered daily in the practice setting. Through this knowledge nurses can help clients become aware of available services and link clients to these services. The nurse must understand how health and welfare resources are organized to enhance service delivery, familiarize clients with the service delivery system, link clients to services, and facilitate client care. Knowledge of health and welfare resources and services is essential for the community health nurse. The nurse needs to work in partnership with health care professionals and community resources to promote health.

## CRITICAL THINKING
*exercise*

LHDs all over the United States have historically provided public health services to local communities, and as national health care reform emerges, these agencies could play a much greater role in service provision. Envision new and innovative ways for these LHDs to provide and market their services to the community.

1. How could existing LHD services be expanded and marketed?
2. What specific services could they provide to facilitate meeting *Healthy People 2010* goals and objectives, and how could these services be funded?
3. What roles do you see for a nursing role in public health service delivery?

## REFERENCES

Agency for Toxic Substances and Disease Registry (ATSDR): *CDC/ATSDR public health workforce development initiative*, Washington, DC, 2000, USDHHS, Public Health Service.

American Nurses Association (ANA): *Standards of community health nursing practice*, Washington, DC, 1986, American Nurses Publishing.

American Nurses Association (ANA): *Nursing's agenda for health care reform*, Kansas City, Mo, 1991, ANA.

Anderson E, Mejer AT: *Consensus conference on the essentials of public health nursing practice and education*, Rockville, Md, 1985, USDHHS, Public Health Service.

Centers for Disease Control and Prevention: *Prevention Research Centers: investing in the nation's health*, Washington, DC, 2000, US Department of Health and Human Services.

Division of Nursing: *50 years at the Division of Nursing: United States Public Health Service*, Washington, DC, 1997, The Division.

44.3 million in U.S. lack health insurance, *Public Health Rep* 114: 491, 1999.

Gillis L, Thomas D: *Developing clinical systems for working in a managed care environment*, Washington, DC, June 7-9, 1996, Conference on Health Care for the Homeless.

Harrington C: A national health care program: has its time come? *Nurs Outlook* 36:214-216, 225, 1989.

Health Care Financing Administration: *1999 HCFA statistics*, Washington, DC, 2000, US Department of Health and Human Services.

Health Insurance Association of America (HIAA): *Source book of health insurance data 1983-84*, Washington, DC, 1983, HIAA.

Health Insurance Association of America (HIAA): *Source book of health insurance data 1995*, Washington DC, 1995, HIAA.

Health Insurance Association of America (HIAA): *Source book of health insurance data 1999*, Washington DC, 1999, HIAA.

Health Resources and Services Administration (HRSA): *Child health USA 2000*, Washington, DC, 2000, US Government Printing Office.

Institute of Medicine (IOM), Committee for the Study of the Future of Public Health: *The future of public health*, Washington, DC, 1988, National Academy Press.

Jones DC, Davis JA, Davis MC: *Public health nursing education and practice*, Springfield, Va, 1987, National Technical Information.

Kalisch BJ, Kalisch PA: *Politics of nursing*, Philadelphia, 1982, Lippincott.

Kerns WL, Glanz MP: Private social welfare expenditures, 1972-88, *Social Sec Bull* 54(2):2-11, 1991.

Leviss PS: Financing the public's health. In Novick LF, Mays GO, editors: *Public health administration. Principles for population-based management*, Gaithersburg, Md, 2001, Aspen.

Mays G: Organization of the public health delivery system. In Novick LF, Mays GO, editors: *Public health administration. Principles for population-based management*, Gaithersburg, Md, 2001, Aspen.

National Association of County and City Health Officials (NACCHO): *National profile of local health departments*, Washington, DC, 1998, NACCHO.

National Center for Health Statistics (NCHS): *Health, United States, 2000*, Hyattsville, Md, 2000, US Public Health Service.

National Commission on Community Health Services: *Health is a community affair*, Cambridge, Mass, 1966, Harvard University Press.

Needleman J: Nonprofit to for-profit conversions by hospitals, health insurers, and health plans, *Public Health Rep* 114:108-119, 1999.

Office of the Federal Register: *United States government manual, 2000-2001*, Washington, DC, 2000, US Government Printing Office.

Pew Health Professions Commission: *Critical challenges: revitalizing the health professions for the twenty-first century*, San Francisco, 1995, UCSF Center for the Health Professions.

Pickett G, Hanlon JJ: *Public health administration and practice*, ed 9, St Louis, 1990, Mosby.

Public Health Foundation (PHF): Budget woes force SHAs to make cuts, *Public Health Macroview* 5(1):2, 1992.

Public Health Foundation (PHF): State health agency and local health department spending in 1991 by source of funds, *Public Health Macroview* 7(1):2, 1995.

Public Health Functions Project: *The public health workforce: an agenda for the 21st century*, Washington, DC, 1998, USDHHS.

Public Health Practice Program Office (PHPPO): *National public health performance standards program*, Atlanta, 1999, Centers for Disease Control and Prevention.

Social Security Administration (SSA): *Understanding Social Security*, Washington, DC, 1993, SSA.

Social Security Administration: *Annual statistical supplement to the Social Security Bulletin, 1995*, Washington, DC, 1995, SSA.

Social Security Administration: *Annual statistical supplement to the Social Security Bulletin, 1999*, Washington, DC, 1999, SSA.

Turner C, Campbell E: Counting the uninsured using state-level hospitalization data, *Public Health Rep* 114:149-156, 1999.

US Department of Health and Human Services (USDHHS): *Healthy People 2000: midcourse review and 1995 revisions*, Washington, DC, 1995, US Government Printing Office.

US Department of Health and Human Services (USDHHS): *Healthy People 2010: conference edition*, Washington, DC, 2000, US Government Printing Office.

Wall S: Transformation in public health systems, *Health Affairs* 5(2):64-80, 1998.

Wilner DM, Walkley RP, O'Neill EJ: *Introduction to public health*, ed 7, New York, 1978, Macmillan.

## SELECTED BIBLIOGRAPHY

Association of State and Territorial Directors of Nursing: *Public health nursing. A partner for healthy populations*, Washington, DC, 2000, American Nurses Publishing.

Association of State and Territorial Health Officials (ASTHO): *Building our nation's public health systems. State instrument*, Atlanta, 2000, Centers for Disease Control and Prevention.

Cohen WJ: Current problems in health care, *N Engl J Med* 281:193-197, 1969.

Doner L, Siegel M: Public health marketing. In Novick LF, Mays GO, editors: *Public health administration. Principles for population-based management*, Gaithersburg, Md, 2001, Aspen.

Hatcher MT, Nicola R: Building constituencies for public health. In Novick LF, Mays GO, editors: *Public health administration. Principles for population-based management*, Gaithersburg, Md, 2001, Aspen.

Health Resources and Services Administration: *United States health workforce personnel factbook*, Washington, DC, 2000, US Department of Health and Human Services.

Kennedy EM: *In critical condition: the crisis in American health care*, New York, 1973, Pocket Books.

Mays GP, Miller CA, Halverson PK: *Local public health practice: trends and models*, Washington, DC, 1999, American Public Health Association.

National Association of County and City Health Officials (NACCH): *Building our nation's public health systems. Local instrument*, Atlanta, 2000, Centers for Disease Control and Prevention.

National Association of Local Boards of Health (NALBOH): *Building our nation's public health systems. Governance instrument*, Atlanta, 2000, Centers for Disease Control and Prevention.

National Public Health Performance Standards Program: *National Public Health Performance Standards Program. Program overview*, Atlanta, 2000, Centers for Disease Control and Prevention.

Nicola RM, Hatcher MT: A framework for building effective public health constituencies, *J Public Health Manage Practice* 6(2):1-10, 2000.

Novick LF: A framework for public health administration and practice. In Novick LF, Mays GO, editors: *Public health administration. Principles for population-based management*, Gaithersburg, Md, 2001, Aspen.

# 6

# Environmental Health and Disaster Nursing

*Sandra L. McGuire*

## OBJECTIVES

*Upon completion of this chapter, the reader should be able to:*

1. Discuss environmental health as a major public health concern.
2. Discuss the origins of environmental health in the United States.
3. Be knowledgeable concerning the *Healthy People 2010* national health objectives that relate to environmental health.
4. Describe the nurse's role in environmental health.
5. Name major pieces of environmental health legislation in the United States.
6. Discuss the role of federal, state, and local governments in environmental health.
7. Discuss selected environmental diseases.
8. Discuss areas of environmental concern.
9. Describe the nurse's role in disasters.
10. Discuss the phases of disaster management.

## KEY TERMS

Acid rain
Agency for Toxic Substances and Disease Registry (ATSDR)
Air pollution
American Red Cross (ARC)
Clean Air Act
Clean Water Act
Deforestation
Desertification
Disaster management phases
Disaster nurses
Endangered Species Act

Energy depletion
Environmental diseases
Environmental health
Environmental health competencies
Environmental Protection Agency (EPA)
Federal Emergency Management Agency (FEMA)
Greenhouse effect
Hazardous waste
Loss of biologic diversity
National Center for Environmental Health (NCEH)

National Environmental Policy Act
Nightingale Institute for Health and the Environment (NIHE)
*Nursing, Health, and the Environment*
Overpopulation
Ozone depletion
*Standards of Occupational and Environmental Health Nursing*
Water pollution
Wetlands destruction

*We did not inherit the earth from our ancestors. We borrow it from our children.*

OLD PENNSYLVANIA DUTCH SAYING

Environmental health was one of the earliest public health concerns. Maintenance of safe food and water, proper sewage disposal, and interment of the dead became matters of law and custom. Archaeologists and historians have indicated that the Minoans (3000-1430 BC) and the Myceneans (1430-1150 BC) built drainage systems, toilets, and water-flushing systems (Pickett, Hanlon, 1990, p. 21). About 1500 BC the Hebrews had a written hygienic code with environmental practices, Athenians of 1000-400 BC had elaborate environmental sanitation measures, and early Egyptians constructed drainage systems and earth privies for sewage (Pickett, Hanlon, 1990, p. 21).

During the Middle Ages, 500 to 1500 AD, environmental health practices often were ignored, and epidemics of leprosy, typhus, and bubonic plague ravaged the civilized world (Kalisch, Kalisch, 1995, p. 11). Known as the "Black

Death," bubonic plague is a bacterial disease spread by rodents and their fleas, and when left untreated has a case fatality rate of 50% to 60% (Chin, 2000, p. 381). In the mid-1300s bubonic plague killed as many as 60 million people (Kalisch, Kalisch, 1995, p. 12). Diseases and conditions related to environmental factors continue to be contemporary health issues.

The link between the environment and health is becoming increasingly evident. In *Healthy People*, the Surgeon General stated that "there is virtually no major chronic disease to which environmental factors do not contribute, either directly or indirectly" (USDHEW, 1979, p. 105) and noted that 20% of the deaths in the United States could be attributed to environmental factors such as pollution and toxic chemicals. The Healthy People Initiative (see Chapter 4) has consistently addressed environmental health as a national public health concern. Unfortunately, the twentieth century created countless environmental health problems that contributed to illness, disability, and death, and this century will doubtless present countless others. Poor environmental quality is estimated to be directly responsible for 25% of all the world's preventable health conditions (USDHHS, 2000; WHO, 1997a).

## Stop and Think About It

What are some of the things that occurred during the twentieth century that created problems with the world's environment. What are some of the environmental problems that you have noted in the community in which you live or work?

## ENVIRONMENTAL HEALTH IN THE UNITED STATES

Environmental health has biologic, chemical, physical, and sociologic components and includes the immediate and future conditions in which people live. Definitions of environmental health are identified in Box 6-1.

In the colonial United States (1607-1797) little attention was paid to community hygiene and sanitation, and there was almost a complete lack of community organization for health services (Smillie, 1955, pp. 15, 72). During this time epidemics of cholera, smallpox, yellow fever, measles, dysentery, influenza, pneumonia, scarlet fever, diphtheria, malaria, and syphilis continually occurred (Smillie, 1955, pp. 21-60). Although such epidemics were attributed to environmental health hazards such as inadequate ventilation, overcrowding, impure water, and inadequate housing, little was done to improve these conditions (Clark, 1972, pp. 30-36).

Early attempts to ensure environmental health included a 1610 Virginia law that stated no man or woman dare throw out water or suds from foul clothes into the open street, clean pots or kettles within 20 feet of a well or pump, or do the necessities of nature within a quarter mile of the town (Smillie, 1955, p. 61). Those who violated the law

## BOX 6-1
### *Environmental Health Defined*

**Environmental Health: The Science**
Environmental health compromises those aspects of human health, disease, and injury that are determined or influenced by factors in the environment. This includes the study of both the direct pathologic effects of various chemical, physical, and biologic agents, as well as the effects on health of the broad physical and social environment, which includes housing, urban development, land use and transportation, industry, and agriculture.*

The systematic development, promotion, and conduct of measures that modify or otherwise control those external factors in the indoor and outdoor environment that might cause illness, disability, or discomfort through interaction with the human system.†

**Environmental Health: A Personal Perspective**
Freedom from illness or injury related to exposure to toxic agents and other environmental conditions that are potentially detrimental to human health.‡

Environmental health is the interaction between the individual and environmental factors.§

*World Health Organization (WHO): Indicators for policy and decision making in environmental health (draft), Geneva, Switzerland, 1997, WHO; USDHHS: *Healthy People 2010*, conference edition, Washington, DC, 2000, USDHHS.
†USDHHS: *Evaluating the environmental health workforce* [HRP #0907160], Rockville, Md, 1988, USDHHS, p. 11.
‡Institute of Medicine, Committee on Enhancing Environmental Health Content in Nursing Practice; Pope AM, Snyder MA, Mood LH, editors: *Nursing, health and the environment: strengthening the relationship to improve the public's health*, Washington, DC, 1995, National Academy Press, p. 15.
§American Association of Occupational Health Nurses (AAOHN): *Advisory: environmental health: expanding dimensions of practice*, Atlanta, 1998, AAOHN.

could be whipped and punished (Smillie, 1955, p. 61). Such measures were often more concerned with the aesthetics of the environment than with related health consequences, and environmental practices frequently were directed at keeping the environment "sightly" and controlling "ill airs."

Early measures to control contagious disease often involved the use of isolation and quarantine (Smillie, 1955, p. 62). Quarantine was accepted by the general public as a legitimate governmental function (Hill, 1976, p. 9). Sanitary police enforced quarantine measures and special "quarantine" physicians were employed to make home visits (Clark, 1972, pp. 8-10). As early as 1796 the federal government passed a quarantine act to enforce health and quarantine regulations at U.S. ports of entry.

The beginnings of organized environmental health activities in the United States started with the *Shattuck Report* in 1850. This report made numerous recommendations regarding environmental sanitation and emphasized the need for controlling overcrowded housing, providing safe factories and buildings, ensuring food and water sanitation, and vaccinating against disease (Smillie, 1955, p. 252). Early environmental sanitation activities in the United States included safeguarding community water supplies; proper sewage, refuse, and waste disposal; food and milk sanitation; disinfection and fumigation during epidemics; pest and vector control; and building safety. These activities would later become functions of state and local boards of health (Smillie, 1955, pp. 340-375).

When the American Public Health Association (APHA) was founded in 1872, only three states (California, Massachusetts, and Virginia) and the District of Columbia had established boards of health, and most states were not actively involved in environmental health issues. Dr. Stephen Smith, APHA's first president and one of its founders, wrote *The City That Was*, a shocking description of the unsanitary conditions prevailing in New York City. He was a staunch supporter of the need for environmental health activities (Ravenel, 1921, p. 32), and APHA has continued to have a strong emphasis on environmental health issues.

Safeguarding the environment has been a mainstay of public health practice since 1878 (USDHHS, 2000). The short-lived National Board of Health (1879-1883) instituted many environmental health activities in an effort to control epidemics and communicable disease. From its original focus on sanitation and controlling communicable disease, environmental health has expanded to include protecting and preserving the environment in which we live and ensuring personal environmental health.

Public awareness and interest in the environment has gained impetus in recent years. The publication of Rachel Carson's book *Silent Spring* in 1962 is considered to be the beginning of the modern environmental health movement in this country. From that time on, numerous environmental health groups and advocacy efforts have been prominent in American politics and communities.

Efforts by the American people have helped preserve the environment and promote environmental health (Box 6-2). State and national park systems have been established, laws and agencies exist to safeguard the environment, consumer groups address environmental issues, and efforts have been made to protect endangered wildlife. Environmental health is now being looked at in a global perspective, realizing that environmental issues affecting one country or region affect another (Gochfeld, Goldstein, 1999; USDHHS, 2000).

Actions in every country affect the environment and influence events around the world (USDHHS, 2000). Our nation has expanded its efforts to improve environmental conditions in developing countries. This global scope will help develop and achieve effective ways to prevent disease, disability, and death throughout the world. Since its inception, the Healthy People Initiative (see Chapter 4) has consistently addressed these and other environmental health is-

**BOX 6-2**

### Selected U.S. Environmental Health Activities

The *Shattuck Report* was published in 1850 and outlined numerous environmental health activities necessary to ensure community health.

In 1872 the American Public Health Association was founded and became an advocate for environmental health activities.

On September 10, 1875, the first U.S. conservation organization, the American Forestry Association, was established. This organization remains active today.

On September 25, 1890, Yosemite Park was established by the U.S. Congress in an effort to preserve our natural lands and forests.

The Wilderness Society was founded on January 21, 1935. It remains an important conservation policy group that works primarily on issues involving federal public lands (national forests, national parks, national wildlife refuges). The group was instrumental in persuading Congress to create a national wilderness system.

The National Wildlife Federation was founded on February 5, 1936, and has the largest membership of any U.S. conservation organization. Its publications include *National Wildlife, International Wildlife,* and the children's magazines *Your Big Backyard, Ranger Rick,* and *Animal Baby.*

Rachel Carson published the environmental classic *Silent Spring* in 1962. This book about the effects of pesticide use is considered by many to have provided the impetus for the modern environmental movement in the United States.

In 1964 America's first permanent national wilderness system was established.

In 1970 the first annual Earth Day was held. On Earth Day professionals and the lay public focus on activities to promote an awareness of the environment, address environmental health issues, and develop strategies to preserve the environment.

On December 2, 1970, the Environmental Protection Agency (EPA) was established.

In 1979 *Healthy People* assessed environmental health in the United States, and national health objectives relating to environmental health were written in 1980.

In 1989 *50 Simple Things You Can Do to Save the Earth* was published. It sold more than 1.5 million copies. A sequel has now been published.

In 1990 more than 200 million people around the world celebrated the twentieth anniversary of Earth Day.

In 1991 *Healthy People 2000* established environmental health as a national health priority area and set national environmental health objectives.

In 2000 *Healthy People 2010* continued environmental health as a focus area and reestablished national environmental health objectives.

sues and made environmental health a national health priority. *Healthy People 2010* has environmental health as a focus area for the nation's health.

## ENVIRONMENTAL HEALTH AND THE HEALTHY PEOPLE INITIATIVE

National objectives for environmental health were established as part of the Healthy People Initiative. These objectives were based on data presented in *Healthy People* (USDHEW, 1979) and were targeted to be achieved by 1990. Progress toward almost 75% of these objectives could not be measured because states did not have adequate surveillance and monitoring systems (USDHHS, 1992, pp. 68, 103).

*Healthy People 2000* listed environmental health as one of its 22 priority areas and reestablished national environmental health objectives targeted to be achieved by the year 2000. These objectives challenged the nation to promote environmental health and preserve the global environment. Progress toward achieving the objectives was mixed. Substantial progress was made in decreasing the incidence of childhood lead poisoning, lowering the incidence of outbreaks of waterborne diseases, increasing the proportion of people who lived in counties where EPA air standards were met, and with the recycling of household and hazardous waste (USDHHS, 2000). Moderate progress was made in testing American homes for radon and lead-based paint and in the number of states with laws to track environmental diseases and improved environmental surveillance systems. Mixed progress or movement away from target was seen in the increased incidence of environmental asthma and the provision of safe drinking water. Data showed that the nation regressed over the decade of 1990 to 2000 in the percentage of Americans who have safe drinking water—90% of the population had safe drinking water in 1980, approximately 80% in 1990 (USDHHS, 1992, p. 66), and only 68% by 1995 (USDHHS, 1995, p. 82). Between 1990 and 2000 an increasing number of U.S. lakes

and rivers became polluted, and the number of waterborne disease outbreaks from infectious agents and chemical poisoning increased.

*Healthy People 2010* continued the national emphasis on environmental health, and environmental health was one of its 28 focus areas. The main areas under which *Healthy People 2010* environmental health objectives are organized is given in Figure 6-1. The document's national objectives for environmental health for the decade of 2000-2010 are given in Box 6-3. *Healthy People 2010* suggests improvements are necessary in the nation's public health infrastructure in order to deal effectively with environmental health problems (Box 6-4). Unfortunately, infectious and chemical

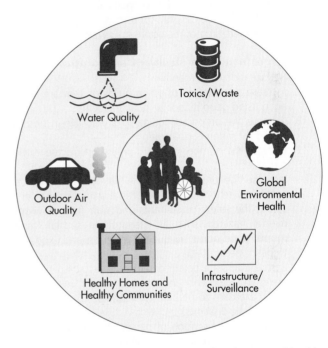

**FIGURE 6-1** *Healthy People 2010* and environmental health. (USDHHS: *Healthy People 2010*, conference edition, Washington, DC, 2000, US Government Printing Office, p. 8-3.)

### BOX 6-3
### *Objectives for Environmental Health*

*Outdoor Air Quality*
1. Reduce the proportion of persons exposed to air that does not meet the U.S. Environmental Protection Agency's (EPA) health-based standards for harmful air pollutants.
2. Increase use of alternative modes of transportation to reduce motor vehicle emissions and improve the nation's air quality.
3. Improve the nation's air quality by increasing the use of cleaner alternative fuels.
4. Reduce air toxic emissions to decrease the risk of adverse health effects caused by airborne toxics.

*Water Quality*
5. Increase the proportion of persons served by community water systems who receive a supply of drinking water that meets the regulations of the Safe Drinking Water Act.
6. Reduce waterborne disease outbreaks arising from water intended for drinking among persons served by community water systems.
7. Reduce per capita domestic water withdrawals.
8. Increase the proportion of assessed rivers, lakes, and estuaries that are safe for fishing and recreational purposes.

From USDHHS: *Healthy People 2010, conference edition*, Washington, DC, 2000, US Government Printing Office, pp. 8-15 to 8-34.

*Continued*

## BOX 6-3
### *Objectives for Environmental Health*

9. Reduce the number of beach closings that result from the presence of harmful bacteria.
10. Reduce the potential human exposure to persistent chemicals by decreasing fish contaminant levels.

### *Toxics and Waste*
11. Eliminate elevated blood lead levels in children.
12. Minimize the risks to human health and the environment posed by hazardous sites.
13. Reduce pesticide exposures that result in visits to a health care facility.
14. Reduce the amount of toxic pollutants released, disposed of, treated, or used for energy recovery.
15. Increase recycling of municipal solid waste.

### *Healthy Homes and Healthy Communities*
16. Reduce indoor allergen levels.
17. Increase the number of office buildings that are managed using good indoor air quality practices.
18. Increase the proportion of persons who live in homes tested for radon concentrations.
19. Increase the number of new homes constructed to be radon resistant.
20. Increase the proportion of the nation's primary and secondary schools that have official school policies ensuring the safety of students and staff from environmental hazards, such as chemicals in special classrooms, poor indoor air quality, asbestos, and exposure to pesticides.
21. Ensure that state health departments establish training plans and protocols and conduct annual multiinstitutional exercises to prepare for response to natural and technologic disasters.
22. Increase the proportion of persons living in pre-1950s housing that have tested for the presence of lead-based paint.

23. Reduce the proportion of occupied housing units that are substandard.

### *Infrastructure of Surveillance*
24. Reduce exposure to pesticides as measured by blood and urine concentrations of metabolites.
25. Reduce exposure of the population to pesticides, heavy metals, and other toxic chemicals, as measured by blood and urine concentrations of the substances or their metabolites.
26. Improve the quality, utility, awareness, and use of existing information systems for environmental health.
27. Increase the number of Territories, Tribes, and States, and the District of Columbia that monitor diseases or conditions that can be caused by exposure to environmental hazards.

### *Global Environmental Health*
28. Increase the number of local health departments or agencies that use data from surveillance of environmental risk factors as part of their vector control programs.
29. Reduce the global burden of disease due to poor weather quality, sanitation, and personal and domestic hygiene.
30. Increase the proportion of the population in the U.S.–Mexican border region that have adequate drinking water and sanitation facilities.

Other objectives related to environmental health are found in the following focus areas: Access to Quality Health Services; Cancer; Chronic Kidney Disease; Disability and Secondary Conditions; Food Safety; Health Communication; Heart Disease and Stroke; Immunization of Infectious Diseases; Injury and Violence Prevention; Maternal, Infant, and Child Health; Occupational Safety and Health; Physical Activity and Fitness; Public Health Infrastructure; Respiratory Diseases; Tobacco Use; and Vision and Hearing.

## BOX 6-4
### *Preventing Health Problems Caused by Environmental Hazards*

Preventing health problems caused by environmental hazards requires:
1. Having enough personnel and resources to investigate and respond to disease and injuries potentially caused by environmental hazards
2. Monitoring the population and its environment to detect hazards, exposures of the public and individuals to hazards, and diseases potentially caused by these hazards
3. Monitoring the population and its environment to assess the effectiveness of prevention programs
4. Educating the public and select populations on the relationship between health and the environment

5. Ensuring that laws, regulations, and practices protect the public and the environment from hazardous agents
6. Providing public access to understandable and useful information on hazards and their sources, distribution, and health effects
7. Coordinating the efforts of all government agencies and nongovernmental groups responsible for environmental health
8. Providing adequate resources to accomplish these tasks

Development of additional methods to measure environmental hazards in people will permit more careful assessments of exposures and health effects.

From USDHHS: *Healthy People 2010, conference edition*, Washington, DC, 2000, US Government Printing Office, p. 8-7.

agents still contaminate food and water, animals continue to carry disease to human populations, and outbreaks of preventable communicable disease still occur. Environmental health is now being looked at in a global perspective, realizing that environmental issues affecting one country or region affect everyone.

## THE NURSE AND ENVIRONMENTAL HEALTH

The environment has been a central concept in the domain of nursing since the days of *Florence Nightingale*. Environment is a core concept in Nightingale's model of nursing, and it was her contention that the environment could be altered in such a way as to improve conditions and assist in curing the patient (Selanders, 1993). Nightingale's regard for the patient's environment is traced to her work with soldiers in the Crimea where she attributed sickness and death to unsanitary environmental conditions. She stressed the importance of developing sanitary codes for hospitals and identified five factors for nurses to consider in optimizing the physical environment of the ill person: (1) pure air, (2) pure water, (3) efficient drainage, (4) cleanliness, and (5) light (Nightingale, 1859). As the *Healthy People 2010* objectives show, these factors are considered important today.

*Lillian Wald*, the founder of public health nursing and the Henry Street Nursing Settlement in New York City in 1893, was well aware of the environment and the effect it had on community health. She regularly admonished anyone who did not observe city sewage and sanitation laws and established milk stations to provide safe milk for infants and children (Coss, 1993, pp. 134, 137; Wald, 1915). To allow children safe places to play, she had playgrounds built behind the nursing settlement houses. She was instrumental in the establishment of city parks and helped children get away from the environmental pollutants and hazards of the city by starting "fresh air" camps at the country homes of her friends and supporters.

*Mary Breckinridge*, the founder of the Frontier Nursing Service (FNS) in 1925, also used environmental health principles in her work (Breckinridge, 1952; Salazar, Primomo, 1994; Wilkie, Moseley, 1969, p. 131). When building a rural hospital, she ensured that the building site had a source of clean water, was at a safe distance from outdoor privies that could contaminate wells, was away from noise, and had adequate light (Wilkie, Moseley, 1969, p. 131). She accomplished her renowned success in reducing infant mortality in the areas where FNS nurses worked by incorporating principles of environmental health into nursing practice (Salazar, Primomo, 1994).

Modern nursing scholars still consider the concept of environment to be central to the development of nursing knowledge and maintenance of health. Nurses are well positioned to help ameliorate the adverse impact of environmental hazards on the health of individuals and communities (Bellack, Musham, Hainer, et al., 1996, p. 74; Institute

of Medicine [IOM], 1995, p. 15). Today, as a major focus in community health, nurses emphasize examining the interrelationship of environment, health, and disease.

### The Contemporary Role of the Nurse

Nursing somehow strayed from the environmental teachings of leaders such as Nightingale, Wald, and Breckinridge. In the early twentieth century, many nurses worked predominantly in the community and saw firsthand the role the environment played in health and disease (Gerber, McGuire, 1999). However, as hospitals assumed a greater role in the care of ill people and nurses worked more frequently in such settings, less emphasis came to be placed on the importance of environmental health (IOM, 1995).

Nursing education has not adequately prepared nurses to understand the impact of the environment on health or to implement environmental interventions (Gerber, McGuire, 1999; IOM, 1995; Rogers, Cox, 1998). In fact, "environmental health hazards have come to be perceived as something separate from the usual practice of nursing, rather than as a set of concerns integral to its mission" (IOM, 1995, p. 14). There has been a consistent lack of nursing literature and research on environmental health. Over a period of almost 30 years, from 1961 to 1990, only 53 articles were found in the nursing literature that addressed the environment (Kleffel, 1991, p. 43). This has not changed significantly since then. A landmark report in 1995 provided guidelines for what the contemporary nursing role in environmental health should be.

NURSING, HEALTH, AND THE ENVIRONMENT: STRENGTHENING THE RELATIONSHIP TO IMPROVE THE PUBLIC'S HEALTH. In 1995, *Nursing, Health and the Environment: Strengthening the Relationship to Improve the Public's Health* was published by the Institute of Medicine's Committee on Enhancing Environmental Health Content in Nursing Practice. This landmark report is commonly called *Nursing, Health, and the Environment* and is still used to guide nursing involvement in environmental health. The report noted that nurses had the potential to be leaders in environmental health and suggested that nurses receive education and training in environmental health hazards. The report noted that more research needs to be done in relation to nursing interventions and environmental health, and environmental health content should be routinely integrated into nursing curriculum. This recommendation is supported by the American Association of Colleges of Nursing (1993) and authors in the field (Gerber, McGuire, 1999; McGuire, Gerber, 1999; Rogers, Cox, 1998; Snyder, Ruth, Sattler, et al., 1994). *Nursing, Health and the Environment* stated that:

Nurses are well positioned to address environmental health hazards, both on an individual and community level, for a number of reasons: they are the largest group of health care providers in the United States (2.2 million), and generally speaking they have more opportunities than other health care providers to talk in depth with patients. In addition, they are often the only health care providers who visit patients in their homes, workplaces and local communities, thus gaining firsthand knowledge of the potential environmental hazards present in these settings (Institute of Medicine [IOM], 1995, p. 2).

General environmental health competencies for nurses recommended by the IOM are given in Box 6-5. IOM recommendations for nursing practice, education, and research in relation to environmental health are given in the Box 6-6. Nurses need to acquire the knowledge and skills to identify potential and actual environmental health problems, treat environmentally induced disease, become advocates for envi-

### BOX 6-5

## *General Environmental Health Competencies for Nurses*

### I. Basic Knowledge and Concepts

All nurses should understand the scientific principles and underpinnings of the relationship between individuals or populations and the environment (including the work environment). This understanding includes the basic mechanisms and pathways of exposure to environmental health hazards, basic prevention and control strategies, the interdisciplinary nature of effective interventions, and the role of research.

### II. Assessment and Referral

All nurses should be able to successfully complete an environmental health history, recognize potential environmental hazards and sentinel illnesses, and make appropriate referrals for conditions with probable environmental etiologies.

An essential component of this is the ability to access and provide information to patients and communities, and to locate referral sources.

### III. Advocacy, Ethics, and Risk Communication

All nurses should be able to demonstrate knowledge of the role of advocacy (case and class), ethics, and risk communication in patient care and community intervention with respect to the potential adverse effects of the environment on health.

### IV. Legislation and Regulation

All nurses should understand the policy framework and major pieces of legislation and regulations related to environmental health.

From Institute of Medicine (Committee on Enhancing Environmental Health Content in Nursing Practice, Pope AM, Snyder MA, Mood LH, editors): *Nursing, health, and the environment: strengthening the relationship to improve the public's health*, Washington, DC, 1995, National Academy Press, p. 5.

### BOX 6-6

## *Recommendations on Environmental Health and Nursing Practice, Education, and Research*

### Nursing Practice

Environmental health should be reemphasized in the scope of responsibilities for nursing practice.

Resources to support environmental health content in nursing practice should be identified and made available.

Nurses should participate as members and leaders in interdisciplinary teams that address environmental health problems.

Communication should extend beyond counseling individual patients and families to facilitating the exchange of information on environmental hazards and community responses.

Nurses should conduct research regarding the ethical implications of occupational and environmental health hazards and incorporate findings into curricula and practice.

Although the environment as a domain in nursing has not been well developed, it is an important aspect of nursing practice and research.

### Nursing Education

Environmental health concepts should be incorporated into all levels of nursing education.

Environmental health content should be included in nursing licensure and certification examinations.

Expertise in various environmental health disciplines should be included in the education of nurses.

Environmental health content should be an integral part of lifelong learning and continuing education for nurses.

Professional associations, public agencies, and private organizations should provide more resources and educational opportunities to enhance environmental health in nursing practice.

### Nursing Research

Multidisciplinary and interdisciplinary research endeavors should be developed and implemented to build the knowledge base for nursing practice in environmental health as it relates to the practice of nursing.

The number of nurse researchers should be increased to prepare to build the knowledge base in environmental health as it relates to the practice of nursing.

Research priorities for nursing in environmental health should be established and used by funding agencies for resource allocation decisions and to give direction to nurse researchers.

Current efforts to disseminate research findings to nurses, other health care providers, and the public should be strengthened and expanded.

From Institute of Medicine (Committee on Enhancing Environmental Health Content in Nursing Practice, Pope AM, Snyder MA, Mood LH, editors): *Nursing, health, and the environment: strengthening the relationship to improve the public's health*, Washington, DC, 1995, National Academy Press, pp. 10-11.

ronmental issues, conduct environmental research, and work in partnership with communities to promote environmental health (Bellack, Musham, Hainer, et al., 1996, p. 75; Gerber, McGuire, 1999; IOM, 1995; McGuire, Gerber, 1999).

Nursing needs to play a much more important role in environmental health issues. Recently initiatives have evolved such as the one sponsored by the W.K. Kellogg Foundation at the University of Maryland School of Nursing to educate nurses about environmental health. The program has helped educate nursing faculty around the country in environmental health and facilitated placement of environmental health content in nursing school curricula. The University of Maryland School of Nursing publishes *enviRNews* as a biannual publication that serves as a forum for nurses to share environmental health issues (Sattler, 1999). The National Institutes of Health offers fellowships for nurses to gain additional training in environmental health sciences. Nursing organizations are taking a more active role in environmental health issues.

## Nursing Organizations

Professional nursing organizations, including the American Association of Occupational Health Nurses, American Nurses Association, International Council of Nurses, American Holistic Nurses Association, the Nightingale Institute for Environmental Health, and the Public Health Nursing Section of the APHA are addressing environmental health issues. The American Association of Occupational Health Nurses (AAOHN) (*http://www.aaohn.org*) is possibly the organization that has addressed environmental health issues most thoroughly. AAOHN recently has added the word *environment* to many of their position statements and into the organizations standards of practice.

Position statements on environmental health have been developed by the American Holistic Nurses Association and the International Council of Nurses (ICN) (Boxes 6-7 and 6-8). The ICN has addressed the need for nurses to assist in environmental assessment, educate the public about environmental health, and assist in formulating environ-

### BOX 6-7

## *The Nurse's Role in Safeguarding the Human Environment*

The preservation and improvement of the human environment has become increasingly important for humankind's survival and well-being. The vastness and urgency of the task places on every individual and every professional group the responsibility to participte in the efforts to safeguard humankind's environment, to conserve the world's resources, and to study how their use affects humankind and how adverse effects can be avoided.

### *The Nurse's Role Is To:*
*Help detect ill effects of the environment on the health of man, and vice-versa.*

The nurse should:
- apply observational skills for the detection of ill effects of environment on the individual;
- observe individuals in all settings for effects of pollutants in order to advise on protective and/or curative measures;
- record and analyze observations made of ill effects of environment and/or pollutants on individuals;
- be informed and report observations of the ecological consequences of pollutants and their adverse effects on the human being.

*Be informed and apply knowledge in daily work with individuals, families and/or community groups as to the data available on potential health hazards and ways to prevent and/or reduce them.*

The nurse should be informed about:
- the studies and identification of the environmental problems at local, national, and international levels;
- their effects on man;
- the standards for the protection of the human organism, especially from pollutants;
- ways to prevent and/or reduce health hazards.

*Be informed and teach preventive measures about health hazards due to environmental factors as well as about conservation of environmental resources to the individual, families, and/or community groups.*

The nurse can:
- request and attend continuing education programs about the study of the environment and the application of this knowledge in daily life and work;
- provide health education for both the general public and health personnel in order to create awareness of environmental issues and to involve the public with environmental management and control;
- apply knowledge in areas where nursing intervention may prevent or reduce health hazards;
- report on steps taken to control the significant environmental problems of the area.

*Work with health authorities in pointing out health care aspects and health hazards in existing human settlements and in the planning of new settlements.*

The nurse can:
- participate in exchange of information and experience about similar environmental problems with authorities in other areas;
- cooperate with health authorities in the preparation of programs to enable national and local authorities to influence their own environments;
- participate in the promotion of legislation to improve health care and reduce/prevent health hazards, and encourage the enforcement of such legislation where/when appropriate;
- participate in national/local pre-disaster planning; and cooperate in international programs in case of disasters in other countries.

From International Council of Nurses: *The nurse's role in safeguarding the human environment: position statement,* Geneva, Switzerland, 1986, The Council.

*Continued*

### BOX 6-7

## *The Nurse's Role in Safeguarding the Human Environment—cont'd*

*Assist communities in their action on environmental health problems.*

The nurse can assist communities in programs to:

- reduce harmful pollutants (chemical, biological or physical, e.g. noise) in air, soil, water and food by industries or other human efforts;
- improve nutrition;
- encourage family planning;
- assess environmental factors in work situations and pursue activities for the elimination or reduction of hazards;
- educate the general public and all levels of nursing personnel in environmental and other health hazards, especially those related to unacceptable levels of contamination.

*Participate in research providing data for early warning and prevention of deleterious effects of the various environmental agents to which man is increasingly exposed and research conducive to discovering ways and means of improving living and working conditions.*

The nurse, as principal investigator or in collaboration with other nurses or related professions, can carry out epidemiological and experimental research designed to provide data for:

- early warning for prevention of health hazards;
- improving living and working conditions;
- monitoring the environmental levels of pollutants;
- measuring the impact of nursing intervention on environmental hazards.

### BOX 6-8

## *Environmental Health Nursing Philosophy*

Believing that human beings and the physical environment, both as open systems, are continuously exchanging matter and energy with one another, Environmental Health Nursing (EHN) is concerned with the effects of environmental degradation on human health. EHN's goal is to decrease, avoid, or eliminate environmental exposures which are determined by research and consensus in the scientific community to constitute an unacceptable risk to human health.

EHN maintains the basic tenants of the nursing profession—promotion and restoration of health and the prevention of illness using the nursing process—assessment, planning, implementation, and evaluation—in this expanded arena.

In assessing the environmental conditions to identify existing or potential exposures associated with the health of the community, EHN integrates knowledge from the natural and behavioral sciences. EHN collaborates with industry, government agencies, other scientific disciplines, and the public.

EHN believes that individuals and communities have a right to know the environmental risks to which they are exposed, as well as a right to participate in decisions of risk acceptance. To assist the community in logical decision making, EHN interprets research and communicates risks of exposures to the community.

EHN assesses communities' perception of risk and helps them cope with disturbances in their environment that they perceive have diminished their health. EHN teaches changes in lifestyle that can decrease, avoid, or eliminate exposures. EHN assists communities in interfacing with agencies and industry in planning and implementing efforts to reduce exposures.

When involved in planning and implementation efforts to remove or prevent exposures, EHN considers research findings, perception of risk, susceptible populations, law, and the cost-benefit ratio in decision making.

From Portman C: Environmental health nursing philosophy, *Nurses for Environmental and Social Responsibility Newsletter* 1(3):3, 1995.

mental health policy and legislation. ICN also proposed that nurses form collaborative interdisciplinary and community relationships for environmental health and be actively involved in environmental health research.

The American Nurses Association (ANA) (*http://www.ana.org*) publishes the *Pollution Prevention Kit for Nurses*. This kit is designed to assist nurses to become active in reducing the toxic pollution created as a health care industry by-product. The kit contains resources and materials for nurses to create environmental change in their communities.

The **Nightingale Institute for Health and the Environment (NIHE)** (*http://www.nihe.org*) is a relatively new organization that provides resources, education, and training to health care professionals to help them recognize the inextricable link between human and environmental health (NIHE, 2001). Its Clinicians Initiative is designed to educate nurses and other clinicians to recognize the impact of their clinical practice on the environment and empower them to promote resource conservation and healthy environmental conditions.

## Standards of Practice

Standards of practice are the hallmark of a profession and guide a profession in its practice. Until recently there were no standards of practice for environmental health nursing. In 1999 the AAOHN published *Standards of Occupational and Environmental Health Nursing*. Before this publication, the word *environmental* had not been in the title of the standards. These standards can be obtained by contacting AAOHN (*http://www.aaohn.org*).

## ENVIRONMENTAL HEALTH LEGISLATION

As previously discussed, the Social Security Act of 1935 serves as umbrella legislation, consolidating U.S. health and welfare legislation under one law, and the Public Health Service Act of 1944 does the same for public health legislation. However, there is no umbrella legislation for environmental health, and numerous environmental health laws exist. The scope of this legislation and its lack of consolidation make it difficult and time consuming to locate and become knowledgeable about the range of environmental health issues that need to be addressed.

Environmental legislation has tended to be reactive and responsive to the demands and crises of the moment rather than preventive (Rabe, 1990, p. 320). The environmental awareness that evolved in the United States in the 1960s marked the advent of numerous pieces of legislation.

Environmental legislation is diverse and encompasses areas such as the Superfund (the environmental fund created to finance the cleanup of hazardous substances), water and air quality, toxic substances in the environment, pesticides, soil conservation, solid waste disposal, radiation, ocean dumping, environmental research, noise pollution, endangered species, and nuclear waste. The **National Environmental Policy Act** (Public Law 91-190) of 1969 is one of the most significant and best-known pieces of U.S. environmental health legislation. This act established the Environmental Protection Agency (EPA). Other important pieces of legislation include the **Clean Air Act** and **Clean Water Act.** An overview of these and other selected U.S. environmental health legislation is given in Box 6-9.

## FEDERAL, STATE, AND LOCAL ROLES IN ENVIRONMENTAL HEALTH

Many of the public health successes that have occurred in relation to controlling communicable disease, improving the quality of life, and reducing mortality across the life span (especially infant mortality) have come about as a result of environmental health practices. The private sector has been involved in environmental health activities, often from the standpoint of serving as an advocate for safeguarding and preserving the nation's lands and wildlife. Traditionally the federal government has enacted national environmental health legislation, while state health authorities (SHAs) and local health departments (LHDs) have been involved in direct provision of environmental health services, policies, and regulations.

### Federal Government and Environmental Health

The federal government is involved in promoting environmental health, and some federal agencies involved in environmental health are discussed here. The federal government assists in protecting the public from the adverse consequences of exposure to harmful environmental agents and protecting and preserving the nation's natural resources. The federal government is involved in direct provision of emergency and disaster services, but direct provision of day-to-day environmental health services is usually carried out through SHAs and LHDs.

ENVIRONMENTAL PROTECTION AGENCY. The **Environmental Protection Agency (EPA)** (*http://www.epa.gov*),

a freestanding agency of the federal government, was created on December 2, 1970, and has regional offices across the nation. It is the federal government's foremost environmental agency and is the single largest employer of environmental health professionals in the world. The agency's mission is to control and abate environmental pollution. The EPA is well known for its efforts to protect and enhance the American environment and enforce national environmental health legislation. It works to control air, water, solid waste, noise, radiation, and toxic substances pollution and manages the Superfund toxic waste cleanup program. The agency works in cooperation with state and local governments. Its National Service Center for Environmental Publications (*http://www.epa.gov/ncepi*) offers 5000 EPA publications free of charge. Its National Center for Environmental Health Assessment (*http://www.epa.gov/ncea*) is a resource center for human health and ecologic risk assessments. The EPA coordinates and supports research in environmental health.

FEDERAL EMERGENCY MANAGEMENT AGENCY. The **Federal Emergency Management Agency (FEMA)** (*http://www.fema.gov*) was established in 1979. It is an independent agency and reports directly to the President. It is the central federal agency for emergency planning, preparedness, and response. FEMA works closely with state and local governments and the American Red Cross to prepare for disasters and take actions when disasters strike. FEMA is the agency called in to help when the President declares a disaster after hurricanes, tornadoes, floods, earthquakes, or other events that pose a threat to American communities. FEMA has a specific link at its website, FEMA for Kids, that presents environmental health issues and activities for children.

FEMA's numerous activities include producing training programs, publications, and technical guidance; managing the President's Disaster Relief Fund (which is the source of most federal funding assistance after major disasters); sponsoring the U.S. Fire Administration; carrying out national emergency management and multihazard response planning; doing flood-plain management and dam safety; planning for emergencies at commercial nuclear power plants and military chemical stockpile sites; providing emergency food and shelter; ensuring federal government continuity during national security emergencies; and coordinating federal response to the consequences of major terrorist incidents.

NATIONAL CENTER FOR ENVIRONMENTAL HEALTH. The **National Center for Environmental Health (NCEH)** (*http://www.cdc.gov/nceh*) is part of the Centers for Disease Control and Prevention (CDC) of the U.S. Department of Health and Human Services. The mission of the NCEH is to provide national leadership, through science and service, that promotes health and quality of life by preventing or controlling those diseases, birth defects, disabilities, or deaths that result from interactions between people and their environment (NCEH, 2001). It carries out activities related to the health effects of environmental hazards (including birth defects and developmental disabilities) and

**BOX 6-9**

## Selected Environmental Health Legislation: United States*

1948 *Water Pollution Control Act (Public Law 80-845)*—Authorized the Public Health Service to help states develop water pollution control programs and to aid in the planning of sewage treatment plants.

1963 *Clean Air Act (Public Law 88-206)*—Authorized direct grants to states and localities for air pollution control; provided for federal enforcement of interstate air pollution; directed major research efforts for control of motor vehicle exhaust, removal of sulfur from fuel, and the development of air quality criteria.

1965 *Solid Waste Disposal Act (Public Law 89-272)*—Established a program of grants to states to develop solid waste disposal programs.

1966 *Disaster Relief Act of 1966 (Public Law 89-769)*—Authorized assistance to U.S. communities suffering a major natural disaster. Significant amendments in 1970.

1969 *National Environmental Policy Act (Public Law 91-190)*—One of the best-known and most significant pieces of U.S. environmental health legislation. Established national environmental policy and authorized formation of the Environmental Protection Agency (EPA).

1970 *Environmental Education Act (Public Law 91-516)*—Authorized the establishment of education programs to encourage public understanding of policies and environmental activities designed to enhance environmental quality. Established the Office of Environmental Education.

*Lead-Based Paint Poisoning Prevention Act (Public Law 91-695)*—Provided federal assistance to help cities and communities combat lead-based paint poisoning. Established demonstration and research projects.

1973 *Endangered Species Act (Public Law 93-205)*—The first federal law to protect endangered and threatened species of U.S. fish, wildlife, and plants.

1974 *Safe Drinking Water Act (Public Law 93-523)*—Amended the Public Health Service Act to require the EPA to set national drinking water standards and to aid states and localities in enforcement.

1976 *Toxic Substances Control Act (Public Law 94-469)*—Regulated toxic chemicals already in existence and tried to prevent new hazardous chemicals from entering the market. Required EPA to test existing hazardous chemicals, gather and disseminate information about these chemicals, and prevent future chemical risks by premarket screening and tracking. An overall goal of the act was to prevent unreasonable injury to individual health or harm to the en-

vironment associated with the manufacture, processing, distribution, use, or disposal of hazardous chemical substances.

1980 *Asbestos School Hazard Detection and Control Act (Public Law 96-270)*—Established a program for the inspection of schools to detect the presence of hazardous asbestos materials; provided for loans to states or local educational agencies to contain or remove hazardous asbestos materials from schools and replace such materials with suitable building materials.

*Comprehensive Environmental Response, Compensation and Liability Act of 1980 (Public Law 96-510)*—Known as the "Superfund," this act provided for liability, compensation, cleanup, and emergency response for hazardous substances released into the environment and cleanup of inactive hazardous waste disposal sites. The EPA was to oversee the programs of the act. It established the Agency for Toxic Substances and Disease Registry and the Hazardous Substance Response Trust Fund.

1990 *Global Change Research Act of 1990 (Public Law 101-606)*—Required the establishment of a United States Global Change Research program aimed at understanding and responding to global change. Encouraged international discussion toward protocols in global change research.

*Environmental Research Geographic Local Information Act (Public Law 101-617)*—Provided a method of locating private and governmental research on environmental issues by specific geographic locations. The EPA will identify major environmental research relating to a specific geographic area, compile and maintain the research, and make it available to the public. The EPA is authorized to enter into contractual agreements to obtain the data.

*America the Beautiful Act of 1990 (Public Law 101-624)*—This act was Title XII, Subtitle C of the Food, Agriculture, Conservation, and Trade Act of 1990. Authorized the President to designate a private nonprofit foundation to be eligible for a grant to be used to create public awareness and a spirit of volunteerism in relation to tree-planting projects in U.S. communities and urban areas.

*Global Climate Change Prevention Act of 1990 (Public Law 101-624)*—This act was Title XIV of the Food, Agriculture, Conservation, and Trade Act of 1990. Established, within the Department of Agriculture, a global climate change program to coordinate all issues and activities relating to climate change, including policy analysis and research.

*Note:* Many of these acts are frequently amended.

works extensively with childhood lead poisoning prevention, improving air pollution and respiratory health, improving environmental health surveillance programs, and providing technical assistance to the National Park System in matters of environmental health. The center collaborates with state and LHDs, federal and state regulatory agencies, research institutions, private groups, and international organizations to promote environmental health.

AGENCY FOR TOXIC SUBSTANCES AND DISEASE REGISTRY. The Agency for Toxic Substances and Disease Registry (ATSDR) (*http://www.atsdr.cdc.gov*) is part of the U.S. Department of Health and Human Services. It assists the federal government in registering toxic substances and providing information about community health risks. The ATSDR has been discussed in Chapter 5.

## State Government and Environmental Health

SHAs historically have been involved in environmental health activities and provide many environmental health services (see Chapter 5). Some SHAs administer federal environmental health legislation including the Clean Air Act, the Clean Water Act, the Safe Drinking Water Act, the Resource Conservation and Recovery Act, and the Superfund.

The SHA is the lead environmental agency in some states and other states have a separate state level agency, such as the *Department of Environment*. This trend toward removing environmental health authority from SHAs has led to diffuse patterns of responsibility, lack of coordination, and inadequate handling of environmental problems (IOM, 1988, p. 150). The state agency in charge of environmental health activities collects information on environmental pollution in local communities, maintains an environmental disease registry, takes part in environmental monitoring activities, and provides consultation to LHDs.

### Stop and Think About It

Does your state have a separate Department of the Environment? How does your state monitor environmental health issues? What agencies in your local communities address environmental health issues?

## Local Government and Environmental Health

LHDs have traditionally offered numerous environmental health services to the local communities they serve (see Chapter 5). Such services are often provided through the department's environmental engineers or sanitarians. Community health nurses work cooperatively with them to implement nursing interventions.

Environmental health personnel work to prevent, eliminate, and control environmental hazards. LHDs are often responsible for testing community water and air, overseeing solid and hazardous waste disposal, performing food and restaurant inspections, monitoring noise pollution, ensuring

sanitation of public swimming and recreational facilities, implementing vector (e.g. skunk, rat, and mosquito) control measures, and ensuring safe housing (Table 6-1).

## Private Sector Environmental Health Activities

Shortly after the establishment in 1872 of Yellowstone, our first national park, the first private U.S. conservation organization, the American Forestry Association, was established. Other organizations such as the National Wildlife Federation, Sierra Club, Wilderness Society, World Wildlife Federation, Environmental Action, Greenpeace, Worldwatch Institute, and Nature Conservancy are actively involved in promoting environmental health worldwide. These groups have many interesting magazines and publications (e.g., National Wildlife Federation publishes the magazines *National Wildlife*; *International Wildlife*; and for children, *Animal Baby*, *Your Big Backyard*, and *Ranger Rick*). The efforts of the American Red Cross, an international voluntary agency, are discussed later in this chapter under disaster nursing.

Millions of Americans each year participate in activities to support the environment. In local communities people are taking part in environmentally safe activities and donating time to plant trees and clean up parks, lakes, and rivers. Every year in the United States, on the third Saturday in September, people of all ages spend the day cleaning up trash from beaches and waterways. Each year millions of people around the world celebrate Earth Day on April 22. We can be proud of such efforts to support our environment—after all, there is only one earth.

Private corporations are helping too. Each year corporations across the nation make financial donations and sponsor environmental projects. One such project, *EarthQuest*, a traveling exhibit sponsored by the Ford Motor Company, the Hertz Corporation, and IBM, is a giant video game where children try to avoid Toxicus, the monster of waste, and learn about making choices that environmentally help the planet. Businesses often work with communities on hazardous waste and environmental cleanup. They also encourage their employees to adopt roads for cleanup and to sponsor community beautification projects.

## THE ENVIRONMENTAL HEALTH WORKFORCE

Almost 80% of all environmental health practitioners are employed by government agencies at the federal, state, and local levels (USDHHS, 1988, p. 3). The federal government is the largest employer of environmental health professionals in the United States.

For half a century the title *sanitarian* has been used to describe the environmental health practitioner who applies technical knowledge obtained from the biologic and chemical sciences to promote and protect environmental health (USDHHS, 1988). Nationwide, LHDs employ sanitarians

**TABLE 6-1**

*Environmental Health Programs within Local Health Departments (LHDs)*

| CATEGORIES OF ENVIRONMENTAL CONCERN | PROGRAMS | PROGRAM PURPOSE |
| --- | --- | --- |
| Air | Air quality management | To ensure a community air resource conducive to good health that will not injure plant or animal life or property and will be esthetically desirable |
| Water | Water supply sanitation | To ensure the provision of safe public and private water supplies, adequate in quantity and quality for every person |
|  | Water pollution control | To ensure the cooperation with state water pollution control agencies and that surface and subsurface water supplies meet all state and local standards and regulations for water quality |
| Waste | Solid waste management | To ensure that all solid wastes are stored, collected, transported, and disposed of in a manner that does not create health, safety, or esthetic problems |
|  | Liquid waste management | To ensure the treatment of liquid wastes in such a manner as to prevent problems of sanitation, public health nuisances, or pollution |
|  | Toxic and hazardous waste management | To ensure that toxic and hazardous wastes are stored, collected, transported, and disposed of in a manner that does not create health or safety problems |
| Food | Food protection | To ensure that all people are adequately protected from unhealthful or unsafe food or food products. This necessitates a comprehensive food protection program covering every facility where food or food products are stored, transported, processed, packaged, served, or vended and regulating sanitation, wholesomeness, adulteration, advertising, labeling weights and measures, and fill of containers |
| Recreational areas | Swimming pool sanitation and safety | To ensure the safety and sanitation of public, semipublic, and private swimming pools |
|  | Recreational sanitation | To ensure that all public recreational areas are operated so as to prevent health and safety problems |
| Product safety | Consumer product safety | To ensure that all people are adequately protected from unhealthful or unsafe substances or products in the home, business, and industry |
| Radiation | Radiation control | To prevent unnecessary or hazardous radiation exposure from the transportation, use, or disposal of all types of radiation-producing devices and products |
| Occupational | Occupational health and safety | To ensure, in cooperation with state officials, the health and safety of workers in places of employment through controlling relevant environmental factors |
| Vectors | Vector control | To control all insects, rodents, and other animals that adversely affect health, safety, or comfort |
| Noise | Noise pollution control | To prevent hazardous or annoying noise levels in residential, business, industrial, and recreational structures and areas |
| Accidents | Environmental injury prevention | To influence or regulate planning, design, and construction in such a manner as to reduce the possibility of accidents through proper management of the environment |
| Buildings | Housing sanitation, safety, and rehabilitation | To ensure programs that will provide decent, safe, and healthful housing for all people |
|  | Institutional sanitation, safety, and rehabilitation | To ensure that institutions such as hospitals, schools, nurseries, jails, and prisons are operated so as to prevent sanitation and safety problems |

Modified from American Public Health Association: Position paper on the role of official local health agencies, *Am J Public Health* 65:189-193, 1975; and USDHHS: *Evaluating the environmental health workforce* (HRP#0907160), Rockville, Md, 1988, USDHHS, p. 3.

to design and implement environmental health programs. Today more contemporary titles include *environmental engineer, environmental health specialist,* and *environmentalist.* Historically, the environmental health work force has focused on reducing the incidence of communicable diseases spread by vectors and contaminated food and water. It is estimated that thousands of additional environmental health specialists are needed to meet the nation's demands.

## Environmental Health Teamwork

Community health nurses work collaboratively with other health professionals on environmental health concerns. For example, interdisciplinary teams of personnel, including nurses, sanitarians, and health educators, work together to combat lead poisoning in children. On such a team the nurse might teach about lead poisoning prevention, complete risk assessments on targeted aggregates, do lead screenings in well-baby and women, infants, and children (WIC) clinics, and participate in community education activities at a local health fair.

Numerous other interdisciplinary efforts are carried out to improve environmental health conditions. The environmental health sanitarian may make joint home visits with the community health nurse to conduct an environmental assessment, complete mapping programs to identify clusters of cases within a local community, enforce housing codes to eliminate lead in the home environment, and participate in community education activities. The health educator may develop and organize community education activities. Together they might write grants to obtain funds for program development.

Another example of a cooperative interaction between nurses and environmental health personnel is the collaboration that occurs during an epidemiologic investigation of serious outbreaks of foodborne diseases such as botulism and *Salmonella*. During these investigations both disciplines interview affected persons, investigate sources of contamination, and may conduct house-to-house surveys to identify ill people (see Chapter 11). Nurses are becoming increasingly involved in aggregate- and community-based environmental health activities and aware of the importance of environmental health. Individually and as part of a team, community health nurses must have an active role in environmental health issues.

## SELECTED ENVIRONMENTAL DISEASES AND CONDITIONS

Environmental diseases are caused by biologic, chemical, physical, and sociologic hazards and most are highly preventable. Biologic hazards include infectious agents such as bacteria, viruses, and protozoa; plants; insects; fungi; and molds. Chemical hazards include toxicants, irritants, asphyxiants, poisons, carcinogens, mutagens, and teratogens. Physical hazards include radiation, dust, vibration, noise, heat, and cold. Sociologic hazards include stress, violence, inadequate housing, and terrorism. Many of these hazards enter the environment through direct discharge into air or water, inadequate landfills, and dumping sites.

For today's nurse, addressing the problems of environmental disease requires systematic environmental assessment. Nurses need to assess the public health implications of environmental hazards. To aid in determining environmental etiology an *environmental health history* should be routinely taken by the nurse as part of a client's health history (Box 6-10). An excellent reference for obtaining information on environmental and communicable diseases is the APHA's classic publication, *Control of Communicable Diseases Manual,* that has been published since 1917 (Chin, 2000). The American Academy of Pediatrics (AAP) has published the *Handbook of Pediatric Environmental Health* that addresses many environmental diseases and conditions of children (AAP, 1999). Selected waterborne, foodborne, soilborne, vectorborne, and zoonoses diseases; lead poisoning; environmental lung dis-

**BOX 6-10**

*Environmental History*

- Occupation of family members and potential hazards in the work setting
- Home:
  - Age of home (homes built before 1950 are likely to have leaded paint)
  - Type of dwelling
  - Building materials used and stored in the home (e.g., asbestos, formaldehyde)
  - Exposure to smoke in the home (e.g., environmental tobacco smoke [ETS], combustion smoke from fireplaces/wood stoves)
  - Procedures for storing chemicals/poisons
  - Poison Control information
  - Source of water (e.g., well, municipal)
  - Source of fresh fruits and vegetables
  - Home heating and ventilation system
  - Sewage disposal system (e.g., septic, municipal)
  - Home pesticide use
  - Pets
- Contact with animals
- Hobbies (especially hobbies that might increase exposure to chemicals, sunlight, or waste products)
- Types of industry in the neighborhood
- Known exposures to lead or other chemicals
- Vector exposure
- Exposure to known or suspected sources of contaminated air, soil, or water

ease; environmental cancers; and environmental birth defects are discussed in this chapter.

### Waterborne Diseases

Waterborne diseases are a result of water that is biologically and/or chemically polluted (water pollution is discussed later in this chapter). In most countries of the world, contaminated drinking water and food are responsible for large outbreaks of infectious disease (Goldman, 2000, p. 58). Sewage contamination of drinking water remains a worldwide problem and the World Health Organization (WHO) estimates 7% of deaths and disease worldwide can be attributed to fecally contaminated drinking water (Nadakavukaren, 2000, p. 602). In developing countries, infectious diarrhea, caused by contaminated drinking water, is the leading cause of infant mortality (Goldman, 2000, p. 61). Some scientists believe that perhaps 80% of all the illnesses in the world could be prevented if people had access to safe water supplies (Nadakavukaren, 1995, p. 611).

Hundreds of biologic agents and thousands of chemical agents can be found in water (AAP, 1999, p. 251). Agents responsible for waterborne diseases include bacteria such as *Shigella, Salmonella,* and *Campylobacter;* viruses such as Hepatitis A, poliomyelitis, and rotavirus; protozoan parasites such as *Giardia;* and chemicals such as lead, nitrates, and copper. Waterborne diseases include gastroenteritis, typhoid, cholera, polio, hepatitis, giardiasis, bacterial dysentery, and chemical poisoning.

Outbreaks of epidemic waterborne disease were prevalent in the United States up through the late nineteenth century. In 1885 a major outbreak of typhoid disease in Chicago had a death toll of 90,000 people and was the impetus needed for city officials to divert the flow of city sewage from Lake Michigan, which was also the source of city drinking water (Nadakavukaren, 2000, p. 601). Today, most Americans obtain drinking water from a public water system that is regulated under federal standards, but outbreaks of waterborne disease still occur. In 1993 in Milwaukee a waterborne epidemic caused by a protozoan parasite, *Cryptosporidium*, sickened more than 400,000 people and resulted in 4,000 hospitalizations and an estimated 104 deaths. Thousands of individual cases of waterborne diseases are reported each year in the United States, and the number of waterborne epidemics has recently increased. People living in rural areas, or areas where untreated well water is used, are at greater risk for contracting waterborne diseases than people using city water.

In the United States it is estimated that more than 30% of the population does not have safe drinking water (USDHHS, 1995, p. 82). *Healthy People 2010* objectives address improving the integrity of the water supply and control of waterborne disease. The CDC and the EPA have a collaborative surveillance system for collecting and reporting data on U.S. waterborne disease outbreaks. Waterborne pathogens are suspected to be responsible for as many as 30 million cases of waterborne disease each year in the United States (Morris, Naumova, Levin, et al., 1996, p. 237).

As the safety of our national drinking water becomes less sure, the incidence of waterborne diseases can be expected to increase. To counteract the threat of unsafe drinking water Americans are spending billions of dollars each year on bottled water. Unfortunately, research has shown that up to one fourth of bottled water brands have chemical or biologic contaminants that violate water quality regulations (Nadakavukaren, 2000, p. 616; National Resources Defense Council, 1999).

In many countries a heavy financial burden is placed on families because they must buy drinking water. In Port-au-Prince, Haiti, 20% of a typical slum-dweller's household budget is spent on purchasing drinking water (Nadakavukaren, 2000, p. 532). Many of the world's nations are experiencing water shortages. Egypt is almost entirely dependent on water resources beyond its own borders. With countries becoming more desperate for sources of drinking water, the potential for "water wars" looms. Unless water quality is substantially upgraded, it will continue to be a threat to national and international health.

## Foodborne Diseases

Foodborne diseases are diseases transmitted by food. There are hundreds of known causes of foodborne illness. How-

**BOX 6-11**

*Consumer Tips for Safe Food Handling*

**When You Shop.** Buy cold food last, get it home fast.
**When You Store Food.** Keep it safe; refrigerate and freeze fresh meat, poultry, or fish immediately if you can't use it within a few days.
**When You Prepare Food.** Keep everything clean; wash hands in hot soapy water before preparing food and after using the bathroom, changing diapers, and handling pets; avoid contact between raw and cooked food; protect food from insects, rodents, and other animals.
**When You're Cooking.** Cook thoroughly. Generally cook red meat to 160° F and poultry to 180° F.
**When You Serve Food.** Never leave it out over 2 hours; use clean dishes and utensils; pack lunches and picnics in insulated carriers with a cold pack.
**When You Handle Leftovers.** Use small containers for quick cooling of the leftover food and remove stuffing from meats and poultry.
**When You Reheat.** Bring sauces, soups, and gravy to a boil, and heat other leftovers to 165° F.
**Kept It Too Long?** When in doubt, throw it out!

Modified from U.S. Department of Agriculture: *A quick consumer guide to safe food handling* (Home and Garden Bulletin No. 248), Washington, DC, 1995, USDA.

ever, the etiology of many foodborne outbreaks is unknown. For those of known etiology, the greatest number are bacterial in origin. Estimates on the frequency of foodborne illness each year in the United States are as high as 81 million cases, 9000 deaths, and a cost of as much as $37 billion (Nadakavukaren, 2000, p. 331). Worldwide, foodborne diseases are very prevalent, especially in developing countries. Food contamination is best prevented by the use of good agricultural and manufacturing techniques and careful food preparation, handling, and storage (Goldman, 2000, p. 64).

*Healthy People 2010* has objectives to reduce infections caused by foodborne pathogens, reduce the incidence of outbreaks of foodborne diseases, and increase the percentage of American households where safe food handling occurs. Factors that may be implicated in outbreaks of foodborne illness include improper holding temperatures for food, inadequate cooking, contaminated equipment, contaminated food, and infected food handlers.

Bacteria that cause foodborne illness include, *Campylobacter jejuni, Salmonella, Escherichia coli, Listeria monocytogenes, Staphylococcus aureus, Clostridium botulinum, Helicobacter pylori,* and *Shigella* (Chin, 2000; Nadakavukaren, 2000, pp. 334-343). In Japan, food poisoning caused by *E. coli* sickened more than 6000 children after they ate school-prepared lunches—the same strain of bacteria that just a few years before affected 500 people who ate undercooked hamburgers in the state of Washington (Wasson, 1996, p. 9A). Consumer tips for safe food handling are given in Box 6-11.

**TABLE 6-2**

*Examples of Food Defect Action Levels*

| PRODUCT | DEFECT | ACTION LEVEL |
|---------|--------|--------------|
| Apricots, canned | Insect filth | Average of 2% or more by count insect-infested or insect-damaged |
| Beets, canned | Rot | Exceeds average of 5% by weight of pieces with dry rot |
| Broccoli, frozen | Insects and mites | Average of 60 aphids, thrips, and/or mites per 100 g |
| Corn, canned | Insect larvae (corn ear worms, corn borers) | Two or more 3 mm or longer larvae, cast skins or cast skin fragments of corn ear worm or corn borer, the aggregate length exceeding 12 mm in 24 pounds |
| Curry powder | Insect filth | Average of more than 100 insect fragments per 25 g |
| | Rodent filth | Average of more than 4 rodent hairs per 25 g |
| Peanut butter | Insect filth | Average of 30 or more insect fragments per 100 g |
| | Rodent filth | Average of 1 or more rodent hairs per 100 g |
| | Grit | Gritty taste and water insoluble inorganic residue is more than 25 mg per 100 g |
| Tomatoes, canned | Drosophila fly | Average of 10 fly eggs per 500 g; or 5 fly eggs and 1 maggot per 500 g; or 2 maggots per 500 g |

Source: Nadakavukaren A: *Our global environment: a health perspective*, ed 5, Prospect Heights, Ill, 2000, Waveland Press, p. 321.

Contributors to foodborne disease are *food contaminants*. These contaminants include dirt, hairs, feces, fungi, insect eggs and fragments, pesticide residues, and chemical substances. Growth hormones in meat and poultry and pesticide residues on fruits and vegetables are well-known food contaminants. The Food and Drug Administration (FDA) has established *defect action levels* that specify the maximum limit of contamination the agency permits before legal action is taken to remove the product from the market (Table 6-2).

## Soilborne Parasitic Diseases

Soilborne parasitic diseases are the most common infectious diseases in the world and are primarily transmitted by the fecal-oral route. Community health nurses regularly assess for exposure to soilborne diseases when working with children.

PINWORM. Pinworm (enterobiasis) is the most common worm infection in the United States. Climate helps make these infections more prevalent in the southeastern part of the country. Prevalence of the disease is highest in school-age children. Infection often occurs in more than one family member, reinfections are common, and the disease can be difficult to control.

TAPEWORM. Tapeworm (Taeniasis) is an infection caused by a large roundworm. Clinical manifestations of the disease include nervousness, weight loss, abdominal pain, and digestive disturbances (Chin, 2000, p. 488). The disease is rarely fatal but can be difficult to cure.

ASCARIASIS. Ascariasis is a large, roundworm disease. In tropical climates half of the population may actually be infected with *Ascaris lumbricoides* (Chin, 2000, p. 58). Prevalence and intensity of this infection is usually greatest in children 3 to 8 years old (Chin, 2000). A single female *Ascaris* can produce 200,000 eggs per day (Chin, 2000, p. 59).

HOOKWORM. Hookworm is widely endemic in tropical and subtropical countries, and millions of persons are infected with hookworm worldwide. The bloodletting activity of the worm can lead to anemia and children with mental, physical, and developmental delays.

## Vectorborne Diseases

Vectorborne diseases are diseases transmitted by vectors to humans. A *vector* is a nonhuman carrier of disease organisms that can transmit these organisms directly to humans. Vector transmission is an indirect form of biologic or mechanical disease transmission. *Mechanical transmission* includes the disease spread by a crawling or flying insect (e.g., mosquitoes, ticks, and houseflies) that does not require multiplication or development of the transmitted organism (Chin, 2000, p. 578). *Biologic transmission* involves multiplication (propagation) or development of the organism before the vector can transmit the infective agent (Chin, 2000).

Health professionals' lack of training in the etiology, diagnosis, and treatment of such diseases has hampered disease control efforts. The use of protective clothing and insect and tick repellants helps prevent these diseases. The use of insecticides and mosquito control measures has decreased the occurrence of vectorborne diseases worldwide. Some insect vectors and the diseases transmitted by them are given in Table 6-3. The vectorborne diseases of malaria, yellow fever, Lyme disease, and Rocky Mountain spotted fever are discussed briefly.

MALARIA. Malaria is transmitted by mosquitoes and remains a major illness in many tropical and subtropical areas. This disease often manifests with fever. Infections may persist for life. Prompt treatment is essential because irreversible complications may suddenly appear, and case fatality rates among untreated children and nonimmune adults can be 40% or higher (Chin, 2000, p. 310).

YELLOW FEVER. Yellow fever also is transmitted by mosquitoes and was prevalent in the United States until the

**TABLE 6-3**

*Some Insect Vectors and Diseases They Transmit*

| VECTOR | DISEASE |
|---|---|
| *Mosquitoes* | Malaria |
| | Yellow fever |
| | Filariasis |
| | Encephalitis |
| | Dengue fever |
| *Biting Flies* | |
| Deer fly | Filariasis |
| Black fly | River blindness |
| Tsetse fly | Sleeping sickness |
| Sand fly | Tropical ulcer |
| | Phlebotomus fever |
| *Other Insects* | |
| Gnats | Filariasis |
| Rat flea | Plague |
| | Murine typhus |
| Body louse | Pediculosis |
| | Epidemic typhus |
| | Trench fever |
| Tick | Rocky Mountain spotted fever |
| | Colorado tick fever |
| | Lyme disease |
| Mite | Rickettsial pox |
| | Scabies |

early 1900s. It is an acute, viral disease of short duration and varying severity (Chin, 2000, p. 553). Mild cases may be indeterminate and symptoms often include sudden onset of fever, chills, headache, backache, muscle pain, nausea, and vomiting (Chin, 2000). It was an epidemic of this disease originating in the port of New Orleans that precipitated the formation of a National Board of Health in 1879. It remains an important health problem in tropical regions of Africa and Latin America. Its case fatality rate can be as high as 40% in individual outbreaks (Chin, 2000, p. 583).

LYME DISEASE. Lyme disease is a vectorborne disease transmitted by ticks, and thousands of cases occur each year in the United States. It was diagnosed in 1975 in Lyme, Connecticut, after the Connecticut State Health Department was notified of an abnormally high incidence of juvenile arthritis, a relatively rare condition. Epidemiologists investigated and found that the causative agent was a spirochete bacterium, *Borrelia burgdorferi*, which was transmitted to humans, dogs, and horses by the bite of an infected deer tick. There are three stages of Lyme disease. The first is a spreading red rash that begins as a red bump at the site of the tick attachment and expands outward in a circular fashion. It is often accompanied by headache, fever, chills, backache, and fatigue. If the disease is not treated, it can progress to the second stage, where there may be evi-

dence of central nervous system dysfunction, muscle pain, and cardiac abnormalities. The third stage can begin months or years after the initial lesion and usually involves recurrent bouts of arthritis, often in the knees. Vaccination exists for the disease.

ROCKY MOUNTAIN SPOTTED FEVER. Rocky Mountain spotted fever is a vectorborne disease transmitted by ticks. Its causative agent is *Rickettsia rickettsii*. It seldom occurs in the Rocky Mountains but is common in the Southeast. Symptoms include sudden onset of moderate-to-high fever (which can persist for 2 to 3 weeks in untreated cases), malaise, deep muscle pain, severe headache, chills, deep muscle pain, and chills (Chin, 2000, p. 430). Frequently a maculopapular rash occurs that starts on the extremities and spreads to the rest of the body. In untreated cases, the case fatality rate can reach 25%. Prompt antibiotic treatment is critical for disease control. No vaccine is available for the disease, but one infection probably results in lifelong immunity.

## Zoonoses

Zoonoses are infections transmitted under natural conditions from vertebrate animals to humans (Chin, 2000, p. 579). Methods of transmission include inhalation, ingestion, and animal bites. Some of the better known zoonoses are *rabies, toxoplasmosis,* and *cat scratch fever.*

RABIES. Rabies is probably the best known of the zoonoses. The causative agent is a virus that is transmitted in the bite of an infected animal. Bats are the most frequent transmitter of rabies in the United States. No treatment is successful for rabies once symptoms occur, it is almost always fatal and death is often due to respiratory paralysis. Postexposure prophaylaxis is extremely important to survival. It is estimated that 40,000 rabies deaths occur worldwide each year (Chin, 2000, p. 411). Animals can be vaccinated for rabies; however, many wild and domestic animals are infected with the rabies virus. To prevent rabies, the wound should be treated immediately with a thorough cleansing with soap or detergent and flushing of all wounds with water (Chin, 2000, p. 415). If possible, the wound should not be sutured. Human rabies immune globulin (HRIG) should be used as soon as possible after exposure to neutralize the virus at the bite wound site and then the vaccine should be given at a different site to elicit active immunity.

TOXOPLASMOSIS. Toxoplasmosis is caused by *toxoplasma gondii*, a protozoa, and the definitive host is cats. Primary infection during early pregnancy can result in fetal brain damage, hydrocephaly, microcephaly, or death. Infection later in pregnancy results in mild or subclinical fetal disease (Chin, 2000, p. 501).

CAT SCRATCH FEVER. Cat scratch fever is caused by *Bartonella benselae*, a bacteria. Domestic cats are the reservoir. It is a subacute, usually self-limited bacterial disease that is characterized by malaise, lymphadenitis, and fever, and more than 90% of cases are preceded by a cat scratch, lick, or bite that produces a red, papular lesion (Chin, 2000, pp. 87-88). Although cats are the reservoir for the bacteria, they do not evidence clinical illness with the disease.

## Lead Poisoning

Lead poisoning is a preventable environmental disease. Lead can be inhaled, ingested, or transmitted in utero. It is an extremely toxic substance to the cardiovascular, renal, reproductive, and neurologic systems. Chronic lead poisoning and exposure to high levels of lead are potentially fatal. Even low levels of exposure can cause central nervous system damage, hearing impairments, and growth deficits. If a calcium or iron deficiency exists, even more lead is absorbed from the gastrointestinal tract (Preventing lead poisoning, 1992, p. 1). Higher rates of lead absorption and the immature central nervous system of children make them highly susceptible to lead poisoning.

Over time the lead that is not excreted by the body is deposited in the bones (estimated half-life of 27 years). Lead that has accumulated in children's deciduous "baby" teeth has been used to indicate a child's lead burden (Nadakavukaren, 2000, p. 254). High lead levels in deciduous teeth has been associated with a much higher rate of failure to graduate from high school, reading disabilities, greater absenteeism, and behavioral deficits (AAP, 1999, p. 136; Needleman, Schell, Bellinger, et al., 1990). Also, lead stored in bones can be suddenly released back into the bloodstream during times of disease or distress (e.g., pregnancy, osteoporosis, and illness) and result in cases of acute lead poisoning.

Lead poisoning is an important environmental health concern. It has been documented throughout history. Hippocrates described the symptoms of lead poisoning as early as 370 B.C. Some historians theorize that it was one of the conditions leading to the fall of the Roman Empire. Many wealthy and influential Romans could afford to use leaded pipes to have water brought to their homes and ate from expensive lead-glazed dishes. It is believed that this lead to a high incidence of lead poisoning in the ruling class and their offspring. The effects of such exposure resulted in children being unable to meet their full mental and physical potential and adults suffering from neurotoxicity, bizarre behavior, stillbirths, and sterility.

Lead poisoning was a serious problem in the early days of the American automobile industry because of the extensive use of lead in the automobile frames. Automobile workers inhaled lead throughout the day and ingested lead when they sat around the assembly line to eat their meals. *Dr. Carey P. McCord* of the University of Michigan conducted research studies on lead poisoning in the automobile industry, and his research resulted in regulations to protect workers from lead inhalation, protective measures for workers, and the first lunchrooms and cafeterias in industry—places for workers to eat that were away from lead particles (McCord, 1976). The Occupational Safety and Health Act of 1970 has helped monitor the use of lead in the workplace. Today, many Americans are still at risk of exposure to lead in their workplaces.

Lead can be found in many products. World production of lead is estimated at 3 million tons annually (Nadakavukaren, 2000, p. 250). Virtually every car on the road in America uses a lead storage battery containing up to 20 pounds of lead, and disposal of these batteries is an environmental concern. Before the use of unleaded gas in the United States was mandated, automobile emissions were a major source of environmental lead. Researchers estimate that the use of leaded gas in the United States for more than 50 years has left a residue of almost 5 million metric tons of lead dust along American highways (Nadakavukaren, 2000). Children living along lead-contaminated highways and in neighborhoods where soil lead content is high frequently exhibit high blood lead levels (Mielke, 1999).

In 1971 Congress passed the Lead-Based Paint Poisoning Prevention Act, which banned the usage of lead-based paint in interior paints and on furniture and toys. However, it is estimated that 3 million tons of lead from paint remains in the 57 million U.S. homes and apartment complexes built before the law went into effect (Nadakavukaren, 2000, p. 252).

Over the last three decades the Healthy People Initiative (see Chapter 4) has lead a strong national effort to eradicate childhood lead poisoning (USDHHS, 1980, 1991, 1995, 2000). These efforts have resulted in a remarkable decline in childhood exposure to lead in the United States (AAP, 1999, p. 131). Today, air lead levels are 98% lower than they were 25 years ago, and the number of American children with elevated lead levels has dramatically decreased (Goldman, 2000, p. 52). In 1995, 3 million U.S. children under the age of 6 had elevated lead levels (USDHHS, 1995); today less than 1 million do (AAP, 1999; USDHHS, 2000). The ANA has a position statement that supports lead poisoning prevention activities to reduce children's blood lead levels (ANA, 1996, p. 193). Casefinding and eliminating sources of lead poisoning in the home and community are major challenges for community health nurses.

## Environmental Lung Diseases

Pollutants in the air contribute to numerous environmental lung diseases, including lung cancer, chronic obstructive pulmonary disease, asthma, acute respiratory conditions, pneumoconiosis, and asbestosis. Reducing human exposure to air pollutants such as smoke, carbon monoxide, nitrogen dioxide, sulfur dioxide, and particulates is important in reducing the incidence of environmentally linked lung diseases. Occupational lung diseases are discussed in Chapter 21.

The incidence of adult and childhood *asthma* is on the rise. The greatest increase has been observed for children younger than 5 years of age, and rates in this age group rose 160% over a 15-year period (Goldman, 2000, p. 76). Asthma is being increasingly linked to passive inhalation of smoke and other environmental pollutants and it affects millions of Americans (USDHHS, 1991; USDHHS, 2000). Asthma incidence rises in the summertime, with peak levels of atmospheric ozone.

Children with asthma have shown marked improvements in their conditions just by having their parents quit smoking. In inner cities, asthma is a leading cause of hospital admissions for children. School nurses and advanced practice nurses in nurse-run school clinics see a large number of asthma cases.

The EPA estimates that asthmatic children who are exposed to significant levels of environmental tobacco smoke suffer up to 80% more asthma attacks and that there are at least 150,000 serious respiratory ailments among young children each year from environmental tobacco smoke (Nadakavukaren, 2000, p. 219). It is estimated that more than 113 million Americans live in areas that do not reach EPA air quality standards (USDHHS, 2000). Significant gains have been made in reducing air pollution from motor vehicles and other sources. Additional gains are needed to promote the public's health.

### Environmental Cancers

Environmental cancers have been documented for centuries. In 1775 Sir Percival Pott, an English physician, made an association between cancer of the scrotum in chimney sweeps and exposure to soot, an early determination of an environmental carcinogen. Cancer is the second leading cause of death in the United States and, although the etiology of many cancers is unknown, some cancers are linked to environmental carcinogens.

Several environmental agents such as cigarette smoke, radon, sunlight, and x-rays are known to be carcinogenic. Environmental factors, coupled with an individual's genetic predisposition to cancer and acquired susceptibility, are believed to be responsible for an estimated 80% to 90% of human cancers (Nadakavukaren, 2000, p. 208).

Researchers have identified more than 4000 chemicals in tobacco smoke, and of these at least 43 cause cancer in humans. Environmental tobacco smoke has been estimated to account for 30% of all cancers in the United States (USDHHS, 1991, p. 72). The EPA estimates that approximately 20,000 cases of lung cancer each year occur as a result of radon exposure (USDHHS, 1991, p. 322). The National Institute of Occupational Safety and Health estimates that millions of American workers are exposed to chemicals that are potential carcinogens on their jobs. Environmental exposures to carcinogens are generally preventable.

### Birth Defects

Birth defects are technically not an environmental disease, but they are conditions that are being increasingly linked to environmental factors. Between 3% to 5% of all pregnancies in the United States result in a serious birth defect

(Goldman, 2000, p. 76). Birth defects are the leading cause of infant mortality in the United States. Embryos that are genetically normal may be seriously damaged by environmental hazards—teratogens that cause birth defects.

Fetal vulnerability is most acute from the eighteenth day after conception to the sixtieth day, with a peak around the thirtieth day (Nadakavukaren, 2000, p. 202). Spina bifida, blindness, deafness, mental retardation, and phocomelia are some examples of birth defects known to have linkages to environmental teratogens. When infants survive birth defects, they usually are left with chronic, lifelong, debilitating problems that often prevent them from living independent lives. Some known teratogens are presented in Chapter 21.

## PRESERVING THE ENVIRONMENT

Increasing concern about the global environment and the ability of the planet to maintain future generations has resulted in worldwide environmental initiatives to preserve and protect Earth's environment. Environmental issues have become a part of every major political campaign, and Americans are demanding ecologically sound products, legislation, and activities. We need to work together to protect the environment and make the world a healthier place to live. Some contemporary environmental health concerns are discussed here.

### Greenhouse Effect

Natural gases in the atmosphere form a blanket around the earth and keep the planet warm. These natural gases are predominantly carbon dioxide ($CO_2$), methane, and nitrous oxide. Without this natural thermal insulation, the entire earth would be covered with ice and life as we know it would not exist (Miller, 2000, p. 499).

A problem occurs when technologic gases (often $CO_2$) thicken this blanket. When this occurs, these gases trap excess heat around the earth, and this results in global warming known as the **greenhouse effect**. The majority of these greenhouse gases have been caused by burning fossil fuels, agriculture, deforestation and the use of chlorofluorocarbons (CFCs) (Miller, 2000, p. 501). CFCs are especially troublesome because once they reach the stratosphere they trap up to 1700 times as much heat per molecule as $CO_2$ (Miller, 2000, p. 500). As global warming occurs, the temperature of the earth's surface will warm enough to cause climatic and environmental changes that can be detrimental to health and existence.

An international panel of scientists estimate that the earth's temperature could change as much as 10° over the next 100 years—the most rapid change in 10 millennia and more than 60% higher than predicted a few years ago (Washington Post, 2001). It is estimated that more than a 4° increase will occur over the next 50 years. A 4° change would be as great as the drop in temperature that caused the last Ice Age (Doll, 1992, p. 939). Scientists predict that over the next century rising temperatures will melt polar ice caps, raise ocean levels, flood and destroy coastal areas and wetlands, cause brutal and frequent droughts, alter weather patterns and change rain distribution, result in violent storms, and create deserts.

If these estimates are accurate, rising temperature will raise sea levels as much as 34 inches, causing floods that would displace millions of people and engulf coastal areas such as the Florida Everglades. Glacier National Park in the United States has already lost 113 of its 150 glaciers and it is anticipated that the remainder will disappear within the next 30 years (Stolzenburg, 2001).

Temperature changes will affect the length of the seasons. In the northern United States, spring is now arriving a week earlier than it did in the 1970s and autumn lasts 2 to 4 days longer (Nadakavukaren, 2000, p. 430). Climate changes resulting from global warming result in "habitats on the move" for humans, plants, and animals and agricultural changes.

Global warming can result in diminished crop yields and food shortages. Such warming can result in the loss of biodiversity (discussed later in this chapter) and the creation of conditions more conducive to the spread of communicable diseases (Harte, 2000, p. 510). Such warming results in the extension of areas favorable to vectorborne and parasitic disease, increased incidence of fungal skin diseases, skin cancer, heat stroke and exhaustion, and changing patterns of human migration. The enlargement of tropical climates would bring diseases such as malaria, encephalitis, and yellow fever to formerly temperate climates.

## Air Pollution

Air pollution results when one or more chemicals exist in the air in concentrations high enough to harm plants, animals, or humans. Particulate matter and excess heat and noise are also considered to be air pollutants. Air pollution has always occurred through natural occurrences in the environment, including volcanoes, forest fires, pollination, dust storms, swamp gas, and methane gas in mines.

Concern for the effects of air pollution on public health dates back to at least the thirteenth century, when government commissions were established in England to investigate sources of air pollution and "the fouling of air" (Blumenthal, Greene, 1985, p. 117). In 1257 the queen of England moved away from the city of Nottingham because the heavy smoke from wood burning was unendurable (Miller, 2000, p. 475). The Industrial Revolution greatly added to the problem of air pollution, and gas-powered vehicles, power plants, and industry continue to contribute to this problem today. Early community efforts to minimize air pollution in the United States included local regulations to control unpleasant "airs," limiting outdoor burning and controlling smoke.

The Clean Air Act has worked to reduce air pollution in the United States and mandated establishment of national ambient air quality standards for suspended particulates, sulfur oxides, carbon monoxide, nitrogen oxide, artificial ozone, hydrocarbons, and lead. Unfortunately, according to the EPA, millions of Americans today live in areas where the Clean Air Standard is exceeded (USDHHS, 2000).

An example of how the Clean Air Act has assisted communities in combating air pollution is seen in Rothschild, Wisconsin. When students in Rothschild began suffering from asthma attacks brought on by sulfur dioxide emissions from a local paper mill, parents protested. The EPA used the Clean Air Act to enforce mill emission standards, and the number of school children experiencing medical emergencies from asthma declined (Monks, 1996, p. 27). Another air pollution success story is that of Chattanooga, Tennessee. The city's air was so polluted in the 1950s that when women wearing nylon stockings walked outside the legwear would sometimes disintegrate (Glick, 1996, p. 44). The citizens engaged in a successful environmental cleanup, and Chattanooga serves as a model for other cities trying to recover from air pollution.

*Healthy People 2010* addressed the need for more American communities to comply with air quality standards. In order for this to occur, additional educational methods focusing on air pollution control and improved coordination between health and environmental agencies is needed. The *American Lung Association* tries to educate the American public about the importance of clean air and respiratory health. Air pollution is often classified as indoor or outdoor.

**INDOOR AIR POLLUTION.** Indoor air pollution is a significant concern and may actually pose a greater risk to human health than outdoor air pollution. Levels of 11 common pollutants can be found in American homes and businesses at concentrations as high as 70 times greater than they are found outdoors (Miller, 2000, p. 483). Because people spend much of their time indoors, this has significant health implications.

Indoor air pollution is commonly caused by tobacco smoke, radon, asbestos, formaldehyde, infectious agents (e.g., mold, bacteria, viruses), dust, combustion smoke (e.g., furnaces, fireplaces, and woodstoves), and household chemicals (e.g., pesticides). Symptoms of indoor air pollution include dizziness, headaches, coughing, sneezing, nausea and vomiting, burning eyes, and flulike symptoms. Indoor air pollutants have been linked to acute and chronic respiratory infections and conditions, allergic reactions, headaches, and cancer.

Research conducted by the National Aeronautics and Space Administration (NASA) has indicated that the use of houseplants can actually help absorb contaminants in the air. When NASA found that plants helped remove benzene, formaldehyde, and carbon monoxide and put oxygen back into the environment, the agency started to use plants as part of the biologic life support system aboard orbiting space stations.

The term *sick building syndrome* (SBS) has been used to describe commercial buildings that have been linked to human illness from indoor air pollution. With SBS, building occupants experience various forms of illness and discomfort. Common characteristics of this syndrome are chest tightness, muscle aches, cough, fever, chills, and headache; respiratory infections, hoarseness, nausea, and dizziness; and eye, nose, and throat irritation (Jaakkola, Tuomaala, Seppanen, 1994, p. 422; Nadakavukaren, 2000, p. 501). Often times no causative agent can be found. The symptoms become better or disappear when the occupants of the building go outside.

Newer buildings are more likely to be "sick" because of reduced air exchange to save energy or emission of chemicals from new carpeting and furniture (Miller, 2000, p. 483). WHO estimates that up to 30% of the world's new and remodeled buildings may be generating complaints (Nadakavukaren, 2000, p. 501). The EPA estimates that at least 17% of the 4 million commercial buildings in the United States are "sick"—including the EPA's Washington, D.C., headquarters (Miller, 2000, p. 483). Some common indoor air pollutants are discussed.

*Radon.* Radon is a colorless, odorless, cancer-producing gas formed by radioactive decay of the radium and uranium found in natural soil. Since the 1980s, radon has been recognized as a serious form of indoor air pollution and a national health problem (Box 6-12). The EPA has ranked radon as one of the most dangerous cancer risks in the environment. It is the second leading cause of lung cancer in the United States.

Radon can be found all over the United States, but some areas are "hot spots" for radon. The *National Council on Radiation Protection and Measurement* estimates that the average individual receives at least 55% of their yearly dose of ionizing radiation from radon inside homes (Nadakavukaren, 2000, p. 491).

Radon particles are carried deep into the lung where they release small bursts of energy and damage lung tissue, resulting in possible lung damage, lung disease, and lung cancer. Lung damage from radon has no early warning symptoms. Smokers are much more vulnerable to the effects of radon and have higher death rates from it than nonsmokers.

Radon silently seeps into American homes, schools, and businesses through cracks in basement walls, floors, foundations, and joint spaces between walls and floors; well water; and openings around pipes and sump pumps. The EPA estimates that 4 to 5 million American homes have elevated radon levels (Miller, 2000, p. 486). Radon can hide undetected in the American home. Elevated radon levels in buildings pose health threats, but there are simple, inexpensive ways to fix a radon problem. EPA recommends that homeowners across the nation test their homes for radon. However, only a small percentage of all American homes have been tested for radon. If a home has a radon problem and the home has well water, the well also should be tested for radon.

The federal government is educating the American public on the dangers of radon. The EPA has numerous publications on radon, including *Radon Reduction Methods*. To get more information on radon and to find out about state radon programs phone 1-800-SOS-RADON.

### BOX 6-12
## *Is Radon Gas Hiding In Your Home?*

When Stanley Watras arrived for work at the Limerick nuclear power plant on a December morning in 1984, he started radiation-detection alarms ringing. The radioactive contamination that was detected on Watras that fateful winter morning obviously had come from outside the nuclear facility, so Watras requested Philadelphia Electric, the utility company that owned the plant to check his home.

To everyone's amazement, tests revealed that the Watras home had levels of radon gas approximately 1000 times higher than normal. Investigators estimated that the Watras family was receiving radiation exposure equivalent to 455,000 chest x-rays a year just by living in their house. The Watras family had been unaware of the radon in their home.

Further investigation showed that radon was "hiding" in thousands of American homes. It was determined that large sections of eastern Pennsylvania, New Jersey, and New York, which are underlain by a uranium geologic formation, had thousands of homes where elevated levels of radon existed. Since that time, the threat of radon in American homes has become a growing concern, and families around the country have been urged to test their homes for radon. Is radon gas hiding in your home?

Modified from Nadakavukaren A: *Our global environment: a health perspective,* ed 5, Prospect Heights, Ill, 2000, Waveland Press, p. 490.

### Stop and Think About It
Do you live in a part of the country that is a hot spot for radon? Do you know where materials for testing radon could be purchased in your community? Has your home been tested? How would you explain the risks of radon to a client?

*Environmental tobacco smoke (ETS).* Environmental tobacco smoke (ETS) is a major indoor air pollutant and health risk. ETS is a complex mixture of thousands of chemicals, many of which are toxic or carcinogenic. ETS has been estimated to account for 30% of all cancers in the United States (USDHHS, 1991, p. 72). Thousands of lung cancer deaths occur each year in the United States as a result of ETS. ETS represents a major source of exposure to benzene, a carcinogen. Researchers have calculated that 45% of Americans' total exposure to benzene comes from inhaling tobacco smoke and only 3% is due to industrial emissions (Nadakavukaren, 2000, p. 494; Otto, Roberts, 1998). For years the Occupational Safety and Health Administration has considered a ban on workplace smoking but that ban has not occurred. Many restaurants and other public facilities have put smoking bans in place.

Children's lungs are especially susceptible to the harmful effects of ETS. Forty-three percent of American children aged 2 months to 11 years live in a home with at least one person who smokes (AAP, 1999, p. 97). Infants whose mothers smoke are 38% more likely to be hospitalized during the first year of life with pneumonia than those infants whose mothers do not smoke (AAP, 1999, p. 98). Conditions such as cancer, bronchitis, pneumonia, asthma, sudden infant death syndrome (SIDS), and acute respiratory infections occur up to twice as often during the first 2 years of life in children who are exposed to ETS, and there is strong evidence of increased middle ear infections, reduced growth, and reduced lung function. A study by researchers at Harvard University found that household ETS is the main source of indoor air pollution for most children (Nadakavukaren, 2000, p. 494). The more smoking in the home, the higher the prevalence of respiratory symptoms in children.

*Asbestos.* Asbestos is a fibrous form of silica. It is virtually indestructible and resists destruction by heat, fire, and acid. Exposure is primarily through inhalation, but some people are exposed through drinking water. Unless completely sealed within a product, asbestos easily disintegrates into particles that can be suspended in the air and inhaled into the lungs (Miller, 2000, p. 484). Smokers are much more susceptible to the effects of asbestos than nonsmokers and have higher rates of lung cancer than nonsmokers.

Diseases caused by asbestos include asbestosis, lung cancer, mesothelioma, and gastrointestinal cancer. It is estimated that of the 11 million current and retired asbestos workers exposed to large amounts of asbestos, up to 40% can expect to die of asbestos-related cancer (Nadakavukaren, 2000, p. 243).

Asbestos has been used extensively in roofing shingles, ceiling and floor tiles, clutches, brakes and transmission parts, fireproofing, and thermal insulation. Between 1920 and the early 1970s millions of tons of asbestos were used in the construction of homes, schools, and public buildings across the United States (AAP, 1999, p. 35).

A federal ban in 1988 on the use of asbestos in many products severely limited its use. However it remains in place in thousands of American buildings (Miller, 2000, p. 484). The federal government has provided funding to help schools become asbestos free. Many people are not aware that asbestos was used in their home's construction.

Inhaled asbestos fibers do not cause acute toxicity; instead they go deep into the lungs where they remain "dormant" for many years. Decades after exposures, asbestosis and a rare form of cancer, mesothelioma, often occur. In the past, miners, pipefitters, shipyard employees, demolition workers, brake-drum workers, and firefighters were groups that had exposures to high levels of asbestos. Asbestos fibers can be brought home on clothing and other items and have

the potential to contaminate family members. Communities in which asbestos industries have resided have residents who have been exposed to high levels of asbestos. Because these fibers are too small to be seen by the human eye, they can easily go undetected in the ambient air.

*Other indoor air pollutants.* These pollutants include *biologic air pollutants* (e.g., dust, mites, molds, and animal dander), *volatile organic compounds* (VOCs) (e.g., benzene, carbon tetrachloride, and formaldehyde), and *combustion products* (e.g., carbon monoxide, nitrogen dioxide, sulfur dioxide, and particulates). Biologic agents are known to cause infections, hypersensitivity, and toxicoses. Many biologic agents have been discussed previously in this chapter.

The health effects of VOCs include irritation of the skin, eyes, and respiratory system; liver and kidney damage; cancer; and birth defects. Formaldehyde is an extremely volatile compound that can be emitted from building materials such as plywood, particleboard, and paneling; household furnishings such as furniture, drapes, and upholstery; and adhesive in carpeting and wallpaper. Levels of formaldehyde are often high in mobile homes (Nadakavukaren, 2000, p. 494). It is suspected of being carcinogenic.

Combustion products can reach high levels inside homes where fireplaces, kerosene heaters, wood-burning stoves, and gas appliances are used; when automobile or other motor emissions can enter the house; or when there are cigarette smokers in the home (Nadakavukaren, 2000, p. 493). Carbon monoxide emission from wood, coal, or gas stoves often exceed Clean Air Act standards for outside air (Nadakavukaren, 2000). Exposure to high levels of carbon monoxide can result in death. Carbon monoxide detectors are recommended for use in American homes. For more information on indoor air pollutants call the EPA's Indoor Air Quality Information Clearinghouse at 1-800-438-4318.

**OUTDOOR AIR POLLUTION.** Outdoor or "ambient" air pollution is prevalent in the United States. Major ambient air pollutants are carbon oxides, sulfur oxides, nitrogen oxides, volatile organic compounds (e.g., methane, benzene, and formaldehyde), suspended particles, photochemical oxidants (e.g., ozone and hydrogen peroxide), radioactive substances, heat, and noise.

Lung damage from polluted air is a risk for millions of Americans and is a serious problem in many American cities. Outdoor air pollution can result in health conditions such as lung cancer, bronchial asthma, acute respiratory illnesses and conditions, and skin and eye conditions. It damages agriculture and vegetation and adds to the problem of deforestation (pine trees are very susceptible). It also damages property; creates esthetic problems; incurs property damage and loss; and contributes to increased morbidity, mortality, and absenteeism from work.

*Smog* is a combination of the words *smoke* and *fog* and is a major form of outdoor air pollution. The word was coined in 1911 in the aftermath of an air pollution disaster in London,

England, that claimed more than 1000 lives (Miller, 2000, p. 475). All major American cities suffer from some level of smog. It is more prevalent in industrial areas with dense population; large numbers of motor vehicles; and a sunny, dry climate. The Los Angeles metropolitan area suffers the worst levels of smog in the nation. Smog harms plants, animals, and people. Over the years, smog has been blamed for numerous outbreaks of respiratory illness and death.

### Ozone Depletion

An invisible layer of natural ozone shields and protects the earth's surface against ultraviolet radiation and allows life to develop. Ozone depletion occurs when this natural layer is damaged. People are destroying this natural ozone shield through the use of CFCs and other man-made chemicals. Tons of CFCs are used annually worldwide. CFCs are compounds made up of carbon, chlorine, and fluorine. They are routinely used in refrigeration and air conditioning (e.g., freon), aerosol sprays, and cleaning agents. CFCs deplete the ozone layer when they rise into the stratosphere and their chlorine atoms react with ozone.

Sherwood Rowland, of the University of California at Irvine, issued the first ozone depletion alert in 1974 (Lemonick, 1992, p. 62). A hole in the ozone layer over Antarctica was confirmed in 1984 when researchers analyzing satellite data found seasonal ozone depletion of between 40% and 50% in the upper stratosphere over Antarctica, and since then, this depletion has expanded (Miller, 2000, p. 521). Ozone depletion is worsening worldwide, and researchers have now found signs of ozone depletion in North America.

Holes in the ozone layer deplete our natural protection from the sun, making it increasingly important to wear sunglasses, protective clothing, and sunscreen when exposed to the sun for prolonged periods. It is crucial to minimize the time spent in the sun during the peak period of 10 AM to 3 PM, minimize sunbathing, and avoid being in the sun for long periods of time.

The countries of New Zealand, South Africa, Argentina, and Chile, where the ozone layer is very thin for several months a year, are seeing increased incidence of skin cancer and cataracts. Other health hazards linked to ozone depletion are suppression of the immune system; an increase in eye-burning; and accelerated skin aging, eye cataracts, and mutations in deoxyribonucleic acid (DNA). Ozone depletion also causes hazards to vegetation and threatens the world's food supply. It can cause depletion of food crops by interference with the process of photosynthesis, and phytoplankton depletion (phytoplankton is important in the ocean food chain). Scientists are concerned about the warming effects of ozone depletion on climate.

### Water Pollution

Water pollution occurs when water becomes contaminated. The human body's dependence on a regular intake of water is second only to its need for oxygen, and human beings need 1 to 3 L of water daily just to maintain body functions (Nadakavukaren, 2000, p. 531). As amazing as it may seem, less than 3% of the Earth's water is fresh, and only 1% is available for drinking. The greatest amount of drinking water is found beneath the surface of the soil in the form of groundwater. Americans are the largest users of water in the world and use billions of gallons of fresh water every day.

Existing U.S. water supplies are rapidly being polluted and depleted. According to the EPA, 30% of the nation's rivers and 42% of its lakes are polluted, 40% of the nation's fresh water is unusable, and toxic chemicals are still being discharged into the nation's waters (The 27th environmental quality review, 1995, p. 38). Sources of potential water pollution are construction activities, industrial wastes, human and animal wastes, landfill waste, accidental spills, mining operations, leaking underground storage tanks, agricultural waste and runoff, fallout of airborne pollutants, urban street runoff, fertilizers, and pesticides.

Homeowners add to groundwater contamination through the use of septic tanks and by dumping household chemicals down the drain or on the ground. Household septic tanks, used by millions of American families, have the potential to add to water pollution.

Although water is a renewable resource, in the near future, water supply could become a serious crisis in many areas of the United States. Water resources in the United States are not evenly distributed. Areas in the Pacific Northwest can receive 80 inches of rainfall annually, whereas the driest state, Nevada, may receive less than 10 inches annually. Even where there are abundant sources of water, serious problems result if the water is unfit for human consumption. We need to conserve and protect our nation's water supplies (Figure 6-2).

Worldwide, 1.5 billion people do not have access to safe drinking water and the number is growing (Nadakavukaren, 2000, p. 536). Each year millions of people worldwide become ill and die from preventable waterborne diseases discussed previously in this chapter such as polio, typhoid, cholera, hepatitis, and bacterial dysentery. *Healthy People 2000* set a goal that 85% of Americans would have safe drinking water by the year 2000. This goal was not met. *Healthy People 2010* again has set a goal to improve the nation's drinking water, and progress toward this goal will be carefully monitored.

### Hazardous Waste

Hazardous wastes pose serious health problems. **Hazardous waste** is any discarded material that may pose a substantial threat or potential danger to human health or the environment (Box 6-13). Such wastes have properties that make them hazardous to human health such as toxicity, flammability, explosiveness, radioactivity, reactivity, corrosiveness, and communicability (the presence of pathogens). The EPA estimates that 6 billion tons of hazardous waste are produced each

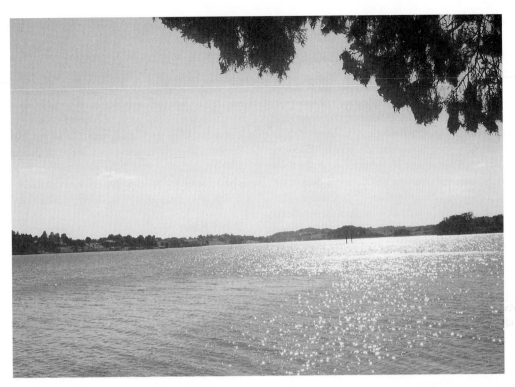

**FIGURE 6-2** Safeguarding our natural resources is a major public health concern. Even with modern technology our nation has not been able to control disease outbreaks related to environmental pollutants. Ensuring adequate, safe drinking water is an important national health concern. (Courtesy Ed Richardson.)

year in the United States—an average of 23 tons of hazardous waste for every U.S. citizen (Miller, 2000, p. 580). However, only 6% of this is legally defined as hazardous waste.

Many hazardous waste sites are "abandoned" industrial sites, with the waste having been left for years. Many communities are not aware of the hazardous wastes within their midst. The increasing amount of hazardous wastes, transporting of hazardous wastes, and hazardous waste sites are prompting Americans to become more concerned about environmental health issues. People want hazardous wastes managed in a way that is safe for the environment; on the other hand, few people want to live near the site selected for its storage, treatment, or disposal (Nadakavukaren, 2000, p. 664). Phrases such as "Not in My Back Yard" (NIMBY), "Put it in Their Back Yard" (PIITBY), and "Locally Unwanted Land Use" (LULU) are commonly heard in American communities (Nadakavukaren, 2000, p. 668; Rhodes, Odell, 1992). Improper disposal of hazardous industrial waste has led to numerous health problems, communities being evacuated and relocated, and community coalitions for environmental health.

*Superfund legislation* was enacted in 1980 in response to public demands that something be done to alleviate the problems of hazardous waste in American communities. This fund has authorized monies for cleanup activities in American communities and long-term containment of

 **BOX 6-13**
### What is Hazardous Waste?

In the United States hazardous waste is legally defined as any discarded solid or liquid material that:
1. Contains one or more of 39 toxic, carcinogenic, mutagenic or teratogenic compounds at levels that exceed established limits, including many solvents, pesticides, and paint stripper
2. Catches fire easily (gasoline, paints, and solvents)
3. Is reactive or unstable enough to explode or release toxic fumes (acids, bases, ammonia, chorine bleach)
4. Is capable of corroding metal containers such as tanks, drums, and barrels (industrial cleaning agents and oven and drain cleaners)

This definition does not include radioactive wastes, hazardous and toxic substances discarded by households, mining wastes, oil and gas drilling wastes (routinely discharged into surface waters or dumped into unlined pits and landfills), liquid wastes containing organic hydrocarbon compounds (80% of all liquid hazardous waste), cement kiln dust, and wastes from the thousands of small businesses and factories that generate less than 220 pound of hazardous waste per month.

From: Miller GT: *Living in the environment: principles, connections, and solutions*, ed 11, Pacific Grove, Calif, 2000, Brooks/Cole Publishing Company, p. 580.

hazardous waste dump sites. The EPA has compiled a National Priority List of hazardous sites. Sixty million Americans live within 4 miles of a Superfund site (Nadakavukaren, 2000, p. 672).

Some innovative and environmentally sound ways to deal with selected hazardous wastes have been developed. An environmentally sound process called *bioremediation* has been used to devour waste products and unwanted hazardous waste materials. In bioremediation special bacteria are used to break down hazardous waste into nonhazardous compounds. Such safe, innovative methods to deal with hazardous waste materials need to be developed and used.

Nurses need to be aware of hazardous wastes in the community, consider whether community members have been exposed, and determine the effect on public health. Hazardous and toxic wastes have been linked to deaths, poisoning, acute and chronic illness, cancer, birth defects, blindness, and sterility. Communities such as Love Canal in New York have been declared federal disaster areas, and residents were relocated. Cleanup of such areas is expensive and sometimes not possible. Hazardous wastes have serious effects on human life and health.

## Garbage and Solid Waste

The United States has the dubious distinction of being the world's biggest solid waste producer. With only 4.6% of the world's population, Americans produce 33% of the world's solid wastes—11 billion tons each year amounting to an average of 44 tons per person each year (Miller, 2000, p. 579). Every day each person in every American household tosses away an average of 4.3 pounds of refuse (EPA, 1998).

Mining waste is the largest category of solid waste. However, Americans throw away an amazing amount of solid waste, including enough aluminum to rebuild the country's entire commercial airline fleet every 3 months, enough tires each year to encircle the planet almost three times, and 18 billion disposable diapers each year that would reach the moon and back 7 times (Miller, 2000, p. 589).

Where to put garbage and solid waste is becoming a major problem. More than two thirds of the nation's landfills have been full since the late 1970s, and many will be full in the near future. Trash, landfills, piles of refuse, and unsightly and unsanitary conditions are becoming a regular part of the American landscape. "America the beautiful" may soon be a phrase from the past. Adequate garbage disposal is especially important in summer months, when pests such as flies breed and garbage can be an increased source of communicable disease.

Today the three *R*s of waste control are *Reuse, Recycle,* and *Reduce.* Americans need to practice the three *R*s more. Recycling is becoming more popular in the United States, but still less than 32% of municipal solid waste (including composting) is recycled (Nadakavukaren, 2000, p. 634). This percentage could increase as recycling becomes revenue-producing business (Young, 1996, p. 246) and as legis-

lation changes to mandate recycling. For example, New York City earns millions of dollars from selling its newsprint, and Madison, Wisconsin, receives over a million dollars a year from recyclables (Young, 1996, p. 246).

Using "reusables" and reducing the amount of garbage and solid waste has been slow to gain momentum in the United States; just look at how disposable items are used in everyday life—including health care settings. The best way to manage garbage and waste is to not produce it in the first place. Garbage and solid waste produce health risks such as the possibility of soil and water pollution, spread of communicable disease, and accidental illness and injury.

## Acid Rain

The term **acid rain** was coined by an English chemist, Robert Angus Smith, to describe corrosive rain falling on industrial Manchester, England, more than 100 years ago (Nadakavukaren, 2000, p. 479). By the 1960s the term was being used to describe conditions in Canadian lakes.

Natural rain is slightly acidic with a pH of 5.0 to 5.6. Acid rain has a much more acidic pH. Today the average pH of rainfall in the United States east of the Mississippi River is 4.4 (Nadakavukaren, 2000, p. 479).

Sulfur dioxide is the primary component of acid rain. It mixes with nitrogen oxides in the atmosphere to chemically form sulfuric acid and nitric acid. These acids fall back to earth in the form of acid rain or snow. Sulfur dioxide is discharged into the atmosphere in amounts averaging 15 million tons each year in the United States (Nadakavukaren, 2000, p. 480). Electric utilities are responsible for the majority of sulfur dioxide emissions in the United States. Nitrogen oxide emissions in the United States are primarily from auto emissions. You can help prevent acid rain by conserving energy, car pooling, and driving less.

Typical rain in the eastern United States is about 10 times more acidic than normal rain, and in some areas it is 100 times more acidic with a pH of 3—as acidic as vinegar (Miller, 2000, p. 478). Rain that had a pH value almost equivalent to that of battery acid once fell on Wheeling, West Virginia (Miller, 1996, p. 436). Areas along the Appalachian Mountains have had rain that has the acidic content of lemon juice—a pH of 2.3. Acid rain can destroy aquatic life in lakes, rivers, and streams. Reports of disappearance of once abundant fish, amphibians, and aquatic insects are becoming common across the country. Although increased acidity levels seldom kill fish directly, it can induce reproductive failure and declining fish populations. Also, increased acidity of lakes apparently converts moderately toxic inorganic mercury compounds found in lake-bottom sediments into highly toxic methylmercury (Miller, 2000, p. 481).

It is estimated that the effects of acid rain in the United States cost billions of dollars each year. Acidic lakes, rivers, and streams can upset the ecologic balance needed to sustain fish, plant, and animal life. Acid causes dermatologic conditions, kills aquatic life, can result in crop depletion, and results in the loss of plant and animal diversity. Acid rain is detrimental to human health.

Forests are also vulnerable to acid rain. Pine trees at high elevations are especially vulnerable (Nadakavukaren, 2000, p. 485). In Vermont over half of the red spruce have died since 1960 and forests in Germany have been so ravaged that German scientists have coined the word *wald-sterben*, "forest death," in relation to the phenomena (Nadakavukaren, 2000).

## Loss of Biologic Diversity

Loss of biologic diversity involves losing forms of life on the planet. It is a serious threat to global health and existence. Extinction is forever. Once a plant, animal, or insect species is gone, we can never get it back. It is estimated that up to 73,000 animal and plant species become extinct each year, far surpassing the expected extinction rate of 3 to 30 species a year (Miller, 2000, p. 684). The rate of extinction grows as the human species takes over more space on the planet. We are living through the greatest mass extinction since the die-off of the dinosaurs 65 million years ago (Raven, 1995, p. 38). For the first time in millions of years, species are vanishing more rapidly than new ones are evolving (Nadakavukaren, 2000, p. 164). "According to a 1998 survey, 70% of biologists polled believe that we are in the midst of a mass extinction and that this loss of species will pose a major threat to human existence" (Miller, 2000, p. 686).

To protect endangered species, the **Endangered Species Act** was passed. It gave the United States one of the most far-reaching laws ever enacted by any country to prevent the extinction of imperiled animals and plants. Hundreds of native mammals, birds, reptiles, crustaceans, plants, and other life forms were officially protected. In addition, more than 500 foreign species are now protected under the act. The U.S. Fish and Wildlife Service of the Department of the Interior is charged with protecting American wildlife and endangered species.

Conservation biologists estimate that each day up to 200 species of plants and animals become extinct worldwide (Miller, 2000, p. 683). In tropical areas alone, home to an estimated 10 million species, we are losing 27,000 species each year (74 each day) to extinction, and if the present rate of extinction continues, up to 20% of all rain forest species will be extinct within the next 20 years (Nadakavukaren, 2000, p. 167; Wilson, 1992). If poaching, animal exploitation, environmental pollution, and destruction of critical habitats continue at the present rate, many of the world's plant, animal, and insect species could be lost forever within the next few decades.

Plants are especially important to health—more than 60% of the world's people depend directly on plants for their medicines, and plants play a role in the derivation of the top 20 pharmaceutical products sold in the United States (Raven, 1995, p. 40). Preserving critical habitats and land is crucial to preserving plant and animal species.

We are in the process of eliminating many biologically diverse environments such as rain forests, coral reefs, and wetlands (Miller, 2000, p. 685). Groups such as the *Nature Conservancy* and *World Wildlife Foundation* have launched campaigns to save endangered species. Individuals around the world are doing their part to save endangered species. For example, the people living in the Poconos Mountains in Pennsylvania are working with the Podocarpos National Park in Ecuador to protect the migration patterns and habitat of a dozen-plus migratory birds known to frequent both areas (Green, 2001).

We need to remember that everything in nature is interlinked. Species diversity is a major determinant of ecologic stability and human survival. As we lose plant and animal species, we increase the risk of our own extinction. With the loss of each plant species, we could possibly be losing a cure for acquired immunodeficiency syndrome (AIDS), cancer, or numerous other diseases or conditions.

## Desertification

According to the United Nations Environment Programme (UNEP), desertification is one of the most serious global environmental problems (Stopping the dry destruction, 1996, p. 194). At a United Nations conference desertification was defined as land degradation in arid, semiarid, and dry subhumid areas resulting from various factors including climatic variations and human activities (Nadakavukaren, 2000, p. 160). Today desertification affects the lives and well-being of almost 1 billion people worldwide (Nadakavukaren, 2000). Most desertification occurs naturally at the edges of existing desert as a result of dehydration of the top layers of soil, but desertification also can result from abusive land use practices such as overgrazing, improper soil management, and use of water resources, and deforestation. Worldwide, 3 million square miles (an area the size of Brazil, or 12 times the size of Texas) have become desert during the past 50 years, each year 23,000 square miles become desert (an area the size of West Virginia), and yearly 77,000 square miles (an area the size of Kansas) undergoes desertification to the point of not being viable for farming or agriculture (Miller, 2000, p. 356). In the American Southwest, overgrazing is largely responsible for the formation of Arizona's Sonoran Desert (Nadakavukaren, 2000, p. 161).

Once land has become desert, it is difficult to reclaim. Restoration efforts often involve reforestation. Loss of land previously used for food production has a direct impact on nutrition and quality of human life. Also, migration of people and animals resulting from "habitats on the move" can result in overcrowding and other undesirable social conditions.

## Wetlands Destruction

*Wetlands* include marshes, swamps, ponds, floodplains, bogs, tidal marshlands, wet arctic tundra, wet meadows, and mudflats. **Wetlands destruction** is the loss of these areas. Some wetlands are covered with water yearlong and some are seasonal. U.S. wetlands are rapidly being depleted and destroyed. Over half of America's wetlands are gone. Today, wetlands cover just 5% of the land surface in the contiguous 48 states, and Alaska has more wetlands than the 48 states combined (Nadakavukaren, 2000, p. 162).

Wetlands play important ecologic and economic roles, such as providing food and habitats for fish, migratory waterfowl, and other wildlife and improving water quality by filtering and degrading toxic wastes and other pollutants (Miller, 2000, p. 203). Wetlands have been called "nature's kidneys" and "living filters." Wetlands help replenish groundwater supplies and are a primary water source for over 50% of the U.S. population (Miller, 2000). Their ability to retain large amounts of water make them natural floodplains, which helps prevent floods.

We have built on wetland floodplains and have made many cities vulnerable to flooding. Recent flooding along the Mississippi River has shown this to be true and demonstrated the serious loss of life and property destruction that can occur in floods. When left intact, wetlands serve as natural floodplains.

Until recently many wetland areas were seen as nuisances because of water accumulation and insects, and many wetlands were drained for agricultural, industrial, and residential purposes. However, environmentalists and the general public are now recognizing their value, and legislation has been passed to help preserve and protect America's remaining wetlands.

Of special concern is protecting the Florida Everglades, the world's largest freshwater marsh. The Everglades is one of the most threatened ecosystems in the United States and has already lost half of its 4 million acres (Nadakavukaren, 2000, p. 165). Efforts to restore and revitalize the Everglades are underway, but this will be a slow and expensive task. Americans need to protect their remaining wetlands.

## Deforestation

Ralph Waldo Emerson said, "In the woods, is perpetual youth . . . In the woods, we return to reason and faith." Emerson believed that the outdoors offered a cleansing of both mind and spirit and that through nature people can find knowledge and self-discovery (Seeing beauty: thoughts from Emerson, 1996, p. 50). Unfortunately our woods are being rapidly depleted, and the beauty of many forests is lost forever. Protected state and national forests are helping save trees. However, even protected forests are threatened by pollution. **Deforestation** is loss of a forested area.

We have reduced the world's original forest land area by about one quarter, and each year there is a net loss of 62,000 square miles of forest (Miller, 2000, p. 644). The World Wildlife Fund (WWF) has launched a global campaign to protect the world's forests. It is encouraging nations to set aside at least 10% of their representative original forests as protected areas and to work to slow forest loss and degradation (WWF, 1996). In many underdeveloped countries,

forests are being cleared and burned to make way for farms and industry. In the United States, it takes over 500,000 trees to supply Americans with their Sunday papers each week (The Earthworks Group, 1990). Although trees are a renewable resource, like water, they are renewable at a slow rate.

Rainforests are forests that receive at least 100 inches of rain each year (Rainforests, 1990, p. 3). Tropical rainforests are located in a narrow region near the equator in Africa, South and Central America, and Asia. Haiti has lost all of its original primary forest, and Bangladesh has lost 95% of its original tropical rainforest (Hinrichsen, 1994, p. 38). Once there were more than 5 billion acres of rainforest; today there is less than half that amount (Rainforests, 1990, p. 3).

Although rainforests make up only 6% to 7% of the Earth's surface, over half of the world's plant, animal, and insect species live in them (Myers, 1992, p. 282). If the current rate of rainforest destruction continues, up to 2 million species of plants, animals, and insects will become prematurely extinct in the next 30 years—presently we are losing 74 species per day (3 species per hour), and the rate is accelerating (Nadakavukaren, 2000, p. 167).

One in four pharmaceuticals has components from a rainforest plant, and 70% of the plants identified by the National Cancer Institute as being helpful in the treatment of cancer are found only in the rainforests. Recently a potent anticancer drug, paclitaxel (Taxol), was derived from the bark of the Pacific yew. Rainforests include plants from which analgesics, antibiotics, heart drugs, cancer drugs, hormones, diuretics, tranquilizers, laxatives, dysentery treatments, and anticoagulants are made (Carr, Pederson, Ramaswamy, 1996, p. 135). Examples of plants that are pharmaceuticals are the serpentine root (reserpine) used in tranquilizers, Mexican yam (diosgenin) for infertility drugs, cinchona tree (quinine) for malaria, and rosy periwinkle (vincristine and vinblastine) to fight cancer (Carr, Pederson, Ramaswamy, 1996, p. 135).

Carbon dioxide is removed from the atmosphere by green plants during photosynthesis. Cutting down forests destroys the natural process of removing carbon dioxide from the atmosphere. Forested watersheds act as giant sponges and help regulate water flow and availability. Through transpiration and evaporation, forests influence climate (Miller, 2000, p. 646), and deforestation accelerates global warming. Deforestation results in "habitats on the move" and loss of plant and animal life. It has been estimated that a typical tree provides $196,250 worth of ecologic benefits during its lifetime and sold as timber, the same tree is worth only about $590 (Miller, 2000, p. 646).

## Energy Depletion

**Energy depletion** involves depleting the world's renewable and nonrenewable energy resources. The United States has the distinction of being the world's largest energy user and waster. The largest users and wasters of energy in the United States are energy-inefficient buildings, factories, and vehicles. At least 43% of all energy used in the United States is unnecessarily wasted, and this waste equals all the energy consumed by two thirds of the world's population (Miller, 2000, p. 397). Such unnecessarily wasted energy has been estimated to cost about twice as much as the annual U.S. federal budget deficit, or more than the entire military budget.

Major sources of U.S. energy are the nonrenewable resources of petroleum, coal, and natural gas. Renewable sources of energy include thermal, electric, hydroelectric, wind, solar (photovoltaic cells), geothermal, and biomass power. Heating, cooling, and lighting buildings consumes about one third of the energy we use, and we need to increase the energy efficiency of buildings. Every winter the energy equivalent of all the oil that flows through the Alaskan pipeline in a year leaks through American windows (The Earthworks Group, 1990).

Superinsulated homes cost slightly more to build, but save the owners money over the years and save energy. The energy efficiency of existing houses can be improved significantly by adding insulation, filling cracks and leaks, and installing energy efficient windows and lighting (Miller, 2000, p. 405). Solar power, a renewable energy resource, is being used as a power source in more homes.

## Overpopulation

The human species has had a population explosion in the last 50 years. **Overpopulation** contributes to depletion of natural resources and increased sewage and solid wastes. The world population is almost 6 billion, and it is expected to reach 10 to 11 billion by the year 2050 (Miller, 2000, pp. 2, 265). Many undeveloped countries have fertility reduction programs. Millions of people in the world are hungry or malnourished and lack safe drinking water. Rapid population growth in developing countries is a major reason for unemployment and economic woes.

Overpopulation places a strain on world food supplies and causes overcrowding and unsafe health conditions. Population growth is already outstripping food production and water supply. Already more than 900 million people in developing countries do not get enough calories to maintain normal levels of physical development, and 36% of preschool children in developing countries are below expected weight for their age (Brown, 1995). Poverty, malnutrition, overcrowding, increased susceptibility to disease, and shortened life span are all health-related conditions that are affected by overpopulation.

## DISASTER NURSING

Throughout history natural and man-made disasters have disrupted food and water supplies and sanitation, causing communicable disease, injury, illness, and death. Natural disasters have claimed approximately 3 million lives worldwide over the last 20 years and have had a direct impact on the lives of almost a billion people (Noji, 1997). Every state and territory in the United States has communities at risk for one or more natural hazards. In the United States approximately 2 million households experience injuries and physical damage each year from fire, floods, hurricanes, tornadoes, tropical storms, windstorms, and earthquakes (Meichenbaum, 1995).

Media coverage of man-made disasters such as the 1995 Oklahoma City bombing and natural disasters such as hurricanes, droughts, and floods has shown the devastating effects these events impose on human life, property, and the environment. Nurses need to be able to respond quickly and effectively to disaster and emergency situations.

Disasters can be natural or man-made. *Natural disasters* include droughts, earthquakes, tsunamis, forest fires, landslides and mudslides, blizzards, hurricanes, tornadoes, floods, and volcanic disruptions. *Man-made disasters* include hazardous substance accidents (e.g., chemicals, toxic gases), radiologic accidents, dam failures, resource shortages (e.g., food, electricity, and water), structural fire and explosions, and domestic disturbances (e.g., terrorism, bombing, and riots). Bioterroism as a man-made disaster threat is discussed in Chapter 11.

Although little can be done to prevent natural disasters, much can be done to prevent man-made ones. The United Nations (UN) declared the 1990s as the "International Decade for Natural Disaster Reduction," with emphasis on disaster prevention and preparedness. WHO and FEMA have developed guidelines and procedures to aid in disaster preparedness and response efforts. It is important to remember that individual preparedness is critical to community response to a disaster.

## Legislation

Legislation has been enacted to provide federal assistance to individuals and communities to aid recovery from devastation caused by disasters to human life and property. The *Disaster Relief Act of 1966* (Public Law 89-769) was a landmark piece of legislation that affected disaster relief efforts and funding and mandated a Disaster Assistance Study. In response to this study, the *Disaster Relief Act of 1970* (Public Law 91-606) was passed. This act repealed and replaced most previous disaster relief legislation. It defined *disaster* and provided direction for coordinating disaster assistance, ranging from early disaster warnings to relocation. The *Disaster Relief Act Amendments of 1974* (Public Law 93-288) distinguished between the terms *disaster* and *emergency* (Box 6-14). These amendments expanded coverage under the act, clarified the administration of disaster relief efforts, mandated immediate federal disaster relief, and provided for long-term economic assistance for disaster areas. The federal government has given authority to the American Red Cross to provide disaster relief.

**BOX 6-14**

### Defining Emergency and Major Disaster

*Emergency*

Any hurricane, tornado, storm, flood, high water, wind-driven water, tidal wave, tsunami, earthquake, volcanic eruption, landslide, mudslide, snowstorm, drought, fire, explosion, or other catastrophe in any part of the United States that requires federal emergency assistance to supplement state and local efforts to save lives and protect property, public health, and safety or to avert or lessen the threat of a disaster.

*Major Disaster*

Any hurricane, tornado, storm, flood, high water, wind-driven water, tidal wave, tsunami, earthquake, volcanic eruption, landslide, mudslide, snowstorm, drought, fire, explosion, or other catastrophe in any part of the United States that in the determination of the President, causes damage of sufficient severity above and beyond emergency services by the federal government, to supplement the efforts and available resources of states, local governments, and disaster relief organizations in alleviating the damage, loss, hardship, or suffering caused thereby.

From US Congress: *Disaster Relief Act Amendments of 1974* (Public Law 93-288), Section 102.

**BOX 6-15**

### Selected Publications from the American Red Cross

*Emergency/Disaster Plan for Business and Industry*
*Are You Ready? Your Guide to Disaster Preparedness*
*Emergency Preparedness Checklist*
*Preparing for Emergencies. A Checklist for People with Mobility Problems*
*Disaster Preparedness for Seniors by Seniors*
*Family Survival Guide. Preparing Your Family for Times of Emergency*
*Your Family Disaster Supplies Kit*
*Helping Children Cope With Disaster*
*Coping with Disaster. Emotional Health Issues for Victims*
*Pets and Disaster: Get Prepared*
*Hurricane*
*Tornado*
*Fires. Family Survival Guide*
*Safe Living in Your Manufactured Home*
*Flashfloods and Floods...the Awesome Power. A Preparedness Guide*
*Thunderstorms and Lightning...the Underrated Killers: A Preparedness Guide*
*Winter Storms...a Deceptive Killer: A Guide to Survival*

## The American Red Cross

The **American Red Cross** (ARC) (*http://www.redcross.org*) was founded in 1881 by Clara Barton. The ARC is not a government agency, but the government formalized its authority to provide disaster relief in 1905. At that time it was chartered by Congress to "carry on a system of national and international relief in time of peace and apply the same in mitigating the suffering caused by pestilence, famine, fire, floods and other great national calamities, and to devise and carry on measures for preventing the same" (ARC, 2001a, p. 2).

The ARC is known all over the world for its disaster relief efforts, and each year the ARC responds to more than 60,000 disasters worldwide (ARC, 2001a). Recently the Red Cross has responded to disasters such as Hurricanes George and Floyd and the earthquakes in India and El Salvador. Red Cross disaster relief focuses on meeting people's immediate emergency disaster-caused needs (ARC, 2001a). All ARC disaster relief assistance is free. There are local offices of the ARC across the country.

The ARC works with FEMA to develop guidelines for community disaster preparation, and numerous publications are available for families and communities to use to prepare for disasters. An especially helpful publication for families is the *Emergency Preparedness Checklist*, which is a joint FEMA and ARC publication. The ARC also publishes a grade K-8 curriculum, *Masters of Disaster*, to educate children about

disasters. Box 6-15 has a listing of selected ARC publications. Historically nurses have played an important role in Red Cross provision of services.

RED CROSS NURSING. The ARC provides disaster training for nurses. Historically nurses have been a cornerstone for services provided by the ARC. Red Cross nurses have provided their assistance during times of disaster and conflict beginning with the 1880 Johnstown floods and the 1888 Yellow Fever epidemic (ARC, 2001b). A separate service with the ARC, the *Red Cross Nursing Service*, was started by *Jane Delano* in 1909. In honor of Delano's service to the Red Cross, the *Jane Delano Society* was founded in 1990 and works to ensure active nursing involvement at all levels of the Red Cross and to document the history of Red Cross nursing (ARC, 2001c). Today, more than 40,000 nurses are involved in paid or volunteer activities with the ARC (ARC, 2001b). These nurses provide direct services such as disaster relief and blood collection drive efforts, and they also develop and teach courses (e.g., first aid, disaster preparedness, disaster relief). These nurses also carry out management and supervisory roles.

For more than half a century, student nurses have been involved in helping the Red Cross deliver services (ARC, 2001d). These students volunteer their efforts and assist in teaching courses; serving on disaster action teams; and taking part in health fairs, immunization clinics, blood drives,

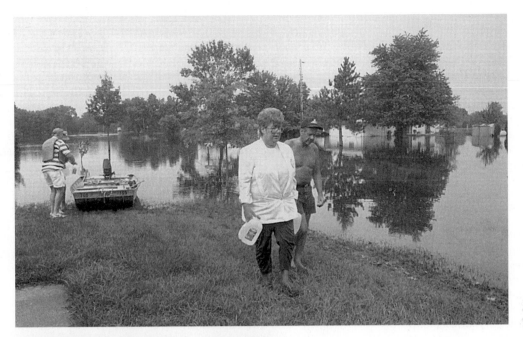

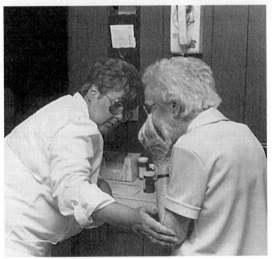

**FIGURE 6-3** A disaster worker boats out to a flooded area and assists an 86-year-old widow who refused to leave her home. Nurses often provide relief services in disaster areas and use skills such as crisis intervention to help individuals and families cope with the stresses they are experiencing. (Courtesy Kathy Kuper.)

and screening clinics. The Red Cross publishes a guidebook, *Make a Difference. Guidelines for Student Nurse Involvement in the American Red Cross*, that can be downloaded from the Red Cross website.

## The Nursing Role in Disasters

**Disaster nurses** play key leadership and service provision roles in planning and implementing disaster relief efforts, preventing technologic disasters, and addressing problems that occur during a disaster, such as the physical and emotional stress of disaster victims (Figure 6-3). The ANA and the ARC recognize the need to have an adequate supply of nurses trained for disaster relief, and ANA collaborates with the Red Cross, federal and civilian agencies, and nursing specialty organizations to enhance nurses' contributions in disaster management.

During a disaster many environmental health problems emerge. The scope and magnitude of these problems determines the nursing role. Nurses collaborate with community agencies and officials to recognize and reduce disaster risks and maximize the health and safety of individuals involved in disaster crises. Some community disaster strategies for nurses are given in Box 6-16.

Following a disaster, nurses make numerous referrals to community agencies for a variety of needs including psychologic care, emotional support services, and treatment for victims and their families. Recovery encompasses dealing with many disaster effects such as loss of life, income, and

**BOX 6-16**

*Community Disaster Strategies for Nurses\**

---

*Assess the Community*

Is there a current community disaster plan in place?

What previous disaster experiences has the community been involved with locally, statewide, nationally?

How is the local climate conducive to disaster formation (e.g., hurricanes, tornadoes, blizzards)?

How is the local terrain conducive to disaster formation (e.g., earthquakes, flooding, forest fires, avalanches, mudslides)?

What are the local industries?

Are there any community hazards (e.g., toxic waste and chemical spills, industrial or agricultural pollutants, mass transportation problems)?

What personnel are available for disaster interventions (e.g., nurses, doctors, dentists, pharmacists, clergy, volunteers, emergency medical teams)?

What are the locally available disaster resources (e.g., food, clothing, shelter, pharmaceutical)?

What are the local agencies and organizations (e.g., hospitals, schools, churches, emergency medical, Red Cross)?

What is immediately available for infant care (e.g., formula, diapers) and care of the elderly and disabled?

What are the most salient chronic illnesses in the community that will need immediate attention (e.g., diabetes, arthritis, cardiovascular)?

*Diagnose Community Disaster Threats*

Determine actual and potential disaster threats (e.g., toxic waste spills, explosions, mass transit accidents, hurricanes, tornadoes, blizzards, floods, earthquakes).

*Community Disaster Planning*

Develop a disaster plan to prevent or deal with identified disaster threats.

Identify a local community communication system.

Identify disaster personnel, including private and professional volunteers, local emergency personnel, agencies, and resources.

Identify regional backup agencies, personnel.

Identify specific responsibilities for various personnel involved in disaster coping and establish a disaster chain of command.

Set up an emergency medical system and chain for activation.

Identify location and accessibility of equipment and supplies.

Check proper functioning of emergency equipment.

Identify outdated supplies and replenish for appropriate readiness.

*Implement Disaster Plan*

Focus on primary prevention activities to prevent occurrence of man-made disasters.

Practice community disaster plans with all personnel carrying out their previously identified responsibilities (e.g., emergency triage, providing supplies such as food, water, medicine, crises and grief counseling).

Practice using equipment; obtaining and distributing supplies.

*Evaluate Effectiveness of Disaster Plan*

Critically evaluate all aspects of disaster plans and practice drills for speed, effectiveness, gaps, and revisions.

Evelute the disaster impact on community and surrounding regions.

Evaluate response of personnel involved in disaster relief efforts.

---

\*See Chapters 3 and 14 for specific guidelines for community assessment.

home. The communicable disease implications of disasters are also immense. Other conditions, such as domestic violence and depression, can become rampant. Nurses need to realize that the emotional effects of disasters may persist for many years and that a person's initial response to the traumatic event is often predictive of future response (Cardena, Spiegel, 1993; Meichenbaum, 1995, p. 35). Nurses work in all phases of disaster management.

## PHASES OF DISASTER MANAGEMENT

FEMA has described four **disaster management phases:** mitigation, preparedness, response, and recovery, which serve as a model for community disaster preparations and nursing interventions (Figure 6-4). Some preparedness, response, and recovery activities by local communities and the American Red Cross are given in Table 6-4.

### Mitigation

Mitigation includes any activities that prevent a disaster, reduce the chance of a disaster happening, or reduce the damaging effects of unavoidable disasters. Nurses have a key role in disaster mitigation by working with local, state, and federal agencies in identifying disaster risks and developing disaster prevention strategies through extensive public education in disaster prevention and readiness. Effective mitigation includes recognizing and preventing potential technologic disasters and being adequately prepared should such events occur.

To plan effectively for disaster prevention the nurse needs to have community assessment information (see Chapter 14), including knowledge of community resources (e.g., emergency services, hospitals, and clinics), community health personnel (e.g., nurses, doctors, pharmacists, emergency medical teams, dentists, and volunteers), community

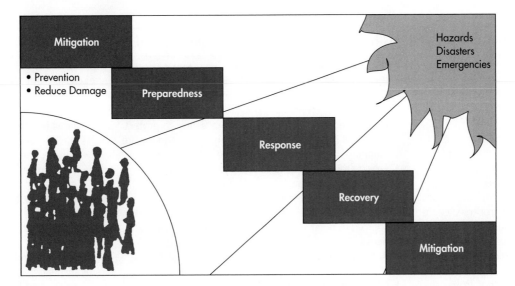

**FIGURE 6-4** Phases of disaster management. (From Federal Emergency Management Agency [FEMA]: *Emergency management U.S.A.,* Washington, DC, 1986, FEMA, p. 1.5.)

**TABLE 6-4**

*Disaster Management Responsibilities: Preparedness, Response, and Recovery*

| RED CROSS | OTHER VOLUNTARY ORGANIZATIONS | BUSINESS AND LABOR ORGANIZATIONS | LOCAL GOVERNMENT |
|---|---|---|---|
| *Preparedness* | | | |
| • Participates with government in developing and testing community disaster plan. Designates persons to serve as representatives at government emergency operations centers and command posts.<br>• Develops and tests local Red Cross disaster plans.<br>• Identifies and trains personnel for disaster response.<br>• Collaborates with other voluntary agencies in developing and maintaining a local Voluntary Organizations Active in Disaster group to promote cooperation and coordinate resources for disasters.<br>• Works with business and labor organizations to identify resources and people for disaster work.<br>• Educates the public about hazards and ways to avoid, prepare for, and cope with their effects.<br>• Acquires material resources needed to ensure effective response. | • Collaborate in developing and maintaining a local Voluntary Organizations Active in Disaster group to identify roles, resources, and plans for disasters.<br>• Identify and train personnel for disaster response.<br>• Identify community issues and special populations for consideration in disaster preparedness.<br>• Make plans to continue to serve regular clients following a disaster.<br>• Identify facilities, resources, and people to serve in time of disaster.<br>• Educate specific client groups on disaster preparedness. | • Develop disaster plans for business locations and integrate their plans with the community disaster plan.<br>• Develop procedures to facilitate continuity of operations in time of disaster.<br>• Develop plans for assisting business employees following a disaster.<br>• Identify union and business facilities, resources, and people that may be able to support community disaster plans.<br>• Provide volunteers, financial contributions, and in-kind gifts to the Red Cross and other voluntary organizations to support disaster preparedness.<br>• Educate employees and union members about disaster preparedness. | • Coordinates the development of the community plan and conducts evaluation exercises.<br>• Trains staff to carry out the plan.<br>• Passes legislation to mitigate the effects of potential disasters.<br>• Designs measures to warn the population of disaster threats.<br>• Conducts building safety inspections.<br>• Develops procedures to facilitate continuity of public safety operations in time of disaster.<br>• Identifies public facilities, resources, and public employees for disaster work.<br>• Educates the public about disaster threats in the community and safety procedures. |

*Continued*

**TABLE 6-4**

*Disaster Management Responsibilities: Preparedness, Response, and Recovery—cont'd*

| RED CROSS | OTHER VOLUNTARY ORGANIZATIONS | BUSINESS AND LABOR ORGANIZATIONS | LOCAL GOVERNMENT |
|---|---|---|---|
| *Response* | | | |
| • Operates shelters.<br>• Provides feeding services.<br>• Provides individual and family assistance to meet immediate emergency needs. Services include providing the means to purchase groceries, clothing, and household items.<br>• Provides disaster health services, including mental support.<br>• Handles inquiries from concerned family members outside the area.<br>• Coordinates relief activities with other agencies, business, labor, and government.<br>• Informs the public of services available.<br>• Seeks and accepts contributions from those wishing to help. | • Provide services that are identified in predisaster planning.<br>• Provide regular services to ongoing client groups.<br>• Identify unanticipated needs and provide resources to meet those needs.<br>• Act as advocates for their client groups.<br>• Coordinate services with all other groups involved with the disaster response.<br>• Seek and accept donations from those wishing to help. | • Take action to protect employees and ensure the safety of the facility.<br>• Advise public safety forces of hazardous conditions.<br>• Identify resources like union halls, generators, and heavy equipment that are available to support the disaster response.<br>• Provide volunteers, financial contributions, and gifts of goods and services to the relief effort. | • Provides for coordination of the overall relief effort.<br>• Advises the public on safety measures such as evacuation.<br>• Provides public health services.<br>• Provides fire and police protection to the disaster-affected area.<br>• Inspects facilities for safety and health codes.<br>• Provides ongoing social services for the community.<br>• Repairs public buildings, sewage and water systems, streets, and highways. |
| *Recovery* | | | |
| • During recovery, all of the segments represented here pull together with one goal—the restoration of the economic and civic life of the community.<br>• Government takes the lead in rebuilding roads, bridges public works, and buildings, and providing services to citizens.<br>• Business returns to operation to provide economic support to the community.<br>• Voluntary agencies, including the Red Cross, work together to identify and meet the remaining needs of individuals and families. | | • The Red Cross remains available to support those with long-term needs by helping people access vital services and apply for assistance from local, state, and federal disaster programs. However, if such relief assistance is not available, the Red Cross also can provide assistance to promote the recovery of individuals.<br>• All of the groups involved work in partnership with the people affected by disasters, who are ultimately responsible for their own recovery. | |

From American Red Cross: *Disasters happen*, Washington, DC, 1993, American Red Cross.

government officials, and local industry. Disasters such as floods, tornadoes, hurricanes, and earthquakes can have devastating effects (Figure 6-5). Long before a disaster strikes, communities need to have disaster prevention measures in place (Noji, 1997). In planning for disasters, health care professionals and disaster response agencies need to be prepared to mobilize resources, provide care, and minimize chaos and confusion.

## Preparedness

Preparedness includes plans or preparations made to save lives and to help response and rescue operations in the event of a natural or technologic disaster. Long before a dis-

aster strikes, communities need to have disaster preparedness measures in place and conduct disaster education and training programs (Noji, 1997). Nurses have a key role in maximizing the health and safety of all individuals affected by a disaster.

Disaster preparedness involves developing plans for rescue; evacuation; caring for disaster victims; training disaster response personnel; and gathering resources, equipment, and materials necessary for coping with disaster. Community-focused planning skills are discussed in Chapter 15. Establishing an effective public communication system is essential for successful disaster emergency communication and community safety. Community officials need to be able

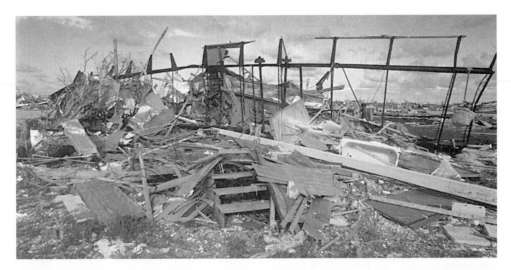

**FIGURE 6-5** Hurricanes and other environmental disasters cause many community-wide health problems. (Courtesy U.S. Department of Agriculture.)

to issue timely warnings and take life-saving, preventive actions and conduct evacuations as necessary (Noji, 1997). Making anticipatory provisions for food, water, clothing, shelter, and medicine is also an important preparedness activity. It is crucial for the nurse to understand effective disaster preparedness. Through community assessment, nurses can identify disaster risks and collaborate in developing disaster plans for the particular disaster risks (e.g., tornadoes, chemical spills, floods, earthquakes, and explosions).

## Response

Response includes actions taken to save lives and prevent further damage in a disaster or emergency situation and puts pre-disaster planning services into action. Nurses play a key role in disaster response. Nurses have skills in triage and crisis intervention and are involved in acute care, triage, first aid, rescue and evacuation procedures, managing life-threatening events, recognizing and preventing communicable illnesses, assessment, and providing immediate health care needs during disaster impact.

Nurses work with community disaster teams in emergency rescue and care operations with a focus on lessening the effect on victims. This includes triage of disaster victims, providing immediate health care (e.g., first aid), providing food and shelter, maintaining effective channels of communication, and minimizing chaos and panic.

In disaster response a primary concern for nurses is safety—safety for themselves, the rescue team, and victims. Nurses are involved in promoting not only safety and physical health but also the mental health of all involved in the disaster. The nurse works to reduce fear, panic, and hysteria by encouraging victims to express their fears and concerns. Helping people cope with the disaster situation involves caring, listening, encouraging people to express their feel-

ings, and providing emotional support to the victims and their families.

## Recovery

Recovery includes actions taken to return to a normal, or even safer, situation following a disaster. The recovery period may last for an extended period of time. It is a period of reconstruction and rehabilitation (Noji, 1997). The goal of recovery is to prevent debilitating effects and restore personal, economic, and environmental health and stability to the community. Disaster relief activities may be provided by local, state, regional, national, and international efforts.

A wide range of emotional responses including fear, anxiety, depression, sadness, grief and shock, and posttraumatic stress disorder occur in a disaster (Meichenbaum, 1995; Noji, 1997). During the recovery phase, mental health services have a key role. From a mental health viewpoint, there are phases of emotional reaction during a disaster (Box 6-17).

Rescue personnel should be included in the mental health efforts of the recovery process. Prevention and control of stress among emergency workers is important. Rescuers are vulnerable to emotional crises in relation to disaster events (Craft, 1996), and as a result, debriefings are important interventions for rescue personnel (Stuhlmiller, 1996).

Community health nurses have unique skills for assisting communities in planning for disaster relief efforts and addressing problems that occur during a disaster. Community health nurses' knowledge of community resources, community assessment and organization, epidemiology, health planning, and family health promotion provides a background for organizing and participating in community relief efforts.

**BOX 6-17**

*Phases of Emotional Reaction During a Disaster*

From a mental health viewpoint, work with victims of disasters has suggested the following classifications related to emotional reactions:

- **HEROIC PHASE**

  This phase appears at the time of the disaster and is characterized by people working together to save each other and their property. Excitement is intense, and people are concerned with survival.

- **HONEYMOON PHASE**

  This is a relatively short (2 weeks to 2 months) postdisaster period in which the victims feel buoyed and supported by the promises of governmental and communal help and see an opportunity to reconstitute quickly. Optimism continues high, losses are counted, and plans to reestablish are made.

- **DISILLUSIONMENT PHASE**

  Lasting anywhere from several months to a year or more, this phase contains unexpected delays and failures, which emphasize the frustration from bureaucratic confusion. Victims turn to rebuilding their own lives and solving their own individual problems.

- **RECONSTRUCTION PHASE**

  This phase may last for several years. It is characterized by a coordinated individual and community effort to rebuild and reestablish normal functioning.

From Farberow NL, Gordon NS: *Manual for child health workers in major disasters,* Washington, DC, 1986, USDHHS (Substance Abuse and Mental Health Services Administration), p. 3.

## SUMMARY

*Healthy People 2010* has a focus area on environmental health and national environmental health. Environmental health legislation supports public health professionals in their efforts to resolve environmental health problems. Environmental health remains a major, worldwide public health concern. Man-made and natural disasters in recent years have caused tremendous economic instability and extensive personal suffering in communities across the United States and the world. The threat of terrorism is an emerging disaster concern.

Since the days of Florence Nightingale, nursing leaders have recognized the importance of the environment on health and the important role environment played in nursing care. Today nurse scholars reinforce this importance. Nursing organizations such as the AAOHN and the NIHE are addressing environmental health issues. Worldwide, nurses are being encouraged to safeguard the human environment and specific environmental health roles for nurses have been identified.

Community health nurses have unique skills to deal with environmental health issues. They provide care and consultation for clients with conditions that originate in the environment, including injuries and illnesses resulting from disasters and exposure to toxic wastes, chemicals, and water and air pollution; malnutrition; and overcrowding. They work collaboratively with environmental health professionals to reduce the incidence of environmental diseases and conditions. They are advocates for safe environmental health practices. We all need to focus on preserving and protecting the environment, something we cannot create. Remember, pollution is unhealthy and difficult to eradicate, and extinction is forever.

## CRITICAL THINKING
*exercise*

Examine the local community in which you live.
1. What types of environmental hazards exist?
2. What types of environmental disasters have occurred or have the potential to occur?
3. What are some agencies that would respond to a disaster?
4. What disaster provisions has the community made?
5. Describe some of the activities you see nurses being responsible for in a disaster. What actions could nurses take to promote environmental health?

## REFERENCES

American Academy of Pediatrics (AAP): *Handbook of pediatric environmental health,* Elk Grove Village, Ill, 1999, AAP.

American Association of Colleges of Nursing (AACN): *Addressing nursing's agenda for health care reform,* Washington, DC, 1993, AACN.

American Association of Occupational Health Nurses (AAOHN): *Advisory. Environmental health: expanding dimensions of practice,* Atlanta, 1998, AAOHN.

American Association of Occupational Health Nurses (AAOHN): *Standards of occupational and environmental health nursing,* Atlanta, 1999, AAOHN.

American Nurses Association (ANA): *American Nurses Association position statement on lead poisoning and screening: compendium of American Nurses Association position statements,* Washington, DC, 1996, ANA.

American Public Health Association (APHA): Position paper on the role of official local health agencies, *Am J Public Health* 65:189-193, 1975.

American Red Cross (ARC): *Disasters happen,* Washington, DC, 1993, ARC.

American Red Cross (ARC): *FACTS. Disaster services,* Washington, DC, 2001a, ARC. Retrieved from the internet Feb, 2001. *http://www.redcross.org*

American Red Cross (ARC): *About Red Cross Nursing,* Washington, DC, 2001b, ARC. Retrieved from the internet Feb, 2001. *http://www.redcross.org*

American Red Cross (ARC): *Jane Delano Society,* Washington, DC, 2001, ARC. Retrieved from the internet Feb, 2001. *http://www.redcross.org*

American Red Cross (ARC): *Student nurses*, Washington, DC, 2001d, ARC. Retrieved from the internet Feb, 2001. *http://www.redcross.org*

Bellack JP, Musham C, Hainer A, et al: Environmental health competencies: a survey of U.S. nurse practitioner programs, *J Nurs Educ* 35(2):74-81, 1996.

Blumenthal DS, Greene M: Air pollution. In Blumenthal DS, editor: *An introduction to environmental health*, New York, 1985, Springer.

Breckinridge M: *Wide neighborhoods: a story of the Frontier Nursing Service*, New York, 1952, Harper and Brothers.

Brown LR: Reassessing the earth's population, *Society* May/June:7-10, 1995.

Cardena E, Spiegel D: Dissociative reactions to the San Francisco bay earthquake of 1989, *Am J Psych* 150:474-478, 1993.

Carr TA, Pederson HL, Ramaswamy S: Rain forest entrepreneurs. In Allen JL, editor: *Environment: annual edition 96/97*, Guilford, Conn, 1996, Dushkin.

Chin J: *Control of communicable disease manual*, ed 17, Washington, DC, 2000, American Public Health Association.

Clark HG: Origins of public health in America: superiority of sanitary measures over quarantines. An address delivered before the Suffolk District Medical Society at its third anniversary meeting, Boston, April 24, 1852. In Rosenberg CE, editor: *Medicine and society in America*, New York, 1972, Arno Press.

Coss C: Lillian D. Wald: progressive activist, *Public Health Nurs* 10(3):134-138, 1993.

Craft M: The many graces of Oklahoma nurses, *Reflections* 22(1):10-13, 1996.

Doll R: Health and the environment in the 1990s, *Am J Public Health* 82(7):923-941, 1992.

Earthworks Group: *Simple things you can do to save the earth: 1991 tip a day calendar*, New York, 1990, Andrews and McNeel.

Environmental Protection Agency (EPA): *Characterization of municipal solid wastes in the United States: 1997 update*, No. EPAA530-R-98-007, Office of Solid Waste, Washington, DC, 1998, EPA.

Farberow NL, Gordon NS: *Manual for child health workers in major disasters*, Washington, DC, 1986, US Department of Health and Human Services (Substance Abuse and Mental Health Services Administration).

Gerber DE, McGuire SL: Teaching students about nursing and the environment: part 1—nursing role and basic curricula, *J Community Health Nurs* 16:69-79, 1999.

Glick D: Cinderella story, *Natl Wildlife* 34(2):42-46, 1996.

Gochfeld M, Goldstein BD: Lessons in environmental health in the twentieth century. *Annu Rev Public Health* 20:35-53, 1999.

Goldman LR: Environmental health and its relationship to occupational health. In Levy BS, Wegman DH, editors: *Occupational health. Recognizing and preventing work-related disease and injury*, ed 4, Philadelphia, 2000, Lippincott Williams & Wilkins.

Green MH: Leap of faith. How birds—and instinct—led the Pennsylvanians to Ecuador, *Nature Conservancy* 51(3):12-18, 2001.

Harte J: The scientific consensus about global warming. In Miller GT, editor: *Living in the environment: principles, connections, and solutions*, ed 11, Pacific Grove, Calif, 2000, Brooks/Cole Publishing Company.

Hill L: Health in America: a personal perspective. In US Department of Health, Education, and Welfare: *Health in America 1776-1976*, DHEW Pub. No (HRA) 76-616, Washington, DC, 1976, US Government Printing Office.

Hinrichsen D: Putting the bite on planet earth, *International Wildlife* Sept/Oct:36-45, 1994.

Institute of Medicine (Committee for the Study of the Future of Public Health): *The future of public health*, Washington, DC, 1988, National Academy Press.

Institute of Medicine (Committee on Enhancing Environmental Health Content in Nursing Practice: In Pope AM, Snyder MA, Mood LH, editors): *Nursing, health, and the environment: strengthening the relationship to improve the public's health*, Washington, DC, 1995, National Academy Press.

International Council of Nurses: *The nurse's role in safeguarding the human environment: position statement*, Geneva, Switzerland, 1986, The Council.

Jaakkola JJK, Tuomaala P, Seppanen OL: Air recirculation and sick building syndrome: a blinded crossover, *Am J Public Health* 84(3):422-428, 1994.

Kalisch PA, Kalisch BJ: *The advance of American nursing*, Boston, 1995, Little, Brown.

Kleffel D: Rethinking the environment as a domain of nursing knowledge, *Adv Nurs Sci* 14(1):40-51, 1991.

Lemonick MD: The ozone vanishes, *Time* 139(7):60-63, 1992.

McCord CP: *Conversation with author regarding industrial lead poisoning*, Ann Arbor, Mich, 1976, University of Michigan.

McGuire SL, Gerber DE: Teaching students about nursing and the environment: part 2—legislation and resources, *J Community Health Nurs* 16:81-94, 1999.

Meichenbaum D: Disasters, stress and cognition. In Hobfoll SE, deVries MW, editors: *Extreme stress in communities: impact and intervention*, 1995, Boston, Kluwer Academic Publishers.

Mielke HW: Lead in the inner cities, *Am Scientist* 86:62, 1999.

Miller GT: *Living in the environment: principles, connections, and solutions*, ed 9, Pacific Grove, Calif, 1996, Brooks/Cole Publishing Company.

Miller GT: *Living in the environment: principles, connections, and solutions*, ed 11, Pacific Grove, Calif, 2000, Brooks/Cole Publishing Company.

Monks V: Environmental regulations: who needs them? *Natl Wildlife* 34(2):24-31, 1996.

Morris RD, Naumova EN, Levin R, et al.: Temporal variation in drinking water turbidity and diagnosed gastroenteritis in Milwaukee, *Am J Public Health* 86(2):237-242, 1996.

Myers N: Guest essay: tropical forests and their species, going, going . . . ? In Miller GT, editor: *An introduction to environmental science: living in the environment*, ed 7, Belmont, Calif, 1992, Wadsworth.

Nadakavukaren A: *Our global environment: a health perspective*, ed 4, Prospect Heights, Ill, 1995, Waveland Press.

Nadakavukaren A: *Our global environment: a health perspective*, ed 5, Prospect Heights, Ill, 2000, Waveland Press.

National Center for Environmental Health (NCEH): *Message from the NCEH director*. Retrieved from the internet Feb, 2001. *http://www.cdc/gpv/nceh/Information/about.htm*

National Resources Defense Council [NRDC]: *Bottled water: pure drink or pure hype*, New York, 1999, NRDC.

Needleman HL, Schell A, Bellinger D, et al: The long-term effects of exposure to low doses of lead in childhood: an 11-year follow-up report, *N Engl J Med* 332:83-88, 1990.

Nightingale F: *Notes on nursing: what it is and what it is not*, New York, 1859, Dover.

Nightingale Institute for Health and the Environment (NIHE): *The Nightingale Institute for Health and the Environment: about us*. Retrieved from the internet Feb, 2001. *http://www.nihe.org*

Noji EK: The nature of disaster: general characteristics and public health effects. In Noji EK, editor: *The public health consequences of disasters*, New York, 1997, Oxford University Press.

Otto WR, Roberts JW: Everyday exposure to toxic pollutants, *Scientific Amer* 268:86-91, 1998.

Pickett G, Hanlon JJ: *Public health administration and practice*, ed 9, St Louis, 1990, Mosby.

Preventing lead poisoning, *Health Watch* 12(1):1-3, 1992.

Rabe B: Environmental health policy. In Pickett G, Hanlon JJ: *Public health administration and practice*, ed 9, St Louis, 1990, Mosby.

Rainforests, *Kids for Saving Earth News* Fall:3, 1990.

Raven P: A time of catastrophic extinction: what we must do, *The Futurist* Sept/Oct:38-41, 1995.

Ravenel MP: *A half century of public health: jubilee historical volume of the American Public Health Association,* New York, 1921, American Public Health Association.

Rogers B, Cox AR: Expanding horizons. Integrating environmental health in occupational health nursing, *AAOHN J* 46:9-13, 1998.

Salazar MK, Primomo J: Taking the lead in environmental health: defining a model for practice, *AAOHN J* 42(7):317-324, 1994.

Sattler B: Welcome to enviRNews, *enviRNews* 1(1):1, 1999.

Seeing beauty: thoughts from Emerson, *Int Wildlife* 26(4):50, 1996.

Selanders LC: *Florence Nightingale: an environmental adaptation theory,* Newbury Park, 1993, Sage.

Smillie WG: *Public health: its promise for the future,* New York, 1955, Macmillan.

Snyder M, Ruth V, Sattler B, et al.: Environmental and occupational health education, *AAOHN J* 42(7):325-328, 1994.

Stolzenburg W: Glacier-less park? *Nature Conservancy,* 51(2):6, 2001.

Stopping the dry destruction. In Allen JL, editor: *Environment: annual edition 96/97,* Guilford, Conn, 1996, Dushkin.

Stuhlmiller C: Studying the rescuers, *Reflections* 22(1):18-19, 1996.

The 27th environmental quality review, *Natl Wildlife* 33(2):34-41, 1995.

United States Department of Agriculture: *A quick consumer guide to safe food handling* (Home and Garden Bulletin No. 248), Washington, DC, 1995, USDA.

United States Department of Health, Education and Welfare (USDHEW): *Healthy people,* Washington, DC, 1979, US Government Printing Office.

United States Department of Health and Human Services (USDHHS): *Promoting health, preventing disease: objectives for the nation,* Washington, DC, 1980, US Government Printing Office.

United States Department of Health and Human Services (USDHHS): *Evaluating the environmental health workforce* (HRP #0907160), Rockville, Md, 1988, USDHHS.

United States Department of Health and Human Services (USDHHS): *Healthy People 2000: national health promotion and disease prevention objectives for the nation, full report, with commentary,* Washington, DC, 1991, US Government Printing Office.

United States Department of Health and Human Services (USDHHS): *Health United States 1991 and prevention profile,* Washington, DC, 1992, US Government Printing Office.

United States Department of Health and Human Services (USDHHS): *Healthy People 2000: midcourse review and 1995 revisions,* Washington, DC, 1995, US Government Printing Office.

United States Department of Health and Human Services (USDHHS): *Healthy People 2010: conference edition,* Washington, DC, 2000, US Government Printing Office.

Wald L: *The house on Henry Street,* New York, 1915, Henry Holt and Company.

Washington Post: Warning on earth warming is most ominous yet, *Knoxville News-Sentinel,* January 23, 2001, p. A5.

Wasson N: *E. coli* illness fells 6,000 children, *USA Today,* July 18, 1996, p. 9A.

Wilkie KE, Moseley ER: *Frontier nurse Mary Breckinridge,* New York, 1969, Julian Messner.

World Health Organization (WHO): *Indicators for policy and decision making in environmental health* (draft), Geneva, Switzerland, 1997a, WHO.

World Health Organization (WHO): *Fact sheet 170,* Geneva, Switzerland, 1997b, WHO.

World Wildlife Fund (WWF): WWF launches global campaign to protect world's forests, *Focus* 18(4):1, 1996.

Young JE: The sudden new strength of recycling. In Allen JL, editor: *Environment: annual review 96/97,* Guilford, Conn, 1996, Dushkin.

## SELECTED BIBLIOGRAPHY

American Red Cross (ARC): *History: The history and organization of the Red Cross Nursing Service,* Washington, DC, 2001, ARC. http://www.redcross.org

Clunn P: The nurse's kit for survivors, *Reflections* 22(1):8-9, 1996.

Durkin MS, Khan N, Davidson LL, et al.: The effects of a natural disaster on child behavior: evidence for posttraumatic stress, *Am J Public Health* 83(11):1549-1553, 1993.

Garcia LM: *Disaster nursing: planning, assessment and intervention,* Rockville, Md, 1985, Aspen.

General Accounting Office (GAO): *Environmental protection issues,* Washington, DC, 1993, GAO.

Graves JS: Emotional aftermath of a major earthquake, *AAOHN J* 43(2):95-100, 1995.

Komnenich P, Feller C: Disaster nursing. In Fitzpatrick JJ, Taunton RL, Jacox AK: *Annual review of nursing research,* vol 9, New York, 1991, Springer.

Landrigan R: Commentary: environmental diseases—a preventable epidemic, *Am J Public Health* 82(7):941-943, 1992.

Martin F: Volunteering for disaster nursing, *Imprint* 41(2):45-46, 1994.

Pickens S: The decade for natural disaster reduction: the role of health care workers, *Nurs Health Care* 13(4):192-195, 1992.

Schuster EA, Brown CL: *Exploring our environmental connections,* New York, 1995, National League for Nursing.

Shalauta NM, Burke TA, Gordon LJ, et al.: An examination of the educational needs for environmental health and protection, *J Public Health Management Prac* 5(6):1-12, 1999.

Worthington K, Cary A: Primary health care: environmental challenges, *Am Nurse* 25(10):10-11, 1993.

# Family Assessment and Cultural Diversity: Concepts and Tools

*Ella M. Brooks*

## OBJECTIVES

*Upon completion of this chapter, the reader should be able to:*

1. Construct a definition for the term *family*.
2. Identify variations in family structure in the United States.
3. Describe the cultural diversity among American families.
4. Discuss the meaning of the phrase *the family is the unit of service*.
5. Explain how the use of a theoretical framework for family study promotes family-focused nursing practice.
6. Discuss the structural and process parameters for family assessment and their relevance to community health nursing practice.
7. Discuss how cultural factors influence health and health behaviors.
8. Formulate guidelines for completing a cultural assessment.
9. Describe tools used to facilitate the family assessment process.

## KEY TERMS

Cultural assessment
Culture schema
Cultural sensitivity
Developmental approach
Ecomap
Family
Family assessment
Family boundaries

Family-centered approach
Family communication patterns
Family functions
Family-life chronology model
Family nursing theory
Family rituals and symbols
Family roles
Genogram

Interactional frame of reference
Intracultural diversity
Nontraditional family
Power
Role strain
Structural-functional framework
Systems theory
Traditional family

---

*The ancient trinity of father, mother, and child has survived more vicissitudes than any other relationship. It is the bedrock underlying all other family structures. Although more elaborate family patterns can be broken from without or may even collapse of their own weight, the rock remains. In the Götterdammerung, which otherwise science and overfoolish statesmanship are preparing for us, the last man will spend his last hours searching for his wife and child.*

LINTON (1959, P. 52)

The composition of American households has shifted dramatically over the last three decades and the traditional family structure has drastically declined (Wellner, 2000). Even though **traditional family** structure has declined as a result of such events as divorce, single parenthood, stepfamilies, a growing number of mothers in the workforce, cohabitating relationships, domestic partnerships, and other alternate family forms, the family is still the basic social unit in society. "Families are America's most precious resource and most important institution. The strength of our families is the key determinate of the health and well-being of our nation, of our communities, and of our lives as individuals" (White

### BOX 7-1

## Select Alternative Family Structures in the United States

### Traditional Family Structures

- *Nuclear family*—legally married couple with children in a common household with one or both partners gainfully employed
- *Reconstituted nuclear family*—blended or stepfamily household with children with one or both partners gainfully employed
- *Dyadic nuclear family*—childless, legally married couple with one or both partners gainfully employed; family may never have had children or children may be "launched"
- *Single-parent family*—one-parent family as a consequence of divorce, abandonment, separation, or death; parent may or may not be working
- *Single adult*—living alone, usually with a career, who may or may not desire to marry
- *Three-generation family*—extended family with three or more generations living in a common household
- *Kin network*—nuclear households or unmarried members living in close geographic proximity and operating within a reciprocal system of exchange of goods and services

### Nontraditional Family Structures

- *Binuclear family*—coparenting and joint custody family system in which the child is part of two nuclear households
- *Unmarried single family*—one-parent family where marriage is not desired or possible
- *Unmarried couple family with children*—usually a common-law marriage
- *Voluntary childless nuclear family*—a legally married couple who has chosen not to have children
- *Heterosexual cohabiting family*—unmarried couple living together
- *Commune family*—household of more than one monogamous couple with children, sharing common facilities and resources; socialization of children is a group activity
- *Lesbian/gay family*—a male or female couple living together with or without children

Modified from Sussman MB, chairperson: *Changing families in a changing society: 1970 White House Conference on Children,* Forum 14 report, Washington, DC, 1971, US Government Printing Office, pp. 228-229; Macklin ED: Nontraditional family forms. In Sussman MB, Steinmetz SK, editor: *Handbook of marriage and the family,* New York, 1987, Plenum Press, pp. 317-353.

### BOX 7-2

## Selected Trends that Have Altered Traditional Family Patterns in the United States

Increase in divorce rate
Multiple remarriages
Increased number of intergenerational families
Growth in number of blended families (stepfamilies)
Increased number of mothers in workforce
Both parents in workplace
Rise in single-parent families
Increase in cohabitating relationships
Increased life expectancy
Rise in elderly population

House Conference on Families, 1978, p. 286). Politicians, religious leaders, scholars, community members, and leaders have engaged in vibrant efforts and discussion regarding the importance of family to our society (Stranton, 2000). Consumers and health care professionals are examining how to strengthen the family to promote health action.

"On June 1, 1996, over 250,000 people of every race, faith, age, and state gathered at the Lincoln Memorial to Stand For Children in the largest and most uplifting demonstration of commitment to children in American history" (Children's Defense Fund, 1997, p. xvii). This na-

tional mobilization effort was a day for spiritual, family, and community renewal. It was a call for action to help children by strengthening families and communities.

Child advocates are reconfirming the importance of the family in providing a healthy start for children. However, they are recognizing that rapid societal changes and the changing definitions of family are making it more difficult for many families to provide a nurturing environment. All Americans are being urged to help eliminate societal conditions that increase a family's vulnerability to stress and crises. Nurses play a vital role in promoting family and community wellness.

## THE AMERICAN FAMILY: CULTURALLY AND STRUCTURALLY DIVERSE

*Diversity* and *change* are the terms that best describe today's American family. Cultural backgrounds, socioeconomic levels, and family structures differ nationwide. The two-parent nuclear family unit—mother, father, and child(ren)—established through the legal sanction of marriage is less prevalent, and alternative family structures, as shown in Box 7-1, are more common. Box 7-2 presents trends that have altered traditional family patterns.

Household composition has changed significantly in the past several decades (Figure 7-1). Although the number of U.S. households has almost doubled in less than 40 years, the share of households headed by married couples has notably decreased. During this same period, the proportion of children living with one parent more than doubled, and

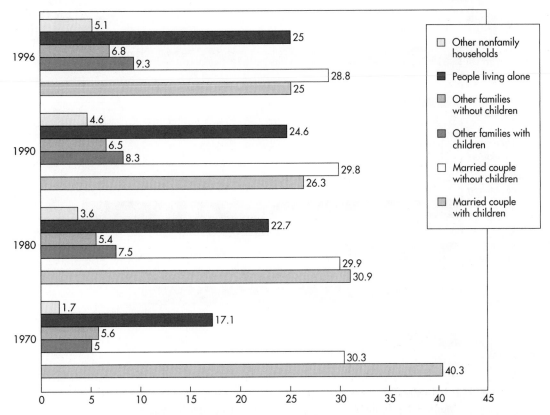

**FIGURE 7-1** Household composition in the United States: 1970-1996. (Modified from US Bureau of the Census: *Population profile of the United States:1997,* current population report, series P23-194, Washington, DC, 1998, US Government Printing Office, p. 24.)

household size has shrunk from an average of 3.3 persons to 2.6 persons (Box 7-3) (Francese, 1996).

In 1998 there were almost 99 million households in the United States. It is projected that by the year 2010 there will be 115 million households. It is also anticipated that the overall composition of households will shift (Figure 7-2), reflecting a decreasing proportion of family households with children and an increasing proportion of family households having no children and people living alone. Aging cohorts of empty-nest, post–World War II baby boomers will influence this shift (Day, 1996).

The wide variety of ethnic and racial groups in the United States enriches the diversity of family life (Figure 7-3). It is projected that the U.S. population will become more diverse by race and Hispanic origin. By the middle of the twenty-first century, it is anticipated that the black population will almost double, the Asian and Pacific Islander population will increase to more than five times its current size, and the Hispanic-origin population will triple its current size. "Demographers predict that by the year of 2056, today's ethnic and racial minorities will be the majority of the U.S. population" (Demo, 2000, p. 16).

Future fertility and immigration will significantly influence the country's population characteristics in the next 60 years. It is projected that after the year 2015 there will be more births every year than ever before in American

 **BOX 7-3**

*Number of Households and Size of Households in the United States: 1960 to 2010*

| Households in— | |
| --- | --- |
| 1960 | 53 million |
| 1970 | 63 million |
| 1980 | 81 million |
| 1990 | 93 million |
| 1996 | 99 million |
| 2010 | 115 million (projected) |

| Persons Per Household In— | |
| --- | --- |
| 1960 | 3.30 |
| 1970 | 3.14 |
| 1980 | 2.76 |
| 1990 | 2.63 |
| 1996 | 2.65 |
| 2010 | 2.53 (projected) |

From Day JC: *Projections of the number of households and families in the United States: 1995 to 2010,* US Bureau of the Census, current population reports, series P25-1129, Washington, DC, 1996, US Government Printing Office, p. 8; US Bureau of the Census: *Population profile of the United States: 1997,* current population reports, series P23-194, Washington, DC, 1998, US Government Printing Office.

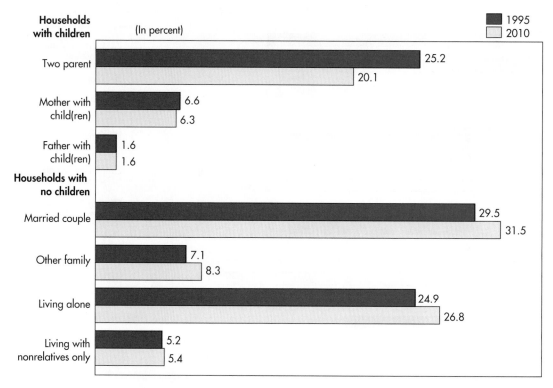

**FIGURE 7-2** Projections of changing household composition: 1995 and 2010. (From Day JC: *Projections of the number of households and families in the United States: 1995 to 2010*, US Bureau of the Census, current populations reports, series P25-1129, Washington, DC, 1996, US Government Printing Office, p. 11.)

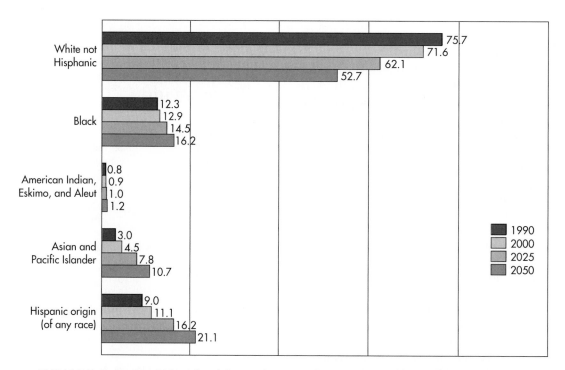

**FIGURE 7-3** Race and Hispanic-origin populations in the United States, percent of the total population: 1990, 2000, 2025, 2050. (From US Bureau of the Census: *Population profile of the United States: 1993*, current population reports, series P23-185, Washington, DC, 1993, US Government Printing Office, p. 5.)

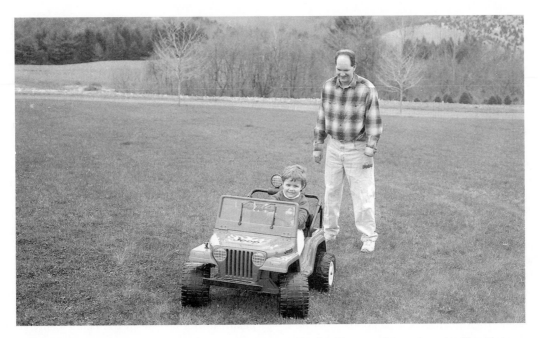

**FIGURE 7-4** Increasingly, fathers are becoming more involved in parenting and are significantly influencing a child's socialization.

history (Day, 1993). "Fertility is assumed to increase steadily, from close to 2.1 live births per woman in 1995 to 2.2 births in 2050" (U.S. Bureau of the Census, 1998, p. 8). Since 1980, between 27% and 29% of the nation's population growth has been the result of net international immigration, and it is anticipated that immigration will be higher in the future (U.S. Bureau of the Census, 1993, pp. 3, 5). Between 1980 and 1990 the foreign-born in the United States increased by 40.4%, from 14.1 million to 19.8 million persons. The number of foreign-born persons in the United States in 1990 was the largest number of foreign-born individuals in the history of the United States (U.S. Bureau of the Census, 1998). The net immigration is expected to remain constant at approximately 820,000 per year, and future immigration will be determined by development of national policy on immigration and refugee admissions to the United States (U.S. Bureau of the Census, 1998).

With increasing diversity and change, new opportunities and challenges have emerged for families and society. In recent years, emphasis has been placed on increasing family values and the responsibility of fatherhood (Coltrane, 2000). Men increasingly enjoy the opportunities associated with parenthood (Figure 7-4) and women value the career options available to them in the job market. However, the institutions and its support systems that make up American society have been slow to adapt to these changes (Coontz, 2000; Levitan, Conway, 1990; Tiedje, Darling-Fisher, 1996). With both parents in the workforce, families need to deal with complicated child care and elder care arrangements and have to coordinate family and work roles as well

as intergenerational and stepfamily extended relationships (Coleman, Ganong, 2000; Oliker, 2000).

In the coming years, society must address child care and elder care concerns as well as other social issues such as increasing poverty, the dramatic rise in premarital childbearing, rising health care costs, and maintaining the viability of social support organizations as volunteer workers become less available (Coleman, Ganong, 2000; Hooyman, 1992; Levitan, Conway, 1990). Social policy must take into consideration the needs of varying family structures and lifestyles because the American family is changing.

## DEFINING THE FAMILY

What actually constitutes a **family** is no longer easy to define. Various family organizational structures have made the concept of the family an elusive one, open to numerous definitions, depending on one's value system. The traditional definition of this term—a group of two or more persons related by blood, marriage, or adoption who reside together—is no longer adequate for understanding and studying the needs of the American family. The increase in family diversity highlights the difficulty in defining family (Coleman, Ganong, 2000). A much broader definition is needed to portray the significant commitments individuals can make to each other, even though they may choose an alternative family form outside of the bonds of marriage. A family in its broadest sense is *a group of two or more persons related by blood, marriage, adoption, or emotional commitment who have a permanent relationship and who work together to meet life goals and needs.*

Practitioners in the helping professions must remain flexible in their interpretation of the word *family* so that the development of social policies are sensitive to the growth of all types of families. Families who are not legally bound together by marriage have the same needs as families who are. They need health services, social and educational opportunities, and financial resources to meet their basic needs. Community health nurses must be sensitive to the needs of the diverse family forms.

Practitioners in the helping professions must also carefully identify their attitudes and values about family life. Although community health nurses may not choose a particular mode of living for themselves, their personal preferences should not influence their clinical judgments about the adequacy of family functioning. Data collected from the family should be the key factor the community health nurse uses to determine family strengths and needs. A single-parent mother, for instance, may be meeting the needs of her child much more appropriately than a married couple who has endless conflicts in their marriage. Assumptions about how well a family is providing for its members should not be made solely on the basis of the family's organizational structure.

## *Stop and Think About It*

What is your personal definition of family? Does this definition include your client family? How might your definition of family influence your interactions with clients?

## THE FAMILY AS A UNIT OF SERVICE

Despite the changing nature of the American family, community health nurses still subscribe to the philosophy that the family is the *basic unit of service* in community health nursing practice. They believe that the family, as the major socializing unit of society, determines how its individual members relate and act in our culture. They recognize that the family greatly influences the beliefs, values, attitudes, and health behaviors of its members and realize that the health of individual family members affects the health of the entire family unit. They see that the family provides support and encouragement at times of stress and joy. They value the role the family has in facilitating the physical and psychosocial growth of its members.

Over 20 years ago, Ronald Peterson (1978) put into very simple but impressive terms the significance of the family in promoting the growth of its individual members. He presented the following concept of the family at a national conference on the chronic mentally ill client, which is still relevant today:

A family is a place where I think a lot of things go on. You really don't feel you're being "raised," that people are doing things to you, to raise you. Your life seems "real" and most of the time, almost everything that happens to you, you talk about it. Sometimes you have good news, sometimes you have bad news. But most of the time, it's just talking about what is going on.

It's a place you go from, to the doctor or to the hospital or the dentist, or school, or to the movies or to a job. But it's a place where you belong, where you somehow learn a lot. You change I'm sure, but usually without knowing it. And you certainly are not looked at as a patient or one who is being rehabilitated. You don't get discharged or terminated, and even when you grow up and get a job of your own and move away, it's a place you keep in touch with and visit. There's always an interest, and that's what makes the difference (p. 1).

Families do make a difference. They provide supportive and nurturing services in a way no other social institution does. They often extend themselves much further in providing assistance than would friends or health care professionals. Families influence health beliefs and attitudes even when they are not physically present. For blended families, their beliefs, attitudes, interactions, and rituals may become more complex because each family brings their own attributes to the new family (Braithwaite, Baxter, Harper, 1998). It is for these reasons that community health nurses believe in the family-centered approach to nursing care.

### Historical Perspectives

Historically the family-centered approach to community health nursing practice grew out of the recognition that the physical care of an individual client could not be divorced from all other aspects of a client's functioning. Innovative community health nursing leaders of the early 1900s recognized that a preventive, holistic approach to the delivery of nursing services was essential if the health of an individual, the family, and the community was to be maintained and enhanced. They saw the need to work with the family and the community in order to achieve their goals with individual clients.

The concept of family-centered care has evolved over time. Initially emphasis was on analyzing how the family could assist its members to achieve health and well-being. Gradually the enhancement of the health and well-being of the entire *family unit* became the primary objective for community health nursing visits, with a focus on examining family dynamics and identifying the health status of all family members.

Over time, clinical practice and research have sufficiently demonstrated the value of the family-centered approach to community health nursing practice. "The family constitutes perhaps the most important social context within which illness occurs and is resolved. It consequently serves as a primary unit in health and medical care" (Litman, 1974, p. 495). In recent years, practitioners have been faced with new challenges in understanding the family member's responsibilities in relation to the changing family structures. The family influences the development of health behavior, the use of health services, and health outcomes for individuals (Danielson, Hamel-Bissell, Winstead-Fry, 1993; Friedman, 1998; Loveland-Cherry, 1996).

Although the family-centered approach to nursing care is valued, it is not fully realized in the clinical setting. Lack of knowledge regarding family processes, federal legislation that financially supports individual services, insufficient criteria for judging family health, and heavy caseload demands impede nurses' efforts to implement family care. However, a renewed focus on the family is emerging as institutional health care is significantly decreasing and home care is rapidly growing. Understanding family roles and responsibilities in relation to health and illness is a priority for practitioners in the twenty-first century (Hinshaw, 2000).

Community health nursing leaders of the past were truly creative and innovative. They were far ahead of their time when they subscribed to the belief that family care was a key principle in community health nursing practice. It was not until the 1950s that most professional disciplines actually began to focus attention on working with families rather than with individual clients. It was only at this time that social scientists initiated systematic theory building in relation to family processes.

Knowledge gained about family functioning since the 1950s has made it easier for nurses to analyze family strengths and needs and to intervene appropriately with families. Theoretical frameworks that have emerged from the study of the family assist nurses in organizing the family assessment process and in identifying the range of variables essential for understanding family relationships. To successfully implement family-centered care, the community health nurse must internalize the belief that working with the family as a unit is important.

## THEORETICAL FRAMEWORKS FOR FAMILY NURSING

Use of a theoretical framework for guiding the family assessment process is essential in the clinical setting. A theory—"a set of relatively specific and concrete concepts and propositions that describe, explain, or predict something of interest" (Whall, Fawcett, 1991, p. 4)—helps the practitioner assess family structure and process in an organized and logical fashion. Theories provide boundaries to consider when collecting data about client situations and facilitate the synthesis of data so family strengths, needs, and interventions can be identified. Theories help organize data and derive a sound rationale for the actions nurses take (Ellis, Hartley, 2001). When a theoretical framework is lacking, it is difficult to group data and to identify relationships between all of the variables that influence family health.

The development of *explicit* family nursing theory was just beginning in the 1980s (Artinian, 1991). The original thrust of the major nursing theorists was centered on the individual. Recent expansion of some of the major conceptual models of nursing (e.g., King, Neuman, Orem, and Roy; see Chapter 9) to include a focus on the family is evident and is providing an explicit impetus for formal family nursing the-

ory development (Loveland-Cherry, 1996; Whall, Fawcett, 1991). The Family Nursing Continuing Education Project, a 3-year project begun in 1987, was designed to foster a nationwide network of family nurses who hoped to achieve a common knowledge and research base for their practice (Krentz, 1989).

"Theoretical frameworks from other disciplines have guided the evolution of family nursing science" (Hanson, Boyd, 1996, p. 43). "Family theories developed in disciplines other than nursing provide direction for identifying characteristics of optimal families" (Loveland-Cherry, 1996, p. 24). Illustrative of this is the developmental framework that emerged from theorists in the social sciences. The developmental framework delineates life-cycle stages and specific family tasks that need to be accomplished during each stage. Families who are able to achieve their stage-specific developmental tasks while maintaining the integrity of the family unit and promoting the growth of individual family members have been defined as healthy, or optimal, families (Loveland-Cherry, 1996).

Select theoretical frameworks from the social sciences that are particularly relevant to family nursing are briefly summarized. These frameworks were first outlined by Hill and Hansen (1960) in their classic writing during the 1960s. Practitioners generally find that an eclectic approach, or one that integrates concepts from several frameworks, best meets their needs when completing a family assessment. When nurses conduct a family assessment, emphasis is on identifying the health promotion needs of the family.

### Structural-Functional Framework

The **structural-functional framework** was developed by social scientists from sociology and social anthropology. It views the family as a social system that interacts with other social systems within society. It focuses on the analysis of family interplay between collateral systems such as school, work, or health care worlds and the transactions between the family and its subsystems (husband-wife dyad, sibling cliques, and personality systems of individual family members). With this approach, emphasis is on examining the functions society performs for the family, as well as the functions the family performs for society and its individual family members. In addition, this framework looks at how the structure (organizational parameters) of systems affects family functioning (Hill, Hansen, 1960). The family in the structural-functional approach is seen as open to outside influences and transactions.

The structural-functional approach to family study helps the practitioner systematically assess family structure and function. A family's structure (organization) influences what is viewed as important to the family and facilitates or inhibits the family's ability to carry out its functions. The family carries out several functions to promote family growth, provide a nurturing environment for individual family members, and meet the needs of society.

Friedman (1998) has identified five **family functions** that are especially important for nurses to consider when assessing and intervening with families. These are (1) the *affective* function, which addresses the psychologic needs of family members, including the need for companionship and love; (2) the *socialization and social placement* function, which helps children to prepare for and assume adult social roles; (3) the *reproductive* function, which ensures the continuity of the family across generations and society survival; (4) the *economic* function, which involves securing adequate resources for survival and decision-making processes focused on the appropriate allocation of these resources; and (5) the *health care* function, which entails obtaining physical necessities such as food, shelter, and clothing and health care for all family members (Friedman, 1998, p. 102).

Over several decades, the structural-functional approach has provided a meaningful framework for guiding family assessment in the clinical setting. The broad scope of this framework has allowed for the analysis of the multiple environmental forces that influence family functioning in addition to family interactions and transactions (Aldous, 1978, p. 14). The changing nature of the American family makes it increasingly critical for the practitioner to examine the interplay between the family and its external environment. Many functions once assumed primarily by the family system, such as child-rearing responsibilities, are now being shared by collateral systems in the community.

## Interactional Approach

Frequently labeled as the *symbolic* **interactional frame of reference**, this approach comes from sociology and social psychology. The interactionalist views the family as a unity of interacting personalities within which individual family members occupy a position or positions, such as husband-father, wife-mother, and daughter-sister. A cluster of roles—such as provider, homemaker, companion, and sex partner—are assigned to each of these positions, and a set of social norms or behavioral role expectations is perceived for each of these roles by the individual fulfilling them. Perceptions about role expectations emerge from an individual's self-concept and from an individual's reference group. As each individual carries out the various roles, role expectations are retained, modified, or discarded based on the reactions of others within the family environment (Aldous, 1978, pp. 10, 14).

Interactionalists viewed the family as being relatively closed to outside systems. Family members are seen as actors and reactors who interact with their environment through symbolic communication. As a reactor, an individual does not simply respond to stimuli from the external environment. Symbolic communication evolving from the self and the environment helps individuals interpret and select the environment to which they respond. Based on this assumption, interactionalists stressed that investigators or clini-

cians must see the world from the point of view of the individual (Stryker, 1964, pp. 134-135). This viewpoint is still relevant today.

The interactional framework emphasizes analysis of the internal aspects of family functioning but neglects the family's relationships with other social systems. This framework identifies how relationships with others affect an individual's functioning. In addition to role analysis, interactionalists examine communication, decision-making and problem-solving processes; conflict; reactions to stress; and other family situations such as divorce and domestic violence that are influenced by family interactions and interactive processes (Aldous, 1978; Hill, Hansen, 1960). This approach helps the practitioner identify if family interactions promote or inhibit effective family functioning.

## Developmental Approach

Concepts from various disciplines and approaches (rural sociology, child psychology, human development, sociology, and structural-functional and interactional approaches) were synthesized to create the **developmental approach** to family study. Classically (Hill, Hansen, 1960), this approach looked at family development throughout its generational life cycle. It examined developmental tasks and role expectations for children, parents, and the family as a unit and traced these changes during a series of specific stages in the family life cycle (Hill, Hansen, 1960). This classic emphasis laid a foundation from which theorists have refined the developmental approach to family study.

Duvall has focused her scholarly efforts on defining normal family development. She identified eight stages in the two-parent, nuclear family life cycle that highlight critical periods of family growth, development, and change (Duvall, Miller, 1985). These stages address family events related to the comings and goings of family members: marriage, birth and rearing of children, launching children from the household, and retirement and death (Carter, McGoldrick, 1988). The developmental framework helps practitioners assess what a given family is going through at any particular time and provides a basis for forecasting role transition issues throughout a family's life span (Duvall, Miller, 1985). This, in turn, aids the professional in predicting potential educational and resource needs of families. For example, new childbearing families often desire information about child care and growth and development patterns of children and may need help in obtaining adequate supplies for infant care. Additionally, they frequently need assistance in achieving a balance between family and personal needs. Reconciling conflicting developmental tasks and needs of various family members is a major task for childbearing families (Carter, McGoldrick, 1988; Duvall, Miller, 1985).

In recent years, family theorists have focused attention on examining how variables such as changing family structures, social and economic factors, and cultural and ethnic differences influence the family life cycle. Family life-cycle patterns have changed dramatically as a result of the lower birth rates, longer life expectancy, the changing role of women, postponement of marriage, and the increasing divorce and remarriage rate (Carter, McGoldrick, 1988). To address these changes, Carter and McGoldrick have added an additional stage to the family life cycle. They begin the new family life cycle at the stage of young adulthood (Table 7-1). This is in contrast to the traditional sociologic depiction of the family life cycle, which commences at courtship or marriage. During the young adulthood, or "between families," stage, young men and women formulate personal life goals and differentiate themselves from their family of origin. In the past this phase was never considered necessary for women, because "their identities were determined primarily by their family

functions as mother and wife" (Carter, McGoldrick, 1988, p. 11).

When using the developmental framework for guiding family assessment, practitioners should realize that there are major variations in the family life cycle. Socioeconomic and cultural factors influence the timing (Table 7-2) of the life cycle phases and the importance given to different life cycle transitions (Fulmer, 1988; McGoldrick, 1988). For example, funerals are a significant occurrence for African-American and Irish families, who go to considerable expense to bury their loved ones. In contrast, Italian and Polish families place the greatest emphasis on weddings and often celebrate this occurrence over a considerable period of time (McGoldrick, 1988). The professional who understands that there are significant variations in the family life-cycle can more effectively evaluate family functioning during critical transition periods.

**TABLE 7-1**

*The Stages of the Family Life Cycle*

| FAMILY LIFE CYCLE STAGE | EMOTIONAL PROCESS OF TRANSITION: KEY PRINCIPLES | SECOND-ORDER CHANGES IN FAMILY STATUS REQUIRED TO PROCEED DEVELOPMENTALLY |
|---|---|---|
| 1. Leaving home: single young adults | Accepting emotional and financial responsibility for self | Differentiation of self in relation to family of origin<br>Development of intimate peer relationships<br>Establishment of self regarding work and financial independence |
| 2. The joining of families through marriage: the new couple | Commitment to new system | Formation of marital system<br>Realignment of relationships with extended families and friends to include spouse |
| 3. Families with young children | Accepting new members into the system | Adjusting marital system to make space for child(ren)<br>Joining in childrearing, financial, and household tasks<br>Realignment of relationships with extended family to include parenting and grandparenting roles |
| 4. Families with adolescents | Increasing flexibility of family boundaries to include children's independence and grandparents' frailties | Shifting of parent-child relationships to permit adolescent to move in and out of system<br>Refocus on midlife marital and career issues<br>Beginning shift toward joint caring for older generation |
| 5. Launching children and moving on | Accepting a multitude of exits from and entries into the family system | Renegotiation of marital system as a dyad<br>Development of adult-to-adult relationships between grown children and their parents<br>Realignment of relationships to include in-laws and grandchildren<br>Dealing with disabilities and death of parents (grandparents) |
| 6. Families in later life | Accepting the shifting of generational roles | Maintaining own and/or couple functioning and interests in face of physiologic decline; exploration of new familial and social role options<br>Support for a more central role of middle generation<br>Making room in the system for the wisdom and experience of the elderly, supporting the older generation without overfunctioning for them<br>Dealing with loss of spouse, siblings, and other peers and preparation for own death; life review and integration |

Modified from Carter B, McGoldrick M, editors: *The changing family life cycle: a framework for family therapy,* ed 2, New York, 1988, Gardner Press, p. 15.

**TABLE 7-2**

## Comparison of Family Life Cycle Stages

| AGE | PROFESSIONAL FAMILIES | LOW-INCOME FAMILIES |
|-----|----------------------|---------------------|
| 12-17 | Prevent pregnancy<br>Graduate from high school<br>Parents continue support while permitting child to achieve greater independence | First pregnancy<br>Attempt to graduate from high school<br>Parent attempts strict control before pregnancy. After pregnancy, relaxation of controls and continued support of new mother and infant |
| 18-21 | Prevent pregnancy<br>Leave parental household for college<br>Adapt to parent-child separation | Second pregnancy<br>No further education<br>Young mother acquires adult status in parental household |
| 22-25 | Prevent pregnancy<br>Develop professional identity in graduate school<br>Maintain separation from parental household; begin living in serious relationship | Third pregnancy<br>Marriage—leave parental household to establish stepfamily<br>Maintain connection with kinship network |
| 26-30 | Prevent pregnancy<br>Marriage—develop nuclear couple as separate from parents<br>Intense work involvement as career begins | Separate from husband<br>Mother becomes head of own household within kinship network |
| 31-35 | First pregnancy<br>Renew contact with parents as grandparents<br>Differentiate career and child-rearing roles between husband and wife | First grandchild<br>Mother becomes grandmother and cares for daughter and infant |

Modified from Fulmer R: Lower-income and professional families: a comparison of structure and life cycle process. In Carter B, McGoldrick M, editors: *The changing family life cycle: a framework for family therapy,* ed 2, New York, 1988, Gardner Press, p. 551.

## Systems Approach

First introduced by biologist Ludwig von Bertalanffy (1968), **systems theory** is currently used by many disciplines. General systems theory is a science of wholeness. An underlying assumption of system theory is the belief that the whole is greater than the sum of its parts. From a family perspective, this implies that the family unit has a unique character that is different from that of its individual parts (family members) (Boss, 1988). However, change in one part of the family system affects the system as a whole, as well as all individual family members. For example, when a family member becomes ill and is unable to carry out his or her role responsibilities, the whole family unit needs to change to successfully cope with the demands of the stress encountered.

A system consists of two or more connected components or subsystems that form an organized whole and that interact with each other to achieve desired goals. A family is a social system of interdependent members (components) possessing two fundamental system features: *structure,* or organization, and *function,* or interaction. Family members engage in continual interaction according to roles and norms that evolve over time and make it possible for the family to survive and achieve desired goals (Janosik, Green, 1992).

An input-process-output feedback model (Figure 7-5) commonly is used to depict the structural relationships of a

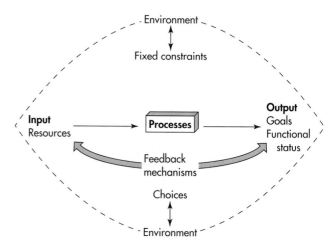

**FIGURE 7-5** Structural arrangements of a system. (Modified from Clemen [Parks] SJ: *Introduction to health care facility: food services administration,* University Park, Penn, 1974, Pennsylvania State University Press, p. 24.)

system. In simplistic terms, this model illustrates that all systems have *inputs,* or resources that, when *processed,* help the system achieve its goals, or *outputs.* The processing of inputs (resources) received from the environment requires a series of dynamic, interrelated transactions. These transactions link together the environment, the system inputs, and the system outputs. Transactions or processes used by families to maintain healthy family functioning are discussed in a later section of this chapter.

The feedback mechanism is a major attribute of a system. This mechanism assists the family system in identifying its strengths and needs and in evaluating how well it is accomplishing its goals. Feedback provides data essential for effective adaptation to internal and external system changes. It provides information that helps the system select corrective actions when problems exist. A system needs a mechanism that facilitates the sharing of both positive and negative feedback. A family system that discourages negative input often remains static or develops ineffective family patterns.

No system can function in a vacuum. The environment in which a system exists greatly influences how the system is able to function. The environment imposes constraints (e.g., rules that require school attendance or prohibit drinking and driving) on the family system and provides resources for effective family functioning. However, every system has filtering mechanisms, or *boundaries*, that regulate the flow of energy to and from the environment and between family subsystems. Boundaries in a system are not physical barriers. Rather, they are abstract entities such as norms, values, attitudes, and rules that inhibit or facilitate human transactional processes between systems.

Energy transport is crucial to the survival of any system. An effectively functioning family system uses energy to obtain resources from the outside, to process resources to achieve its goals, and to release outputs into the environment. "The most important factor governing the amount of energy needed is the rate of utilization of energy within the system itself. Systems with high levels of activity utilize large quantities of energy, and therefore must receive greater amounts of input from the environment in order to meet their energy demands" (Friedman, 1998, p. 159). Family systems that are ineffectively dealing with stress and crisis frequently lack the energy to obtain input from the environment.

A system that exchanges energy and resources with other systems is an open system. "Depending on the nature of family boundaries, a family system may be fully open, entirely closed, or somewhere in between" (Janosik, Green, 1992, p. 13). Families generally interact with the environment to obtain resources (e.g., information, financial, and health care) necessary for family growth and survival and to reduce stress within the family system. "The key to successful family adaptation is selective permeability of family boundaries" (Friedman, 1998, p. 162). This implies that a family can be too open or too closed. Boundary maintenance issues are addressed further in a later section of this chapter.

Systems theory provides a framework for family assessment that is consistent with the holistic nature of humankind and professional practice. It offers a logical way to integrate all of the factors that influence family functioning and link the family together into a meaningful whole. It provides a humanistic philosophy of professional care that negates individual blame and addresses family strengths as well as needs. "Approaching the family as a system in which parents, children, extended family members, and the community influence each other in reciprocal ways means that whatever occurs is a shared responsibility" (Janosik, Green, 1992, p. 15).

## USE OF THEORETICAL FRAMEWORKS

Table 7-3 summarizes select characteristics of the four family theories just discussed. Because only an introductory description is presented, the reader will find it useful to explore the literature in depth when selecting a conceptual framework for guiding practice. Of particular interest is literature that helps readers examine the application of concepts in nursing practice (Bomar, 1996; Friedman, 1998; Hanson, Boyd, 1996; Whall, 1991; Wright, Leahey, 1994).

It is important to remember that no one theory focuses attention on all aspects of family functioning. An example is a situation in which a nurse visits a young married couple in their twenties who have just had their first child. Using a developmental framework, the nurse would direct his or her evaluation of family health on how well the family and individual members were accomplishing stage-specific development tasks. On the other hand, systems-oriented nurses would focus their analysis on how the change in the family system (the addition of a new family member) has affected system functioning as a whole (e.g., its resources and goals, family processes, subsystems—especially the spouse relationships—and the family's interactions with its external environment).

Community health nurses generally use a combination of several theoretical frameworks to guide the family assessment process. This is appropriate because client situations vary and because no one framework explains all family phenomena. In the clinical setting it is essential for the nurse to examine the multiple aspects of family functioning, including the family's structure, its relationships with other social systems, and its interactions with the environment. All of these areas must be assessed before an effective management plan can be developed.

### Stop and Think About It

Analyze a client family according to each of the four family theories (use Table 7-3 as a guide). Do you agree with the advantages and disadvantages described in the table? Did those frameworks help you organize your data?

**TABLE 7-3**

*Select Characteristics of Four Family Theories*

| THEORY | FOCUS OF ANALYSIS | ADVANTAGES | DISADVANTAGES |
|---|---|---|---|
| Structural-functional | Family interplay between collateral systems<br>Transactions between the family and its subsystems | Allows for analysis of the multiple forces that influence family functioning. Handles well-family interactions and transactions | Family and its individual family members are considered to be reactive, passive elements of systems; deals poorly with social change processes and dynamics |
| Interactional | Internal aspects of family functioning, including role analysis, communication, decision making, problem solving and conflict resolution processes, reactions to stress, and other family dynamics (e.g., divorce and domestic violence) influenced by family interactions | Views family members as having control over their environment (e.g., family members interpret and select the environment to which they respond); focuses on seeing the world from the client's perspective | Neglects family relationships with other systems |
| Developmental | Accomplishment of individual and family developmental tasks throughout the generational life cycle; change in the family system over time | Highlights critical periods of family growth and development; keeps the traditionally defined family in focus throughout its life span; recognizes and helps predict what a given family is experiencing at any particular time | Data that examine socio-economic, cultural, and ethnic variations in the family life cycle are limited |
| Systems | Analysis of the family as a whole; interdependence of the various parts of the family system and change; interactions of the family system and its external environment | Unites scientific thinking across disciplines; provides a holistic perspective for analyzing family functioning that negates blame; allows for analysis of family relationships with other systems and environmental influences on health; examines family change and adaptation processes | Complex theory can make it difficult for an inexperienced practitioner to fit all family dynamics into the specific categories defined within the system |

## PARAMETERS TO CONSIDER DURING THE FAMILY ASSESSMENT PROCESS

During the family assessment process, parameters related to both family structure and process should be considered regardless of the theoretical framework used to guide family assessment. These parameters assist the nurse in obtaining a holistic view of the family, helping the nurse identify how the family is organized and how it interacts to carry out family functions.

### Structural Parameters for Family Assessment

Structural components of a family are those variables that provide organization for the family system. They assist the family in coordinating their activities so that family and individual needs are met. In his classic article on family organization, Briar (1964) identified eight major structural characteristics of families: (1) division of labor, (2) distribution of power and authority, (3) communication, (4) boundaries of the family's world, (5) relations with other groups and

systems, (6) ways of obtaining and giving emotional support, (7) rituals and symbols, and (8) a set of personal roles (pp. 251-254). These, as well as cultural values and attitudes and religious beliefs, are described in the following sections. Briar's delineation of the structural components of a family continues to be consistent with recent notions about the structural parameters of family life.

### Division of Labor

More mothers are in the workforce than in previous decades and working parents are challenged with fair division of domestic responsibilities (Polatnick, 2000). Families allocate leadership responsibilities for maintaining their household in a variety of ways. Some follow traditional norms, with the man assuming major responsibility for the provider role and the woman the homemaker role, regardless of the other role responsibilities each person has in the partnership. Some divide tasks according to their likes and dislikes or the level of competence each person has in relation to a particular task. Others share responsibilities equally, based on the demands each person has from other role positions.

Cultural background is an important variable to consider when the nurse examines family role performance. Ethnicity significantly influences the development of attitudes about the division of labor within the family unit. For example, within the traditional nuclear family, it is common for Navajo Indian (Hanley, 1991) and Italian (Bowen, 1991) women to be responsible for the domestic duties associated within the home and for the men from these ethnic groups to be responsible for any outside work needed to maintain the family and its home. However, **intracultural diversity** also exists, and individuals may not practice or possess all the characteristics of the ethnic group with which they identify (Fong, 1985).

Families who rigidly define either the provider or homemaker role tend to experience more stress when family members are unable to perform their expected tasks than do families who have a flexible division of labor (Beavers, 1977; Lewis, Beavers, Gossett, et al., 1976; Otto, 1963; Pratt, 1976). It is also extremely difficult for families with rigid patterns of functioning to mobilize new coping mechanisms when experiencing a crisis. Health care professionals, for instance, often observe confusion and disorganization when a spouse dies. This confusion is heightened if the man or woman has not been prepared to deal with the demands of daily living. Assuming responsibilities for tasks one is not accustomed to performing is difficult at any time, but especially when one is experiencing a crisis.

Identifying how the division of labor is handled by a family helps the community health nurse understand the stresses family members are experiencing when changes have occurred. **Role strain** results when families do not take into consideration that role responsibilities change over time. Mothers, for example, are often confronted with excessive role demands after the birth of a child. This is especially true if husbands do not share the responsibility for housekeeping and child care tasks. Role strain also occurs when family members are unable to perform the activities related to a given role. This is particularly noticeable when role modifications are needed because of the prolonged absence of one family member. Role strain often becomes even more complex in the case of remarriage and the added family responsibilities related to the blended families with stepparents and stepchildren (Coleman, Ganong, 2000).

In some instances, "fatherhood is the single biggest cause of our most pressing social problems" (Coltrane, 2000, p. 26). Parental absences that are a result of illness, divorce, separation, or vocational responsibilities frequently require drastic modifications in a family's division of labor and result in role strain. As a result, recent religious and political crusades have promoted responsible fatherhood as one way to strengthen the family unit (Coltrane, 2000).

*All* family members can experience role strain when the division of labor is inappropriately balanced. Children may be required to assume adult responsibilities excessive for their age and level of growth and development. This most often occurs during times of crisis or when parents have not assumed adult leadership responsibilities required to maintain their household. It is important for community health nurses to recognize that children experience role strain when they assume parental functions and to avoid reinforcing role-reversal patterns. It is easy to praise a child who is functioning beyond his or her chronologic age. This praise, however, may support the continuance of family patterns that are unhealthy and that adversely affect a child's emotional growth and development.

## Distribution of Power and Authority

**Power** was conceptualized by Bredemeir and Stephenson (1965) as "the capacity to carry out, by whatever means, a desired course of action despite the resistance of others and without having to take into consideration their needs. When power is institutionalized through respect, fear, esteem, or position, it is referred to as **authority**" (p. 50).

Several variables affect who will have power in the family system. The position of power can be culturally prescribed, usually with the father being in a position of authority by virtue of his role as a male. This is frequently seen in Spanish-American and Asian cultures, where male dominance is the norm. Power also can be prescribed situationally when family members do not necessarily follow cultural norms but develop a power structure based on their circumstances and personal interactions.

The continuum of family power based on cultural and situational variables ranges from complete dominance to complete absence of power, both of which can produce ineffective family patterns. Complete dominance by one family member poses a threat to the self-esteem of other family members and makes it difficult for individuals to resolve the independence-dependence conflicts that arise during adolescence and young adulthood. Complete absence of power in a family system tends to produce confusion, disorganization, and chaos. This also can occur when the gender roles are unclear, thereby contributing to uncertain expectations (Sollie, 2000). Vulnerable families frequently exhibit power structures on either end of the continuum. In healthy families, power is frequently articulated and shared by adult members, and children are involved in the decision-making process.

Understanding the relationship between issues of power and decision making is essential to effect permanent changes within a family system. If the power and authority structure of a family is ignored, nursing interventions are often inappropriate and place additional stress on family members who lack the power to make decisions about needed health actions. Family members who have power must be consulted if changes in health behavior are to occur. One community health nurse, for instance, realized after several home visits to a Spanish-American family that the only way she would influence the family to obtain needed surgery for their 4-year-old preschooler was to talk with the child's father. Although the mother stated frequently that she felt it was important for her son to have surgery, no action was taken. When the mother was questioned regarding her husband's perceptions of this matter, the nurse discovered that he felt surgery was unnecessary and that he was the one who made the final decision about needed health care.

In situations where the dominant family member is temporarily immobilized, it is extremely important for the community health nurse to recognize that the family may reassign the dominant position to the nurse. Because of the nurse's professional status, families under stress may initially allow a nurse to assume a position of authority within the family structure. They may follow the nurse's suggestions without questioning the pros and cons to reduce their level of stress. These suggestions may not necessarily be appropriate for the family. Taking over decision making for a family is not therapeutic.

## Communication Patterns

Verbal and nonverbal interactions within a family usually display significant regularities or patterns. Norms involving what is shared and not shared with whom are implicitly, if not explicitly, known by all family members. Messages are provided in a variety of ways to let family members know how to communicate within and outside the family system.

The ability to communicate accurately and effectively is essential to all aspects of family functioning because communication is an integral part of daily living. It helps the family carry out its functions, meet the needs of individual family members, and move toward achieving its goals.

Communication is an extremely complex process, involving not only what is said but also how it is said and the *behavioral interactions* that occur during the course of a conversation. An individual can communicate even when verbal information is not shared. In their classic book, Watzlawick, Beavin, and Jackson (1967) noted that because all behavior in an interactional situation has message value, it is impossible for a person not to communicate. They believe that "activity or inactivity, words or silence, all have message value which influence others; others, in turn, cannot avoid responding to these communications and are thus, themselves communicating" (p. 49). Even silence conveys a message to an individual who is sharing thoughts, ideas, or feelings. Understanding communication patterns may be a complex task, particularly when blended families are in a state of flux with members moving in and out of the households and mixed messages abound (Braithwaite, Baxter, Harper, 1998).

Braithwaite, Baxter, and Harper (1998) conducted in-depth interviews with 53 members of blended families in an attempt to discern how they communicated through established rituals. The researchers focused on rituals that (1) ceased when the family became blended, (2) were im-

ported to the blended family and successfully continued without changing, (3) were begun in the blended family and successfully continued, and (4) were begun in the new blended family and failed. They found that blended families brought communication patterns from previous family structures to the new blended family and these practices were often a source of strength for the children learning to adjust in the new family. Conversely, when the old family communication rituals were dropped, it created a sense of loss or grief to the children. As nurses assess the communication patterns and rituals of families, it is essential for them to understand the family boundaries and structure. "Sometimes the nurse's ability to be outside the family and observe more accurately what goes on makes it easier to transmit information about family communication patterns that family members cannot observe" (Arnold, 1999, p. 317). To facilitate healthy family communication, nurses must be able to recognize when those patterns are unhealthy.

Communication-oriented theorists believed that family communication patterns need to be analyzed along several dimensions (Haley, 1971; Jackson, 1968; Satir, 1972; Watzlawick, Beavin, Jackson, 1967). Verbal, nonverbal, and behavioral processes should be observed to identify the content of communication, how the content is shared and received, and linguistic characteristics that influence interpretation of communication.

CONTENT OF COMMUNICATION. What actually is conveyed is known as the *content* of communication. Observations should be made to determine what is being shared and what is not. It is not unusual for individuals to feel uncomfortable about sharing information concerning personal topics such as sexuality, finances, and troubled relationships with significant others. A health care professional needs to "listen between the lines" to help clients verbalize areas of concern beyond those that are explicitly expressed.

TRANSMISSION OF CONTENT. How content is shared can significantly influence its meaning to the receiver. The sharing of content does not necessarily convey to the receiver accurate information or help the receiver understand the message a person is attempting to send. Content becomes functional when there is clarity of thought, organization of ideas, and accuracy and completeness of facts. It is difficult for the receiver to understand what is being said when information is being withheld or unintentionally not shared, when too much information is shared in an unorganized manner, or when conflicting messages are being conveyed. These problems tend to distort reality and confuse the listener. They can lead to a lack of responsiveness or hostile interchange.

BEHAVIORAL INTERACTIONS. How an individual responds, either verbally or nonverbally, during a conversation provides clues to others about how this individual views what is being said and how he or she regards the sender or receiver. Body mannerisms, eye contact, silence or responsiveness to content, vocal characteristics, and ways of eliciting information all provide behavioral messages that guide the course of a conversation. Behavioral messages are often far more meaningful from a positive or negative perspective than verbal content. They may provide *double-level messages* "with the voice saying one thing and the rest of the person saying something else" (Satir, 1972, p. 60). Healthy families tend to share fewer double-level messages than unhealthy families.

INTERPRETATION OF COMMUNICATION. How content and behavioral interactions are interpreted varies from one individual to another. Perceptions about messages being conveyed are influenced by several factors, including things such as previous experiences between the sender and receiver, the motivations of the persons involved in the communication process, feelings about oneself, and current stresses being experienced. For example, families who have low self-esteem frequently find it difficult to interpret messages positively; praise is often not heard or is negated.

The interpretation of messages is a key factor that determines the difference between effective and ineffective communication. When assessing family communication patterns, it is essential to notice if the content of communication, feelings, and behavioral transactions are accurately perceived. When healthy communication patterns exist, family members seek clarification if they do not understand the content, and they validate their interpretations of feelings and behavioral interactions.

MODES OF COMMUNICATION DURING STRESS. Satir's (1975) classic writings have guided the analysis of communication patterns over time. She noted that individuals use five major transactional modes to communicate when they are under stress. These are placating, blaming, super-reasonable, irrelevant, and congruent (Table 7-4). Congruent transactions are the most functional. When the other transactional modes of communication become patterned, psychosomatic and other illnesses often result (Satir, 1975).

When nurses work with families under stress, they help these families clarify the facts in the situation, express feelings and emotions, and avoid fault-finding or blame. The content of communication and behavioral interactions are frequently distorted during times of stress and crisis. Chapter 8 elaborates on family assessment and intervention when stress and crisis exist.

LINGUISTIC CHARACTERISTICS OF COMMUNICATION. Families have varying dialects or language differences based on their cultural background, their socialization process, and their geographic location. It is essential for a community health nurse to note these differences because they may adversely influence the communication process. Generally, clients are more than willing to help a health care professional understand language differences if the professional shows genuine interest in learning about them.

Cultural differences among families are reflected in all aspects of verbal and nonverbal communications. Gestures, posture, facial expression, eye contact, touch, vocabulary, grammatical structure, voice qualities, and silence all send important messages to members of a specific ethnic group. For example, in some cultures (e.g., Mexican and some Native American) touch is considered magical and healing; in other cultures (e.g., Vietnamese), touch produces anxiety because it is believed that the soul can leave the body on physical contact (Giger, Davidhizar, 1999; Roccereto, 1981). During the family assessment process, it is important to determine whether the client practices cultural behaviors or styles of communication. The nurse must be prepared to communicate in a manner that meets clints' cultural needs (Giger, Davidhizar, 1999).

**TABLE 7-4**

*Modes of Communication During Stress*

| COMMUNICATION MODE | DESCRIPTION |
|---|---|
| Placating | Family members outwardly agree with each other to avoid conflict in the family unit. There is an inconsistency between what a family member outwardly shares and what is inwardly felt. |
| Blaming | Family members fear assuming accountability for their feelings and actions and, thus, resort to fault-finding, blaming behaviors and other ineffective communication patterns to hide their insecurities. |
| Super-reasonable | Family members avoid the sharing of feelings and emotions by focusing on intellectual issues during the communication process. Avoidance of feelings and emotions makes it difficult to address ineffective family functioning and to reduce anxiety in the family system. |
| Irrelevant | Family member's mode of communication is illogical from the perspective of what is happening in the family environment. Irrelevant communication patterns affect the flow of a conversation, as well as problem-solving and decision-making processes. |
| Congruent | Family member's mode of communication is consistent between what the individual outwardly shares and what is inwardly felt and is logical in relation to what is happening in the environment. |

Modified from Satir V: You as a change agent in helping families to change. In Satir V, Stachowiak J, Taskman H, editors: *Helping families to change,* New York, 1975, Jason Aronson, pp. 141-149.

The primary goal of observing family communication patterns is to determine if the patterns established by a particular family are functional. In assessing communication patterns, the nurse should ask what the patterns are and whether they help the family carry out its functions, relate effectively to the environment, meet the needs of individual family members, and achieve its goals. It is important to remember that ways of achieving functional communication between family members can vary from one family to another.

## Boundaries of the Family World

Boundary development and maintenance is essential for family survival and growth. Families must have effective filtering mechanisms so that the exchange of energies corresponds to the needs of the family. Energy exchanges that occur too rapidly or too slowly can be disruptive to the family system. Families need to bring inputs into their system and release outputs into the environment so that they can carry out their functions. However, they also need to limit the amount of input from the environment to prevent system overload and to limit the release of outputs to prevent energy depletion.

The rate of energy flow between the family and the environment must vary in order for the family to maintain the integrity of its system. Families who do not adjust their energy flow to correspond to their current circumstances have difficulty handling stress and change. In times of family stress and change, limiting the exchange of inputs and outputs conserves energy needed to carry out activities of daily living. A new mother or father, for instance, may need to reduce working hours (output) to conserve energy for child care activities and to provide emotional support for others in the family system.

It is not uncommon for community health nurses to work with families who are having difficulty adjusting energy flow to and from their family system. When boundaries are too open or too closed, not agreed upon, or ambiguous, stress occurs in the family system. Families dealing with these types of boundary maintenance issues find it difficult to achieve family goals and to adapt during periods of stress and crisis.

BOUNDARIES TOO OPEN. Disorganized, multiproblem, and crisis-prone families tend to take little control over what enters or exists in their environment. They have numerous outsiders (inputs), such as health care professionals or legal authorities, working with them, and often they do not set rules about how and when family members should interact outside the family system. These families usually come to the attention of health care professionals because their outputs are not acceptable to the suprasystem (community). It is not unusual for such families to be referred to the community health nurse when their children enter school. Frequently, families lack the energy to fulfill the health requirements (immunizations and physical examina-

tions) mandated for school entry. In these situations, families' energies are often used to deal with outsiders or crises while the needs of individual family members are neglected.

BOUNDARIES TOO CLOSED. Some families allow few inputs to cross their boundaries. They isolate themselves from the larger community, and as a consequence, may not obtain the resources needed for family growth. Families from differing cultural backgrounds or families who have members with a mental or physical handicap, for example, may limit inputs from the environment because they fear that their differences will not be accepted. Conflicts between these families and their environment arise when they do not release outputs (e.g., do not send their children to school) or when their outputs are inadequate (e.g., children are not prepared to handle environmental demands and pressures).

BOUNDARIES NOT AGREED UPON. At times, community health nurses find a discrepancy between the views of one family member and another regarding boundary maintenance. Families may have some boundaries that are well defined and others that are unclearly defined. For example, they may use community resources appropriately but may not agree on how often and when they should interface with friends and the extended family. In these situations it is important for the community health nurse to help family members address their differences and work toward a mutually satisfying solution. Lack of agreement on boundary maintenance issues can lead to conflict, disequilibrium, and system disintegration.

BOUNDARY AMBIGUITY. Boss (1988) believes that boundary ambiguity is a major barrier to stress management in families. In simple terms, she defines boundary ambiguity as "not knowing who is in and who is out of the family" (p. 73). Two types of boundary ambiguity exist. Boundary ambiguity occurs when a family member is *physically absent with psychologic presence* or *physically present with psychologic absence* (Boss, 1988). When a member of the family is physically absent as a consequence of kidnapping, a run-away incident, or other situations (e.g., divorce) that the family cannot control, the family becomes preoccupied with the absent member. This preoccupation prevents grieving and family restructuring (Boss, 1988).

Family members are frequently physically present but psychologically absent when they have an illness such as alcohol addiction or Alzheimer's disease, or when work and other demands consume a significant amount of time (Boss, 1988). In these situations, the family is intact, but family members find it difficult to work together to achieve important family goals or to carry out family functions.

## Relations with Other Groups and Systems

The development of relationships with other groups, such as extended kin or neighbors, and other systems, such as church, school, or health care agencies, is directly related to the way the family handles its boundary maintenance functions. Family boundaries can facilitate or inhibit the establishment and maintenance of interpersonal relationships with others outside the family system. Families with rigid boundaries have few contacts with persons outside their family system; families with flexible boundaries evaluate their needs for social support.

When assessing family relationships outside the family system, it is important to look at the *type* of relationships they have, as well as the contact allowed. Interaction with numerous people does not necessarily mean that the family is meeting their support, companionship, and growth needs. Some families develop relationships that involve more giving than receiving. In these situations, family energies are devoted to helping others, but the family receives little support in return. In other families, interactions with others in the environment are not evaluated and may result in negative outcomes. For example, children may encounter legal difficulties when no controls are placed on their relationships with people who engage in illegal activity such as drug selling.

## Ways of Obtaining and Giving Emotional Support

Families need to achieve a balance between their relationship with others and their relationship with family members. If the family excludes itself from its external environment, they may lack support during times of stress and crisis. If, on the other hand, the family devotes all its energy to helping others, it is highly unlikely that the family will be able to meet the emotional needs of individual family members.

Families meet their emotional needs in a variety of ways. They develop norms that regulate sources of support, provide guidelines for giving support, and define when support will be given. When assessing the ways a family obtains and gives emotional support, it is important to examine who receives emotional support and when and how it is given.

DISTRIBUTION OF EMOTIONAL SUPPORT. All family members need support, encouragement, and praise. If support is not evenly distributed, family members may seek support from their environment or isolate themselves from the family system. Or they may withdraw and limit contact with others outside the family, as well as within the family system.

How an individual member is viewed by other family members greatly affects the amount of emotional support this individual receives. Family norms and rules and the emotional maturity of the family influence how well individual members are accepted by others in the family system. Individual members who do not conform to family norms usually receive less support than those who do. Illustrating this is the teenager from a family with high educational aspirations who does not share these same views and decides not to go to college. This teenager very quickly receives a message from the family that this is an inappropriate decision. If she or he does not alter these views, the family may withdraw its support.

WHEN AND HOW EMOTIONAL SUPPORT IS PROVIDED. Some families provide emotional support only during times of stress and crisis. Other families provide this type of support on a regular basis or neglect the emotional needs of family members all together. All human beings need ongoing emotional care and nurturing. "Having at least one strong intimate relationship is an important predictor of good health" (Heaney, Israel, 1997, p. 186). Family members who lack consistent emotional support often experience physical or psychosocial difficulties. Frequently, individuals who do not receive effective support from the family system will seek this support from others in the external environment.

Families use both verbal and nonverbal communication to provide emotional support for their members. Some families share support spontaneously, whereas others are more reserved with their emotional interchanges. Neither pattern of functioning is right or wrong. The important thing to consider during the family assessment process is the perceptions of family members concerning the quality of emotional support they are receiving. Chapter 8 discusses how perceptions influence an individual's interpretation of what is occurring in their environment.

## Set of Personal Roles

Every family has the task of organizing its roles in a way that helps the family achieve its goals and carry out its functions. No one role-allocation pattern works for all families. Families must allocate and differentiate roles in a manner that facilitates their functioning.

Personal roles as well as family roles evolve when families organize their role structure. Some common examples of personal roles are "the 'baby' in the family; the 'good' child; the 'bad' child; the scapegoat; the strict parent; and the 'sickest' member of the family. Such roles, even when they emerge fortuitously, can become patterned very quickly. As a result, the person may be 'locked' in the role, with important consequences for how others will treat him and what they will expect of him" (Briar, 1964, p. 254). When assessing family dynamics it is extremely important to identify how personal role allocation has influenced the behavior of all family members. The "sick" member of the family, for example, is often not allowed to do things that he or she is capable of doing. Frequently family members "take care" of this person so well that he or she never learns how to function independently.

## Rituals and Symbols

Family rituals and symbols come from two major sources. Some are adopted from the culture as a whole or a subculture within the wider culture. Others develop from human transactional processes that have occurred within the family system (Briar, 1964).

Family rituals and symbols develop around multiple aspects of family life. They help family members and outsiders identify

**TABLE 7-5**

*Examples of Rituals and Symbols in Family Systems*

| RITUAL/SYMBOL | EXAMPLES |
|---|---|
| Mealtime activity | Designating times for meals, seating arrangements during meals, and conversation shared |
| Naming of family members | Giving nicknames to all family members or naming children after specific relatives |
| Holiday events | Serving specific types of food (see Figure 7-6) or carrying out certain kinds of activities such as religious ceremonies (see Figure 7-7) |
| Religious observances | Saying prayers at mealtime or bedtime or engaging in specific activities when a family member dies |

what the family views as important. They provide structure for activities of daily living and for special occasions.

Examples of the types of rituals and symbols that develop in family systems are shared in Table 7-5. Although some of the rituals within a family appear very similar to societal ones, family rituals usually have some very specific, unique characteristics.

Family rituals and symbols are extremely significant and are usually valued highly by families. They are often continued even when individual family members do not view them as important. In the case of blended families, the rituals are continued successfully when both families embrace them (Braithwaite, Baxter, Harper, 1998). Frequently pressure is placed on family members to conform to family rituals and symbols until the entire family unit alters its views about them. When rituals are imposed, particularly in blended families, without other members' consent or cooperation, conflict may result and thereby contribute to alienation amongst its family members (Braithwaite, Baxter, Harper, 1998).

## Cultural Values and Attitudes

Numerous factors influence the biologic, psychosocial, and spiritual development of all human beings. Human growth and development begins with genetic characteristics inherited from parents but then branches off in different directions as one interacts with one's environment. Within this environment, caring and nurturing by significant others greatly affects how growth progresses and what decisions are made about handling activities of daily living. Through environmental conditioning, people learn patterns of behavior that influence how they relate to others, how they act in social situations, and how they make decisions about significant issues. Because these patterns of behavior provide stability and security, they are not easily altered; they contin-

uously influence the direction of one's life. They shape beliefs and values that provide a foundation for future decision making.

*Culture* is the term used to describe the values, attitudes, and patterns of behavior that are transmitted to all individuals in a particular social environment. Social scientists have defined culture in many ways, but most of these definitions have three central themes: (1) beliefs, values, and patterns of behavior are learned and passed on from one generation to the next; (2) culture provides a prescription for daily living and decision making; and (3) the components of a culture are valued by members of the culture and are considered to be right and not open to questioning.

Every culture has a *schema*, composed of specific components, that shapes such things as family structure; dietary habits; religious practices; the development of art, music, and drama; ways of communicating; dress; and health behavior (Figures 7-6 and 7-7). A **culture schema,** for instance, affects how one perceives health and illness and when and from whom one seeks health care. For example, because the Jewish culture values the sacredness of human life and health, members of this particular cultural group have traditionally respected health care providers and have engaged in activities to restore health, regardless of the expense. The value the Jewish culture places on health is reflected in a favorite Yiddish parting phrase, *Sei gesund,* "be well" (Kensky, 1977). In contrast to the health values held by the Jewish culture are the beliefs and values transmitted by the Mexican-American culture. Many individuals from this culture are influenced by a folk system that encourages the use of folk medicine and supports the belief that one has very little control over one's life. These individuals believe that supernatural forces cause disease and that one can do very little to prevent illness. Mexican healers, *curanderos(as)*, rather than health care professionals are used by some Mexican-American families when health care services are needed (Andrews, Boyle, 1998).

A rich diversity of cultural values and attitudes exists in our nation. In community health nursing practice, encountering clients who have beliefs that differ from those of the health care professional is a common occurrence. For a community health nurse to work effectively with such clients, he or she must develop an appreciation for the inherent worth of different cultural patterns. This involves a process that not only increases knowledge about various cultural schemata but also increases acceptance of all human beings.

Developing **cultural sensitivity** in clinical practice enriches and broadens the nurse's approach to diverse families and can lead to a more effective delivery of care. Crucial to this process is being aware of one's own cultural background, values, and beliefs. Health care professionals are influenced by their own social conditioning, which has a long-lasting effect on everything they do. Social conditioning can positively or negatively influence the therapeutic relationship. Cultural patterns subtly influence the professional's

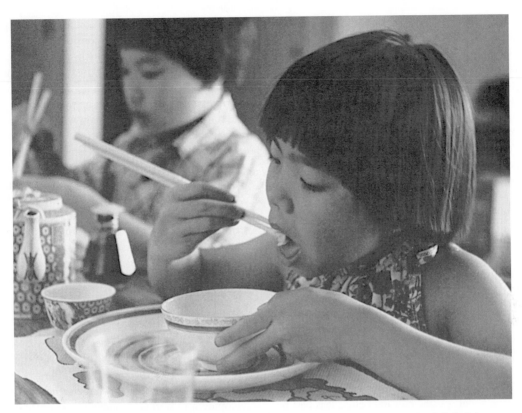

**FIGURE 7-6** Cultural values and attitudes provide a foundation for activities of daily living.

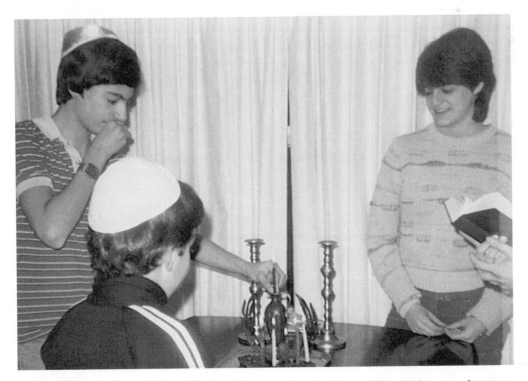

**FIGURE 7-7** For centuries, religious systems have significantly influenced the development of customs and rituals within family systems and have preserved and transmitted these traditions from one generation to another. Hanukkah, a festive Jewish holiday lasting for 8 days in early December, has been celebrated for centuries in memory of the rededication of the temple of Jerusalem under the Maccabees in 164 BCE. Hanukkah is a celebration of freedom: freedom to practice one's own religion. It is a joyous time that includes a symbolic lighting of candles, the sharing of gifts, and the serving of special foods.

perceptions about the appropriateness of a family's health beliefs, practices, and family relationships.

CULTURAL VARIATIONS. Select characteristics of some ethnic and racial groups are presented in Appendix 7-1. They illustrate cultural variations in relation to health beliefs and practices, family relationships, and communication processes. *However, nurses must understand that there are also intracultural variations based on socioeconomic factors and generational differences within groups* (Fong, 1985; Wong, 1999).

Cherry and Giger (1995) discuss intracultural variations in how African-Americans view descriptive terminology regarding their race. They have determined that some African-American individuals and groups encourage the use of the term *Black Americans,* whereas others prefer the term *African-Americans.* The latter term brings together the cultural heritage of Africa and America, whereas the emphasis in the former term is on biologic and racial identity (Cherry, Giger, 1995). In keeping with these findings and what is commonly used in the literature, the term *African-American* will be used throughout this text with the following exceptions: (1) when necessary to preserve the integrity of another author's work and (2) when there is a specific intent to delineate between black and nonblack biologic and racial variations.

When learning about specific cultural beliefs it is best to seek information from members of the particular culture being studied. Many cultural patterns are not written or recorded. Most, in fact, are transmitted from one generation to another through oral communication and behavioral transactions. Even when receiving input from individuals who represent a given cultural group, it is extremely important to remember that not all individuals within a cultural group have similar characteristics. Knowledge about cultural values and attitudes helps nurses identify factors to consider when collecting data about family functioning. This knowledge, however, *never* replaces the need to obtain specific data from individual families during the assessment process. When working with families in the community setting, a **cultural assessment** should be done to determine their unique characteristics and needs.

Cultural assessments assist nurses in individualizing family care. When conducting a cultural assessment, community health nurses need to focus on collecting basic cultural data that identify major family values, beliefs, customs, and behaviors that influence and relate to health needs, health care practices, and family attitudes about health and illness, health care providers, and health care systems (Orque, Bloch, Monrroy, 1983; Tripp-Reimer, Brink, Saunders, 1984, p. 79). According to Tripp-Reimer, Brink, and Saunders (1984), "basic cultural data include: ethnic affiliation, religious preference, family patterns, food patterns, and ethnic health care practices" (p. 79).

Appendix 7-2 displays a classic cultural assessment tool developed by Bloch (1983) to facilitate cultural assessments in the clinical setting. This tool identifies content areas

such as race, language and communication processes, and nutritional variables to be considered when making a cultural assessment. Orque, Bloch, and Monrroy (1983) and Giger and Davidhizar (1999) examine factors to consider when providing nursing care for specific ethnic groups. Referring to these writings will help the reader plan appropriate nursing interventions when working with families from different ethnic groups.

When using a cultural assessment guide, it is important to remember that a barrage of questions related to the cultural content areas on this tool is inappropriate. This type of interviewing inhibits communication and adversely affects the nurse-client relationship. When collecting data during the assessment phase of the nursing process, the community health nurse focuses on building a therapeutic relationship. The Giger and Davidhizar (1999) textbook provides some valuable guidelines to consider when collecting cultural data.

## Religious Beliefs

Cultural values and attitudes are often shaped and maintained by religious systems. From earliest times, religious systems have preserved and transmitted traditions from one generation to another and have greatly influenced the development of norms for social behavior. *Spiritual beliefs* valued by these systems have provided a foundation for moral behavior in societies. These beliefs also have helped maintain order and cohesiveness in social groups.

Despite major changes in religious systems in the past two decades, spiritual beliefs still affect the lives of most individuals. They influence such things as contraceptive practices, dietary habits, developmental transitions through rites of passage, selection of marriage partners, reactions to health and illness, and the development of customs and rituals (see Figure 7-7). Appendix 7-3 presents religious beliefs that affect nursing care.

Spiritual beliefs of clients are often neglected in the clinical setting. Involving spiritual leaders in a client's care and allowing clients to verbalize their feelings about their religious values can strengthen the relationships between health care professionals and clients and can promote effective decision making about needed health care services. Religious beliefs frequently comfort distressed individuals and help them cope with illness and crisis.

## Process Parameters for Family Assessment

Basic to the understanding of family functioning is the analysis of family processes. Family processes are methods families use to determine how their structure evolves, how decisions are made, and how the family carries out its functions to maintain stability and to promote growth within the family unit. Parameters to consider when assessing family processes can be found in Box 7-4.

Family health is a function of process rather than outcome. It is family process that helps the family manage

## BOX 7-4

*Select Process Parameters to Consider During Family Assessment*

- How the family integrates its role relationships
- How the family uses information from the environment
- How the family adapts to change within the family system and its environment
- How the family deals with conflict or disagreement
- How the family maintains the integrity of the family unit
- How the family promotes the personal autonomy of family members

stress, survive crises, deal with conflict, and organize itself so that it can achieve its goals. Usually, however, a family comes to the attention of the health care professional because its outputs are inadequate or because the family perceives difficulty in meeting its goals. When assessing family functioning, it is extremely important to examine process variables as well as outcomes desired by a family. Family processes frequently need to be altered before desired outcomes can be reached.

Direct observation of the family system is the best way to gain an understanding of family processes. This is especially true during times of crisis, because it is during these periods that functional or dysfunctional behaviors become more evident. Decision-making and communication patterns should be analyzed carefully in an assessment of family processes. Chapter 8 presents the concepts of stress and crisis and examines some of the factors that affect decision making when people are distressed. Parameters to observe when looking at family communication patterns have been discussed previously in this chapter. Classic writings by Ackerman (1959, 1970); Bowen (1973); Haley (1971); Jackson (1968); Minuchin (1974); Satir (1972); and Watzlawick, Beavin, and Jackson (1967) provide an in-depth analysis of family processes and are very useful references for practitioners who view the family as their unit of service.

Characteristics that reflect dysfunctional processes in a family unit are presented in Box 7-5. These behaviors were identified by the North American Nursing Diagnosis Association (NANDA), a national organization established to develop standard nursing diagnoses for the profession. Having an understanding of these behaviors assists the community health nurse in identifying families who need nursing intervention.

### Stop and Think About It

What does culture and cultural variation mean to you? How does your understanding influence your actions with your client family? How does your cultural background influence your perception about family processes?

## BOX 7-5

*NANDA Nursing Diagnosis: Altered Family Processes (Specify Processes)*

**Definition**

Inability of family system (household members) to meet needs of members, carry out family functions, or maintain communications for mutual growth and maturation

**Defining Characteristics**

- Inability of family members to relate to each other for mutual growth and maturation
- Failure to send and receive clear messages
- Poorly communicated family rules, rituals, symbols; unexamined myths
- Unhealthy family decision-making processes
- Inability of family members to express and accept wide range of feelings
- Inability to accept and receive help
- Does not demonstrate respect for individuality and autonomy of members
- Rigidity in functions and roles
- Fails to accomplish current (or past) family developmental tasks
- Inappropriate (nonproductive) boundary maintenance
- Inability to adapt to change
- Inability to deal with traumatic or crisis experience constructively
- Parents do not demonstrate respect for each other's views on child-rearing practices
- Inappropriate (nonproductive) level and direction of energy
- Inability to meet needs of members (physical, security, emotional, spiritual)
- Family uninvolved in community activities

**Etiologic or Related Factors**

- Situational crisis or transition (e.g., alcoholism of a member)
- Developmental crisis or transition

From Gordon M: *Manual of nursing diagnosis*, ed 9, St Louis, 2000, Mosby, p. 441.

## TOOLS THAT FACILITATE THE FAMILY ASSESSMENT PROCESS

A community health nurse can use a variety of tools to facilitate family assessment. Some of these tools are discussed in the following text. They are designed to help the practitioner elicit data about certain aspects of family structure, function, and process and to aid the health professional in determining major family concerns, needs, and strengths. Assessment tools, however, are only guides, and before using them one needs to have an understanding of family theory and of communication processes that enhance effective nurse-client relationships.

## Family Assessment Guides

Many community health agencies have developed family assessment guides so that staff members can focus attention on family functioning in addition to the health status of individual family members. Appendix 7-4 is an example of such a tool. When completed, it provides a quick visual summary of family strengths, family behaviors that need to be altered, and anticipated guidance needs.

Generally, family assessment guides examine both the family's relationships with its environment and its internal functioning. It is extremely important when designing guides to facilitate the data collection process to take into consideration the need to identify both effective and ineffective behaviors within a family system. It is easy to focus only on family problems. When this is done, ineffective family functioning may be overemphasized. This can lead to frustration, discouragement, and a feeling of hopelessness. Nurses who are unable to see family strengths "burn out" quickly. Families who never receive positive feedback for what they are handling well question their ability to adequately maintain themselves and often become dependent on others for decision making.

A family assessment guide should be consistent with one's philosophy of practice. For example, in the community health setting, nurses firmly believe that a preventive health approach is important. This belief would be operationalized if staff members were encouraged to discern anticipatory guidance needs and then to plan nursing interventions that may prevent future health problems. An assessment guide that identifies the need to address anticipatory guidance issues would support staff in implementing a preventive approach to practice.

Family assessment tools are only helpful when the practitioner has the theoretical background to use them. Knowledge of role theory, cultural values and attitudes, family decision making, and concepts of stress and crisis is essential for effective use of an assessment guide. Assessment tools can never replace an understanding of theories that analyze family functioning or that describe how nurse-client interactions affect the therapeutic process.

## Genograms

A **genogram** is a tool that aids the community health nurse in collecting generational information about family structure and processes. It visually portrays to the nurse and the family how the family has evolved. It quickly helps the community health nurse identify the relationships between family members, the health status of individual family members, and the family's reactions to sociocultural and spiritual variables that have affected their lives. The genogram provides a picture that clearly connects events and relationships. This makes it easier for the nurse to more objectively evaluate the family system over time. "There are three parts to constructing a genogram: (1) mapping the family structure; (2) recording the family

information; and (3) delineating family relationships" (Arnold, 1999, p. 306).

Figure 7-8 is a partial genogram constructed by a community health nurse during her sixth home visit to the Z. family. Before completing the genogram, the nurse had been helping the family to deal with their feelings about the son's recent diagnosis of allergies and had identified a discrepancy in how each parent viewed the son's health status. Wondering whether this was related to previous life experiences, the nurse believed that a genogram could help her and the family address how social conditioning can influence perceptions of health and illness. The nurse was able to trace each parent's attitudes about health and illness and discovered that all family members had unresolved feelings about the death of two children in the family. These feelings distorted the mother's perceptions about the seriousness of the son's health problems. Genograms can help family members focus more clearly on current stressful events and gain an appreciation for how past events influence present health problems.

Genograms schematically depict a family tree (Hartman, 1995). A family tree drawn by a professional differs from one drawn by a family in that the professional uses theory as a basis to elicit data about family structure, function, and process. The interview process is the most critical component to consider when completing a genogram. If information concerning child-rearing practices, health beliefs and attitudes, significant social data, and traditions passed on from one generation to another is not assessed, the genogram has little meaning. Completing the actual drawing of a genogram takes minimal skill; focusing the conversation on relevant aspects of family functioning requires not only interviewing skill but also knowledge of family dynamics.

## Ecomap

An ecomap is another tool health care professionals use to schematically portray factual data about family relationships. The ecomap visually diagrams a family's relationship with external resources (Arnold, 1999, p. 308). It provides a picture for both a family and the nurse to visually analyze a family's interactions with its external environment. Presented in Figure 7-9 is an ecomap developed by Dr. Ann Hartman (1978), one of the forerunners to use this tool effectively in practice. Based on a systems theoretical framework, Hartman's tool examines boundary-maintenance aspects of family functioning. It dramatically illustrates the amount of energy used by a family to maintain its system, as well as the presence or absence of situational supports and other family resources. The ecomap continues to be a viable family assessment tool that addresses family relationships with the external environment and the energy the family uses to support its system (Arnold, 1999; Hartman, 1995; Hodge, 2000).

An ecomap helps families identify how their energies are being used and when relationships with the external environment are positively or negatively influencing family

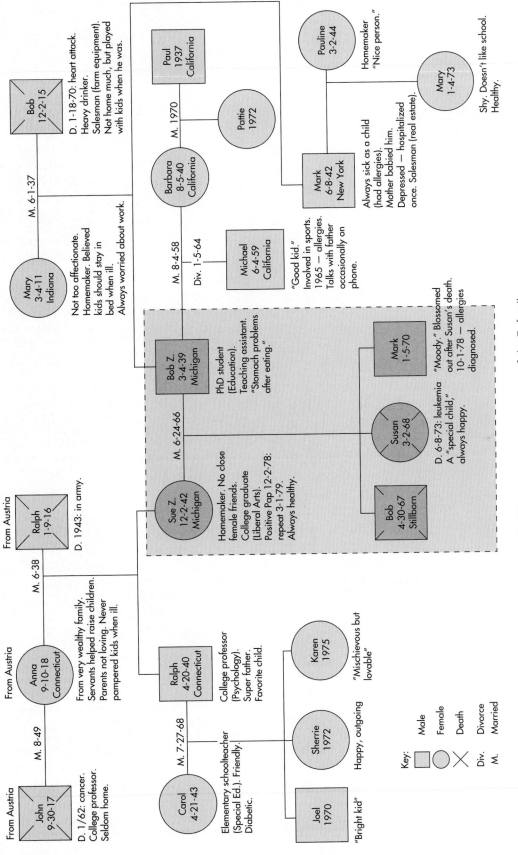

**FIGURE 7-8** Sample genogram of the Z. family.

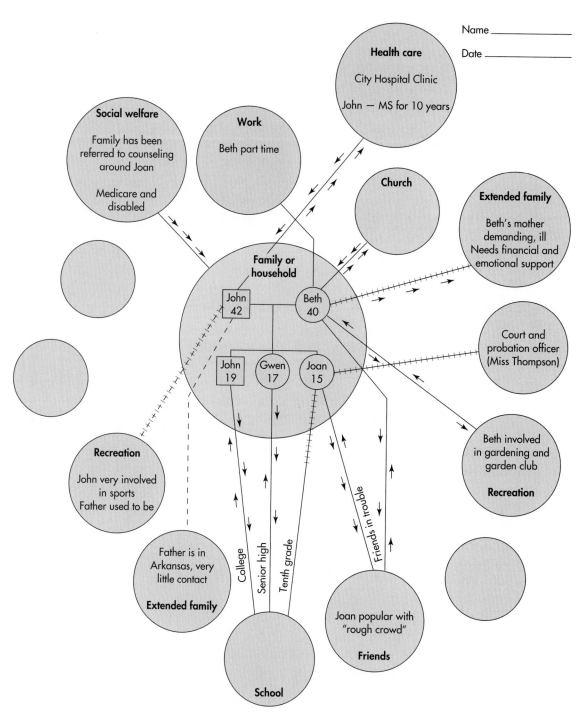

**FIGURE 7-9** Ecomap. Fill in connections where they exist. Indicate nature of connections with a descriptive word or by drawing different kinds of lines: —— for strong; – – – for tenuous; ׀+׀+ for stressful. Draw arrows (→—→—→) along lines to signify flow of energy, resources, and so on. Identify significant people and fill in empty circles as needed. (From Hartman A: Diagrammatic assessment of family relationships, *Social Casework* 59:470, 1978.)

functioning. For example, if a family's flow of energy as depicted on the ecomap reflects only an outward directional process (→→→), the family may have difficulty providing a nurturing environment for family members and achieving its goals.

It is impossible to function effectively in the community health setting without looking at how the family interfaces with its external environment. The ecomap enhances the community health nurse's ability to gain this type of information. It is an especially useful tool because it summarizes

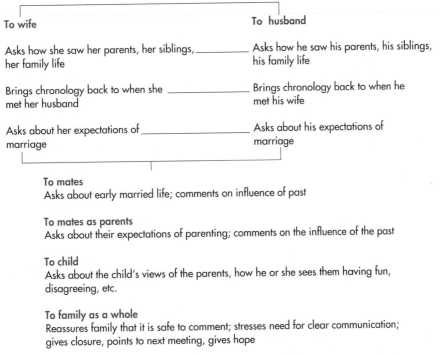

**To mates**

Asks about how they met, when they decided to marry, etc.

**To wife**

Asks how she saw her parents, her siblings, her family life

Brings chronology back to when she met her husband

Asks about her expectations of marriage

**To husband**

Asks how he saw his parents, his siblings, his family life

Brings chronology back to when he met his wife

Asks about his expectations of marriage

**To mates**
Asks about early married life; comments on influence of past

**To mates as parents**
Asks about their expectations of parenting; comments on the influence of the past

**To child**
Asks about the child's views of the parents, how he or she sees them having fun, disagreeing, etc.

**To family as a whole**
Reassures family that it is safe to comment; stresses need for clear communication; gives closure, points to next meeting, gives hope

**FIGURE 7-10** Main flow of family-life chronology. (From Satir V: *Conjoint family therapy: a guide to theory and technique*, Palo Alto, Calif, 1967, Science & Behavior Books, p. 135.)

on one page family strengths, conflicts, and stresses in relation to its interactions with individuals and agencies outside the family system. Community health nurses have found the use of the ecomap particularly beneficial when clients are involved with numerous community systems or when clients perceive a lack of support from significant others.

## Family-Life Chronology

Community health nurses may encounter families who are experiencing relationship problems, a situation that makes it difficult for them to concentrate on health concerns or to take needed health actions. These families can find it hard to examine objectively what is happening in their relationships or to make a decision about seeking counseling. Satir's (1967) **family-life chronology model** (Figure 7-10) helps the community health nurse and the family identify interactive processes that have evolved. Families that have had long-standing relationship difficulties should be referred for counseling. However, it is not unusual for significant family stress (e.g., illness or financial difficulties) to strain family relationships. The family-life chronology can help these families identify the strengths in their relationships over time and the need to alter family functioning to reduce stress.

A community health nurse cannot ignore relationship problems when working with families in their homes. Such

difficulties can disrupt all parameters of family functioning and are often the key factor in preventing a family from taking needed health action. If these difficulties are ignored, nursing intervention strategies can be ineffective. Dealing with the symptoms of distress such as physical health problems, complaints about lack of time for leisure activities, or feelings of depression, rather than with the relationship difficulties themselves will not alter a family's functioning in any lasting way. One mother, for example, complained to the community health nurse that she had no time for herself and that she found caring for three children, 4, 6, and 8 years old, very restrictive. Suggestions by the community health nurse on how she might care for her children and still have time for leisure activities were ignored. The mother finally shared with the nurse that her husband felt that "a woman's place was in the home. Even if I enrolled my 4-year-old son in a nursery school, I still could not get out of the house. My husband gets very upset if I am gone from home without him." This woman was depressed and discouraged. Although she loved her children, she also wanted to explore adult interests. To fulfill this need she had to address relationship conflicts with her husband.

When addressing relationship difficulties with a family, it is important for the nurse to facilitate the development of effective family processes. This implies that the nurse avoids forming an alliance with an individual family member and encourages family members to find ways to discuss their differences. "Taking sides" in family conflicts is nontherapeutic and can adversely affect family functioning and the therapeutic relationship.

## Videotaping

Videotaping is another tool that helps the community health nurse assess individual and family functioning. Community health nurses find this tool especially useful when they want to assess family interactions and/or functional abilities of a family member. For example, videotaping can be used to examine how a disabled child is performing activities of daily living. Community health nurses use videotaping in this situation to observe simultaneously the actions of a child and family, as well as the functional capabilities of the client being assessed. It is important to observe both the client and significant others during a functional assessment because the behavior of significant others either inhibits or enhances functional development.

Videotaping provides specific data about family dynamics and an individual's functional abilities that are often missed during a home visit. For example, it is easy to overlook a child's small accomplishments when other activities are occurring in the environment. It is equally easy to miss nurse or family behaviors that adversely affect a child's performance. Families are usually receptive to videotaping, especially when the community health nurse explains that a more accurate evaluation of a child's abilities may be obtained through the use of this tool. Obtaining written, informed consent from clients and assuring them that confidentiality will be maintained also relieves their anxiety.

A videotaped child assessment can be very motivating to families because it dramatically illustrates a child's strengths and needs. Videotaping helps a family identify positive and negative behaviors that are promoting or inhibiting a child's growth. The impact of seeing actual behaviors is not quickly forgotten.

A unique program, "A Star is Born," uses videotaping to help teenage parents learn about child growth and development through the first year of life. This parent education program also helps mothers and fathers identify how their interactions influence their child's emotional and physical development. The "A Star is Born" program is a creative way to help teenagers identify their strengths and needs in relation to parenting and to facilitate parent-infant bonding. It actively engages parents in the learning process and provides a way to role model effective parent-child interactions.

## SUMMARY

Despite its changing nature, the family is still considered the basic unit of service in community health nursing settings.

Historical evidence from clinical practice and research has sufficiently demonstrated that family-centered nursing services more effectively meet the needs of individuals, families, and communities than do services delivered only to individual clients. However, viewing the family from the traditional perspective is no longer appropriate because alternative family structures and culturally diverse family forms are more prevalent in our society. The nuclear family unit is no longer the only acceptable form of family life.

It is essential for community health nurses to have an understanding of family theory in order to implement a family-centered preventive health approach to nursing care. Theory helps the practitioner assess family structure, function, process, and communication patterns in an organized and logical fashion. It provides parameters to consider when collecting data about client situations. It assists in explaining the phenomena that are occurring within a family, which in turn helps one plan effective intervention strategies.

Tools such as the genogram, the ecomap, and family assessment guides are available for facilitating the family assessment process. These tools do not, however, take the place of a genuine understanding of family dynamics. They only provide guidelines for the organization and collection of data.

*Ella M. Brooks acknowledges the work from previous editions of this text in the development of this chapter.*

## CRITICAL THINKING
*exercise*

Given the following case situations, discuss how a nursing assessment from a holistic family perspective would differ from a nursing assessment directed toward the identified client (Sally Huling/Cissy Jones).

1. You are visiting Sally Huling, a 16-year-old teenager recently referred to the Visiting Nurse Association following her hospitalization for regulation of an unstable diabetic condition. Sally lives with her parents, a 10-year-old brother, and a 5-year-old sister in a four-bedroom, well-kept home in a middle-class neighborhood. While she was hospitalized both Sally and her family expressed anxiety about Sally's diabetic condition.

2. You are visiting Cissy Jones, age 2, and her family. Cissy was referred for community health nurse follow-up by the nurse in the well-child clinic because of notable strabismus. The Jones family's income is minimal. They have inadequate furniture and clothing for their son, age 1 month. Although Mrs. Jones appears tired upon your first home visit, she is anxious to talk about resources for obtaining eye care for Cissy.

# REFERENCES

Ackerman NW, editor: *The psychodynamics of family life: diagnosis and treatment of family relationships*, New York, 1959, Basic Books.

Ackerman NW, editor: *Family process*, New York, 1970, Basic Books.

Aldous J: *Family careers: developmental change in families*, New York, 1978, Wiley.

Anderson P, Fenichel D: *Serving culturally diverse families of infants and toddlers with disabilities*, Washington, DC, 1989, National Center for Clinical Infant Programs.

Andrews MM, Boyle JS: *Transcultural concepts in nursing care*, Philadelphia, 1998, JB Lippincott.

Arnold E: Communicating with families. In Arnold E, Boggs K: *Interpersonal relationships: professional communication skills for nurses*, ed 3, Philadelphia, 1999, WB Saunders.

Artinian NT: Philosophy of science and family nursing theory development. In Whall AL, Fawcett J: *Family theory development in nursing: state of the science and art*, Philadelphia, 1991, FA Davis.

Beavers WR: *Psychotherapy and growth: a family systems perspective*, New York, 1977, Brunner/Mazel.

Bloch B: Bloch's assessment guide for ethnic/cultural variations. In Orque MS, Bloch B, Monrroy LSA, editors: *Ethnic nursing care: a multicultural approach*, St Louis, 1983, Mosby.

Bomar PJ, editor: *Nurses and family health promotion: concepts, assessment, and interventions*, ed 2, Philadelphia, 1996, WB Saunders.

Boss P: *Family stress management*, Newbury Park, Calif, 1988, Sage.

Bowen M: Toward the differentiation of a self in one's own family. In Framo JL, editor: *Family interaction: a dialogue between family researchers and family therapists*, New York, 1973, Springer.

Bowen M: Italian Americans. In Giger JN, Davidhizar RE: *Transcultural nursing: assessment and intervention*, St Louis, 1991, Mosby.

Braithwaite DO, Baxter LA, Harper AM: The role of rituals in the management of dialectical tension of "old" and "new" in blended families, *Communication Studies* 49(2):101-120, 1998.

Bredemeir HC, Stephenson RN: *The analysis of social systems*, New York, 1965, Holt.

Briar S: The family as an organization: an approach to family diagnosis and treatment, *Soc Service Rev* 38:247-255, 1964.

Carpenito LJ: *Nursing diagnosis: application to clinical practice*, ed 4, Philadelphia, 1992, JB Lippincott.

Carter B, McGoldrick M, editors: *The changing family life cycle: a framework for family therapy*, ed 2, New York, 1988, Gardner Press.

Cherry B, Giger JN: African-Americans. In Giger JN, Davidhizar RE: *Transcultural nursing: assessment and intervention*, ed 3, St Louis, 1995, Mosby.

Children's Defense Fund: *The state of America's children, yearbook 1992*, Washington, DC, 1997, The Fund.

Clark AL, editor: *Culture and childrearing*, Philadelphia, 1981, FA Davis.

Clemen (Parks) SJ: *Introduction to health care facility: food services administration*, University Park, Penn, 1974, Pennsylvania State University Press.

Coleman M, Ganong LH: Changing families, changing responsibilities? *National Forum* 80(3):34-37, 2000.

Coltrane S: Fatherhood and marriage in the 21st century, *National Forum* 80(3):25-28, 2000.

Conley L: Childbearing and childrearing practices in Mormonism, *Neonatal Network* 9(3):41-48, 1990.

Coontz S: Marriage: then and now, *National Forum* 80(3):10-15, 2000.

Danielson C, Hamel-Bissell B, Winstead-Fry P: *Families, health and illness: perspectives on coping and intervention*, St Louis, 1993, Mosby.

Day JC: *Population projections of the United States, by age, sex, race, and Hispanic origin: 1993 to 2050*, US Bureau of the Census, current population reports, P 25-1104, Washington, DC, 1993, US Government Printing Office.

Day JC: *Projections of the number of households and families in the United States: 1995 to 2010*, US Bureau of the Census, current population reports, series P25-1129, Washington, DC, 1996, US Government Printing Office.

Demo D: Children's experience of family diversity, *National Forum* 80(3):16-20, 2000.

DeSantis L: Cultural factors affecting newborn and infant diarrhea, *J Pediatric Nurs* 3(6):391-398, 1988.

Duvall EM, Miller BC: *Marriage and family development*, ed 6, New York, 1985, Harper & Row.

Ellis JR, Hartley CL: *Nursing in today's world*, ed 7, Philadelphia, 2001, JB Lippincott.

Fong CM: Ethnicity and nursing practice, *TCN* 7:1-10, 1985.

Francese P: The 100 millionth household, *American Demographics* 18:15-16, 1996.

Friedman MM: *Family nursing: theory and practice*, Norwalk, Conn, 1998, Appleton & Lange.

Fulmer R: Lower-income and professional families: a comparison of structure and life cycle process. In Carter B, McGoldrick M, editors: *The changing family life cycle: a framework for family therapy*, ed 2, New York, 1988, Gardner Press.

Geissler EM: *Pocket guide to cultural assessment*, St Louis, 1994, Mosby.

Giger JN, Davidhizar RE: *Transcultural nursing: assessment and intervention*, ed 2, St Louis, 1995, Mosby.

Giger JN, Davidhizar RE: *Transcultural nursing: assessment and intervention*, ed 3, St Louis, 1999, Mosby.

Gordon M: *Manual of nursing diagnosis*, ed 9, St Louis, 2000, Mosby.

Haley J, editor: *Changing families*, New York, 1971, Grune & Stratton.

Hanley CH: Navajo Indians. In Giger JN, Davidhizar RE: *Transcultural nursing assessment and intervention*, St Louis, 1991, Mosby.

Hanson SM, Boyd ST: *Family health care nursing: theory, practice, and research*, Philadelphia, 1996, FA Davis.

Hartman A: Diagrammatic assessment of family relationships, *Social Casework* 59:465-476, 1978.

Hartman A: Diagrammatic assessment of family relationship, *Families in Society* 76(2):111-112, 1995.

Heaney CA, Israel BA: Social networks and social support. In Glanz K, Lewis FM, Rimer BK, editors: *Health behavior and health education: theory, research and practice*, ed 2, San Francisco, 1997, Jossey-Bass.

Hill R, Hansen DA: The identification of conceptual frameworks utilized in family study, *Marriage Family Living* 22:299-311, 1960.

Hinshaw AS: Nursing knowledge for the 21st century: opportunities and challenges, *Nursing Scholarship* 32(2):117-123, 2000.

Hodge DR: Spiritual ecomap: a new diagrammatic tool for assessing marital and family spirituality, *Marital and Family Therapy* 26(2):217-228, 2000.

Holland S, Sweeney E: *Vietnamese children and families: the impact of culture*, Washington, DC, 1985, Association for the Care of Children's Health.

Hollingsworth AO, Brown LP, Brooten DA: The refugees and childbearing: what to expect, *RN* 43(11):45-48, 1980.

Hooyman NR: Social policy and gender inequities in caregiving. In Dwyer J, Coward R, editors: *Gender, families, and elder care*, Newbury Park, Calif, 1992, Sage.

Jackson DD, editor: *Communication, family and marriage*, vol 1, Palo Alto, Calif, 1968, Science & Behavior Books.

Janosik E, Green E: *Family life: process and practice*, Boston, 1992, Jones & Bartlett.

Kensky AD: Cultural influences on the Jewish patient. In Clemen SA, Will M, editors: *Family and community health nursing: a workbook*, Ann Arbor, 1977, University of Michigan Press.

Kozier B, Erb G: *Fundamentals of nursing*, ed 5, Menlo Park, Calif, 1995, Addison-Wesley.

Krentz LG: *Nursing of families and the health care delivery system: workshop proceedings*, Portland, Ore, 1989, Oregon Health Sciences University.

Levitan SA, Conway EA: *Families in flux: new approaches to meeting workforce challenges for child, elder, and health care in the 1990s*, Washington, DC, 1990, The Bureau of National Affairs.

Lewis J, Beavers R, Gossett JT, et al.: *No single thread: psychological health in family systems*, New York, 1976, Brunner/Mazel.

Linton R: The natural history of the family. In Anshen RN, editor: *The family: its function and destiny*, revised ed, New York, 1959, Harper & Row.

Litman TJ: The family as a basic unit in health and medical care: a social-behavioral overview, *Soc Sci Med* 8:495-519, 1974.

Loveland-Cherry C: Family health promotion and health protection. In Bomar PJ, editor: *Nurses and family health promotion: concepts, assessments, and interventions*, ed 2, Philadelphia, 1996, WB Saunders.

Macklin ED: Nontraditional family forms. In Sussman MB, Steinmetz SK, editors: *Handbook of marriage and the family*, New York, 1987, Plenum Press.

McGoldrick M: Ethnicity and the family life cycle. In Carter B, McGoldrick M: *The changing family life cycle: a framework for family therapy*, ed 2, New York, 1988, Gardner Press.

McQuay JE: Cross cultural customs and beliefs related to health crisis, death, and organ donation/transplantation, *Crit Care Nurs Clin North Am* 7(3):581-594, 1995.

Minuchin S: *Families and family therapy*, Cambridge, Mass, 1974, Harvard University Press.

Oliker S: Family care after welfare ends, *National Forum* 80(3):29-33, 2000.

Orque MS, Bloch B, Monrroy LSA, editors: *Ethnic nursing care: a multicultural approach*, St Louis, 1983, Mosby.

Otto H: Criteria for assessing family strengths, *Family Process* 2:329-338, 1963.

Peterson R: *What are the needs of the chronic mental patients?* Presented at the APA Conference on the Chronic Mental Patient, Washington, DC, January 11-14, 1978.

Polatnick MR: Working Parents, *National Forum* 80(3):38-41, 2000.

Pratt L: *Family structure and effective health behavior: the energized family*, Boston, 1976, Houghton Mifflin.

Randall-David E: *Strategies for working with culturally diverse communities and clients*, Washington, DC, 1989, Association for the Care of Children's Health.

Roccereto L: Selected health beliefs of Vietnamese refugees, *J Sch Health* 51:63-64, 1981.

Satir V: *Conjoint family therapy: a guide to theory and technique*, Palo Alto, Calif, 1967, Science & Behavior Books.

Satir V: *Peoplemaking*, Palo Alto, Calif, 1972, Science & Behavior Books.

Satir V: You as a change agent in helping families to change. In Satir V, Stachowiak J, Taskman H, editors: *Helping families to change*, New York, 1975, Jason Aronson.

Sodetaini-Shibata AE: The Japanese American. In Clark AL, editor: *Culture and childrearing*, Philadelphia, 1981, FA Davis.

Sollie DL: Beyond Mars and Venus, *National Forum* 80(3):42-45, 2000.

Spector RE: *Cultural diversity in health and illness*, ed 2, Stamford, Conn, 1985, Appleton & Lange.

Spector RE: *Cultural diversity in health and illness*, ed 4, Stamford, Conn, 1996, Appleton & Lange.

Stranton GT: The spiritual significance of family, *National Forum* 80(3):21-24, 2000.

Stryker SL: The interactional and situational approaches. In Christensen HT, editor: *Handbook of marriage and the family*, Chicago, 1964, Rand McNally.

Sussman MB, chairperson: *Changing families in a changing society: 1970 White House Conference on Children*, Forum 14 report, Washington, DC, 1971, US Government Printing Office.

Tiedje LB, Darling-Fisher C: Fatherhood reconsidered: a critical review, *Res Nurs Health* 19:471-484, 1996.

Tripp-Reimer T, Brink PJ, Saunders JM: Cultural assessment: content and process, *Nurs Outlook* 32:78-82, 1984.

US Bureau of the Census: *Population profile of the United States: 1993*, current population reports, series P23-185, Washington, DC, 1993, US Government Printing Office.

US Bureau of the Census: *Population profile of the Unites States: 1997*, current population reports, series P23-194, Washington, DC, 1998, US Government Printing Office.

von Bertalanffy L: *General systems theory*, New York, 1968, George Braziller.

Watzlawick P, Beavin JH, Jackson DD: *Pragmatics of human communication: a study of interactional patterns, pathologies, and paradoxes*, New York, 1967, Norton.

Wellner AS: Who is in the house? *American Demographics* 31(2):48-51, 2000.

Whall AL: Family system theory: relationship to nursing conceptual models. In Whall AL, Fawcett J, editors: *Family theory development in nursing: state of the science and art*, Philadelphia, 1991, FA Davis.

Whall AL, Fawcett J: *Family theory development in nursing: state of the science and art*, Philadelphia, 1991, FA Davis.

Wong DL: *Whaley and Wong's nursing care of infants and children*, ed 6, St Louis, 1999, Mosby.

Wright LM, Leahey M: *Nurses and families: a guide to family assessment and intervention*, ed 2, Philadelphia, 1994, FA Davis.

## SELECTED BIBLIOGRAPHY

Allen ML, Brown P, Finlay B: *Helping children by strengthening families: a look at family*, Washington, DC, 1992, Children's Defense Fund.

Anderson P, Fenichel D: *Serving culturally diverse families of infants and toddlers with disabilities*, Washington, DC, 1989, National Center for Clinical Infant Programs.

Bomar PJ: *Nurses and family health promotion: concepts, assessment, and interventions*, ed 2, Philadelphia, 1996, Saunders.

Burr WR, Leigh GK: Famology: a new discipline, *J Marriage Family* 45:467-480, 1983.

Cherlin A, Furstenburg F: The American family in the year 2000. In Cornish E, editor: *The 1990s and beyond*, Bethesda, Md, 1990, World Future Society.

Fine MA: Families in the United States: their current status and future prospects, *Family Relations* 41:430-434, 1992.

Friedman MM: *Family nursing theory: theory and practice*, Norwalk, Conn, 1997, Appleton-Century-Crofts.

Hanson SMH, Boyd ST: *Family health care nursing: theory, practice and research*, Philadelphia, 1996, FA Davis.

Jung M: Family-centered practice with single-parent families, *Families in Society: J Contemporary Human Services* 77:583-591, 1996.

Leininger M: Culture care theory, research, and practice, *Nurs Sc Q* 9:71-78, 1996.

Neuman B, editor: *Neuman systems model*, ed 3, New Jersey, 1999, Prentice Hall.

Roy SC, Andrews HA: *Roy adaptation model*, ed 2, New Jersey, 1999, Prentice Hall.

# Cultural Characteristics Related to Health Care of Children and Families

| CULTURAL GROUP | HEALTH BELIEFS | HEALTH PRACTICES |
| --- | --- | --- |
| **Asians**<br>**Chinese** | A healthy body viewed as gift from parents and ancestors and must be cared for<br>Health is one of the results of balance between the forces of **yin** (cold) and **yang** (hot)—energy forces that rule the world<br>Illness caused by imbalance<br>Believe blood is source of life and is not regenerated<br>**Chi** is innate energy<br>Lack of chi and blood results in deficiency that produces fatigue, poor constitution, and long illness | Goal of therapy is to restore balance of yin and yang<br>Acupuncturist applies needles to appropriate meridians identified in terms of yin and yang<br>Acupressure and **tai chi** replacing acupuncture in some areas<br>**Moxibustion** is application of heat to skin over specific meridians<br>Wide use of medicinal herbs procured and applied in prescribed ways<br>Folk healers are herbalist, spiritual healer, temple healer, fortune healer<br>Meals may or may not be planned to balance hot and cold<br>Milk intolerance relatively common<br>Use of condiments (e.g., monosodium glutamate and soy sauce) may create difficulty with some diet regimens (e.g., low-salt diets) |
| **Japanese** | Three major belief systems:<br>  **Shinto** religious influence<br>    Humans inherently good<br>    Evil caused by outside spirits<br>    Illness caused by contact with polluting agents (e.g., blood, corpses, skin diseases)<br>  Chinese and Korean influence<br>    Health achieved through harmony and balance between self and society<br>    Disease caused by disharmony with society and not caring for body<br>  Portuguese influence<br>    Upholds germ theory of disease | Believe evil removed by purification<br>Energy restored by means of acupuncture, acupressure, massage, and moxibustion along affected meridians<br>**Kampō** medicine—use of natural herbs<br>Believe in removal of diseased parts<br>Trend is to use both Western and Oriental healing methods<br>Care for disabled viewed as family's responsibility<br>Take pride in child's good health<br>Seek preventive care, medical care for illness<br>May avoid some food combinations (e.g., milk and cherries, watermelon and crab) and believe pickled plums to have special properties |
| **Vietnamese** | Good health considered to be balance between yin and yang<br>Believe person's life has been predisposed toward certain phenomena by cosmic forces<br>Health believed to be result of harmony with existing universal order; harmony attained by pleasing good spirits and avoiding evil ones | Family uses all means possible before using outside agencies for health care<br>Fortune-tellers determine event that caused disturbance<br>May visit temple to procure divine instruction<br>Use astrologer to calculate cyclic changes and forces<br>Regard health as family responsibility; outside aid sought when resources run out |

From Wong DL: *Whaley and Wong's nursing care of infants and children,* ed 6, St Louis, 1999, Mosby, pp. 64-68.
Sources: Anderson and Fenichel, 1989; Clark, 1981; DeSantis, 1988; Geissler, 1994; Giger, Davidhizar, 1995; Holland, Sweeney, 1985; Hollingsworth, Brown, Brooten, 1980; Orgue, Bloch, Monrroy, 1983, Randall-David, 1989; Sodetaini-Shibata, 1981.

# Cultural Characteristics Related to
# Health Care of Children and Families (cont'd)

| FAMILY RELATIONSHIPS | COMMUNICATION | COMMENTS |
|---|---|---|
| Extended family pattern common<br>Strong concept of loyalty of young to old<br>Respect for elders taught at early age—acceptance without questioning or talking back<br>Children's behavior a reflection on family<br>Family and individual honor and "face" important<br>Self-reliance and self-restraint highly valued; self-expression repressed<br>Men valued more highly than women; women submissive to men in family | Open expression of emotions unacceptable<br>Often smile when do not comprehend | Do not react well to painful diagnostic workup; are especially upset by drawing of blood<br>Deep respect for their bodies and believe it best to die with bodies intact; therefore may refuse surgery<br>Believe in reincarnation<br>Older members fear hospitals; often believe hospital is a place to go to die<br>Children sometimes breastfed for up to 4 or 5 years* |
| Close intergenerational relationships<br>Family provides anchor<br>Family tends to keep problems to self<br>Value self-control and self-sufficiency<br>Concept of *haji* (shame) imposes strong control; unacceptable behavior of children reflects on family<br>Many adopt practices of contemporary middle class<br>Concern for child's missing school may result in sending to school before fully recovered from illness | Issei—born in Japan; usually speak Japanese only<br>Nisei, Sansei, and Yonsei have few language difficulties<br>New immigrants able to read and write English better than able to speak or understand it<br>Make significant use of nonverbal communication with subtle gestures and facial expression<br>Tend to suppress emotions<br>Will often wait silently | Generational categories:<br>**Issei**—1st generation to live in U.S.<br>**Nisei**—2nd generation<br>**Sansei**—3rd generation<br>**Yonsei**—4th generation<br>Issei and Nisei—tolerant and permissive childrearing until 5 or 6, then emphasis on emotional reserve and control<br>Cleanliness highly valued<br>Time considered valuable and used wisely<br>Tendency to practice emotional control may make assessment of pain more difficult |
| Family is revered institution<br>Multigenerational families<br>Family is chief social network<br>Children highly valued<br>Individual needs and interests are subordinate to those of a family group<br>Father is main decision maker<br>Women taught submission to men | Many immigrants are not proficient in speaking and understanding English<br>May hesitate to ask questions<br>Questioning authority is sign of disrespect; asking questions considered impolite<br>Use indirectness rather than forthrightness in expressing disagreement | Consider status more important than money<br>Children taught emotional control<br>Time concept more relaxed—consider punctuality less significant than other values (i.e., propriety)<br>Place high value on social harmony |

*Most Asian cultures consider the child 1 year old at the time of birth. Traditional Chinese custom adds 1 year on January 1 regardless of the birthday—a child born in December is 2 years old the next January.

*Continued*

# Cultural Characteristics Related to Health Care of Children and Families (cont'd)

| CULTURAL GROUP | HEALTH BELIEFS | HEALTH PRACTICES |
|---|---|---|
| **Asians**—cont'd<br>**Vietnamese**—cont'd | Belief in ***am duc,*** the amount of good deeds accumulated by ancestors<br>Many use rituals to prevent illness<br>Practice some restrictions to prevent incurring wrath of evil spirits | Certain illnesses considered only temporary (such as pustules, open wounds) and ignored<br>Seek generalist health healers<br>May use special diets to prevent illness and promote health<br>Lactose intolerance prevalent |
| **Filipinos** | Believe God's will and supernatural forces govern universe<br>Illness, accidents, and other misfortunes are God's punishment for violations of His will<br>Widely accept "hot" and "cold" balance and imbalance as cause of health and illness | Some use amulets as a shield from witchcraft or as good luck pieces<br>Catholics substitute religious medals and other items |
| **African-American Blacks** | Illness classified as:<br>    Natural—affected by forces of nature without adequate protection (e.g., cold air, pollution, food and water)<br>    Unnatural—evil influences (e.g., witchcraft, voodoo, hoodoo, hex, fix, root work); symptoms often associated with eating<br>Believe serious illness sent by God as punishment (e.g., parents punished by illness or death of child)<br>Believe serious illness can be avoided<br>May resist health care because illness is "will of God" | Self-care and folk medicine prevalent<br>Folk therapies usually religious in origin<br>Attempt home remedies first; poorer people do not seek help until illness serious<br>Usually seek help from:<br>    "Old lady"—woman in community with a common knowledge of herbs; consulted regarding pediatric care<br>    Spiritualist—has received gift from God for healing incurable diseases or solving personal problems; strongly based in Christianity<br>    Priest (voodoo priest/priestess)—most powerful healer<br>    Root doctor—meets need for herbs, oils, candles, and ointments<br>Prayer is common means for prevention and treatment |
| **Haitians*** | Illnesses have a supernatural or natural origin<br>Supernatural illnesses are caused by angry voodoo spirits, enemies, or the dead, especially deceased ancestors | Health is a personal responsibility<br>Foods have properties of "hot"/"cold" and "light"/"heavy" and must be in harmony with one's life cycle and bodily states |

*This section was written by Lydia DeSantis, RN, PhD.

# Cultural Characteristics Related to
# Health Care of Children and Families (cont'd)

| FAMILY RELATIONSHIPS | COMMUNICATION | COMMENTS |
|---|---|---|
| Parents expect respect and obedience from children | May avoid eye contact with health professionals as a sign of respect | |
| Family is highly valued, with strong family ties<br>Multigenerational family structure common, often with collateral members as well<br>Personal interests are subordinated to family interests and needs<br>Members avoid any behavior that would bring shame on the family | Immigrants and older persons may not be able to speak or understand English | Tend to have a fatalistic outlook on life<br>Believe time and providence will solve all |
| Strong kinship bonds in extended family; members come to aid of others in crisis<br>Less likely to view illness as a burden<br>Augmented families common (unrelated persons living in same household)<br>Place strong emphasis on work and ambition<br>Sex-role sharing among parents<br>Elderly members respected | Alert to any evidence of discrimination<br>Place importance on nonverbal behavior<br>May use nonstandard English or "Black English"<br>Use "testing" behaviors to assess personnel in health care situations before seeking active care<br>Best to use simple, direct, but caring approach | High level of caution/distrust of majority group<br>Social anxiety related to tradition of humiliation, oppression, and loss of dignity<br>Will elect to retain dignity rather than seek care if values are compromised<br>Strong sense of peoplehood<br>High incidence of poverty<br>Black minister a strong influence in black community<br>Visits by family minister are sought, expected, and valued in helping to cope with illness and suffering |
| Maintenance of family reputation is paramount<br>Lineal authority supreme; children in a subordinate position in family hierarchy | Recent immigrants and older persons may speak only Haitian creole<br>May prefer family/friends to act as translators and confidants | Will use biomedical and ethnomedical (folk) systems simultaneously<br>Resistant to dietary and work restrictions |

*Continued*

# Cultural Characteristics Related to Health Care of Children and Families (cont'd)

| CULTURAL GROUP | HEALTH BELIEFS | HEALTH PRACTICES |
|---|---|---|
| Haitians—cont'd | Natural illnesses are based on conceptions of natural causation:<br>Irregularities of blood volume, flow, purity, viscosity, color, and/or temperature (hot/cold)<br>Gas *(gaz)*<br>Movement and consistency of mother's milk<br>"Hot/cold" imbalance in the body<br>Bone displacement<br>Movement of diseases<br>Health is maintained by good dietary and hygienic habits | Natural illnesses are treated by home remedies first<br>Supernatural illness treated by healers: voodoo priest *(houngan)* or priestess *(mambo)*, midwife *(fam saj)*, and herbalist or leaf doctor *(dokte fey)*<br>Amulets and prayer used to protect against illness due to curses or willed by evil people |
| Hispanics<br>Mexicans<br>(Latinos,<br>Chicanos,<br>Raza-Latinos) | Health beliefs have strong religious association<br>Believe in body imbalance as a cause of illness, especially imbalance between **caliente** ("hot") and **frio** ("cold") or "wet" and "dry"<br>Some maintain good health is a result of "good luck"—a reward for good behavior<br>Illness prevented by performing properly, eating proper foods, and working proper amount of time; accomplished through prayer, wearing religious medals or amulets, and sleeping with relics at home<br>Illness is a punishment from God for wrongdoing, forces of nature, and the supernatural | Seek help from **curandero** or **curandera**, especially in rural areas<br>Curandero(a) receives his/her position by birth, apprenticeship, or a "calling" via dream or vision<br>Treatments involve use of herbs, rituals, and religious artifacts<br>Practice for severe illness—make promises, visit shrines, offer medals and candles, offer prayers<br>Adhere to "hot" and "cold" food prescriptions and prohibitions for prevention and treatment of illness |
| Puerto Ricans | Subscribe to the "hot-cold" theory of causation of illness<br>Believe some illness caused by evil spirits and forces | Infrequent use of health care systems<br>Seek folk healers—use of herbs, rituals<br>Consult spiritualist medium for mental disorders<br>**Santeria** is system, and practitioners are called **santeros**<br>Treatments classified as "hot" or "cold" |
| Cubans* | Prevention and good nutrition are related to good health | Diligent users of the medical model<br>Eclectic health-seeking practices, including preventive measures, and, in some instances, folk medicine of both religious and nonreligious origins; home remedies; in many instances seek assistance of santeros and spiritualists to complement medical treatment |

*This section was written by Mercedes Sandaval, PhD.

# Cultural Characteristics Related to
# Health Care of Children and Families (cont'd)

| FAMILY RELATIONSHIPS | COMMUNICATION | COMMENTS |
|---|---|---|
| Children valued for parental social security in old age and expected to contribute to family welfare at an early age<br>Children viewed as "gifts from God" and treated with indulgence and affection | Often smile and nod in agreement when do not understand<br>Quiet and gentle communication style and lack of assertiveness lead health care providers to falsely believe they comprehend health teaching and are compliant<br>Will not ask questions if health care provider is busy or rushed | Adherence to prescribed treatments directly related to perceived severity of illness |
| Traditionally men considered breadwinners and key decision makers in matters outside the home; women considered homemakers<br>Males considered big and strong **(macho)**<br>Strong kinship; extended families include **compadres** (godparents) established by ritual kinship<br>Children valued highly and desired, taken everywhere with family<br>Many homes contain shrines with statues and pictures of saints<br>Elderly treated with respect | May use nonstandard English<br>Some bilingual; many only speak Spanish<br>May have a strong preference for native language and revert to it in times of stress<br>May shake hands or engage in introductory embrace<br>Interpret prolonged eye contact as disrespectful | High degree of modesty—often a deterrent to seeking medical care and open discussions of sex<br>Youngsters often reluctant to share communal showers in schools<br>Relaxed concept of time—may be late for appointments<br>More concerned with present than with future and therefore may focus on immediate solutions rather than long-term goals<br>Magicoreligious practices common<br>May view hospital as place to go to die |
| Family usually large and home centered—the core of existence<br>Father has complete authority in family—family provider and decision maker<br>Wife and children subordinate to father<br>Children valued—seen as a gift from God<br>Children taught to obey and respect parents; corporal punishment to ensure obedience | May use nonstandard English<br>Spanish speaking or bilingual<br>Strong sense of family privacy—may view questions regarding family as impudent | Relaxed sense of time<br>Pay little attention to *exact* time of day<br>Suspicious and fearful of hospitals |
| Strong family ties with mother and father kinships<br>Children supported and assisted by parents long after becoming adults<br>Elderly cared for at home | Most are bilingual (English/Spanish) except for segments of the senior population | In less than 30 years Cubans have been able to obtain a higher standard of living than other Hispanic groups in U.S. |

*Continued*

# Cultural Characteristics Related to Health Care of Children and Families (cont'd)

| CULTURAL GROUP | HEALTH BELIEFS | HEALTH PRACTICES |
|---|---|---|
| **Hispanics**—cont'd<br>**Cubans**—<br>cont'd | | Nutrition is important; parents show overconcern with eating habits of their children and spend a considerable part of the budget on food; traditional Cuban diet is rich in meat and starch; consumption of fresh vegetables added in U.S. |
| **Native Americans** (numerous tribes) | Believe health is state of harmony with nature and universe<br>Respect of bodies through proper management<br>All disorders believed to have aspects of supernatural<br>Violation of a restriction or prohibition thought to cause illness<br>Fear of witchcraft<br>May carry objects believed to guard against witchcraft<br>Theology and medicine strongly interwoven | Medicine persons:<br>Altruistic persons who must use powers in purely positive ways<br>Persons capable of both good and evil—perform negative acts against enemies<br>Diviner-diagnosticians—diagnose but do not have powers or skill to implement medical treatment<br>Specialists—use herbs and curative but nonsacred medical procedures<br>Medicine persons—use herbs and ritual<br>Singers—cure by the power of their song obtained from supernatural beings; effect cures by laying on of hands |

# Cultural Characteristics Related to
# Health Care of Children and Families (cont'd)

| FAMILY RELATIONSHIPS | COMMUNICATION | COMMENTS |
|---|---|---|
| | | Have been able to retain many of their former social institutions: bilingual and private schools, clinics, social clubs, the family as an extended network of support, etc.<br>Many do not feel discriminated against or harbor feelings of inferiority with respect to Anglo-Americans or "mainstream" population |
| Extended family structure—usually includes relatives from both sides of family<br>Elder members assume leadership roles | Most continue to speak their Native American language, as well as English<br>Nonverbal communication | Time orientation—present<br>Respect for age<br>Going to hospital associated with illness or disease; therefore may not seek prenatal care because pregnancy viewed as natural process<br>Tend to take time to form an opinion of professionals<br>Sexual matters not openly discussed with members of opposite sex |

# Bloch's Ethnic/Cultural Assessment Guide

| CATEGORIES | GUIDELINE QUESTIONS/INSTRUCTIONS | DATA COLLECTED |
|---|---|---|
| *Cultural* | | |
| Ethnic origin | Does the patient identify with a particular ethnic group (e.g., Puerto Rican, African)? | |
| Race | What is the patient's racial background (e.g., Black, Filipino, American Indian)? | |
| Place of birth | Where was the patient born? | |
| Relocations | Where has he or she lived (country, city)? During what years did patient live there and for how long? Has he or she moved recently? | |
| Habits, customs, values, and beliefs | Describe habits, customs, values, and beliefs patient holds or practices that affect his or her attitude toward birth, life, death, health and illness, time orientation, and health care system and health care providers. What is degree of belief and adherence by patient to his or her overall cultural system? | |
| Behaviors valued by culture | How does patient value privacy, courtesy, respect for elders, behaviors related to family roles and sex roles, and work ethics? | |
| Cultural sanctions and restrictions | *Sanctions*—What is accepted behavior by patient's cultural group regarding expression of emotions and feelings, religious expressions, and response to illness and death? | |
| | *Restrictions*—Does patient have any restrictions related to sexual matters, exposure of body parts, certain types of surgery (e.g., hysterectomy), discussion of dead relatives, and discussion of fears related to the unknown? | |
| Language and communication processes: | What are some overall cultural characteristics of patient's language and communication process? | |
| Language(s) and/or dialect(s) spoken | Which language(s) and/or dialect(s) does patient speak most frequently? Where? At home or at work? | |
| Language barriers | Which language does patient predominantly use in thinking? Does patient need bilingual interpreter in nurse-patient interactions? Is patient non–English-speaking or limited English-speaking? Is patient able to read and/or write in English? | |
| Communication process | What are rules (linguistics) and modes (style) of communication process (e.g., "honorific" concept of showing "respect or deference" to others using words only common to specific ethnic/cultural group)? | |
| | Is there need for variation in technique of communicating and interviewing to accommodate patient's cultural background (e.g., tempo of conversation, eye/body contact, topic restrictions, norms of confidentiality, and style of explanation)? | |
| | Are there any conflicts in verbal and nonverbal interactions between patient and nurse? | |
| | How does patient's nonverbal communication process compare with other ethnic/cultural groups, and how does it affect patient's response to nursing and medical care? | |

Modified from Bloch B: Bloch's assessment guide for ethnic/cultural variations. In Orque MS, Bloch B, Monrroy LSA, editors: *Ethnic nursing care: a multicultural approach,* St Louis, 1983, Mosby, pp. 63-69.

# Bloch's Ethnic/Cultural Assessment Guide (cont'd)

| CATEGORIES | GUIDELINE QUESTIONS/INSTRUCTIONS | DATA COLLECTED |
|---|---|---|
| Communication process—cont'd | Are there any variations between patient's interethnic and interracial communication process or intracultural and intraracial communication process (e.g., ethnic minority patient and Caucasian middle-class nurse, ethnic minority patient and ethnic minority nurse; beliefs, attitudes, values, role variations, stereotyping [perceptions and prejudice])? | |
| **Healing beliefs and practices** Cultural healing system | What cultural healing system does the patient predominantly adhere to (e.g., Asian healing system, Raza/Latina Curanderismo)? What religious healing system does the patient predominantly adhere to (e.g., Seventh Day Adventist, West African voodoo, Fundamentalist sect, Pentacostal)? | |
| Cultural health beliefs | Is illness explained by the germ theory or cause-effect relationship, presence of evil spirits, imbalance between "hot" and "cold" (yang and yin in Chinese culture), or disequilibrium between nature and man? Is good health related to success, ability to work or fulfill roles, reward from God, or balance with nature? | |
| Cultural health practices | To what types of cultural healing practices does the person from ethnic/cultural group adhere? Does he or she use healing remedies to cure *natural* illnesses caused by the external environment (e.g., massage to cure *empacho* [a ball of food clinging to stomach wall], wearing of talismans or charms for protection against illness)? | |
| Cultural healers | Does patient rely on cultural healers [e.g., medicine men for American Indian, Curandero for Raza/Latina, Chinese herbalist, hougan (voodoo priest), spiritualist, or minister for African-American]? | |
| Nutritional variables or factors | What nutritional variables or factors are influenced by the patient's ethnic/cultural background? | |
| Characteristics of food preparation and consumption | What types of food preferences and restrictions, meaning of foods, style of food preparation and consumption, frequency of eating, time of eating, and eating utensils are culturally determined for patient? Are there any religious influences on food preparation and consumption? | |
| Influences from external environment | What modifications if any did the ethnic group that the patient identifies with have to make in its food practices in White dominant American society? Are there any adaptations of food customs and beliefs from rural setting to urban setting? | |
| Patient education needs | What are some implications of diet planning and teaching to patient who adheres to cultural practices concerning foods? | |
| *Sociological* Economic status | Who is principal wage earner in patient's family? What is total annual income (approximately) of family? What impact does economic status have on lifestyle, place of residence, living conditions, and ability to obtain health services? | |
| Educational status | What is highest educational level obtained? Does patient's educational back-ground influence his or her ability to understand how to seek health services, literature on health care, patient teaching experiences, and any written material patient is exposed to in health care setting (e.g., admission forms, patient care forms, teaching literature, and laboratory test forms)? | |

*Continued*

# Bloch's Ethnic/Cultural Assessment Guide (cont'd)

| CATEGORIES | GUIDELINE QUESTIONS/INSTRUCTIONS | DATA COLLECTED |
|---|---|---|
| Educational status—cont'd | Does patient's educational background cause him to feel inferior or superior to health care personnel in health care setting? | |
| Social network | What is patient's social network (kinship, peer, and cultural healing networks)? How do they influence health or illness status of patient? | |
| Family as supportive group | Does patient's family feel need for continuous presence in patient's clinical setting (is this an ethnic/cultural characteristic)? How is family valued during illness or death? | |
| | How does family participate in patient's nursing care process (e.g., giving baths, feeding, using touch as support [cultural meaning], supportive presence)? | |
| | How does ethnic/cultural family structure influence patient response to health or illness (e.g., roles, beliefs, strengths, weaknesses, and social class)? | |
| | Are there any key family roles characteristic of a specific ethnic/cultural group (e.g., grandmother in African-American and some Native American families), and can these key persons be a resource for health personnel? | |
| | What role does family play in health promotion or cause of illness (e.g., would family be intermediary group in patient interactions with health personnel and making decisions regarding his or her care)? | |
| Supportive institutions in ethnic/cultural community | What influence do ethnic/cultural institutions have on patient receiving health services (e.g., institutions such as Organization of Migrant Workers, NAACP, Black Political Caucus, churches, schools, Urban League, community clinics)? | |
| Institutional racism | How does institutional racism in health facilities influence patient's response to receiving health care? | |
| *Psychological* | | |
| Self-concept (identity) | Does patient show strong racial/cultural identity? How does this compare to that of other racial/cultural groups or to members of dominant society? | |
| | What factors in patient's development helped to shape his or her self-concept (e.g., family, peers, society labels, external environment, institutions, racism)? | |
| | How does patient deal with stereotypical behavior from health professionals? | |
| | What is impact of racism on patient from distinct ethnic/cultural group (e.g., social anxiety, noncompliance to health care process in clinical settings, avoidance of utilizing or participating in health care institutions)? | |
| | Does ethnic/cultural background have impact on how patient relates to body image change resulting from illness or surgery (e.g., importance to appearance and roles in cultural group)? | |
| | Any adherence or identification with ethnic/cultural "group" identity? (e.g., solidarity, "we" concept)? | |

# Bloch's Ethnic/Cultural Assessment Guide (cont'd)

| CATEGORIES | GUIDELINE QUESTIONS/INSTRUCTIONS | DATA COLLECTED |
|---|---|---|
| Mental and behavioral processes and characteristics of ethnic/cultural group | How does patient relate to his or her external environment in clinical setting (e.g., fears, stress, and adaptive mechanisms characteristic of a specific ethnic/cultural group)? Any variations based on the life span? What is patient's ability to relate to persons outside of his or her ethnic/cultural group (health personnel)? Is he or she withdrawn, verbally or nonverbally expressive, negative or positive, feeling mentally or physically inferior or superior? How does patient deal with feelings of loss of dignity and respect in clinical setting? | |
| Religious influences on psychological effects of health/illness | Does patient's religion have a strong impact on how he or she relates to health/illness influences or outcomes (e.g., death/chronic illness, cause and effect of illness, or adherence to nursing/medical practices)? Do religious beliefs, sacred practices, and talismans play a role in treatment of disease? What is role of significant religious persons during health/illness (e.g., African-American ministers, Catholic priests, Buddhist monks, Islamic imams)? | |
| Psychological/cultural response to stress and discomfort of illness | Based on ethnic/cultural background, does patient exhibit any variations in psychological response to pain or physical disability of disease processes? | |
| *Biological/ Physiological* (Consideration of *norms* for different ethnic/cultural groups) | | |
| Racial-anatomical characteristics | Does patient have any distinct racial characteristics (e.g., skin color, hair texture and color, color of mucous membranes)? Does patient have any variations in anatomical characteristics (e.g., body structure [height and weight] more prevalent for ethnic/cultural group, skeletal formation [pelvic shape, especially for obstetrical evaluation], facial shape and structure [nose, eye shape, facial contour], upper and lower extremities)? How do patient's racial and anatomical characteristics affect his or her self-concept and the way others relate to him or her? Does variation in racial-anatomical characteristics affect physical evaluations and physical care, skin assessment based on color, and variations in hair care and hygienic practices? | |
| Growth and development patterns | Are there any distinct growth and development characteristics that vary with patient's ethnic/cultural background (e.g., bone density, fat folds, motor ability)? What factors are important for nutritional assessment, neurological and motor assessment, assessment of bone deterioration in disease process or injury, evaluation of newborns, evaluation of intellectual status, or capacity in relationship to motor/sensory development in children? How do these differ in ethnic/cultural groups? | |

*Continued*

# Bloch's Ethnic/Cultural Assessment Guide (cont'd)

| CATEGORIES | GUIDELINE QUESTIONS/INSTRUCTIONS | DATA COLLECTED |
|---|---|---|
| Variations in body systems | Are there any variations in body systems for patient from distinct ethnic/cultural group (e.g., gastrointestinal disturbance with lactose intolerance in African Americans, nutritional intake of cultural foods causing adverse effects on gastrointestinal tract and fluid and electrolyte system, and variations in chemical and hematological systems [certain blood types prevalent in particular ethnic/cultural groups])? | |
| Skin and hair physiology, mucous membranes | How does skin color variation influence assessment of skin color changes (e.g., jaundice, cyanosis, ecchymosis, erythema, and its relationship to disease processes)? | |
| | What are methods of assessing skin color changes (comparing variations and similarities between different ethnic groups)? | |
| | Are there conditions of hypopigmentation and hyperpigmentation (e.g., vitiligo, mongolian spots, albinism, discoloration caused by trauma)? Why would these be more striking in some ethnic groups? | |
| | Are there any skin conditions more prevalent in a distinct ethnic group (e.g., keloids in African Americans)? | |
| | Is there any correlation between oral and skin pigmentation and their variations among distinct racial groups when doing assessment of oral cavity (e.g, leukoedema is normal occurrence in African Americans)? | |
| | What are variations in hair texture and color among racially different groups? Ask patient about preferred hair care methods or any racial/cultural restrictions (e.g., not washing "hot-combed" hair while in clinical setting, not cutting very long hair of Raza/Latina patients). | |
| | Are there any variations in skin care methods (e.g., using petroleum jelly on African-American skin)? | |
| Diseases more prevalent among ethnic/cultural group | Are there any specific diseases or conditions that are more prevalent for a specific ethnic/cultural group (e.g., hypertension, sickle cell anemia, G6-PD, lactose intolerance)? | |
| | Does patient have any socioenvironmental diseases common among ethnic/cultural groups (e.g., lead paint poisoning, poor nutrition, overcrowding [prone to tuberculosis], alcoholism resulting from psychological despair and alienation from dominant society, rat bites, poor sanitation)? | |
| To which diseases ethnic/cultural group has increased resistance | Are there any diseases that patient has increased resistance to because of racial/cultural background (e.g., skin cancer in African Americans)? | |

# Religious Beliefs that Affect Nursing Care

| BELIEFS ABOUT BIRTH AND DEATH | BELIEFS ABOUT DIET AND FOOD PRACTICES | BELIEFS REGARDING MEDICAL CARE | COMMENTS |
|---|---|---|---|
| **Adventist (Seventh-Day Adventist; Church of God; Christian Church)** | | | |
| **Birth:** Opposed to infant baptism; baptism in adulthood<br>**Death:** Believe the dead are asleep until the return of Jesus Christ, at which time final rewards and punishments will be given<br>**Organ donation/transplantation:** Individual and family have the right to receive or donate those organs that will restore any of the senses or will prolong life | Meat is prohibited in some groups<br>No alcohol, coffee, or tea | Some believe in divine healing and practice anointing with oil and use of prayer<br>May desire Communion or baptism when ill<br>Believe in man's choice and God's sovereignty<br>Some oppose hypnosis as therapy | Saturday is the biblical day of worship |
| **Baptist (27 Groups)** | | | |
| **Birth:** Opposed to infant baptism; believers are baptized by immersion as adults<br>**Death:** Clergy seeks to minister by counsel and prayer with patient and family<br>**Organ donation/transplantation:** Both organ donation and transplantation are generally approved of when they do not seriously endanger donor and when they offer medical hope for recipient; a transplant must offer possibility of physical improvement and extension of human life | Some groups discourage coffee, tea, and alcohol | "Laying on of hands" (some)<br>May encounter some resistance to some therapies, such as abortion<br>Believe God functions through physician<br>Some believe in predestination; may respond passively to care | Fundamentalist and conservative groups accept Bible as inspired word of God |
| **Black Muslim** | | | |
| **Birth:** No baptism<br>**Death:** Have a carefully prescribed procedure for washing and shrouding the dead and performing funeral rites<br>**Organ donation/transplantation:** To Muslims, life is precious; will accept a transplant if they need it to live | Prohibit alcohol, pork, and foods traditional among African Americans (e.g., corn bread, collard greens) | Faith healing is unacceptable<br>Always maintain personal habits of cleanliness | General adherence to Moslem tenets is overlaid, in many instances, by antagonism to whites, especially Christians and Jews<br>Do not indulge in activities (such as sleeping) more than is necessary to health |

Sources: Carpenito, 1992; Conley, 1990; Kozier, Erb, 1995; McQuay, 1995; Spector, 1985.
From Wong DL: *Whaley and Wong's nursing care of infants and children,* ed 6, St Louis, 1999, Mosby, pp. 57-62.

*Continued*

# Religious Beliefs that Affect Nursing Care (cont'd)

| BELIEFS ABOUT BIRTH AND DEATH | BELIEFS ABOUT DIET AND FOOD PRACTICES | BELIEFS REGARDING MEDICAL CARE | COMMENTS |
|---|---|---|---|
| **Buddhist Churches of America** | | | |
| **Birth:** No infant baptism; infant presentation<br>**Death:** "Last rite" chanting is often practiced at bedside soon after death; the deceased's Buddhist priest should be contacted, or family should contact him<br>**Organ donation/transplantation:** Believe that organ donation is a matter of individual conscience; there is no written resolution on the issue | No requirements or restrictions<br>Some sects are strictly vegetarian<br>Discourage use of alcohol and drugs | Illness is believed to be a trial to aid development of soul; illness due to Karmic causes<br>May be reluctant to have surgery or certain treatments on holy days<br>Cleanliness is believed to be of great importance<br>Family may request Buddhist priest for counseling | Optimistic outlook; teach ways to overcome fears, anxieties, apprehension |
| **Church of Christ Scientist (Christian Science)** | | | |
| **Birth:** No baptism<br>**Death:** No "last rites"; autopsy is not permitted except in cases of sudden death; it is an individual's decision to choose burial or cremation<br>**Organ donation/transplantation:** Church takes no specific position on transplantation or donation as distinct from other medical or surgical procedures; members normally rely on spiritual rather than medical means for healing, but they are free to choose whatever form of medical treatment they desire, including organ transplantation | No requirements or restrictions | Deny the existence of health crisis; see sickness and sin as errors of the mind that can be altered by prayer<br>Oppose human intervention with drugs or other therapies; however, accept legally required immunizations<br>Many adhere to belief that disease is human mental concept that can be dispelled by "spiritual truth" to extent that they refuse all medical treatment | Many desire services of practitioner or reader; will sometimes refuse even emergency treatment until they have consulted a reader<br>Unlikely to donate organs for transplant |
| **Church of Jesus Christ of Latter Day Saints (Mormon)** | | | |
| **Birth:** No baptism at birth; infant is "blessed" by church official at first opportunity after birth (in church); baptism by immersion at 8 years<br>**Death:** Believe that it is proper to bury the dead in the ground, and cremation is discouraged; baptism of the dead is held as essential, although a living person may serve | Prohibit tea, coffee, alcohol<br>Some individuals avoid chocolate and other products that contain caffeine<br>Encourage sparing use of meats<br>Fasting for 24 hours on first Sunday of each month (from after | Devout adherents believe in divine healing through anointment with oil and "laying on of hands" by church officials (appointed church members)<br>Medical therapy is not prohibited | May request **Sacrament** on Sunday while in hospital<br>Financial support for sick is available through well-funded welfare system<br>Discourage cremation<br>Discourage use of tobacco<br>Married adults wear special undergarments |

# Religious Beliefs that Affect Nursing Care (cont'd)

| BELIEFS ABOUT BIRTH AND DEATH | BELIEFS ABOUT DIET AND FOOD PRACTICES | BELIEFS REGARDING MEDICAL CARE | COMMENTS |
|---|---|---|---|
| *Church of Jesus Christ of Latter Day Saints (Mormon)—cont'd* | | | |
| as proxy; preaching of the gospel to the dead is also practiced<br>**Organ donation/transplantation:** Question of whether one should will his or her organs to be used as transplants or for research after death must be answered from deep within conscience of the individual involved | evening meal Saturday until evening meal Sunday) | | |
| *Eastern Orthodox (Turkey, Egypt, Syria, Rumania, Bulgaria, Cyprus, Albania, etc.)* | | | |
| **Birth:** Most believe in infant baptism by immersion 8 to 40 days after birth<br>**Death:** "Last rites" are obligatory if death is impending; cremation is discouraged<br>**Organ donation/transplantation:** No religious conflict; both are permitted | Restrictions depend on specific sect | Anointment of the sick<br>No conflict with medical science | Discourage cremation |
| *Episcopal (Anglican)* | | | |
| **Birth:** Infant baptism is mandatory; urgent if poor prognosis<br>**Death:** "Last rites" (Rite for Anointing of the Sick) are not mandatory for all members; when death is imminent, family and pastor are gathered, and it is usually highly desirable to have Litany at the Time of Death read; infant baptism is mandatory and especially urgent if prognosis is poor, although aborted fetuses and stillborns are not baptized<br>**Organ donation/transplantation:** Find nothing offensive in organ donation/transplantation as long as moral integrity of donor is not violated | Abstain from meat on fast days<br>May fast on Wednesday, Friday, during Lent, and before Christmas<br>Some fast for 6 hours before receiving Holy Communion | Some believe in spiritual healing<br>Rite for anointing of the sick is available but not mandatory | Religious icons are very important<br>Communion four times yearly: Christmas, Easter, June 30, and August 15; may be mandatory for some |
| *Friends (Quakers)* | | | |
| **Birth:** No baptism; infant's name is recorded in official book | No requirements or restrictions<br>Most practice moderation | No special rites or restrictions | Believe in plain speech and dress<br>Pacifists |

*Continued*

# Religious Beliefs that Affect Nursing Care (cont'd)

| BELIEFS ABOUT BIRTH AND DEATH | BELIEFS ABOUT DIET AND FOOD PRACTICES | BELIEFS REGARDING MEDICAL CARE | COMMENTS |
|---|---|---|---|
| *Friends (Quakers)—cont'd* **Death:** Do not believe in life after this life; God is in every person and can be approached directly **Organ donation/transplantation:** Are in agreement with philosophy and concepts of organ donation/ transplantation; both are permitted | Avoid alcohol and illicit drugs | | |
| *Greek Orthodox* **Birth:** Baptism is considered important; performed 40 days after birth; if not possible to baptize by sprinkling or immersion, church allows child baptism "in the air" by moving child in the form of a cross as appropriate words are said **Death:** "Last rites" are Sacrament of Holy Communion; death rituals play a crucial role in life of family; death must be properly mourned, or else dead person may not be fully incorporated in world of the dead and may return to world of the living and inflict harm on close relatives **Organ donation/transplantation:** Organ transplantation such as skin grafting and blood transfusions from one human to another have always been acceptable; this is extended to include kidney transplants, heart transplants, etc.; life of donor, however, is of equal importance | Church-prescribed fast periods—usually occur on Wednesday, Friday, and during Lent; consist of avoiding meat and (in some cases) dairy products If health is compromised, priest may be contacted to convince family to forego fasting | Each health crisis is handled by ordained priest; deacon may also serve in some cases Holy Communion is administered in hospital Some may desire Sacrament of the Holy Unction performed by priest | Oppose euthanasia Believe every reasonable effort should be made to preserve life until termination by God Discourage autopsies that may cause dismemberment Prefer burial to cremation |
| *Hindu* **Birth:** No ritual **Death:** Certain prescribed rites are followed after death; priest may tie thread around neck or wrist to signify blessing, and this should not be removed; immediately after | Many dietary restrictions Beef and veal are not eaten Some are strict vegetarians | Illness or injury is believed to represent sins committed in previous life Accept most modern medical practices | Cremation is preferred |

# Religious Beliefs that Affect Nursing Care (cont'd)

| BELIEFS ABOUT BIRTH AND DEATH | BELIEFS ABOUT DIET AND FOOD PRACTICES | BELIEFS REGARDING MEDICAL CARE | COMMENTS |
|---|---|---|---|
| *Hindu—cont'd* <br> death, priest will pour water into the mouth of the corpse, and family will wash the body; are particular about who touches their dead; bodies are to be cremated <br> **Organ donation/transplantation:** According to Hindu Temple of North America, they are not prohibited by religious laws from donating their organs; this is an individual decision | | | |
| *Islam (Muslim/Moslem)* <br> **Birth:** No baptism <br> **Death:** Must confess sins and beg forgiveness before death, and family should be present; family washes and prepares the body and then turns it to face Mecca; only relatives and friends may touch the body, and unless required by law, there should be no autopsy; no body part should be removed unless for donation <br> **Organ donation/transplantation:** Moslem Religious Council initially rejected organ donation by followers of Islam, but it has since reversed its position, provided that donors consent in advance in writing; organs of Moslem donors must be transplanted immediately and not stored in organ banks | Prohibit all pork products and any meat that is not ritually slaughtered <br> Daylight fasting is practiced during ninth month of Muhammadan year (Ramadan) <br> Strict Muslims do not use alcohol or mind-altering drugs | Faith healing is not acceptable unless psychologic condition of patient is deteriorating; performed for morale <br> Ritual washing after prayer; prayer takes place five times daily (on rising, midday, afternoon, early evening, and before bed); during prayer, face Mecca and kneel on prayer rug | Older Muslims often have a fatalistic view that may interfere with compliance to therapy <br> May oppose autopsy |
| *Jehovah's Witness* <br> **Birth:** No baptism <br> **Death:** No official "last rites" practiced when death occurs <br> **Organ donation/transplantation:** No definite statement related to this issue; do not encourage organ donation but believe it is a matter for individual conscience, according to Watch Tower Society (legal | Eat nothing to which blood has been added; can eat animal flesh that has been drained | Adherents are generally absolutely opposed to transfusions of whole blood, packed red blood cells, platelets, and fresh or frozen plasma, including banking of own blood; individuals can sometimes | Often possible to obtain a court order appointing a hospital official as temporary guardian to consent to a child's transfusion when parents refuse consent <br> Autopsy is approved only as required by law |

*Continued*

# Religious Beliefs that Affect Nursing Care (cont'd)

| BELIEFS ABOUT BIRTH AND DEATH | BELIEFS ABOUT DIET AND FOOD PRACTICES | BELIEFS REGARDING MEDICAL CARE | COMMENTS |
|---|---|---|---|
| *Jehovah's Witness—cont'd* corporation for the religion); all organs and tissues, however, must be completely drained of blood before transplantation | | be persuaded in emergencies<br>May be opposed to use of albumin, globulin, factor replacement (hemophilia), vaccines<br>Not opposed to nonblood plasma expanders | No restrictions on giving blood sample |
| *Judaism (Orthodox and Conservative)*<br>**Birth:** No baptism; ritual circumcision of male infants on eighth day; performed by Mohel (ritual circumciser familiar with Jewish law and aseptic technique); reform Jews favor ritual circumcision, but not as a religious imperative<br>**Death:** According to tradition, during last moments of life, relatives and close friends remain with the deceased; it is considered a matter of great respect to watch over a person as he or she passes from this world to the next<br>**Organ donation/transplantation:** Donation or transplantation of organs requires rabbinical consultation; sanctity of the human body covers each of its members and organs, so where any part of the body is separated from the corpus it, too, requires burial; where an organ is to be transplanted to save the life of a patient or improve his or her health, however, it is permitted; saving a human life takes precedence over maintaining sanctity of the human body | Numerous dietary kosher laws exist that may be influenced by local practices and family and cultural tradition<br>Are allowed only meat from animals that are vegetable eaters, are cloven hoofed, chew their cud, and are ritually slaughtered; fish that have scales and fins<br>Prohibit any combination of meat and milk; milk products served first can be followed by meat in a few minutes, but milk may not be consumed for several hours after eating meat<br>Fasting for 24 hours is part of Yom Kippur observance<br>Matzo replaces leavened bread during Passover week | May resist surgical procedures during Sabbath, which extends from sundown Friday until sundown Saturday<br>Seriously ill and pregnant women are exempt from fasting<br>Illness is grounds for violating dietary laws (e.g., patient with congestive heart failure does not have to use kosher meats, which are high in sodium) | Oppose all forms of mutilation, including autopsy; amputated limbs, organs, or surgically removed tissues should be made available to family for burial<br>Donation or transplantation of organs requires rabbinical consent<br>May oppose prolongation of life after irreversible brain damage |
| *Lutheran*<br>**Birth:** Baptize only living infants shortly after birth | No requirements or restrictions | Church or pastor is notified of hospitalization | Accept scientific developments |

# Religious Beliefs that Affect Nursing Care (cont'd)

| BELIEFS ABOUT BIRTH AND DEATH | BELIEFS ABOUT DIET AND FOOD PRACTICES | BELIEFS REGARDING MEDICAL CARE | COMMENTS |
|---|---|---|---|
| *Lutheran—cont'd*<br>**Death:** "Last rites" are optional<br>**Organ donation/transplantation:** Ability to transplant organs from a deceased person to a living person is considered a genuine medical advancement; both are acceptable and encouraged | | Communion may be given before or after surgery or similar crisis | |
| *Mennonite (Similar to Amish)*<br>**Birth:** No baptism in infancy; baptism during early or middle teens<br>**Death:** No formal prescribed action; personal assistance and prayer as appropriate while patient is still conscious is necessary<br>**Organ donation/transplantation:** No religious conflict, so both organ donation and transplantation are acceptable | No requirements or restrictions | No illness rituals<br>Deep concern for dignity and self-determination of individual that would conflict with shock treatment or medical treatment affecting personality or will | |
| *Methodist*<br>**Birth:** No baptism at birth; performed on children or adults<br>**Death:** Believe in divine punishment after death; good will be rewarded and evil punished<br>**Organ donation/transplantation:** Church encourages "people of ethical concern in various relevant fields to get together to engage in study and direction of these developments," recognizing that they offer great potentialities for enhancing health while at the same time raising serious issues for traditional views of human nature and value | No requirements or restrictions | Communion may be requested before surgery or similar crisis | Encourage donations of body or body parts to medical science |
| *Nazarene*<br>**Birth:** Baptism optional<br>**Death:** No last rites | No requirements or restrictions<br>Alcohol is prohibited | Church official administers Communion and laying on of hands<br>Adherents believe in divine healing but not exclusive of medical treatment | Cremation is permitted |

*Continued*

# Religious Beliefs that Affect Nursing Care (cont'd)

| BELIEFS ABOUT BIRTH AND DEATH | BELIEFS ABOUT DIET AND FOOD PRACTICES | BELIEFS REGARDING MEDICAL CARE | COMMENTS |
|---|---|---|---|
| *Pentecostal (Assembly of God, Four-Square)* | | | |
| **Birth:** No baptism at birth; baptism by complete immersion after age of accountability | Abstain from alcohol, eating blood, strangled animals, or anything to which blood has been added | No restrictions regarding medical care | Some insist illness is divine punishment; most consider it an intrusion of Satan |
| **Death:** No official "last rites" practiced when death occurs | Some individuals may resist pork | Deliverance from sickness is provided for in atonement; may pray for divine intervention in health matters and seek God in prayer for themselves and others when ill | Practice glossolalia (speaking in tongues) |
| **Organ donation/transplantation:** No official position on organ donation/transplantation | | | |
| *Orthodox Presbyterian* | | | |
| **Birth:** Infant baptism by sprinkling | No requirements or restrictions | Communion is administered when appropriate and convenient | Full forgiveness is granted for any illness connected with a sin |
| **Death:** "Last rites" are not a sacramental procedure and are not performed; instead, they read scripture and pray | | Blood transfusion is accepted when advisable | |
| **Organ donation/transplantation:** Encourage and endorse organ donation; respect individual conscience and a person's right to make decisions regarding his or her own body | | Pastor or elder should be called for ill person. Believe science should be used for relief of suffering | |
| *Roman Catholic* | | | |
| **Birth:** Infant baptism is mandatory; especially urgent if poor prognosis, when it may be performed by anyone | Fasting (eating only one full meal and no eating between meals) and abstaining from meat are mandatory on Ash Wednesday and Good Friday; fasting is optional during Lent; no meat on Fridays during Lent as a general rule | Encourage anointing of the sick, although this may be interpreted by older members of church as equivalent to old terminology "extreme unction" or "last rites"; they may require careful explanation if reluctance is associated with fear of imminent death | Family may request that major amputated limb be buried in consecrated ground |
| **Death:** Rite for Anointing of the Sick is a sacrament for the living; if prognosis is poor while patient is alive, patient or his or her family may request it. | Children and most hospital patients are exempt from fasting | Traditional church teaching does not approve of contraceptives or abortion | Transplant is accepted as long as loss of organ does not deprive donor of life or functional integrity of body |
| **Organ donation/transplantation:** Transplantation of organs is viewed by Catholics as ethically and morally acceptable to Vatican; organ donation is an act of charity, fraternal love, and self-sacrifice; transplantation of organs from living donors is permissible when anticipated benefit to recipient is proportionate to harm done | Some older Catholics may adhere to older rule of no meat on Friday | | Autopsy is acceptable. Religious articles are important |

# Religious Beliefs that Affect Nursing Care (cont'd)

| BELIEFS ABOUT BIRTH AND DEATH | BELIEFS ABOUT DIET AND FOOD PRACTICES | BELIEFS REGARDING MEDICAL CARE | COMMENTS |
|---|---|---|---|
| *Roman Catholic—cont'd* to donor (provided that loss of such organ[s] does not deprive donor of life itself or of functional integrity of his or her own body) | | | |
| *Russian Orthodox* **Birth:** Baptism by priest only **Death:** Traditionally after death, arms are crossed, fingers set in a cross | No meat or dairy products on Wednesday, Friday, and during Lent | Cross necklace is important and should be removed only when necessary and replaced as soon as possible Adherents believe in divine healing, but not exclusive of medical treatment | Opposed to autopsy, embalming, or cremation |
| *Unitarian Universalist* **Birth:** Some practice infant baptism; most consider it unnecessary **Death:** No ritual | No requirements or restrictions | Most believe in general goodness of their fellow humans and appreciate expression of that goodness by visits from clergy and fellow parishioners during times of illness | Cremation is preferred to burial Believe in fully living this life as they know and understand it |

# Family Assessment Guide

Family name _____ Family ID no. _____

Source of referral _____

Reason for referral _____

Occupational status _____

Health insurance _____

Medical emergency plan _____

Preventive health care _____

Community agencies involved with family _____

*Family composition:* Map family constellation; include health problems of individual members.

| DATE | | | RATING | | |
|------|------|-------------------|------|------|----------------|
| **1ST** | **2ND** | **ASSESSMENT PARAMETERS** | **1ST** | **2ND** | **SIGNIFICANT DATA** |
| | | 1. *Structural characteristics*<br>  a. Family composition<br>  b. Financial resources<br>  c. Educational experiences<br>  d. Allocation of family and personal roles<br>  e. Division of labor<br>  f. Distribution of power and authority<br>  g. Cultural influences<br>    • Health beliefs and attitudes<br>    • Family goals<br>    • Norms for social behavior<br>    • Spiritual beliefs<br>    • Beliefs about folk diseases and medicine<br>  h. Activities of daily living<br>    • Dietary habits<br>    • Child-rearing practices<br>    • Housekeeping<br>    • Sleeping arrangements<br>    • Laundry facilities<br>    • Transportation<br>    • Child care arrangements<br>  i. Family health status/practices<br>    • Health history<br>    • Health status of family members (relevant diagnoses and treatment regimens)<br>    • Knowledge of health problems<br>    • Health risk factors (e.g., dietary, substance abuse, or current stressors)<br>    • Prevention practices (primary, secondary, and tertiary)<br>    • Care arrangements for ill family members | | | |

*Note:* Code for recording assessment data—use a different color ink for the first and second assessment or rating (generally it takes several home visits to complete a family assessment). Rating scale: 1 = strength; 2 = problem; 3 = anticipatory guidance warranted; 4 = problem—family does not wish to change this area of functioning at this time; 5 = not applicable. Family functioning should be rated every 4 months to assist in evaluating family progress and nursing intervention strategies.

# Family Assessment Guide (cont'd)

| DATE | | ASSESSMENT PARAMETERS | RATING | | SIGNIFICANT DATA |
|------|------|------|------|------|------|
| **1ST** | **2ND** | | **1ST** | **2ND** | |
| | | 1. *Structural characteristics—cont'd*<br> i. Family health status/practices—cont'd<br>  • Source of preventive and curative health care<br>  • Barriers to health care<br>2. *Process characteristics*<br> a. Atmosphere of home<br> b. Communication patterns<br> c. Decision-making processes<br>  • How decisions are made<br>  • How decisions are implemented<br> d. Conflict negotiation<br> e. Achievement of developmental tasks<br> f. Adaptation to change<br> g. Autonomy of individual family members<br>3. *Relationships with external systems*<br> a. How family boundaries are established<br> b. Use of information from environment<br> c. Contact with extended families<br> d. Interactions with friends and neighbors<br> e. Attitudes about community systems<br>  • Health<br>  • Welfare<br>  • Educational<br>  • Others (describe)<br> f. Use of the referral process<br>  • Ability to seek assistance<br>  • Level of independence<br>4. *Environmental characteristics*<br> a. Neighborhood<br>  • Accessibility of facilities to meet basic needs<br>  • Availability of recreational, educational, religious, and other resources<br>  • Safety (physical and psychosocial)<br> b. Housing<br>  • Suitability in relation to family needs<br>  • Condition of structural components<br>  • Suitability of home furnishings<br>  • Sanitation (water source, sewage and garbage disposal, and housekeeping practices)<br>  • Accident hazards<br>  • Barriers to family mobility | | | |

Professionals and volunteers working with family (identify person and agency) _____

Summary of family strengths (based on categories rated No. 1) _____

Description of family priorities and assistance desired _____

Specific factors to consider when developing and implementing a family care plan _____

Assessor _____ Date _____

Assessor _____ Date _____

Assessor _____ Date _____

# 8

# Foundations for Family Intervention: Families Under Stress

*Susan Clemen-Stone*

---

## OBJECTIVES

*Upon completion of this chapter, the reader should be able to:*

1. Discuss the concepts of stress and crisis as they relate to family functioning.
2. Describe factors that affect the outcome of a family crisis.
3. Identify characteristics that signal ineffective individual or family coping during periods of stress and crisis.
4. Differentiate between normative and nonnormative stressors and give examples of each type of stressor.

5. Describe general principles that the community health nurse should apply when giving constructive assistance to families during periods of stress and crisis.
6. Explain nursing intervention strategies used by community health nurses to promote effective family functioning during periods of stress and crisis.
7. Describe how cultural factors influence perceptions of stress and crisis.

---

## KEY TERMS

ABCX Model of Family Stress
Adaptation
Crisis sequence
Distress
Eustress
Evil eye phenomenon
Family coping
Family coping strategies
Family crisis

Family health promotion
Family Inventory of Life Events and Changes (FILE)
Family perception
Family stress
Family system resources
General adaptation syndrome (GAS)
Health education process
Homeostasis

Natural explanations of illness
Nonnormative stressors
Normative stressors
Resiliency Model of Family Stress, Adjustment, and Adaptation
Social networks
Social support
Stressor
Unnatural explanations of illness

---

*Accept me as I am so I may learn what I can become.*

---

A major responsibility of the community health nurse is to help individuals and families handle stressful life events so that their energies can be used to achieve self-fulfillment and extend themselves to others. Although stress is normal and essential for life and growth, too much stress prevents people from seeing what they can become.

Stress provides the stimulus needed to adapt to the ever-changing conditions of life. When Selye (1976) examined individual stress, he found that any emotion or activity, whether it produces joy or sadness, causes stress. He noted

that stressful life events often result in disease and unhappiness when individuals are not prepared to handle these events. Persons frequently are not prepared to handle unexpected stressors, such as a new diagnosis of a chronic illness or the accidental death of a close family member. Individuals who encounter these types of stressors often do not recognize the signals of distress that reflect a need to mobilize different coping mechanisms.

Boss (1988) focuses on examining the concept of stress from a family perspective. She defines family stress as "pressure or tension in the family system. It is disturbance in the steady state of the family" (p. 12). This disturbance results from events or situations that have potential to cause change, and it is normal and even desirable at times (Boss, 1988). Stress is a dynamic state that can assist families in mobilizing stress management processes that promote growth for the family as a whole, as well as for individual family members. Boss contends that when addressing stress within a family system "the focus on the family system should not come at the expense of individuals within that system" (Boss, 1988, p. 19). However, she does believe that the stress level of the family unit, as well as individual family members, should be assessed when a change occurs in the family system. Both the family unit and individual family members may need assistance in coping with this change.

Community health nurses are in a key position to help individuals and families adapt to new or threatening life changes. In their work in the home and other settings they encounter clients who are experiencing various degrees of stress. Many times these clients have not had life experiences or exposure to knowledge that would assist them in achieving patterns of functioning that would help them minimize stress. Most parents, for instance, have not been prepared to handle children whose growth and development significantly deviate from the norm. Hence, they experience heightened distress and are frequently open to professional intervention. Illustrative of this is the scenario encountered by a community health nurse when she visited the Slavovi family for the first time.

The Slavovi family was referred to the community health nurse for health supervision follow-up after the birth of their fourth child, Stephanie, who had multiple disabilities. Even though this was the family's first exposure to community health nursing service, Mr. and Mrs. Slavovi talked freely when the nurse visited. Both manifested high levels of anxiety and confusion about how to care for their newborn infant. Mr. and Mrs. Slavovi had always taken great pride in being good parents. Stephanie's physical and mental disabilities were particularly distressing to them: "We don't know how to help her. She continues to cry even when we hold her and seems to hurt all the time. Children need loving. Why doesn't Stephanie want us to hold her? We must be doing something wrong."

Having an understanding of the concept of stress helps the community health nurse intervene more effectively with clients like the Slavovis. Stress theory provides the foundation for identifying signs and symptoms of distress and for recognizing potential stressors. It also provides clues about how to bring about change when a client's usual methods of coping are no longer effective.

## THE STRESS PHENOMENON

Although the term *stress* dates back to the fourteenth century, Hans Selye's work during the twentieth century on the physiological and psychological effects of stress on the human body (Box 8-1) played a major role in strengthening the scientific nature of this concept (Lazarus, Folkman,

### BOX 8-1

*Examples of Physiological and Psychological Signals of Stress*

*Physiological signals*
- Pounding of the heart
- Dryness of the throat and mouth
- Sweating
- Frequent need to urinate
- Diarrhea, indigestion, vomiting
- Migraine headaches
- Missed menstrual period
- Loss of or excessive appetite
- Increased smoking and alcohol and drug use
- Increased use of legally prescribed drugs (e.g., tranquilizers or amphetamines)
- Pain in neck or lower back

*Psychological signals*
- General irritability, hyperexcitation, or depression
- Impulsive behavior, emotional instability
- Overpowering urge to cry or run and hide
- Inability to concentrate, flight of thoughts, and general disorientation
- Floating anxiety
- Trembling, nervous tics
- Nightmares
- Neurotic or psychotic behavior
- Accident proneness

From Selye H: *The stress of life*, New York, 1976, McGraw-Hill, pp. 174-177.

1984). Selye (1976) defined stress as "the nonspecific response of the body to any demand" (p. 1). A demand that produces stress is known as a **stressor**. A stressor can produce unpleasant or disease-producing stress, known as distress, or good, pleasant, or curative stress, known as eustress (Selye, 1976).

A nonspecific set of responses in the nervous and endocrine systems alerts individuals to the occurrence of distress or eustress. This set of responses evolves in the following three stages, which Selye (1976) labeled the ***general adaptation syndrome* (GAS):**
1. The *alarm reaction*, during which defense mechanisms are mobilized;
2. The *stage of resistance*, when adaptation is acquired because optimum channels of defense were developed; and
3. The *stage of exhaustion*, which reflects a depletion of adaptation energy necessary to cope with prolonged and intensified stress (p. 163).

Stress theory is based on the concepts of homeostasis (state of physiological balance) and adaptation. Because stress is an inherent and integral part of life, individuals must constantly readjust to maintain themselves. A state of balance is maintained when a person learns to recognize the signals of distress and then adapts or changes functioning to meet the demands of the stressor encountered. Individuals differ significantly in how they respond to and cope with these demands.

Lazarus's (1966) classic work on psychological stress highlighted the importance of examining individual responses to environmental demands and pressures. He believed that "although certain environmental demands and pressures produce stress in a substantial number of people, individual and group differences in the degree and kind of reaction are always evident" (Lazarus, Folkman, 1984, p. 22). For example, many people perceive job loss as a significant threat to their financial security, but some individuals view this event as a challenging opportunity for growth. This difference is influenced by a person's cognitive appraisal of a stressor event. "Psychological stress is a particular relationship between the person and the environment that is appraised by the person as taxing or exceeding his or her resources and endangering his or her well-being" (Lazarus, Folkman, 1984, p. 19). The factors that influence an individual's cognitive appraisal of a stressor event are discussed in a later section of this chapter.

## FAMILY STRESS

Boss (1988) believes that families "have a distinctive quality apart from the individuals making up the family" (p. 18). In keeping with this view, she assumes "that a family system has a character of its own and that this unity produces the variable, **family perception**" (Boss, 1988, p. 19). This perception influences the family's appraisal of stressful events or change in the family system and the coping processes mobilized by the family to deal with those events. Like individuals, families differ significantly in how they respond to and cope with stressor events in their environment.

Family stress is manifested by ineffective family patterns, as well as by the occurrence of physiological and psychological signs and symptoms of stress in its individual family members. Strained communication patterns and difficulty carrying out activities of daily living are examples of ineffective family patterns that may result when a family is experiencing stress. Other examples are shared in Chapter 7. All individuals and families have the capacity to deal with stress. To do so, they need to learn the boundaries of stress that they can tolerate and the nurturing, coping, and adaptive resources that promote growth and homeostasis.

### Family Stress Models

Complex and dynamic interactions between multiple variables influence a family's abilities to effectively mobilize resources to prevent crisis. Hill (1949, p. 9; 1965), the father of family stress theory, illustrated this complexity in his classic **ABCX Model of Family Stress.** He proposed that the interactions between the following factors influence whether

a family under stress experiences a crisis: **A** (the event and associated hardships) interacting with **B** (the family's crisis-meeting resources; its role structure, flexibility, and previous history with crisis) interacting with **C** (the definition the family makes of the event) produces **X** (crisis).

Hill believed that a crisis-prone family was one who experienced stressor events with great frequency and severity (A), defined these events more frequently as crisis-provoking (C), had meager crisis-meeting resources (B), and had failed to learn from past experience with crises (Hill, 1965, p. 40).

In addition to identifying the variables that lead to a family crisis, the ABCX Model of Family Stress examines family adjustment during a crisis. During a crisis, families go through a period of disorganization, a period or "angle" of recovery, and lastly a period of reorganization where a new level of family function evolves (Hill, 1965). This new level of family functioning may be at a level the same as, better than, or worse than the precrisis level.

Most family stress theorists have built on the work of Reuben Hill and confirm and expand his theories about the dynamic and complex nature of family stress and coping (Boss, 1987, 1988; McCubbin, McCubbin, 1987, 1991, 1993; McCubbin, Patterson, 1983, 1991). McCubbin and McCubbin's (1993) **Resiliency Model of Family Stress, Adjustment, and Adaptation** (Figure 8-1) proposes that seldom is a single stressor at the root of family crisis. Rather, a "pile up of stressors" causes crisis situations in families. Family vulnerability to stress, "ranging from high to low, is determined by (1) the accumulation, or pile up, of demands on or within the family unit, such as financial debts, poor health status of relatives, and changes in a parent's work role or work environment, and (2) the trials and tribulations associated with the family's particular life-cycle stage with all of its demands and changes" (p. 28).

McCubbin, Thompson, and McCubbin (1996) focus on family change and adaptation over time and examine adaptation-oriented components during and beyond the initial crisis. They believe that a family's adjustment during periods of stress is influenced by several variables: (1) the severity of the stressor, (2) the family's vulnerability or pile up of stressors, (3) the family's definition or appraisal of a stressor, (4) the family's problem-solving and coping abilities, (5) the family's resistance resources or strengths the family uses to cope, (6) the family's established patterns of functioning, and (7) the family's abilities and capabilities to address and manage the stressor without introducing major changes in the family system (McCubbin, Thompson, McCubbin, 1996, p. 16).

The Resiliency Model of Family Stress, Adjustment, and Adaptation has two phases: the adjustment phase and the adaptation phase (see Figure 8-1). During the adjustment phase, if minor changes in established patterns of family functioning are not adequate to deal with current family stressors, a crisis evolves and the adaptation phase of the model begins. "Family crisis is conceptualized in the model

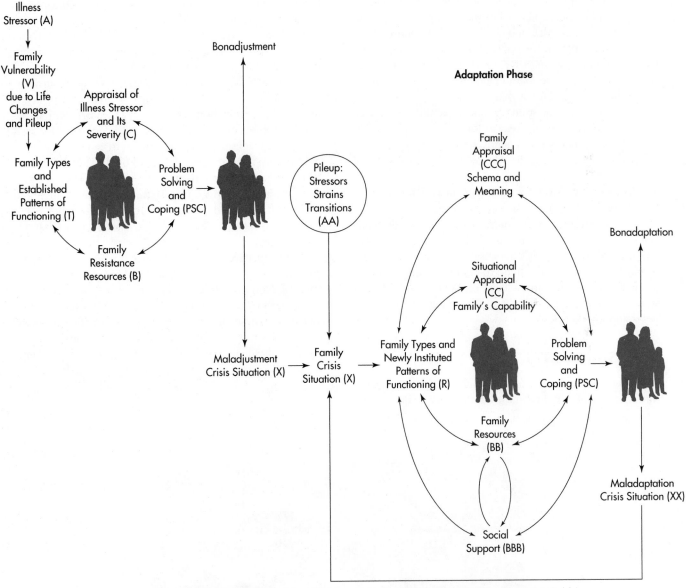

**FIGURE 8-1** The Resiliency Model of Family Stress Adjustment and Adaptation. (From McCubbin MA, McCubbin HI: Families coping with illness: the resiliency model of family stress, adjustment, and adaptation. In Danielson CB, Hamel-Bissell BP, Winstend-Fry P, editors: *Families, health, and illness: perspectives on coping and intervention,* ed 3, St Louis, 1993, Mosby, p. 23.)

as a continuous condition of disruptiveness, disorganization, or incapacitation in the family social system" (Burr, 1973, cited in McCubbin, McCubbin, 1993, p. 31; Friedman, Svavarsdottir, McCubbin, 1998, p. 443).

During the adaptation phase of the Resiliency Model of Family Stress, Adjustment, and Adaptation, the family needs to make change in its patterns of functioning to adapt to the crisis situation. **Adaptation** is defined as "the outcome of family efforts to bring about a new level of balance, harmony, coherence, and functioning to a family-crisis situation" (McCubbin, McCubbin, 1993, p. 35). During a crisis, adaptation may have positive or functional outcomes (bonadaptation) or negative or dysfunctional outcomes (maladaptation). "The main emphasis of this model is on the resiliency of families or their ability to recover from adverse events and what strengths and capabilities influence this process" (Friedman, Svavarsdottir, McCubbin, 1998, p. 441). The processes and family strengths that influence positive family outcomes are discussed in a later section of this chapter.

The Resiliency Model provides a framework for assessing the strengths and needs of families experiencing stress. When using this model, the nurse would examine the variables that influence a family's adjustment during periods of stress, such as the family's appraisal of the event. Having this knowledge assists the nurse to obtain information from the family about its current level of functioning. This, in turn, provides a foundation for developing nursing diagnoses and interventions.

## STRESSOR EVENTS

"A stressor event is an occurrence that is of significant magnitude to provoke change in the family system" (Boss, 1988, p. 36). Although stress and crisis are basically matters of individual perceptions, certain life events have frequently been found to increase a family's risk for stress and crisis. These events are viewed as normative or developmental, nonnormative or situational, or a combination of the two. Stressor events produce change in a family system that necessitates mobilizing the family's coping processes. *Stressor events lead to crisis only when the family is unable to adapt effectively to the changes brought about by the event* (Boss, 1988; Friedman, Svavarsdottir, McCubbin, 1998).

*Normative* stressors occur across the life spectrum. They relate to critical transition points in the course of normal human development that involve many physical, psychological, and social changes. These transition stages, such as entry into school, puberty, starting a career, moving from home (Figure 8-2), marriage, parenthood, middlescence, retirement, and facing one's own death from aging, promote change in a family system. Normative stressors were identified by the developmental family theorists (see Chapter 7). Although they are predictable, they often require significant role change and produce heightened stress. The role changes that occur during these *anticipated* events are discussed in Chapters 16 through 21.

*Nonnormative* stressors also occur across the life span, but they are usually *not anticipated* and frequently are highly stressful. Nonnormative stressors are events such as divorce, illness, accident, change in social status, cultural relocation, and premature death of a significant other. Because nonnormative stressor events often *occur suddenly* and *are unexpected*, individuals and families must deal with these events without benefit of anticipatory problem solving. This makes individuals and families more vulnerable to crisis or negative outcomes.

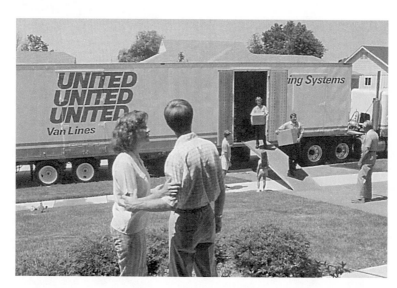

**FIGURE 8-2** Moving is a normal transition event, but it can cause a great deal of stress. (Courtesy United Van Lines.)

Sometimes normative and nonnormative stressor events occur simultaneously. When this happens, individual and family adjustment and adaptive energies become seriously overtaxed. Multiple stressors make it more difficult for persons to realistically appraise the changes that are occurring and to adjust their coping style to accommodate them. For example, a 5-year-old child who has recently changed cultural settings must deal with stresses related to school entry in addition to those related to living in a new environment. School entry in itself is often very traumatic. This, coupled with the pressures that result from relocation such as learning a different language, developing all new friendships, and adjusting to an unfamiliar lifestyle, can be overwhelming.

American families are experiencing a number of nonnormative stressors (Box 8-2). Environmental conditions and lifestyle patterns are placing them at risk for situations such as domestic violence, criminal victimization, unexpected disasters, economic distress, and infectious diseases. Supportive family intervention can assist families in dealing with these stressors.

## BOX 8-2
### Stress and Crisis Among America's Families

#### Victims of Crime and Violence[c,f,g]
- The United States ranks first among industrialized nations in violent death rates for young people.
- On average, 10 children under age 19 are homicide victims daily in the United States.
- Although there has been an overall decline in homicide mortality, homicide continues to be the leading cause of death for young African-American men 15 to 24 years of age.

#### Widespread Unintended Pregnancies[d]
- The rate of unintended pregnancies in the United States is higher than that of many other industrialized countries.
- Fifty-seven percent of all pregnancies and 44% of all births are unintended.
- The proportion of unintended births is significantly higher among women in poverty (60%), among African-American women (62%), among never-married women (73%), and among unmarried teenagers (86%).

#### Poverty Is Prevalent[a,b,c]
- In 1999, a total of 32.3 million people were poor.
- The poverty rate for Native Americans and Alaskan Natives (25.9%), African Americans (23.6%), Hispanics (22.8%), and Asians and Pacific Islanders (10.7%) was significantly higher than the poverty rate for Caucasian non-Hispanics (7.7%) in 1999.
- Almost 10 million young children live in low-income families.
- Young children under age 6 living with single mothers are significantly more likely to be poor than those living with both parents.
- Over half of African-American children (55%) and Hispanic children (60%) who live with a single mother live below the federal poverty level.

#### Homelessness Is Prevalent[h]
- On any given night, up to 400,000 Americans are literally homeless.
- Homeless families with children, over 80% of whom are headed by a single mother, make up about one-fifth of homeless persons.
- A significant number of vulnerable persons on public housing waiting lists and involuntarily doubled up with friends and relatives are on the edge of homelessness.

#### Disparities in Health Care Access[e,g]
- More than 40 million Americans, including over 11 million children, had no health insurance at any given time during 1998.
- Over one fourth, or 3 million, of the people living near the United States–Mexico border are uninsured.
- One in five African-American children and one in three Hispanic children have no health insurance, compared with one in nine white children.
- Hispanic and African Americans are more likely than Caucasian Americans to be uninsured, to lack a usual source of care and to be in fair or poor health.

#### Ineffective Stress Management[d,g,i]
- Almost one third of women in the United States have been kicked, punched, hit, choked, or otherwise physically abused by a spouse or partner in their lifetime.
- Approximately 903,000 children were victims of substantiated child abuse or neglect in 1998.
- An estimated 14.8 million Americans were current users of illicit drugs in 1999.
- About 40 million American adults, or 22% of the population, had a diagnosis of mental disorder in the past year.

Data from (a) Bennett N, Li J, Song Y, et al.: *Young children in poverty: a statistical update, June 1999 edition,* New York, 1999, National Center for Children in Poverty; (b) Dalaker J, Proctor B: *Poverty in the United States, 1999,* Current population reports (series P60-210), Washington, DC, 2000, US Government Printing Office; (c) Federal Interagency Forum on Child and Family Statistics: *America's children: key national indicators of well-being, 2000,* Washington, DC, 2000, US Government Printing Office; (d) Grason HA, Hutchins JE, Silver GB, editors: *Charting a course for the future of women's perinatal health, Volume 1: concepts, findings, and recommendations,* Baltimore, Md, 1999, Women's and Children's Health Policy Center; (e) Kass BL, Weinick RM, Monheit AC: *Racial and ethnic differences in health, 1996,* MEPS chartbook No. 2, Rockville, Md, 1999, Agency for Health Care Policy and Research; (f) Murphy SL: Deaths: final data for 1998, *National Vital Statistics Report* 48(11):1-13, 2000; (g) Maternal and Child Health Bureau: *Child health USA 2000,* Washington, DC, 2000, US Government Printing Office; (h) Nunez R: A snapshot of family homelessness across America, *Political Science Quarterly* 114(2):289-307, 1999; (i) US Department of Health and Human Services (USDHHS): *Healthy people 2010: with understanding and improving health and objectives for improving health* (2 volumes), ed 2, Washington, DC, 2000, US Government Printing Office.

## MEASUREMENT OF STRESSOR EVENTS

Research since the early 1960s has documented that significant life changes can adversely affect the health status of individuals (Rahe, 1972). The Life Change Questionnaire (Table 8-1), developed by Holmes, Rahe, Masuda, and others, has been used to demonstrate the relationships between a cluster of events requiring life changes and illness. It has been shown that individuals whose life change units (LCU) are greater than the value of 150 in a year's time are more susceptible to illness than individuals whose life change units are below this value. Studies conducted by Rahe demonstrated that 50% of the individuals whose life change units ranged from 150 to 300 LCU had an illness within the following year. In addition, 70% of those individuals whose LCU values exceeded 300 had an illness the following year (Rahe, 1972).

Based on the recognition that the types of life change events that produce stress vary across the life span, research has been conducted to increase the relevance of the life event questionnaire for a particular age group or for specific population groups. For example, Norbeck (1984) modified the life event questionnaire to address the needs of adult women of childbearing age. Norbeck's modified tool deals with significant concerns of women, such as having difficulties with contraception, changing child care arrangements, being the victim of violent acts (e.g., rape and assault), and parenting conflicts.

Barnard's (1988) Difficult Life Circumstance (DLC) scale was designed to ascertain the existence of chronic family problems among high-risk families dealing with pregnancy. The items on the DLC scale address such things as domestic violence, child abuse, long-term illness, and problems with alcohol and drug use. Barnard found that families with a high DLC score (a score reflecting the existence of several difficult life circumstances) had less favorable maternal and family outcomes than families with a low DLC score.

Beall and Schmidt (1984) developed a tool for use with adolescents (Table 8-2). The Youth Adaptation Rating Scale is not designed to be used as a predictor of illness. Rather, it was developed "to measure the causes of adolescent adaptation and stress during the adolescent years" (Beall, Schmidt, 1984, p. 197). This tool was tested in a variety of settings and by six ethnic groups. Adolescents were

**TABLE 8-1**

*Life Change Events*

| EVENTS | LCU VALUES | EVENTS | LCU VALUES |
|---|---|---|---|
| *Family* | | *Personal—cont'd* | |
| Death of spouse | 100 | Changing to a new school | 20 |
| Divorce | 73 | Change in residence | 20 |
| Marital separation | 65 | Major change in recreation | 19 |
| Death of a close family member | 63 | Major change in church activities | 19 |
| Marriage | 50 | Major change in sleeping habits | 16 |
| Marital reconciliation | 45 | Major change in eating habits | 15 |
| Major change in health of family | 44 | Vacation | 13 |
| Pregnancy | 40 | Christmas | 12 |
| Addition of new family member | 39 | Minor violations of the law | 11 |
| Major change in arguments with spouse | 35 | | |
| Son or daughter leaving home | 29 | *Work* | |
| In-law troubles | 29 | Being fired from work | 47 |
| Spouse starting or ending work | 26 | Retirement from work | 45 |
| Major change in family get-togethers | 15 | Major business adjustment | 39 |
| | | Changing to different line of work | 36 |
| *Personal* | | Major change in work responsibilities | 29 |
| Detention in jail | 63 | Trouble with boss | 23 |
| Major personal injury or illness | 53 | Major change in working conditions | 20 |
| Sexual difficulties | 39 | | |
| Death of a close friend | 37 | *Financial* | |
| Outstanding personal achievement | 28 | Major change in financial state | 38 |
| Start or end of formal schooling | 26 | Mortgage or loan over $10,000 | 31 |
| Major change in living conditions | 25 | Mortgage foreclosure | 30 |
| Major revision of personal habits | 24 | Mortgage or loan less than $10,000 | 17 |

From Rahe RH: Subjects' recent life changes and their near-future illness reports, *Ann Clin Res* 4:250-265, 1972. This study report was supported by the Bureau of Medicine and Surgery, Department of the Navy, under Research Work Unit MF51.524.002-5011-DD5G (Report No. 72-31). Opinions expressed are those of the author and are not to be construed as necessarily reflecting the official view or endorsement of the Department of the Navy.

asked to rank each item on the tool using a 5-point descriptive scale, with 0 indicating that the event was not stressful at all and 5 reflecting a very stressful event that would require a major change in one's life. No significant differences existed between the ethnic groups or the adolescents from communities of different sizes. It was found, however, that the need for adaptation or the recognition of that need becomes more evident as the adolescent grows older and matures (Beall, Schmidt, 1984).

Practitioners as well as researchers use life change questionnaires to identify *individuals* at risk for illness. When they discover individuals who are dealing with significant life changes, they discuss the effect of these changes on one's health status and the importance of not making other major life changes at this time.

## Family Life Events and Changes

As previously discussed, "families have a distinctive quality apart from the individuals making up the family" which is known as a *"family perception"* (Boss, 1988). To capture a family's perception of stress, McCubbin, Patterson, and Wilson (1996) developed the Family Inventory of Life Events and Changes (FILE). FILE examines a family's perception of a range of normative and nonnormative life events (see Appendix 8-1) and identifies how many of the specified 71 stressors have occurred within the family unit in the past year. Standardized family weights ranging from 21 to 99 have been assigned to each item on FILE to indicate the relative stressfulness of a life event or family change. These weights are included on the file instrument (McCubbin, Thompson, McCubbin, 1996).

### TABLE 8-2

## *Youth Adaptation Rating Scale*

| EVENT | DEGREE OF SEVERITY | EVENT | DEGREE OF SEVERITY |
|---|---|---|---|
| • Graduation | .57 | • Getting a bad report card | .59 |
| • Pet dies | .55 | • Getting fired from a job | .63 |
| • Fights with parents | .67 | • Going into debt | .72 |
| • Getting pressure about having sex | .63 | • Being stereotyped/discriminated [against]/ having bad rumors spread about you | .70 |
| • Caught cheating or lying repeatedly | .73 | • Death of a close family member | .94 |
| • Getting a major illness/injury/car accident | .81 | • Death of a boy/girlfriend/close friend | .94 |
| • Becoming religious or giving up religion | .63 | • Getting an STD | .86 |
| • Referral to the principal's office | .47 | • Getting someone pregnant/getting pregnant | .92 |
| • Getting acne/warts | .45 | • Taking finals/SAT test | .61 |
| • Trouble getting a date when it was not a problem before | .61 | • Moving to a different town/school/making new friends | .67 |
| • Problems developed with teachers/ employers | .59 | • Getting a car | .35 |
| • Making career decisions (college, majors training, etc.) | .64 | • Trying to get a job/job interview | .49 |
| | | • Getting an award, office, etc. | .36 |
| • Starting to go to weekend parties/ rock concerts | .35 | • Making a team (drill, athletic, debate) | .44 |
| • First day of school | .37 | • Getting married | .73 |
| • Going on first date/starting to date | .53 | • Getting beat up by parents | .86 |
| • Death of a parent/guardian | .95 | • Taking the driver license test | .55 |
| • Not getting promoted to next grade | .76 | • Getting a new addition to the family | .45 |
| • Getting caught using drugs | .86 | • Going to the dentist or doctor | .37 |
| • Getting attacked/raped/beat up | .84 | • Going to jail/reform school | .88 |
| • Getting a ticket or other minor problems with law | .58 | • Starting to use drugs | .82 |
| | | • Getting braces | .45 |
| • Parents getting a divorce/separation | .83 | • Going on a diet | .41 |
| • Getting expelled/suspended | .71 | • Losing or gaining weight | .49 |
| • Fad pressure | .43 | • Changing exercise habits | .21 |
| • Breaking up with boy/girlfriend | .57 | • Pressure to take drugs | .71 |
| • Getting minor illness (cold, flu, etc.) | .30 | • Moving out of the house | .56 |
| • Arguments with peers/brothers/sisters | .46 | • Falling in love | .66 |
| • Starting to perform (speeches, presentations, musical or drama performances) | .60 | • Getting a bad haircut | .57 |
| | | • Getting glasses | .49 |
| | | • Family member moving out | .47 |

From Beall S, Schmidt G: Development of a youth adaptation rating scale, *J Sch Health* 54(5):197-200, 1984.
*Note:* The ratio value or degree of severity was determined by dividing the total value for each item by the highest possible score. Events with a high ratio value produce greater stress and require a greater degree of adaptation than do events with a lower ratio value.

In clinical practice, FILE is used to assist practitioners in identifying families who are experiencing a pile up of stressors, which makes families more vulnerable to crisis or negative outcomes (McCubbin, Patterson, 1991). The FILE is either completed by the adult family members together, or separately by each partner. If either or both partners record a *yes* on an item, the family couple score is a *yes*. A high total family/couple score implies high stress. Low-, moderate-, and high-stress scores vary across the seven stages of the family life cycle (McCubbin, Patterson, 1991). Scores considered high by family stage are: couple stage (720+), preschool stage (840+), school-age stage (735+), adolescent stage (850+), launching stage (950+), empty nest stage (690+), and retirement stage (700+). The reader is encouraged to review scoring procedures in McCubbin and Patterson (1991) and McCubbin, Thompson, and McCubbin (1996) before using FILE.

FILE provides a guide for quickly assessing a family's level of stress. Families with high-stress scores are helped to analyze their current family situation and how they can mobilize family resources to reduce the demands in their lives. Although families with moderate stress scores fall within the normal range of stressors, these families are particularly vulnerable to future stressful events. They should be counseled about their vulnerability and helped to identify family capabilities that can help them eliminate or mediate the impact of demands in their lives (McCubbin, Patterson, 1991; McCubbin, Thompson, McCubbin, 1996).

*Stop and Think About It*

What type of stressors are your families in the clinical setting experiencing? How are they dealing with these stressors? Might some of your families be experiencing a crisis?

## EFFECTS OF CULTURE ON PERCEPTIONS OF STRESS AND CRISIS

Cultural patterns of the family must be considered when assessing client situations during periods of stress and crisis. Cultural characteristics of families influence their perceptions about the causes of sickness and stress, the meaning and treatment of illness, appropriate coping behaviors, self-care activities, relationships with health care providers and significant others, and expression of stress and discomfort (Andrews, Boyle, 1999; Bomar, 1996; Davidhizar, Giger, 1998; Davitz, Sameshima, Davitz, 1976; Dehn, 1997; Giger, Davidhizar, 1999; Lipson, Dibble, Minarik, 1996; Murray, Zentner, 2000; Villarruel, Ortiz de Montellano, 1992).

When considering the effects of culture on perceptions of stress, it is important to understand that scientists and anthropologists have distinguished between the terms *illness* and *disease* to help them explain why health professionals and clients can differ in their views of a hazardous event. Illness does not necessarily correlate with the biomedical interpretation of disease. In Western culture, what an individual or family feels and expresses in terms of stress and discomfort is labeled *illness*. *Disease*, on the other hand, is a physician-diagnosed condition that deviates from clearly defined norms. In terms of these culturally defined definitions, illness can occur in the absence of disease and vice versa (Giger, Davidhizar, 1999; Twaddle, 1981). It is important to differentiate between these concepts because "where only disease is treated, care will be less satisfactory to the patient and less clinically effective than where both disease and illness are treated together" (Kleinman, Eisenberg, Good, 1978).

In their classic writings, Kleinman, Eisenberg, and Good (1978, p. 252) contend that illness is culturally shaped in the sense that it is individually perceived—that is, how individuals and families experience and cope with disease is based on their explanations of sickness. In clinical practice it is not uncommon to encounter a wide variation in families' and individuals' explanations of sickness. While community health nurses encounter many clients whose beliefs are consistent with the Western biomedical model, which focuses on scientific explanations for disease and illness occurrence, they also work with many families whose beliefs about health and illness have evolved from the folk medicine system.

Snow (1974), in his seminal work on folk medical beliefs, noted that these beliefs promote both natural and unnatural explanations for illness. **Natural explanations of illness** emphasize that there is a direct connection between the body and the forces of nature, and that there is safety in harmony and balance and danger in anything that is done to interfere with natural processes. *Natural illnesses* occur when the individual is inadequately protected against the forces of nature such as cold air and impurities in food, water, and air, or when there is an imbalance between natural forces (Snow, 1974). Community health nurses find that families holding these beliefs will take measures to protect themselves against dangerous elements in nature. For example, Chinese families may overdress their infants to prevent cold air from entering their children's bodies (Wong, 1999).

A commonly held natural imbalance supported by the Hispanic, Filipino, and Arab cultures is that which exists between "cold" and "hot," or yin (cold) and yang (hot) in the Chinese culture (Chang, 1995; Wong, 1999). This belief classifies illnesses, foods, areas of the body, and medicines according to intrinsic hot and cold properties (Snow, 1974). These properties can both cause illnesses and treat them and must be kept in balance to maintain health. Persons holding those beliefs will eat yin/cold foods such as honey, vegetables, and fruits when they have a disease with excessive yang/hot forces such as infections, fever, and hypertension (Ludman, Newman, 1984). Crucial to these beliefs are the implications they hold for nursing practice. Community health nurses who respect cultural differences work with families within the context of their cultural perspectives. They may, for instance, assist families in maintaining the harmony of nature by planning a balanced diet with them that avoids hot or cold food at given times.

Not all illnesses have folk explanations involving the disruption of forces in nature. Some result when individuals fall out of favor with the Lord and an evil influence or the devil takes over. Others are caused by witchcraft. "Witchcraft is based on the belief that there are individuals with the ability to mobilize unusual powers for good or evil" (Snow, 1974, p. 85). Snow found that belief in witchcraft as a cause of illness is widespread among Haitians, Trinidadians, Puerto Rican Americans, African Americans, and Mexican Americans. This belief continues to exist among some cultural groups.

Snow (1974) has labeled illnesses that result from supernatural evil influences or forces beyond nature as **unnatural explanations of illness.** Evil forces can cause all types of physical and mental health stresses that are frightening to families because they cannot be cured by natural remedies or health personnel. A common health belief found among people from Latin American, South Asian, Near Eastern, and some African societies is the belief in the evil eye (Pasquale, 1984). This phenomenon involves the belief that the gaze of the human eye can bring illness and misfortune to people. "Envy is the pivotal emotion that activates people's ability to cause harm and misfortune to others" (Pasquale, 1984, p. 32).

The **evil eye phenomenon** is a cluster of beliefs that associates people's internal strength-weakness states with the power of the evil eye (Pasquale, 1984). When these states are in balance, individuals are not likely to cast or fall victim to the evil eye. However, when people have an excess of envy their strength increases and they are capable of casting the evil eye intentionally or unintentionally.

Children are particularly vulnerable to the gaze of the evil eye because their internal strength-weakness states are immature. People exposed to the evil eye often have a sudden onset of illness and may have a variety of symptoms such as fever, nausea, diarrhea, and nervousness. Preventive and treatment measures for the evil eye phenomenon usually involve supernatural rituals carried out by the client or approved healers (Pasquale, 1984). For example, Hindus paint a spot of lamp-black on children's foreheads as a precautionary measure against the evil eye (Andrews, Boyle, 1999).

A knowledge of folk health beliefs can assist the community health nurse in understanding clients from the client's perspective and can prevent a client from being labeled noncompliant. This knowledge also can help the nurse avoid unintentional involvement in spell-casting, such as giving the evil eye when admiring a new baby during a home visit. Lack of understanding can create barriers to therapeutic nursing intervention. Box 8-3 presents nursing interventions that are used "to bridge or mediate between the patient's culture and the biomedical health care system" (McCloskey, Bulechek, 2000).

When visiting clients from differing cultures, it is important to remember that folk explanations for sickness are not limited to the poor and uneducated. Clients from all socioeconomic levels believe in folk explanations for ill-

**BOX 8-3**

## NIC Nursing Intervention: Culture Brokerage

### Definition
Deliberately using culturally competent strategies to bridge or mediate between the patient's culture and the biomedical health care system

### Activities
- Determine the nature of the conceptual differences that the patient and nurse have of the health problem or treatment plan
- Promote open discussion of cultural differences and similarities
- Identify, with the patient, cultural practices that may have a negative impact on health so the patient can make informed choices
- Discuss discrepancies openly and clarify conflicts
- Negotiate, when conflicts cannot be resolved, an acceptable compromise of treatment based on biomedical knowledge, knowledge of the patient's belief systems, and ethical standards
- Allow more than the usual time to process the information and work through a decision
- Appear relaxed and unhurried in interactions with the patient
- Use nontechnical language
- Arrange for cultural accommodation (e.g., late kitchen during Ramadan)
- Include the family, when appropriate, in the plan for adherence with the prescribed regimen
- Accommodate involvement of family to give support or direct care
- Translate the patient's symptom terminology into health care language that other professionals can more easily understand
- Facilitate intercultural communication (e.g., use of a translator, bilingual written materials/media, accurate nonverbal communication; avoid stereotyping)
- Provide information to the patient about the health care system
- Provide information to the health care providers about the patient's culture
- Assist other health providers to understand and accept patient's reasons for nonadherence
- Alter the therapeutic environment by incorporating appropriate cultural elements
- Modify typical interventions (e.g., patient teaching) in culturally competent ways

From McCloskey JC, Bulechek GM, editors: *Nursing interventions classification (NIC)*, ed 3, St Louis, 2000, Mosby, p. 241.

ness (Pasquale, 1984). It is also important to remember that there is significant intracultural variation in relation to health beliefs and practices. As families from different cultures assimilate Western beliefs, some of their traditions are relinquished and others are retained (Louie, 1985).

However, folk medical beliefs continue to be documented in the client–health care professional relationship (Andrews, Boyle, 1999; Eckholm, 1990; Kay, Yoder, 1987).

Because the meaning of illness and stress is individually perceived within a person's cultural context and self-concept, serious stressful events may or may not evolve into a crisis. Individuals and families who interpret these events as challenges to accomplish significant life goals are often able to develop coping mechanisms to effectively deal with their distress. However, if they perceive stressful events as the will of God, a spirit possession, or events out of their control, a crisis may emerge.

## THE CRISIS PHENOMENON

Like stress, crisis is identified by recognizing the manifestations or characteristic signs and symptoms of the crisis state. Having an understanding of the concepts of crisis helps the practitioner to quickly recognize clients who need to adjust their coping mechanisms to manage the demands of a stressful event. Boss (1988) defines "family coping to mean the management of a stressful event or situation by the family as a unit with no detrimental effects on any individual in that family" (p. 60).

It is especially critical for community health nurses to be well grounded in crisis theory. They frequently encounter clients, such as the Slavovi family discussed earlier in this chapter, who are dealing with new, different, or threatening stressful events. Early identification of those clients who are having difficulty coping with these events could prevent an intensified crisis state.

A preventive health philosophy stimulated the development of crisis theory and intervention. Erich Lindemann (1944), in his classic study of grief reactions, identified the need for preventive counseling with clients experiencing loss through death or separation. After investigating the responses of clients who had lost a relative in the famous Coconut Grove night club fire in Boston, he concluded that appropriate psychiatric intervention with clients who were experiencing grief could prevent prolonged and serious social maladjustment (Lindemann, 1944). He further concluded, after observing clients who experienced an "anticipatory grief reaction," that prophylactic counseling could prevent family crisis (Lindemann, 1944, p. 148). Anticipatory grief reactions occur when there is a threat of death, such as when soldiers engage in war activities. Clients in these situations can go through all the stages of grief. It has been found in some cases that wives of soldiers in the war, for example, handle the grief process so effectively that they emancipated themselves from their spouses. This precipitates a crisis when husbands return from the war, because their wives need to reestablish their marital relationships before they can express feelings of love and caring. Husbands in these situations can feel that their wives no longer love them and frequently ask for a divorce (Lindemann, 1944).

Crisis reactions such as those previously described can be predicted and often prevented. Crisis theorists have delin-

eated a sequence of events that occur when a client is experiencing a crisis, as well as factors that intensify the crisis state. They also have identified therapeutic processes that have a positive influence on client functioning during a family crisis. A community health nurse who understands the nature of a crisis and therapeutic crisis intervention can assist families under stress and crisis to adapt and grow.

## THE CRISIS SEQUENCE

Gerald Caplan (1961), the founder of preventive psychiatry, describes *crisis* as a state provoked when a person faces an obstacle to important life goals that is, for a time, insurmountable through the utilization of customary methods of problem solving. A period of disorganization ensues, a period of upset, during which many different abortive attempts at solution are made. Eventually some kind of adaptation is achieved, which may or may not be in the best interests of that person and his fellows.

When describing the normal sequence of events that occur during a crisis, Caplan (1964) identified four characteristic phases during the **crisis sequence:**

1. In the initial phase, an individual's tension rises as he or she uses habitual problem-solving responses to achieve emotional homeostasis.
2. In the second stage, tension increases and the individual becomes ineffective and upset because coping mechanisms were not effective in resolving the state of crisis.
3. A third threshold occurs when tension mounts and stimulates the mobilization of new and emergency problem-solving mechanisms. The problem may be resolved if an individual can redefine the situation in order to cope with it and can adjust to role changes that have occurred.
4. The final phase occurs when tension mounts beyond the limits an individual can tolerate, and major disorganization results.

Inherent in Caplan's description of a crisis are several key concepts. These are delineated in Box 8-4. The concepts have remained viable over time.

**BOX 8-4**

### *Concepts Inherent in Crisis Theory*

- Change that threatens an individual's ability to meet life goals disrupts the individual's homeostasis.
- Crisis results when an individual's customary methods of adaptation are ineffective in handling change.
- Disorganization occurs during the crisis state.
- Crisis is self-limiting, with a subsequent reduction of emotional tension (adaptation).
- Biopsychosocial homeostasis following a crisis may be at a level the same as, better than, or worse than the pre-crisis level.

From Caplan G: *Principles of preventive psychiatry*, New York, 1964, Basic Books.

## FAMILY CRISIS

Boss (1988) defines a family crisis as "(a) a disturbance in the equilibrium that is so overwhelming, (b) a pressure that is so severe, or (c) a change that is so acute that the family system is blocked, immobilized, and incapacitated" (p. 50). During a crisis a family is no longer able to maintain its structural boundaries, is ineffective in carrying out family roles and tasks, and family members have difficulty functioning, physically or psychologically (Boss, 1988). Crisis causes disorganization and ineffective functioning within the family unit and among individual family members. Hence the needs of both the family system and individual family members should be assessed when a family is experiencing a crisis.

Family crisis is self-limiting and can promote either growth within the family system or ineffective patterns of family functioning. The goal of crisis intervention is to help the family and individual family members to maintain a level of functioning equal to or better than the precrisis level. Characteristics of families that show potential for growth during stress or crisis are identified in Box 8-5.

Multiple factors affect how well a family handles stress and deals with crises. Community health nurses who understand these variables are better able to help families achieve successful resolution and growth during a crisis state.

### BOX 8-5

*NANDA Nursing Diagnosis: Family Coping: Potential for Growth*

#### Definition
Effective management of adaptive tasks involved with the client's health challenge by family member, who now exhibits desire and readiness for enhanced health and growth in regard to self and in relation to the client.

#### Defining Characteristics
- Family member is moving in direction of health-promoting and enriching lifestyle that (1) supports and monitors maturational processes, (2) audits and negotiates treatment programs, and (3) generally chooses experiences that optimize wellness
- Individual expresses interest in making contact on a one-to-one basis or on a mutual-aid group basis with another person who has experienced a similar situation
- Family member attempts to describe growth impact of crisis on his or her own values, priorities, goals, or relationships

#### Etiological or Related Factors
- Readiness for seeking goals related to self-actualization

From Gordon M: *Manual of nursing diagnosis*, ed 9, St Louis, 2000, Mosby, p. 527.

## FACTORS AFFECTING THE OUTCOME OF STRESS AND CRISIS

It has been well established that there is significant variation in how families and individuals respond to stress and crisis. This variation is influenced by several critical variables that can be categorized under three major headings: *perception of the event, family and individual resources,* and *family and individual coping mechanisms.* These variables affect how clients appraise stressful events and how they mobilize resources to achieve successful adaptation during periods of disequilibrium.

### Perception of the Event

Crisis is the emotional reaction that occurs in relation to a new, different, or threatening event, not the event itself. Basically, the extent of this emotional reaction is determined by how the client (individual, family, aggregate) defines his or her particular circumstances (Aguilera, 1994; Boss, 1988; Burr, Klein, Associates, 1994; Caplan, 1964; Glanz, Lewis, Rimer, 1997; Hansen, Hill, 1964; McCubbin, McCubbin, 1993).

Perception of a hazardous event is a multidimensional phenomenon. McCubbin and McCubbin (1993) noted that "the assessments families make include many components of the stressor, such as the intensity, the degree of controllability of the situation, the amount of change expected of the family system, and whether or not the family is capable of responding to the situation" (p. 50).

Consistent with McCubbin and McCubbin's view, Glanz, Lewis, and Rimer (1997) contend that when a person is faced with a stressor he or she "evaluates the potential threat or harm [primary appraisal], as well as his or her ability to alter the situation and manage negative emotional reactions [secondary appraisal]" (p. 116). During the primary appraisal process, individuals make judgments about the severity of the threat and their susceptibility to the threat. Additionally, they examine what impact the stressor has on their goals or concerns and the cause of the stressor. During the secondary appraisal process, individuals examine their coping resources and options and assess such things as their perceived ability to change the situation, their perceived ability to manage the emotional reactions to the threat, and expectations about the effectiveness of their coping resources (Glanz, Lewis, Rimer, 1997).

During the clinical family assessment process, it is important to guide the interview to obtain data about the multiple variables that influence how a client perceives a hazardous situation. Box 8-6 identifies factors to be considered when assessing a client's response to current stressors. Information about the structural and process parameters of family functioning is presented in Chapter 7. This information helps the practitioner examine the impact of the stressful situation on the family system. For example, it would be important to assess how the family was handling its division of labor when a family member is ill and unable to carry out his or her normal patterns of functioning. Families experi-

### BOX 8-6

*Factors Influencing a Family's Perception of a Stressful Event*

- Number of stressors family is experiencing
- Family's past experiences in handling current stressor(s)
- Biopsychosocial status of the client before encountering stressful event(s)
- Duration of exposure to current stressor(s)
- Magnitude or seriousness of current event(s)
- Suddenness of the event
- Family's understanding of the stressor event(s)
- Impact of event on family structure, process, and goals
- Family's perceptions about its ability to manage the demands of the stressful event, including an appraisal of family resources
- Family's perceptions about its ability to change the stressful situation

encing a crisis are no longer able to perform their customary roles and tasks (Boss, 1988).

Even though the responses of individuals and families to hazardous events are highly variable, evidence suggests that distress increases when multiple stressors are encountered (McCubbin, McCubbin, 1993; McCubbin, Patterson, 1983; Rahe, 1974), the stressor or stressors are experienced for a prolonged length of time (Gaynor, 1990; Rowat, Knafe, 1985; Selye, 1976), or the stressful event presents hardship or a threat to life's goals or has serious consequences such as death (Glanz, Lewis, Rimer, 1997; Hill, 1949). Distress also increases if families or their individual family members believe that they have little control over the stressful event (Boss, 1988; McCubbin, McCubbin, 1993). When distress heightens, clients are more likely to have a distorted view of the current stressor. They may experience feelings such as helplessness, hopelessness, anxiety, fatigue, or depression.

Factors influencing a family's perception of a stressful event only place individuals more at risk for developing crisis. Caplan (1964), in his classic work on crisis, has found that for a stressor to become problematic "it must be perceived as a threat or loss to need satisfaction or as a challenge" (pp. 42-43). He believes that two major variables, personality and sociocultural factors, significantly affect how one perceives life events. These variables determine the type of life experiences one has, prescribe the limits of acceptable behavior when dealing with stress, and influence how one feels about one's abilities to handle changes in life. Case scenarios can best illustrate how the variables of personality and sociocultural influences affect one's perception of an event.

**CASE Scenario**    Mrs. Farias was 34 years old and left with two sons, 8 and 10 years old, and one daughter, age 14, when her husband was killed in a car ac-

cident. The community health nurse had encountered the Farias family before Mr. Farias's death because Carmelina, their 14-year-old daughter, needed orthopedic follow-up for a scoliosis problem discovered through health screening at her high school. During a home visit 8 months after Mr. Farias's death, the community health nurse became concerned about Mrs. Farias's physical and psychological health. She looked uncared for, her home was untidy, and she had no interest in talking about Carmelina's health problems. Weeping, Mrs. Farias shared with the nurse that "nothing was going right lately; the children don't obey, I can't get my husband's life insurance, and my friends haven't visited lately." She became particularly distressed when she talked about how she was going to feed her family in the future. "Our savings are almost gone. I can't get a job. What will I do? I have never worked, because Julio thought that a wife should stay at home. My folks thought that girls should marry and raise a family. I never was good at much except maybe cooking, housekeeping, and loving the kids.

My family thinks it is wrong to take money from the welfare department. They say they will help me until I remarry, but I know they don't have anything extra. Besides, I am too old to remarry. Most men I know want their own children, not someone else's. You can't meet men when you are my age."

Another case scenario illustrates different family reactions to the death of its male provider.

**CASE Scenario**    Mrs. Ulisses was a 33-year-old widow with two daughters, 2 and 6 years of age, and two sons, ages 8 and 11. Her husband was killed while hunting. The community health nurse started visiting Mrs. Ulisses after she brought her 2-year-old to the well-baby clinic 6 weeks after her husband's death. At that time she expressed a desire to obtain information about day-care centers. The nurse visited regularly for a year to help Mrs. Ulisses sort out what she would like to do in the future. She and her husband were never able to save much, so Mrs. Ulisses applied for financial assistance from the Department of Social Service. She did not like receiving Temporary Assistance to Needy Families but felt that she needed time to make child care arrangements before she went back to work. Seven and a half months after her husband's death, Mrs. Ulisses enrolled in college. "I know I can find a job, because I have worked off and on since age 15. If I had some training, however, I would be more secure in the future. I am still not sure if I want to get married again, so I better prepare myself to care for my family."

Both Mrs. Farias and Mrs. Ulisses were facing similar situations. They experienced the loss of a significant other who had assumed the provider role in their family system when he was living. Mrs. Farias, however, was more threatened by her circumstances because past and current cultural influences affected her ability to be flexible when role changes were needed. In addition, Mrs. Farias lacked confidence (personality factor) in her abilities to succeed in work and social settings. Her life experiences were focused on preparing her for traditional female roles only.

Mrs. Ulisses, on the other hand, was discouraged at times but was actively involved in planning for a future career. She was better prepared to assume the provider role, having worked off and on since her teenage years. She felt more confident about her abilities to succeed outside the home setting. Her life experiences provided her with a different perception of her female role.

## Family and Individual Resources

Families may have both family system resources and social supports that can assist them during periods of stress and crisis. Family system resources such as economic stability, cohesiveness, effective problem-solving abilities and communication patterns, and an adequate knowledge base help families deal with the harmful health effects of stress and crisis (Boss, 1988; Burr, Klein, Associates, 1994; McCubbin, McCubbin, 1993). Chapter 9 expands on family system resources or strengths that help families adjust and adapt during periods of stress and crisis.

Family system resources are the economic, psychological, and physical assets and strengths upon which family members can draw in response to a stressful event or events (Boss, 1988; Burr, Klein, Associates, 1994). "Having resources, however, does not imply whether or how a family will use them. For example, a family may use a resource such as money to deal with the event of unemployment in a dysfunctional way (e.g., buy more liquor or a larger television set) or, more functionally, to train for another job" (Boss, 1988, p. 68). During the family assessment process it is important to collect data about how family resources are being used, as well as about the type of resources available to the family. "The greater the breadth, depth, and efficacy of the available personal and family resources, the greater the ease with which the family is able to adapt to the illness situation" (McCubbin, McCubbin, 1993, p. 48).

It has been well established over time that social support can assist families and individuals to cope with the stresses of life (Caplan, Robinson, French, et al., 1976; Cassel, 1976; Cobb, 1976; Hamburg, Killilea, 1979; Heaney, Israel, 1997). It has been demonstrated that social support can play a significant role in buffering the impact of stress and in influencing positive health behaviors, such as the use of health services and adherence to medical regimens. Social support also can stimulate the development of coping strategies and promote mastery or control over one's situation (Cassel, 1976; Cobb, 1976; Hamburg, Killilea, 1979; Pilisuk, Parks, 1983).

Heaney and Israel (1997) distinguish between social networks and social support. They see **social networks** as the "linkages between people that may (or may not) pro-

vide social support and that may serve other functions in addition to that support" (p. 180). In contrast, Heaney and Israel (1997) see **social support** as the aid and assistance exchanged through social relationships and interpersonal transactions that is always intended to be helpful, is consciously provided by the sender, and is provided within an interpersonal context of caring, trust, and respect for each person's right to self-determination (pp. 180-181). Examples of social support are tangible assistance like financial aid and help with daily maintenance activities, the provision of information that helps clients under stress clarify and address the stressful event, and emotional support that conveys trust, caring, and empathy (House, 1981).

Although it has been shown that social support can positively influence the outcome of a stressful event or crisis, research also has demonstrated that the *nature* of social support is significant to consider when evaluating this variable during the family assessment process (Gottlieb, 1983; Krause, 1986). Thus it is important to ascertain from families their perceptions about the *quality* as well as the *quantity* of support that exists in their environment. Use of a genogram and/or an ecomap (see Chapter 7) often helps the practitioner assess clients' perceptions about the quality of their internal and external social resources.

During periods of disequilibrium, persons need supportive relationships that allow them to verbalize feelings and encourage them to sort out the realities of their situation. Clients also need assistance with problem solving. In addition, clients frequently need concrete help in obtaining resources, such as financial assistance from their environment. Behaviors that support a client's distorted perception of the event are not helpful. A friend, for example, who reinforces a client's blaming behaviors inhibits client growth and successful resolution of a crisis. This type of behavior supports the client's current ineffective coping style, and as a result, prevents the client from mobilizing more effective coping mechanisms.

When working with clients who are experiencing a crisis, it is extremely important to remember that their significant others also may be in crisis. Often the practitioner finds that others in a client's social network are experiencing as much or more distress than the client. Thus they are unable to provide the assistance needed by the client to achieve healthy adaptation and may, in fact, be reinforcing maladaptive behaviors. Because of this, significant others are often included in the therapeutic process so that they do not inhibit a client's growth and they themselves receive the help needed to cope with the stressful event.

## Family and Individual Coping Strategies

The stress-crisis sequence evolves when a family's or an individual's usual coping mechanisms are inadequate to deal with the threatening event(s) being encountered. A major task for a family or an individual who is experiencing stress is to recognize when customary coping mechanisms are ineffective and new patterns for coping must be established. "Coping strategies play a critical role in adaptation" (McCubbin, McCubbin, 1993, p. 57).

**Family coping strategies** are the active *processes* and *behaviors* families actually try to help them manage, adapt, or deal with stressful events (McCubbin, Dahl, 1985). Examples of specific strategies for managing family stress are gaining useful knowledge about the stressful event; building and enhancing trusting relationships with others; seeking help from relatives, friends, and community agencies; and maintaining family adaptability and flexibility (Burr, Klein, Associates, 1994, pp. 134-136).

Coping with stress and crisis is a complex process that may require changes in the basic structure of the family (e.g., family priorities and beliefs about life) as well as specific patterns of family functioning (e.g., allocations of role responsibilities). For example, as Maria and Angel Slavovi (discussed in the beginning of this chapter) were dealing with the demands of the stressors associated with caring for their child who had disabilities, they changed how the family carried out child care responsibilities and the family's expectations and goals. Mr. Slavovi assumed more responsibility for meeting the basic care needs of his children, and both parents came to realize that their disabled child would never meet the family's educational aspirations. Angel and Maria Slavovi wanted all of their children to go to college so that the children would have a better life than they themselves had. A conflict between expectations and what is realistic is distressing to families. In these situations they must compromise or accept a less-than-perfect solution to successfully manage the demands of their stressful event (McCubbin, McCubbin, 1993).

"No (one) coping strategy has been found to be a cure-all" (Burr, Klein, Associates, 1994, p. 147). Rather, the literature suggests that families are able to deal with stressors more effectively if they have a rich repertoire of coping strategies (Burr, Klein, Associates, 1994; McCubbin, McCubbin, 1993). However, Burr, Klein, and associates (1994) stress that "it is important to help families understand that not all coping strategies are helpful for everyone in every situation" (p. 203) and that professional intervention must be individualized to the specific concerns and needs of each family. Their research suggests that the nature of stressors influences family's perceptions about the helpfulness of specific types of coping strategies and that the type of coping strategies used varies by gender. Men appear to use more harmful strategies (e.g., using alcohol or withdrawing) and women tend to reach out to others. Women also tend to use a wider range of coping strategies (Burr, Klein, Associates, 1994).

## Recognizing Inadequate Coping Patterns

Boss (1988) believes that "sometimes it may be better for a family to give up, to let go, to fail to cope even if that precipitates crisis" (p. 63), particularly if maladaptative coping strategies (e.g., social isolation or domestic violence) are used by the family to adapt. These types of coping strategies can cause psychological and physical harm to individual family members and the family unit. The following case scenario illustrates how psychological distress can evolve in a seemingly stable family situation and how maladaptive coping strategies were causing harm to one of the family members.

**CASE Scenario** Sally Himes called the county health department and requested nursing service for her mother. Without emotion, she stated, "Someone needs to show me how to care for her. I don't know what to do any longer." Sally Himes was a 50-year-old, single woman who lived with her 85-year-old mother. Her mother had a cerebrovascular accident 15 years previously that left her paralyzed and unable to speak. Before her father's death, Ms. Himes had promised him that she would always care for her mother.

When the community health nurse arrived at the Himes home, Sally immediately took her to her mother's bedroom. Although the mother appeared very comfortable and well cared for, Sally insisted that the nurse check her over carefully. "I am doing something that is not right. The doctor needs to visit more frequently to give mother water shots." When the nurse's assessment revealed that the mother's condition was stable, she decided to spend time talking with Sally. Very abruptly in the conversation, Sally replied, "The mailman came today." It took several probing questions like, "Was there something special about the mailman's visit?" before Sally identified that she had received an invitation to her niece's wedding. She was distressed because her mother had not also been invited. "They don't care about her anymore."

Further interviewing revealed that for the past 2 years Sally had isolated herself from family and friends because she felt her mother's condition was deteriorating and that her significant others were too busy to assist her. Sally also shared that she was really discouraged because she wondered if her family cared about her or her mother. "If they cared, they would have invited mother to Sue's wedding."

Disrupting the status quo when she received an invitation to her niece's wedding was a very positive coping strategy for Sally. "Letting go" and asking for help from others assisted Sally in reevaluating her current situation and seeing that she needed to make changes in her current pattern of functioning. Isolating herself from family and friends and "toughing it out" or keeping feelings to herself resulted in depression and made it more stressful for Sally to care for her mother. Nursing intervention helped Sally alter her perceptions about her mother's condition, the type of support she needed, and the nature of support her family desired to provide, and helped Sally realize she was using ineffective coping strategies. One nursing intervention, arranging a conference with the entire family, resulted in a plan in which Sally's brothers and sisters would share responsibility for the care of their mother.

When nurses work with clients who are experiencing stress, they often find that a triggering event (e.g., the invitation to Sue's wedding) stimulates the development of a crisis. This event produces a "pile up" of stress beyond the point where the client is able to adapt. Frequently the event appears to be a minor occurrence, which makes it difficult for professionals and significant others to recognize the seriousness of the client's situation. For example, a child who comes sobbing into the health clinic at school because of being shoved by peers on the playground may need just a little extra attention. However, if this child perceives the push to mean that he or she is not liked, the child may need help in evaluating social relationships. It is usually wise for a community health nurse to obtain information about the client's daily functioning, support systems, and recent life changes when she or he believes that an emotional reaction to an event is disproportionate to what one would normally expect.

Having an awareness of behaviors that are commonly observed when individuals and families have developed ineffective coping mechanisms enhances the community health nurse's ability to quickly identify clients who are experiencing distress, crisis, or dysfunctional family dynamics. The North American Nursing Diagnosis Association (NANDA) has identified characteristics of individuals and families who have ineffective coping patterns. These characteristics are displayed in Boxes 8-7, 8-8, and 8-9 and can assist community health nurses in determining when individuals and families are having difficulty handling stress. The ineffective behaviors presented in the family coping boxes are primarily identified in terms of how a family relates to a client with an identified problem. During times of distress and crisis families also may develop dysfunctional patterns of functioning that affect the entire family unit. Examples of such patterns are deceptive, confused, or secretive communication processes; inability to meet basic needs of family life (e.g., impaired home management); inappropriate or lack of decision making and problem solving; and family interactions characterized by constant conflict. Other examples are shared in Chapter 7.

When community health nurses work with families, particularly those who tend to perceive all difficulties as crisis, they often find that problems from the past are reactivated during the crisis state. This occurs because these families

---

## BOX 8-7
### *NANDA Nursing Diagnosis: Ineffective Coping (Individual)*

#### *Definition*
Impairment of adaptive behaviors to meet life's demands and roles (valid appraisal, choice of response, and/or inability to use resources). Methods of handling stressful life situations are insufficient to prevent or control anxiety, fear, or anger. Specify stressor(s) (e.g., situational or maturational crises, uncertainty).

#### *Defining Characteristics*
**DIAGNOSTIC CUES**
- Reports presence of life stress/problems (specify)
- Reports feeling anxious, apprehensive, fearful, angry, and/or depressed
- Expresses inability to cope or ask for help
- Ineffective or inappropriate use of defense mechanisms (forms of coping that impede adaptive behavior, e.g., see avoidance coping, denial)

**SUPPORTING CUES**
- Disturbance in pattern of tension release
- Disturbance in pattern of threat appraisal
- Inadequate resources (financial, etc.)
- Change in usual communication patterns
- Decrease in use of social support

- Poor concentration
- Lack of goal-directed behavior and resolution of problem (e.g., inability to attend to problem; difficulty organizing information)
- Inability to meet role expectations
- Inability to meet basic needs
- Destructive behavior toward self or others
- Sleep disturbance
- Fatigue
- Risk taking
- High illness rate
- Abuse of chemical agents
- High degree of perceived or actual threat

#### *Etiological or Related Factors*
- Inadequate problem solving
- Inadequate confidence in coping ability
- Inadequate perception of control
- Social support deficit or characteristics of relationships
- Inability to conserve adaptive energies

#### *High-Risk Populations*
- Inadequate opportunity to prepare for stressor

From Gordon M: *Manual of nursing diagnosis*, ed 9, St Louis, 2000, Mosby, pp. 507-509.

have previously used inadequate coping strategies when dealing with stressful situations (Caplan, 1964). Although the resurfacing of old issues can compound the impact of current stressors, it also can provide an opportunity for client growth. Clients can be helped to resolve old as well as new problems during times of crisis and to learn effective ways to address stressful events. Even families who experience extreme types of stress can successfully find new levels of satisfaction and fulfillment in their family lives (Burr, Klein, Associates, 1994, p. 204).

### BOX 8-8

## NANDA Nursing Diagnosis: Compromised Family Coping

### Definition

Usually supportive primary person (family member or close friend) providing insufficient, ineffective, or compromised support, comfort, assistance, or encouragement, which may be needed by client to manage or master adaptive tasks related to health challenge.

### Defining Characteristics

**DIAGNOSTIC CUES**

Client or another person expresses concern or complaint about significant other's response to health problem and one or more of the following:

- Significant person displays protective behavior disproportionate (too little or too much) to client's abilities or need for autonomy
- Significant person describes preoccupation with personal reactions (e.g., fear, guilt, anticipatory grief, anxiety) to client's illness, disability, or other situational or developmental crises
- Significant person describes or confirms inadequate understanding of knowledge base that interferes with effective assistive or supportive behaviors (specify)
- Significant person withdraws or enters into limited or temporary personal communication with client at time of need
- Significant person attempts assistive or supportive behaviors with less than satisfactory results

### Etiological or Related Factors

- Knowledge deficit (specify area)
- Emotional conflicts (specify)
- Exhaustion of supportive capacity
- Role changes (family)
- Temporary family disorganization
- Developmental or situational crises (specify)

### High-Risk Populations

- 24-hour home care
- Home care with periodic health crises
- History of family life stresses

From Gordon M: *Manual of nursing diagnosis*, ed 9, St Louis, 2000, Mosby, pp. 517, 519.

### BOX 8-9

## NANDA Nursing Diagnosis: Disabling Family Coping

### Definition

Behavior of significant person (family member or primary person) disables own capacities and client's capacities to effectively address tasks essential to either person's adaptation to the health challenge.

### Defining Characteristics

**DIAGNOSTIC CUES**

Neglectful care of client in regard to basic human needs and/or illness treatment and one or more of the following:

- Distortion of reality regarding client's health problem, including extreme denial about existence or severity
- Intolerance
- Rejection
- Abandonment
- Desertion
- Carrying on usual routines, disregarding client's needs
- Psychosomaticism
- Taking on illness signs of the client
- Decisions and actions by family that are detrimental to economic or social well-being
- Agitation, depression, aggression, hostility
- Impaired restructuring of a meaningful life for self, impaired individuation, prolonged overconcern for client
- Neglectful relationships with other family members
- Client's development of helpless, inactive dependence

### Etiological or Related Factors

- Chronically unexpressed guilt/anxiety/hostility by significant other
- Dissonant discrepancy of coping styles (for dealing with adaptive tasks by the significant person and client or among significant people)
- Highly ambivalent family relationships
- Arbitrary handling of family's resistance to treatment (tends to solidify defensiveness as it fails to deal adequately with underlying anxiety)

### High-Risk Populations

- 24-hour home care
- History of family life stresses
- Home care with periodic health crises

From Gordon M: *Manual of nursing diagnosis*, ed 9, St Louis, 2000, Mosby, pp. 521, 523.

## SUPPORTIVE FAMILY SERVICES AND INTERVENTIONS

The type of services and interventions needed by families to address stressful situations varies, based on the nature of the stressor(s) encountered and the level of family functioning.

The Children's Defense Fund (1992) believes that most families can change when offered the right kind of help and that most families in crisis want to be helped to better provide for their family members. This organization advocates for a pyramid (Figure 8-3) of family-focused services in

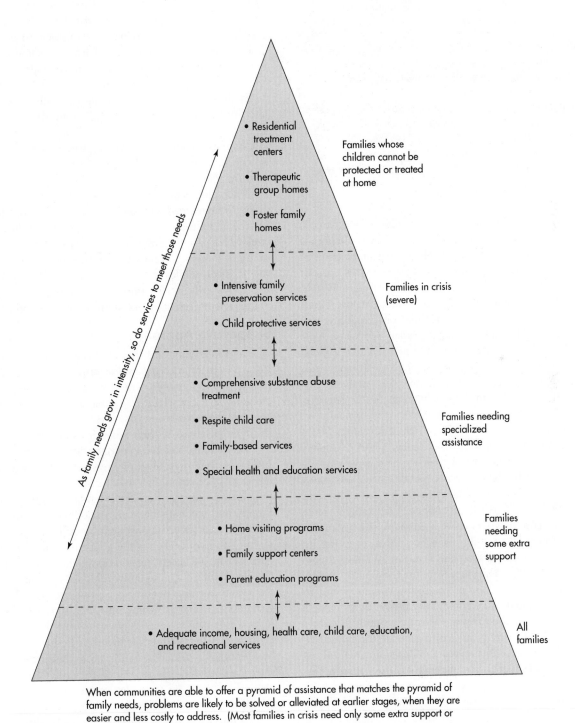

**FIGURE 8-3** Building a pyramid of family-focused services. (From Children's Defense Fund [CDF]: *The state of America's children 1992*, Washington, DC, 1992, CDF, p. 68.)

### BOX 8-10

*Effective Approaches for Working with Families Under Stress*

- Emphasize the family unit instead of focusing narrowly on an individual child or other family member.
- Build on family strengths instead of emphasizing deficits.
- Offer preventive services to avert crises instead of merely reacting to emergencies.
- Address family needs comprehensively instead of merely reacting to emergencies.
- Treat families with respect, and honor cultural differences.
- Offer flexible, responsive services instead of rigid, single-purpose services.

From Children's Defense Fund (CDF): *The state of America's children 1992*, Washington, DC, 1992, CDF, p. 65.

every community that matches the pyramid of family needs and a holistic approach to family stress management that honors cultural variations and reflects respect of families (Box 8-10). Supportive family services and interventions build on family strengths, emphasize prevention, and help families through difficult times (Children's Defense Fund, 1992). "When a community is focused on promoting the health of its families, a rich array of primary services [are offered]. A healthy community offers a network of contacts, widely available to families, that contribute to emotional security" (Weissbourd, 2000). Chapters 9, 10, and 16 elaborate on how families might benefit from the services displayed in Figure 8-3.

*Families are especially amenable to outside assistance during periods of disequilibrium or crisis* (Caplan, 1964). Caplan found that intervention at this time can be the critical balancing factor in helping clients achieve positive outcomes during crisis states. Most families in crisis need only some extra support or specialized assistance. For example, refer once again to the Slavovi family discussed in the beginning of this chapter. This family was successful in adapting its family functioning to address the needs of all family members, with supportive assistance from the community health nurse and specialized early intervention workers from the public school system. The community health nurse helped the parents express their feelings about their child's disabilities, assisted the parents in learning about the nature of their child's health condition (cerebral palsy and mental retardation), and helped the parents identify appropriate community resources (e.g., early intervention program in the school system). Additionally, the nurse helped the family establish a pattern of functioning that addressed the needs of all family members. The early intervention workers aided the parents in promoting their child's growth and development and in identifying effective ways to care for their child's needs.

## NURSING INTERVENTION STRATEGIES

Community health nurses use a variety of intervention approaches to facilitate adaptation during times of stress and to enhance successful resolution of crisis. Some of these approaches are briefly summarized under three major categories: *supportive, educative,* and *problem-solving.* Separating strategies into categories is an artificial technique that is used here only to focus discussion about ways to effect client change. In reality community health nurses find that often they must integrate several intervention approaches to effectively assist clients under stress.

Establishing rapport and collecting adequate data to identify the task to be accomplished are the essential first steps in any intervention process. These steps are discussed in Chapters 7 and 9 and are not repeated here. They should, however, be kept in mind when selecting a particular intervention approach.

When clients are experiencing crisis, they may express a desire to be rescued and request that others make decisions for them. *Rescue behavior* only temporarily reduces client stress. This type of behavior prevents the client from developing new ways of coping with threatening events. Adhering to the principles of crisis intervention (Box 8-11) assists the community health nurse in avoiding rescue activities and in selecting an appropriate intervention approach.

### Supportive Approach

The multiple symptoms that clients experience when dealing with stressful events and/or crises were previously discussed in this chapter. These symptoms can be very unpleasant and can create considerable discomfort. Clients can fear that something is seriously wrong with them, and this tends to increase their anxieties and fears.

Often clients who are experiencing symptoms of distress need to reduce their level of stress before they can actively engage in activities that will lead to problem resolution. Supportive intervention by significant others (family, friends, and professionals) can assist clients in stress reduction. Three types of support are especially helpful: (1) providing an opportunity for the client to share feelings with persons who are accepting and nonjudgmental; (2) assisting the client with concrete daily tasks, such as home management and keeping health appointments; and (3) support system enhancement. Community health nurses frequently help clients who are experiencing crisis with concrete tasks by making referrals for homemakers or home health aides or by helping the client mobilize family resources. At times they also provide this assistance themselves during home visits. They may, for example, feed an infant while talking to a distressed mother.

It is important to remember that clients who are experiencing high levels of stress often need time to deal with their feelings. They also need time to reevaluate their perceptions of the stressful event before they can actively engage in problem solving and in learning new knowledge. Ig-

### BOX 8-11
*Principles of Crisis Intervention*

- *Help the client confront the crisis* by supporting expression of feelings and emotions such as fear, guilt, and crying.
- *Help the client confront the crisis in manageable doses* without dampening the impact of the crisis to a point where the client no longer recognizes the need to alter coping mechanisms. Drugs and diversional activities are helpful when they are used to decrease unmanageable stress. They are harmful when they prevent the client from looking at the realities of his or her situation.
- *Help the client find the facts* because truth is less frightening than the unknown. Clients may need frequent visits during periods of crisis because they may not have the energy to analyze all the stresses they are experiencing during one home visit.
- *Do not give client false reassurance* because this leads to mistrust and maladaptive coping behaviors. To succeed in resolving a crisis, a client needs reassurance that supports his or her ability to handle the crisis situation.
- *Do not encourage the client to blame others* because blaming only reduces the tension momentarily and can help the client suppress feelings. This can result in maladaptive behaviors that decrease the client's level of functioning after crisis resolution.
- *Help the client accept help* because some clients avoid confronting a crisis by denying that they need help and that a problem exists. If the client does not face the crisis, he or she will not mobilize coping mechanisms that will enhance growth.
- *Help the client with everyday tasks* in a manner that reflects kindness and thoughtfulness rather than one that gives a message that the client is weak or incompetent. Clients need help with everyday tasks because it takes considerable energy to resolve a crisis; thus clients often lack sufficient energy to handle daily activities as well.

From Cadden V: Crisis in the family. In Caplan G, editor: *Principles of preventive psychiatry,* New York, 1964, Basic Books, pp. 293-296.

### BOX 8-12
*NIC Nursing Intervention: Support System Enhancement*

**Definition**
Facilitation of support to patient by family, friends, and community

**Activities**
- Assess psychologic response to situation and availability of support system
- Determine adequacy of existing social networks
- Identify degree of family support
- Identify degree of family financial support
- Determine support systems currently used
- Determine barriers to using support systems
- Monitor current family situation
- Encourage the patient to participate in social and community activities
- Encourage relationships with persons who have common interests and goals
- Refer to a self-help group, as appropriate
- Assess community resource adequacy to identify strengths and weaknesses
- Refer to a community-based promotion/prevention/treatment/rehabilitation program, as appropriate
- Provide services in a caring and supportive manner
- Involve family/significant others/friends in the care and planning
- Explain to concerned others how they can help

From McCloskey JC, Bulechek GM, editors: *Nursing interventions classification (NIC),* ed 3, St Louis, 2000, Mosby, p. 624.

### Stop and Think About It
Taking into consideration the families you have seen in the clinical setting, identify signs of stress you have observed. What type of support is available to these families? From your observations or personal experiences, what type of interventions have you found to be helpful in reducing stress and preventing a crisis?

### Educative Approach

Health education is a major component of community health nursing practice. Health education is a strategy used to facilitate behavior change in individuals, families, groups, or communities (McCloskey, Bulechek, 2000). It is a process that involves much more than finding and addressing a problem (Doyle, Ward, 2001). The health education process or educative approach is defined as "the continuum of learning which enables people, as individuals, and as members of social structures, to voluntarily make decisions, modify behaviors, and change social conditions in ways that are health enhancing" (Joint Committee on

noring the feeling levels of clients during these times can disrupt the therapeutic relationship and may result in the client withdrawing. Following the principles of crisis intervention shared in Box 8-11 helps develop a caring, trusting, professional relationship with clients in crisis.

Families with a limited support system may need assistance in expanding their support base. Nursing interventions that help enhance family support are displayed in Box 8-12. One strategy important to all social network intervention is to increase awareness among members of the client group of the health-enhancing qualities of social relationships (Heaney, Israel, 1997). "Someone who fully appreciates the importance of social relationships to good health is more likely to be motivated to engage in the processes of providing and receiving support" (Heaney, Israel, 1997, p. 191).

Health Education Terminology, 1991, p. 105). Health education during periods of stress and/or crisis can prevent a crisis from evolving or assist individuals and families to adapt during a crisis. For example, teaching a family how to care for a child or adult with disabilities could prevent a crisis related to caregiver burn out.

The key focus of health education is health behavior (Glanz, Lewis, Rimer, 1997). Theoretical perspectives related to health education, including models of individual and community health behavior change, are discussed extensively in Chapter 12. The educative process is also addressed in that chapter.

Models of health behavior change provide an organizing framework for identifying determinants influencing health behavior and factors that promote healthy behavior outcomes. Most health behavior models have focused on the individual or community as client (see Chapter 12). Loveland-Cherry (1996) has proposed a preliminary model for family health promotion (Figure 8-4) based on Pender's (1996) revised model for health promoting behavior, family theory, and research. This model illustrates that general, health-related, and behavioral-specific influences affect health promotion outcomes from a family perspective. During periods

of stress and crisis, these influences may need to be altered to increase the family's quality of life.

A major role of community health nurses during periods of stress and crisis is to "teach health promoting and health protecting behaviors to enhance family adjustment and adaptation to stress" (Bomar, Cooper, 1996). When working with families, it is important to identify and address educative needs of the family unit as well as individual family members. Educative needs of families under stress relate to the normative and nonnormative stressors discussed previously. For example, community health nurses commonly work with pregnant families and teach about needs of families during pregnancy and the childrearing stages of family life. This, in turn, can assist families to deal with family role and relationship changes. The steps used by the community health nurse to plan, implement, and evaluate educative activities are discussed in Chapter 12.

## Problem-Solving Approach

In the community health setting, nurses encounter clients who are having difficulty making decisions about a variety of personal life events. Specifically, community health nurses help clients make decisions about such things as ca-

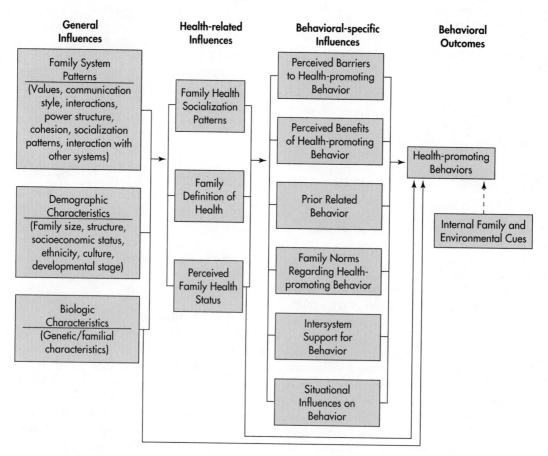

**FIGURE 8-4** Family health promotion model. (Modified from Loveland-Cherry CJ: Family health promotion and health protection. In Bomar PJ, editor: *Nurses and family health promotion: concepts, assessment, and interventions*, ed 2, Philadelphia, 1996, WB Saunders, p. 27.)

reer choices, maintaining or establishing intimate relationships with others, when and where to obtain preventive and curative health care services, how to deal with family conflicts, how to handle financial crisis, or how to provide needed care for aging family members. Clients dealing with situations such as these may have difficulty identifying why they cannot make a decision about what to do or may not recognize that they are not effectively dealing with stress.

At times a family's or an individual's problem-solving capabilities are ineffective in addressing the demands of the stressors encountered. "Problem solving refers to the family's ability to organize a stressor into manageable components, to identify alternative courses of action to deal with each component, to initiate steps to resolve the discrete issues, as well as the interpersonal issues, and to develop and cultivate patterns of problem-solving communication needed to bring about family problem-solving efforts" (McCubbin, McCubbin, 1993, p. 30).

A variety of internal and external factors influence why clients are unable to identify and develop solutions that effectively resolve their stress. The following case scenarios identify select factors that influence problem-solving capabilities of families and individuals under stress.

**CASE**
*Scenario*
### Client Has Not Identified the Nature of the Problem
Barb Lehi, a 28-year-old wife and the mother of two children, returned to work when her youngest child entered school. Her family adjusted well to her role change because joint decision-making occurred before Barb's employment. Barb was enjoying what she was doing but began to have tension headaches two months after she started her new job. She felt her headaches were related to the adjustments she had to make in her daily routine and assumed that they would go away shortly. However, her headaches continued until she was able to identify that she was having guilt feelings about being a working mother.

### Client Reaps Benefits from Illness Behavior
Mrs. Jackson, a 68-year-old widow living by herself, kept finding reasons why she should not see a physician after she started having "fainting spells." Her family became frustrated and worried and asked the community health nurse to visit. Referral for medical evaluation was successfully implemented only when Mrs. Jackson was able to verbalize that being ill was the only way she could get attention from her family. Her family visited sporadically when she was well but daily when she was ill.

### Client Is Using Disabling Coping Strategies
Gail Hayes, a 31-year-old mother and wife, provided no stimulation for her 2-year-old daughter who was disabled as a result of rubella exposure in utero. The community health nurse became involved after hearing from a neighbor that Gail left her daughter alone in the house when she visited friends and neighbors. After several home visits, the nurse discovered that Gail did so because, "I can't stand to be

with her. She is such a fussy child and wants attention all of the time. I hate seeing her so deformed and feel guilty because if I hadn't gotten measles while pregnant she would be all right." Gail had never before acknowledged these feelings. When she did, she was able to use the help offered by others and to relate more effectively to her daughter.

### Client Avoids Accountability for Feelings
Bob Woodrow, a 40-year-old construction worker, was referred to the community health nurse for rehabilitative services after a myocardial infarction. Because of the strenuous nature of construction work, it was recommended that he seek other employment. He verbalized an interest in obtaining job training through the Division of Vocational Rehabilitation but took no action. When the community health nurse questioned why, he responded by placing the blame on others. "My wife thinks it is too soon and nags me about not going back to work. I am not sure if my physician thinks I should, because he is always so vague about what is happening with my heart. My car needs fixing before I can use it regularly, and we don't have the money to get it fixed." It took several months for Bob to see that he was not taking action because of his own fears about having another heart attack and about not being able to succeed in a new line of work.

### Client Perceptions of Stress Are Distorted
Carol Strang, a 17-year-old junior in high school, repeatedly visited the school nurse for minor physical concerns. Assessments made by the nurse revealed that this occurred when Carol felt that she was not performing well academically. In reality Carol was very successful in her schoolwork, ranking in the top 5% of her class. In addition, she had several close friends who provided praise for her academic achievements. However, Carol perceived that she could only be successful if she obtained straight As. When she received anything less than an A, she expressed feelings associated with failure.

### Client Lacks Problem-Solving Experience
Mrs. Raabe, a 71-year-old widow, became confused and severely upset after her husband's death. All her life she had been cared for by others. Her parents and her brothers anticipated her needs because she was the "baby" of the family and "helpless." Because her husband assumed the same role as her family, Mrs. Raabe felt lost when he died. She found managing her finances particularly stressful because she had never taken care of the family budget. She needed help with such basics as writing a check, depositing money in the bank, and balancing her income and expenses.

### Client Energy Is Depleted Because of Undetected Health Problems
Mrs. La Rosa, a 37-year-old divorced mother of six children, was referred to the health department by her caseworker from the Department of Family Independence. Her caseworker believed that Mrs. La Rosa was neglecting her children and felt that environmental conditions were dangerous to the family's health. Mrs. La Rosa told the community health nurse, "I know I should keep my home more tidy, but

I am just too tired to keep up with things that need to be done around the house. Sometimes all I want to do is sleep." The community health nurse assisted her in obtaining a medical evaluation. It was found during this evaluation that Mrs. La Rosa had hypertension and diabetes. When both of these conditions were under control, home management and child care skills improved significantly.

### Client Has Knowledge and Skill Deficits

Mr. and Mrs. Lueck were extremely upset when their 10-year-old disabled son was sent home from camp because he could not handle activities of daily living such as bathing and toileting. "Tommie always does these things at home. They just don't know how to work with retarded kids." Upon talking with the Luecks, the community health nurse discovered Tommie did wash himself when bathing at home, but that family members helped him with most of the activities necessary for completing a bath. For example, the family ran his bath water for him; assembled the materials he needed to take a bath, including soap, washcloth, and towel; and selected the clothing he would wear afterward. It was obvious to the nurse but not the parents that Tommie had missed essential steps in skill development. He had skill in washing body parts, but lacked decision-making skill about how and when to carry out these activities.

### Client Is Unable to Generate or Fears Consequences of Alternative Options

Amy Schmidt, wife and mother of two preschoolers, was physically abused by her husband regularly and expressed a desire to leave him. She found it difficult to take this action because she thought that it was impossible for her to do so. She felt trapped because she had no job skills and her family and friends were unable to assist her financially. In addition, she felt that the abuse would not stop even if she left home because her husband could always find her. The community health nurse assisted Mrs. Schmidt in identifying ways to obtain financial aid and legal assistance to control her husband's behavior. Mrs. Schmidt was also helped to see that living alone could be less frightening for her and her children than being physically abused.

A community health nurse has two major goals when using the problem-solving approach: (1) to assist the client in solving immediate problems and (2) to help the client increase independent problem-solving abilities. Implicit in these goals is the belief that clients can learn skills that will help them make decisions wisely and to alter behavior accordingly. A community health nurse who has difficulty internalizing this belief will find it hard to move a client toward independence. This nurse is more likely *to do for* the client than *to work with* the client.

A variety of nursing interventions can be used to help a client enhance his or her problem-solving abilities, including such things as individual counseling, group work, role modeling, referral to community resources, client contracting, and behavioral modification. When using any one of these techniques, the community health nurse should focus on helping the client identify the nature of the problem(s), discover alternative options for problem solving, make decisions about which option is most appropriate, and take action to resolve the problem(s). The community health nurse should not assume that the client will take action after making a decision about the most appropriate option and prematurely close the family to service. Taking action is often the most difficult step in the problem-solving process because it is at this point that the client is giving up the secure familiar for the threatening unknown. Clients may need supportive intervention to maintain their commitment to action.

Problem-solving takes time. Both the client and the community health nurse must guard against expecting change too rapidly. When progress is slow a client may question if the nurse can really help, and the nurse often begins to wonder whether or not the client really wants to change. At times, both of these feelings are justified. More frequently, however, the need is for the client and nurse to recognize that well-established patterns of behavior cannot be changed immediately.

Most clients experiencing stress and crisis do not need intensive counseling. Instead, they need someone who cares and who will provide supportive guidance and positive reinforcement for the strength they have. Families and individuals have tremendous capabilities for "weathering the storms of stress" (Burr, Klein, Associates, 1994).

## SUMMARY

The community health nurse is often the primary source of assistance when an individual or a family is experiencing stress. Stress is a normal human phenomenon necessary for survival and growth. It triggers the general adaptation syndrome that helps people adapt to the demands and pressures of life. Although stress is essential for survival and growth, individuals and families have limits beyond which stress is no longer tolerated. Prolonged and intensified stress results in crisis, especially when an individual's coping mechanisms are inadequate to reduce disequilibrium.

Families and individuals in crisis experience disorganization and heightened stress. Crisis is self-limiting, but biopsychosocial homeostasis following a crisis may be at a level equal to, better than, or lower than the precrisis level. Timely supportive intervention may be the critical factor that determines if an individual or family has a positive or negative outcome during periods of crisis.

Millions of American families are under stress. Environmental conditions and lifestyle patterns are placing them at risk for situations such as domestic violence, criminal victimization, and economic distress. To address the needs of families from a holistic perspective, every community needs to provide a range of family-focused supportive services and interventions. Most families under stress and crisis want to be helped and can achieve new levels of functioning. The community health nurse plays a key role in helping families to prevent a crisis situation and to adapt when crisis occurs.

# CRITICAL THINKING
*exercise*

You are the community health nurse visiting the Slavovi family described on page 225. Shortly after arriving at their home for your first home visit, it becomes obvious that Mr. and Mrs. Slavovi want you to tell them "the right way to do things with Stephanie" and that they are hoping to find someone who can "cure her." (Hospital personnel had shared with the family that Stephanie has cerebral palsy and mental retardation and needs long-term health and educational follow-up.) Considering the factors that influence the outcome of a crisis, discuss with a peer the type of assessment data you would collect on your first home visit and how you would apply the principles of crisis intervention in this situation. Additionally, identify at least three resources in your local community that could assist this family in dealing with its current situation.

# REFERENCES

Aguilera DC: *Crisis intervention: theory and methodology,* ed 7, St Louis, 1994, Mosby.

Andrews MM, Boyle JS: *Transcultural concepts in nursing care,* ed 3, Philadelphia, 1999, JB Lippincott.

Barnard KE: Difficult life circumstances (DLC). In Krentz LG, editor: *Nursing and the promotion/protection of family health: work-shop proceedings,* Portland, Ore, 1988, Oregon Health Sciences University.

Beall S, Schmidt G: Development of a youth adaptation rating scale, *J Sch Health* 54(5):197-200, 1984.

Bennett N, Li J, Song Y, et al.: *Young children in poverty: a statistical update, June 1999 edition,* New York, 1999, National Center for Children in Poverty.

Bomar PJ, editor: *Nurses and family health promotion: concepts, assessment, and interventions,* Philadelphia, 1996, WB Saunders.

Bomar P, Cooper S: Family stress. In Bomar P, editor: *Nurses and family health promotion: concepts, assessment and interventions,* Philadelphia, 1996, WB Saunders.

Boss P: *Family stress management,* Newburg Park, Calif, 1988, Sage.

Boss PG: Family stress. In Sussman M, Steinmetz S, editors: *Handbook on marriage and the family,* New York, 1987, Plenum.

Burr WR: *Theory construction and the sociology of the family,* New York, 1973, John Wiley & Sons.

Burr WR, Klein SR, et al.: *Reexamining family stress: new theory and research,* Thousand Oaks, Calif, 1994, Sage.

Cadden V: Crisis in the family. In Caplan G, editor: *Principles of preventive psychiatry,* New York, 1964, Basic Books.

Caplan G: *An approach to community mental health,* New York, 1961, Grune and Stratton.

Caplan G: *Principles of preventive psychiatry,* New York, 1964, Basic Books.

Caplan RD, Robinson EAR, French JRP Jr, et al.: *Adhering to medical regimens: pilot experiments in patient education and social support,* Ann Arbor, Mich, 1976, University of Michigan, Institute for Social Research.

Cassel JC: The contribution of the social environment to host resistance, *Am J Epidemiol* 104:107-128, 1976.

Chang K: Chinese Americans. In Giger JN, Davidhizar RE: *Transcultural nursing: assessment and intervention,* St Louis, 1995, Mosby.

Children's Defense Fund (CDF): *The state of America's children 1992,* Washington, DC, 1992, CDF.

Cobb S: Social support as a moderator of life stress, *Psychosomatic Medicine* 38:300-314, 1976.

Dalaker J, Proctor B: *Poverty in the United States, 1999,* Current population reports (series P60-210), Washington, DC, 2000, US Government Printing Office.

Davidhizar RE, Giger JN: *Canadian transcultural nursing: assessment and intervention,* St Louis, 1998, Mosby.

Davitz LJ, Sameshima Y, Davitz J: Suffering as viewed in six different cultures, *AJN* 76:1296-1297, 1976.

Dehn MA: Cactus juice, copper bracelets and garlic: self-care issues facing community health nurses. In Spradley BW, Allender JA: *Readings in community health nursing,* ed 5, Philadelphia, 1997, JB Lippincott.

Doyle E, Ward S: *The process of community health education and promotion,* Mountain View, Calif, 2001, Mayfield Publishing.

Eckholm E: AIDS and folk healing, a Zimbabwe encounter, *New York Times,* October 5, 1990, 1-2.

Federal Interagency Forum on Child and Family Statistics: *America's children: key national indicators of well-being, 2000,* Washington, DC, 2000, US Government Printing Office.

Friedman M, Svavarsdottir E, McCubbin M: Family stress and coping processes: family adaptation. In Friedman M: *Family nursing: research, theory, and practice,* ed 4, Stamford, Conn, 1998, Appleton & Lange.

Gaynor SE: The long haul: the effects of home care on caregivers, *Image J Nurs Sch* 22:208-212, 1990.

Giger JN, Davidhizar RE: *Transcultural nursing: assessment and intervention,* ed 3, St Louis, 1999, Mosby.

Glanz K, Lewis FM, Rimer BK, editors: *Health behavior and health education: theory, research and practice,* ed 2, San Francisco, 1997, Jossey-Bass.

Gordon M: *Manual of nursing diagnosis,* ed 9, St Louis, 2000, Mosby.

Gottlieb BH: *Social support strategies: guidelines for mental health practice,* Beverly Hills, Calif, 1983, Sage.

Grason HA, Hutchins JE, Silver GB, editors: *Charting a course for the future of women's perinatal health, volume 1: concepts, findings, and recommendations,* Baltimore, Md, 1999, Women's and Children's Health Policy Center.

Hamburg A, Killilea M: Relation of social support, stress, illness, and use of health services. In Hamburg D, editor: *Healthy people: the Surgeon General's report on health promotion and disease prevention,* DHEW PHS Pub. No. 79-55071A, Washington, DC, 1979, US Department of Health, Education, and Welfare.

Hansen DA, Hill R: Families under stress. In Christensen HT, editor: *Handbook of marriage and the family,* Chicago, 1964, Rand McNally.

Heaney CA, Israel BA: Social networks and social support. In Glanz K, Lewis FM, Rimer BK, editors: *Health behavior and health education: theory, research, and practice,* ed 2, San Francisco, 1997, Jossey-Bass.

Hill R: *Families under stress: adjustment to the crises of war separation and reunion,* New York, 1949, Harper.

Hill R: Generic features of families under stress. In Parad HJ, editor: *Crisis intervention: selected readings,* New York, 1965, Family Service Association of America.

House JS: *Work stress and social support,* Reading, Mass, 1981, Addison-Wesley.

Joint Committee on Health Education Terminology: Report of the 1990 Joint Committee on Health Education terminology, *J Health Educ* 22(2):105-106, 1991.

Kass BL, Weinick RM, Monheit AC: *Racial and ethnic differences in health, 1996,* MEPS Chartbook No. 2, Rockville, Md, 1999, Agency for Health Care Policy and Research.

Kay M, Yoder M: Hot and cold in women's ethnotherapeutics: the American Mexican west, *Soc Sci Med* 25:347-355, 1987.

Kleinman A, Eisenberg L, Good B: Culture, illness, and care: clinical lessons from anthropologic and cross-cultural research, *Ann Intern Med* 88:251-258, 1978.

Krause N: Social support, stress and well-being among older adults, *J Gerontol* 41:512-519, 1986.

Lazarus RS: *Psychological stress and the coping process,* New York, 1966, McGraw-Hill.

Lazarus RS, Folkman S: *Stress, appraisal and coping*, New York, 1984, Springer.

Lindemann E: Symptomatology and management of acute grief, *Am J Psychiatry* 101:141-148, 1944.

Lipson JG, Dibble SL, Minarik PA, editors: *Culture and nursing care: a pocket guide*, San Francisco, 1996, UCSF Nursing Press.

Louie KB: Providing health care to Chinese clients, *ICN* 7:18-25, 1985.

Loveland-Cherry CJ: Family health promotion and health protection. In Bomar PJ: *Nurses and family health promotion: concepts, assessment, and interventions*, ed 2, Philadelphia, 1996, WB Saunders.

Ludman EK, Newman JM: The health-related food practices of three Chinese groups, *J Nutr Educ* 16:4, 1984.

Maternal and Child Health Bureau: *Child health USA 2000*, Washington, DC, 2000, US Government Printing Office.

McCloskey JC, Bulechek GM, editors: *Nursing interventions classification (NIC)*, ed 3, St Louis, 2000, Mosby.

McCubbin H, Dahl B: *Marriage and family: individuals and life cycles*, New York, 1985, John Wiley.

McCubbin HI, McCubbin MA: Family system assessment in health care. In McCubbin HI, Thompson AI, editors: *Family assessment inventories for research and practice*, Madison, Wis, 1991, University of Wisconsin-Madison.

McCubbin HI, Patterson JM: Family stress adaptation to crises: a double ABCX model of family behavior. In Olson DH, Miller BC, editors: *Family studies review year book*, vol 1, Beverly Hills, Calif, 1983, Sage.

McCubbin HI, Patterson JM: FILE: Family Inventory of Life Events and Changes. In McCubbin HI, Thompson AI, editors: *Family assessment inventories for research and practice*, Madison, Wis, 1991, University of Wisconsin-Madison.

McCubbin H, Patterson J, Wilson L: FILE: Family Inventory of Life Events and Changes. In McCubbin HI, Thompson AI, McCubbin MA, editors: *Family assessment: resiliency, coping and adaptation—inventories for research and practice*, Madison, Wis, 1996, University of Wisconsin System.

McCubbin HI, Thompson AI, McCubbin MA: *Family assessment: resiliency, coping and adaptation—inventories for research and practice*, Madison, Wis, 1996, University of Wisconsin System.

McCubbin MA, McCubbin HI: Family stress theory and assessment: the T-Double ABCX model of family adjustment and adaptation. In McCubbin HI, Thompson A, editors: *Family assessment inventories for research and practice*, Madison, Wis, 1987, University of Wisconsin-Madison.

McCubbin MA, McCubbin HI: Families coping with illness: the resiliency model of family stress, adjustment, and adaptation. In Danielson CB, Hamel-Bissell BP, Winstead-Fry P, editors: *Families, health, and illness: perspectives on coping and interventions*, ed 3, St Louis, 1993, Mosby.

Murphy SL: Deaths' final data for 1998, *National Vital Statistics Report*, 48(11):1-13, 2000.

Murray RB, Zentner JP: *Health promotion strategies through the life span*, ed 7, Upper Saddle River, NJ, 2000, Prentice Hall.

Norbeck J: Modification of life event questionnaires for use with female respondents, *Res Nurs Health* 7:61-71, 1984.

Nunez R: A snapshot of family homelessness across America, *Political Science Quarterly* 114(2):289-307, 1999.

Pasquale EA: The evil eye phenomenon: its implications for community health nursing, *Home Health Nurse* 2:32-37, 1984.

Pender N: *Health promotion in nursing practice*, ed 3, Stamford, Conn, 1996, Appleton & Lange.

Pilisuk M, Parks S: Social support and family stress. In McCubbin H, Sussman M, Patterson J, editors: *Social stress and the family: advances and developments in family stress theory and research*, New York, 1983, Haworth.

Rahe RH: Subjects' recent life changes and their near-future illness reports, *Ann Clin Res* 4:250-265, 1972.

Rahe RH: The pathway between subjects' recent life changes and their near-future illness reports: representative results and methodological issues. In Dohrenwend BS, Dohrenwend BP, editors: *Stressful life events*, New York, 1974, Wiley.

Rowat KM, Knafe KA: Living with chronic pain: the spouse's perspective, *Pain* 3:259-271, 1985.

Selye H: *The stress of life*, New York, 1976, McGraw-Hill.

Snow LF: Folk medical beliefs and their implications for care of patients: a review based on studies among Black Americans, *Ann Intern Med* 81:82-96, 1974.

Twaddle AC: Sickness and the sickness career: some implications. In Eisenberg L, Kleinman A, editors: *The relevance of social science for medicine*, Dordrecht, Holland, 1981, D. Reidel.

US Department of Health and Human Services (USDHHS): *Healthy people 2010: with understanding and improving health and objectives for improving health* (2 volumes), ed 2, Washington, DC, 2000, Government Printing Office.

Villarruel AM, Ortiz de Montellano B: Culture and pain: a Mesoamerican perspective, *Adv Nurs Sci* 15:21-32, 1992.

Weissbourd B: Supportive communities for children and families, *Public Health Rep* 115:167-173, 2000.

Wong DL: *Whaley and Wong's nursing care of infants and children*, ed 6, St Louis, 1999, Mosby.

## SELECTED BIBLIOGRAPHY

Ammerman R, Hersen M: *Case studies in family violence*, ed 2, Norwell, Mass, 2000, Kluwer Academic Publishers.

Bogen-Schneider K: Has family policy come of age? A decade review of the state of US family policy in the 1990s, *J of Marriage and the Family* 62(11):1136-1159, 2000.

Burke S, Kauffmann E, Harrison M, Wiskin N: Assessment of stressors in families with a child who has a chronic condition, *MCN Am J Matern Child Nurs* 24(2):98-106, 1999.

Carter B, McGoldrick M: *The expanded family life cycle: individual, family, and social perspectives*, ed 3, Boston, 1999, Allyn and Bacon.

Gillis CL, Knafl KA: Nursing care of families in non-normative transitions: the state of science and practice. In Hinshaw AS, Feetham SL, Shaver JL, editors: *Handbook of clinical nursing research*, Thousand Oaks, Calif, 1999, Sage.

James K, Scotti J: The educative approach to intervention with child excess behavior: toward an application to parent training packages, *Child and Family Behavior Therapy* 22(3): 1-37, 2000.

Mealey AR, Richardson H, Dimico G: Family stress management. In Bomar PJ, editor: *Nurses and family health promotion: concepts, assessment, and interventions*, ed 2, Philadelphia, 1996, WB Saunders.

McCubbin M: Normative family transitions and health outcomes. In Hinshaw AS, Feetham SL, Shaver JL, editors: *Handbook of clinical nursing research*, Thousand Oaks, Calif, 1999, Sage.

Purnell LD, Paulanka BJ, editors: *Transcultural healthcare: a culturally competent approach*, Philadelphia, 1998, FA Davis.

Strader T, Collins D, Noe T: *Building healthy individuals, families, and communities: creating lasting connections*, Norwell, Mass, 2000, Kluwer Academic Publishers.

Teachman J, Tedrow L, Crowden K: The changing demography of America's families, *J Marriage Fam* 62:1234-1246, 2000.

Zarit SH, Stephens MA, Townsend A, et al.: Stress reduction for family caregivers: effects of adult day care use, *Journal of Gerontology: Social Science* 53B(5):S267-S277, 1998.

Zimmerman S: A family policy agenda to enhance families' transactional interdependencies over the life span, *Families in society: J Contemp Human Services* 81:557-567, 2000.

# FILE
## Family Inventory of Life Events and Changes©

## PURPOSE

Over their life cycle, all families experience many changes as a result of normal growth and development of members and external circumstances. The following list of family life changes can happen in a family at any time. Because family members are connected to each other in some way, a life change for any one member affects all the other persons in the family to some degree.

*"Family" means a group of two or more persons living together who are related by blood, marriage or adoption. This includes persons who live with you and to whom you have a long-term commitment.*

## DIRECTIONS

*"Did the change happen in your family?"*

Please read each family life change and decide whether it happened to any member of your family—**including you**—during the past 12 months and check **Yes** or **No**.

| *Did the Change Happen in Your Family?* | DURING THE LAST 12 MONTHS | | SCORE |
| --- | --- | --- | --- |
| | YES | NO | |
| **I. INTRAFAMILY STRAINS** 1. Increase of husband/father's time away from family | ○ | ○ | **46** |
| 2. Increase of wife/mother's time away from family | ○ | ○ | **51** |
| 3. A member appears to have emotional problems | ○ | ○ | **58** |
| 4. A member appears to depend on alcohol or drugs | ○ | ○ | **66** |
| 5. Increase in conflict between husband and wife | ○ | ○ | **53** |
| 6. Increase in arguments between parent(s) and child(ren) | ○ | ○ | **45** |
| 7. Increase in conflict among children in the family | ○ | ○ | **48** |
| 8. Increased difficulty in managing teenage child(ren) | ○ | ○ | **55** |
| 9. Increased difficulty in managing school age child(ren) (6-12 yr) | ○ | ○ | **39** |
| 10. Increased difficulty in managing preschool age child(ren) (2.5-6 yr) | ○ | ○ | **36** |
| 11. Increased difficulty in managing toddler(s) (1-2.5 yr) | ○ | ○ | **36** |
| 12. Increased difficulty in managing infant(s) (0-1 yr) | ○ | ○ | **35** |
| 13. Increase in the amount of "outside activities" that the children are involved in | ○ | ○ | **25** |
| 14. Increased disagreement about a member's friends or activities | ○ | ○ | **35** |
| 15. Increase in the number of problems or issues that don't get resolved | ○ | ○ | **45** |

From McCubbin H, Patterson J, Wilson L: FILE: Family Inventory of Life Events and Changes. In McCubbin HI, Thompson AI, McCubbin MA, editors: *Family assessment: resiliency, coping and adaptation—inventories for research and practice*, Madison, Wis, 1996, University of Wisconsin System, pp. 142-145. © H. McCubbin

*Continued*

# FILE
# Family Inventory of Life Events and Changes©

| *Did the Change Happen in Your Family?* | DURING THE LAST 12 MONTHS | | SCORE |
|---|---|---|---|
| | YES | NO | |
| 16. Increase in the number of tasks or chores that don't get done | ○ | ○ | 35 |
| 17. Increased conflict with in-laws or relatives | ○ | ○ | 40 |
| **II. MARITAL STRAINS** | | | |
| 18. Spouse/parent was separated or divorced | ○ | ○ | 79 |
| 19. Spouse/parent had an "affair" | ○ | ○ | 68 |
| 20. Increased difficulty in resolving issues with a "former" or separated spouse | ○ | ○ | 47 |
| 21. Increased difficulty with sexual relationship between husband and wife | ○ | ○ | 58 |
| **III. PREGNANCY AND CHILDBEARING STRAINS** | | | |
| 22. Spouse had unwanted or difficult pregnancy | ○ | ○ | 45 |
| 23. An unmarried member became pregnant | ○ | ○ | 65 |
| 24. A member had an abortion | ○ | ○ | 50 |
| 25. A member gave birth to or adopted a child | ○ | ○ | 50 |
| **IV. FINANCE AND BUSINESS STRAINS** | | | |
| 26. Took out a loan or refinanced a loan to cover increased expenses | ○ | ○ | 29 |
| 27. Went on welfare | ○ | ○ | 55 |
| 28. Change in conditions (economic, political, weather) that hurts the family investments | ○ | ○ | 41 |
| 29. Change in agriculture market, stock market, or land values that hurts family investments and/or income | ○ | ○ | 43 |
| 30. A member started a new business | ○ | ○ | 50 |
| 31. Purchased or built a home | ○ | ○ | 41 |
| 32. A member purchased a car or other major item | ○ | ○ | 19 |
| 33. Increased financial debts due to overuse of credit cards | ○ | ○ | 31 |
| 34. Increased strain on family "money" for medical/dental expenses | ○ | ○ | 23 |
| 35. Increased strain on family "money" for food, clothing, energy, home care | ○ | ○ | 21 |
| 36. Increased strain on family "money" for child(ren)'s education | ○ | ○ | 22 |
| 37. Delay in receiving child support or alimony payments | ○ | ○ | 41 |

# FILE
# Family Inventory of Life Events and Changes©

| *Did the Change Happen in Your Family?* | DURING THE LAST 12 MONTHS | | SCORE |
|---|---|---|---|
| | YES | NO | |
| **V. WORK-FAMILY TRANSITIONS AND STRAINS** | | | |
| 38. A member changed to a new job/career | ○ | ○ | **40** |
| 39. A member lost or quit a job | ○ | ○ | **55** |
| 40. A member retired from work | ○ | ○ | **48** |
| 41. A member started or returned to work | ○ | ○ | **41** |
| 42. A member stopped working for extended period (e.g., laid off, leave of absence, strike) | ○ | ○ | **51** |
| 43. Decrease in satisfaction with job/career | ○ | ○ | **45** |
| 44. A member had increased difficulty with people at work | ○ | ○ | **32** |
| 45. A member was promoted at work or given more responsibilities | ○ | ○ | **40** |
| 46. Family moved to a new home/apartment | ○ | ○ | **43** |
| 47. A child/adolescent member changed to a new school | ○ | ○ | **24** |
| **VI. ILLNESS AND FAMILY "CARE" STRAINS** | | | |
| 48. Parent/spouse became seriously ill or injured | ○ | ○ | **44** |
| 49. Child became seriously ill or injured | ○ | ○ | **35** |
| 50. Close relative or friend of the family became seriously ill | ○ | ○ | **44** |
| 51. A member became physically disabled or chronically ill | ○ | ○ | **73** |
| 52. Increased difficulty in managing a chronically ill or disabled member | ○ | ○ | **58** |
| 53. Member or close relative was committed to an institution or nursing home | ○ | ○ | **44** |
| 54. Increased responsibility to provide direct care or financial help to husband's and/or wife's parents | ○ | ○ | **47** |
| 55. Experienced difficulty in arranging for satisfactory child care | ○ | ○ | **40** |
| **VII. LOSSES** | | | |
| 56. A parent/spouse died | ○ | ○ | **98** |
| 57. A child member died | ○ | ○ | **99** |
| 58. Death of husband's or wife's parent or close relative | ○ | ○ | **48** |
| 59. Close friend of the family died | ○ | ○ | **47** |
| 60. Married son or daughter was separated or divorced | ○ | ○ | **58** |
| 61. A member "broke up" a relationship with a close friend | ○ | ○ | **35** |

*Continued*

# FILE
# Family Inventory of Life Events and Changes©

| *Did the Change Happen in Your Family?* | DURING THE LAST 12 MONTHS | | SCORE |
|---|---|---|---|
| | YES | NO | |
| **VIII. TRANSITIONS "IN AND OUT"**<br>62. A member was married | ○ | ○ | **42** |
| 63. Young adult member left home | ○ | ○ | **43** |
| 64. Young adult member began college (or post–high school training) | ○ | ○ | **28** |
| 65. A member moved back home or a new person moved into the household | ○ | ○ | **42** |
| 66. A parent/spouse started school (or training program) after being away from school for a long time | ○ | ○ | **38** |
| **IX. FAMILY LEGAL VIOLATIONS**<br>67. A member went to jail or juvenile detention | ○ | ○ | **68** |
| 68. A member was picked up by police or arrested | ○ | ○ | **57** |
| 69. A member experienced physical or sexual abuse or violence in the home | ○ | ○ | **75** |
| 70. A member ran away from home | ○ | ○ | **61** |
| 71. A member dropped out of school or was suspended from school | ○ | ○ | **38** |

# 9

# Use of Family-Centered Nursing Process with Culturally Diverse Clients

*Ella M. Brooks*

## OBJECTIVES

*Upon completion of this chapter, the reader should be able to:*

1. Understand the interrelationship between the phases of the family-centered nursing process.
2. Use the nursing process to plan family-centered nursing care.
3. Articulate the influence of cultural phenomena on client functioning and clinical decision making.
4. Analyze the concept of family health from a holistic perspective.
5. Understand nursing responsibilities and client rights in a provider/client relationship.
6. Understand the significance of using a theoretical base for guiding practice.

## KEY TERMS

Bonadaptation
Contracting
Corrupt contract
Cultural phenomena
Ethnocentrism
Ethnorelativity
Family-centered nursing process
Family dynamics
Health risk appraisal

Heritage consistency
Intracultural variations
Levels of prevention (primary, secondary, tertiary)
Maladaptation
Metaparadigm
Nursing Interventions Classifications (NIC)

Nursing Outcomes Classifications (NOC)
Omaha Classification System
Right of privacy
Right of self-determination
Salad bowl trend
Systematic approach
Theory-guided practice

*For a green plant to survive, it must reach sunlight. So nature provides that if the plant's growth is blocked in one direction, it can grow in another.*

CONOCO OIL COMPANY

People, like green plants, can grow in multiple directions. Barriers to growth do not necessarily stop growth. Barriers may delay growth or may actually strengthen the root system. In spite of obstacles, with enough nurturing and sunlight the plant eventually grows (Figure 9-1). This is also true for individuals and families. When barriers are inhibiting the growth process, caring, support, and assistance from significant others can help people grow and change the course of their development. A significant support system for many individuals is the family.

The family has long been considered the social unit of our society. The family unit influences the successes or failures of its members (Friedman, 1998). "The health of society is integral with the health of families, where each family assumes responsibility and advocacy for the expression of its health" (Phillips, 1993, p. 113). There are times when families need guidance in identifying behaviors that support and facilitate the growth, development, health and success of its members.

Community health nurses often facilitate the family growth process. They work to develop trusting, supportive relationships so that clients can reach out and use their help when it is needed. Some clients will not seek assistance from community health nurses because they have found other support systems more relevant to them. However, when a client does accept the help offered by community

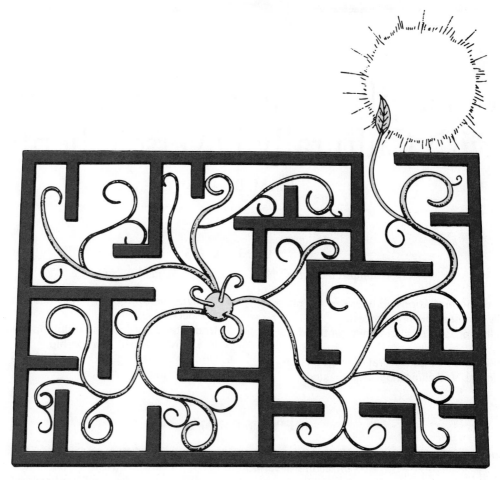

**FIGURE 9-1** Nature doesn't explore just one path to reach a goal. Neither should people. (Courtesy Conoco Oil Company.)

health nurses, it is important for nurses to recognize that their role is to work *with* the client in making choices that will promote family health. Nurses who encourage families to make decisions about life choices are more likely to facilitate growth than those who impose their beliefs on client choices.

Increasingly, health care professionals are encouraging active family involvement in health care decision making. They have identified that doing *for* clients instead of working *with* them can result in client dependence, rather than independence. Health care professionals can influence family change, but only families can alter their behavior. Clients must perceive the need for change before they will alter their actions.

To function effectively in the community setting, a nurse must accept the fact that clients are responsible for their health behavior choices regardless of what those choices may be. Nurse-defined goals for clients are seldom achieved. Goals defined by the client are more likely to be accomplished.

Effective use of the nursing process helps community health nurses facilitate client goal setting. "The nursing process provides a tool for nurses in all settings to use to continually evaluate and improve the quality of nursing care" (Murray, Atkinson, 2000, p.5). In the community health setting, the nursing process is labeled the *family-centered nursing process* because community health nurses use it to analyze family functioning and to extend services to the family as a whole. This focus is based on the belief that the family, as the basic unit, is the client. Family functioning establishes values, attitudes, and beliefs about health practices (Figure 9-2). How the family functions may inhibit or facilitate family growth and influence its members to accept or reject help from community systems. Consequently, how the family functions affects the health of all its members. The family-centered nursing process helps community health nurses analyze family functions; this process can be enhanced through theory-guided practice.

## THEORY-GUIDED PRACTICE

The American Nurses Association (ANA) (1986) standards of community health nursing practice specify that "the nurse applies theoretical concepts as a basis for deci-

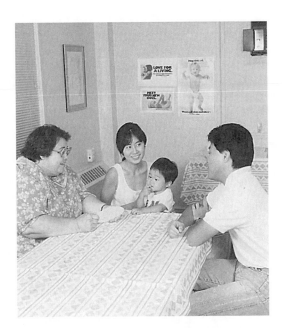

**FIGURE 9-2** The family-centered approach to nursing care focuses on the family as the unit of service. When using the nursing process in the community setting, nurses assess family dynamics as well as individual functioning and establish client-centered goals relevant to the needs of the entire family unit. (From Barkauskas VH, Stoltenberg-Allen C, Baumann LC, et al.: *Health and physical assessment*, St Louis, 1994, Mosby.)

sions in practice. Theoretical concepts define the context within which the community health nurse understands phenomena and their interrelationships, thereby providing a framework for assessment, intervention, and evaluation" (p. 5). Therefore, **theory-guided practice** requires the nurse to translate concepts into actions.

To function effectively in community health, the nurse must use skills and knowledge relevant to both nursing and public health (ANA, 1986, 1999; APHA, 1996). Public health knowledge includes concepts from epidemiology, biostatistics, environmental health, social sciences, and public health administration. Core concepts from the epidemiological model (host, agent, and environment) and **levels of prevention (primary, secondary, and tertiary)** guide public health practice. These concepts are discussed in Chapter 11.

Concepts from epidemiology help the nurse identify at-risk clients (individuals, families, and aggregates) for the purposes of promoting health and preventing disease. During the assessment phase of the family-centered nursing process, nurses complete a family health risk appraisal. A **health risk appraisal** is a process whereby data are collected and analyzed to identify characteristics that may make clients vulnerable to illness, premature death, or unhealthy conditions. Examples of such characteristics are unhealthy family patterns that may result in child, spousal, or elder abuse; lifestyle patterns such as smoking

or a high-cholesterol diet that increase the potential for disease occurrence; and hereditary links to disease such as sickle cell anemia. When a health risk is identified, the community health nurse suggests interventions that could reduce this risk. For example, family counseling and caregiver support might decrease the potential for child or elder abuse.

Nursing theoretical conceptualizations also help the nurse focus on the client. Several nursing models have been developed in an attempt to capture a comprehensive, holistic view of clients. Although these models vary in their approach to client, they all have four essential concepts (client, health, environment, and nursing) in common. These concepts are collectively known as nursing's **metaparadigm** and are used to organize nursing theories and models (Fawcett, 1989). Each concept is uniquely defined within that respective theoretical perspective. Examples of such models include Johnson's Behavioral System Model, King's Conceptual Framework of Nursing, Neuman's Health Care Systems, Orem's Self-Care Framework, Rogers' Science of Unitary Human Beings, Roy's Adaptation Model, White's Model for Public Health Nursing Practice, and Anderson's Community as Client Model. Although most of the nursing models focus on the individual as the unit of analysis, rather than the family and the community, some models have been advanced to address family and community. Table 9-1 provides examples of selected nursing theoretical models applicable to community health nursing practice and potential community health nursing interventions based on these models.

Theory development is an ongoing effort to expand nursing's knowledge base and articulate nursing's uniqueness. Theory-based nursing practice in homes and communities "offers a unique and invaluable opportunity for enrichment of the human health experience across continents, cultures, socioeconomic levels, and life spans" (Cody, 1997, p. 4). For the nursing discipline to continue its development, nurses must practice from a *nursing perspective*. "There can be no nursing language until the features of humankind specific to nursing are conceptualized and named and their structure uncovered" (Orem, 1997, p. 29).

Nursing family and community theories are still in their infancy. Although most of the models were developed with individuals as the primary focus, some have been expanded to include the family (Chin, 1985; Clements, Roberts, 1983; Friedemann, 1989a, 1989b; Gonot, 1986; Hanson, 1984; Johnston, 1986; Riehl-Sisca, 1985; Whall, 1981, 1986; Whall, Fawcett, 1991), group or aggregate, and community (Hanchett, 1988).

Because a comprehensive discussion about nursing theory is beyond the scope of this text, the reader is encouraged to examine writings by the primary author to obtain an accurate understanding of the theoretical and conceptual bases of each nursing model. Examining how others have discussed the application of these models in practice, research, and education also can be beneficial.

**TABLE 9-1**

*Examples of Selected Nursing Theoretical Models Applicable to Community Health Nursing*

| APPLICABLE CONTENT | OREM'S SELF-CARE/DEFICIT THEORY | ROY'S ADAPTATION MODEL | NEUMAN'S SYSTEMS MODEL | KING'S THEORY OF GOAL ATTAINMENT |
|---|---|---|---|---|
| Client | Self-Care Agency: may be individuals or multiperson units such as family, aggregate, community, populations (Orem, 2001). | Adaptive System: may be individuals, groups, or community (Roy, Andrews, 1999). | Client or Client System: may be "individuals, families, groups, communities and organizations, or collaborative relationships between two or more individuals" (Neuman, 1996, p. 67). | Personal, Interpersonal and Social System: may be individuals, groups or society (King, 1992). |
| Environment | People exist in their environments. Environments include chemical, physical, biological, and social features that are interactive and can "positively or negatively affect lives, health and well-being of individuals, families, communities" (Orem, 2001, p. 79). | "All conditions, circumstances and influences surrounding and affecting the development and behavior of persons and groups" (Roy, Andrews, 1999, p. 19). | "All internal and external factors or influences surrounding the client or client system" (Neuman, 1989, p. 31). | "Immediate environment, spatial and temporal reality, in which two individuals establish a relationship to cope with events in the situation (King, 1995, p. 27). |
| Health | "A state of a person that is characterized by soundness or wholeness of developed human structures and of bodily and mental functioning" (Orem, 2001, p. 186) that enhances or impedes the power of self-care agency. | "A process and state of being and becoming whole and integrated in a way that reflects person and environment mutuality (Roy, Andrews, 1999, p. 19). | Optimal stability of the client system where there is a dynamic equilibrium of the normal line of defense (Neuman, 1995). | "Dynamic life experience... which implies continuous adjustment to stressors in the internal and external environment through optimal use of one's resources to achieve maximum potential for daily living" (King, 1981, p. 5). |
| Nursing | Help self-care agents "with health-associated self-care deficits to know and meet with appropriate assistance the components of their therapeutic self-care demands and to regulate the exercise and development of their powers of self-care agency" (Orem, 1997, p. 27). | Focuses on the "promotion of adaptation for individuals and groups in each of the four adaptive modes, thus contributing to health quality of life and dying with dignity" (Roy, Andrews, 1999, p. 19). | Identify and reduce "actual or potential environmental stressors [through] use of primary, secondary, and tertiary levels of prevention interventions for retention, attainment, and maintenance of optimal client system wellness" (Neuman, 1996, p. 67). | Focuses on nurse and client system interactions that foster attainment of mutually defined goals (King, 1997). |

**TABLE 9-1**

*Examples of Selected Nursing Theoretical Models Applicable to Community Health Nursing—cont'd*

| APPLICABLE CONTENT | OREM'S SELF-CARE/DEFICIT | ROY'S ADAPTATION MODEL | NEUMAN'S SYSTEMS MODEL | KING'S THEORY OF GOAL ATTAINMENT |
|---|---|---|---|---|
| Possible Community Health Nursing Family-Centered Interventions | Assess physical, chemical, biological aspects (e.g., air, water, pollutants) that influence self-care agency. Determine universal, developmental, and health-deviation requisites needed to improve family self-care agency. Determine a family dependent care agent's abilities and limitations (Gaffney, Moore, 1996; Taylor, 2001). Assess basic conditioning factors (e.g., environmental conditions, sociocultural/ spiritual orientation, available resources) needed to improve family self-care agency. | Evaluate the coping processes, adaptive modes, and adaptation levels of a family system (Hanna, Roy, 2001). Assess contextual stimuli and adaptation of a family experiencing grief (Robinson, 1995). Design interventions that promote adaptive abilities for family who has member with chronic illness (Pollock, 1993). Design interventions that enhance family systems' interactions with environment. Assess environmental focal and contextual stimuli affecting the development of family adaptive system. Perform a community assessment on focal and contextual stimuli related to resources needed for family adaptation. | Gather data on a family system's flexible line of defense, normal line of defense, and line of resistance (Reed, 1993). Assess internal and external environmental stressors of a traditional family system. Evaluate internal and external stressors of a single-parent family system. Develop interventions to strengthen the family system's line of defense. Conduct a parenting class on ways to reduce environmental stressors to strengthen the family system's line of defense. | Develop communication patterns that foster interaction and eventual transaction between nurse and parents (Norris, Hoyer, 1993). Assess the interactions between community and family that fosters or impedes mutually defined goal attainment. Determine how the interpersonal interactions among family groups in the community influence their health behavior choices. Develop mutually defined interventions with a family that facilitates interpersonal communication between and among its members. |

*Stop and Think About It*

Analyze two nursing theoretical models that interest you. Apply the theoretical concepts to a client family in the clinical setting. Compare and contrast the differences in goals and outcomes according to the theoretical perspectives.

## FAMILY-CENTERED NURSING PROCESS DEFINED

The **family-centered nursing process** is a systematic approach to scientific problem solving, involving a series of dynamic actions—assessing, analyzing, planning, implementing, evaluating, and terminating—for the purpose of facilitating optimum client functioning. This definition has four key elements:

- *Systematic approach.* This process enables the community health nurse to approach clients in an orderly, logical manner. The nurse plans his or her actions to achieve

specific goals and recognizes that time and efforts are often wasted if a "hit-or-miss" approach is used.

- *Scientific problem solving.* Decisions made about client needs and appropriate nursing interventions are based on scientific principles. The problem-solving approach is used in everyday life. The nursing process differs from simple problem solving: scientific knowledge gained from advanced study assists the nurse in refining the data analysis process in relation to health, illness, and prevention, and in expanding intervention options that aid clients in maximizing their self-care capabilities. McCain (1965, p. 82), in her classic article on the nursing process, stressed that this process helps nurses function in a deliberative rather than an intuitive way. This notion has been supported in recent literature (Gordon, 2000; Weber, 1991) and Orem's Self-Care Framework (Orem, 2001).

- *Dynamic actions.* Dynamic implies change and movement. The nursing process facilitates change and growth.

No one action alone helps the community health nurse enhance client growth. Regardless of the length of interaction between nurse and client, the nurse uses all phases of the nursing process in *every* interaction with clients (Murray, Atkinson, 2000). All phases of the nursing process must be carried out in order for sound decision making and effective nursing intervention. The nursing process is dynamic in nature because each phase provides data that either validate or alter original nursing diagnoses, goals, and plans. From a dynamic perspective, care plans are revised when assessment and evaluation data reflect changes needed to facilitate client growth.

- *Purpose of facilitating optimum client functioning.* Nursing interventions should help the client resolve his or her health care needs and achieve specific, client-defined goals and expected outcomes. A helping, interactive process, through which the client and the nurse share data and work together to define goals, facilitates achievement of goals and outcomes.

To achieve defined outcomes in a family situation, the nurse must recognize that having knowledge only about a disease process is insufficient to adequately address the impact of illness on the family system. Illustrative of this are the factors nurses take into consideration when they work with a family who has a child with insulin-dependent diabetes. Based on scientific knowledge from the biological sciences, the nurse knows that this child requires an appropriate diet, proper hygiene, insulin injections, regular blood glucose testing, and adequate exercise. However, teaching about these needs may be ineffective unless the nurse applies knowledge from the behavioral and social sciences to gain an understanding of how environmental, lifestyle, and family factors are influencing the child's health behaviors. This is illustrated in the following case scenario:

**CASE Scenario** One community health nurse frequently visited the family of a 6-year-old child who had an unstable diabetic condition. The child did not follow her prescribed diabetic regimen and one consequence was frequent hospitalization for treatment of diabetic coma. When the nurse discussed with the parents their perceptions of their child's health condition, she learned that they were not ready to accept the diagnosis as permanent. Denying the diagnosis was their way of coping with it. The parents needed assistance in dealing with their feelings of guilt and anger before they could address appropriate treatment plans for their child.

## CULTURAL FACTORS INFLUENCE PRACTICE

As significant demographic changes have altered the ethnic and racial composition of our nation's population (see

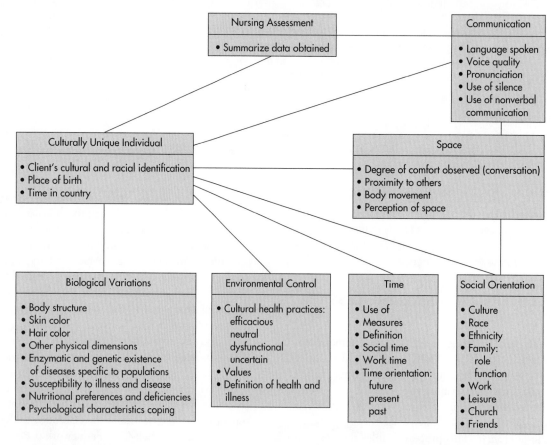

**FIGURE 9-3** Giger and Davidhizar's transcultural assessment model. (Modified from Giger JN, Davidhizar RE: *Transcultural nursing: assessment and intervention*, ed 3, St Louis, 1999, Mosby, p. 8.)

Chapter 7), an increased appreciation for cultural diversity has emerged. The concept of the melting pot, now outmoded, has been replaced with the "**salad bowl trend**" (Catalano, 2000, p. 324) in which culturally different individuals retain their cultural customs and beliefs without accepting customs of the dominant culture. "Some cultural groups manage to blend the melting pot and the salad bowl together through a complex process called *heritage consistency*" (Catalano, 2000, p. 325). In **heritage consistency,** members may outwardly appear to acculturate into the dominant culture, but privately, they retain their own cultural customs and beliefs (Catalano, 2000, p. 325).

Viewing clients from an ethnocentric perspective negates the value of cultural differences and leads to ineffective nursing practice. "**Ethnocentrism** is the belief that one's own cultural values and beliefs are right" (Murray, Atkinson, 2000, p. 13). Nurses must move beyond ethnocentrism and understand clients within their respective cultures if they expect to facilitate healthy family growth and outcomes.

It has been well documented that clients bring to the helping relationship values, attitudes, beliefs, and priorities that have developed over generations and that influence health beliefs and practices (Hines, Preto, McGoldrick, et al., 1999). Cultural patterning influences lifestyle patterns and

families' decisions about when to obtain care and whom they should consult when care is needed. Regardless of the nurse's knowledge of culture, the community health nurse must always assess clients "in a manner that considers cultural aspects and uniqueness" (Murray, Atkinson, 2000, p. 14).

"Cultural knowledge in community nursing practice begins with a careful assessment of clients and families in their home environment" (Boyle, 1999, p. 309). Nurses in the community health setting are privileged to enter the homes and lives of culturally diverse families in very intimate ways. They show respect for this privilege by seeking information that increases their awareness of a family's situation from its perspective. The effective community health nurse takes into account cultural factors throughout the helping process. The ability of nurses to "communicate effectively with [clients] and their families incorporates the use of meaningful language and other forms of communication, knowledge of sociocultural practices and willingness to search out the meaning of what persons receiving care are endeavoring to communicate" (Orem, 1997, p. 29).

Giger and Davidhizar (1999) have identified **cultural phenomena** (Figure 9-3) that are evident in all cultural groups but have unique cross-cultural variations. These phenomena, summarized briefly in Box 9-1, are further de-

---

### BOX 9-1

## *Cultural Phenomena to Be Considered Throughout the Nursing Process*

### Communication
Communication includes all verbal and nonverbal behavior between people, including things such as vocabulary, grammatical structure, silence, touch, facial expressions, eye and body movements, and expression of warmth and humor.

### Space
Providing culturally competent care involves examining how families use and control their interpersonal space, including objects in the environment and spatial behavior. Families control their environment to protect themselves from harm, to maintain privacy, to control what occurs in their interpersonal space, and to promote self-identity.

### Social Organization
A variety of social organizations (e.g., family, religious groups, ethnic and racial groups, kinship groups, and special interest groups) in a client's environment influences the patterning of cultural behaviors. All of these organizations develop structural and process characteristics that promote specific values, attitudes, beliefs, and norms about growth and development processes, health practices, life goals, and family functioning (refer to Chapter 7).

### Time
Both clock time (an interval of time) and social time influence family behavior. Clock time directs regularity in our lives. So-

cial time refers to patterns and orientations (e.g., past, present, future) that relate to social processes and to the conceptualization and ordering of social life.

### Environmental Control
This term refers to the ability of a family from a particular cultural group to plan activities that control nature or to direct factors in the environment. Health practices and actions taken by families when a family member is ill are affected by how the environment is viewed. Families' views about the environment are influenced by things such as their beliefs about locus of control (internal or external), causes of health and illness (natural or unnatural), and people-to-nature orientation (dominate nature, live in harmony with nature, or subjugate to nature). Views about the environment are also influenced by families' relationships with systems in their environment (e.g., folk medicine or religious system).

### Biological Variations
This phenomena involves examining norms for different cultural/ethnic groups in relation to anatomical characteristics, skin and hair physiology, growth and development patterns, susceptibility and resistance to disease, variations in body systems, and nutritional preferences and deficiencies.

Modified from Giger JN, Davidhizar RE: *Transcultural nursing: assessment and intervention,* ed 3, St Louis, 1999, Mosby.

**TABLE 9-2**

*Cross-Cultural Examples of Cultural Phenomena Affecting Nursing Care*

| NATIONS OF ORIGIN | COMMUNICATION | SPACE | TIME ORIENTATION | SOCIAL ORGANIZATION | ENVIRONMENTAL CONTROL | BIOLOGICAL VARIATIONS |
|---|---|---|---|---|---|---|
| *Asian*<br>China<br>Hawaii<br>Philippines<br>Korea<br>Japan<br>Southeast Asia (Laos, Cambodia, Vietnam) | National language preference<br>Dialects, written characters<br>Use of silence<br>Nonverbal and contextual cuing | Noncontact people | Present | Family: hierarchical structure, loyalty<br>Devotion to tradition<br>Many religions, including Taoism, Buddhism, Islam, and Christianity<br>Community social organizations | Traditional health and illness beliefs<br>Use of traditional medicines<br>Traditional practitioners: Chinese doctors and herbalists | Liver cancer<br>Stomach cancer<br>Coccidioidomycosis<br>Hypertension<br>Lactose intolerance |
| *African*<br>West Coast (as slaves)<br>Many African countries<br>West Indian Islands<br>Dominican Republic<br>Haiti<br>Jamaica | National languages<br>Dialect: Pidgin, Creole, Spanish, and French | Close personal space | Present over future | Family: many female, single parent<br>Large, extended family networks<br>Strong church affiliation within community<br>Community social organizations | Traditional health and illness beliefs<br>Folk medicine tradition<br>Traditional healer: root-worker | Sickle cell anemia<br>Hypertension<br>Cancer of the esophagus<br>Stomach cancer<br>Coccidioidomycosis<br>Lactose intolerance |
| *Europe*<br>Germany<br>England<br>Italy<br>Ireland<br>Other European countries | National languages<br>Many learn English immediately | Noncontact people<br>Aloof<br>Distant<br>Southern countries: closer contact and touch | Future over present | Nuclear families<br>Extended families<br>Judeo-Christian religions<br>Community social organizations | Primary reliance on modern health care system<br>Traditional health and illness beliefs<br>Some remaining folk medicine traditions | Breast cancer<br>Heart disease<br>Diabetes mellitus<br>Thalassemia |
| *Native American*<br>170 Native American tribes<br>Aleuts<br>Eskimos | Tribal languages<br>Use of silence and body language | Space very important and has no boundaries | Present | Extremely family oriented<br>Biological and extended families<br>Children taught to respect traditions<br>Community social organizations | Traditional health and illness beliefs<br>Folk medicine tradition<br>Traditional healer: medicine man | Accidents<br>Heart disease<br>Cirrhosis of the liver<br>Diabetes mellitus |
| *Hispanic Countries*<br>Spain<br>Cuba<br>Mexico<br>Central and South America | Spanish or Portuguese primary language | Tactile relationships<br>Touch<br>Handshakes<br>Embracing<br>Value physical presence | Present | Nuclear family<br>Extended families<br>*Compadrazzo*: godparents<br>Community social organizations | Traditional health and illness beliefs<br>Folk medicine tradition<br>Traditional healers: *Curandero, Espiritista, Partera, Senora* | Diabetes mellitus<br>Parasites<br>Coccidioidomycosis<br>Lactose intolerance |

Compiled by Rachel Spector, RN, PhD. Modified from Potter PA, Perry AG: *Fundamentals of nursing: concepts, process, and practice*, ed 4, St Louis, 1997, Mosby, p. 356.

lineated in Appendix 9-1. The phenomena described by Giger and Davidhizar influence family health factors such as how clients interact with health care providers and others in their environment, clients' beliefs about health and illness and their susceptibility to disease, nutritional preferences and deficiencies, role relationships and communication patterns within a family unit, and time management.

Table 9-2 provides specific examples of how cultural phenomena vary across cultures. These variations influence the use of the nursing process throughout all of its stages. For example, ethnic differences have been found in how members of a specific culture communicate symptoms and how they respond to these symptoms. Simply knowing the language is not enough. Nurses must understand and respect the cultural differences in terms of health behaviors (Chwedyk, 2000). Research has shown that response to pain varies cross-culturally (Calvillo, Flaskerud, 1993). For instance, the Navajo Indians have very few words for describing the nature of pain, and their value system supports bearing pain in silence (Simons, 1985). This can result in an inaccurate assessment and diagnosis regarding the severity of a client's pain, which in turn can influence the nature of interventions (e.g., amount of pain medication given) and evaluation (e.g., relief of pain) of the client's status.

Community health nurses must always remember that people are continuously influenced by their culture (Hines, Preto, McGoldrick, et al., 1999). If nurses function within an ethnocentric perspective, these cultural differences can adversely affect the therapeutic process. For example, it is not unusual for health care providers and clients to have different time perceptions and for the professional to label the client irresponsible when he or she does not keep or is late for appointments. "It is important for the nurse to discern carefully if the client's time is attributable to cultural phenomena or to some biochemical or psychosocial manifestation" (Giger, Davidhizar, 1999, p. 102). This does not necessarily reflect a disregard for others. Rather, it may reflect differences in lifestyle patterns that have not been addressed during the therapeutic process.

Box 9-2 describes situations that illustrate how disparity in health beliefs can adversely affect the therapeutic process. In these situations, Eliason (1993) identifies how *ethnocentrism* can adversely influence clients' acceptance of the health care professional and health teaching. Eliason also has identified ethnorelative solutions for reducing cultural barriers to the therapeutic process in the case examples shared in this box. "*Ethnorelativity* is the ability to conceive of alternative viewpoints and to respect the beliefs of another culture even though they are different from one's own" (Eliason, 1993, p. 226).

Even though specific incidents can be provided that illustrate how cultural patterning differs across ethnic and racial groups, *it is critically important to mention again that intracultural variations exist and that an individualized assessment is necessary to identify family values, attitudes, beliefs, and norms.* Awareness of cultural differences provides a framework for nursing assessment, intervention, and evaluation. Use of the nursing process assists practitioners to individualize their care.

## Stop and Think About It

Recall an experience in which you prejudged someone from an ethnocentric perspective. Write out the ethnocentric experience and describe how this experience could be changed by applying an ethnorelative perspective.

---

 **BOX 9-2**

*Examples of Disparity in Health Beliefs*

### Example #1

Carlos is a 15-year-old from a poor urban area where drugs proliferate and many young men trade sex for drugs or money. You are fairly certain that Carlos does not use intravenous (IV) drugs but know that he often has sex with men for money. Carlos believes that only homosexual men are at risk for acquired immunodeficiency syndrome (AIDS). Because he considers his prostitution a job not associated with his sexual identity, he does not consider himself as being at risk for AIDS.

**ETHNOCENTRIC SOLUTIONS**

1. Convince Carlos that he is homosexual because he has sex with men and, therefore, is at risk for AIDS.
2. Diagnose Carlos as "noncompliant" because he does not alter his behavior after you inform him of the risks.

**ETHNORELATIVE SOLUTIONS**

3. Respect Carlos's beliefs and try to teach him about risky behaviors without discussing sexual identities or applying a label to his behavior.

### Example #2

Harold and Sarah are expecting their first child. Sarah comes to a prenatal clinic for her first visit. The nurse notes that Sarah is 26 years old, well educated, and healthy. Sarah is informed that she has no unusual risks for her pregnancy. The infant is born healthy, but 10 months later the clinic is being sued because the baby has Tay-Sachs disease, and Harold and Sarah were not told that they, as Ashkenazi Jews, were at risk.

Modified from Eliason MS: Ethics and transcultural nursing care, *Nurs Outlook* 41(5):227-228, 1993.

*Continued*

**BOX 9-2**

*Examples of Disparity in Health Beliefs—cont'd*

**ETHNOCENTRIC SOLUTIONS**

1. Blame Sarah for not informing the clinic, because she did not "look Jewish."
2. Blame the clinic administrators, who did not include "Jewish" as a racial identity as well as a religion.

**ETHNORELATIVE SOLUTIONS**

3. Alter clinic health assessment records to ensure reporting of racial/ethnic identity. Educate staff on health and risk-for-illness factors that differ by race or ethnicity.

*Example #3*

June, a 35-year-old surgical nurse, grew up in a fundamentalist religion, although she rarely attends church now. June admits a middle-aged female patient who is to undergo major surgery the next day. The patient, Barbara, insists that her companion, Alicia, be present for the preoperative teaching and any discussions of her health. June explains that only spouses or biological family members will be allowed to visit Barbara in the recovery room or the intensive care unit (ICU) after surgery. When Barbara explains that she considers Alicia her spouse, June leaves the room. Later she comments to coworkers, "It wouldn't be so bad if she didn't throw her homosexuality in my face like that! It really bothers me when those people flaunt their sexuality!" She avoids Barbara's room for the rest of the shift.

**ETHNOCENTRIC SOLUTIONS**

1. Uphold hospital policy and do not allow Alicia to visit or make decisions with Barbara.
2. Refuse to care for Barbara, or, if giving her care, avoid any discussion of her sexual identity.

**ETHNORELATIVE SOLUTIONS**

3. Reconsider hospital policies. Must "significant others" be so narrowly defined? What are the purposes of the restrictions?
4. Examine personal beliefs. How did June come to be so negative about lesbians? Does her religious background—much of which she has already rejected—affect her current views?
5. Find out more information about the health care needs of lesbians. Ask Barbara about her wishes and include Alicia in her care.

*Example #4*

Tammi is a 75-year-old woman who was born in China and immigrated to the United States when she was 40. She lives in a predominantly Chinese neighborhood and maintains her traditional values and customs. Although the nurse introduced himself as Tony several times and has asked Tammi to call him by his first name, she continues to call him "doctor." Whenever Tony addresses her as Tammi, she looks away but does not say anything to explain her behavior. Tony is finding it increasingly difficult to communicate with Tammi. Later Tony learns from Tammi's daughter that in her mother's culture it is not proper to address strangers by their first name, and it is disrespectful for 25-year-old Tony to call an elder by her first name. It is also not considered polite to make demands on authority figures but rather to take what they offer.

**ETHNOCENTRIC SOLUTIONS**

1. Diagnose an alteration in communication or lack of assertiveness because Tammi failed to inform Tony of her wishes.
2. Tell Tammi that in this country, we call people by their first names.

**ETHNORELATIVE SOLUTIONS**

3. Ask her how she would like to be addressed. Offer your whole name and let her choose how to address you.
4. Offer her choices instead of asking open-ended questions.

*Example #5*

Clara is an 82-year-old African-American woman from a small rural community. She has arthritis and congestive heart failure. She recently has experienced considerable knee pain, and Ruth is following up on her prescription for an antiinflammatory medication. Ruth, a community health nurse, discovers that Clara never filled the prescription but is using a "mustard plaster" made of various greens from her garden. She states that the pain is gone and she has no need for expensive pills.

**ETHNOCENTRIC SOLUTIONS**

1. Label her as "noncompliant" and encourage her to fill the prescription.
2. Try to persuade her that the greens have no therapeutic value. She should use "real" medicine.

**ETHNORELATIVE SOLUTIONS**

3. Try to determine whether there are other reasons for her rejecting the medication, such as not being able to afford the prescription.
4. Believe her when she says she has no pain and encourage her to continue the mustard plaster treatments.

Modified from Eliason MS: Ethics and transcultural nursing care, *Nurs Outlook* 41(5):227-228, 1993.

## PHASES OF THE FAMILY-CENTERED NURSING PROCESS

The family-centered nursing process has six phases: assessing, analyzing, planning, implementing, evaluating, and terminating. Although each phase is discussed separately, they are dynamically interrelated and overlap. The interdependent nature of these phases, along with nursing activities during each phase, is presented in Table 9-3.

**TABLE 9-3**

*Relationships Among the Phases of the Family-Centered Nursing Process*

| Assessing ⟶ | Analyzing ⟶ | Planning ⟶ | Implementing ⟶ | Evaluating ⟶ | Terminating ⟶ |
|---|---|---|---|---|---|
| Process for obtaining a database | A critical thinking process that results in the identification of nursing diagnoses | Formulation of desired family outcomes (goals) and identification of actions (intervention strategies) to achieve goals | A systematic approach to action used by the family and nurse to achieve desired family outcomes | A continuous, concurrent process used to critique each component of the nursing process | A therapeutic process that helps the client and the nurse end their relationship |

| ASSESSING | ANALYZING | PLANNING | IMPLEMENTING | EVALUATING | TERMINATING |
|---|---|---|---|---|---|
| 1. Develop a trusting relationship:<br>a. Explain purpose of community health nursing visit<br>b. Describe what community health nurse has to offer<br>c. Facilitate the sharing of thoughts, feelings, and data<br>d. Set time parameters for evaluation and frequency and length of visits<br>2. Collect data in variety of ways:<br>a. Observation<br>b. Interview<br>c. Inspection<br>d. Physical assessment<br>e. Contact with secondary sources<br>f. Review of records | 1. Make differential conclusions about family needs by:<br>a. Using theoretical knowledge to identify significant signs and symptoms<br>b. Grouping data to show relationships between assessment categories and to identify *patterns* of behavior<br>c. Relating family data to relevant clinical and research findings<br>d. Comparing nursing diagnoses with diagnoses of other health professionals | 1. Formulate client-centered goals and expected outcomes:<br>a. Establish realistic goals consistent with the database and nursing diagnoses<br>b. State goals and outcomes in measurable terms<br>c. Develop family and individual goals and expected outcomes in collaboration with the family<br>2. Identify intervention strategies:<br>a. Identify direct and indirect care interventions consistent with client needs | 1. Base nursing actions on client needs, lifestyle patterns, level of knowledge, and motivation<br>a. Determine client readiness<br>b. Demonstrate awareness of proper timing for nursing activities<br>c. Adapt or alter nursing interventions if client situation changes<br>d. Modify nursing activities to accommodate lifestyle patterns, level of knowledge<br>2. Address barriers (e.g., cultural or financial) to client action | 1. Elicit ongoing feedback from client to determine if goals, plans, and interventions are appropriate<br>2. Identify the results of intervention activities taken by:<br>a. Client<br>b. Community health nurse<br>c. Other health care professionals<br>3. Determine why intervention activities have been ineffective, if warranted<br>4. Modify the management plan when appropriate<br>5. Use a variety of methods to evaluate:<br>a. Obtain feedback from client | 1. Deal with feelings associated with termination<br>2. Review client achievements<br>3. Discuss what the therapeutic process has meant<br>4. Plan carefully the termination of visits<br>5. Share with client how to reestablish contact if needed<br>6. Discuss with client self-care requirements upon discharge |

*Continued*

**TABLE 9-3**

*Relationships Among the Phases of the Family-Centered Nursing Process—cont'd*

| ASSESSING | ANALYZING | PLANNING | IMPLEMENTING | EVALUATING | TERMINATING |
|---|---|---|---|---|---|
| 3. Assess all parameters of family functioning:<br>a. Family dynamics<br>b. Health status: family and individual members<br>c. Physiological data<br>d. Psychosocial data<br>e. Sociocultural data<br>f. Environmental data<br>g. Preventive health practices<br>4. Obtain data from multiple sources:<br>a. Client, family<br>b. Health team members<br>c. Community agencies<br>d. Significant others<br>e. Relevant records<br>5. Use standards of care to focus the interviewing process | 2. Formulate specific nursing diagnoses:<br>a. Base diagnoses on a strong database<br>b. Identify the functional aspects of a client's current health status<br>c. Determine various levels of family functioning<br>(1) Strengths<br>(2) Needs<br>(3) Anticipatory guidance warranted<br>d. Identify when data are insufficient to make a nursing diagnosis | b. Determine activities that the client, the nurse, and other health care professionals might carry out to achieve expected outcomes<br>c. Assist the client in identifying the pros and cons of each intervention and in making decisions about the appropriate course of action<br>3. Identify priority needs, goals, and interventions:<br>a. Use theory to differentiate between problems that need immediate action and those that can wait<br>b. Identify potential crisis situations<br>c. Consider client safety<br>4. Identify evaluation criteria | a. Explore with family reasons for progress or lack of it<br>b. Assist family in overcoming barriers to action<br>3. Carry through with planned interventions<br>a. Keep appointments with the family<br>b. Carry out nursing activities in a timely manner<br>c. Discuss with the family the need for altering interventions if necessary<br>d. Assist the family in carrying out planned interventions<br>4. Base intervention activities on scientific knowledge<br>a. Review scientific literature<br>b. Use acceptable standards (e.g., growth and development or nutritional)<br>c. Consult with peers, supervisors, and other health care providers | b. Consult with peers, supervisors, and other health care professionals<br>c. Summarize records<br>d. Conduct nursing audits | |

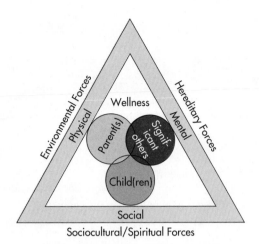

**FIGURE 9-4** Triangle of family health.

A comprehensive family assessment initiates the process and evaluates multiple components of family health (Figure 9-4). In the community setting, the family is the central focus throughout the nursing process, and assessment data are always validated with the family. The family should be active participants in planning, implementing, and evaluating interventions that are designed to promote family growth. The family-centered nursing process is a client-oriented, not a nurse-oriented, process. This process focuses on strengthening the family's self-care capacities.

## ASSESSING

The assessment phase involves a systematic data collection process that provides the foundation for making nursing diagnoses. During this phase the community health nurse places emphasis on collecting specific data about client (family) functioning so that objective conclusions regarding the client's health status can be made. Inferences about a client's level of functioning should be made only after a sufficient database has been obtained.

The primary responsibilities of the community health nurse during the assessment phase are threefold: (1) developing a trusting, therapeutic relationship; (2) using a variety of data collection methods to obtain client information from all available resources; and (3) assessing all parameters of family health, including family dynamics, family resources, health status of individual family members, and environmental factors that influence family health. **Focused assessment** includes careful attention to all three of these activities, which helps the community health nurse more clearly delineate client needs and goals and interventions that may enhance client growth.

### First Home Visits

Home visiting is a long-established method for promoting family health at all levels of prevention (General Account-

ing Office [GAO], 1990; Weiss, 1993). In the home health care setting, it is the principal means by which community health nurses provide services for clients and their families. Recent laws, in particular those dealing with Medicaid prenatal care expansions and services to developmentally delayed and at-risk infants and toddlers and their families, include provisions that provide a new impetus for home visiting (GAO, 1990, p. 24).

Making first home visits to families initially can be stressful, especially for a nurse entering an unknown environment controlled by the client rather than the health care professional. First home visits can also be rewarding, particularly if the nurse recognizes that he or she is providing a valuable service. In general, families are receptive and interested in the services community health nurses have to offer. There may be times, however, when a family prefers to handle its health care needs within the family unit without assistance from others. The community health nurse must respect the family's preference. Sometimes families do not appear interested in home visits because they are unaware of how a community health nurse may assist them. Educating a family about community health nursing services may provide the family with the information needed to make an informed decision regarding continued visits.

### First Home Visits: Nursing Responsibilities

First home visits can influence families' receptivity to future home visits. Carefully planned first visits can facilitate relationship building and assist nurses in demonstrating the contributions they can make in helping families deal with current health needs. Table 9-4 outlines how to prepare for a first home visit, tasks to initiate during the visit, and postvisit activities. The goals for the first visit should be to establish a positive client/nurse working relationship, obtain baseline data on the family situation, and address the immediate concerns of the family. The extent to which the nurse carries out the tasks identified in Table 9-4 during the initial visit will vary depending on the family's circumstances. Some tasks will not be done at all because they are not appropriate for the client's situation. For example, doctor's orders are not required for families receiving only health promotion services. On the other hand, nurses do not provide home health or care of the sick services without a doctor's order. It is critical to remember that the assessment phase of the nursing process is ongoing and should extend throughout the length of the nurse-client relationship. It is not feasible or appropriate to obtain all needed data during the initial contact.

Community health nurses encounter a variety of situations on first home visits, such as families who want parenting education or elderly couples who have requested assistance with care of an ill family member. Although the major focus on these visits may vary from care of the sick to health teaching, the *delivery of primary prevention services is a major component of all community health nursing visits.*

**TABLE 9-4**

*First Home Visits: Responsibilities and Tasks*

| RESPONSIBILITY | TASKS |
| --- | --- |
| I. Previsit preparation | Review available family data, including referral information and previous family records. |
| | Clarify data with others (e.g., contact family physician and/or other referral sources or talk with intake nurse). |
| | Establish a plan for the visit. |
| | Consider appropriate community resources. |
| | Review theory related to identified family problems. |
| | Prepare for a safe visit (e.g., identify exact location of home, consider safety issues in relation to the neighborhood being visited, and request escort or shared visit services if needed). |
| II. Establish contact with family | Contact family via phone, if available. |
| | Identify self, including name and agency you are representing. |
| | Explain who referred family to agency and purpose of referral. |
| | Discuss briefly services the community health nurse (CHN) can provide, such as sharing data about available community resources. |
| | Identify family's need for CHN services and willingness to have nurse visits. |
| | Schedule home visit at a time convenient for family. |
| III. Home visit intervention | |
| A. Relationship-building period | Introduce self and role. |
| | Introduce agency, agency obligations, and programs and services. |
| | Explain purpose of home visit. |
| | Build a nurse-client relationship. |
| | Discuss client rights and responsibilities. |
| | Assess safety of care plan: is a primary caregiver present and available if needed? |
| | Consider safety issues for the health care provider (e.g., park near the home, don't enter the house if the client is not home, and dress professionally, avoiding expensive jewelry and suggestive clothing). |
| B. Intervention period | Carry out an *initial* client assessment.* |
| | Carry out an *initial* family assessment.* |
| | Carry out an *initial* environmental assessment;* pay particular attention to client safety and health needs. |
| | Elicit physician's perceptions of how a CHN can assist. |
| | Assess doctor's orders and need for changes if appropriate. |
| | Assess appropriateness of stated third-party reimbursement. |
| | Assess need for other services such as physical therapy or referral to a community agency for parenting classes. |
| | Assess need for equipment and supplies. |
| | Confirm medication orders, dosages, and client knowledge of medications. |
| | Identify client's knowledge base related to identified problems (e.g., disease process or care of infant). |
| | Discuss estimated length of service, including limits set by third-party payers, if appropriate. |
| C. Closing period | Summarize visit activities with family. |
| | Together decide what the client/family will be doing between now and the next visit. |
| | Inform client/family how to reach nurse between visits. |
| | Set time for next visit. |
| IV. Postvisit activities | Begin the nursing care plan. |
| | Document visit. |
| | Make contacts on behalf of client/family if needed (e.g., initiate other services, contact physician regarding needed change in order, or inform vendors about needed equipment and supplies). |
| | Complete agency reporting forms and paperwork for third-party reimbursement. |
| | Evaluate visit progress. |

*On the first home visit it is not feasible to complete a comprehensive family assessment. Priority should be given to assessing the family's major concerns and influencing factors. Referral data can assist a nurse in focusing the initial family assessment.

Examples of these types of interventions are teaching to increase the client's self-care capabilities, environmental assessment to promote safety and prevent home accidents, and making referrals for respite services to prevent caregiver burnout.

## Safety in the Community

As in any situation, it is important to consider issues of environmental safety when visiting an unfamiliar area. Statistical data reflect that crime is prevalent in all types of socioeconomic neighborhoods and in a variety of health and welfare organizations. Although reports of crime involving community health nurses are unusual, nurses need to take precautions to avoid unsafe or potentially unsafe situations.

It is important to carefully observe environmental safety conditions and to leave a home or neighborhood if you "sense" that it could be unsafe. Experienced nurses watch for such things as an unusually large number of people congregating in the neighborhood, violent exchanges between family members or individuals in the community, people who appear to be abusing alcohol or drugs, and individuals suspiciously hanging around cars or doorways. Numerous websites offer practical safety tips and crime prevention tips for individuals, families, and communities. Logging on to *http://www.go.com* and searching for information provides a variety of safety and crime prevention topics.

Most community health agencies have safety guidelines to follow, including refusing rides from strangers, dressing professionally, not wearing expensive jewelry and suggestive clothing, planning ahead to avoid appearing lost, leaving an established visit plan in the agency, and not entering an environment where safety is questionable. In some cases, it is appropriate to make visits with a partner. Families being visited also may provide the nurse with safety guidelines such as where to park one's car in the neighborhood and best times during the day to visit. The nurse may consult with a family by phone if she has questions about environmental conditions. Seeking consultation from colleagues also helps when a nurse has concerns about environmental safety.

## Relationship Building

The type of relationship established during the assessment phase can be the critical factor in helping the client determine whether to accept the assistance offered by the community health nurse. It is natural for clients to evaluate their interactions with community health nurses. It takes time for most people to develop a trusting relationship.

Trust between the nurse and the client can be established by taking the time to explain the purpose of the community health nursing visits, describing the services that can be provided, and creating a nonthreatening atmosphere that allows the client to share data at his or her own pace. Clarifying why the community health nurse is visiting is essential. When clients do not understand the purpose of nursing visits, the therapeutic relationship may not get established. This can result in frustration and mistrust and inhibit the expression of thoughts, feelings, and data.

Clients usually do not share information freely until they understand why the information is needed. Sharing with clients their rights and responsibilities and agency obligations can help clarify the purpose of home visits. All clients have the right to be active participants in the care process, including continuity of care decisions, and to have their privacy and property respected. They also have the right to voice complaints without fear of reprisal. Table 9-5 delineates specific client rights and responsibilities and related agency obligations as defined by the Health Care Financing Administration (HCFA) (HCFA, 1991; 1994). The HCFA's name was changed to the Centers for Medicare and Medicaid Services (CMS) in 2001.

## Family Interviews

Working with families presents special interviewing challenges for the community health nurse because families are composed of unique individuals who have varying needs, concerns, and communication styles. The goal of community health nursing is to enhance the well-being of the family unit (Bomar, McNeely, 1996). This involves working with individual family members as well as the family as one unit. It also includes examining their patterns of communication, cultural influences, and societal expectations in relation to life events (Carter, McGoldrick, 1999; Hines, Preto, McGoldrick, et al., 1999). For example, when nurses work with a family that is dealing with an unexpected stressful event, such as the birth of a premature infant or a diagnosis of cancer, it is crucial to explore how well the family unit is carrying out its role responsibilities (e.g., maintaining work and school schedules and nurturing all family members). During times of stress, it is not uncommon for the family to neglect these responsibilities. This can significantly alter family functioning. When this occurs, the community health nurse problem-solves with the family to determine ways to achieve a balance in family dynamics (see Chapter 8 for interventions that enhance family problem-solving abilities during times of stress).

When a nurse is allowed to cross the family boundaries and is accepted by the family system, the influences the nurse has on that system must be examined carefully. The nurse must remain cognizant of professional boundaries, be aware of his or her own interactions between individual family members, and avoid establishing alliances during the family decision-making process. Establishing an alliance with an individual family member impedes the therapeutic process and can lead to, or reinforce, ineffective family patterns. For example, a nurse who firmly believes that all women need a career outside the home may strongly support a female client's desires to work without allowing her husband or significant other to verbalize his concerns. In situations like these, the nurse needs to help the family

**TABLE 9-5**

*Client Rights and Responsibilities and Related Agency Obligations*

| RIGHTS/OBLIGATIONS | CLIENT RIGHTS | AGENCY OBLIGATIONS |
|---|---|---|
| Notice of rights | To be fully informed of all his or her rights and responsibilities | Provide client with a written notice of rights in advance of initiating care<br>Obtain signed verification from client or client's caregiver that they have received written notice of rights |
| Exercise of rights and respect for property and person | To have property treated with respect<br>To voice grievances and suggest change in service without fear of reprisal or discrimination<br>To have family or guardian voice grievances when judged incompetent<br>To have privacy respected | Investigate complaints made by client or client's family or guardian<br>Document existence of complaint and resolution of complaint |
| To be informed and to participate in planning care and treatment | To receive appropriate and professional care related to physician orders<br>To choose care provided<br>To receive information necessary to give informed consent before the start of any care<br>To know how to reach agency staff 24 hours a day, 7 days a week, and what to do in an emergency<br>To refuse treatment within the confines of the law and be informed of the consequences of this action<br>To reasonable continuity of care<br>To be informed in reasonable time of anticipated termination of service and plans for transfer to another agency | Admit client for service only if the agency has the ability to provide safe professional care at the level of intensity needed<br>Share with client physician orders<br>Advise client in advance of care, the disciplines that will furnish care, and the frequency of visits<br>Advise client in advance of any changes in care<br>Involve client in the planning of care<br>Inform client of agency policies and procedures |
| Confidentiality of medical record | To have agency maintain confidentiality of the clinical records | Advise client of agency's policies and procedures regarding disclosure of information in clinical records |
| Liability for payment | To receive information regarding charges for services, the client's potential liability for these charges, and client's eligibility for third-party reimbursements<br>To referral if service denied solely on the inability to pay for service | Inform client orally and in writing and in advance of care the extent to which third-party reimbursement may pay for care and charges client may have to pay<br>Notify client orally and in writing of changes in eligibility for services from third-party reimbursement |
| Home health hotline | To know about the availability of a toll-free home health hotline in the state to voice complaints about agency services or to have questions answered about home care | Inform client in writing how to reach the home health hotline |

Data from Health Care Financing Administration (HCFA): *Conditions of participation: home health agencies,* 42 CFR Part 484, Section 484.10 through 484.52, Washington, DC, October, 1994, HCFA, Section 484.10.

evaluate the pros and cons of taking a certain action, and then encourage decision making between the couple.

The values, attitudes, and beliefs held by the community health nurse also can disrupt the nurse-family interview. Professionals bring to the therapeutic process cultural patterning that influences thinking about variables such as how roles should be implemented, how a home should be managed, and how children should be raised. The nurse may inappropriately label family behavior as ineffective if it is not consistent with his or her beliefs. The guidelines presented in Box 9-3 can assist the nurse in avoiding barriers to therapeutic communication and relating effectively with clients from different cultures.

## Sources and Methods for Collecting Data

During the assessment phase both primary and secondary data are collected from all available sources. Primary data are those data that the community health nurse directly ob-

**BOX 9-3**

## Guidelines for Relating to Clients from Different Cultures

1. Assess your personal beliefs surrounding persons from different cultures.
   - Review your personal beliefs and past experiences.
   - Set aside any values, biases, ideas, and attitudes that are judgmental and may negatively affect care.
2. Assess communication variables from a cultural perspective.
   - Determine the ethnic identity of the client, including generation in America.
   - Use the client as a source of information when possible.
   - Assess cultural factors that may affect your relationship with the client and respond appropriately.
3. Plan care based on the communicated needs and cultural background.
   - Learn as much as possible about the client's cultural customs and beliefs.
   - Encourage the client to reveal cultural interpretation of health, illness, and health care.
   - Be sensitive to the uniqueness of the client.
   - Identify sources of discrepancy between the client's and your own concepts of health and illness.
   - Communicate at the client's personal level of functioning.
   - Evaluate effectiveness of nursing actions and modify the nursing care plan when necessary.
4. Modify communication approaches to meet cultural needs.
   - Be attentive to signs of fear, anxiety, and confusion in the client.
   - Respond in a reassuring manner in keeping with the client's cultural orientation.
   - Be aware that, in some cultural groups, discussion concerning the client with others may be offensive and may impede the nursing process.
5. Understand that respect for the client and communicated needs is central to the therapeutic relationship.
   - Communicate respect by using a kind and attentive approach.
   - Learn how listening is communicated in the client's culture.
   - Use appropriate active listening techniques.
   - Adopt an attitude of flexibility, respect, and interest to help bridge barriers imposed by culture.
6. Communicate in a nonthreatening manner.
   - Conduct the interview in an unhurried manner.
   - Follow acceptable social and cultural amenities.
   - Ask general questions during the information-gathering stage.
   - Be patient with a respondent who gives information that may seem unrelated to the client's health problem.
   - Develop a trusting relationship by listening carefully, allowing time, and giving the client your full attention.
7. Use validating techniques in communication.
   - Be alert for feedback that the client is not understanding.
   - Do not assume meaning is interpreted without distortion.
8. Be considerate of reluctance to talk when the subject involves sexual matters.
   - Be aware that, in some cultures, sexual matters are not discussed freely with members of the opposite sex.
9. Adopt special approaches when the client speaks a different language.
   - Use a caring tone of voice and facial expression to help alleviate the client's fears.
   - Speak slowly and distinctly, but not loudly.
   - Use gestures, pictures, and play acting to help the client understand.
   - Repeat the message in different ways if necessary.
   - Be alert to words the client seems to understand and use them frequently.
   - Keep messages simple and repeat them frequently.
   - Avoid using medical terms and abbreviations that the client may not understand.
   - Use an appropriate language dictionary.
10. Use interpreters to improve communication.
    - Ask the interpreter to translate the message, not just the individual words.
    - Obtain feedback to confirm understanding.
    - Use an interpreter who is culturally sensitive.

Modified from Giger JN, Davidhizar RE: *Transcultural nursing: assessment and intervention,* ed 3, St Louis, 1999, Mosby, p. 34.

tains from the client—data that the nurse actually sees, hears, feels, or smells in the client's environment. An astute community health nurse carefully notes observations and verbal information received from the client. Significant clues about the client's level of coping and functioning can be obtained by observing how the client interacts within the environment. For example, during home visits, it is not unusual for the community health nurse to discern a child discipline problem by repeatedly watching parents interact

with their children. It is important to remember that inferences about client problems should be based on patterns of behavior rather than isolated incidents. Labeling behavior ineffective after one observation is a dangerous practice and can adversely affect the nurse-family relationship.

In the community health setting, secondary data are obtained from a variety of sources such as significant others, personnel from health and social agencies, the family's physician, spiritual leaders, and health records. Generally the community health nurse receives either verbal or written permission from the client before making contact with other secondary sources. This practice not only protects the client's **right of privacy** but also promotes honesty and trust in the therapeutic relationship. In addition, seeking a client's permission to obtain information from others demonstrates to the client that the nurse respects the client's **right of self-determination.** The nurse should keep in mind that secondary data may not accurately reflect clients' perceptions of themselves or their needs. Instead, secondary data may reflect others' perceptions of what is needed. The sources of information should always be indicated when the data are documented.

Various assessment methodologies should be used to collect primary and secondary data. Interview, observation, direct examination (auscultation, percussion, palpation, inspection, and measurement), contact with secondary sources of data, and review of relevant records are methods used by the community health nurse to obtain an accurate and complete profile of a family's situation. These methods are used to identify client strengths as well as client limitations or needs.

The significance of using a variety of methods to collect data about family functioning cannot be overstated. No one data collection method provides the community health nurse with all the information needed to formulate accurate nursing diagnoses. The Daniels' family case scenario that follows illustrates this fact by showing the contrast between the type of data one nurse obtained from an interview and from direct observation.

**CASE**
*Scenario* Following hospitalization of Mr. Daniels for an acute exacerbation episode of multiple sclerosis, the Daniels' family was referred to the health department for health supervision follow-up. Ms. Garitt, hospital social worker, requested that a community health nurse assess this family's needs in relation to its understanding of multiple sclerosis, its ability to handle activities of daily living, its knowledge of community resources, and the impact of Mr. Daniels' illness on family functioning. While community health nurse, Jane Mathews, was interviewing the family and collecting data on the entire family situation, she asked Mr. and Mrs. Daniels how they were managing Mr. Daniels' exercises. Both related that they were doing them regularly. Mrs. Daniels accurately described how the exercises should be done and verbalized that she felt comfortable handling them because she had been instructed how to do so by hospital staff. While Mrs. Daniels was demonstrating what she had learned it was found that she did have an understanding about the proper exercises for her husband. However, her body mechanics were inappropriate, and this caused severe backache that she failed to mention during the interviewing process. In addition to Mrs. Daniels' poor body mechanics, the nurse also discovered that Mr. Daniels was very demanding of his wife, expecting her to do exercises for him that he could do independently. Further exploration revealed that Mr. Daniels was doing very little for himself. Before his illness he had been the "man of the house. Now I can't do anything." Through demonstration and return demonstration the nurse showed Mr. Daniels that he was not helpless and assisted Mrs. Daniels in learning how to position herself appropriately when helping her husband. The nurse also helped the family identify family patterns that were fostering dependency. Observing family interactions provided this nurse with data about family functioning that were not obtained through interview.

## Assessing All Parameters of Family Health

The family-centered approach to nursing care focuses on the family as a unit rather than a collection of individual family members. This implies that the family is viewed as a system in which the actions and health status of one family member always affect the behavior and health status of all other family members. Thus when community health nurses assess family health, they not only examine the health status of individual family members but also look at family dynamics (Figure 9-5). Chapter 7 presents guidelines for examining **family dynamics** and includes a family assessment guide (see Appendix 7-4) that facilitates data col-

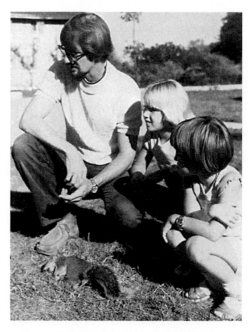

**FIGURE 9-5** Family dynamics influence how well individual family members handle critical life events. The ability to provide support and security during times of stress (exposure to death) is a family strength that should be reinforced.

lection for the purpose of evaluating a family's health status. Hanson and Mischke (1996) have identified a range of family assessment and measurement instruments that have been developed by nonnurses and nurses. Several of these instruments are discussed more extensively in Berkey and Hanson's *Pocket Guide to Family Assessment and Intervention* (1991).

## Family Health Status

As previously discussed, a major goal of nurses working with families in the community is to enhance the well-being of the family unit. Inherent in this goal is the belief that it is important for families to maintain the integrity of the family unit while meeting the needs of individual family members. It is crucial for both families and nurses to recognize that if the health status of the family unit is neglected, it will be difficult for families to assist individual family members, particularly during periods of stress.

"Family health is the family's quality of life from a holistic perspective as it is affected by such variables as spirituality, nutrition, stress, environment, recreation and exercise, sleep, and sexuality" (Bomar, 1996, p. ix). Nurses must be able to evaluate and assess the total needs of families (Ericksen, 2000). During the assessment phase of the nursing process, the community health nurse evaluates the health status of the family unit from a holistic perspective to identify both family strengths and needs. Table 9-6 delineates criteria to consider when assessing family strengths.

Several themes emerge when reviewing the literature that addresses characteristics of healthy families (Beavers, 1977; Curran, 1983; Lewis, Beavers, Gossett, et al., 1976; Otto, 1963; Pratt, 1976). Healthy families have flexible role patterns, maintain growth-producing relationships within the family unit and between the family and the broader community, have active problem-solving mechanisms, have an ability to accept help, and are responsive to the needs of individual members. Healthy families also have effective communication patterns; provide a warm, caring atmosphere; and have a strong sense of family in which rituals and traditions are shared. "Overall, a well-functioning family is a flexible one that can shift roles, levels of responsibilities, and patterns of interaction as it passes through periods of varying stressful life changes" (Danielson, Hamel-Bissell, Winstead-Fry, 1993, p. 201).

Community health nurses encounter families with varying states of health. Most families visited by nurses in the community setting are dealing with some type of stressor such as the birth of a child, a newly diagnosed health problem, or inadequate resources to meet the family's basic needs. Danielson, Hamel-Bissell, and Winstead-Fry (1993) use a multifaceted framework (Figure 9-6) to assess whether family behavior during these periods of stress is bonadaptive or maladaptive. **Bonadaptation** is "the ability of the family

to stabilize with instituted patterns in place, promote the individual development of its members, and achieve a sense of coherence and congruency even when stressors and substantive changes threaten established patterns of family functioning" (Danielson, Hamel-Bissell, Winstead-Fry, 1993, p. 413).

**Maladaptation** occurs when a family is unable to achieve a balance in family functioning during periods of stress (see Chapter 8). Danielson, Hamel-Bissell, and Winstead-Fry's multifaceted assessment framework assists the community health nurse in evaluating the health of the family from three perspectives: "the result of the interaction between individual members and the family unit, between the family unit and the larger social system, and between sociocultural subsystems and individual members" (Danielson, Hamel-Bissell, Winstead-Fry, 1993, p. 201).

Because culture affects how a person perceives health and illness and the manner in which clients seek health care, it is important to examine the family's cultural beliefs, values, and practices when assessing a family's health status. "Cultural assessments are performed to identify patterns that may assist or interfere with a nursing intervention or treatment regimen" (Tripp-Reimer, Brink, Saunders, 1984, p. 81). Cultural assessments help the community health nurse individualize the nursing care plan for each family. Appendix 7-2 provides guidelines for completing a cultural assessment.

HEALTH STATUS OF FAMILY MEMBERS. The purpose of a family health assessment is to obtain pertinent data about the functioning of family members as individuals and the family as a system. In keeping with the view of family health just presented, family members are viewed from an integrated, holistic, individual perspective. Biological, psychological, sociocultural, spiritual, developmental, and environmental parameters of functioning are assessed to determine the client's perception of his or her health status. Select cultural and biopsychosocial characteristics to consider when completing an individual health assessment are presented in Box 9-4. In general, clients do not think systematically about all of the variables that affect their health. A major role of the community health nurse when completing an individual health assessment is to increase the client's awareness of all the factors that influence healthy functioning.

The vehicles used for organizing an individual functional assessment are the health history and the physical examination. Exploring the techniques of physical appraisal is beyond the scope of this text. Barkauskas, Stoltenberg-Allen, Baumann, and Darling-Fisher (2002) extensively discuss the physical examination process. It is essential for community health nurses to have skill in completing a gross physical appraisal because clients may lack a regular source of medical care even though they have health problems. Community health nurses must have the ability to distin-

**TABLE 9-6**

*Criteria to Consider When Assessing Family Strengths: Three Authors' Viewpoints*

| ASSESSMENT PARAMETERS | AUTHORS | | |
| --- | --- | --- | --- |
| | OTTO (1963): FAMILY STRENGTHS | PRATT (1976): FAMILY STRUCTURE AND HEALTH BEHAVIOR CHARACTERIZING THE ENERGIZED FAMILY | CURRAN (1983): TRAITS OF A HEALTHY FAMILY |
| Adaptive abilities | The ability to provide for the physical, emotional, and spiritual needs of a family<br>The ability to use a crisis or seemingly injurious experience as a means of growth<br>The ability for self-help and ability to accept help when appropriate<br>An ability to perform family roles flexibly<br>The ability to communicate effectively | Combined health behaviors of all family members are energized; all family members tend to care for their health<br>Actively and energetically attempt to cope with life's problems and issues<br>Flexible division of tasks and activities | The healthy family admits to and seeks help with problems<br>The healthy family communicates and listens |
| Atmosphere and affect | The ability to be sensitive to the needs of family members<br>The ability to provide support, security, and encouragement | Responsive to the particular interests and needs of individual family members<br>Regular and varied interaction among family members | The healthy family teaches respect for others<br>The healthy family has a sense of play and humor<br>The healthy family shares leisure time<br>The healthy family fosters table time and conversation |
| Individual autonomy and integrity of family system | Mutual respect for the individuality of family members<br>A concern for family unity, loyalty, and interfamily cooperation | Egalitarian distribution of power<br>Provide autonomy for individual family members | The healthy family respects the privacy of individual members<br>The healthy family affirms and supports individual members<br>The healthy family maintains a balance of interaction among members<br>The healthy family has a strong sense of family in which rituals and traditions abound<br>The healthy family exhibits a sense of shared responsibility<br>The healthy family develops a sense of trust<br>The healthy family has a shared religious core |
| Relationships with others | The ability to initiate and maintain growth-producing relationships and experiences within and without the family<br>The capacity to maintain and create constructive and responsible relationships in the neighborhood, school, town, and local and state government | Provide regular links with the broader community through active participation in community activities | The healthy family values service to others<br>The healthy family teaches a sense of right and wrong |

Modified from Otto H: Criteria for assessing family strength, *Family Process* 2:333-336, 1963; Pratt L: *Family structure and effective health behavior: the energized family,* Boston, 1976, Houghton Mifflin, pp. 84-92; Curran D: *Traits of a healthy family,* Minneapolis, 1983, Winston Press, pp. 23-24.

*Questions*

• Is family flexible in regard to roles?
• How high is anxiety?
• Are individual members' needs being met?
• Is family as a unit participating?
• What is the family type and pattern of functioning?

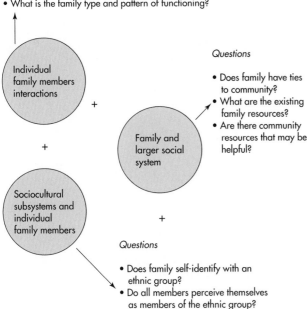

*Questions*

• Does family have ties to community?
• What are the existing family resources?
• Are there community resources that may be helpful?

*Questions*

• Does family self-identify with an ethnic group?
• Do all members perceive themselves as members of the ethnic group?
• What is the family appraisal and values related to the situations?

**FIGURE 9-6** Multifaceted family assessment framework. (From Danielson CB, Hamel-Bissell B, Winstead-Fry P: *Families, health and illness: perspectives on coping and intervention*, St Louis, 1993, Mosby, p. 202.)

guish between *abnormal* and *normal* health findings. When abnormal findings are identified, community health nurses need skill in the use of the referral process (see Chapter 10) to help clients obtain needed health care services.

HEALTH HISTORY. In the community setting, the health history is an important vehicle for assessing the health status of individual family members from a holistic perspective. It has long been recognized that a health assessment from a nursing perspective differs from the health assessment conducted by other disciplines. For example, "a nursing health history differs from a medical health history in that it focuses on the meaning of illness and hospitalization [health care] to the patient [client] and his family as a basis for planning nursing care. The medical history is taken to determine whether pathology is present as a basis for planning medical care" (McPhetridge, 1968, p. 68). When completing a health history, the community health nurse carefully explores the client's perceptions of his or her health status and how current stressors are affecting functioning. Emphasis is placed on identifying the client as a unique individual rather than as a person who has a specific disease process.

Components included in a health history vary slightly from one author to another. Basically the goal of a health history is to determine how well the client is meeting health needs and how activities of daily living have been altered to meet these needs. A comprehensive review of the client's past and current health status is elicited to identify an accurate and complete composite of the client's health functioning. With this information, the client and the nurse can explore ways for increasing the client's self-care capabilities.

The health history framework developed by Mahoney, Verdisco, and Shortridge (1982) is commonly used in the practice setting. These authors identified seven components of an individual health history, which are presented in Table 9-7. Every nurse must decide on a systematic format that facilitates data collection.

A commonly used framework for organizing a health status assessment is Gordon's (2000) Functional Health Patterns Typology. Gordon (1987) stated that "all human beings have in common certain functional patterns that contribute to their health, quality of life, and achievement of human potential" and that "these common patterns are the focus of nursing assessment" (p. 92). Table 9-8 provides abbreviated definitions for Gordon's functional health patterns. Expanded definitions of these functional health patterns can be found in Gordon's (2000) *Manual of Nursing Diagnoses*.

When completing a health history, it is important to elicit the client's expectations of the health care provider. If the client's and the professional's expectations are inconsistent, frustration results for all parties involved. For instance, a client who has diabetes and is expecting a cure will likely have difficulty working with a health care professional whose goal is to help the client live a normal life within the limitations of his or her condition. If the discrepancy between these two goals is not resolved, neither of these goals will be reached.

Assessment guides can help the community health nurse collect health data in an orderly fashion. Assessment tools designed to collect information about the health status of individual family members should help the nurse examine multiple aspects of a client's functioning. Appendixes 9-2 and 9-3 are examples of assessment forms that help community health nurses organize this beginning phase of the nursing process. These tools aid the nurse in identifying psychosocial as well as physical components of a client's health status. In addition, they help a nurse integrate individual and family functioning data by raising issues pertinent to the needs of all family members. Other examples of assessment guides, based on the 11 functional health pattern areas, can be found in Gordon's *Manual of Nursing Diagnosis* (2000). When using these guides, a skilled interviewer learns to ask probative questions that yield comprehensive data with minimal questioning.

## BOX 9-4

### Select Cultural and Biopsychosocial Characteristics of an Individual

**Physical Appearance (Body)**
Age and developmental stage
Sex and gender identity
Size, height, weight
Skin color
Hair color, configuration, presence/absence
Race (self-identified, perceived by others)
Posture, facial expression
Grooming, personal hygiene
Dress: style, condition
Presence of physical disability
Other characteristics not previously listed

**Mental Characteristics, Psychological Orientation (Mind)**
Cognitive ability, intelligence
Level of consciousness
Emotional disposition, temperament
Aptitude, ability
Sensory acuity (visual, auditory)
Personal traits
Mental health
Other characteristics not previously listed

**External Influences (Social and Physical Environment)**
Family history, ancestry, geographic origin
Strength of family unit, lines of authority
Role in family, birth order
Languages, communication patterns
Expectations and behavioral norms for age, sex, role

Format (rituals) for major life events (birth, marriage, illness, death)
Economic and work opportunities, access to resources
Housing, living arrangements
Dominant religion, other religions
Theories of disease causation
Availability, quality, variety of health care services
Political, governmental structure
Dietary customs, access to food
Community resources in education, art, music, recreation
Geographic and climatic features
Other influences not previously listed

**Internal Synthesis of Body, Mind, and Environment (Self)**
Self-concept, self-perception, expectations of self
Beliefs, values, spirituality, religious affiliation
Affect, mood, congruity between words and affect
Attitudes toward health and self-care: health history, use of health services
Personal goals, short- and long-term
Work role, economic contribution to self, others
Areas of accomplishment, achievement, sources of pride
Knowledge base, use of educational opportunities
Response to stress, coping strategies, ability to adapt
Language usage: formal, slang, dialect
Food preferences, dietary restrictions
Interests in applied and fine arts, crafts, hobbies, music, literature
Reading ability and preferences
Other characteristics not previously listed

Modified from Sibley BJ: Cultural influences on health and illness. In Long BC, Phipps WJ, Cassmeyer VL: *Medical-surgical nursing,* ed 3, St Louis, 1992, Mosby, p. 32.

## TABLE 9-7

### Seven Components of an Individual Health History

| COMPONENT | DATA COLLECTED |
| --- | --- |
| Reason for contact | Why the client is seeking help at this time |
| Biographical data | Structural variables common to all clients such as name, age, sex, marital status, religious preference, ethnic background, educational level, occupational status, health insurance, and social security information |
| Current health status | The client's perceptions of his or her health with a specific delineation of current complaints and activities of daily living |
| Past health history | Data relative to the previous health or illness state of the client and contact with health care professionals, including a description of developmental accomplishments, health practices, known illnesses, allergies, restorative treatment, and social activities, such as foreign travel, that might be related to the client's current health status |
| Family history | A description of the current health status of each family member, relationships among family members, and a genetic history in relation to health and illness |
| Social history | An accounting of intrapersonal and interpersonal factors that influence the client's social adjustment, including environmental stressors that may be increasing or decreasing the client's vulnerability to crisis during times of stress |
| Review of systems* | A systematic assessment of biological functioning from head to toe |

From Mahoney EA, Verdisco L, Shortridge L: *How to collect and record a health history,* ed 2, Philadelphia, 1982, Lippincott, pp. 6-7.
*Gordon's (2000) Functional Health Patterns Typology is a commonly used method for examining biological functioning and other aspects of a client's health status.

**TABLE 9-8**

*Gordon's Functional Health Patterns Typology: Abbreviated Definitions for the Eleven Health Patterns*

| HEALTH PATTERN | ABBREVIATED DEFINITION |
|---|---|
| Health perception–health management pattern | Describes the client's perceived pattern of health and well-being and how health is managed. |
| Nutritional-metabolic pattern | Describes pattern of food and fluid consumption relative to metabolic need and pattern indicators of local nutrient supply. |
| Elimination pattern | Describes patterns of excretory function (bowel, bladder, and skin). |
| Activity-exercise pattern | Describes pattern of exercise, activity, leisure, and recreation. |
| Sleep-rest pattern | Describes patterns of sleep, rest, and relaxation. |
| Cognitive-perceptual pattern | Describes sensory-perceptual and cognitive pattern. |
| Self-perception–self-concept pattern | Describes self-concept pattern and perceptions of mood state. |
| Role-relationship pattern | Describes pattern of role engagements and relationships. |
| Sexuality-reproductive pattern | Describes patterns of satisfaction or dissatisfaction with sexuality; describes reproductive pattern. |
| Coping–stress tolerance pattern | Describes general coping pattern and effectiveness of the pattern in terms of stress tolerance. |
| Value-belief pattern | Describes patterns of values, goals, or beliefs (including spiritual) that guide choices or decisions. |

Modified from Gordon M: *Manual of nursing diagnosis*, ed 9, St Louis, 2000, Mosby, pp. 2-5.

## ANALYZING

Once individual and family data are collected, the analysis phase of the nursing process begins. This phase encompasses a deliberative critical thinking process, which results in the formation of *nursing diagnoses*. A nursing diagnosis is "a clinical judgment about an individual, family, or community response to actual or potential health problems/life processes. A nursing diagnosis provides the basis for selection of nursing interventions to achieve outcomes for which the nurse is accountable" (approved at the ninth conference, 1990) (North American Nursing Diagnosis Association [NANDA], 1999, p. 149).

### Formulating Nursing Diagnoses

Nursing diagnoses are based on patterns reflected in assessment data and identify actual or potential client problems amenable to nursing interventions (Gordon, 2000). They also delineate client strengths that should be reinforced when the nurse is helping the client enhance his or her self-care capabilities. In the community health setting, nursing diagnoses examine the needs and strengths of family units in addition to the needs and strengths of individual clients. If the identified needs of a family or individual clients are not amenable to nursing intervention, the community health nurse makes a referral to an appropriate care provider (see Chapter 10).

To formulate nursing diagnoses, the community health nurse groups data so that relationships between assessment categories can be analyzed and patterns of behavior can be identified. Establishing relationships between assessment categories involves looking at all parameters of individual and family functioning. It requires a synthesis of data and an application of scientific knowledge to determine the unique combination of biological, psychosocial, developmental, spiritual, and environmental factors that are making an impact on a specific family unit. It is important to synthesize data collected from a family because client needs vary, even when clients are experiencing similar situations. The following case scenarios illustrate this situation:

CASE *Scenario*   One community health nurse was visiting two different families, both of whom were concerned about a child's leaving for school. In one family situation, the nurse's diagnosis of this behavior was "anticipatory anxiety related to the family's inability to address the father's health status with all family members." This nursing diagnosis was derived from the following assessment data:

- Susie had enjoyed school until her father had a heart attack.
- Susie's father had his heart attack while she was at school.
- Susie had been asking lately if her father was going to die.
- The family believed it was important to assure the children that everything was fine with the father even though he was unable to work or participate in strenuous family activities at this time.

In the other family situation, the nursing diagnosis in relation to the child's difficulty in leaving for school was quite different. Based on the following assessment data, the nursing diagnosis was "altered growth and development, social skills, related to the family's inability to adjust to normative developmental transitions":

- Bonnie started school a year late because she was "immature" for her developmental age.
- Bonnie has never enjoyed school.
- Bonnie spends most of her free time with her mother, even when children her own age are around.
- Bonnie clings to her mother when baby-sitters come to the home.

Nursing diagnoses are derived from assessment data (ANA, 1991) that have been validated by the client and synthesized. Formulating diagnoses without adequate information, or in relation to fragmented pieces of data, leads to invalid diagnoses and inappropriate client goals and nursing interventions. For example, a nursing diagnosis that is based only on environmental observations yields inadequate data. Similarly, a nursing diagnosis that focuses on "unsafe housekeeping practices" provides very little direction for client and nursing intervention. Unsafe housekeeping practices can result from several factors, including lack of home management skill, energy depletion resulting from normative and nonnormative situational crises, and differing values about environmental safety. How a community health nurse would intervene when focusing on unsafe housekeeping practices is greatly influenced by the database obtained and associated nursing diagnosis. For instance, an educative strategy is used when a client "lacks home management skill," whereas a crisis intervention approach is initiated when a "family's energies are depleted due to crisis." Chapter 8 aids the nurse in determining when a client may be in a state of crisis or vulnerable to stress and crisis.

When comparing clinical data with relevant clinical and research findings, it is important to identify nursing diagnoses in relation to client strengths as well as client needs. Discerning client strengths helps the community health nurse reinforce self-sufficiency skills, which in turn aids the nurse in avoiding dependency-building nursing activities. In the community health nurse setting, special emphasis is also placed on identifying nursing diagnoses that relate to situations or potential problems that warrant anticipatory guidance counseling. This emphasis is based on the belief that primary prevention should be a major focus in community health nursing practice. Situations throughout the life span that warrant anticipatory guidance are covered in Chapters 16 through 22.

## Nursing Classification Systems

Using a nursing classification system can help practitioners refine their diagnostic skills and document the effectiveness of nursing interventions. In addition, these systems facilitate the collection of assessment data and assist in organizing these data. Two such systems, one developed by NANDA and the other by the Visiting Nurse Association

of Omaha, Nebraska, are commonly used in the community setting.

### NANDA's Nursing Diagnoses Classification

NANDA was established in St. Louis, Missouri, in 1973 for the purpose of developing a standard nomenclature for describing health problems amenable to treatment by nurses (Kim, Moritz, 1982, p. xvii). Since its inception, this association has sponsored several National Nursing Diagnosis Conferences, which have resulted in the identification of appropriate nursing diagnostic categories for practitioners. Numerous nursing diagnoses have been accepted for clinical testing by NANDA and endorsed by the ANA. Gordon (2000) has grouped these diagnoses under the 11 functional health patterns to facilitate the linking of assessment data and nursing diagnoses (Appendix 9-4). Gordon's *Manual of Nursing Diagnosis* (2000) explicates in more detail how to use the Functional Health Patterns Typology to facilitate nursing assessments and the identification of nursing diagnoses.

NANDA's nursing diagnoses taxonomy revisions and development are ongoing. It is expected that nurses will modify, delete, and add to the currently accepted classifications. Nurses are continuously encouraged to submit refinements of diagnoses to the North American Nursing Diagnosis Association, 1211 Locust Street, Philadelphia, Pennsylvania 19107 or email *NANDA@nursecominc.com* (NANDA, 1999). Further work is needed in the development of family and health promotion nursing diagnoses. Donnelly (1990) noted that only seven of the NANDA diagnostic categories described family-focused needs and only one of these seven addressed the family from a health promotion perspective. Leninger (1990) believes that the NANDA diagnostic taxonomy needs to be refocused to adequately address the health and well-being of people from varying cultures.

### The Omaha Classification System

The Omaha Classification System developed by the Visiting Nurse Association of Omaha was designed to provide an organizing framework for client problems diagnosed by nurses in the community health setting. This classification system, based on the ANA definition of community health nursing, addresses the needs of families as well as individuals. This system has three major components: Problem Classification Scheme, Intervention Scheme, and Problem Rating Scale for Outcomes (Martin, Scheet, 1992). The Problem Classification Scheme is a taxonomy of nursing diagnoses that is structured at four levels: domains, problems, modifiers, and signs/symptoms. The 40 client problems are grouped into four major domains: environmental, psychosocial, physiological, and health behaviors (Martin, 1994). Definitions for each of these domains are displayed in Table 9-9. Within each of these domains are the names of identified problems that are referenced by two sets of

**TABLE 9-9**

## The Omaha System: Definitions of Domains

| DOMAIN | DEFINITIONS |
|---|---|
| Environmental | Refers to the material resources and physical surroundings both internal and external to the client, home, neighborhood, and broader community. |
| Psychosocial | Refers to patterns of behavior, communications, relationships, and development. |
| Physiological | Refers to the functional status of processes that maintain life. |
| Health-related behaviors | Refers to activities that maintain or promote wellness, promote recovery, or maximize rehabilitation. |

From Martin K, Scheet N: *The Omaha System: a pocket guide for community health nursing,* Philadelphia, 1992, Saunders, pp. 18-19, 24, 30.

**TABLE 9-10**

## The Omaha System: Organization of Classification Scheme for Client Problems, Select Examples

| DOMAIN | PROBLEM LABEL | MODIFIERS | SIGN OR SYMPTOM* |
|---|---|---|---|
| Environmental | Income | Deficit, family | Low/no income<br>Uninsured medical expenses<br>Inadequate money management<br>Able to buy only necessities<br>Difficulty buying necessities<br>Other (specify) |
| Psychosocial | Communication with community resources | Impairment, family | Unfamiliar with options/procedures for obtaining services<br>Difficulty understanding roles/regulations of service provider<br>Unable to communicate concerns to service provider<br>Dissatisfaction with services<br>Language barrier<br>Inadequate/unavailable resources<br>Other (specify) |
| Physiological | Hearing | Impairment, individual | Difficulty hearing normal speech tones<br>Absent/abnormal response to sound<br>Abnormal results of hearing screening test<br>Other (specify) |
| Health-related behaviors | Health care supervision | Impairment, family | Fails to obtain routine medical/dental evaluation<br>Fails to seek care for symptoms requiring medical/dental evaluation<br>Fails to return as requested to physician/dentist<br>Inability to coordinate multiple appointments/regimens<br>Inconsistent source of medical/dental care<br>Inadequate prescribed mental/dental regimen<br>Other (specify) |

From Martin K, Scheet N: *The Omaha System: a pocket guide for community health nursing,* Philadelphia, 1992, Saunders, pp. 18, 20, 24, 32.
*Only those signs or symptoms that apply to the family situation are referenced in the client's record.

modifiers: each problem is referenced as health promotion, potential (deficit/impairment) or actual (deficit/impairment), as well as family or individual. "When an actual problem modifier is used, a cluster of problem-specific signs and symptoms provides the diagnostic clues to problem identification" (Martin, 1994, p. 41). Table 9-10 provides examples of how the Omaha Problem Classification

Scheme is organized according to domain, problem label, modifier, and sign or symptom.

Directly related to the problem scheme in the Omaha Classification System and the nursing process is a Likert-type problem-rating scale that helps nurses evaluate client outcomes at regular intervals and a nursing intervention scheme consisting of nursing activities aimed at addressing

**TABLE 9-11**

*The Omaha System: Definitions of the Intervention Categories*

| CATEGORIES | DEFINITIONS |
| --- | --- |
| I. Health teaching, guidance, and counseling | Health teaching, guidance, and counseling are nursing activities that include giving information, anticipating client problems, encouraging client action and responsibility for self-care and coping, and assisting with decision making and problem solving. The overlapping concepts occur on a continuum with the variation due to the client's self-direction capabilities. |
| II. Treatments and procedures | Treatments and procedures are technical nursing activities directed toward preventing signs and symptoms, identifying risk factors and early signs and symptoms, and decreasing or alleviating signs and symptoms. |
| III. Case management | Case management includes nursing activities of coordination, advocacy, and referral. These activities involve facilitating service delivery on behalf of the client, communicating with health and human service providers, promoting assertive client communication, and guiding the client toward use of appropriate community resources. |
| IV. Surveillance | Surveillance includes nursing activities of detection, measurement, critical analysis, and monitoring to indicate client status in relation to a given condition or phenomenon. |

From Martin K, Scheet N: *The Omaha System: a pocket guide for community health nursing,* Philadelphia, 1992, Saunders, p. 48.

specific nursing problems. Four nursing intervention categories are delineated in the Omaha System: health teaching, guidance, and counseling; treatments and procedures; case management; and surveillance. Definitions of these categories are presented in Table 9-11. Martin and Scheet's (1992) book, *The Omaha System: A Pocket Guide For Community Health Nursing,* discusses the Omaha System in depth, including how to individualize nursing interventions to client needs, how to use the problem-rating scale, and how to link nursing diagnoses, interventions, and client outcomes.

## PLANNING

After nursing diagnoses are established and validated with the client, the community health nurse and the client move into the planning phase of the nursing process. Three major activities occur during this phase: (1) client-centered goals and expected outcomes for evaluating goal attainment are formulated; (2) interventions and evaluation criteria are identified; and (3) goals, outcomes, and interventions are prioritized. A *goal* is a broad desired outcome toward which behavior is directed, such as "the family will value preventive health care services." An *expected outcome* or behavioral objective delineates client behaviors that reflect when a goal has been reached. "The family will obtain a regular source of care for preventive medical and dental services by September" might be one outcome established to determine if the above goal has been accomplished. *Interventions* are activities that may be implemented by the client, the nurse, and other health care professionals to help the client

achieve the desired goals. For example, in relation to the previously mentioned expected outcome, the nurse might discuss with the family its beliefs about health care, the services of all the available health care resources in the community, and barriers to health care utilization. If barriers to health care utilization exist, the nurse would identify with the family strategies for reducing these barriers (see Chapter 10 for a discussion of these strategies).

All goals and expected outcomes should be stated in specific and realistic terms and linked to the nursing diagnoses that have been established. They should not include expectations that are beyond the professional's or client's resources or capabilities. A goal of a severely retarded child achieving normal growth and development is extremely unrealistic. It is very appropriate to state that the family will work toward maximizing this child's potential, but inappropriate to expect that this child will reach normal growth and development parameters. Expecting that the family of this child will continue to function exactly as they did before the child's birth is also unrealistic. During times of stress and crisis, change is necessary and unavoidable. A goal statement that focuses on the family demonstrating constructive behavior to reduce stressors related to the care of their developmentally disabled child is more appropriate.

Goal statements and expected outcomes that are written in positive terms provide direction for nursing interventions more effectively than those that have a negative orientation. Negative goal statements such as "parents will not use harsh disciplinary measures with their children" tend to focus on family weaknesses rather than on family strengths. It is through its strengths that a family mobilizes energies to reduce current stresses. Positive goal statements, such as "parents will talk with their children when the children act out," lead to the development of more positive interventions for achieving goals.

The nurse may find that, after client-centered goals are developed, the client finds it impossible to work on all of them immediately. When this happens, the nurse and the client should work together to differentiate between problems that require immediate action and those that are of less concern to the client. When establishing priorities in relation to client goals, the nurse must keep in mind that the client has the right to make the final decision about goals on which to focus. The nurse does have a responsibility to share concerns when she or he believes that client actions are unsafe or are precipitating a crisis situation.

After client-centered, positively stated goals have been established and priorities determined, expected outcomes that can be measured should be written. The importance of formulating specific outcomes for evaluating goal attainment must be stressed. Broad, general goals do not provide sufficient direction for planning intervention strategies. "Maximizing the potential" of a child who has a developmental lag, for example, does not specifically identify needed areas of improvement. Expected outcomes such as those listed below more appropriately facilitate the identification of intervention strategies because they focus on specific developmental needs of the child and the family.

- Joel's family will help him achieve daytime bladder and bowel control by December.
- Joel's family will help him learn how to eat solid foods by October.
- Joel's family will share their feelings about Joel's condition.
- Joel's family will verbally identify how their feelings about Joel's condition positively or negatively affect his growth and development.
- Joel's family will identify strategies to reduce the stress associated with his care.
- Joel's parents will share ways to maintain a healthy spouse relationship.

Interventions, like expected outcomes, should be specific and based on sound scientific knowledge. "Teaching about growth and development" or "provide support to the family" are not specifically stated interventions. They are extremely global and do not take into account the individual needs of a particular family. A community health nurse might better prepare for family visits if the interventions were stated as follows: "implement a urinary habit training program" and "teach caregiver stress management techniques" (McCloskey, Bulechek, 2000, pp. 200, 689).

A research team at the University of Iowa has developed the **Nursing Interventions Classification (NIC)** that outlines a "comprehensive standardized language that describes the treatments that nurses perform" (McCloskey, Bulechek, 2000, p. ix). This classification identifies numerous nursing interventions and associated actions for each intervention

that helps nurses benefit clients. "Each intervention has a label name, a definition, a list of activities that a nurse does to carry out the intervention, and a short list of background readings" (McCloskey, Bulechek, 2000, p. ix). Box 9-5 presents a sample intervention and illustrates the format for each intervention. "Nursing interventions include both direct and indirect care, both nurse-initiated, physician-initiated, and other provider-initiated treatments" (McCloskey, Bulechek, 2000). The definitions for these different types of nursing interventions and nursing activities are presented in Box 9-6.

When delineating a plan for intervention, both family and nurse activities should be identified. If only nursing actions are established, the client cannot be an active participant in the therapeutic process. Family resources are

---

 **BOX 9-5**

## *Nursing Interventions Classification (NIC) Intervention: Family Integrity Promotion*

### *Definition*
Promotion of family cohesion and unity

### *Activities*
Be a listener for the family members
Establish trusting relationship with family members
Determine family understanding of causes of illness
Determine guilt family may feel
Assist family to resolve feelings of guilt
Determine typical family relationships
Monitor current family relationships
Identify typical family coping mechanisms
Identify conflicting priorities among family members
Assist family with conflict resolution
Counsel family members on additional effective coping skills for their own use
Respect privacy of individual family members
Provide for family privacy
Tell family members it is safe and acceptable to use typical expressions of affection
Facilitate a tone of togetherness within/among the family
Provide family members with information about the client's condition regularly, according to client preference
Collaborate with family in problem solving
Assist family to maintain positive relationships
Facilitate open communications among family members
Provide for care of client by family members, as appropriate
Provide for family visitation
Refer family to support group of other families dealing with similar problems
Refer for family therapy, as indicated

From McCloskey JC, Bulechek GM, editors: *Nursing interventions classification (NIC)*, ed 3, St Louis, 2000, Mosby, p. 328.

## BOX 9-6

*Nursing Interventions Classification (NIC): Definitions of Nursing Intervention and Nursing Activities*

### Nursing Intervention

*Any treatment, based upon clinical judgment and knowledge that a nurse performs to enhance patient/client outcomes.* Nursing interventions include both direct and indirect care; both nurse-initiated, physician-initiated, and other provider-initiated treatments.

A *direct care intervention* is a treatment performed through interaction with the client(s). Direct care interventions include both physiological and psychosocial nursing actions; both the "laying on of hands" actions and those that are more supportive and counseling in nature.

An *indirect care intervention* is a treatment performed away from the client but on behalf of a client or group of clients. Indirect care interventions include nursing actions aimed at management of the client care environment and interdisciplinary collaboration. These actions support the effectiveness of the direct care interventions.

A *community (or public health) intervention* is targeted to promote and preserve the health of populations. Community interventions emphasize health promotion, health maintenance, and disease prevention of populations. Community intervention includes strategies to address the social and political climate in which the population resides.

A *nurse-initiated treatment* is an intervention initiated by the nurse in response to a nursing diagnosis; an autonomous action based on scientific rationale that is executed to benefit the client in a predicted way related to the nursing diagnosis and projected outcomes. Such actions would include those treatments initiated by advanced nurse practitioners.

A *physician-initiated treatment* is an intervention initiated by a physician in response to a medical diagnosis but carried out by a nurse in response to a "doctor's order." Nurses may also carry out treatments initiated by other providers, such as pharmacists, respiratory therapists, or physician assistants.

### Nursing Activities

The specific behaviors or actions that nurses do to implement an intervention and that assist patients/clients to move toward a desired outcome. Nursing activities are at the concrete level of action. A series of activities is necessary to implement an intervention.

From McCloskey JC, Bulechek GM, editors: *Nursing interventions classification (NIC)*, ed 3, St Louis, 2000, Mosby, p. ix.

frequently overlooked when intervention strategies are developed. For instance, plans are too often made to involve community resources in the client's care even though friends or family members are available and would be more than willing to assist the client in achieving goals.

## Guiding Principles of the Therapeutic Process

Several key principles must be taken into consideration during all phases of the nursing process. These are (1) individualization of client care, (2) respect of diverse values, (3) active family participation, (4) the family's right of self-determination, (5) confidentiality, and (6) maintenance of therapeutic focus. Adherence to these principles is basic to a trusting nurse-client relationship and reflects a respect for the worth and dignity of human beings.

Inherent in these principles is the belief that clients have unique needs, values, and ways of functioning that should be determined before diagnoses, goals, expected outcomes, and interventions are established. Actively involving the client in the therapeutic process helps community health nurses discover the uniqueness of the families they are serving. Active client participation in all phases of the nursing process also promotes client commitment to goal attainment and decreases resistance to change.

Individualizing client care does not negate the value of using standardized assessment tools and nursing diagnoses and intervention classification systems. Rather, this principle focuses on the need to use sound clinical judgment when tools for facilitating data collection and the planning of client care are utilized. McCloskey and Bulechek (1994) believe that "the use of standardized language will allow nurses more time and opportunity to focus on the unique aspects of each patient's care" (p. 59). They see the Nursing Intervention Classification as "a tool that makes it easier to select interventions for a particular patient" (p. 60), but stress that selecting an intervention and carrying out that intervention needs to be tailored for each client. Actively involving the client in the planning process helps the nurse appropriately select and implement interventions and adhere to the principle of confidentiality. The principle of confidentiality is most often violated when goals are not mutually established and the nurse shares or seeks data to validate nurse-focused goals.

For clients to fully participate in the therapeutic process, they must have the right to refuse any course of action they deem inappropriate. Community health nurses can help a client examine the pros and cons of certain health actions or the consequences of continuing a particular pattern of functioning, but they also recognize that a client's right of self-determination must be respected when decisions are made. The nurse should not make decisions for the client or expect the client to make decisions in the way the nurse would make them. A community health nurse may intervene without a client's consent if the client is a threat to others (e.g., child abuse, spread of communicable disease) or to herself or himself (suicidal). Even in these situations, the community health nurse works with the client, if possible, to help reduce the distress being experienced and to develop new patterns of coping.

## Professional Contracting

Contracting is an intervention designed to promote active client participation in decision making. A contract—a mutual agreement between two or more persons for a specific purpose—provides a framework for establishing a facilitative client approach that supports and enhances a client's self-care capabilities. Basic to contracting is a philosophical belief that professional intervention should focus on assisting clients to act effectively on their own behalf. The professional using the contracting method of intervention must feel comfortable with the philosophy that clients have the potential for growth and that they are capable of effective decision making.

**Contracting** actively engages the client in the therapeutic process for the purpose of developing mutually acceptable goals, expected outcomes, and therapeutic interventions. Simply stated, a professional contract may be defined as a mutually agreed-upon working understanding that relates to the terms of treatment and is continuously negotiable between the nurse and the family (Boehm, 1989; Maluccio, Marlow, 1974; Seabury, 1976). The community health nurse guides the client through the process by facilitating informed decision making, assessing client needs, exploring alternatives for need resolution, assisting clients in carrying out actions that support need resolution, and evaluating expected outcomes.

CONTRACTING PROCESS. The community health nurse who believes in contracting involves the client in all aspects of care. She or he makes an agreement with the client that spells out explicitly, mutually defined, client-centered goals. The quality of explicitness implies that both the client and the nurse clearly understand the terms of intervention. When contracting occurs, all involved parties have a mutual understanding regarding the following aspects of care:

1. The purpose of client-nurse interactions
2. Nursing diagnoses
3. Desired outcomes (goals) toward which behavior is directed
4. Priority needs in relation to client goals
5. Methods of intervention
6. Specific activities each party will carry out to achieve stated goals
7. Established time parameters for evaluation and the frequency and length of visits

Contracting is a dynamic, complex process that gradually evolves as the therapeutic relationship is strengthened. It should not be viewed as a simple procedure, involving only a discussion about goals, intervention strategies, and time limits. To successfully engage a family in the contracting process, the community health nurse must help the family gain a clear understanding of its needs and the nature of a therapeutic relationship.

Initially a contract may be very general and include only an agreement to explore the nature of the client's needs.

The terms of a contract become more inclusive as the therapeutic relationship evolves and specific data are obtained. Asking clients questions about what they feel they need, what they have been doing to resolve their needs, and how they would like their current situation to change, can elicit specific data that help the client and the nurse structure the therapeutic relationship. Establishing time parameters is important even when a general contract is developed because these parameters emphasize the need for reviewing progress made in relation to goal attainment.

Contracting increases the clarity in nurse-client interactions. Specific commitments are made orally so that each party is aware of its role in the therapeutic process. Increased clarity often enhances the therapeutic relationship. This is especially true when clients have multiple problems or are unable to identify the nature of their problems. A case scenario can best illustrate this point.

**CASE *Scenario*** The Beech family, two parents with five children, had been visited by community health nurses for years. The family folder reflected many problems: marital stress, financial difficulties, poor nutrition, lack of preventive health care for family members, irregular school attendance, and frequent childhood infections were the primary problems with which the family was dealing. The community health nurse made infrequent visits because the family continually failed to deal actively with health care needs. Because they moved frequently, the Beech family never had consistent contact with one nurse for any length of time. Finally the community health nurse decided to talk with Mrs. Beech about terminating nursing service because she believed that the family did not desire assistance. To her surprise, Mrs. Beech verbalized that her family did need help and that she really wanted the nurse to continue visiting. She further shared that she had difficulty concentrating on anything because the family had so many problems to handle. The nurse agreed with Mrs. Beech that it was an impossible task to solve all the family problems at once. She proposed that it might be helpful if the family and the nurse could work together to resolve the one health problem Mrs. Beech felt was most distressing at that time. Mrs. Beech had trouble focusing on one particular concern because she had never before attempted to do so. Because she spent a considerable amount of time talking about Mary, her 10-year-old who had recently failed a hearing test at school, the nurse asked Mrs. Beech if she might want to explore ways to resolve this health care problem. The nurse also suggested that it might be helpful to prioritize the family's health problems from most significant to least significant. Because these suggestions were acceptable to Mrs. Beech, a sample contract was established (Box 9-7).

Mary saw the physician within the appropriate time frame. It was determined that she would need ear surgery. Because the contracting method of intervention helped

**BOX 9-7**

*Sample Nurse-Client Contract—*
*Beech Family*

- *Purpose of client-nurse interactions:* The community health nurse will help the family establish priorities in relation to their health problems and to handle their problems in manageable doses.
- *Priority need:* Mary's failure of hearing test at school.
- *Mutual goal:* Mary's hearing problem will be evaluated by a physician.
- *Method of intervention:* Family will take Mary to the hearing specialist she had seen before. (This decision was made after the nurse discussed all the possible resources where Mary could obtain care, and Mrs. Beech shared that Mary had had hearing problems in the past.)
- *Responsibilities of family:* (1) Make appointment with the physician; (2) arrange for child care for the two preschoolers for the afternoon of the appointment; (3) arrange for transportation; and (4) together with the nurse, make list of questions to ask the physician during the visit.
- *Responsibilities of nurse:* Contact the physician to share the results of Mary's hearing test and Mrs. Beech's fears about health care professionals. (In the past, health care professionals had frequently criticized Mrs. Beech for waiting too long before she sought medical help.) Visit weekly to evaluate how plans for Mary's care are progressing and to help the family establish priorities for health care action.
- *Time limits:* Mary is to see the physician by the end of the month.

Mrs. Beech achieve her first goal, Mrs. Beech and the nurse agreed to renegotiate for follow-up, based on the physician's recommendation. Many other contracts were made before this family case record was closed. Accomplishing resolution of one problem helped family members see that their situation was not hopeless. Setting priorities in relation to goal attainment decreased the family's anxiety about all the problems they had to handle.

Contracting is one effective way to involve families in their own health care. However, contracting can reinforce ineffective family patterns if the nurse does not carefully analyze family dynamics. When a contract supports unhealthy family functioning it is labeled a *corrupt contract* (Beall, 1972, p. 77). A corrupt contract might evolve, for instance, when a community health nurse is working with a family who would like their aging parents to move to a nursing home. Sometimes families push for nursing home placement to meet their own needs rather than the needs of their elderly family members. If the community health nurse supports the family's decision and encourages the parents to move without talking to them about their needs and desires,

he or she is violating the rights of these family members and the principles of contracting.

During the contracting process a community health nurse may identify problems, such as lack of protection against communicable diseases or inadequate dental care, that do not seem to be of concern to the family. In these situations a nurse-centered goal rather than a client-centered goal is formulated. A nurse-centered goal should be stated as such and should not emphasize family action like "the family will make an appointment at the immunization clinic." Instead it should focus on increasing the family's awareness of the problem and be stated in terms such as "the family will verbalize an understanding of immunizations." Distinguishing carefully between nurse goals and family goals helps the community health nurse prevent imposing personal values on clients. It also helps the nurse focus on the problems and goals important to the family. Generally, families do not explore problems identified by the nurse that they do not see as problems until they have achieved their own client-centered goals.

## IMPLEMENTING

The implementation phase of the nursing process deals specifically with how activities are carried out to achieve client goals. Together the client and the nurse select and test intervention strategies to determine their appropriateness in helping the client move toward need resolution. Priorities concerning when actions will be taken are established so that the client can deal with his or her needs in manageable doses. If needed, other resources are mobilized to help the client handle the change process.

The community health nurse uses various intervention strategies to help clients alter those aspects of life they desire to change. Some of these are discussed in Chapter 8, which explores supportive, educative, and problem-solving strategies. Nursing actions should be based on sound scientific principles and knowledge. For example, if a planned intervention is nutritional counseling, the activities the nurse carries out to implement this intervention should reflect knowledge of acceptable nutritional standards and appropriate application of the principles of teaching and learning. Because one principle of teaching and learning is to provide for individual differences (Redman, 1997), effective nursing activities reflect that the nurse took into consideration client characteristics that influence nutritional habits such as cultural preferences in relation to food likes and dislikes, financial resources, and the demands on the homemaker's time.

All other phases of the nursing process are usually carried out during the implementation phase. While clients are actively participating in the intervention process, they share data verbally or nonverbally through action taken or not taken. The community health nurse must analyze these new data carefully to determine if care plans need to be revised.

Nursing care plans should never be static. Rather, they should be continuously open to renegotiation as the client's situation changes or new data are discovered.

During the implementation phase, it is not unusual to discover that clients do not wish to pursue a particular goal, even though they previously expressed a desire to work on that goal. Sometimes clients verbalize an *awareness* that a problem exists but are not ready to change their behavior in the way necessary to resolve that problem. Clients may not recognize the difference between awareness and readiness until concrete plans have been made to alter their current situation. If this happens, it can be difficult for these clients to verbally convey to the nurse that they are not ready for change. Frequently they share this message nonverbally by not taking action. That is why it is so important for the community health nurse to find out why clients are not meeting commitments that had been mutually agreed upon. Goals and plans should be modified if clients are not ready to alter their behavior.

Some clients are resistant to change because all their alternatives for change have negative consequences. A woman, for example, who has limited financial resources, no preparation for a job, and few support systems may be very hesitant to divorce her husband even though their marital relationship is destructive to her emotional health. The fear of not being able to support herself and being alone might be far more stressful to her than the emotional pain she is experiencing in the marital relationship. When community health nurses encounter such a situation, they must remain empathic and guard against feeling that the woman has no options. Clients in these situations can be assisted by helping them identify their strengths, obtain needed resources to achieve their goals, and recognize that they can achieve control over their lives.

## Documentation

For a variety of reasons, the nurse clearly documents relevant data on the agency record throughout all phases of the nursing process. Accurate record keeping provides direction for the planning, implementation, and evaluation of client care; assists the health care team in coordinating services provided; and helps practitioners substantiate the quality of care rendered for reimbursement, legal, and certification purposes (Della Monica, 1994). Accurate record keeping also helps agency administrators analyze the characteristics of clients served by the agency, including a demographic profile and a profile of client health care needs and service requirements. Having this knowledge assists an agency in analyzing community needs, planning appropriate staffing patterns, and identifying staff competencies needed to provide care to clients served by the agency.

Accurate record keeping is an essential responsibility of the community health nurse. It demonstrates professional accountability and assists the nurse in providing individualized, quality care. To successfully carry out that responsibil-

ity, the nurse must have a clear understanding of the agency's documentation policy and the nursing process. A quality client service record reflects appropriate implementation of the nursing process.

## EVALUATING

Evaluation is the continuous critiquing of each aspect of the nursing process. Although it is discussed as a separate phase, it must take place concurrently with all phases of the nursing process. Ongoing feedback should be elicited from the client to determine whether goals, plans, and intervention strategies are appropriately focused. When expected outcomes are established, defining how they will be evaluated is a necessity. A well-written expected outcome will contain the potential for evaluation. For example, "John will learn how to give his own insulin injection by the end of the month" is a concise statement that can be used to determine whether John has achieved a desired goal.

Evaluation criteria, which help the family and the nurse to determine if expected client outcomes are being reached, should be established very early in the nurse-client relationship. Developing evaluation criteria early in the helping relationship validates the importance of evaluation and provides direction for client and nurse actions. Presented in Table 9-12 is a care plan for the Lopez family (see the accompanying case scenario) that illustrates how one community health nurse *initially* established evaluation criteria to determine whether expected outcomes were achieved. When reviewing these criteria, note how they relate to each stage of the nursing process.

**CASE** *Scenario* The Lopez family consists of Juan, age 35, Elena, his 30-year-old wife, five children, and Mr. Lopez's mother, Teresa. The family is second-generation Mexican-American from Texas, representative of a stream of Spanish-speaking families who yearly migrate north to harvest a variety of crops. Six months ago, the family decided to stay in a northern midwestern community when Mr. Lopez was offered a permanent job as a farmhand. The family made this decision because they felt the children could have a better education and life than the parents had experienced. Spanish is spoken in the home. Mr. Lopez speaks some English but is unable to read or write it. Mrs. Lopez has limited comprehension of English and has had no education beyond the fourth grade. Mr. Lopez's mother speaks only Spanish. The children speak English but are behind in school achievement as a result of frequent family moves.

The family lives in a five-room house that is on the farm property. Although housekeeping practices are adequate, the home is in poor condition and in need of paint and repairs. It has running water, the source of which is a well. A septic system is used for sewage disposal. There is electricity for lighting and heating, and bottled gas is used for cooking.

**TABLE 9-12**

## Lopez Family: Initial Care Plan

| ASSESSMENT DATA | NURSING DIAGNOSES | EXPECTED CLIENT OUTCOMES | NURSING INTERVENTIONS | EVALUATION CRITERIA |
|---|---|---|---|---|
| Children behind in school achievement because of frequent family moves. Family moved north so "children could have a better education." | Family coping, potential for growth as evidenced by family's desire to obtain a better education and life for their children. | Children will succeed in the educational system. | 1. Verbally, positively reinforce the family's decision to obtain an education for its children. 2. Identify barriers to successful school achievement. 3. Provide family with information about school policies and procedures. | 1. All children will attend school regularly. 2. Children will report satisfying school experiences. 3. Children will obtain passing grades in school. |
| Family has no regular source of medical care. Family cannot afford to go to the physician. Family members have obvious health needs. Difficult for family to obtain medical care during daytime hours. Family expresses a desire to follow up on the children's health needs. | Health maintenance, altered, due to limited financial resources and access problems. | Family will obtain the resources needed to follow up on family members' health needs. Family will obtain a regular source of medical and preventive health care. | 1. Discuss family's beliefs about health, illness, and health care. 2. Share with family resources in community to assist them in meeting their health needs (e.g., Lions' Club and MSS). 3. Discuss barriers to the use of the referral process. 4. Discern family's interest in obtaining a regular source of care. 5. Advocate for the family as needed. 6. Provide opportunities for breadwinner to meet work responsibilities while obtaining health care for the family. | 1. Family members' health needs will be corrected: a. Mr. Lopez will obtain dentures. b. Mrs. Lopez will obtain prenatal care. c. Juanita will obtain an eye examination. d. Francesca will obtain medical care for her ear infection. e. All of the children will obtain dental care. f. All family members' immunizations will be up-to-date. |

*Continued*

The family lives rent-free in the house, which is provided by the owner of the farm. The owner also provides utilities. Family income is limited to Mr. Lopez's income of $100 per week and his mother's income of $65 per month from Supplemental Security Income (SSI). Only Grandmother Lopez has health insurance, on the basis of SSI. The tenant farm on which the family lives is 10 miles from the nearest town. Mr. Lopez has a pickup truck that the family uses for transportation when necessary. However, Mr. Lopez finds it difficult to get off work during daytime hours to take the family in for medical care.

Health problems are evident in the family. Mr. Lopez is in need of dentures, and all of the school-age children are in need of dental care, as reported by their teachers. Juanita, age 7, was recently referred for ophthalmologic examination following vision screening at school. Francesca, age 3,

**TABLE 9-12**

*Lopez Family: Initial Care Plan—cont'd*

| ASSESSMENT DATA | NURSING DIAGNOSES | EXPECTED CLIENT OUTCOMES | NURSING INTERVENTIONS | EVALUATION CRITERIA |
|---|---|---|---|---|
| Only grandmother has health insurance. Children have limited clothing for school. Total family income is $465/month. | Income deficit as evidenced by uninsured medical needs and difficulty buying necessities. | Family will be able to obtain the necessities of life. | 1. Discuss with the family expectations regarding their needs. 2. Share with family community resources that could help expand the family income (e.g., food stamps, health department immunization clinic, and clothing closet). 3. Provide assistance in meeting basic family needs. | 1. Family will have adequate food and clothing. 2. Family will obtain needed medical care. 3. Family is able to maintain its home. |
| Mr. Lopez speaks some English but is unable to read or write it. Mrs. Lopez has limited comprehension of English, as does the grandmother. | Communication with community systems impaired, related to an insufficient number of care providers who speak Spanish. | Family will be able to communicate basic needs with care providers in the community. | 1. Use culturally appropriate visual aids to facilitate family understanding. 2. Seek a translator to discuss critical health issues. 3. Show respect for the family's cultural differences (e.g., seek information about family customs, traditions, and health beliefs). 4. Keep language simple and talk slowly. 5. Involve the father in the conversation. 6. Show respect to all family members. 7. Use nonverbal communication (e.g., pictures, drawings, or gestures) to clarify situations with the family. | 1. Family will obtain adequate food and clothing. 2. Family will express satisfaction with their encounters in the community. |
| Home in need of repairs and lead paint removal. Nitrates in well water potentially harmful to a new infant. | Environment impaired, due to presence of lead paint in home and nitrates in well water. | Lead paint will be removed from the environment. Family will use a safe alternative source of water for the new infant. | 1. Elicit the family's understanding of lead poisoning and its effects. 2. Assist family in obtaining community resources for repair of home if desired. 3. Help the family obtain testing to discern safety of water for all family members. | 1. Well water is tested. 2. Family verbalizes an understanding of lead poisoning. 3. Family takes action to protect children from lead poisoning. |

is in need of medical care for a draining ear. All of the children are behind in their immunizations. The adults in the family do not know which "shots" they have had. Mrs. Lopez is in her seventh month of pregnancy and has had no medical care. The family expresses a desire to obtain care for their children but "we have no extra money to pay a doctor. We can hardly afford to buy food and clothing for the kids."

Although evaluation is one of the most significant aspects of the nursing process, it is the one most frequently neglected or haphazardly done. When developing the nursing care plan, intervals should be established for the systematic review of all aspects of the nursing process. Some community health agencies have a policy stating that all records should be summarized and analyzed after a given number of visits have been made or when the family case is being transferred to another nurse. A well-written summary helps the community health nurse synthesize data and vividly identify what has or has not been accomplished in a specified period of time.

## Evaluating Outcomes

Evaluating outcomes is an evaluation of the effectiveness of nursing interventions (Johnson, Maas, Moorhead, 2000). When evaluating outcomes, the effectiveness of all interventions implemented by the family, the nurse, and other health care professionals must be closely examined. For example, some of the interventions evaluated may include analyzing ongoing interventions, new interventions, and revised interventions; evaluating strategies and processes involved in the management of the problem; evaluating appropriateness of problem-solving strategies and processes; and analyzing effectiveness of communication techniques among individuals involved in the intervention process (Johnson, Maas, Moorhead, 2000). When evaluating the outcomes, the nurse may find that clients are not reaching their expected outcomes. This happens for various reasons that are not always obvious to either the client or the nurse. Outlined in Box 9-8 are some factors for the nurse to consider as guidelines when examining why client outcomes have not been reached.

## BOX 9-8

*Common Reasons for Lack of Outcome Achievement*

- Database is inadequate to identify the *actual* needs of the family.
- Goals and expected outcomes are too broad and not tailored to the needs of the family.
- Goals and expected outcomes are not mutually established; nurse's goals being imposed on the family.
- Family priorities in relation to goals and expected outcomes are not ascertained.
- Family energies are not focused on priority family needs; the family is attempting to deal with all needs at once.
- Family energies are depleted as a result of normative and nonnormative crises.
- Barriers to care are not identified because follow-up on client and nurse actions is neglected.
- Nursing diagnoses, goals, and expected outcomes are not revised as the family situation changes.
- Interventions are not tailored to the needs of the family.
- Family lacks the support it needs to reduce anxiety during the change process.
- Coordination of care among all health professionals is neglected; family is receiving inconsistent messages about appropriate interventions, or gaps in services exist.

Noting only that the family has kept an appointment at a clinic provides very little data about the effectiveness of this client behavior. Identifying what happened when the family went to the clinic and what motivated them to do so is far more significant. These types of data provide the key for future interventions. Finding out, for instance, if the family was satisfied with the care they received or if the family understood the recommendations for follow-up can help the nurse identify barriers to the utilization of health care services. Data obtained from these types of questions also can assist the nurse in planning interventions specific to the current needs of the family. Evaluating outcomes can be scientifically done through use of the Nursing Outcomes Classification (NOC) process.

## Nursing Outcomes Classification

The **Nursing Outcomes Classification (NOC)** process provides a standardized systematic format to evaluate client outcomes (Johnson, Bulechek, Dochterman, et al., 2001). The client "outcomes serve as the criteria against which to judge the success of a nursing intervention. Outcomes describe a [client's] state, behaviors, responses and feelings in response to the care provided" (Johnson, Bulechek, Dochterman, et al., 20001, p. 8). In the NOC system each outcome "has a label name, a definition, a list of indicators to evaluate [client] status in relation to the outcome" (p. 9). The effectiveness of each outcome is evaluated on a 5-point Likert Scale. Table 9-13 provides an example of an NOC outcome evaluation applied to anxiety. More than 250 outcomes have been grouped into seven domains: functional health, physiological health, psychosocial health, health knowledge and behavior, perceived health, family health, and community health. This work is an ongoing effort and nurses are encouraged to contribute to these efforts through use, evaluation, and development of the classifications.

Use of the NOC classification system enhances the ability to define outcomes and to articulate what nursing does in a health care delivery system in which cost containment is an ongoing priority. "Developing nursing knowledge requires the use of outcome measures" (Johnson, Maas, Moorhead, 2000, p. 15). Establishing linkages between what is known and what is expected provides a common language for nurses in their practice.

The first step in establishing linkages is determining the nursing diagnosis. "Once a nursing diagnosis is determined, the nurse can locate the diagnosis in the linkages and determine if any of the suggested outcomes are appropriate for the individual [client or client group]" (Johnson, Bulechek, Dochterman, et al., 2001, p.18). Currently more than 250 linkages have been made between NANDA (nursing diagnosis), NIC (nursing interventions), and NOC (nursing outcomes). Table 9-14 provides an example of how NANDA-NIC-NOC linkages were applied to a case study. The NANDA-NIC-NOC linkages can be used to develop

**TABLE 9-13**

*Example of an NOC Outcome Evaluation*

*Anxiety Control*

**Definition:** Personal actions to eliminate or reduce feelings or apprehension and tension from an unidentifiable source.

| ANXIETY CONTROL | NEVER DEMONSTRATED 1 | RARELY DEMONSTRATED 2 | SOMETIMES DEMONSTRATED 3 | OFTEN DEMONSTRATED 4 | CONSISTENTLY DEMONSTRATED 5 |
|---|---|---|---|---|---|
| Monitors intensity of anxiety | 1 | 2 | 3 | 4 | 5 |
| Eliminates precursors of anxiety | 1 | 2 | 3 | 4 | 5 |
| Decreases environmental stimuli when anxious | 1 | 2 | 3 | 4 | 5 |
| Seeks information to reduce anxiety | 1 | 2 | 3 | 4 | 5 |
| Plans coping strategies for stressful situations | 1 | 2 | 3 | 4 | 5 |
| Uses effective coping strategies | 1 | 2 | 3 | 4 | 5 |
| Uses relaxation techniques to reduce anxiety | 1 | 2 | 3 | 4 | 5 |
| Reports decreased duration of episodes | 1 | 2 | 3 | 4 | 5 |
| Reports increased length of time between episodes | 1 | 2 | 3 | 4 | 5 |
| Maintains role performance | 1 | 2 | 3 | 4 | 5 |
| Maintains social relationships | 1 | 2 | 3 | 4 | 5 |
| Maintains concentration | 1 | 2 | 3 | 4 | 5 |
| Reports absence of sensory perceptual distortions | 1 | 2 | 3 | 4 | 5 |
| Reports adequate sleep | 1 | 2 | 3 | 4 | 5 |
| Reports absence of physical manifestations of anxiety | 1 | 2 | 3 | 4 | 5 |
| Behavioral manifestations of anxiety absent | 1 | 2 | 3 | 4 | 5 |
| Controls anxiety response | 1 | 2 | 3 | 4 | 5 |
| Other _____ (Specify) | 1 | 2 | 3 | 4 | 5 |

Modified from: Johnson M, Bulechek G, Dochterman JM, et al., editors: *Nursing diagnoses, outcomes, and interventions, NANDA, NOC, and NIC linkages,* St Louis, 2001, Mosby, p. 10.

individualized care plans and clinical pathways (Johnson, Bulechek, Dochterman, et al., 2001).

## Clinical Pathways

Clinical pathways are used in some community health agencies to monitor the achievement of clinical outcomes. A clinical pathway identifies key activities that must occur in a time-sequenced order to achieve specified client goals (Maturen, Zander, 1993). "They define the process (actions) most likely to yield the desired outcomes" (Murray, Atkinson, 2000, p. 150). Clinical pathways resemble standardized care plans, but in addition to identifying client needs, expected outcomes and interventions, pathways identify very specific timelines for implementing care activities and outcome achievement. They also include a variance record that identifies "any difference between what was planned and what actually occurred" (Marrelli, Hilliard, 1996, p. 27). Variance records portray whether goals are met in a specified time frame and within a cost limit allocation.

Clinical pathways are managed care tools "designed to streamline [client] care, emphasize the achievement of predetermined expected outcomes, minimize length of stay, and control costs while maintaining acceptable quality"

**TABLE 9-14**

*Case Study with Example of NANDA-NIC-NOC Linkage*

| CASE STUDY: MRS. C | NANDA-NIC-NOC LINKAGES DEMONSTRATED IN MRS. C'S PLAN OF CARE | | |
| --- | --- | --- | --- |
| | NURSING DIAGNOSIS BODY IMAGE DISTURBANCE | NURSING INTERVENTION BODY IMAGE ENHANCEMENT | NURSING OUTCOME BODY IMAGE |
| Mrs. C, a 38-year-old woman, is married and has two adult stepchildren. She maintains a healthy lifestyle and has no family history of cancer. She performs breast self-examinations routinely and has never identified a lump or any unusual finding during her monthly examination. Mrs. C works full-time as a magazine publisher. One day at work as she was going down a flight of stairs, her high heel caught on the rung of the step, and she fell to the next landing. She received multiple bruises, including one in the chest area where she hit a metal railing. Ignoring her injuries because she was embarrassed about the fall, she continued to work throughout the day. That evening she told her family about her fall at work. Everyone was concerned, but she downplayed the incident because she was still more embarrassed about falling than concerned about the injuries she sustained. Subsequently Mrs. C experienced localized pain in her left breast. The pain started out as dull ache and did not improve over time. For several days Mrs. C was aware of the breast pain but disregarded it as simply being a bruise resulting from the accident. The pain gradually became worse and, ultimately, Mrs. C could feel a lump in her breast. The biopsy was done a week later and confirmed the presence of a malignant tumor. Mrs. C had a radical mastectomy of the left breast several days later.<br><br>Mr. C was at the hospital during the surgery but left for work after Mrs. C entered postanesthesia recovery. After work, Mr. C, an alcoholic, decided to go to the bar for a few drinks. He phoned Mrs. C from the bar and told her he would call her again once he reached home. Mrs. C was concerned about her husband driving home from the bar and worried a great deal about this during the evening. Several hours later he phoned her from home. While talking to her he "passed out" on the other end, and she could not disconnect from him. This upset Mrs. C because she knew he was not dealing well with the mastectomy. She needed his support to deal with her recovery, and he needed her to help him cope with her surgery. Mrs. C relied on the nursing staff for support with accepting her body image changes and also for emotional support. The staff located Reach for Recovery, a breast cancer support group, to help Mrs. C through this difficult time in her life. | *Defining Characteristics*<br>Nonverbal response to actual or perceived change in structure and/or function; verbalization of feelings that reflect an altered view of one's body in appearance, structure, or function<br><br>*Objective*<br>Missing body part; not touching body part; not looking at body part<br><br>*Subjective*<br>Negative feelings about body; fear of rejection or reaction by others<br><br>*Related factors*<br>Surgery; illness treatment | *Nursing Activities*<br>Assist client to discuss changes caused by illness or surgery.<br>Assist client to separate physical appearance from feelings of personal worth.<br>Assist client to discuss stressors affecting body image due to surgery.<br>Monitor frequency of statements of self-criticism.<br>Monitor whether client can look at the changed body part.<br>Monitor for statements that identify body image perceptions concerned with body shape and body weight.<br>Determine client's and family's perception of the alteration in body image versus reality.<br>Determine if a change in body image has contributed to increased social isolation.<br>Assist client to identify actions that will enhance appearance.<br>Facilitate contact with individuals with similar changes in body image.<br>Identify support groups available to client. | *Indicators*<br>Congruence between body reality, body ideal, and body presentation<br>Description of affected body part<br>Willingness to touch affected body part<br>Satisfaction with body appearance<br>Adjustment to changes in physical appearance<br>Adjustment to changes in health status<br>Willingness to use strategies to enhance appearance and function |

Modified from: Johnson M, Bulechek G, Dochterman JM, et al., editors: *Nursing diagnosis, outcomes, and interventions, NANDA, NOC, and NIC Linkages,* St Louis, 2001, Mosby, pp. 19-20.

(Marrelli, Hilliard, 1996, p. xi). Clinical pathways are standardized care plans that address the needs and service requirements of *homogenous, high-volume* client case types. For example, a home health care agency might develop a clinical pathway to sequence health care provider activities for clients that have diabetes or hypertension, because these diagnoses are common among home health care clients. In contrast, staff in a public health agency would be more likely to develop clinical pathways for their high-volume maternal-child health families or clients that have a communicable disease such as tuberculosis.

A sample clinical pathway is displayed in Appendix 9-5. Agencies using this pathway establish a timeline for interventions and expected outcomes based on the characteristics of the clients served by the agency. For example, if 90% of their diabetic clients required 8 weeks of service, the time frame used would be 8 weeks. Like other types of standardized care plans, clinical pathways are individualized to meet the unique needs of clients. Additional care activities and expected outcomes are added to their pathway based on data obtained during the assessment phase of the nursing process. The reader is referred to Marrelli and Hilliard's (1996) book for a comprehensive discussion of how agencies develop clinical pathways and how pathways are individualized to meet client needs. Clinical pathways can assist the health care team in determining when to prepare clients for termination based on identified client needs.

## TERMINATING

Terminating is seldom identified as a separate phase in the nursing process. It is alluded to during the evaluation phase, but little attention is devoted to discussing the effect termination has on the nurse and the client in the community health setting. Frequently, feelings associated with the separation process are not handled by the client or the nurse. The inability to deal with these feelings can stifle the development of close, caring professional relationships. For this reason terminating is labeled as a separate phase in the family-centered nursing process in this text.

Terminating is the period when the client and nurse deal with feelings associated with separation and when they distance themselves (Kelly, 1969, p. 2381). Ending a meaningful relationship with a client should be planned carefully. Clients, as well as nurses, need time to deal with the strong emotions that are often evoked by separation. Anger, sadness, denial, withdrawal, and regression are some normal reactions associated with termination. The type of reaction that occurs depends, to a great extent, on how the nurse and the client have dealt with separation in the past.

### The Termination Process

The family should be adequately prepared for termination. The family's readiness for ending the therapeutic relationship should be ascertained. Factors the nurse considers when assessing readiness include the family's desire to terminate, progress made in goal achievement, the family's ability to identify personal health care needs and to take action to resolve these needs, and the family's ability to identify and access needed family resources.

The family should be involved in making the decision about how and when the therapeutic relationship will end. Some families find a gradual process, in which the nurse decreases the frequency of visits but continues to maintain contact with the family, the most helpful way to terminate. Other families decide when it is time to terminate nursing services and establish a specific time for ending the relationship.

From a realistic perspective, the nurse may find that, because of financial constraints, the number of visits that can be made is limited. When agencies have contracts with managed care companies to provide nursing services, the company decides when termination will occur. The number of visits should be clearly identified during the nurse's initial visit to the client's home. The nurse may need to advocate for additional nursing services when the specified number of visits does not meet client needs, or the nurse may need to assist the client to access additional resources in the community.

When ending a therapeutic relationship, the nurse assists the client in analyzing what has been accomplished and the client's strengths in handling his or her health care needs. The nurse also assists the client in determining how to access nursing services or other community resources in the future.

## SUMMARY

The family-centered nursing process is a systematic approach to scientific problem solving, involving several dynamic actions—assessing, analyzing, planning, implementing, evaluating, and terminating—for the purpose of facilitating optimum client functioning. Nurses in all settings use this process to individualize care for clients in an orderly, deliberative, and logical manner. In the community health setting, emphasis is on meeting the needs of the family unit, as well as the needs of individual family members.

The principles of individualization, active participation, self-determination, confidentiality, and values clarification must be applied in all phases of the nursing process. Contracting is used with clients to promote active client participation in the therapeutic process and to support the client's right of self-determination. *Contracting* is a term used to denote a process that involves the establishment of mutually defined goals and intervention strategies. It is a working agreement between client and nurse, explicitly stated, in which all parties involved are working together to achieve a common goal.

Use of the family-centered nursing process is rewarding and challenging. The family-centered nursing process assists the nurse in helping clients from diverse cultural and ethnic backgrounds to mobilize personal strengths that will enhance their self-care capabilities. It provides the nurse with a framework for facilitating client decision making about health care matters. It also enables the nurse to become truly involved with other human beings in a supportive, therapeutic way.

*Ella M. Brooks acknowledges the work from previous editions of this text in the development of this chapter.*

## CRITICAL THINKING
*exercise*

Based on The Athen family data provided below, develop an initial care plan for the Athen family by including:
- Assessment data
- Nursing diagnosis
- Expected outcomes/goals
- Nursing interventions/actions
- Evaluation criteria

### The Athen Family

You are the public health nurse from the Pottsville County Health Department and are visiting Mr. and Mrs. Athen, an elderly couple (89 and 85, respectively) who were referred by their family physician for monitoring of a wound on Mrs. Athen's right arm. Mr. Athen dresses this wound twice a day but is concerned because it is healing slowly. Mr. Athen wears glasses and a hearing aid but is in good health considering his age. He does admit that he "tires faster these days." Mr. Athen is the primary caregiver for his wife and caretaker of the household. Mrs. Athen has left-sided hemiplegia from a cerebrovascular accident 3 years ago. She uses a wheelchair for mobility and a guard rail for walking and range-of-motion exercises. The family lives in a well-kept home that is wheelchair accessible. Their daughter and her husband live 30 miles away and are available for emergency help and specific projects. However, they do not visit often because of caregiver responsibilities for their 40-year-old son, who is severely disabled from cerebral palsy. The Athens are devoted to each other and will do everything they can to stay out of a nursing home. They are concerned about what will happen to their grandson should his parents die or become unable to care for him.

## REFERENCES

American Nurses Association (ANA): *Standards of community health nursing practice*, Kansas City, Mo, 1986, ANA.

American Nurses Association (ANA): *Standards of clinical nursing practice*, Kansas City, Mo, 1991, ANA.

American Nurses Association (ANA), Quad Council of Public Health Nursing Organizations: *Scope and standards of public health nursing practice*, Washington, DC, 1999, ANA.

American Public Health Association (APHA): *The definition and role of public health nursing: a statement of APHA Public Health Nursing Section*, Washington, DC, 1996, APHA.

Barkauskas VH, Stoltenberg-Allen C, Baumann LC, et al.: *Health and physical assessment*, St Louis, 1994, Mosby.

Barkauskas VH, Stoltenberg-Allen C, Baumann LC, et al.: *Health and physical assessment*, ed 3, St Louis, 2002, Mosby.

Beall L: The corrupt contract: problems in conjoint therapy with parents and children, *Am J Orthopsychiatry* 42(1):77-81, 1972.

Beavers WR: *Psychotherapy and growth: a family systems perspective*, New York, 1977, Brunner/Mazel.

Berkey KM, Hanson SMH: *Pocket guide to family assessment and intervention*, St Louis, 1991, Mosby.

Boehm S: Patient contracting. In Fitzpatrick JJ, Taunton RL, Benoliel JQ, editors: *Annu Rev Nurs Res*, vol 7, New York, 1989, Springer.

Bomar PJ: *Nurses and family health promotion: concepts, assessment, and interventions*, ed 2, Philadelphia, 1996, Saunders.

Bomar PJ, McNeely G: Family health nursing role: past, present, and future. In Bomar PJ: *Nurses and family health promotion: concepts, assessment, and interventions*, ed 2, Philadelphia, 1996, Saunders.

Boyle JS: Culture, family, and community. In Andrew MM, Boyle JS: *Transcultural concepts in nursing care*, Philadelphia, 1999, Lippincott.

Calvillo EF, Flaskerud JH: The adequacy and scope of Roy's adaptation model to guide cross-cultural pain research, *Nurs Sci Q* 6(3):118-129, 1993.

Carter B, McGoldrick M: Coaching at various stages of the life cycle. In Carter B, McGoldrick M, editors: *The expanded family life cycle, individual family, and social perspectives*, ed 3, Boston, 1999, Allyn & Bacon.

Catalano JT: Cultural diversity. In Catalano JT: *Nursing now today's issues, tomorrow's trends*, ed 2, Philadelphia, 2000, FA Davis.

Chin S: Can self-care theory be applied to families? In Riehl-Sisca J, editor: *The science and art of self-care*, Norwalk, Conn, 1985, Appleton-Century-Crofts.

Chwedyk P: Speaking of cultural competence, *Minority Nurse* (Spring 2000):28-31.

Clements IW, Roberts FB, editors: *Family health: a theoretical approach to nursing care*, New York, 1983, Wiley.

Cody WK: Of tombstones, milestones, and gemstones: a retrospective and prospective on nursing theory, *Nurs Sci Q* 10(1):3-5, 1997.

Curran D: *Traits of a healthy family*, Minneapolis, 1983, Winston Press.

Danielson CB, Hamel-Bissell B, Winstead-Fry P: *Families, health and illness: perspectives on coping and intervention*, St Louis, 1993, Mosby.

Della Monica E: Home health care documentation and record keeping. In Harris MD: *Handbook of home health care administration*, Gaithersburg, Md, 1994, Aspen.

Donnelly E: Health promotion, families, and the diagnostic process, *Fam Community Health* 12:12-20, 1990.

Eliason MS: Ethics and transcultural nursing care, *Nurs Outlook* 41(5):225-228, 1993.

Ericksen AB: Separate identities, *Minority Nurse* (Summer 2000): 20-23.

Fawcett J: *Conceptual models of nursing*, ed 2, Philadelphia, 1989, FA Davis.

Friedemann ML: Closing the gap between grand theory and mental health practice with families, Part 1: the framework of systemic organization for nursing of families and family members, *Arch Psychiatr Nurs* 3:10-19, 1989a.

Friedemann ML: Closing the gap between grand theory and mental health practice with families. Part 2: the control-congruence model for mental health nursing of families, *Arch Psychiatr Nurs* 3:20-28, 1989b.

Friedman MM: *Family nursing, research, theory and practice*, ed 4, Stamford, Conn, 1998, Appleton & Lange.

Gaffney KF, Moore JB: Testing Orem's theory of self-care deficit: dependent care agent performance for children, *Nurs Sc Q* 9(4):160-164, 1996.

General Accounting Office (GAO): *Home visiting: a promising early intervention strategy for at-risk families*, GAO/HRD-90-83, Washington, DC, 1990, GAO.

Giger JN, Davidhizar RE: *Transcultural nursing: assessment and intervention*, ed 3, St Louis, 1999, Mosby.

Gonot PW: Family therapy as derived from King's conceptual model. In Whall AL, editor: *Family therapy for nursing: four approaches*, Norwalk, Conn, 1986, Appleton-Century-Crofts.

Gordon M: *Nursing diagnosis: process and application*, ed 2, New York, 1987, McGraw-Hill.

Gordon M: *Manual of nursing diagnosis*, ed 9, St Louis, 2000, Mosby.

Hanchett ES: *Nursing frameworks and community as client: bridging the gap*, Norwalk, Conn, 1988, Appleton-Lange.

Hanna DR, Roy SC: Roy adaptation model and perspectives on the family, *Nurs Sci Q* 14(1):9-13, 2001.

Hanson J: The family. In Roy C, editor: *Introduction to nursing: an adaptation model*, ed 2, Englewood Cliffs, NJ, 1984, Prentice-Hall.

Hanson SMH, Mischke KB: Family health assessment and intervention. In Bomar PJ: *Nurses and family health promotion: concepts, assessment, and interventions*, ed 2, Philadelphia, 1996, WB Saunders.

Health Care Financing Administration (HCFA): Medicare Program: home health agencies—conditions of participation, *Federal Register* 56:32967-32975, July 18, 1991.

Health Care Financing Administration (HCFA): *Conditions of participation: home health agencies*, 42 CFR Part 484, Section 484.10 through 484.52, Washington, DC, October 1994, HCFA, Section 484.10.

Hines PM, Preto NG, McGoldrick M, et al.: Culture and the family life cycle. In Carter B, McGoldrick M, editors: *The expanded family life cycle, individual, family and social perspectives*, ed 3, Boston, 1999, Allyn and Bacon.

Johnson M, Bulechek G, Dochterman JM, et al., editors: *Nursing diagnoses, outcomes, and interventions, NANDA, NOC, and NIC linkages*, St Louis, 2001, Mosby.

Johnson M, Maas M, Moorhead S, editors: *Nursing outcomes classification (NOC)*, St Louis, 2000, Mosby.

Johnston RL: Approaching family intervention through Rogers' conceptual model. In Whall AL, editor: *Family therapy theory for nursing: four approaches*, Norwalk, Conn, 1986, Appleton-Century-Crofts.

Kelly HS: The sense of an ending, *Am J Nurs* 69:2378-2381, 1969.

Kim MJ, Moritz DA: *Classification of nursing diagnoses: proceedings of the third and fourth national conferences*, New York, 1982, McGraw-Hill.

King IM: *A theory for nursing systems, concepts, process*, Albany, NY, 1981, Delmar.

King IM: King's theory of goal attainment, *Nurs Sci Q* 5(1):19-26, 1992.

King IM: The theory of goal attainment. In Frey MA, Sieloff CL, editors: *Advancing King's systems framework and theory of nursing*, Thousand Oaks, Calif, 1995, Sage.

King IM: Reflections on the past and a vision for the future, *Nurs Sci Q* 10(1):15-17, 1997.

Leninger M: Issues, questions, and concerns related to the nursing diagnoses cultural movement from a transcultural nursing perspective, *J Transcult Nurs* 2:23-32, 1990.

Lewis J, Beavers R, Gossett JT, et al.: *No single thread: psychological health in family systems*, New York, 1976, Brunner/Mazel.

Mahoney EA, Verdisco L, Shortridge L: *How to collect and record a health history*, ed 2, Philadelphia, 1982, Lippincott.

Maluccio AN, Marlow W: The case for the contract, *Soc Work* 19:28-36, 1974.

Marrelli TM, Hilliard LS: *Home care and clinical paths: effective care planning across the continuum*, St Louis, 1996, Mosby.

Martin K: The Omaha System: a data base for ambulatory and home care. In Mills MEC, Romano CA, Heller BR: *Information management in nursing and health care*, Springhouse, Penn, 1994, Springhouse.

Martin KS, Scheet NJ: *The Omaha System: a pocket guide for community health nursing*, Philadelphia, 1992, Saunders.

Maturen VL, Zander K: Outcome management in a prospective pay system, *Caring* 12:46-53, 1993.

McCain F: Nursing by assessment—not intuition, *Am J Nurs* 65:82-84, 1965.

McCloskey JC, Bulechek GM: Standardizing the language for nursing treatments; an overview of the issues, *Nurs Outlook* 42:56-63, 1994.

McCloskey JC, Bulechek GM, editors: *Nursing interventions classification (NIC)*, ed 3, St Louis, 2000, Mosby.

McPhetridge LM: Nursing history: one means to personalize care, *Am J Nurs* 68:68-75, 1968.

Murray ME, Atkinson LD: *Understanding the nursing process*, ed 6, New York, 2000, McGraw-Hill.

Neuman B: *The Neuman systems model, application to education and practice*, ed 2, Norwalk, Conn, 1989, Appleton & Lange.

Neuman B: The Neuman systems model. In Neuman B, editor: *The Neuman systems model*, ed 3, Norwalk, Conn, 1995, Appleton & Lange.

Neuman B: The Neuman systems model in research and practice, *Nurs Sci Q* 9(2):67-70, 1996.

Norris DM, Hoyer PJ: Dynamism in practice: parenting within King's framework, *Nurs Sci Q* 6(2):79-85, 1993.

North American Nursing Diagnosis Association (NANDA): *Nursing diagnoses: definitions and classification, 1999-2000*, Philadelphia, 1999, NANDA.

Orem DE: View of human beings specific to nursing, *Nurs Sci Q* 10(1):26-31, 1997.

Orem DE: *Nursing: concepts of practice*, ed 6, St Louis, 2001, Mosby.

Otto H: Criteria for assessing family strength, *Family Process* 2:333-336, 1963.

Phillips JR: Changing family patterns and health, *Nurs Sci Q*, 6(3):113-114, 1993.

Pollock SE: Adaptation to chronic illness: a program of research for testing nursing theory, *Nurs Sci Q* 6(2):86-92, 1993.

Potter PA, Perry AG: *Fundamentals of nursing: concepts, process, and practice*, ed 4, St Louis, 1997, Mosby.

Pratt L: *Family structure and effective health behavior: the energized family*, Boston, 1976, Houghton Mifflin.

Redman EK: *The process of patient education*, St Louis, 1997, Mosby.

Reed KS: Adapting the Neuman systems model for family nursing, *Nurs Sci Q* 6:93-97, 1993.

Riehl-Sisca J, editor: *The science and art of self-care*, Norwalk, Conn, 1985, Appleton-Century-Crofts.

Robinson JH: Grief responses, coping responses, and social support of widows: research with Roy's model, *Nurs Sci Q* 8(4):158-164, 1995.

Roy SC, Andrews HA: *The Roy adaptation model: a definitive statement*, Norwalk, Conn, 1999, Appleton & Lange.

Seabury BA: The contract: uses, abuses and limitations, *Soc Work* 21(8):39-45, 1976.

Sibley BJ: Cultural influences on health and illness. In Long BC, Phipps WJ, Cassmeyer VL: *Medical-surgical nursing*, ed 3, St Louis, 1992, Mosby.

Simons RC: *Understanding human behavior in health and illness*, ed 3, Baltimore, 1985, Williams & Wilkins.

Taylor SG: Orem's general theory of nursing and families, *Nurs Sci Q* 14(1):7-9, 2001.

Tripp-Reimer T, Brink PJ, Saunders JN: Cultural assessment: content and process, *Nurs Outlook* 32:78-82, 1984.

Weber G: Making nursing diagnosis work for you and your client, *Nurs Health Care* 12:424-430, 1991.

Weiss HB: Home visits necessary but not sufficient, *Future of Children* 3(3):113-128, 1993.

Whall AL: Nursing theory and the assessment of families, *J Psychiatr Nurs Mental Health Serv* 19(1):30-36, 1981.

Whall AL, editor: *Family therapy theory for nursing: four approaches*, Norwalk, Conn, 1986, Appleton-Century-Crofts.

Whall AL, Fawcett J: *Family theory development in nursing: state of the science and art*, Philadelphia, 1991, FA Davis.


## SELECTED BIBLIOGRAPHY

Ackley BS, Ladwig GB: *Nursing diagnosis handbook: a guide to planning care*, ed 4, St Louis, 1999, Mosby.

Adams D: Making cultural competency work, *Closing the Gap*, January 2000, p. 3.

Andrews MM, Boyle JS: *Transcultural concepts in nursing care*, ed 3, Philadelphia, 1999, Lippincott.

Fawcett J: The metaparadigm of nursing: present status and future refinements, *Image J Nurs Sch* 16(3):84-87, 1984.

Health Research Service Administration (HRSA) Maternal and Child Health Bureau: *Promoting cultural diversity and cultural competency: self-assessment checklist*, January 2000, pp. 6-7.

Hartweg DL: Self-care actions of healthy middle-aged women to promote well-being, *Nurs Res* 42:221-227, 1993.

Imber-Black E: Creating meaningful rituals for new life cycle transitions. In Carter B, McGoldrick M, editors: *The expanded family life cycle*, ed 3, St Louis, 1999, Mosby.

McCubbin M: Normative family transitions and health outcomes. In Hinshaw AS, Feetham SL, Shaver JL: *Handbook of clinical nursing research*, Thousand Oaks, Calif, 1999, Sage.

Murray RB, Zentner JP: *Health promotion strategies through the life span*, Upper Saddle River, NJ, 2000, Prentice Hall.

Randall-David E: *Strategies for working with culturally diverse communities and clients*, Bethesda, Md, 1989, The Association for the Care of Children's Health.

Whall AL: Family system theory; relationship to nursing conceptual models. In Whall AL, Fawcett J: *Family theory development in nursing: state of the science and art*, Philadelphia, 1991, FA Davis.

World Health Organization: Constitution of the World Health Organization, *WHO Chron* 1:29-43, 1947.

# Giger and Davidhizar's Transcultural Assessment Model

## Culturally Unique Individual

1. Place of birth
2. Cultural definition
   What is . . .
3. Race
   What is . . .
4. Length of time in country (if appropriate)

## Communication

1. Voice quality
   A. Strong, resonant
   B. Soft
   C. Average
   D. Shrill
2. Pronunciation and enunciation
   A. Clear
   B. Slurred
   C. Dialect (geographical)
3. Use of silence
   A. Infrequent
   B. Often
   C. Length
      (1) Brief
      (2) Moderate
      (3) Long
      (4) Not observed
4. Use of nonverbal
   A. Hand movement
   B. Eye movement
   C. Entire body movement
   D. Kinesics (gestures, expression, or stances)
5. Touch
   A. Startles or withdraws when touched
   B. Accepts touch without difficulty
   C. Touches others without difficulty
6. Ask these and similar questions:
   A. How do you get your point across to others?
   B. Do you like communicating with friends, family, and acquaintances?
   C. When asked a question, do you usually respond (in words or body movement, or both)?
   D. If you have something important to discuss with your family, how would you approach them?

## Space

1. Degree of comfort
   A. Moves when space invaded
   B. Does not move when space invaded
2. Distance in conversations
   A. 0 to 18 inches
   B. 18 inches to 3 feet
   C. 3 feet or more
3. Definition of space
   A. Describe degree of comfort with closeness when talking with or standing near others
   B. How do objects (e.g., furniture) in the environment affect your sense of space?
4. Ask these and similar questions:
   A. When you talk with family members, how close do you stand?
   B. When you communicate with coworkers and other acquaintances, how close do you stand?
   C. If a stranger touches you, how do you react or feel?
   D. If a loved one touches you, how do you react or feel?
   E. Are you comfortable with the distance between us now?

## Social Organization

1. Normal state of health
   A. Poor
   B. Fair
   C. Good
   D. Excellent
2. Marital status
3. Number of children
4. Parents living or deceased?
5. Ask these and similar questions:
   A. How do you define social activities?
   B. What are some activities that you enjoy?
   C. What are your hobbies, or what do you do when you have free time?
   D. Do you believe in a Supreme Being?
   E. How do you worship that Supreme Being?
   F. What is your function (what do you do) in your family unit/system (father, mother, child, advisor)?

From Giger JN, Davidhizar RE: *Transcultural nursing: assessment and interventions*, ed 3, St Louis, 1999, Mosby, pp. 11-13.

# Giger and Davidhizar's Transcultural Assessment Model (cont'd)

G. What is your role in your family unit/system (father, mother, child, advisor)?
H. When you were a child, what or who influenced you most?
I. What is/was your relationship with your siblings and parents?
J. What does work mean to you?
K. Describe you past, present, and future jobs.
L. What are your political views?
M. How have your political views influenced your attitude toward health and illness?

## Time
1. Orientation to time
   A. Past-oriented
   B. Present-oriented
   C. Future-oriented
2. View of time
   A. Social time
   B. Clock-oriented
3. Physiochemical reaction to time
   A. Sleeps at least 8 hours a night
   B. Goes to sleep and wakes on a consistent schedule
   C. Understands the importance of taking medication and other treatments on schedule
4. Ask these and similar questions:
   A. What kind of timepiece do you wear daily?
   B. If you have an appointment at 2 PM, what time is acceptable to arrive?
   C. If a nurse tells you that you will receive a medication in "about a half hour," realistically, how much time will you allow before calling the nurses' station?

## Environmental Control
1. Locus-of-control
   A. Internal locus-of-control (believes that the power to affect change lies within)
   B. External locus-of-control (believes that fate, luck, and chance have a great deal to do with how things turn out)
2. Value orientation
   A. Believes in supernatural forces
   B. Relies on magic, witchcraft, and prayer to affect change
   C. Does not believe in supernatural forces
   D. Does not rely on magic, witchcraft, or prayer to affect change

3. Ask these and similar questions:
   A. How often do you have visitors at your home?
   B. Is it acceptable to you for visitors to drop in unexpectedly?
   C. Name some ways your parents or other persons treated your illnesses when you were a child.
   D. Have you or someone else in your immediate surroundings ever used a home remedy that made you sick?
   E. What home remedies have you used that worked? Will you use them in the future?
   F. What is your definition of "good health"?
   G. What is your definition of illness or "poor health"?

## Biological Variations
1. Conduct a complete physical assessment noting:
   A. Body structure (small, medium, or large frame)
   B. Skin color
   C. Unusual skin discolorations
   D. Hair color and distribution
   E. Other visible physical characteristics (e.g., keloids, chloasma)
   F. Weight
   G. Height
   H. Check laboratory work for variances in hemoglobin, hematocrit, and sickle phenomena if African American or Mediterranean
2. Ask these and similar questions:
   A. What diseases or illnesses are common in your family?
   B. Describe your family's typical behavior when a family member is ill.
   C. How do you respond when you are angry?
   D. Who (or what) usually helps you to cope during a difficult time?
   E. What foods do you and your family like to eat?
   F. Have you ever had any usual cravings for:
      (1) White or red clay dirt?
      (2) Laundry starch?
   G. When you were a child what types of food did you eat?
   H. What foods are family favorites or are considered traditional?

# Giger and Davidhizar's Transcultural Assessment Model (cont'd)

### Nursing Assessment

1. Note whether the client has become culturally assimilated or observes own cultural practices.
2. Incorporate data into plan of nursing care:
   A. Encourage the client to discuss cultural differences; people from diverse cultures who hold different world views can enlighten nurses.
   B. Make efforts to accept and understand methods of communication.
   C. Respect the individual's personal need for space.
   D. Respect the rights of clients to honor and worship the Supreme Being of their choice.
   E. Identify a clerical or spiritual person to contact.
   F. Determine whether spiritual practices have implications for health, life, and well-being (e.g., Jehovah's Witnesses may refuse blood and blood derivatives; an Orthodox Jew may eat only kosher food high in sodium and may not drink milk when meat is served).
   G. Identify hobbies, especially when devising interventions for a short or extended convalescence or for rehabilitation.
   H. Honor time and value orientations and differences in these areas. Allay anxiety and apprehension if adherence to time is necessary.
   I. Provide privacy according to personal need and health status of the client (Note: the perception and reaction to pain may be culturally related).
   J. Note cultural health practices.
      (1) Identify and encourage efficacious practices.
      (2) Identify and discourage dysfunctional practices.
      (3) Identify and determine whether neutral practices will have a long-term effect.
   K. Note food preferences.
      (1) Make as many adjustments in diet as health status and long-term benefits will allow and that dietery department can provide.
      (2) Note dietary practices that may have serious implications for the client.

# Antepartum
# Nursing Assessment Guide

Client's name _____

EDC _____ GRAV _____ PARA _____ ABORT _____ DATE MED. CARE STARTED _____

M.D. _____ HOSP. _____ SIGNIFICANT MEDICAL HISTORY OF PREGNANCIES _____

Mother's opinion of previous pregnancy, delivery, and newborn (NB) _____

| CURRENT PREGNANCY | YES | NO | FIRST ASSESSMENT, COMMENTS<br>TRIMESTER 1 2 3 DATE _____ | YES | NO | SECOND ASSESSMENT, COMMENTS<br>TRIMESTER 1 2 3 DATE _____ |
|---|---|---|---|---|---|---|
| *Medical Supervision* | | | | | | |
| Medical appointments made | | | | | | |
|   Plans to keep | | | | | | |
| Dental appointments made | | | | | | |
|   Plans to keep | | | | | | |
| Dental care completed | | | | | | |
| Ct understanding of doctor's orders is: | | | | | | |
| *Signs and Symptoms* | | | | | | |
| Nausea | | | | | | |
| Vomiting | | | | | | |
| Heartburn | | | | | | |
| Spotting | | | | | | |
| Bleeding | | | | | | |
| Edema | | | | | | |
| Leg cramps | | | | | | |
| Varicosities | | | | | | |
| Backache | | | | | | |
| Dyspnea | | | | | | |
| Constipation | | | | | | |
| Hemorrhoids | | | | | | |
| Dysuria | | | | | | |

Printed with permission and modified from the Nursing Division, King County Health Department, 1000 Public Safety Building, Seattle, Washington.

# Antepartum
# Nursing Assessment Guide (cont'd)

| CURRENT PREGNANCY | YES | NO | FIRST ASSESSMENT, COMMENTS<br>TRIMESTER 1 2 3 DATE ____ | YES | NO | SECOND ASSESSMENT, COMMENTS<br>TRIMESTER 1 2 3 DATE ____ |
|---|---|---|---|---|---|---|
| *Signs and Symptoms—cont'd* | | | | | | |
| Urinary frequency | | | | | | |
| Fetal movements | | | | | | |
| Braxton Hicks | | | | | | |
| Other | | | | | | |
| *Personal Management* | | | | | | |
| Weight Gain | | | | | | |
|   Normal | | | | | | |
| Diet—type ____<br>  Breakfast<br>  Lunch<br>  Dinner<br>  Snacks<br>  Dislikes<br>  Fluid intake pattern<br>  Comments | | | | | | |
| Sleep—no. of hours | | | | | | |
| Health Habits | | | | | | |
|   Physical activity | | | | | | |
|   Substance use (specify) | | | | | | |
|   Safety practices | | | | | | |
|   Preventive care | | | | | | |
| Clothing | | | | | | |
|   Supportive | | | | | | |

*Continued*

# Antepartum
# Nursing Assessment Guide (cont'd)

Client's name _____

*Emotional (complete with client's feelings toward)*

| | FIRST ASSESSMENT, COMMENTS | SECOND ASSESSMENT, COMMENTS |
|---|---|---|
| **CURRENT PREGNANCY** | TRIMESTER 1 2 3 DATE _____ | TRIMESTER 1 2 3 DATE _____ |
| *Personal Management—cont'd* | | |
| Pregnancy | | |
| Motherhood | | |
| Changes in self-image | | |
| Mood swings | | |
| Pregnancy and parenthood affecting personal family goals | | |
| Husband-wife social and sexual relationships | | |
| Stresses created by emotional and physical changes of this pregnancy | | |
| Anxiety re: labor and delivery | | |
| Social and financial family stability re: future plans for NB | | |
| Past and present personality difficulties | | |
| Fetus | | |
| Father's awareness of, interest and attitude | | |

# Antepartum
# Nursing Assessment Guide (cont'd)

Client's name _____

| | YES | NO | FIRST ASSESSMENT, COMMENTS TRIMESTER 1 2 3 DATE ____ | YES | NO | SECOND ASSESSMENT, COMMENTS TRIMESTER 1 2 3 DATE ____ |
|---|---|---|---|---|---|---|
| **Plans for Delivery** | | | | | | |
| Made plans for hospitalization | | | | | | |
| Make arrangements for care of family at home | | | | | | |
| Knows what to expect of hospital routine | | | | | | |
| Knows signs of labor | | | | | | |
| Knows what to expect during labor and delivery | | | | | | |
| Knows what to expect PP | | | | | | |
| **Plans for Newborn** | | | | | | |
| Plans to breastfeed | | | | | | |
| Plans to bottle feed | | | | | | |
| Adequate layette and equipment | | | | | | |
| Plans to have help PP | | | | | | |
| Knows what to expect of NB | | | | | | |
| **Family Planning** | | | | | | |
| Knows methods of birth control | | | | | | |
| Wants information on family planning | | | | | | |

What kind of help does family want from CHN?

_____

_____

_____

What kind of help does family want from CHN?

_____

_____

_____

# Postpartum
# Nursing Assessment Guide

Client's name _____

GRAV _____ PARA _____ M.D. _____

HOSPITAL _____ SIGNIFICANT MEDICAL HISTORY OF PREGNANCIES _____

Check items that best describe client or complete with notation.

| POSTPARTUM EXAMINATION | FIRST ASSESSMENT DATE _____ | | SECOND ASSESSMENT DATE _____ | |
|---|---|---|---|---|
| | YES | NO | YES | NO |

Temp _____

### Breasts
Physical Appearance:

| | | | | |
|---|---|---|---|---|
| Normal | | | | |
| Engorgement | | | | |
| Soreness | | | | |
| Soft | | | | |
| Cracked | | | | |
| Redness | | | | |
| Caked | | | | |
| Inverted | | | | |
| Lactation: Leaking | | | | |
| Filling | | | | |
| Nursing | | | | |
| Not nursing | | | | |
| "Dry up" pills | | | | |

### Abdomen

| | | | | |
|---|---|---|---|---|
| Fundus (firmness, position) | | | | |
| C-section (incision) | | | | |

### Rectovaginal

| | | | | |
|---|---|---|---|---|
| Laceration | | | | |
| Episiotomy: | | | | |
| None | | | | |
| Clean | | | | |

Printed with permission and modified from the Nursing Division, King County Health Department, 1000 Public Safety Building, Seattle, Washington.

# Postpartum
# Nursing Assessment Guide (cont'd)

| | FIRST ASSESSMENT DATE ____ | | SECOND ASSESSMENT DATE ____ | |
|---|---|---|---|---|
| **POSTPARTUM EXAMINATION** | **YES** | **NO** | **YES** | **NO** |
| *Rectovaginal—cont'd* | | | | |
| Episiotomy—cont'd | | | | |
|   Healing | | | | |
|   Painful | | | | |
| Hemorrhoids | | | | |
| Other | | | | |
| *Lochia* | | | | |
| Rubra | | | | |
| Serosa | | | | |
| Alba | | | | |
| Clots | | | | |
| No. pads per day | | | | |
| *Voiding* | | | | |
| No difficulty | | | | |
| Anuria | | | | |
| Dysuria | | | | |
| Frequency | | | | |
| Burning | | | | |
| *Bowels* | | | | |
| Constipated | | | | |
| No difficulty | | | | |
| Other | | | | |

First assessment date _____        Second assessment date _____

**Personal Health Practices** (Describe what the client is doing about the following.)

A. Care

    Bathing _____

    Pericare _____

    Breast care _____

B. Rest_____

    Sleep _____

    Recreation _____

    Exercise and activity _____

# Postpartum
# Nursing Assessment Guide (cont'd)

C. Foundation garment _____

D. Diet—Type _____

    Breakfast _____

    Lunch _____

    Dinner _____

    Snacks _____

    Dislikes _____

    Fluid intake _____

      Comments _____

    _____

E. Sexual relations _____

*Psychosocial* (Describe mother's feeling or reaction to the following.)

Pregnancy _____

_____

Labor _____

_____

Delivery _____

_____

Newborn _____

_____

Motherhood _____

_____

Family's reaction to labor, delivery, NB _____

_____

Other _____

| MEDICAL SUPERVISION | YES | NO | | YES | NO |
|---|---|---|---|---|---|
| Medical appointments made | | | | | |
| Plan to keep | | | | | |
| Dental care up to date | | | | | |

Client's understanding of physician's orders is _____

*Family Planning*

Future family plans (method, problems) _____

What kind of help does family want from CHN? _____

_____

_____

# NANDA Nursing Diagnoses Grouped by Gordon's Functional Health Patterns*

## HEALTH-PERCEPTION–HEALTH MANAGEMENT PATTERN

**Health-Seeking Behaviors (Specify)**
**Altered Health Maintenance (Specify)**
**Ineffective Management of Therapeutic Regimen (Specify Area)**
**Risk for Ineffective Management of Therapeutic Regimen (Specify Area)**
**Effective Management of Therapeutic Regimen**
**Ineffective Family Management of Therapeutic Regimen**
**Ineffective Community Management of Therapeutic Regimen**
Health-Management Deficit (Specify Area)
Risk for Health-Management Deficit (Specify Area)
**Noncompliance (Specify Area)**
Risk for Noncompliance (Specify Area)
**Risk for Infection (Specify Type/Area)**
**Risk for Injury (Trauma)**
**Risk for Perioperative Positioning Injury**
**Risk for Poisoning**
**Risk for Suffocation**
**Altered Protection (Specify)**
**Energy Field Disturbance**

## NUTRITIONAL-METABOLIC PATTERN

**Altered Nutrition: More than Body Requirements** or Exogenous Obesity
**Altered Nutrition: Risk for More than Body Requirements** or Risk for Obesity
**Altered Nutrition: Less than Body Requirements** or Nutritional Deficit (Specify Type)
**Adult Failure to Thrive**
**Ineffective Breastfeeding**
**Interrupted Breastfeeding**
**Effective Breastfeeding**
**Ineffective Infant Feeding Pattern**
**Impaired Swallowing** (Uncompensated)
**Nausea**

Risk for Aspiration
**Altered Oral Mucous Membrane (Specify Alteration)**
**Altered Dentition**
**Fluid Volume Deficit**
**Risk for Fluid Volume Deficit**
**Fluid Volume Excess**
**Risk for Fluid Volume Imbalance**
**Impaired Skin Integrity**
**Risk for Impaired Skin Integrity** or Risk for Skin Breakdown
Pressure Ulcer (Specify Stage)
**Impaired Tissue Integrity (Specify Type)**
**Latex Allergy Response**
**Risk for Latex Allergy Response**
**Ineffective Thermoregulation**
**Hyperthermia**
**Hypothermia**
**Risk for Altered Body Temperature**

## ELIMINATION PATTERN

**Constipation**
**Perceived Constipation**
Intermittent Constipation Pattern
**Risk for Constipation**
**Diarrhea**
**Bowel Incontinence**
**Altered Urinary Elimination Pattern**
**Functional Urinary Incontinence**
**Reflex Urinary Incontinence**
**Stress Incontinence**
**Urge Incontinence**
**Risk for Urinary Urge Incontinence**
**Total Incontinence**
**Urinary Retention**

## ACTIVITY-EXERCISE PATTERN

**Activity Intolerance (Specify Level)**
**Risk for Activity Intolerance**

---

From Gordon M: *Manual of nursing diagnosis,* ed 9, St Louis, 2000, Mosby, pp. x-xvi.
*Boldface type indicates diagnoses currently accepted by the North American Nursing Diagnosis Association (NANDA). Others are either diagnoses received by NANDA for development or not accepted by NANDA but found to be useful in clinical practice.

# NANDA Nursing Diagnoses Grouped by Gordon's Functional Health Patterns* (cont'd)

Fatigue
**Impaired Physical Mobility (Specify Level)**
**Impaired Bed Mobility (Specify Level)**
**Impaired Transfer Ability (Specify Level)**
**Impaired Wheelchair Mobility**
**Impaired Walking (Specify Level)**
**Risk for Disuse Syndrome**
Risk for Joint Contractures
**Total Self-Care Deficit (Specify Level)**
**Self-Bathing-Hygiene Deficit (Specify Level)**
**Self-Dressing-Grooming Deficit (Specify Level)**
**Self-Feeding Deficit (Specify Level)**
**Self-Toileting Deficit (Specify Level)**
Developmental Delay: Self-Care Skills (Specify Level)
**Delayed Surgical Recovery**
**Altered Growth and Development**
**Risk for Altered Development**
**Risk for Altered Growth**
**Diversional Activity Deficit**
**Impaired Home Maintenance Management (Mild,**
  **Moderate, Severe, Potential, Chronic)**
**Dysfunctional Ventilatory Weaning Response**
**Inability to Sustain Spontaneous Ventilation**
**Ineffective Airway Clearance**
**Ineffective Breathing Pattern**
**Impaired Gas Exchange**
**Decreased Cardiac Output**
**Altered Tissue Perfusion (Specify)**
**Dysreflexia**
**Risk for Autonomic Dysreflexia**
**Disorganized Infant Behavior**
**Risk for Disorganized Infant Behavior**
**Potential for Enhanced Organized Infant Behavior**
**Risk for Peripheral Neurovascular Dysfunction**
**Decreased Intracranial Adaptive Capacity**

## SLEEP-REST PATTERN

Sleep-Pattern Disturbance (Specify Type)
**Sleep Deprivation**
Delayed Sleep Onset
Sleep Pattern Reversal

## COGNITIVE-PERCEPTUAL PATTERN

**Pain (Specify Location)**
**Chronic Pain (Specify Location)**
Pain Self-Management Deficit (Acute, Chronic)
Uncompensated Sensory Loss (Specify Type/Degree)
Sensory Overload (Sensory-Perceptual Alteration)
Sensory Deprivation (Sensory-Perceptual Alterations)
**Unilateral Neglect**
**Knowledge Deficit (Specify Area)**
**Altered Thought Processes**

## ATTENTION-CONCENTRATION DEFICIT

**Acute Confusion**
**Chronic Confusion**
**Impaired Environmental Interpretation Syndrome**
Uncompensated Memory Loss
**Impaired Memory**
Risk for Cognitive Impairment
**Decisional Conflict (Specify)**

## SELF-PERCEPTION–SELF-CONCEPT PATTERN

**Fear (Specify Focus)**
**Anxiety**
Mild Anxiety
Moderate Anxiety
Severe Anxiety (Panic)
Anticipatory Anxiety (Mild, Moderate, Severe)
**Death Anxiety**
Reactive Depression (Specify Situation)
**Risk for Loneliness**
**Hopelessness**
**Powerlessness (Severe, Moderate, Low)**
**Low Self-Esteem**
**Chronic Low Self-Esteem**
**Situational Low Self-Esteem**
**Body Image Disturbance**
**Risk for Self-Mutilation**
**Personal Identity Disturbance**

# NANDA Nursing Diagnoses Grouped by Gordon's Functional Health Patterns* (cont'd)

## ROLE-RELATIONSHIP PATTERN

Anticipatory Grieving
Dysfunctional Grieving
Chronic Sorrow
Altered Role Performance (Specify)
Unresolved Independence-Dependence Conflict
Social Isolation or Social Rejection
Social Isolation
Impaired Social Interaction
Developmental Delay: Social Skills (Specify)
Risk for Self-Directed Violence
Risk for Other-Directed Violence
Relocation Stress Syndrome
Altered Family Processes (Specify Process)
Altered Family Process: Alcoholism
Altered Parenting (Specify Alteration)
Risk for Altered Parenting (Specify Alteration)
Parental Role Conflict
Weak Parent-Infant Attachment
Risk for Altered Parent-Infant/Child Attachment
Parent-Infant Separation
Caregiver Role Strain
Risk for Caregiver Role Strain
Impaired Verbal Communication
Developmental Delay: Communication Skills (Specify Type)
Risk for Violence

## SEXUALITY-REPRODUCTIVE PATTERN

Altered Sexuality Patterns
Sexual Dysfunction
Rape Trauma Syndrome
Rape Trauma Syndrome: Compound Reaction
Rape Trauma Syndrome: Silent Reaction

## COPING—STRESS-TOLERANCE PATTERN

Ineffective Coping (Individual)
Avoidance Coping
Defensive Coping
Ineffective Denial or Denial
Compromised Family Coping
Disabling Family Coping
Ineffective Community Coping
Family Coping: Potential for Growth
Potential for Enhanced Community Coping
Impaired Adjustment
Posttrauma Syndrome
Risk for Posttrauma Syndrome
Support System Deficit

## VALUE-BELIEF PATTERN

Spiritual Distress (Distress of Human Spirit)
Potential for Enhanced Spiritual Well-Being
Risk for Spiritual Distress

# Sample Clinical Path

CLINICAL PATH  __DIABETES MELLITUS (DM), adult, juvenile, ketoacidosis, PVD__  ICD-9 Code(s) __250.9, 250.91, 250.11, 250.70__

Patient Name _____  Pt. ID No. _____  SOC Date _____  Discharge Date _____

| DATE NOTED | EXPECTED OUTCOMES | ACHIEVED Y | ACHIEVED N | DATE | VARIANCE CODES | DATES NOTED | NURSING/FUNCTIONAL DIAGNOSES | DATE CLOSED |
|---|---|---|---|---|---|---|---|---|
| | 1. Stable endocrine status by visit no. ____ as noted by blood glucose in range of ____ to ____. | | | | | | Cardiac output, decreased <br><br> Outcome(s) no. ____; | |
| | 2. Patient/caregiver demonstrates compliance with treatment regimen, to include dietary and exercise requirements, as well as general health issues by visit no. ____. | | | | | | Coping, ineffective family/patient <br><br> Outcome(s) no. ____; | |
| | 3. Patient/caregiver demonstrates understanding and compliance with blood glucose testing, insulin administration, and medication regimens as evidenced by return demonstration by visit no. ____. | | | | | | Denial, ineffective <br> Outcome(s) no. ____; <br> Knowledge deficit: medication and therapeutic regimen <br> Outcome(s) no. ____; | |
| | 4. Patient/caregiver demonstrates understanding of home safety, general emergency measures related to disease condition, infection control, and proper disposal of contaminated wastes by visit no. ____. | | | | | | Management of therapeutic and medication regimen, ineffective <br> Outcome(s) no. ____; <br> Nutrition, altered: high risk for body requirements <br> Outcome(s) no. ____; | |

| DATE NOTED | EXPECTED OUTCOMES | ACHIEVED Y | N | DATE | VARIANCE CODES | DATE NOTED | NURSING/FUNCTIONAL DIAGNOSES | DATE CLOSED |
|---|---|---|---|---|---|---|---|---|
| | | | | | | | Tissue perfusion, altered: peripheral, renal | |
| | 5. Other: | | | | | | Outcome(s) no. ____: | |
| | 6. Other: | | | | | | Noncompliance (specify) | |
| | | | | | | | Outcome(s) no. ____: | |
| | 7. Other: | | | | | | Other: | |
| | | | | | | | Outcome(s) no. ____: | |
| | | | | | | | Other: | |
| | | | | | | | Outcome(s) no. ____: | |

*Continued*

From Marrelli TM, Hilliard LS: *Home care and clinical paths: effective care planning across the continuum,* St. Louis, 1996, Mosby, pp. 105-106.

# Sample Clinical Path (cont'd)

| ASSESSMENTS/INSTRUCTIONS/INTERVENTIONS | VS NO._ | VS NO._ | VS NO._ | VS NO._ | VS NO._ | VS NO._ | VS NO._ | VS NO._ | VS NO._ | VS NO._ | VS NO._ | VS NO._ |
|---|---|---|---|---|---|---|---|---|---|---|---|---|
| Explain patient rights and responsibilities. | | | | | | | | | | | | |
| Assess for home safety management. | | | | | | | | | | | | |
| Assess vital signs. | | | | | | | | | | | | |
| Assess endocrine status. | | | | | | | | | | | | |
| Assess hydration and nutrition status. | | | | | | | | | | | | |
| Assess weight. | | | | | | | | | | | | |
| Assess coping skills of patient/family/caregiver. | | | | | | | | | | | | |
| Assess patient/caregiver's strengths/weaknesses related to therapeutic regimen. | | | | | | | | | | | | |
| Assess patient/caregiver's willingness and ability to provide home therapeutic regimen. | | | | | | | | | | | | |
| Assess patient/caregiver's understanding of disease process and compliance with therapeutic regimen. | | | | | | | | | | | | |
| Refer to: Dietitian for nutritional needs and safe allowances. | | | | | | | | | | | | |
| Instruct on home safety. | | | | | | | | | | | | |
| Instruct on medication regimen and compliance issues. | | | | | | | | | | | | |
| Instruct patient/caregiver on signs of hypoglycemia and hyperglycemia and emergency measures related to those conditions. | | | | | | | | | | | | |
| Instruct patient/caregiver on blood glucose testing. | | | | | | | | | | | | |

## ASSESSMENETS/INSTRUCTIONS/INTERVENTIONS

| | VS NO._ | VS NO._ | VS NO._ | VS NO._ | VS NO._ | VS NO._ | VS NO._ | VS NO._ | VS NO._ | VS NO._ |
|---|---|---|---|---|---|---|---|---|---|---|
| Instruct patient/caregiver on self/caregiver administration of insulin. | | | | | | | | | | |
| Instruct patient/caregiver on home maintenance program (including exercise and correct nutritional allowances). _____ on visit no. _____ | | | | | | | | | | |
| Venipuncture for ordered laboratory tests. | | | | | | | | | | |
| Other: | | | | | | | | | | |
| Other: | | | | | | | | | | |
| Other: | | | | | | | | | | |

## *Medical Supplies/Home Medical Equipment Needs*

1. Glucometer
2. Insulin syringes/insulin
3. Other _____

Variance codes

1. Patient related
2. Situation related
3. Systems related

Team member signature _____ Initials _____
Team member signature _____ Initials _____
Team member signature _____ Initials _____

Case manager name _____

Patient signature (involved in care planning) _____

# 10

# Continuity of Care Through Care Management and the Referral Process

*Sandra L. McGuire*

## OBJECTIVES

*Upon completion of this chapter, the reader should be able to:*

1. Discuss the process of continuity of care.
2. Discuss the concept of care management.
3. Understand the case management process.
4. Discuss the nurse's role as a case manager.
5. Analyze the steps of the referral process.
6. Discuss the nurse's role in the referral process.
7. Distinguish between the levels of nursing intervention in the referral process.
8. Discuss barriers to the use of the referral process.

## KEY TERMS

Care management
Case management
Case management model

Case manager
Continuity of care
Critical paths

Discharge planning
Referral principles
Referral process

ontinuity of care is a process through which a client's ongoing health care needs are assessed, planned for, coordinated, and met. The process provides for appropriate, uninterrupted care along the health care continuum (American Nurses Association [ANA], 1986a, p. 14) and facilitates the client's transition to different settings and levels of care.

The ANA has emphasized the significant role the community health nurse plays in continuity of care in its *Scope and Standards of Public Health Nursing Practice* (ANA, 1999a), *Standards of Community Health Nursing Practice* (1986a), and *Standards of Home Health Nursing Practice* (1999). In *Standards of Home Health Nursing Practice,* the ANA identified a separate standard for continuity of care that charged the nurse with providing for uninterrupted client care through the use of care management, discharge planning, and coordination of community resources (ANA, 1986b).

Every client should have the opportunity to reach his or her optimum potential for health and recovery; planning for continuity of care helps ensure this. When continuity of care does not occur, the results can be disastrous to the client and costly to the health care system. An integral component of continuity of care is care management.

## CARE MANAGEMENT

The literature does not consistently use or define the term care management. Box 10-1 provides a definition of care management for the community health nurse. **Care management** focuses on provision of care and health outcomes for specific populations. It incorporates population identification and risk assessment, focuses on primary prevention, and utilizes interdisciplinary collaboration and ongoing evaluation (Rowe, 1999, p. 18). It strives to provide quality, cost-effective care and incorporates the client and family into the process.

Care management is practiced in every care setting across the health care continuum. It is a predominant theme in our country's rapidly evolving managed care system, but should not be used interchangeably with managed care. Managed care was discussed in Chapter 5 as both a structure and a process. As a process it manages the care of specific populations. As a structure it represents patient care delivery sys-

### BOX 10-1

## *Care Management for the Community Health Nurse\**

Care management is a population-focused process that promotes holistic, comprehensive, cost-effective, quality care across the health care continuum. It focuses on primary prevention, keeping people healthy, enhanced client outcomes and satisfaction, and efficient use of health care resources (including using the most appropriate provider and level of care). It strives to reduce fragmentation of health care services and encourages interdisciplinary collaboration. It helps ensure that health care needs are met, that health care is coordinated or "seamless," and that clients progress smoothly through the health care system.

\*Case management is part of the care management process.

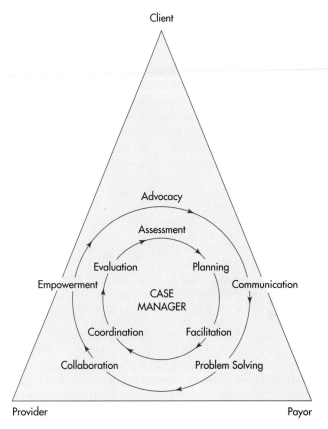

**FIGURE 10-1** Case Management Model. (Case Management Society of America: *Standards of practice for case management,* Little Rock, Ark, 1995, CMSA, p. 9.)

tems such as health maintenance organizations (HMOs), preferred provider organizations (PPOs), point of service plans (POSs), and independent practice associations (IPAs).

Care management activities have resulted in protocols such as standardized plans of care, care maps, disease management, and critical paths. Such protocols help effectively manage the care of populations and guide the care given by practitioners. Critical paths are discussed in this chapter and in Chapter 9.

The national movement toward care management has expanded an already important nursing role, that of case manager. For many nurses, case management is an integrated part of their role, one of the many things that they do. For other nurses, case management is the entirety of their practice; it is what they are employed to do. Some of you reading this text may someday be employed in this specific role.

## NURSES AS CASE MANAGERS

Since the days of Lillian Wald (see Chapter 1), public health nurses have practiced case management (Kaiser, Miller, Hays, et al., 1999, p. 53; Kersbergen, 1996, p. 170; Tahan, 1998). This practice model emphasized coordination of care, education, advocacy, and effective resource utilization (Kaiser, Miller, Hays, et al., 1999, p. 53). Today, nurse case managers are found in every sector of health care (Harris, 1999; Martin, 1999; Tahan, 1998) and at all levels of care. With the advent of managed care, the role of the **case manager** has proliferated, and increasingly more nurses are moving into case management roles (Falter, Cesta, Concert, et al., 1999, pp. 50-51). Nurses provide case management in settings including nursing centers, HMOs, primary care, health departments, community health centers, home health, parish nursing, hospitals, assisted living, and long-term care.

## Case Management Defined

Numerous definitions of case management are found in the literature (Tahan, 1999). The Case Management Society of America (CMSA) has defined **case management** as a collaborative process that assesses, plans, implements, coordinates, monitors, and evaluates options and services to meet an individual's health needs through communication and available resources to promote quality and cost-effective outcomes (CMSA, 1995). The ANA has defined *nurse case management* as a process of care that includes assessing, delivering, coordinating and monitoring services and resources to assure service needs are met (ANA, 1988; Bowers, 1992). The goals of case management include coordination of care, provision of quality health care along a continuum of settings and service, decreased fragmentation of care and enhanced quality of life (May, Schraeder, Britt, 1996). The CMSA's (1995) written standards for case management help nurses operationalize its definition. These standards include a **case management model** (Figure 10-1).

Case management plays a prominent role in managed care and health care reform proposals (Lamb, 1994, p. 149). This process has quality of care, collaboration, advocacy, and fiscal implications (Powell, 1996, pp. 12-15). Case managers coordinate a plan of care that requires interdisci-

**BOX 10-2**

*The Case Management Process*

### Assessment and Diagnosis

A comprehensive assessment of client needs begins the process and is the foundation for effective case management. As a case manager, the nurse gathers relevant data—both physical and psychosocial—by interviewing the client and family and reviewing the treatment plan. The nurse carefully assesses the client's functional status, living situation, financial resources, support systems, coping mechanisms, health values and attitudes, perceptions of health and health care, care preferences, and use of community resources. It is crucial that the nursing assessment be culturally sensitive (Banja, 1994a).

### Planning

Following assessment, the nurse analyzes the data and works collaboratively with the client/family to establish health care needs, a plan of care, and contingency plans. Information provided by the nurse assists the client in making informed decisions; the client is the primary decision maker. Realistic, measurable goals and objectives are formulated and aid in being able to evaluate outcomes. The case management plan strives to minimize overutilization and underutilization of services, inappropriate treatment, and noncompliance (CMSA, 1995, p. 15).

### Interventions

Interventions selected match the care needed with appropriate resources and services and assist clients in achieving their maximum level of functioning. Nursing interventions frequently involve providing direct care, health education, sharing community resource information with clients, coordinating interdisciplinary care management and discharge planning efforts, and alleviating client and family anxiety about continuing care needs. Interventions include referrals to appropriate community agencies and home adaptation strategies. The nurse needs to be knowledgeable about community resources and sensitive to the client's and family's readiness to assume care responsibilities.

### Evaluation

Case management is a goal-directed process that evaluates outcomes (CMSA, 1995, p. 17). Evaluation is ongoing and assesses the effectiveness and outcomes of the process, including client satisfaction. When evaluating, the nurse elicits information from referral agencies, care providers, and the client to determine if care needs were met. In evaluating the process, the nurse should remember that efforts should focus on providing high quality care, facilitating continuity of care, facilitating client independence, and matching the client with appropriate community resources. Results of evaluation assist in revising the care process.

---

plinary expertise and teamwork (Llewellyn, 1999, p. 20). Effective case management results in efficient use of resources, cost-effective interventions, and increased client satisfaction (Hseih, Lee, 1999, p. 6) and assists clients in making appropriate care choices (Lashley, 1993). Ineffective case management can be detrimental to clients' health outcomes.

## The Case Management Process

Case management takes a holistic approach to client care (Powell, 2000, p. 19). It expands on the traditional illness-pathology model often used in clinical settings (Hawkins, Veeder, Pearce, 1998, p. 102) and addresses psychosocial and spiritual health needs as well as physical ones. Its holistic nature involves times and a commitment to quality. The case management process follows the steps of the nursing process and is outlined in Box 10-2.

Nurses are uniquely qualified to be case managers. Their communication skills, knowledge of clinical care, knowledge of community resources, and their readiness to advocate on behalf of clients are all invaluable to case management (Girard, 1994, p. 404). As a case manager, the nurse assists the client in assessing and planning for health care services, facilitates utilization of services, coordinates interdisciplinary care, links clients with community resources,

and monitors the care process. Roles frequently assumed by nurses as case managers are those of educator, caregiver, coordinator, liaison, advocate, and gatekeeper. As advocates, case managers mediate the health of individuals and collective interests of client groups (Meaney, 1999, p. 63). As gatekeepers, nurses allocate resources, ensure care protocols are followed, negotiate services, and evaluate the care given.

Research on nurse case management is in its infancy, and there is a need for more research, especially outcomes research in the field (Lamb, 1994, p. 152). Some activities of nurses as case managers are given in Box 10-3. As a case manager the nurse can help "bring coherence to a chaotic and fragmented system of care" (McCloskey, Grace, 1990, p. 166). An increasing concern to the nurse case manager is that of ethics.

## Ethics and the Nurse Case Manager

The case manager's practice needs to be guided by ethical principles (CMSA, 1995, p. 20). This includes providing service with respect for justice, beneficence, autonomy, informed consent, dignity, privacy, confidentiality, and human rights. Other issues such as withholding and withdrawing care, advance directives, involuntary admissions, medical power of attorney, living wills, and use of restraints arise

## BOX 10-3
### *The Nurse as a Case Manager*

The right service, in the right setting, at the right time, by the right provider:

- Performs casefinding
- Does a comprehensive assessment of the biopsychosocial needs of the client and family
- Develops a plan of care in conjunction with the client and family
- Strives to be culturally sensitive
- Links clients to appropriate community resources through the referral process
- Advocates for necessary and appropriate health care services
- Promotes high-quality care
- Works to promote client satisfaction with the process
- Coordinates and evaluates care
- Provides client education, referral, and direct care
- Promotes client independence and self-care

for the case manager. Taylor and Barnet (1999, p. 30) consider some nonnegotiable issues in moral health care to include a just health system, client-first orientation, health as more than physiologic functioning, trusting professional relationships, and clinical competence.

In our country we are still grappling with the issue of what a just health system is and whether health care is a right or a privilege. We do not have national health insurance, and many people are uninsured or underinsured. In the last few decades we have moved "from an ethic of do anything possible and a high technology approach to care...to rationing of care" (Hawkins, Veeder, Pearce, 1998, p. 174). Many times health care decisions are not made by the consumer or provider but by the for-profit plans or third-party payers (Hawkins, Veeder, Pearce, 1998, p. 174), and this presents numerous ethical dilemmas. Issues such as substandard care, access to care, care rationing, and informing clients of care options have become common concerns for case managers. Ethical questions in relation to autonomy and justice will continue to arise, and even escalate, within the managed care environment.

Managed care and, specifically, for-profit plans "have been criticized as threatening to weaken or displace the professional commitments to beneficence and nonmaleficence that are the foundation of a therapeutic relationship" (Zoloth-Dorfman, Rubin, 1995, p. 341). In today's managed care environment in which a client often is not given everything he or she medically needs, but rather resources are allocated according to what is cost effective, the nurse can easily be put in ethical dilemmas in relation to care management (Banja, 1999, p. 44). The capitation system of managed care "presents what is probably the gravest ethical challenge...that the modern era of medicine has witnessed" (Banja, 1994b, p. 39).

The ANA Code for Nurses states that the nurse "safeguards the client's right to privacy by judiciously protecting information of a confidential nature" (ANA, 1985, p. 3). The courts have granted professional relationships confidentiality provisions. Case managers work with numerous health care providers, interdisciplinary team members, and agencies in the provision of case management. Although it is often difficult, it is necessary to maintain confidentiality. Case managers must obtain client consent before transmitting client information to others (Schetzow, 1994, p. 108). Case managers need to be careful not to share information inappropriately and to maintain confidentiality.

### *Stop and Think About It*

The advocate and gatekeeper roles of the nurse as a case manager often conflict with one another and create ethical dilemmas for the nurse. You work at a managed care organization and are the nurse case manager for Mrs. Tibbell. She came in today and reported having intermittent neurologic symptoms for the past few months, including numbness and tingling in her hands and tremors in her right hand. She has a history of tension headaches and fibromyalgia. You would like to refer her to a neurologist for further follow-up, but your managed care organization requires that you "watch and wait" for at least 6 months before making such a referral. How do you feel about this? What would you do?

### Discharge Planning as Part of Case Management

Discharge planning is an important part of case management. Box 10-4 gives the history of discharge planning. It is a forerunner of today's care management process and remains an integral part of case management. Today, with clients being discharged from health care settings "quicker and sicker" than ever before, their discharge planning needs are increased.

Rorden and Taft (1990, pp. 24-27) described **discharge planning** in acute care settings as occurring in three phases: acute, transitional, and continuing care. In the acute phase, medical attention dominates discharge planning efforts, whereas in the transitional phase, the need for acute care is still present, but its urgency is reduced and clients can begin to address and plan for future health care needs. In the continuing care phase, the client is able to plan and implement continuing care activities. A schema for these phases is given in Figure 10-2.

Some areas for the nurse to assess in discharge planning are identified in Figure 10-3 and Appendix 10-1. Effective discharge planning can reduce morbidity and mortality (e.g., preventing the premature discharge of low-birth-weight infants and arranging appropriate follow-up on infants with congenital anomalies) and readmission rates (Mbweza, 1996, p. 53).

The success of discharge planning activities is largely dependent on how accurately discharge needs are assessed and

### BOX 10-4

## *History of Discharge Planning*

Discharge planning was a forerunner of case management. Historically, discharge planning focused on a single event—the referral of a client to community services or facilities upon discharge from a hospital. Being familiar with community resources, community health nurses frequently worked as hospital liaisons, home care coordinators and discharge planners to make referrals, coordinate care, and "bridge the gap" as the client moved from the hospital to the community.

There is evidence of discharge planning in the late 1800s and early 1900s (O'Hare, Terry, 1988, p. 6; Shamansky, Boase, Horn, 1984, p. 15). Lillian Wald was one of the first to recognize the need for such planning. In 1906 Bellevue Hospital in New York City referred to a nurse whose entire time and care was given to befriending those about to be discharged (O'Hare, Terry, 1988, p. 6).

The 1960s saw the first official use of the term *discharge planning* (Shamansky, Boase, Horn, 1984, p. 16). Discharge planning became a part of many hospital programs, and Edith Wensley's (1963) *Nursing Service Without Walls* urged hospitals to emphasize planning for home care services and referral to community services upon discharge. The National League for Nursing urged hospitals, nursing homes, and home nursing care agencies to have a designated staff person to develop plans for the next stage of nursing care, to implement continuity of care activities, and to develop well-defined, clearly written procedures for client referral (O'Hare, Terry, 1988, p. 7). The passage of Medicaid and Medicare legislation in 1965 placed new emphasis on discharge planning efforts because the home care benefits of these two programs allowed clients to leave hospitals sooner.

In the 1970s discharge planning became inextricably linked with quality assurance. This occurred largely as a result of Medicaid and Medicare legislation in 1972 (Public Law 92-603), which mandated that skilled nursing facilities and hospitals receiving these monies maintain centralized, coordinated programs to ensure that each client had a planned program of continuing care that met postdischarge needs.

In the 1980s federal legislation again shaped the course of discharge planning. A prospective payment system (PPS), aimed at reducing the length of stay in acute care facilities, was enacted for Medicare in 1982. This legislation was instrumental in the development of discharge planning activities across the nation because it gave hospitals a financial incentive to discharge clients as early as possible. Thus discharge planning became a method of cost containment (Willihnganz, 1984).

During the 1980s discharge planning became a hospital priority. The American Hospital Association (AHA) developed guidelines for discharge planning that included early identification of clients likely to need posthospital care; client and family education, assessment, and counseling; discharge plan development, coordination, and implementation; and postdischarge follow-up (AHA, 1984; Corkery, 1989, p. 19). In 1986 Medicare legislation mandated the development of a standardized, uniform needs assessment instrument to evaluate the posthospital "discharge" needs of Medicare clients (Burlenski, 1989, p. 2; McBroom, 1989, p. 1), and required that hospitals receiving Medicare reimbursement notify clients of their right to discharge planning services (Blaylock, Cason, 1992, p. 5; Corkery, 1989, p. 19). Discharge planning is still an important part of individual case management.

---

diagnosed, the extent to which the client and family participate in the planning process, and the availability of community resources to meet discharge planning needs. Risk factors to assess for in discharge planning are presented in Figure 10-4. When discharge planning efforts are unsuccessful, clients can become frustrated and discouraged, and their confidence can be shaken (Glover, King, Green, et al., 1993, p. 40). Community health nurses frequently work with clients to revise discharge planning efforts. The following case scenario of 76-year-old Mrs. Flowers returning home after breaking a hip is an example.

**CASE Scenario** Mrs. Flowers was hospitalized for a broken left hip after a fall in her home. From the day of admission her discharge planning needs were assessed and she was involved in establishing and implementing her discharge plan of care. Mrs. Flowers lives alone but has a son and daughter-in-law who live nearby and friends who are willing to help her with grocery shopping and other errands.

As part of discharge planning efforts, options to assist her, such as homemaker services, friendly visitors, Meals-on-Wheels, the local Visiting Nurse Association, and a more supervised living situation, were discussed with her. Assistive devices she would need at home also were considered. Additionally her support systems, financial resources, and goals for care were considered.

A mutually agreeable discharge plan was established for Mrs. Flowers. The necessary assistive devices were ordered. It was decided that she would have a visiting nurse and homemaker services for housework, and her son would help with transportation and groceries. Mrs. Flowers indicated she would like to take care of her own meal preparation.

After a short period at home, Mrs. Flowers told the community health nurse/case manager that meal preparation was very difficult. She could prepare some simple meals for herself, but total meal preparation was not working out. The nurse worked with Mrs. Flowers to find an acceptable solution to the situation. The combined efforts of family members and a local Meals-on-Wheels program were utilized, and Mrs. Flowers began to feel more confident in her ability to be independent and care for herself at home.

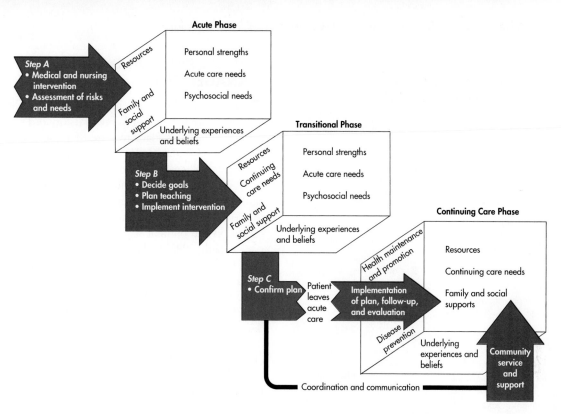

**FIGURE 10-2** Phases of the discharge planning process. (Redrawn from Rorden JW, Taft E: *Discharge planning guide for nurses*, Philadelphia, 1990, Saunders, p. 26.)

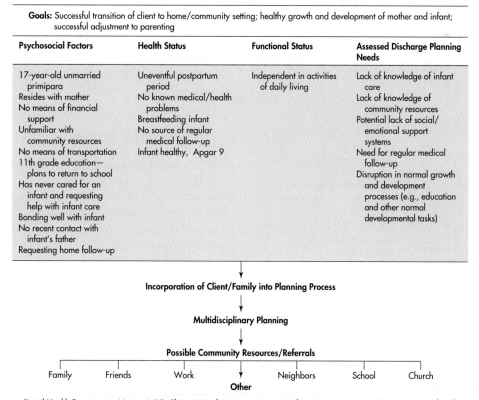

**Goals:** Successful transition of client to home/community setting; healthy growth and development of mother and infant; successful adjustment to parenting

| Psychosocial Factors | Health Status | Functional Status | Assessed Discharge Planning Needs |
|---|---|---|---|
| 17-year-old unmarried primipara | Uneventful postpartum period | Independent in activities of daily living | Lack of knowledge of infant care |
| Resides with mother | No known medical/health problems | | Lack of knowledge of community resources |
| No means of financial support | Breastfeeding infant | | Potential lack of social/emotional support systems |
| Unfamiliar with community resources | No source of regular medical follow-up | | Need for regular medical follow-up |
| No means of transportation | Infant healthy, Apgar 9 | | Disruption in normal growth and development processes (e.g., education and other normal developmental tasks) |
| 11th grade education—plans to return to school | | | |
| Has never cared for an infant and requesting help with infant care | | | |
| Bonding well with infant | | | |
| No recent contact with infant's father | | | |
| Requesting home follow-up | | | |

**Incorporation of Client/Family into Planning Process**

**Multidisciplinary Planning**

**Possible Community Resources/Referrals**

Family   Friends   Work   Neighbors   School   Church

**Other**

(Local Health Department: Nurses, WIC, Clinics; LaLeche League; Young Mothers Support Group; DHHS: TANF, Medicaid; Child and Family Services; Mom's Day Out Programs; Dial-A-Ride)

**FIGURE 10-3** The nurse as a discharge planner: assessing discharge planning needs. (Modified from Siegel H: Nurses improve hospital efficiency through a risk assessment model at admission, *Nurs Manage* 19(10):42, 1988.)

**Circle all that apply and total.
Refer to the risk factor index.\***

Age
 0 = 55 years or less
 1 = 56 to 64 years
 2 = 65 to 79 years
 3 = 80+ years

Living situation/social support
 0 = lives only with spouse
 1 = lives with family
 2 = lives alone with family
   support
 3 = lives alone with friends'
   support
 4 = lives alone with no
   support
 5 = nursing home/
   residential care

Functional status
 0 = independent in activities
   of daily living and
   instrumental activities of
   daily living

Dependent in:
 1 = eating/feeding
 1 = bathing/grooming
 1 = toileting
 1 = transferring
 1 = incontinent of bowel
   function
 1 = incontinent of bladder
   function
 1 = meal preparation
 1 = responsible for own
   medication administration
 1 = handling own finances
 1 = grocery shopping
 1 = transportation

Cognition
 0 = oriented
 1 = disoriented to some
   spheres† some of the time
 2 = disoriented to some
   spheres all of the time
 3 = disoriented to all spheres
   some of the time
 4 = disoriented to all spheres
   all of the time
 5 = comatose

Behavior pattern
 0 = appropriate
 1 = wandering
 1 = agitated
 1 = confused
 1 = other

Mobility
 0 = ambulatory
 1 = ambulatory with me-
   chanical assistance
 2 = ambulatory with hu-
   man assistance
 3 = nonambulatory

Sensory deficits
 0 = none
 1 = visual or hearing
   deficits
 2 = visual and hearing
   deficits

Number of previous
admissions/emergency
room visits
 0 = none in the last
   3 months
 1 = one in the last
   3 months
 2 = two in the last
   3 months
 3 = more than two in
   the last 3 months

Number of active medical
problems
 0 = three medical
   problems
 1 = three to five medical
   problems
 2 = more than five
   medical problems

Number of drugs
 0 = fewer than three
   drugs
 1 = three to five drugs
 2 = more than five
   drugs

**Total score:**

\*Risk factor index: score of 10 = at risk for home care resources;
score of 11 to 19 = at risk for extended discharge planning;
score greater than 20 = at risk for placement other than home.
If the client's score is 10 or greater, refer the client to the
discharge planning coordinator or discharge planning team.
†Spheres = person, place, time, and self.
Copyright 1991 Ann Blaylock.

**FIGURE 10-4** Blaylock Discharge Planning Risk Assessment Screen. (From Blaylock A, Cason CL: Discharge planning predicting patients' needs, *J Gerontol Nurs* 18(7):8, 1992.)

## CRITICAL PATHS AND CARE MANAGEMENT

The term critical path is a relatively recent addition to the managed care literature (A Brief History of Pathways from Case Management Plans to Care Maps, 1998). It is a form of care management and is often used in acute care settings in individual case management. More recently, critical paths are being used in other settings such as home health care agencies (Gartner, Twardon, 1995).

**Critical paths** are protocols for care. They take into consideration the optimal sequencing of health care interventions (Spath, 1995) and function as a map and a time-specific path for interventions and anticipated outcomes (Corbett, Androwich, 1995; Gartner, Twardon, 1995). They incorporate assessment, focused interventions, flexible changes in approach across the life span, and delineation of expected and desired outcomes (Hawkins, Veeder, Pearce, 1998, p. 102).

Critical paths are based on standards of care for a specified client population and identify activities critical to care and involve case consultation and care collaboration (Girard, 1994, p. 408). They are an interdisciplinary approach to care and attempt to control costs through coordination of services. As with other aspects of care management, critical paths link clients with community resources that can meet client needs and provide continuity of care. Clients are linked with community agencies by the referral process.

### Stop and Think About It

Considering the populations served by your clinical agency, what type of critical paths would be useful? How would you individualize these pathways?

## THE REFERRAL PROCESS

The **referral process** is a systematic problem-solving approach involving a series of actions that help clients use resources for the purpose of resolving needs. Clients may be either individuals or groups who require assistance from others in order to achieve their maximum level of functioning (McGuire, Gerber, Clemen-Stone, 1996). The referral process is an integral part of discharge planning (Glover, King, Green, et al., 1993, p. 40), care management, and nursing care.

A wide array of resources are available in the community. Nurses link clients to these resources through use of the referral process (McGuire, Gerber, Clemen-Stone, 1996, p. 222). However, little can be found in the nursing literature on referral.

The community health nurse's major goals for initiating a referral are to promote high-level wellness and to enhance self-care capabilities and quality of care. As clients move from one care setting and one level of care to another, the referral process is frequently used. Referral criteria are helpful in assisting nurses to identify clients who need referrals to community resources (Nash, 1993, p. 707; Townsend, Edwards, Nadon, 1992, p. 203).

To be implemented effectively, the referral process demands knowledge, skill, and experience. It demands knowledge of community resources and an ability to solve problems, set priorities, coordinate care, and collaborate with clients and the interdisciplinary team. It is an integral part of comprehensive, continuous client care and is essential to community health nursing practice.

The community health nurse will make referrals to and receive referrals from health care resources. Referrals can be categorized according to referral initiator, the extent of client contact made with the resource, the level of difficulty of the process, and the source of the referral. Working through the referral process with a client can be an enriching and rewarding experience. Table 10-1 is a chart illustrating different types of referral. Completing a form or telling a client to contact a community agency is only one small aspect of this process.

## Basic Principles of Referral

Wolff's (1962) classic article on referral delineated basic principles to take into consideration when helping clients use the referral process. Others (Combs, 1976; USDHHS, 1982a; Wheeler-Lachowycz, 1983; Wolff, 1968) have reinforced the value of the following referral principles and have expanded on them.

- *There should be merit in the referral.* The referral should meet the needs and objectives of the client and should be necessary and appropriate. Before referring the client to community resources, it is important to assess what resources are available in the client's own environment. Often family, friends, and neighbors can do as much as formal community health resources. If a referral is not necessary or appropriate, it should not be made.
- *The referral should be practical.* The client should be able to use the referral in an efficient, effective manner. The referral should not be a waste of time, money, and effort on behalf of the client, the resource, or the referral facilitator.
- *The referral should be individualized to the client.* A referral that meets the needs of one client may not meet the needs of another. It is essential to assess the individual needs and concerns of clients before decisions about the appropriateness of a referral are made. For example, some clients can learn very well in a group setting, whereas others cannot.

## TABLE 10-1

*Types of Referral by Initiator, Extent of Contact with Resource, Level of Difficulty, and Source*

| | TYPE OF REFERRAL | EXAMPLE |
|---|---|---|
| Initiator | *Primary:* Referral initiated by client, often readily | Client suggesting marriage counseling |
| | *Secondary:* Referral initiated by someone other than client | Community health nurse suggesting marriage counseling |
| Extent of contact with resource | *Formal:* Contact made with a resource on behalf of a client; contact can be made by the client or someone on the client's behalf; contact generally made with client's permission; these referrals are often processed through a system of standardized forms and procedures | Client contacting a local department of social service (DSS) about obtaining food stamps<br><br>or |
| | *Informal:* Discussion of a resource between two or more persons without contact being made with the resource; often the initial step toward a formal referral | Client and community health nurse discussing available DSS services (e.g., food stamps, general assistance, Temporary Assistance to Needy Families, Medicaid) |
| Level of difficulty | *Simple:* Referral reaches need resolution on the initial attempt | On initial attempt, client goes to DSS and obtains food stamps |
| | *Complex:* Referral does not meet need resolution on the initial attempt; process needs to be reworked (see Figure 10-6 for steps in process) | Client goes to DSS seeking food stamps and finds out that she or he is not eligible, but the need for assistance with food budgeting still exists. Other community resources such as the Nutritional Extension Service may be more appropriate |
| Source | *Interresource:* Referrals made from one resource to another | Community health nurse referring client from the local health department to a neighborhood health clinic |
| | *Intraresource:* Referrals made within the resource itself | Community health nurse referring client to local health department sanitarian for water sampling |
| | *Self:* Client refers himself to a resource for service; some agencies will not accept these referrals | Client calls local health department to arrange for community health nursing visits |

- *The referral should be timely.* It should come at a time when the client is ready to work on the health care need and when it is the appropriate time to work on the need.
- *The referral should be coordinated with other activities.* The referral should be congruent with other health care activities that are occurring. This aids in maximizing health care interventions, preventing duplication of service and carrying out contradictory intervention strategies.
- *The referral should incorporate the client and family into planning and implementation.* It has already been stressed that it is critical for the client and family to be involved in health planning and intervention; without this involvement interventions are likely to fail.
- *The client should have the right to say no to the referral.* This principle acknowledges the client's right to self-determination. A competent client has the right to make decisions about health care (ANA, 1986a). The client has the right to refuse a referral unless legal authority dictates otherwise. Cases of law are the exception and vary from state to state. An example of a law that requires the community health nurse to refer a client without his or her consent is a child abuse law that mandates reporting suspected child abuse and neglect cases.

To protect this right of self-determination, the client must be aware of the referral. At times individuals are referred without their knowledge or consent because the referring agency considers them a threat to their own safety or the safety of others. Making referrals for clients without their consent is not good practice. If in following up on a referral the nurse finds that the client was unaware of the referral, the nurse should explain the reason for the referral and the services the nurse can provide, apologize for any inconvenience to the client, and allow the client to accept or reject the referral. The refusal of a referral may be difficult for the nurse to accept, especially if the referral appears to be helpful to the client. However, the client has the right to refuse a referral unless legal authority dictates otherwise.

### Confidentiality and Referral

Confidentiality of client information is an important professional ethical responsibility. Nurses must receive the client's permission to share personal data. Information to be shared should be carefully evaluated. This action should always be in the client's best interest and for the purpose of facilitating optimum care. Many agencies have release-of-information forms for sending and receiving data about clients. It is preferable to obtain written permission to share data.

### Developing a Referral System

Before referral activities occur, a referral system needs to be in place. Developing a referral system involves determining the types of resources necessary to carry out health care activities; locating these resources in the community; collecting information on the resources; developing a referral list, referral protocol, and a follow-up system; training people to make referrals; and periodically updating the referral and re-

source information (USDHHS, 1982a, p. 27). In developing a system, criteria for both sending and receiving referrals would be established.

### Answering a Referral

Answering referrals is an important part of the referral process and helps maintain effective communication between the client, staff, and resources. Prompt, complete, and courteous answering of a referral helps establish and maintain good working relationships, facilitates follow-up, and enhances continuity of client care. In responding to the referring agency, the nurse should include information on the original need(s) that initiated the referral, assessment data, nursing diagnoses, and future plans. If nursing service is to be continued, it is helpful to let the referring agency know that it is needed. Be sure to thank the referring agency for the referral.

## REFERRAL RESOURCES

Once the need for a referral has been established, the appropriate resources must be located in the community. The community health nurse needs to collect information on community resources and be familiar with them (Figure 10-5). Developing a resource "network" can assist the nurse in

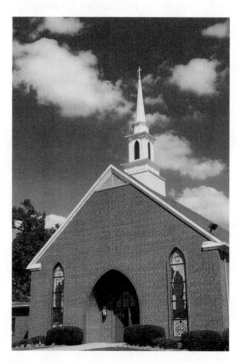

**FIGURE 10-5** Churches are extremely valuable community resources that should not be overlooked by health care professionals. Many churches provide community services, including temporary food, shelter, and clothing; home visiting to ill and disabled persons; home repair services for the needy; and monies to assist families who lack essentials of daily living. Community health nurses frequently find that churches help fill "gaps" in the resource delivery system and provide services that would not otherwise be available. (Courtesy Ed Richardson)

finding resource information and facilitating client care. Ideally, the nurse should independently explore the resource before referring clients.

A resource is defined as an agency, group, or individual that assists a client to meet a need. Resources provide multiple services and have varying requirements for usage. The community health nurse needs to be knowledgeable about community resources, increase client awareness of resources, and assist the client in resource use. Health care resources can be described as formal and informal.

*Formal health care resources* exist primarily for the provision of health care services. They include, but are not limited to, hospitals, extended-care facilities, skilled nursing homes, health departments, outpatient facilities, and the offices of private health care practitioners.

*Informal health care resources* provide health services but do not exist primarily for this purpose. These resources can be relatives in the client's home, service organizations, and self-help groups. They are scattered throughout the community, are minimally coordinated, and are often more difficult to recognize than formal resources. An example of an informal health care resource is the local Lion's Club, which provides free ophthalmology examinations and eyeglasses to children who could not otherwise obtain them. The Lion's Club provides a health care service, but its primary function is not health related. Many such resources within the community are important to the provision of community health services.

Local health departments are excellent sources of information on community health resources. Frequently, compilations of local resources are done by groups such as United Way, chambers of commerce, departments of social service, offices on aging, and health departments. Major service organizations, such as associations for retarded citizens, compile resources specific to the groups they represent. City offices and planning commissions also have local resource information.

## Collecting Information on Resources

When collecting information on referral resources, the nurse needs to develop a systematic way of recording resource information (USDHHS, 1982a, p. 28). Creating an ongoing computer file with a standard format, such as the one shown in Figure 10-6, can be helpful. Such a file should list resources both alphabetically and by service. It should note if the resource has available publications and materials explaining its services. Resources that are frequently used, or used with success, may be coded for easy accessibility. It is necessary that resource information be clear, accurate, and concise.

The following essential information about a resource is readily kept on file cards, in a loose-leaf notebook, or computerized: (1) name of resource (include address, phone number, name and title of person in charge or contact person), (2) purpose and services, (3) eligibility (who may use the resource, including special requirements such as age and income), (4) application procedure, (5) fees, (6) office hours and days, and (7) geographic area served. Resource

files should be dated to aid in updating. Keeping data on clients' perception of the resource is also valuable.

The nurse should be aware of specific information that a resource requests in order to provide service to clients. Information frequently requested by resources includes the following:

1. Name, address, and telephone number of the client
2. Client age, sex, and marital status
3. Names and birthdates of family members and others living in the household
4. Source of medical care and health history
5. Financial status and records
6. Resources with whom the client is presently working
7. Reason for seeking referral

Often resources request that clients bring such information with them to their first appointment to assist in determining eligibility for services. The nurse can assist the clients in finding out what information is necessary. If a client has to return to a resource with additional information, it can be time consuming, costly, and discouraging. It may present a barrier to the client using the referral.

A grid showing frequently used resources can be a helpful reference when one is visiting clients in the community setting. A grid that includes service areas and specific resources is especially helpful. An example of such a grid is

National Foundation March of Dimes
Payne County Office
   Address: 20100 Maplewood, Mio, MI 47236
   Phone:    811-2110 (Area 516)
   Person in charge: Mrs. Nellie Scott, Director

| | |
|---|---|
| Purpose and services: | Through referral and direct aid, assistance is provided in the areas of prenatal care, genetic counseling, diagnosis, and treatment. Offers prevention and treatment services for clients who have congenital malformations or birth defects through research, direct client services, and public education. Sponsors scholarships in related health fields. |
| Eligibility: | No restrictions. |
| Application procedure: | Referrals by private physicians, public health clinics, or health departments. Individuals are encouraged to contact the office for further information. |
| Fees: | None |
| Office hours: | 9 AM to 3 PM, Tuesday-Saturday |
| Geographical area served: | Payne County        Compiled 12/96 |
| Client satisfaction: | Responds immediately to clients' calls. Especially good at obtaining adaptive equipment. |

**FIGURE 10-6** Resource information.

**TABLE 10-2**

*Resource Grid*

| SERVICE NEEDED | TYPES | RESOURCE |
|---|---|---|
| Food | 1. Emergency | 1. Department of Social Services, Salvation Army, local churches, American Red Cross, Goodfellows |
| | 2. Low-cost or free foods | 2. Food stamps, food cooperatives, school lunch programs, WIC |
| | 3. Counseling | 3. Expanded nutrition program, Health Department |
| Financial assistance | 1. Emergency and short-term | 1. Department of Social Services, Salvation Army, Goodfellows, Lion's Club, Traveler's Aid, Volunteers of America, Kiwanis |
| | 2. Long-term | 2. Department of Social Services, Social Security Administration, Veterans Administration |
| Housing | 1. Emergency | 1. Catholic Social Services, Jewish Action League, United Way Community Service, Department of Social Service, American Red Cross, Salvation Army, local churches, domestic violence facilities |
| | 2. Public (low-cost) | 2. Housing Commission, Department of Social Service |

Modified from the University of Michigan, School of Nursing, Family and Community Health Nursing: *Resource grid,* Ann Arbor, undated, University of Michigan, School of Nursing.

presented in Table 10-2. It is not all inclusive, and resources vary from area to area, but it does illustrate how a service resource grid can be organized.

## STEPS OF THE REFERRAL PROCESS

The referral process is systematic and circular. That is, as data are obtained in one step, other steps may need to be repeated, and as the process stops for one referral, another referral may be initiated. These steps are interconnected and interrelated. The steps involved in the referral process are depicted in Figure 10-7. The basic steps of the referral process include:

1. Establish a working relationship with the client
2. Establish the need for a referral
3. Set objectives for the referral
4. Explore resource availability
5. Client decides to use or not use referral
6. Make referral to resource
7. Facilitate referral
8. Evaluate and follow-up

Client participation throughout the process is essential. The community health nurse guides the client through the process by building on client strengths, facilitating informed decision making, assessing client needs and objectives, exploring alternatives for need resolution, assisting the client in using resources, and evaluating the results of the entire process. The client is encouraged to be independent whenever possible.

### Establish a Working Relationship with the Client

The referral process usually evolves after a working relationship with the client has been established. This in-

volves the formation of trust between the nurse and the client. Trust is promoted by nurses when they show respect, empathy, and genuine concern for the client (Rorden, Taft, 1990, p. 46). As a means of building this relationship, the nurse focuses on clients' feelings and perceptions of the situation and starts "where clients are at." A relationship of trust facilitates communication and cooperation in the nurse-client relationship. The nurse needs to be willing to look at the situation from the client's frame of reference and be culturally sensitive. Asking clients questions about the type of services needed, outcomes expected from service use, their perception of the situation, and resources they have utilized can elicit valuable data.

### Establish the Need for a Referral

The community health nurse and client need to thoroughly assess the need for referral.

Unnecessary or unwanted referrals are costly and time consuming, frustrating for clients, may strain relationships between referring agencies, and can adversely affect nurse-client relationships.

It is important to discriminate between problems the community health nurse can and cannot handle. For example, some budgeting problems can be dealt with by a community health nurse and others cannot. A community health nurse can help a family analyze how they can obtain the most for their food dollars by using meal planning, low-cost meals, and inexpensive sources of protein. On the other hand, if the family is having difficulty with creditors and money management, a credit-counseling resource would be more appropriate.

There may be situations in which the nurse finds it difficult to accept clients' decisions about the need for a refer-

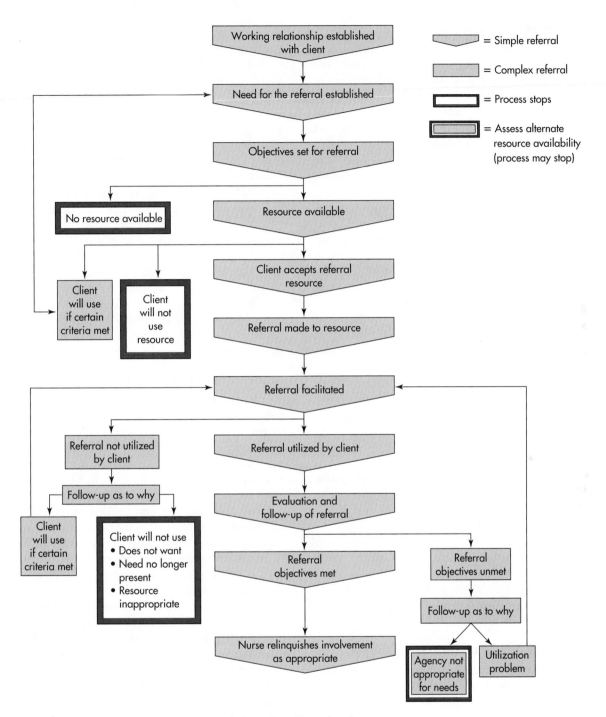

**FIGURE 10-7** The referral process.

ral. People have values, attitudes, and beliefs that may differ from those of the nurse and affect resource use. For example, clients may use folk remedies instead of seeking formal health care, may not value the need for preventive health practices, and may be unwilling to accept assistance programs.

When clients are using denial as a coping mechanism, it can be difficult for them to realistically assess health care and referral needs. The nurse can help the client to realistically assess the situation, share professional observations and concerns, and discuss appropriate community resources. The nurse can help the client view the situation from a different perspective and motivate the client to take action. This is particularly true when a trust relationship has been established, and the client realizes that the nurse is acting in his or her best interests. Once the need for a referral has been established, the nurse and client should establish objectives for the services required and look at which resources in the community can best meet the client's needs.

## Set Objectives for the Referral

What the client would like to see accomplished, tempered with what is realistically feasible, combine to determine the objectives for the referral. It is often helpful to write out objectives with the client in behavioral terms, such as "Mrs. Armstrong will contact the Department of Social Services about obtaining food stamps by March 30." An integral part of setting objectives for the referral is deciding what services are necessary from the referral source, as well as what time frame to use in obtaining these services. Decisions about specific objectives should be made by the client.

In this phase of the referral process, the nurse may find that the client has unrealistic referral expectations. For example, Mrs. Quinn, a single mother, requested counseling for her 16-year-old daughter, who planned to drop out of school and marry her 21-year-old boyfriend. Mrs. Quinn thought a counseling agency could "talk some sense into her." The community health nurse helped Mrs. Quinn to see that a counseling agency would assist the family in working through situations but would most likely not get involved in making family decisions. The nurse helped arrange joint counseling sessions through the local Community Mental Health Center. These sessions helped both mother and daughter to communicate more effectively, understand each other's concerns and needs, and develop skills in problem solving and decision making.

## Explore Resource Availability

A source of aid must be available before a referral can be made. An appropriate resource is one that can meet the client's needs and objectives and is available, acceptable, and accessible to the client. If more than one appropriate resource exists, the client makes the choice about which one to use. If no resource is available, the referral objectives may need to be redefined or a resource developed. Many times resources in the community will reconsider the services they provide to clients, especially if the community health nurse acts as an advocate for certain services.

## Client Decides to Use or Not Use Referral

The client can say *yes*, *no*, or *maybe* when deciding to use a referral resource. If the client says *yes*, the referral process continues. If the client says *no* or *maybe*, the nurse should explore with the client the reasons why. If the client does not want the referral under any condition, the client's right to self-determination must be respected unless legal issues intervene.

In some instances, when clients would use a referral if certain criteria were met, the nurse may be able to assist the client in meeting these criteria. For example, a client might say that she would use a referral to the health department immunization clinic for her 2-year-old if transportation to the clinic could be arranged. The nurse may be able to help this client obtain transportation services from other community resources. However, if a client continues to place conditions on referral use, the nurse and client may want to take a close look at the reasons behind these conditions. It is possible that the client really does not want the referral but fears saying *no*.

Sometimes clients do not want to use one resource to meet a health care need but are willing to use another resource. An example of this is seen in the case scenario on Mrs. Morris.

**CASE Scenario** Mrs. Morris was an elderly client who was eligible for food stamps but would not apply for them. She viewed food stamps as charity and stated, "I do not accept welfare." The community health nurse was frustrated because Mrs. Morris's diet was inadequate, largely for financial reasons. Discussing the food stamp program with Mrs. Morris did not change her mind about using it. The nurse explored alternatives with Mrs. Morris and found that, because she wanted to eat better, she was receptive to learning about how to prepare low-cost, nutritious meals at home and also was interested in applying for a reduced-cost, Meals-on-Wheels program, through which she would "pay" for her meals. Mrs. Morris had refused a referral for food stamps, but she and the nurse were able to use other intervention alternatives that helped meet her nutritional needs.

## Make Referral to Resource

The referral should be specific and informative enough to reflect the client's objectives for the referral. As the demand for community-based care has increased, agencies are developing referral protocols to make the transition from the acute care setting to the community as smooth as possible (Glover, King, Green, et al., 1993, p. 40). The appropriate forms should be filled out and protocols followed (including a release of information form). Clients usually do not hesitate to sign an authorization for information to be released once they have decided that they need a referral. The client should be encouraged to be as independent as possible in contacting the resource and to make an appointment with the agency if one is necessary.

*Timing* influences how the client responds to the referral. Studies have shown that a referral should occur as soon as possible after detecting a need and a well-handled referral can reinforce the importance of taking positive health action to the client (USDHHS, 1982a, p. 27).

Referrals can sometimes be made quickly by telephone or e-mail; a written referral can always follow. An example of a referral form used by a local health department to refer clients is presented in Figure 10-8. This form includes essential referral information, such as data about the person making the referral, the individual or family being referred, the reason for the referral, summary of the client's situation, resources being used by the client, a statement on whether or not the client is aware of the referral, and a place for the receiving resource to share information with the referral agency for follow-up and evaluation.

## Facilitate the Referral

Facilitating a referral involves a number of nursing interventions, including preparing the client for the use of com-

```
Oakland County Health Department
1200 North Telegraph Road                                    27725 Greenfield
Pontiac, Michigan 48053                                      Southfield, Michigan 48075
Telephone 858-1280                                           Telephone 424-7000
```

**Referral Form**

To:_____   From:_____

Address:_____                    ☐ Pontiac Office

_____                         ☐ Southfield Office

Attention:_____   Telephone:_____   Date:_____

Regarding:_____   Aware of referral? ☐ Yes  ☐ No

Address:_____   Telephone:_____

**Family Roster** (Names, birthdates, relationship)

**Reason for Referral**

**Situation**

(over)

**Known Medical, Agency, Community Resources**

Reply Requested:    ☐ No   ☐ Yes        (see back)

**FIGURE 10-8** Sample referral form. (Courtesy Nursing Division, Oakland County Health Department, Pontiac, Mich.)

munity services and identifying and overcoming barriers to the use of these services. It is important to remember that client motivation is critical. If the client is not motivated to make the referral work, the referral process probably will not be successful. Barriers that decrease client motivation are discussed later in this chapter.

## Evaluate and Follow Up

As with all aspects of the nursing process, referrals need to be evaluated. Ongoing evaluation and follow-up are two of the most important aspects in the referral process. Throughout the process the community health nurse evaluates the client's responses to the referral to determine if changes need to be made.

Some clients need support and encouragement during the process, especially if their problems are not resolved immediately. The case scenario of Mr. Connant is an example.

**CASE Scenario** Mr. Connant decided that he was not going back to the community mental health center for counseling after his first visit because his counselor "did nothing but talk." In evaluating this situation, the nurse realized that she needed to discuss more specifically with Mr. Connant his expectations of counseling. She talked to him about his feelings about the session, encouraged him to share his feelings with the counselor, and encouraged him to go back "at least one more time." This interaction with the nurse facilitated Mr. Connant's

Continuation of situation:

Agency reply to Oakland County Health Department:

(Signature) _____

Date: _____

**FIGURE 10-8, cont'd**

return to the mental health center. During a later visit with the nurse, he expressed his gratitude because counseling was helping him to work through many issues that had been troubling him.

The nurse may notice that a client shows evidence of the same problem repeatedly, for example, experiencing the need for frequent emergency food orders. The nurse and client would want to discuss this situation, assess what is happening (e.g., too limited an income, problem with budgeting), use anticipatory guidance, and explore other options.

During evaluation the client's ability to use the process should be assessed, and the client should be encouraged to use the process as independently as possible in the future. Probably the hardest part of evaluation is realizing when it is time for the nurse to relinquish involvement with the client (e.g., the client can use the process independently or expected outcomes have been achieved). This can be an especially difficult task when the client and nurse have developed a strong working relationship.

Effective evaluation of the referral process encompasses reviewing how well client needs are being met. Evaluation looks at referral outcomes and enhances the nurse's competency in using the process. When evaluating, the nurse must realize that there are times when a referral was not appropriate or effective.

A major goal of the nurse in using the referral process is to assist the client to use the process independently. Usually clients are ready to function independently when they can identify personal health care needs, take initiative to contact health care resources, and take action to resolve health care problems.

## BARRIERS TO USE OF THE REFERRAL PROCESS

For each resource and each client, the nurse must identify individual and resource barriers that adversely affect the use of referral services. For example, an agency may have high fees for services (a resource barrier) that the client is unable to afford (a client barrier). In this case, fees are both a resource barrier and a client barrier. Some common barriers are briefly described.

### Resource Barriers

ATTITUDES OF HEALTH CARE PROFESSIONALS. The attitudes of health care professionals affect client use of resources. Clients are quick to sense the attitudes of health care personnel, and if they are not treated with respect and courtesy, they are hesitant to return to the health care setting. Abrupt answers to a client's questions, minimal communication with the client, use of jargon, and conveying frustration when clients ask questions are a few examples of behaviors that impede use of resources. Although the values and attitudes of the nurse may differ from the client's, the nurse must be open to the opinions of others and maintain a nonjudgmental attitude. A good rule of thumb is for the nurse to treat clients the way he or she would like to be treated.

An attitude that became a barrier to the use of a health care resource is shown in the following example.

**CASE *Scenario*** The nurse in charge of an antepartal clinic for low-income mothers refused to make appointments for clinic clients because "these people wouldn't keep appointments anyway." As a result, the clinic operated on a first-come-first-served basis. Clients frequently traveled by bus to get to the clinic. Because no appointments were available, they had to arrive very early to sign in and there were usually long waits to be seen. It was common for clients to leave the clinic before they were seen because of transportation or child-care problems. Many clients became discouraged with the system and did not seek further prenatal care.

Attitudes and practices such as these do not facilitate clients' use of health care services or promote preventive health action.

PHYSICAL ACCESSIBILITY OF RESOURCE. Access, as a barrier to service, has become a national health concern and is a major barrier to the use of health care services (Institute of Medicine, 1993; USDHHS, 1991; USDHHS, 2000). In many communities, necessary health care services are not readily available. This is becoming increasingly evident in rural communities where hospitals and other acute care facilities are closing or cutting back on services at an alarming rate (see Chapter 3). Service access is especially difficult for disadvantaged populations, people who are disabled, and the elderly (see Chapters 13, 18, and 19).

COST OF RESOURCE SERVICES. With today's rapidly escalating health care costs, the cost of a service can make it prohibitive to a client. Even a small or sliding scale fee may be more than a client can pay if their income is at or below the poverty level. Many services considered as "optional" by a client may not be used because of cost. On the other hand, if the client places a high priority on receiving a given service, he or she may make concessions to pay the fees by not buying needed medications and not eating well, for example.

### Client Barriers

PRIORITIES. If the need is not of high priority for the client, he or she may not become actively involved in using the referral services. If other needs are considered to be of higher priority, the nurse should assist the client in meeting these needs first. For example, it may be more important for the family to care for an ill family member than to take a child to the well-baby clinic for immunizations. Or, if the family is having difficulty meeting its basic needs of food, clothing, and shelter, preventive health care services may not be viewed as a priority.

MOTIVATION. If the client is not highly motivated to work on a need, it is not likely that much will be done by the client toward meeting that need. An integral part of client motivation is the concept of *awareness versus readiness*. The fact that the client is aware of a need does not mean that he or she is ready to act on the need. If a differentiation is not made between awareness and readiness, the nurse may feel responsible for the failure of the client to follow through on a referral. Once it is established that the client is not ready to act on a need, the nurse needs to assist the client in prioritizing the needs on which he or she is ready to act. A good example of awareness versus readiness is a client who acknowledges her infant needs to begin immunizations at the local health department, but after numerous nursing visits, much discussion, and ample time, she still has not taken the child for immunizations. The client is aware of the need but is not ready to act on it.

PREVIOUS EXPERIENCE WITH RESOURCES. If a client has not had a positive experience in using a resource in the past, he or she may be hesitant to use this resource again or to use other community resources. *Complaints about resources can be entirely justified.* However, a negative experience can be influenced by a client's readiness to make changes and follow-through. Clients also may have a negative view of the resource because their problems were not resolved. Whatever the reason, it is important to acknowledge the client's feelings and explore ways to make further contacts with community services more meaningful.

LACK OF KNOWLEDGE ABOUT AVAILABLE RESOURCES. Clients need to know about resources before they will use them. Lack of knowledge about resources is a major barrier to the use of health care services. A key role of the community health nurse is to educate clients about health care services in the community.

LACK OF UNDERSTANDING REGARDING NEED FOR REFERRAL. Clients who do not understand the need for a referral frequently do not take action to obtain referral services. This is often true of families who neglect to have their children immunized. Many people know that children need "baby shots" but do not understand why. Clients will be more likely to follow through in obtaining immunizations on a consistent basis if they know the purpose for receiving immunizations and the consequences of not obtaining adequate protection against communicable diseases.

CLIENT SELF-IMAGE. If clients have a negative self-image, they may be hesitant to seek care and may view themselves as unworthy of such care. The nurse should acknowledge these feelings and develop intervention strategies that will help clients increase self-esteem.

CULTURAL FACTORS. Cultural differences can be a barrier to effective use of the referral process. Language is one of the most obvious cultural barriers. In our health care system, clients who do not speak English can have a difficult time using resources and obtaining appropriate health care.

Every culture has beliefs regarding health care practices. Cultural beliefs about the cause of illness, nutrition, preventive health care, and death and dying vary greatly. The norms and values of a culture also affect health care practices. For example, in traditional Arab culture, women are generally not allowed to leave their homes or immediate neighborhoods without a male escort, and health care services are better used if they are located in a neighborhood facility.

For cultural groups who do not routinely seek preventive health services, the nurse may have a difficult time gaining compliance on referrals for immunizations and routine physical examinations. Ethnic and cultural values and attitudes pervade a person's life, and it is important that the nurse identify them in relation to health care practices (Rorden, Taft, 1990, p. 97). However, an effective nurse does *not* use racial, cultural, or ethnic stereotypes in anticipating client preferences and providing client care (Rorden, Taft, 1990, p. 98). Rather, a culturally competent nurse assesses for individual client preferences.

FINANCES. Health care in the United States is expensive. Many clients do not use health care services because they are uninsured or underinsured and cannot afford them. Chapter 5 discussed methods of health care financing in the United States and the cost of health care. The near-poor client, who does not qualify for welfare assistance but may be medically indigent, frequently has difficulty paying for health care. The same is true for families who are uninsured or underinsured. It is a challenge for the nurse to find resources that will assist such clients. Church groups, private foundations, and voluntary organizations are a few examples of resources that frequently assist these families.

ACCESSIBILITY. Clients are less likely to use resources that are not readily accessible. It is well documented that clients frequently do not seek health care because they have problems with transportation to health care facilities. Once a resource is beyond walking distance, other means of transportation must be found. Public transportation is scarce in this country, and even if a family has a car, it may not be available at the time of the appointment, or the family may not have money for gas. The problem is greatly magnified if the resource is at such a distance that the client must make arrangements for overnight stays in order to use its services. Overnight stays often necessitate making arrangements for the care of small children or other members of the family, and they can be very costly to the client. If low-cost public transportation is not available, car pooling, the use of volunteer transportation services, or establishing outreach clinic services in the neighborhood may help reduce transportation barriers. Local churches and departments of human or social services have programs to assist people with transportation needs. Local offices on aging and senior centers may have transportation services available for the elderly.

Although lack of resources can limit service utilization, it is crucial for professionals to examine other concerns when considering the concept of access. "Having insurance or nearby health care providers is no guarantee that people who need services will receive them" (Institute of Medicine, 1993, p. 4). Access is a complex concept that involves structural, personal, and economic issues. Families or aggregates having difficulty accessing services often have a complex set of problems that "require organizational solutions that include continuity of care, integration of services, and other subtle characteristics" (Institute of Medicine, 1993, p. 18). For example, people who are homeless or victims of domestic violence require an interlinked array of personal, social, and public health services that address psychosocial and economic concerns. Chapter 13 discusses these concerns and interventions needed to facilitate need resolution.

## LEVELS OF NURSING INTERVENTION WITH REFERRAL

Clients have varying levels of ability to assume independent functioning when using health care resources, which necessitates different levels of professional intervention by the community health nurse. Identifying the level at which the client is functioning helps community health nurses focus intervention strategies when they use the referral process. Levels of nursing intervention are presented in Box 10-5.

**BOX 10-5**

*Levels of Nursing Intervention with Referral*

*Level I:* At this level the client is largely dependent on the nurse, assumes a passive role, and needs assistance with all aspects of the referral process. These clients need considerable support and encouragement and, often, concrete help from the nurse to follow through on a referral. Community health nursing intervention with these clients involves health teaching and counseling so that they can identify health needs that necessitate referral. In addition, supportive assistance is often necessary while they are learning how to use health care resources.

A major goal at this level is to help clients become more actively involved in taking responsibility for meeting their own health needs. Sometimes it is easier to do for the client than to work with him or her, but it is important to resist this and help the client use health resources independently.

*Level II:* At this level mutual participation is evident. The client actively seeks information to determine what health actions are needed to resolve current health problems or to enhance wellness in the future. Clients at this level may need health teaching to understand the value of preventive health practices, to locate community resources that they can afford, or to learn about community services such as low-cost or free transportation that will help them use needed resources. They are more likely, however, to raise challenging questions, identify health care needs, and suggest resources. At times it may be difficult to recognize when these clients need assistance because they are functioning so well in most aspects of their lives.

*Level III:* At this level the client initiates and implements independent referrals. The nurse may be used as a resource person but otherwise assumes a passive participant role. Reaching this level is a goal for the community health nurse.

## SUMMARY

Clients are moving increasingly "quicker and sicker" from one care setting and level of care to another. Community health nurses help provide client-focused, interdisciplinary, continuous, comprehensive care through care management, case management, and the referral processes. Integral parts of these processes are client participation and satisfaction, interdisciplinary collaboration, continuity of care, quality care, and ongoing evaluation. Effective use of care management, case management, and the referral process helps clients resolve health needs and provides anticipatory guidance about future needs. The role of the nurse in case management is expanding. There are limitless opportunities for the community health nurse in case management.

## CRITICAL THINKING
*exercise*

You are a health department nurse who has been assigned to work with a local hospital's discharge planning team. You are trying to familiarize yourself with community resources and the nursing role in the discharge planning process.

1. How would you begin to gather data about community resources?
2. What types of information would you want to obtain about your role with the discharge planning team?
3. What type of criteria would you use to identify clients in need of continuing care upon hospital discharge?

## REFERENCES

A brief history of pathways from case management plans to care maps, *Hosp Case Manage* 6(4):67, 1998.

American Hospital Association (AHA): *Guidelines: discharge planning,* Chicago, 1984, AHA.

American Nurses Association (ANA): *Code for nurses,* Kansas City, Mo, 1985, ANA.

American Nurses Association (ANA): *Standards of community health nursing practice,* Kansas City, Mo, 1986, ANA.

American Nurses Association (ANA): *Nursing case management.* Publication #NS-32. Kansas City, Mo, 1988, ANA.

American Nurses Association (ANA): *Scope and standards of public health nursing practice,* Washington, DC, 1999a, ANA.

American Nurses Association (ANA): *Scope and standards of home health nursing practice,* Washington, DC, 1999b, ANA.

Banja JD: Ethical dimensions of cultural diversity in case management, *The Case Manager* 5(3):27-29, 1994a.

Banja JD: Ethical challenges of managed care, *The Case Manager* 5(3):37-40, 1994b.

Banja JD: Ethical decision-making: origins, process and applications to case management, *The Case Manager* 10(5):41-47, 1999.

Blaylock A, Cason CL: Discharge planning predicting patients' needs, *J Gerontol Nurs* 18(7):5-10, 1992.

Bowers K: *Case management by nurses,* Washington, DC, 1992, American Nurses Association.

Burlenski M: President's message, *Access* 7(1):2, 4, 1989.

Case Management Society of America (CMSA): *Standards of practice for case management,* Little Rock, Ark, 1995, CMSA.

Combs PA: A study of the effectiveness of nursing referrals, *Public Health Rep* 91:122-126, 1976.

Corbett CF, Androwich IM: Critical paths: implications for improving practice, *Home Healthc Nurse* 12(6):27-34, 1995.

Corkery E: Discharge planning and home health care: what every staff nurse should know, *Orthop Nurs* 8(6):18-27, 1989.

Falter EJ, Cesta TG, Concert C, et al.: Development of a graduate nursing program in case management, *J Care Manage* 5(3):50-56, 72-78, 1999.

Gartner MB, Twardon CA: Care guidelines: journey through the managed care maze, *J WOCN* 22(3):118-121, 1995.

Girard N: The case management model of patient care delivery, *AORN J* 60(3):403-415, 1994.

Glover D, King M, Green C, et al.: The patient care team advantage, *Caring* 12(10):40-42, 1993.

Harris J: Case management evolving into advanced practice, *Inside Case Manage* 6(8):1, 3-5, 1999.

Hawkins JW, Veeder NW, Pearce CW: *Nurse social worker collaboration in managed care*, New York, 1998, Springer.

Hseih S, Lee M: Case management: a collaborative process that enhances outcomes, *Viewpoint* 21(6):5-6, 1999.

Institute of Medicine: *Access to health care in America*, Washington, DC, 1993, National Academy Press.

Kaiser KL, Miller LL, Hays BJ, et al.: Patterns of health resource utilization, cost, and intensity of need for primary care clients receiving public health nursing case management, *Nurs Case Manage* 4(2):53-62, 1999.

Kersbergen AL: Case management: a rich history of coordinating care to control costs, *Nurs Outlook* 44:169-172, 1996.

Lamb GS: Research on nursing case management. In JJ Fitzpatrick, JS Stevenson, NS Polis, *Nursing research and its utilization*, New York, 1994, Springer.

Lashley ML: The hidden benefits of case management, *The Case Manager* 4(3):78-79, 1993.

Llewellyn A: Straight talk: the crucial link, *Rehab Manage* 12(6):20-22, 1999.

Martin CJ: Nursing case management: how the current model is evolving, *Viewpoint* 21(6):1, 4, 1999.

May CA, Schraeder C, Britt T: *Managed care and case management. Roles for professional nursing.* Washington, DC, 1996, American Nurses Association.

Mbweza E: Bridging the gap between hospital and home for premature infants in Malawi, *Int Nurs Rev* 43(2):53-57, 1996.

McBroom A: Uniform needs assessment instrument nearing completion, *Access* 7(1):1, 3-4, 1989.

McClinton DH: Promoting wellness, *Continuing Care* 17(4):6, 1998.

McCloskey JC, Grace HK: *Current issues in nursing*, St Louis, 1990, Mosby.

McGuire SL, Gerber DG, Clemen-Stone S: Meeting the diverse needs of clients in the community: effective use of the referral process, *Nurs Outlook* 44(5):218-222, 1996.

Meaney ME: Building a professional ethical culture in case management, *The Case Manager* 10(5):63-67, 1999.

Nash A: Reasons for referral to a palliative nursing team, *J Adv Nurs* 18:707-713, 1993.

Oakland County Health Department, Nursing Division: *Referral form*, Pontiac, Mich, undated, Oakland County Health Department.

O'Hare P, Terry M: *Discharge planning: strategies for assuring continuity of care*, Rockville, Md, 1988, Aspen.

Powell SK: *Nursing case management. A practical guide to success in managed care*, Philadelphia, 1996, Lippincott.

Powell SK: *Advanced case management. Outcomes and beyond*, Philadelphia, 2000, Lippincott.

Rorden JW, Taft E: *Discharge planning guide for nurses*, Philadelphia, 1990, Saunders.

Rowe RS: Population care management emerging as significant approach to case management. A brave new world for case managers. In Fantle LA, editor: *Case manager's desk reference* (pp.16-19), Gaithersburg, Md, 1999, Aspen.

Schetzow SO: Confidentiality, *The Case Manager* 5(3):108-109, 1994.

Shamansky SL, Boase JC, Horn BM: Discharge planning yesterday, today and tomorrow, *Home Healthc Nurse* 2(13):14-21, 1984.

Siegel H: Nurses improve hospital efficiency through a risk assessment model at admission, *Nurs Manage* 19(10):38-40, 42, 44-45, 1988.

Spath PL: Critical paths: maximizing patient care coordination, *Today's OR Nurse* 17(2):13-20, 34-35, 1995.

Stone M: Discharge planning guide, *Am J Nurs* 79:1445-1447, 1979.

Tahan HA: Case management: a heritage more than a century old, *Nurs Case Manage* 3(2):55-60, 1998.

Tahan HA: Clarifying case management: What is in a label? *Nurs Case Manage* 4(6):268-278, 1999.

Taylor C, Barnet RJ: The ethics of case management. In EL Cohen, V DeBack, editors: *The outcomes mandate. Case management in health care today* (pp. 27-36), St Louis, 1999, Mosby.

Townsend EI, Edwards NC, Nadon C: The hospital liaison process: identifying risk factors in postnatal multiparas, *Can J Public Health* 83(3):203-207, 1992.

United States Department of Health and Human Services (USDHHS): *Source book for health education materials and community resources*, Washington, DC, 1982a, US Government Printing Office.

United States Department of Health and Human Services (USDHHS): *Healthy people 2000: promoting health and preventing diseases. Objectives for the nation, full report, with commentary*, Washington, DC, 1991, USDHHS.

United States Department of Health and Human Services (USDHHS): *Healthy people 2010, conference edition*, Washington, DC, 2000, USDHHS.

University of Michigan, School of Nursing, Family and Community Health Nursing: *Resource grid*, Ann Arbor, undated, University of Michigan, School of Nursing.

Wensley E: *Nursing service without walls*, New York, 1963, National League for Nursing.

Wheeler-Lachowycz J: How to use your VNA, *Am J Nurs* 83:1164-1167, 1983.

Willihnganz G: The next step: pre-admission planning for discharge needs, *Coordinator* 3:20-21, 1984.

Wolff I: Referral—a process and a skill, *Nurs Outlook* 10:253-256, 1962.

Wolff I: Referral—a process and a skill. In DM Stewart, PA Vincent, editors: *Public health nursing*, Dubuque, Iowa, 1968, Wm. C. Brown Company, pp.130-139.

Zoloth-Dorfman L, Rubin S: The patient as commodity: managed care and the question of ethics, *J Clin Ethics* 6:339-357, 1995.

## SELECTED BIBLIOGRAPHY

Harris SJ: Creative discharge planning: a team commitment, *Rehab Nurs* 25(3):86-87, 2000.

Helvie CO: Efficacy of primary care in a nursing center, *Nurs Case Manage* 4(4):201-210, 1999.

Howe RS: Case management in managed care: past, present, and future, *The Case Manager* 10(5):37-40, 1999.

Johnson C, Birmingham J: How to use research information to improve case management practice, *J Care Manage* 5(3):41-46, 1999.

Luker KA, Chalmers KI: The referral process in health visiting, *Int J Nurs Stud* 26(2):173-185, 1989.

Mackey JF: Lack of referral networks: a parent's perspective, *Birth Defects* 26(2):105-108, 1990.

Mullahy CM: *The case manger's handbook*, Gaithersburg, Md, 1995, Aspen.

Mullahy CM: Utilization management: the effective integration of utilization and case management, *The Case Manager* 11(2):53-56, 2000.

Rieve JA: Guidelines and outcomes: proving the value of case management, *The Case Manager* 11(2):42, 2000.

Rose K: Case management as a survival tool, *Home Healthc Nur Manager* 4(1):26-27, 2000.

Sager D: The coming golden age of case management, *The Case Manager* 10(6):4, 1999.

Spath PL: How to measure the value of case management, *Hosp Case Manage* 8(2):29-32, 2000.

Taylor P: Comprehensive nursing case management. An advanced practice model, *Nurs Case Manage* 4(1):2-10, 1999.

Wolfe G: Case management in the millennium: past and future, *J Care Manage* 5(6):8, 1999.

# Discharge Questionnaire

The staff on (unit name) wants to make your return to the community as easy for you as possible. The nurse who is primarily responsible for helping you plan your discharge is _____. He or she will help you and your family reach any resources you may need for your health care at home. There are many agencies, including home care, that assist people in the community with health care problems.

Please complete the following questions with your family as soon as you feel able. Your discharge nurse will be in contact with you within a few days of your admission.

## Data #1

When you get home

1. With whom will you live? _____
2. Will they be able to help with your care if needed? _____
3. Will you have difficulty getting around your home—stairs, small bathroom, low bed, safety problems, to the telephone, to shower, or bathtub? _____
4. Will you have any problems in getting any of the following—transportation, food, medicine, heat, place to stay, child care, pet care, water supply? _____
5. Will you need any of these to function at home—wheelchair, brace, cane, walker, crutches, special equipment? _____
_____

6. How much of the following will you be able to do? (Please mark appropriate column.)

|  | INDEPENDENT | WITH FAMILY | UNABLE TO |
|---|---|---|---|
| Turning in bed |  |  |  |
| Bathing |  |  |  |
| Dressing |  |  |  |
| Eating |  |  |  |
| Sitting |  |  |  |
| Standing |  |  |  |
| Transfers to tub |  |  |  |
| Transfers to toilet |  |  |  |
| Walking |  |  |  |

## Data #2

1. Have you had a problem with any of these areas recently?
   - a. Eyes/ears
   - b. Mouth/throat/teeth
   - c. Skin
   - d. Lungs/breathing
   - e. Breasts
   - f. Heart/blood vessels
   - g. Stomach/bowel
   - h. Bladder/kidneys/urine
   - i. Genitals
   - j. Mental status
   - k. Nerves/muscles
2. Will you have difficulty getting to your physician, nurse, or therapist often enough to have these checked?

## Data #3

Please mark any of the following areas that you would like to know more about:
1. Your disease/illness/accident
   - a. What caused it
   - b. What can be done to prevent a repeat
   - c. How to recognize a repeat
   - d. How it will affect you later

Please mark any of the following areas that you would like to know more about:
2. Your medication
   - a. What it does
   - b. How much to take
   - c. When to take it
   - d. What side effects to be aware of

From Stone M: Discharge planning guide, *Am J Nurs* 79:1445-1447, 1979.

# Discharge Questionnaire (cont'd)

## Data #3—cont'd

3. Your treatments, procedures, or exercises
   - a. What they do for you
   - b. How to do them
   - c. How often to do them
   - d. What difficulties to be aware of
4. Supplies or equipment you'll use at home
   - a. What it does
   - b. When to use it
   - c. How to get more or to get repairs
5. Your nutrition
   - a. How it affects you
   - b. Special diets—how much to eat, when to eat, what to avoid
   - c. How much and what to drink
6. Preventive health practices
   - a. How to examine your breasts
   - b. Pap smears
   - c. Birth control
   - d. Effect of cigarettes
   - e. Effect of alcohol and drugs
   - f. Dental health
   - g. Seat belt
   - h. Immunizations (yourself or children)
   - i. Exercise
7. Other _____

## Data #4

1. Which of these agencies are you involved with?
   - a. VNA/Home Health
   - b. Senior Citizens
   - c. Vocational Rehabilitation
   - d. Social Welfare
   - e. Planned Parenthood
   - f. Mental Health Agency
   - g. Diet Club
   - h. Alcoholics Anonymous
   - i. Cancer Society
   - j. Ostomy Club
   - k. Meals-on-Wheels
   - l. Diabetes Association
   - m. Dialysis Association
   - n. MS Society
   - o. MD Society
   - p. Association for the Blind
   - q. Other _____
2. Please mark any of the areas that you would especially like to discuss with your discharge nurse.
   - a. Finances, jobs
   - b. Drugs, alcohol
   - c. Caring for children or elderly relatives
   - d. Emotional or nerve problem
   - e. Sexuality
   - f. Family or marital relationships
   - g. Grieving
   - h. School or work
   - i. Problem, retirement
   - j. Spiritual needs
   - k. Legal problems
   - l. Other _____

STOP HERE. YOUR DISCHARGE NURSE WILL HELP YOU COMPLETE THE FORM. Ask to see him or her if you haven't met yet, especially if you think you might go home soon.

**Assessments** (To be done by RN and patient)

1. Will there be a need for help with physical care at home?
2. Will there be a need for a nurse or therapist at home to assess physical status, disease process, or exercise and therapy?
3. Will the patient or family need more health education about any of the areas above (Data #3), either during hospitalization or at home?
4. Will the patient or family need more information or assistance with any of the psychosocial areas listed in Data #4?

**Plan** (To be done by patient and nurse together)

Consider the four assessments above. If there are *no* "yes" responses, proceed to section B and complete. If there are any "yes" responses, you *must* select either part 1 or part 2 of section A before completing section B.

A. 1. No referral necessary, but must have further education before discharge regarding _____
   2. Refer to: (see above list of agencies) _____
B. 1. Equipment or supplies to leave with patient _____
   2. Transfer plan _____
   3. Medical follow-up _____
   4. Surgical follow-up _____

# PART TWO

# Planning Health Services for Populations at Risk

The uniqueness of community health nursing practice lies in the nurse's ability to assess the health assets and needs of a community; identify aggregates at risk; and plan, implement, and evaluate population-focused interventions that promote community wellness. Considering the nature of our current health issues, it is important for community health nurses to examine the needs of individuals, families, and populations across the life span. It is also important for them to address health disparity and quality-of-life issues. The increasing number of clients across the life span who have long-term care needs will present significant challenges for consumers and providers throughout the twenty-first century. The *Healthy People 2010* initiative provides the framework for analyzing these challenges.

Part Two explores how community health nurses use knowledge from nursing, public health, and social sciences when they plan interventions for the population as a whole. Emphasis is on how nurses use epidemiology, community diagnoses, health planning, management, quality improvement, and nursing principles to deliver high-quality services in various community settings. Emerging opportunities for health care professionals are highlighted.

Dramatic changes in the health care delivery system and unprecedented societal changes will influence client need and client-provider relationships throughout the twenty-first century. The effect of *health care reform* is in the forefront of the public mind, bringing with it a call for innovation in service delivery and reformulation of health care provider roles. To address these challenges, nurses are becoming politically active, advocating health for all people in need, and engaging in research to test nursing interventions that promote positive health outcomes. Nurses must understand the urgency of keeping pace with changes in the evolving health care system.

# 11

# Concepts of Epidemiology: Infectious and Chronic Conditions

*Diane Gerber Eigsti*

*Timothy Jones*

## OBJECTIVES

*Upon completion of this chapter, the reader should be able to:*

1. Define the term epidemiology and discuss how its scope has expanded over time.
2. Understand how host, agent, and environmental factors influence the natural life history of a disease.
3. Describe how preventive intervention can alter the natural life history of a disease.
4. Characterize the distribution of health and disease by person, place, and time.
5. Discuss the dynamics of infectious disease transmission.
6. Illustrate the use of epidemiological measures and methods in the investigation of infectious disease outbreaks and chronic disease occurrence.
7. Understand how public health surveillance influences the control of disease.
8. Summarize barriers to the epidemiological control of infectious and noninfectious disease.
9. Discuss the use of epidemiological concepts in community health nursing practice.

## KEY TERMS

Agent
Aggregates at risk
Biological/chemical warfare and terrorism
Biostatistics
Casefinding
Chronic disease and the black box
Demographic statistics
Environment

Epidemiology
Era of infectious disease
Germ theory
Herd immunity
Host
Levels of prevention
Miasma
Morbidity statistics
Mortality statistics

Multiple causation of disease
Natural life history of disease
Person, place, time relationships
Risk factors
Sanitary statistics
Screening
Surveillance
Vital statistics

*The Lord will strike thee with a consumption, and with fever, and with an inflammation...and they shall pursue thee until thou perish.*

DEUTERONOMY 28:22

Tuberculosis (TB), known early in the seventeenth century as *consumption*, has been described as the greatest killer in history. In the past 200 years this disease has killed approximately a billion human beings, among them, Chopin, Paganini, Rousseau, Goethe, Chekov, Edgar Allen Poe, Eugene O'Neil, Sir Walter Scott, and Emily and

Charlotte Bronte. TB has inspired great literature including Thomas Mann's *Magic Mountain* and the opera, *La Traviata*. In the late nineteenth century there was fear that TB might destroy European civilization. Today it remains a strange and fascinating disease because new forms continue to emerge. However, the discovery of the cause of, and cure for, TB changed human history. How this was accomplished is a dramatic example of **epidemiology**, an investigative problem-solving process that has two facets: the study of the determinants of health and disease frequencies in populations, and, the planning and implementation of health promotion and disease control programs. Throughout this chapter, the epidemiology of TB is employed to assist readers in understanding the concepts that are involved. If the reader needs to better understand the pathology of TB the Centers for Disease Control and Prevention (CDC) has a website at *http://www.cdc.gov/nchstp/tb* that provides timely and accurate material.

## *Stop and Think About It*

How have computers and the internet affected your life as a student, person, or friend? What criteria do you use to judge the quality of materials found on the internet?

## EPIDEMIOLOGY DEFINED

The word epidemiology is derived from the Greek roots, *epi*, meaning "upon," and *demos*, meaning "people" (collectively). Historically the major focus of the epidemiologist was on analyzing major infectious disease outbreaks (epidemics) so that ways to control and prevent disease occurrence in populations (people, collectively) could be determined. As early as the fifth century, TB was a dreaded scourge called the "King's Evil." Kings were thought to have healing powers from God, and they held audiences to touch and supposedly cure their subjects (Ryan, 1993, pp. 6-7).

Today the definition of epidemiology has been expanded to include the study of variables that affect health and influence disease and condition occurrence.

There are many variations in the definition of the term epidemiology, but most focus on studying determinants of health and disease states among populations. Throughout this chapter the following definition, adapted from MacMahon and Pugh's (1970, p. 1) classic writings, is used: Epidemiology is the systematic, scientific study of the distribution patterns and determinants of health, disease, and condition frequencies in populations for the purpose of promoting wellness and preventing disease/conditions.

Implicit in this definition are two basic assumptions. The first is that patterns and frequencies of health, disease, and conditions in populations can be identified. The second is that factors determining or contributing to the occurrence of health, disease, or conditions can be discovered through systematic investigation.

Community health nurses work with other public health professionals, using the epidemiological process to carry out their systematic investigation of health, disease, and conditions in populations. This process is graphically depicted in Figure 11-1 and is discussed in detail later in this chapter. Note that the epidemiological process shown in Figure 11-1

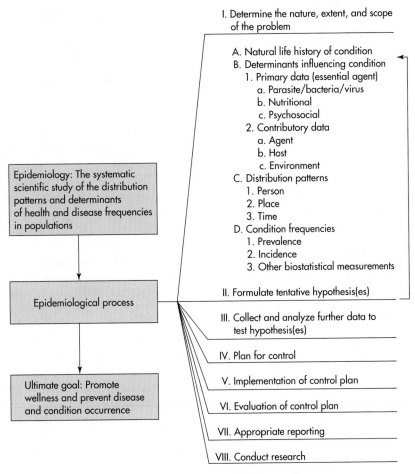

**FIGURE 11-1** Graphic explanation of epidemiology.

**TABLE 11-1**

*Comparison of the Nursing Process and the Epidemiological Process*

| NURSING PROCESS | EPIDEMIOLOGICAL PROCESS |
| --- | --- |
| Assessing (data collection to determine nature of client problems) | I. Determine the nature, extent, and scope of the problem<br>  A. Natural life history of condition<br>  B. Determinants influencing condition<br>    1. Primary data (essential agent)<br>      a. Parasite/bacterium/virus<br>      b. Nutritional<br>      c. Psychosocial<br>    2. Contributory data<br>      a. Agent<br>      b. Host<br>      c. Environment<br>  C. Distribution patterns<br>    1. Person<br>    2. Place<br>    3. Time<br>  D. Condition frequencies<br>    1. Prevalence<br>    2. Incidence<br>    3. Other biostatistical measurements |
| Analyzing (formulation of nursing diagnosis or hypothesis) | II. Formulate tentative hypothesis(es) |
| | III. Collect and analyze further data to test hypothesis(es) |
| Planning | IV. Plan for control |
| Implementing | V. Implement control plan |
| Evaluating | VI. Evaluate control plan |
| Revising or terminating | VII. Make appropriate report |
| Research | VIII. Conduct research |

is similar to the nursing process. The steps are labeled differently but, in essence, they both involve a series of circular, dynamic problem-solving actions. Table 11-1 illustrates this point. Learning the language of epidemiology gives one a distinct advantage, however, because the terminology of epidemiology is used by all community health professionals; the terminology of the nursing process is not.

## History and Scope of Epidemiology

Significant changes in the methodology used in epidemiology have occurred over the past 200 years, including shifts in basic ideas about its purpose, methods of analyzing data, and measuring exposure to disease agents. These changes are significant because they reflect the way that epidemiologists think about health and disease, and they influence the manner in which they study health and disease. Table 11-2 depicts these changes as described by two well-known contemporary epidemiologists (Susser, Susser, 1996a, p. 676). The eras have occurred over time, build on each other, are overlapping, and thus are not discrete time periods. Not every epidemiologist would agree with the interpretation of this material. The following paragraphs discuss the changes as represented in Table 11-2.

In Chapter 1, the efforts of Florence Nightingale to collect data and carry out statistical analysis in relation to nursing care were described. Her work is an example of the first era of epidemiology, **sanitary statistics,** which emphasized controlling **miasma,** poisoning by the foul vapors coming from soil, air, and water. The poor outnumbered the rich in nineteenth century Europe and the United States, and their homes and working conditions were frequently desperate (Figure 11-2). Tracking the high number of sick and dying people was compelling evidence to Nightingale and her contemporaries that the environment caused their suffering. Edwin Chadwick, another reformer discussed in Chapter 1, believed that the environment caused poverty and thus, the solutions were collecting garbage and building sewage drainage systems and public housing. The development of TB sanatoria, resorts devoted exclusively to the care of "consumptives," was another example of this era (Figure 11-3). They were frequently "located in a proper location in the mountains, a liberal diet, wine, fresh air and exercise, graded to prevent fatigue" (Bates, 1992, p.38). Table 11-2 depicts this beginning era of the field of epidemiology: the paradigm or focus was miasma; the analytic approach used by epidemiologists was describing how

**TABLE 11-2**

*Eras in the Evolution of Modern Epidemiology and an Emergent Era*

| ERA | PARADIGM | ANALYTIC APPROACH | PREVENTIVE APPROACH |
|---|---|---|---|
| Sanitary statistics (first half of nineteenth century) | Miasma: poisoning by foul emanations from soil, air, and water | Demonstrate clustering of morbidity and mortality | Introduce drainage, sewage, sanitation |
| Infectious disease (late nineteenth century through first half of twentieth century) | Germ theory: single agents relate one to one to specific diseases | Laboratory isolation and culture from disease sites, experimental transmission and reproduction of lesions | Interrupt transmission (vaccines, isolation of the affected through quarantine and fever hospitals, and ultimately antibiotics) |
| Chronic disease epidemiology (latter half of the twentieth century) | Black box: exposure related to outcome, without necessity for intervening factors or pathogenesis | Risk ratio of exposure to outcome at individual level in populations | Control risk factors by modifying lifestyle (e.g., diet, exercise), agent (e.g., guns, food), or environment (e.g., pollution, passive smoking) |
| Eco-epidemiology (emerging) | Chinese boxes: relations within and between localized structures organized in an hierarchy of levels | Analysis of determinants and outcomes at different levels of organization: within and across contexts (using new information systems) and in depth (using new biomedical techniques) | Apply both information and biomedical technology to find leverage at efficacious levels from contextual to molecular |

From Susser M, Susser E: Choosing a future for epidemiology: II. From black box to Chinese boxes and eco-epidemiology, *Am J Public Health* 86:674-677, 1996b, p. 676.

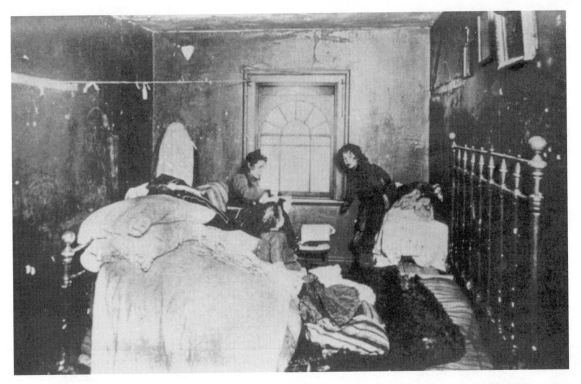

**FIGURE 11-2** "Home Finishers." A consumptive mother and her two children at work. (From the National Library of Medicine, History of Medicine Division; Spargo J: *The bitter cry of children*, New York, 1906, Macmillan.)

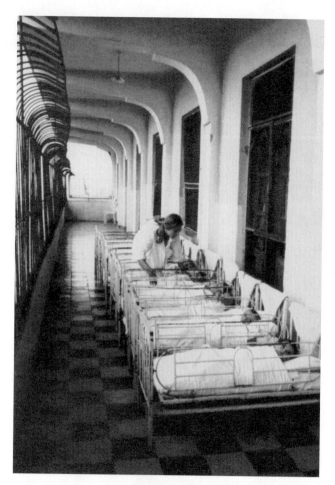

**FIGURE 11-3** Traditional hospitals and sanatoria are now judged unnecessary for most clients with tuberculosis. (From the National Library of Medicine, History of Medicine Division; WHO photo by D. Henrioud.)

groups of ill and dying people clustered in poor areas; and the method they used to deal with the problem was changing the environment with sewage systems, garbage collection, and housing.

The focus of epidemiology changed dramatically with the development of the **germ theory** because the cause of disease could be traced to a single organism. The discovery of the agent that caused TB was understandably dramatic. On March 24, 1882, Robert Koch, a totally unknown country doctor, addressed the Physiological Society in Berlin, Germany. He described how he had selected freshly developed abscesses, called tubercules, from human beings who had just died of TB. He removed pus from the tubercles and spread it on glass slides. Koch's particular genius was to develop a unique stain so that the tubercular bacillus could be seen under a microscope. In his words, "All of these factors taken together can lead to only one conclusion: that the bacilli which are present in the tuberculosis substances not only accompany the tuberculosis process, but are the cause

of it. In the bacilli we have, therefore, the acute infective cause of tuberculosis" (Ryan, 1993, pp. 14-15). Not bad air, not a weakness of a person's body, no longer an unknown, the terrifying killer was a bacterium, "the like of which had never been even suspected before, a most singular life form with a frightening propensity to infect every cat and chicken, pigeon and guinea pig, the white mice and rats and oxen and even the two marmosets, into which Koch had injected it" (Ryan, 1993, p. 15). World TB Day is held annually on March 24, commemorating the day Koch described the discovery of the TB bacillus.

The cure for TB was one of the most urgent medical problems of the twentieth century. Scientists did not know where to begin because at the time of Koch's discovery, not a single medication had been discovered to cure infections. The work of a number of physicians and researchers from Russia, Europe, and the United States led ultimately to streptomycin, the first antibiotic effective against TB, in 1944. In 1952, isoniazid, a synthetic antibiotic was developed and became the decisive treatment for this disease.

In Table 11-2 the **era of infectious disease** is summarized: the paradigm was the germ theory, the analytic approach was to find disease organisms in the laboratory setting. The methods of dealing with the problem of infectious disease involved isolation and quarantine and the development of vaccines. The study of populations, environmental exposures, and the social dynamics of disease that were so crucial to the first epidemiology era were often ignored.

The profound impact of antibiotics and vaccines, along with improved nutrition and higher living standards in the early part of the twentieth century, led to dramatic declines in mortality and morbidity from infectious diseases for people living in the industrialized world. Many people believed that infectious diseases were conquered and funding for TB programs declined dramatically. With the exception of writers like Rene' Dubos (1959), few people anticipated that in the twenty-first century, communicable diseases and global epidemics would once again threaten the lives of many people, particularly in developing countries.

The third epidemiology era, the current one, is that of **chronic disease and the black box.** It gradually came into being with the ending of World War II in 1945. By this time, deaths from TB were down from 70 per 100,000 people in 1930 to a new figure of 40 per 100,000. By 1954, just 10 years after the introduction of streptomycin, the death rate was 10 per 100,000 (Rothman, 1994, p. 248). Today, deaths from this disease in industrialized countries are almost nonexistent.

Major public health problems of this era are chronic conditions including heart disease, cancer, and stroke. In the early 1950s, large-scale studies, usually involving men because of the norms of the day, compared persons with heart disease (called cases) to men who did not have heart disease (controls). Case-control studies helped establish smoking as a risk factor for lung cancer and cholesterol as a risk factor

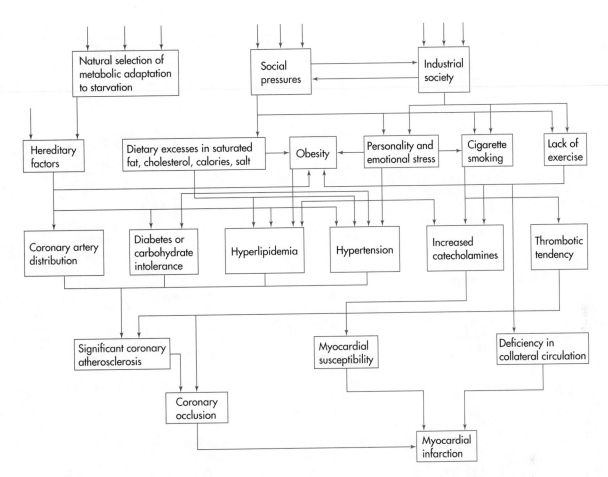

**FIGURE 11-4** The web of causation for myocardial infarction. (From Friedman GE: *Primer of epidemiology,* New York, 1974, McGraw-Hill, p. 5.)

for heart disease. The power of the observation method of epidemiology also was established with these studies; closely following people who were ill and comparing them with those who did not become ill was the hallmark of this period. The development of statistical theories and analysis for use with case-control studies became highly refined.

The use of the term *black box* is a metaphor to describe a situation in which inner processes are unseen by those involved in the outcome. In the era of chronic disease epidemiology, the black box metaphor implied that exposure was related to outcome and there was no need to explain intervening factors or pathogenesis. For example, although men with high cholesterol frequently had heart disease, how this relationship occurred was not explained for many years.

The concept of **multiple causation of disease** has become the basic tenet of this era of epidemiology (Krieger, 1994, p. 887). It is based on the belief that it is the interaction and relationships between persons, called the hosts, their environment, and the causative agent that produce health or disease. For example, a man (host) may develop heart disease because of his inherited risks, obesity, diet, and hypertension (agents) and because of a highly stressful job

(environment). Conversely, he may not develop heart disease if he treats his hypertension, exercises, eats a proper diet, and uses methods to lower his stress. Figure 11-4 depicts the complex *web of causation* for myocardial infarction and the numerous interconnected strands that cause heart disease. It is these strands that are altered by public health professionals in order to change the course of disease or health in populations. Table 11-3 provides examples of how the strands in the web of causation of future disease are used to alter the risk factors and the environment in groups that are at risk. As illustrated in Table 11-3, adolescents and young adults are provided with educational programs about smoking, alcohol, and drug use to prevent the accidents and disease those behaviors lead to. Adults are taught about self-breast examinations and hypertension prevention screening.

### Stop and Think About It

How have you personally used strands in the web of causation for any potential or actual health problem in your own life?

The weakness of the web of causation depicted in Figure 11-4 is that the strands of the web have not been strength-

**TABLE 11-3**

*Epidemiology in Action: Examples of Health Measures Needed to Improve the Health of At-Risk Groups at Each Life Stage*

| INFANTS | CHILDREN | ADOLESCENTS AND YOUNG ADULTS | ADULTS | ELDERLY |
|---|---|---|---|---|
| Education for parenthood | Early comprehensive childhood development programs | Comprehensive injury prevention programs, including roadway safety | Public education about smoking, alcohol, good nutrition, and adequate exercise, including how poor health habits increase risk of disease | Work and social activity for retired persons |
| Genetic counseling | Special support services to aid families under stress (e.g., child abuse, low income, etc.) | Educational programs about smoking, alcohol, and drug use | Protection from environmental health habits | Education about adequate exercise and nutrition |
| Good prenatal care | | Nutrition and exercise guidance | | Preventive multiphasic screening programs |
| Sound prenatal nutritional guidance and services | Injury reduction education | Family planning services | Worksite health and safety programs | Education about proper use of medications |
| Counseling services to decrease adverse maternal habits that affect fetal development (e.g., smoking, drinking, drugs, exposure to radiation) | Comprehensive pediatric care | Sexually transmissible disease services including education, screening, and treatment | Hypertension prevention, screening, and control programs | Immunizations for influenza |
| Amniocentesis | Immunizations | Immunizations | Pap smears | Home safety programs |
| Breastfeeding | Lead poisoning screening | Mental health | Regular breast self-examination | Community and home services that facilitate independent living |
| Regular comprehensive care | Fluoridation of water supplies | Actions to reduce the availability of firearms | Education about cancer signs | |
| Immunizations | Dental care | Comprehensive violence prevention programs | Mental health services | |
| Social services including financial assistance, day care, improved foster and adoption programs, and counseling for families under stress | Nutritional and exercise guidance | | Dental care | |
| Newborn screening and follow-up | Education to prevent and eliminate dysfunctional health habits (smoking, alcohol use, drug use, unprotected sexual activity, poor dietary and exercise patterns) | | Comprehensive violence prevention programs | |

Data from Surgeon General: *Healthy People: the Surgeon General's report on health promotion and disease prevention,* vol II, Washington, DC, 1979, US Government Printing Office, pp. 149-155; USDHHS: *Healthy People 2000: national health promotion and disease prevention objectives, full report with commentary,* Washington, DC, 1991, US Government Printing Office, pp. 9-28; USDHHS: *Healthy People 2010: with understanding and improving health and objectives for improving health* (in 2 volumes), ed 2, Washington, DC, 2000, US Government Printing Office.

ened with research so that they can be counted on to achieve desired results. For example, when or how does education about alcohol and drug use result in their being used or not being used? For adults who are obese and hypertensive, when does counseling about exercise and diet result in desired results? Why does it seemingly "work" for one client and not another? The lack of success with so much intervention is startling: 55% of Americans are overweight or obese (Strawbridge, Walhagen, Shema, 2000, p. 340). Lack of success with changing behaviors mandates that epidemiologists question the basic tenet of the current era of epidemiology, that is, the manipulation of the strands in the web of causation of disease to bring about change.

## A NEW ERA IN EPIDEMIOLOGY

A number of epidemiologists have called for a new era in epidemiology. "Two forces, characteristic of our time and much written about, are blunting the black box paradigm: (1) *a transformation in global health patterns* and (2) *new technology*" (Susser, Susser, 1996a, p. 671).

In less developed countries, the human immunodeficiency virus (HIV), which is responsible for the acquired immunodeficiency syndrome (AIDS) epidemic, has forced public health professionals to question the manner in which epidemiologists have functioned. Although the causative organism (the agent that causes HIV) is well-known and risk factors for AIDS and its host and environment have been described in detail, many countries are being devastated by this disease in the very manner that TB once devastated entire civilizations. In sub-Saharan Africa 10.1 million men and 12.2 million women are infected, and AIDS is the leading cause of death (Susser, Stein, 2000, p. 1043). This horrific epidemic sends the clear message that epidemiologists do not know how to halt its spread. We know what behaviors need to change, *but we do not know how to change them.* We do not understand the forces within society that determine the status of health and disease for groups of people. Public health professionals are learning that solving health problems at the level of an *aggregate,* a group of people, a community, or a country can be difficult. The population or group has its own laws and dynamics, and epidemiologists have not yet begun to understand them.

Another factor in the force for change in epidemiology is technology. For example, in July 2000, scientists announced that the entire genetic code of human beings had been mapped, meaning that the deoxyribonucleic acid (DNA) chemicals that influence the way we walk, talk, think, and sleep, had been deciphered. This advance is already being used in *pharmacogenomics,* the development of medications designed specifically for one person's genes. Other companies are experimenting with blood tests that will reveal disease gene mutations, so that, for example, breast cancer can be predicted and then prevented by adding healthy genes to a person's body. *Imaging,* another development of technology, has been used to examine portions of the body that were heretofore invisible to the eye. These biological systems enable epidemiologists and other scientists to examine diseases with unique approaches. Ultimately these advances will assist public health professionals to clarify disease processes and not just the causal factors of disease, which are strands of the web of causation.

Another crucial aspect of technology that is part of the new era of technology is the global communication network, which provides epidemiologists with immediate access to vital data from across the world. This technology assists epidemiologists to recognize patterns of health and disease, large-scale events, and systems, in their social context. Nursing students have access to at least part of this technology via the internet. Throughout this chapter this technology is referenced because it provides immediate and accurate access to the data being used by epidemiologists on a regular basis.

The field of epidemiology has shifted dramatically from the Era of Sanitary Statistics and the work of Nightingale to change the environment. Koch, in the Era of Infectious Disease, built upon the efforts of those early pioneers. Today, public health professionals see the effects of both the Chronic Disease Era and the emerging Eco-Epidemiology Era. The nature of paradigms is that they change as patterns and technologies emerge. Contemporary epidemiologists face a vital and exciting future as new developments continue to occur. TB, once nearly a vanquished disease, is once again a threat, and multidrug-resistant TB is a particular public health threat. Infectious disease is still the leading cause of death worldwide.

## EPIDEMIOLOGY AND THE COMMUNITY HEALTH NURSE

Effective implementation of the epidemiological process requires a multidisciplinary approach. Nurses, physicians, environmental engineers, laboratory technicians, statisticians, health officers, social workers, laypersons, and others carry out necessary and essential roles in the investigation and control of disease and the promotion of wellness. Any health professional can function as a member of the epidemiological team.

Community health nurses participate on the epidemiological team in a variety of ways. Their contacts with families in the home and with groups in various settings (clinics, schools, and industry) put them in a unique position to carry out many epidemiological activities. They regularly become involved in case finding, health teaching, counseling, and follow-up essential to the prevention of infectious diseases, chronic conditions, and other health-related phenomena. The actions taken by the community health nurse in the following actual case situations illustrate how they work to prevent the spread of TB and lower the levels of lead in the blood.

**CASE**
*Scenario* At a large minimum security prison, nurses administer tuberculin skin tests to prisoners upon their admission to the facility, and again on their birthdays. A conversion from a negative to a positive skin test means that the individual has been exposed to someone with active TB. Persons with positive skin tests are referred for chest radiographs and collection of sputum specimens that are cultured for *Mycobacterium tuberculosis.* In March 2000, a record review revealed that nine inmates had converted from negative to positive skin tests. This was an unusually high number of conversions. The nurses immediately called the county health department to begin an investigation.

Community health nurses also use concepts from epidemiology to address noninfectious health problems. Their work with children who have elevated blood lead levels (BLL) reflects this type of activity.

**CASE**
*Scenario* An 11-month-old child was noted to have a BLL of 43 µg/dl on screening during a routine well-child examination. An evaluation of the home identified no obvious source of exposure to lead. Discussion with the parents revealed that they had applied "surma" to the child's eyes daily for 5 months to "strengthen" them. Surma is a fine powder that resembles

mascara. It is applied to the conjunctival surface of the eyelid for cosmetic or medicinal purposes in many Asian countries (Ali, Smales, Aslam, 1978, p. 915). It had been brought from India by the child's grandmother. Testing of the powder applied to the child's eyes found it to be 25% lead by weight. Application of the material was discontinued, and the child's BLL dropped to 23 $\mu$g /dl within 8 weeks (Jones, Moore, Craig, et al., 1999, p. 1223).

In both of these illustrations, one involving a family and the other involving a much larger group of people, the elements of the epidemiological process were utilized. Refer again to Table 11-1. The nature, extent, and scope of the problem were determined, a conclusion about the problem was reached, treatment was started, and resolution of the problem began. The ultimate goal was prevention of additional TB cases in the prison setting and elimination of lead poisoning in the home setting.

Community health nurses apply the principles of epidemiology to provide preventive health services to aggregates in the community. For example, nurses serving Asian populations might consider the hidden threat of lead poisoning and implement this potential problem into their screening and education programs. The nurse must understand the significance of expanding epidemiological study from individuals and families to efforts with populations. Only in this way will the community health nurse effectively meet the health needs of the community as a whole.

## BASIC CONCEPTS OF EPIDEMIOLOGY

To use the epidemiological process effectively, community health nurses need to have an understanding of the basic concepts, tools, and terms of epidemiology. Because epidemiology is operationally defined in terms of disease measurements, an understanding of the biostatistical concepts is essential. Biostatistics helps describe the extent and distribution of health, illness, and conditions in the community and aids in the identification of specific health problems and community strengths. Biostatistics also facilitates the setting of priorities for program planning.

In addition to biostatistics, several basic concepts guide epidemiological study. These are aggregates at risk, the natural life history of a disease, levels of prevention, host-agent-environment relationships, and person-place-time relationships. In general these concepts provide a foundation for explaining how disease develops and how health is maintained, who is most susceptible to disease, and how disease can be prevented and health promoted.

### Study of Aggregates at Risk

A key concept of epidemiology is that the study of disease in populations is more significant than the study of individual cases of disease. Epidemiological research has demonstrated that using large sampling groups is essential for formulating valid conclusions about the distribution patterns and determinants of health, disease, and condition frequencies in populations. It is by observing large groups that commonalities and differences among people who have or do not have a particular disease or condition can be identified.

The identification of commonalities and differences among groups focuses attention on the essential or contributory factors that produce illness or promote health. For example, TB has been frequently found in prisons and other settings where there is crowding, thus leading to the conclusion that the disease is spread by respiratory droplets. Examining individual cases would not lead one to that conclusion.

A preventive health philosophy has led professionals in community health to emphasize the study of groups. A goal of epidemiological study is to identify *aggregates at risk,* so that preventive health measures such as those presented in Table 11-3 can be used to stop the progression of disease or health-related phenomena. As previously defined in Chapter 3, aggregates at high risk are those who engage in certain activities or who have certain characteristics that increase their potential for contracting an illness, injury, or a health problem. For example, coal miners are daily exposed to dust containing silica, a common mineral. This exposure is known as a *risk factor* for the development of silicosis, a lung disease (Figure 11-5).

### *Stop and Think About It*

As a student, what aggregates have you worked with who are at risk? What factors placed them at risk?

RISK FACTORS. **Risk factors** are determined by a risk estimate process. Risk estimates are derived by contrasting the frequency of a disease or health condition in persons *exposed* to a specific trait or risk factor and the frequency in another group *not exposed* to a risk factor (Jekel, Elmore, Katz, 1996). Risk factors fall into three major categories: (1) behavioral or lifestyle patterns, (2) environmental factors, and (3) inborn or inherited characteristics (Last, 1995). These risk factors increase one's susceptibility to death, disease, and injury. For example, living in homeless shelters (environmental patterns) may expose men who abuse alcohol (lifestyle factors) to active TB. Health problems usually result from multiple interacting factors. When these multiple risk factors come together, they form an interrelated web of forces that increases their potential for causing harm.

McGinnis and Foege (1993) reinforced the significance of addressing lifestyle and environmental determinants of health when they examined the root causes of death in the United States. They proposed that the actual causes of death were not the pathologic disease conditions (e.g., cardiac disease or cancer) existing at the time of death. Rather, the actual causes were external factors such as smoking, diet, and firearms (Box 11-1). The *Behavioral Risk Factor Surveillance System* administered by state health depart-

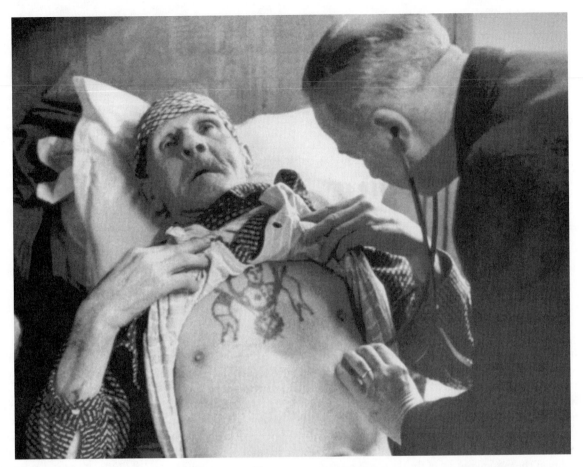

**FIGURE 11-5** Silicosis followed by tuberculosis is the typical story of this miner now pensioned. (From the Library of Medicine, History of Medicine Division; WHO photo by Jean Mohr.)

ments in cooperation with the CDC collects data related to the leading actual causes of death.

Chapters 16 through 22 discuss many health problems related to lifestyle patterns and environmental factors such as accidents, child abuse, suicide, domestic violence, alcoholism, and sexually transmitted diseases (STDs). Anticipatory guidance at each stage across the life span assists individuals, families, and aggregates in developing lifestyle patterns that promote health and reduce the risk of disease and adverse health conditions. Table 11-3 summarizes the measures that help clients at various life stages improve their quality of life.

Health is a part of social, political, and economic justice. During the past 50 years the United Nations has promoted the definition of human rights to include the rights of children, women, and youth; the rights to food and environmental security; the right to safe water; and the right to the highest attainable standard of physical and mental health, including reproductive and sexual health (Rodriguez-Garcia, Akhter, 2000, p. 694). The values that underlie public health are the values of human rights. In a world where there is such gross inequity in the distribution of resources, a firm belief in those values should give the public health professional cause for concern and introspection.

 **BOX 11-1**

## Actual Causes of Death

- Tobacco
- Diet/activity
- Alcohol
- Certain infections
- Toxic agents
- Firearms
- Sexual behavior
- Motor vehicles
- Illicit drug use

From McGinnis MJ, Foege WH: Actual causes of death in the United States, *JAMA* 270:2207-2212, 1993, p. 2208.

## Natural Life History of Disease

In the search for commonalities that may produce disease and health-related phenomena in specific aggregates, epidemiological study focuses on determining the natural life history of these conditions. Observing the natural life history of disease and health-related phenomena aids in

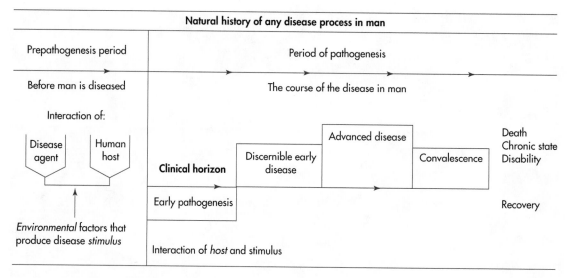

**FIGURE 11-6** Prepathogenesis and pathogenesis periods in the natural history of disease. (From Leavell HR, Clark EG: *Preventive medicine for the doctor in his community: an epidemiological approach*, New York, 1965, McGraw-Hill, p. 18.)

identifying agent-host-environmental factors that influence their development, characteristic signs and symptoms during their different periods of progression, and approaches to preventing and controlling their effects on humans.

The **natural life history of disease** is defined as the course of a disease from onset (inception) to resolution. Many diseases have certain well-defined stages that, taken all together, are referred to as the natural history of the disease in question (Last, 1995, p. 110). In their classic textbook, Leavell and Clark (1965) identified two distinct periods in the natural history of a disease: *prepathogenesis* and *pathogenesis*.

In the *prepathogenesis* period disease has not developed but interactions are occurring between the host, agent, and environment that produce disease stimulus and increase the host's potential for disease. The combination of HIV infection and substance abuse increases the host's potential for developing TB.

The *pathogenesis* period in the natural life history of disease begins when disease-producing stimuli (tubercle bacilli) start to produce changes in the tissues of humans (development of granuloma). Figure 11-6 shows the interrelationship between the prepathogenesis period and the pathogenesis period and how the latter progresses from the presymptomatic stage to advanced, clinical disease. It also shows that disease occurs as a result of processes that happen in the *environment* (prepathogenesis) and processes that happen in *humans* (pathogenesis) (Leavell, Clark, 1965, p. 18). Preventive interventions can alter the natural life history of many diseases.

## Levels of Prevention

The study of the natural life history of disease facilitates the achievement of the ultimate goal of epidemiology—the development of effective methods for preventing and controlling disease or conditions in populations. By identifying significant host-agent-environment relationships that influence

the progression of the natural life history of a condition, the epidemiologist can identify aggregates at risk and develop ways to prevent disease occurrence among them.

A continuum of preventive activities is essential for the promotion of health in any community. Activities can be grouped under three **levels of prevention:** *primary* (health promotion and specific protection), *secondary* (early diagnosis, prompt treatment, and disability limitation), and *tertiary* (rehabilitation). Figure 11-7 identifies preventive activities at all three levels that can alter the natural history of disease. The degree to which preventive activities can be implemented will vary depending on the completeness of knowledge one has about the disease or health problem in question, the complexity of these conditions, and the behavioral and environmental factors influencing the natural life history of the disease (Leavell, Clark, 1965).

## Host-Agent-Environment Relationships

When epidemiologists analyze the natural life history of a disease or a condition for the purpose of identifying preventive measures to eliminate or halt the disease or condition in question, they study the relationships among three variables: **host, agent,** and **environment**. These variables are defined in Table 11-4.

Agents are biological, chemical, or physical and include bacteria, viruses, fungi, pesticides, food additives, ionizing radiation, and speeding objects. The normal habitat in which an infectious (biological) agent lives, multiplies, and/or grows is called a *reservoir*. These habitats include humans, animals, and the environment and are discussed in a later section of this chapter.

A wide variety of characteristics are classified as host factors. Examples of these factors are age, sex, ethnic group, socioeconomic status, lifestyle, and heredity. Four types of environmental factors—physical, social, economic, and family,

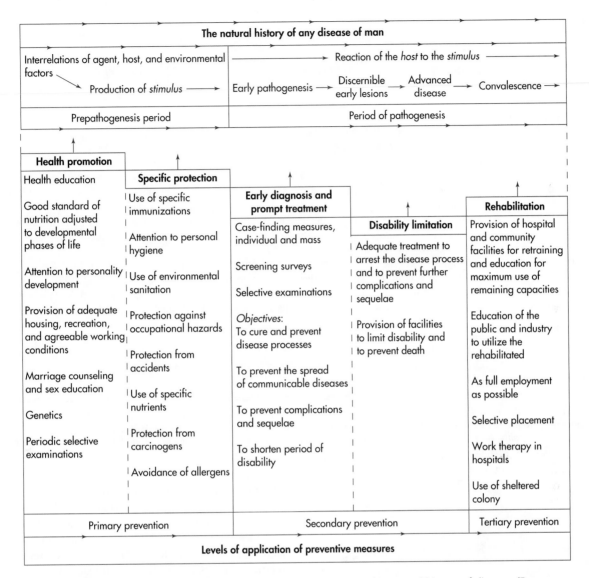

**FIGURE 11-7** Levels of application of preventive measures in the natural history of disease. (From Leavell HR, Clark EG: *Preventive medicine for the doctor in his community: an epidemiological approach*, New York, 1965, McGraw-Hill, p. 21.)

---

**TABLE 11-4**

## Epidemiological Variables: Host, Agent, and Environment

| VARIABLE | DEFINITION |
|---|---|
| HOST | Living species (humans or other animals) capable of being infected or affected by an agent |
|   Primary host | Host in which sexual maturation occurs (e.g., in malaria, the mosquito) |
|   Secondary host | Host in which asexual forms of the parasite develop (e.g., in malaria, a human or other vertebrate mammal or bird) |
|   Transport host | Carrier in which the organism remains alive but does not undergo development |
| AGENT | Factor, such as a microorganism, chemical substance, or form of radiation, whose presence, excessive presence, or (in deficiency diseases) relative absence is essential for the occurrence of a disease |
| ENVIRONMENT | All that which is external to the individual human host; can be divided into physical, biological, social, cultural, etc., any or all of which can influence health status of populations |

Data from Chin J, editor: *Control of communicable diseases manual*, ed 17, Washington, DC, 2000, APHA, p. 570; Last JM: *A dictionary of epidemiology*, ed 3, New York, 1995, Oxford University Press, pp. 5, 53, and 79.

**TABLE 11-5**

*Epidemiological Variables*

| VARIABLE | CHARACTERISTICS |
|---|---|
| **Person:** delineation of group involved | Age, sex, race distribution<br>Socioeconomic status, occupation, education<br>Health habits and behaviors or lifestyle<br>Acquired resistance and susceptibility<br>Health history, natural resistance, hereditary characteristics |
| **Place:** geographic distribution in subdivisions of the area affected | *Physical environment:* weather; climate; geography; radiation; vibration; noise; pressure; animal reservoirs; pollutants; housing facilities; workplace hazards; and sources of air, water, and food contamination<br>*Social environment:* population density and mobility, community groups, occupations and other roles, beliefs and attitudes, technological developments, transportation, educational practices, and health care delivery system<br>*Economic environment:* source of income; income level; employment status; job frustrations; and income for nutrition, housing, and other basic needs<br>*Family environment:* family history; family dynamics; strategies used to handle stress; type, number, and timing of major life changes; home atmosphere; and family health and cultural patterns (see Chapters 7 and 8) |
| **Time:** chronologic distribution of onsets of cases by days, weeks, months | *Incubation period:* determine life cycle; factors affecting multiplication and virulence of organism<br>Seasonal trends<br>Onset of event<br>Duration of event |

Data from MacMahon B, Pugh T: *Epidemiology principles and methods,* Boston, 1970, Little, Brown, pp. 31-32; Centers for Disease Control, Training and Laboratory Program Office: *Principles of epidemiology: agent, host, environment* (self-study course 3030-G, manual 1), Atlanta, 1987a, CDC, pp. 12-30; USDHHS: *Healthy People 2010: with understanding and improving health and objectives for improving health* (in 2 volumes), ed 2, Washington, DC, 2000, US Government Printing Office, pp. 18-20.

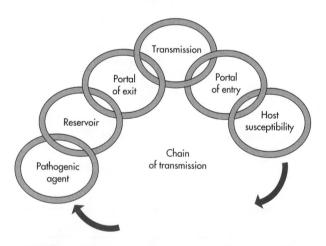

**FIGURE 11-8** Chain of transmission for infection. The chain must be intact for an infection to be transmitted to another host. Transmission can be controlled by breaking any link in the chain. (From Grimes DE: *Infectious diseases,* St Louis, 1991, Mosby, p. 21.)

are discussed in Chapter 6. The dynamic interactions between host-agent-environmental factors and further characteristics of each are discussed later in this chapter.

## Person-Place-Time Relationships

The study of relationships is necessary for the community health professional to formulate valid hypotheses about disease or condition causation. Identification of measurable variables that can facilitate rapid and efficient data collection is essential to this study. In epidemiological study the variables found to be most useful are **person** (who is affected), **place** (where affected), and **time** (when affected) **relationships.** Some of the most frequently analyzed characteristics of these variables are presented in Table 11-5.

TIMING. Timing is a critical factor in disease diagnosis and control. Immediate reporting of a disease outbreak is crucial because the validity of data is often indirectly proportional to the time lapse incurred in obtaining the information. If a significant amount of time is lost in reporting, the ability to formulate valid hypotheses is decreased.

When monitoring incidence of infectious disease, the following terms are used to distinguish relative frequency in time and space:

*Sporadic:* Presence of occasional cases of the event apparently unrelated in time or space

*Endemic:* Constant long-term presence of an event at about the frequency expected from the past history of the community

*Epidemic:* Presence of the event at a much higher frequency than expected from the past history of the community, usually over a short period of time (e.g., one case of cholera would be labeled epidemic in a U.S. community; on the other hand, in some foreign countries, several cases of cholera would be considered an endemic occurrence)

**TABLE 11-6**

*Factors Influencing Infectious Disease Transmission and Progression*

| TERM | DEFINITION |
| --- | --- |
| *Host Characteristics* | |
| Lifestyle factors | Factors (e.g., sanitation practices, sexual habits, food storage, and cooking practices) that facilitate or inhibit agent-host contact |
| Biological factors | Factors that decrease or increase a host's resistance to infection (e.g., general health status, nutritional intake, immune response) |
| General defense mechanisms | External barriers (e.g., skin, nose, and digestive system) that prevent the agent from invading the internal organs of the host and the nonspecific inflammatory response that fights and destroys pathogens |
| Specific defense mechanisms | An immune response that creates host immunity to a specific infectious agent |
| Immunity | Protection from infectious disease associated with the presence of antibodies or cells having a *specific* action on the pathogens that cause a particular infectious disease |
| Passive immunity (temporary, short-duration immunity) | Antibody protection *transferred from another person* either naturally by transplacental transfer from the mother or artificially by inoculation of specific protective antibodies |
| Active immunity (permanent, or long-lasting, immunity) | Antibody and cell protection *produced by the person's own immune system* either naturally by infection with or without clinical manifestations or artificially by inoculation of the agent itself in a killed, modified, or variant form |
| Herd immunity | Resistance of a group or community to invasion and spread of an infectious agent, based on the agent-specific immunity of a high proportion of the population |
| *Agent Characteristics* | |
| Infectivity | The capability of an infectious agent to invade, survive, and multiply in the host |
| Pathogenicity | The power of the agent to produce clinical disease |
| Virulence | The degree of pathogenicity of an infectious agent indicated by the *severity* of disease manifestations (e.g., case-fatality rates and tissue damage) |
| Invasiveness | The capability of an infectious agent to spread and disseminate in the host |
| Toxigenicity | The capability of an infectious agent to produce poisonous products such as exotoxins |
| Antigenicity | The capability of an infectious agent to stimulate the host to produce an immune response (e.g., production of antibodies or antitoxins) |
| *Environmental Characteristics* | |
| Reservoir | Any person, animal, arthropod, plant, soil, or substance in which an infectious agent lives, multiplies, and reproduces itself in a manner that supports survival and transmission |
| Mode of transmission | Any mechanism by which an infectious agent is spread from a source or reservoir to another host |
| Direct transmission | Direct *contact* transmission to a portal of entry, as a result of a host physically touching an infected reservoir, transplacental transfer, or transmission of projected airborne droplet spray |
| Indirect transmission | Transmission through an *intermediate,* contaminated vehicle or vector or an infective vector |

Data from Chin J, editor: *Control of communicable diseases manual,* ed 17, Washington, DC, 2000, APHA, pp. 570-572, 577-579; Grimes DE: *Infectious diseases,* St Louis, 1991, Mosby, pp. 2-3, 20-21; Last JM: *A dictionary of epidemiology,* ed 3, New York, 1995, Oxford University Press, pp. 85, 167-168, 172-174.

*Pandemic:* Presence of an event in epidemic proportions, involving many communities and countries in a relatively short period of time

## THE DYNAMICS OF INFECTIOUS DISEASE TRANSMISSION

Complex interactions between the host, agent, and environment occur before the clinical signs and symptoms of disease are observed. The chain of disease transmission (Figure 11-8) involves a series of events that allows a pathogenic microorganism to come in contact with a host and to invade, multiply, and elicit a physiological response in this host. For infection and subsequent disease to occur, the chain of transmission must remain intact. This requires the presence of a pathogenic agent, an appropriate reservoir, a susceptible host with portals of entry and exit, and favorable environmental conditions that support transmission of the agent. Table 11-6 defines select host, agent, and environmental factors that influence disease transmission and progression.

## Host Characteristics

Host factors affect the ease of contact between the host and agent and the capability of the host to resist the disease-evoking powers of an agent. Lifestyle patterns can significantly influence the host-agent transmission process. Biological characteristics and the host's lines of defense affect how well the host can protect itself against host invasion and dissemination.

A person's (host's) lines of defense (Figure 11-9) can produce inflammatory or immune responses that prevent or contain an infection or destroy the infectious agent. Immunity or protection from infectious disease occurs when an individual's immune response stimulates production of agent-specific antibodies and memory cells (*active immunity*) or when agent-specific antibodies are transferred from one host to another (*passive immunity*). Active immunity is most desirable.

Both passive and active immunity can be acquired either naturally or artificially (Table 11-7). Vaccines produce arti-

ficial immunity. Live attenuated (weakened) and inactivated vaccines are used to produce an immune response in a host. The more similar a vaccine is to the natural disease, the better the immune response to the vaccine. The immune response to a live attenuated vaccine is virtually identical to that produced by a natural infection. In contrast, the immune response to an inactivated vaccine is mostly humoral and little or no cellular immunity results. Table 11-8 identifies the available vaccines by type. Having knowledge of the vaccine type helps predict adverse events, contraindications, and immunization schedule. For example, live attenuated vaccines generally produce long-lasting immunity with a single dose, and adverse reactions to the vac-

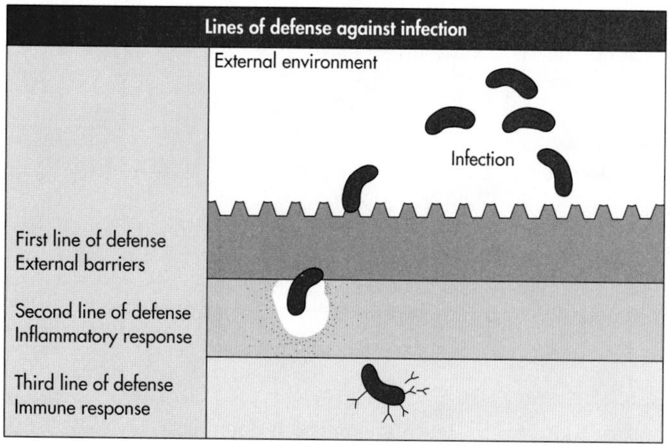

**FIGURE 11-9** Lines of defense against infection. (From Grimes DE: *Infectious diseases*, St Louis, 1991, Mosby, p. 4.)

**TABLE 11-8**

### *Available Vaccines by Type*

#### Live Attenuated Vaccines

| | |
|---|---|
| Viral | Measles, mumps, rubella, polio, yellow fever, vaccinia, varicella |
| Bacterial | Bacille Calmette-Guérin (BCG) |
| Recombinant | Typhoid |

#### Inactivated Vaccines

| | |
|---|---|
| Viral | Influenza, polio, rabies, hepatitis A |
| Bacterial | Pertussis, typhoid, cholera, plague |
| Subunit | Hepatitis B, influenza, acellular pertussis |
| Toxoid | Diphtheria, tetanus |
| Recombinant | Hepatitis B |
| Polysaccharide | Pneumococcal, meningococcal, and *Haemophilus* influenzae type b |

From Atkinson W, Furphy L, Gantt J, et al., editors: *Epidemiology and prevention of vaccine-preventable diseases,* Atlanta, 1995, CDC, pp. 15-17. *Note:* Subunit vaccines are composed of partial bacteria or viruses; toxoids are composed of fractions of bacterial toxins; polysaccharide vaccines are composed of fractions of bacterial cell wall; recombinant vaccines are antigens created by genetic engineering.

**TABLE 11-7**

## *Types of Acquired Immunity*

| TYPE OF IMMUNITY | HOW ACQUIRED | LENGTH OF RESISTANCE |
|---|---|---|
| *Natural* | | |
| Active | Natural contact and infection with the antigen | May be temporary or permanent |
| Passive | Natural contact with antibody transplacentally or through colostrum and breast milk | Temporary |
| *Artificial* | | |
| Active | Inoculation of antigen | May be temporary or permanent |
| Passive | Inoculation of antibody or antitoxin | Temporary |

From Grimes DE: *Infectious diseases,* St Louis, 1991, Mosby, p. 18

cine are usually similar to those produced by a mild form of the natural illness (e.g., fever and rash). Inactivated vaccines always require multiple doses, often require periodic boosting to maintain immunity, and generally produce mostly localized adverse events (e.g., pain at the injection site) with or without fever.

## Agent Characteristics

Agent characteristics influence the likelihood that infection and disease will occur and affect the nature of the disease process. A microorganism that is capable of producing an infection or an infectious disease is commonly referred to as a pathogenic agent. Infection is not synonymous with infectious disease; the result may be inapparent or manifest.

When a pathogenic agent invades a host and multiplies, an inapparent infection occurs. An infection goes through several stages before it produces clinical disease (Figure 11-10). The duration and potential outcomes of each stage vary considerably, depending on agent and host characteristics (Grimes, 1991). Chin (2000) summarizes significant information about the stages of infection for the major communicable diseases in his book *Control of Communicable Diseases Manual*. This book is a valuable reference for any nurse's library.

The concepts that describe the disease-provoking powers of an agent are *infectivity, pathogenicity, virulence, invasiveness, toxigenicity,* and *antigenicity.* These concepts are defined in Table 11-6. Disease-provoking powers of an agent influence a pathogenic agent's ability to invade, multiply, and survive in a host (infectivity) and to produce clinical disease (pathogencity). They also influence the severity of disease (virulence, invasiveness, and toxigenicity). Agents that lack antigenic properties (antigenicity) have a greater chance of surviving in a host than those agents that possess these properties.

The disease-provoking capabilities of an agent vary considerably. While many host-agent relationships result in varying degrees of disease, many others result in inapparent or subclinical infection. From a control perspective, it is important to study asymptomatic individuals exposed to an infectious agent as well as those with visible clinical disease. Individuals with inapparent infection can harbor a specific infectious agent without discernible clinical disease and serve as potential sources of infection. These individuals are *carriers* of disease. Carriers of disease present considerable danger to other hosts because they often do not recognize the need to take action to prevent disease transmission. Individuals for example, can have active TB that is capable of being transmitted to others without realizing that they are ill.

## Environmental Characteristics

Environmental factors influence agent survival and transmission processes. These factors can determine what type of agents is present in a region and may provide reservoirs and

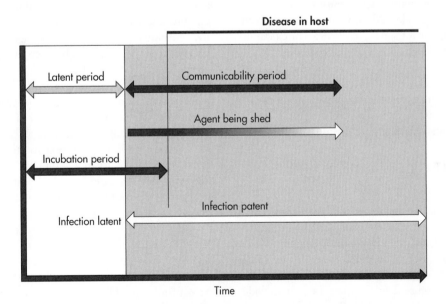

**FIGURE 11-10** Stages of infection. Infection in the host proceeds in identifiable stages; the length of each stage varies with the pathogenic agent and host factors. The *latent period* begins with pathogenic invasion of the body and ends when the agent can be shed (communicability period). The *incubation period* begins with invasion of the agent, during which the organism reproduces, and ends when the disease process begins. The *communicability period* begins when the latent period ends and continues as long as the agent is present. The *disease period* follows the incubation period and ends at variable times. This stage may be subclinical or produce overt symptoms, and it may resolve completely or become latent. (From Grimes DE: *Infectious diseases,* St Louis, 1991, Mosby, p. 19.)

favorable conditions for the spread of disease. For example, malaria is prevalent in tropical and subtropical areas because environmental conditions support the breeding habits of the Anopheles mosquito, the vector that transmits the disease to human hosts. Human reservoirs are also prevalent in these areas and frequently are carriers of the disease. A *reservoir* is any person, animal, arthropod, plant, soil, or substance in which an infectious agent lives, multiplies, and reproduces itself in a manner that supports survival and transmission. The human reservoir may be clinically ill, have a subclinical infection, or be a carrier.

Environmental factors support or inhibit direct or indirect transmission of the pathogenic agent from a reservoir to a susceptible host. *Direct* transmission can occur by actual physical contact with an infected reservoir, by transplacental transfer, or by host inhalation of projected airborne droplet spray. *Indirect* transmission occurs through an intermediate vehicle or vector. A *vehicle* is a contaminated inanimate object or material such as food, water, air, blood, feces, soiled linens, or equipment from a diseased person. Objects contaminated by a diseased individual are referred to as *fomites*. A *vector* is an arthropod or other invertebrate carrier of disease. Vectors may be simple mechanical carriers (flies) or infected nonvertebrate hosts (mosquitos). Vectorborne transmissions have been responsible for major epidemics of disease (e.g., malaria and yellow fever) and have caused extensive morbidity and mortality.

As discussed earlier in this chapter, a balance between host, agent, and environmental factors must be maintained to prevent disease outbreaks. Altering this balance even slightly can cause significant spread of disease. For example, a day-care worker who neglects to wash his or her hands one time after changing an infant's diaper can transmit bacterial diseases such as salmonellosis. Astute community health professionals have been instrumental in preventing bacterial and other types of disease by carefully observing for environmental and host factors that facilitate disease transmission.

## MEASUREMENT OF EPIDEMIOLOGICAL EVENTS

As discussed earlier in this chapter, it is important to monitor the relative *frequency* of an event in time and space to determine health and disease patterns in a community. A variety of methods are used to collect data about these patterns and to identify aggregates at risk in a population. These methods are discussed in Chapter 14 and include such interventions as analyzing all available statistics, carrying out surveys, and interviewing key community informants. Basic statistical concepts used in epidemiology and sources of statistical data are discussed in this chapter.

### Types and Sources of Health Statistics

Statistical data aid health professionals in making comparisons over time and between populations. In community health practice, several terms are used to describe health or health-related data. These are biostatistics, vital statistics, morbidity and mortality statistics, and demographic statistics. **Biostatistics** is the overall broad term used to identify any data that delineate health or population events.

Health statistics that describe birth, adoption, death, marriage, divorce, separation, and annulment patterns are labeled **vital statistics.** CDC's National Center for Health Statistics collects and publishes vital statistics from each state. Despite limitations, these data can assist health professionals in examining trends over time and in establishing health improvement plans. They can be accessed via the internet at *http://www.cdc.gov/scientific.html.*

Vital statistics related to the analysis of death trends are classified as **mortality statistics.** Death certificates are used to obtain demographic information about the deceased as well as the frequency of death, the leading causes of death, and premature mortality. This type of information provides a foundation for assessing the level of wellness in the community. For example, infant and maternal death rates have traditionally been used in community health to make judgments about the health status of a community. Deaths in these two population groups are premature, are considered preventable, and are often associated with poor environmental conditions and inadequate health care. Thus they may reflect not only unmet health needs but also deficiencies in the health care delivery system that need to be corrected.

**Morbidity statistics** are also used to assess the health status of the community. *Morbidity data* describe the extent and distribution of illness and disability in the community, circumstances that affect quality of life as well as productivity. Morbidity in a community is more difficult to evaluate because there is no comprehensive surveillance system that monitors the *incidence* (new cases) of all conditions contributing to morbidity. Hospital discharge records, cancer registry data, and communicable disease surveillance data are used to obtain select information about the extent and distribution of important health problems. Health surveys are selectively conducted to expand the database related to the level of morbidity in a community. As illustrated in the following case scenario, morbidity data can assist the nurse in setting priorities for program planning.

**CASE** *Scenario* One Midwestern community used morbidity statistics to support the need for a neighborhood health clinic in one of its inner-city districts. A comprehensive analysis of these statistics revealed that 52% of all new TB cases, 61% of all new syphilis cases, 72% of all new gonorrhea cases, and 37% of all accidental poisoning cases occurred in one particular section of the city in a given period. It was evident from these data that the health needs in this district were much greater than in other sections of the city. Special funds were allocated to determine if a new approach to delivering health services could alter the morbidity trends; significant positive changes were noted after 3 years. Because morbidity statistics were collected before (known as a baseline for comparison) and during the time the clinic was in existence, city officials responded favorably to a request for additional funds to keep the clinic open. Health professionals in this situation had documented the need for, and the effectiveness of, their pilot-health clinic. The use of statistics assisted these health professionals in establishing a neighborhood health center and in keeping the center functioning after the trial period.

**Demographic statistics** also provide information about significant characteristics of a population that influence community needs and the delivery of health care services. Demographic data describe the number, characteristics, and distribution of people in a given area and socioeconomic changes in the population over time. These data are collected by censuses, special surveys, and registration systems. Census data provide a wealth of information about a community's population characteristics, such as the size and age structure, educational level, economic status, and household composition. These data provide a baseline for analyzing demographic trends over time. Census tracts and census blocks have been established and maintained throughout the country so that social and economic changes can be easily identified from one census to another.

*Census tracts* are small areas in large cities that have a population between 3000 and 6000 persons with fairly homogeneous ethnic and socioeconomic characteristics. *Census blocks* are similar to census tracts but are located almost exclusively in nonmetropolitan areas (Robey, 1989). Census data are analyzed because a significant relationship has been documented between educational background, economic status, and living conditions and the frequency of health needs in specified populations (U.S. Department of Health and Human Services [USDHHS], 2000).

Further sources of health data are shared in Chapter 14. It is important to remember that all data collection systems are subject to error and have limitations. For example, some data collection systems have comprehensive information about a small subset in the population (e.g., cancer registries), whereas others have very selective information regarding 100% of the population (e.g., census). However, both cancer registries and the census are limited by the amount of information respondents remember and are willing to share. The data also can be limited by respondents' interpretations of questions and recording procedures. Users of data systems need to examine strengths and limitations from the perspectives of sample size, characteristics of the population assessed, type of data obtained, and potential sources of inaccuracy (National Center for Health Statistics, 2000). This information is readily available from standardized data sets.

## Use of Relative Numbers

When practitioners analyze the *frequency* of health events in populations, they express absolute numbers or actual counts in terms of relative numbers. Using relative numbers makes it easier to compare results in populations of differing sizes or to visualize what proportion of a given population is affected by the event of interest. A relative number is one that shows a relationship between two absolute numbers; this relationship is expressed in terms of a multiplier or a round number. A percentage is an example of a relative number.

The value of using relative numbers becomes clearer when the nurse actually works with raw data. Raw data from populations of differing sizes cannot be compared unless absolute numbers are converted to relative numbers. For example, knowing the number of students who received free lunches in 2000 in each school in the county becomes relevant only when one summarizes the percentage of children in each school who received free lunches. The following example illustrates how deceptive absolute numbers can be when comparisons of one population with another are made: 250 students receive free lunches at Burns Park High School, while only 75 students receive free lunches at Kent Elementary School. However, even though the number of children (250 vs. 75) receiving free lunches is much higher for Burns Park High School, the proportion of students needing free lunches in Kent Elementary School is two times greater than the proportion of students needing free lunches in Burns Park High School:

75/150 × 100 = 50% of the children in Kent Elementary School received free lunches in 2000

250/1000 × 100 = 25% of the children in Burns Park High School received free lunches in 2000

## Measures of Central Tendency

Descriptive measures, such as averages, are used to organize and characterize health data when a series of measurements or quantitative data are analyzed. Generally, in any series of data, characteristic values tend to cluster near the center of the distribution. Thus averages are often labeled *measures of central tendency.* The most commonly used measures of central tendency in community health nursing practice are the arithmetic mean, the median, and the mode.

The *mean* is the arithmetic average of a set of observations. It is the value in a series of data equivalent to the sum of the measurements divided by the number of measurements.

The formula for calculating the mean is:

$$\text{Arithmetic mean} = \frac{\textit{sum of measurements}}{\text{no. of measurements}}$$

Knowing the mean, or average value of a series of measurements helps the community health nurse quickly identify persons who may have health needs or who are at risk for health problems in the future. Persons who fall far below or far above the average should be comprehensively assessed to determine why this is happening. For example, if the mean weight of children in a second grade classroom is 51 pounds, a community health nurse would examine why one of these children, who weighs 70 pounds, was deviating so far from the norm.

The *median* is the middle value in a series of quantitative data that divides the measurements into two equal parts. That is, 50% of the measurements are less than and 50% are greater than the median value. To calculate the median, the measurements in the distribution must be arranged in order of size.

The median is usually computed when there are very high or very low extremes in a series of measurements, because the mean is distorted by very high or low values but the median is not. For example, when census tract data are reported, median income is usually given because there is such a great variation in family income.

The *mode* is the measurement that appears most frequently in a series of quantitative data. It is identified by counting the number of times a particular value appears. The measurements do not have to be ordered. The mode is helpful when one wants to identify a measure of central tendency value quickly. It is only an estimate, however, and other measurements of central tendency should be used when refining data analysis. The mean is the most frequently used measure of central tendency in community health practice because it is the most stable.

## Rates and Ratios

In addition to percentages and measures of central tendency, rates and ratios are commonly used to analyze the frequency of health events in a community. A *ratio* is a fraction that expresses the size of one number (numerator) in relation to another number (denominator). It is a general term of which a rate, percentage, and proportion are subsets. The number of women to men (sex ratio) and per capita expenditure for health care in a given state are examples of ratios. Per capita ratios are obtained by dividing the amount of money spent for health care (event) by the population in a given state.

A *proportion* is a ratio in which the numerator is included in the denominator, which means that the population affected is a subset of the total population at risk. A *rate* is also a ratio with the additional features of expressing what has happened in terms of a defined time period and the population at risk for a given event. Rates are proportions. Rates delineate the relationship between the number of times an event has occurred to the size of the population at risk. In demographic and epidemiological study, the unit of time for a rate is usually a *year* unless otherwise stated.

A rate is calculated by dividing the number of measured events (numerator) in a specified period by the size of the population at risk (denominator). To adjust for population changes over the year, the estimated midyear population is used as the denominator. A multiplier or a standard base population size is usually used to convert the rate from an awkward fraction or decimal to a whole number: the multi-

plier is one that makes the rate above the value of 1. For example, if an event such as polio occurs infrequently within a large population at risk, the multiplier used would be "per 100,000 population." On the other hand, when an event such as death occurs frequently within a population at risk, the multiplier used would be "per 1000 population." The relationships between the components of a rate are displayed in the following equation:

$$\text{Rate} = \frac{\text{Number of events in specified period} \times \text{multiplier}}{\text{Population at risk during the specified period}}$$

Frequently used rates and ratios in community health nursing practice are displayed in Table 11-9. It is important to note that some of these rates are restricted by a particular characteristic of interest (e.g., age-specific or cause-specific), whereas others include the total population without reference to any characteristics of the individuals in this population. Rates that restrict the dimensions of the numerator and denominator are known as *specific rates*. Rates that include the total population are known as *general* or *crude rates*. At times a specific rate uses the total population as the denominator because the total population is at risk for a specified event (e.g., cause-specific death rate).

Crude death rates must be standardized or adjusted before comparing them across populations because these rates do not take into consideration the profound impact age has on death rates. *Standardized rates* or *adjusted rates* are crude rates that have been modified to control for the effects of age or other characteristics and thereby allow for valid comparisons of rates.

## Morbidity and Mortality Statistics

In epidemiological study, morbidity and mortality data are used to provide a foundation for examining the level of health in a community. Crude, or general, death rates assist a community in identifying leading health problems in the total population. Specific death rates (e.g., age-specific) help target health resources for populations at risk. For example, hypertension screening and educational programs may focus on African Americans because the heart disease mortality rate is higher among African Americans than among the total population. Formulas for calculating crude and specific death rates are identified in Table 11-9.

A major goal in epidemiology is to prevent premature mortality. The impact of premature death is often described in terms of *Years of Potential Life Lost* (YPLL). The YPLL rate is an age-adjusted measure of premature mortality (death before age 65 years) in a population (Johnson, 1995). Major causes of death that primarily affect younger people, such as infant mortality, homicide, and HIV infection significantly influence YPLL rates. Health disparities among Americans in terms of YPLL are significant; they are discussed in Chapter 13.

**TABLE 11-9**

## Frequently Used Rates and Ratios in Community Health Nursing Practice

| RATE OR RATIO | FORMULA | COMMONLY USED MULTIPLIER |
|---|---|---|
| **Mortality Statistics** | | |
| Crude death rate | Number of deaths from all causes during a given year ÷ population estimated at midyear | × 1000 population |
| Age-specific death rate | Number of deaths for a specified age group during a given year ÷ population estimated at midyear for the specified age group | × 1000 population |
| Cause-specific death rate | Number of deaths from a specific condition during a given year ÷ population estimated at midyear | × 100,000 population |
| Maternal mortality rate | Number of deaths from puerperal complications during a given year ÷ number of live births during the same year | × 100,000 live births |
| Infant mortality rate | Number of deaths under 1 year of age during a given year ÷ number of live births during the same year | × 1000 live births |
| Neonatal mortality rate | Number of deaths under 28 days of age during a given year ÷ number of live births during the same year | × 1000 live births |
| Fetal mortality rate | Number of fetal deaths 20 weeks' gestation or more during a given year ÷ number of live births and fetal deaths during the same year | × 1000 live births and fetal deaths |
| Birth-death ratio | Number of live births in a specified population ÷ number of deaths in a specified population | × 100 |
| Case fatality ratio | Number of deaths from specified disease or condition ÷ number of reported cases of the specified disease or condition | × 100 |
| **Morbidity Statistics** | | |
| Incidence rate | Number of new cases of a specified disease or condition occurring during a given time period ÷ population at risk during the same time period | × 100,000 population |
| Prevalence rate (ratio) | Number of old and new cases of specified disease or condition existing at a point ÷ total population at a point | × 100,000 population |
| **Vital and Demographic Statistics Other than Mortality** | | |
| Crude birth rate | Number of live births during a given year ÷ population estimated at midyear | × 1000 population |
| General fertility rate | Number of live births during a given year ÷ population estimated at midyear for females ages 15-44 during the same year | × 1000 female population (15-44 years old) |
| General marriage rate | Number of marriages during a given year ÷ number of persons 15 years of age and over in the population in the same year | × 1000 persons 15 years of age and over |
| General divorce rate | Number of divorces during a given year ÷ persons 15 years of age and over in the population in the same year | × 1000 persons 15 years of age and over |
| Dependency ratio | Persons under 20 years of age and persons 65 years and over ÷ total population ages 20-64 | × 100 |

Significant health disparities among Americans in terms of morbidity (disease) also exist. The concepts of incidence and prevalence are used to identify these disparities as well as to track the frequency of disease occurrence. *Incidence* is the number of *new* cases of a disease in a population over a specified period of time. It is often expressed as a rate that is calculated using the following formula:

$$\text{Incidence Rate} = \frac{\text{Number of new cases in a specified period} \times \text{multiplier}}{\text{Population at risk during the same period}}$$

Bay City, January through December 2000, 25 new cases of diabetes in a population of 50,000.

$$\text{Incidence rate} = \frac{25 \times 100,000}{50,000} = 50$$

Incidence rate for diabetes in Bay City, 2000: 50 new cases of diabetes per 100,000 population.

Incidence rates assist community health professionals in examining the rate of increase or decrease of morbidity during a defined time period.

Prevalence examines the extent of morbidity in a community. *Prevalence* is the number of cases (new and old) of a specified disease or condition existing at a given time. Prevalence is often expressed as a rate that is calculated using the following formula:

Prevalence rate (ratio) = the number of new and old cases of a specified disease or condition existing at a given point divided by the total population estimated at midyear times a multiplier.

Example: Bay City, December 2000, 600 cases of diabetes in a population of 50,000.

$$\text{Prevalence rate (ratio)} = \frac{600}{50,000} \times 100,000 = 1200$$

Prevalence rate (ratio) for diabetes in Bay City, December 2000: 1200 cases of diabetes per 100,000 population.

Prevalence is also expressed as a percentage (e.g., 1.2% of the population had diabetes in Bay City in December 2000).

The prevalence of disease and conditions in a community is influenced by many factors such as the rate of new cases, the number of existing cases, cause-specific mortality

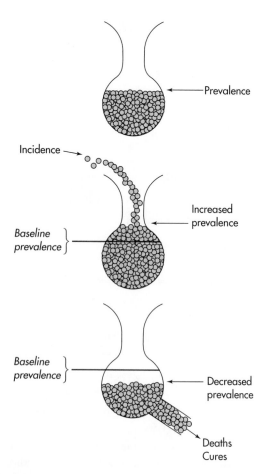

**FIGURE 11-11** Relationship between incidence and prevalence. (Modified from Gordis L: *Epidemiology,* Philadelphia, 1996, Saunders, p. 33.)

trends, population mobility patterns, and an array of factors that promote disease occurrence. Figure 11-11 illustrates the relationship between incidence and prevalence. Monitoring prevalence and incidence of morbidity assists community planners in developing interventions that prevent disease and promote health.

## EPIDEMIOLOGICAL PROCESS AND INVESTIGATION

Basic concepts in epidemiology have been discussed to lay a foundation for epidemiological investigation of community health problems. These concepts aid in identifying variables that public health professionals consider when they describe the distribution patterns and determinants of health, disease, and condition frequencies in populations. They help analyze causal relationships in disease or condition outbreaks. To establish these causal relationships, health professionals use a scientific process known as the *epidemiological process*.

The epidemiological process is a systematic course of action taken to identify (1) who is affected (persons), (2) where the affected persons reside (place), (3) when the persons were affected (time), (4) causal factors of health and disease occurrence (host-agent-environment determinants), (5) prevalence and incidence of health and disease (frequencies), and (6) prevention and control measures (levels of prevention) in relation to the natural life history of a disease or a condition.

The epidemiological process has eight basic steps, which are graphically illustrated in Figure 11-1. Although each step is discussed separately, it is important to remember that these steps overlap and may not always follow a sequential pattern. They are interrelated and dependent on each other. For example, data collected in the initial step provide a foundation for all subsequent steps.

### Step I: Determine the Nature, Extent, and Possible Significance of the Problem

The primary responsibilities during this initial step are twofold: (1) to verify the diagnosis by data collection from multiple sources, and (2) to determine the extent and possible significance of the verified problem. Data gathering begins when an index case is reported or when there is a noticeable change in the incidence rate for a particular disease or condition. The *index case* is the case that brings a household or other group to the attention of community health personnel. Once this case is known to health professionals, data are collected from various sources to determine if a problem really exists.

Clinical observations, laboratory studies, and lay reporting assist the epidemiological team in confirming the homogeneity of the current events. If, for instance, four hospital emergency rooms have reported that several individuals were treated for food poisoning in the last 24 hours, health personnel would want to immediately take the following actions:

1. Interview the affected persons to determine the nature of their symptoms and to identify loci of origin according to person, place, and time.
2. Review laboratory studies to confirm a common causative organism. This process could establish that several events are occurring at the same time.
3. Interview friends, relatives, and lay acquaintances to discern their description of the events that led up to the reported illness and to determine if other individuals have symptoms.

Timely, accurate, and thorough data collection is a critical factor in Step I. Significant data may be destroyed if the data collection process is too slow. In addition, if only the most obvious events—the "tip of the iceberg"—are observed, the extent of the problem will not be identified. The health professional needs to be a detective, beginning by interviewing the affected individual and then branching out into this individual's environment to track down the host-agent-environment factors that influence disease occurrence. As previously discussed, the measurable variables that facilitate rapid and efficient data collection about host-agent-environment factors are person, place, and time.

Analyzing data in terms of person, place, and time helps establish the magnitude of the problem. Data tell the health professional the proportion of the people affected, the seriousness of the effects on the host and the community, improvement or regression over time, and geographic distribution of the disease or condition. They also help in identifying potential sources of infection and causal relationships.

The use of a Geographic Information System (GIS) facilitates pinpointing the exact geographic location of a disease or condition. "A GIS is mapping software that links information about where things are with what things are like. Unlike a paper map where 'what you see is what you get', a GIS map can combine layers of information" (*http://www.gis.com/whatisgis/whatisgis.html*). The software can track sources of diseases and the movement of contagions, and thus, agencies can respond more effectively to outbreaks by identifying at-risk populations and targeting interventions. The website provided gives examples about this innovative technology.

When prevalence and incidence rates are compared, a word of caution is necessary. If there is a distinct departure from normal, it must be ascertained that a problem really exists. It may be that there is only an improvement in reporting, not an actual increase in disease occurrence. If there is an actual increase in the incidence of a particular disease or condition, the health professional makes an educated guess as to the nature of the causative agent, based on the data collected. This formulation of a tentative diagnosis or hypothesis is done to enhance further data collection.

## Step II: Formulate Tentative Hypothesis(es)

When epidemiologists are dealing with infectious diseases, a rapid preliminary analysis of data is imperative. Disease can spread quickly, affecting a large number of people in a short period of time, and can have great ranges in severity. Usually this analysis results in the formulation of several hypotheses. Explanation of the most probable source of infection is made in terms of (1) the agent causing the problem; (2) the source of infection, including the chain of events leading to the outbreak of the problem; and (3) environmental conditions that allowed it to occur. Tentative hypotheses must be tested and may be found to be inappropriate.

Laboratory tests are invaluable in validating hypotheses. For example, different strains of M. *tuberculosis* can be compared on the basis of their genetic content or genotype, called DNA fingerprinting. The DNA is cut up into pieces. Then the number and sizes of these pieces are measured by placing them in a gel-like substance across which a pulsing electrical field is applied. The result is a pattern of bands resembling a bar code, which is the "fingerprint."

These patterns can be compared with others to determine the potential relatedness of bacterial strains. The information can be used to:

- Determine whether bacterial isolates from different clients are potentially related
- Determine if a clinical isolate matches those obtained from samples implicated in an outbreak
- Determine if a particular isolate is being found in other states or regions

PulseNet is a national network of public health laboratories that performs DNA fingerprinting on foodborne bacteria using pulsed field gel electrophoresis (PFGE). The network permits rapid comparison of those "fingerprint" patterns among participating states, through an electronic database at the CDC. The CDC's website* provides detailed information about this innovative technology. Box 11-2 gives examples of the use of PFGE in Tennessee.

**BOX 11-2**

### *Examples of the Use of Pulsed Field Gel Electrophoresis in Tennessee*

Identifying a case of *Salmonella newport* infection in Tennessee as likely being associated with consumption of unpasteurized orange juice while on vacation in a western state

Excluding an unrelated "sporadic" case of *Escherichia coli* O157:H7 from a school-associated outbreak of gastroenteritis

Identifying three different strains of *S. newport* as being part of concurrent, multistate clusters, one of which was associated with a widely distributed processed meat

Confirming that the *Salmonella bareilly* isolated from an ill person matched the bacteria cultured from their private well

Identifying a strain of *S. newport* isolated from a restaurant employee as matching the strain implicated in an outbreak among that establishment's patrons

*Centers for Disease Control and Prevention: *http://www.cdc.gov/ncidod/emergplan/*

The following scenario illustrates how hypotheses are established, using laboratory data as well as other information.

**CASE Scenario** Over a period of 3 years, active TB was diagnosed in 38 inmates and 5 guards from a large urban jail that housed about 2700 inmates. Because jails usually house prisoners awaiting trial or those sentenced to terms of less than a year, inmates are frequently part of the local community. As part of determining the source and extent of this outbreak, medical records of inmates and guards with TB were reviewed and inmates were interviewed. DNA fingerprinting was performed on the M. *tuberculosis* isolates. Nineteen (79%) of the 24 culture-positive inmates had isolates with DNA fingerprints matching those of other inmates. Isolates from both culture-positive guards matched the predominant inmate strain; only 6 (14%) of 43 isolates from infected persons in the community had this pattern. The median length of incarceration of all inmates in the jail was 1 day; the median length of continuous incarceration before diagnosis of TB in inmates was 138 days. Inmates with TB had been incarcerated a median of 15 times. Forty-three percent of persons in the city where the jail was located who had TB diagnosed during a specified time period had been incarcerated in the jail at some time before diagnosis (Jones, Craig, Valway, et al., 1999, p. 557).

## Step III: Collect and Analyze Further Data to Test Hypothesis(es)

A basic starting point in this step is to identify the group affected by the disease or problem under investigation. In the previous scenario, the inmates and guards composed the obvious group of concern; however, people out in the community were also at risk for contracting TB. Individual epidemiological histories should be done to classify persons according to their exposure to suspected or causative agents and to identify the clinical data and bacteriological findings needed to substantiate the diagnosis. Significant variation of incidence in contrasted population groups should be noted. These variations can be identified through study of attack rates. In the jail population, longer and frequent incarceration was related to diagnosis.

An *attack rate* is an incidence rate that identifies the number of people at risk who became ill. In studying a food-borne disease outbreak, the attack rate for persons who ate certain foods would be compared with the attack rate for persons who did not eat certain foods. This is done in an attempt to identify which food was infected by the causative agent. Attack rates are calculated in the following manner:

$$\frac{\text{No. of persons affected}}{\text{No. of persons eating food item}} \times 100$$

$$\frac{\text{No. of persons affected}}{\text{No. of persons not eating food item}} \times 100$$

Table 11-10 illustrates how attack rates are graphically summarized. The attack rates in this table were calculated when people became ill after a banquet. They show that one food item, custard, was probably the infected food (note the differences between the two attack rate percentages). Generally the vulnerable food that shows the greatest differences between the two attack rate percentages is the infected food.

It is essential to remember that attack rates do not positively confirm an infective food. Last (1986, pp. 35-36) has identified the following five reasons why the association of illness with a particular food is often difficult:

1. Some individuals are resistant to the agent and do not become ill even though they are exposed.
2. The employed definition of an ill person may include some who have unrelated illnesses, unless there is a specific test; and even then, if the illness is one that is prevalent, the ill subjects may include some cases not caused by the ingestion of the common vehicle.
3. Contamination of one food by traces of another may take place before or during serving.
4. Errors in history-taking may occur. These may be unbiased errors, caused by memory lapses or misunderstanding, or they may be caused by biases, either on the part of the questioner or the subject. Several kinds of biases

**TABLE 11-10**

## *Attack Rate Table*

| VULNERABLE FOOD | PERSONS WHO DID EAT VULNERABLE FOOD | | | | PERSONS WHO DID NOT EAT VULNERABLE FOOD | | | |
|---|---|---|---|---|---|---|---|---|
| | SICK | WELL | TOTAL | ATTACK RATE (%) | SICK | WELL | TOTAL | ATTACK RATE (%) |
| Baked ham | 19 | 56 | 75 | 25 | 30 | 5 | 35 | 86 |
| Custard | 45 | 15 | 60 | 75 | 4 | 46 | 50 | 8 |
| Gelatin | 20 | 35 | 55 | 36 | 29 | 26 | 55 | 53 |
| Cole slaw | 48 | 58 | 106 | 45 | 1 | 3 | 4 | 25 |
| Baked beans | 45 | 55 | 100 | 45 | 4 | 6 | 10 | 40 |
| Potato salad | 25 | 45 | 70 | 36 | 24 | 16 | 40 | 60 |

From Communicable Disease Center: *Food-borne disease investigation: analysis of field data,* Atlanta, 1964, US Public Health Service, p. 8.

are possible; the questioner may have a preconceived notion of what food was responsible and press the questions more vigorously with respect to that food in the case of ill persons than non-ill persons; or the subject may have preconceived notions leading to the same result. The subject may have reasons for wishing to either claim or disclaim illness. Biases may affect the accuracy either of food histories or illness histories and produce spurious association.

5. Finally, biased sampling also may lead to spurious results.

All of these factors can affect the validity of an attack rate and thereby the choice of the appropriate infective food. Laboratory studies are necessary to identify the etiologic agent and its vehicle or vector. However, identifying the causative agent is not the only step in preventing further spread of disease. Knowing the agent assists in treating ill individuals who seek medical care but does not tell how the disease is being transmitted. The chain of transmission must be broken to stop the spread of disease.

Because one factor alone never causes a disease or condition, it is not sufficient to identify just the causative agent. After the possible agents and the attack group have been identified, the common source(s) to which affected individuals were exposed should be investigated. With foodborne disease, the origin, method, and preparation of suspected foods would be primary factors to examine. Concurrently, environmental conditions should be evaluated. These conditions would include such things as the sanitary status of the restaurant, the area where food was served, and the water and dairy supply. Appendix 11-1 depicts the type of data that one state collects when enteric infections are suspected. Community health nurses frequently are responsible for collecting these data during an epidemiological investigation. In some health departments, nurses also are responsible for collecting specimens for laboratory analysis. The epidemiological division of the state or local health department provides information on how to properly collect, preserve, and ship specimens for epidemiological analysis.

Completing an epidemiological case history form provides an opportunity for health teaching and casefinding. Often the community health nurse identifies new cases during this process and helps clients learn about the nature of the disease and how to prevent its spread.

It is important to use a variety of data-collection methods in determining the extent and source of an epidemiological problem because many individuals frequently do not seek care. Figure 11-12 is the Burden of Illness Pyramid. Using survey data, the CDC has determined the proportion of people in the population having a diarrheal illness and from among them, the number who will seek medical care, as well as the proportion of physicians who order a bacterial stool culture to determine the involved pathogen (CDC, 2000a). The researchers have concluded that for each culture-confirmed

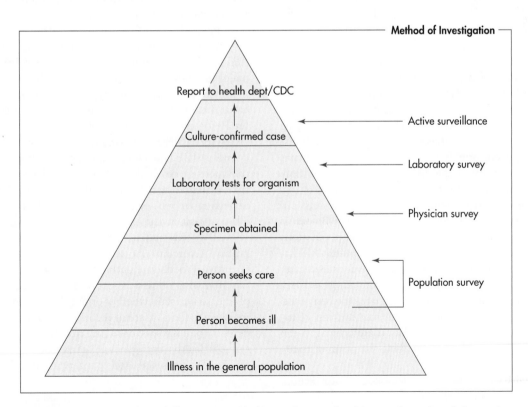

**FIGURE 11-12** Burden of illness pyramid. (From Centers for Disease Control and Prevention (CDC): *FoodNet 1999 surveillance results, preliminary report,* Atlanta, March 2000a, CDC.)

case of illness, there are 38 people who are not reported. The pyramid illustrates the importance of the laboratory in detecting foodborne illnesses.

Tentative hypotheses must be tested; sometimes, however, none of the original hypotheses is appropriate. Testing hypotheses helps determine if the initial control measures were sufficient to resolve the current outbreak. It also aids in identifying the natural life history of the disease and where further action is needed.

## Step IV: Plan for Control

When planning for control, it is essential to identify preventive activities based on the knowledge of the natural history of the disease in question, which can be used to control the further spread of disease occurrence. Host-agent-environment factors should be analyzed to determine the following:

1. Populations at risk
2. Primary, secondary, and tertiary preventive measures available that would
   a. Alter the behavior or susceptibility of the host (e.g., health education, casefinding, immunization, treatment, or rehabilitation)
   b. Destroy the agent (e.g., heat, drug treatment, or spraying with insecticides)
   c. Eliminate the transmission of the agent (e.g., changes in host's health habits or environmental conditions)
3. Feasibility of implementing the control plan, considering such factors as available community resources, time required, cost of control versus partial or no control, facilities, supplies, and personnel needed
4. Priorities in relation to legal mandates, significance of the problem relative to other community needs, and the feasibility of implementing the control plan

BREAKING THE CHAIN OF TRANSMISSION. Control measures are generally directed toward breaking the chain of transmission (see Figure 11-8). This includes destroying or treating the reservoir of infection, interrupting the transmission of the agent from the reservoir to the new host, and decreasing the ability of the agent to adapt and multiply within the host. The concept of multiple causation of disease must be used in breaking the chain of transmission. The TB outbreak in an urban jail illustrates how difficult it can be to break the chain of transmission. Jail populations have a high prevalence of risk factors for communicable diseases, including crowding; lack of intensive health care; rapid turnover in and out into the community; and frequently, substance abuse. Screening inmates for active TB at the time of admission and avoiding introduction of infectious persons into the jail population are critical to the prevention of TB in jails, thus breaking the chain of transmission.

HERD IMMUNITY. When epidemiologists are dealing with infectious diseases and establishing a control plan, the concept of **herd immunity** is important. It is defined as the

"immunity of a group or community. The resistance of a group to invasion and spread of an infectious agent is based on the resistance to infection of a high proportion of individual members of the group" (Chin, 2000, p. 570). Immunity is "that resistance usually associated with the presence of antibodies or cells that have a specific action on the microorganism concerned with a particular infectious disease or on its toxin" (Chin, 2000, p. 571). Characteristics of the different types of immunity are presented in Table 11-6.

If 100% of a given group had received measles vaccine, the herd immunity would be 100%. If 80% had received measles vaccine, the herd immunity would be at least 80%. Some people in the group have natural immunity, raising the percentage higher.

Herd immunity does not have to be 100% to prevent an epidemic or to control a disease, but it is not known just what percentage is safe. A national goal of *Healthy People 2010* is the total elimination of congenital rubella syndrome, diphtheria, *Haemophilus influenzae* type b, measles, mumps, polio, rubella, and tetanus; 41% improvement for pertussis; 99% improvement for hepatitis B; and 99% improvement for varicella (USDHHS, 2000, p. 14-11).

As herd immunity decreases, the chances for epidemics rise. In the United States a major concern is that many school-age children are not receiving immunizations for communicable diseases. Immunization coverage levels vary substantially by state and large urban areas, which greatly decreases the level of herd immunity and is a major barrier to maintaining community health.

Community health nurses are instrumental in helping the public see the need for effective control of disease through active immunization. This will continue to be a major function of the community health nurse because immunizing populations at risk is the most effective way to control many childhood communicable diseases (see Chapter 16 for immunization schedules).

CASEFINDING. **Casefinding** is a major function of epidemiologists. The process focuses on early diagnosis and treatment of newly discovered cases of a disease or condition. Casefinding may evolve through clinical observation, reviewing records, or by mass or individual screening. The TB outbreak in the urban jail was found when nurses reviewed records and found high numbers of inmates with positive tuberculin skin tests. Other examples of casefinding occur with foodborne outbreaks: people who were part of a function where illness is reported are contacted, usually by phone, to ascertain whether or not they became ill after eating specific foods. Careful record keeping assists epidemiologists to quickly spot changing trends in diseases or conditions. Health departments carry out surveillance of reportable diseases at weekly intervals (Box 11-3) to track changes in diseases that can quickly involve large numbers of citizens. These data are then reported to the CDC so that national trends are constantly surveyed.

**BOX 11-3**

*Infectious Diseases Designated as Notifiable at the National Level—United States, 2000\**

| | |
|---|---|
| Acquired immunodeficiency syndrome (AIDS) | Lyme disease |
| Anthrax | Malaria |
| Botulism | Measles |
| Brucellosis | Meningococcal disease |
| Chancroid | Mumps |
| *Chlamydia trachomatis,* genital infections | Pertussis |
| Cholera | Plague |
| Coccidiodomycosis | Poliomyelitis, paralytic |
| Cryptosporidiosis | Psittacosis |
| Cyclosporiasis | Q fever |
| Diptheria | Rabies, animal |
| Ehrlichiosis, human granulocytic | Rabies, human |
| Ehrlichiosis, human monocytic | Rocky Mountain spotted fever |
| Encephalitis, California serogroup viral | Rubella |
| Encephalitis, eastern equine | Salmonellosis |
| Encephalitis, St. Louis | Shigellosis |
| Encephalitis, western equine | Streptococcal disease, invasive, Group A |
| *Escherichia coli* O157:H7 | *Streptococcus pneumoniae,* drug resistant |
| Gonorrhea | Streptococcal toxic-shock syndrome |
| *Haemophilus influenzae,* invasive disease | Syphilis |
| Hansen disease (leprosy) | Syphilis, congenital |
| Hantavirus pulmonary syndrome | Tetanus |
| Hemolytic uremic syndrome, postdiarrheal | Toxic-shock syndrome |
| Hepatitis A | Trichinosis |
| Hepatitis B | Tuberculosis |
| Hepatitis, C/non A, non B | Tularemia |
| HIV infection, adult (≥13 years) | Typhoid fever |
| HIV infection, pediatric (<13 years) | Varicella (deaths only) |
| Legionellosis | Yellow fever |
| Listeriosis | |

From Centers for Disease Control and Prevention (CDC): Changes in national notifiable diseases data presentation, *MMWR* 49(39) October 6, 2000, p. 892.

\*Although not a nationally notifiable disease, the Council of State and Territorial Epidemiologists recommends reporting cases of varicella (chickenpox) through the National Notifiable Diseases Surveillance System.

## Step V: Implement Control Plan

An active effort should be made to elicit and coordinate the cooperation of the lay public, as well as private and official agencies, when control measures are put into operation. A control program that takes into consideration the beliefs, attitudes, and customs of the community is more likely to be accepted by the public than one that ignores community norms.

**CASE Scenario** In one rural area, recent migrants from Mexico are employed by poultry processing plants. The work is difficult and undesirable and the pay often low. The local health department was asked by the plant supervisors to administer tuberculin skin tests to their employees, as company policy (casefinding). The result was that 100 out of the 450 employees had positive tests, not an unexpected result, since the prevalence of TB in many Latino countries is several times greater than in the United States. The employees did not have health insurance; many of them sent 90% of their earnings back to Mexico to their families and did not want to leave work for treatment. Further, the concept of taking medication every day for an extended period of time was difficult: time was limited, planning was hard, and medicine was expensive. Treating and controlling this very serious epidemic depended on a plan that met the personal and work needs of those involved. A plan was developed for the plant nurses to administer the medication at work; the state TB program paid for the medication. Policies to ensure confidentiality were put into place. Their families were brought into clinic for TB skin testing. Although a number of the immigrants were lost to follow-up because of moving away, a high percentage of them received adequate treatment.

Health education programs can help "sell" a control program in the community, especially if they deal with current community attitudes and beliefs. In the situation above, the local Catholic Spanish-speaking churches were contacted, and translators were hired to assist with communication.

**BARRIERS TO CONTROL PLAN.** There are many barriers to the successful implementation of a control plan for both infectious disease and noncommunicable conditions. Barriers to control involve factors such as unknown etiology, no known treatment, unavailable community resources, multifaceted etiology, long latency periods, and lack of reporting. In the preceding scenario, many of the migrants lived in small homes with 15 to 20 other people. Limited resources gave these folks few other choices; however, it put them all at high risk for exposure to TB and other communicable diseases.

An individual without overt disease symptoms but who harbors the disease organism can be a major vehicle in disease transmission. Such individuals are known as *carriers*. Hepatitis C and salmonellosis are examples of diseases that are often transmitted by carriers.

With any disease and for a variety of reasons, some individuals will delay or not seek treatment. Whatever the reason, a delay in confirmation and treatment of the disease can enhance its spread and continuation and impede control plan implementation.

Individuals for whom the diagnosis is not suspected or confirmed are also barriers to the control of disease. Disease may not be confirmed for several reasons. Some people will have atypical symptoms of the disease in question. If clinical symptoms do not fit a disease model, the disease may be missed completely or misdiagnosed. Other individuals are seen too early or too late in the course of the disease process to either suspect or confirm the disease. In these situations, laboratory tests may be falsely negative, or they may not be done at all because the clinical symptoms do not reflect a need. At other times a diagnosis cannot be confirmed because specimens (stools, emesis, or sputum) inadvertently have been destroyed or handled improperly. Epidemiologists are cognizant that specimens are needed for laboratory testing, and often this is the only way that an infectious disease agent is identified. The identified agent often dictates the treatment of the disease and the program of prevention that needs to be instituted.

## Step VI: Evaluate Control Plan

An important part of the epidemiological process is evaluation. This ensures that a process can be improved the next time it is repeated. The first step in evaluation is to determine how well the objectives of the process were met. This implies that, before carrying out the process, objectives were clearly and behaviorally written. The next question to be answered is how the current situation compares to the situation before the investigation. Finally, the practicality of the control measures should be determined. Feasibility and cost in terms of money, time, staff, facilities, and community support should be analyzed.

## Step VII: Make Appropriate Report

Prompt, accurate, and concise epidemiological reporting provide a basis for future investigations and control measures. Reporting should include what was involved in the epidemiological process: diagnosis, factors leading to the epidemic, control measures, process evaluation, and recommendations for preventing similar situations.

For many reasons underreporting of epidemiological investigations occurs. Completion of necessary forms can be tedious and time consuming and, therefore, neglected. There may be no one person assigned the responsibility for seeing that reports are completed, so the responsibility is overlooked. Usually more effective reporting occurs when one person is designated to coordinate the reporting activities of others.

Accurate reporting is essential for the identification of major community health problems and preventive health action that would correct these problems. Treating only individuals with overt symptoms, rather than collecting and reporting data on populations at risk, does very little to prevent future health problems. Appendix 11-2 is an actual report of a foodborne outbreak epidemiological investigation written by a community health nurse epidemiologist.

## Step VIII: Conduct Research

If health services to populations are to be improved, epidemiological research is essential. Health professionals must be prepared to collect and analyze data systematically so that the gaps in knowledge relative to disease causation, prevention, and control are eliminated. The ultimate goal of epidemiology, "the prevention and control of infectious diseases, chronic conditions, and other health-related phenomena in populations" is far from being realized. It is unfortunate that research in the practice setting is often lacking; it can be exciting and challenging, especially when one discovers significant data that will aid a community to improve its health status.

*Stop and Think About It*

Name a health problem in your community that you believe should be investigated. How would you use the epidemiological process to investigate this problem?

## PUBLIC HEALTH SURVEILLANCE

Epidemiological **surveillance** is an essential public health function at all levels of government. "Public health surveillance is the ongoing, systematic collection, analysis, interpretation, and dissemination of health data, including information on clinical diagnoses, laboratory-based diagnoses, specific syndromes, health-related behaviors, and other indicators related to health outcomes. Epidemiologists use these data to detect outbreaks; characterize disease transmission patterns by time, place, and person; evaluate prevention and control programs; and project future health care needs"(CDC, 1998, p. viii).

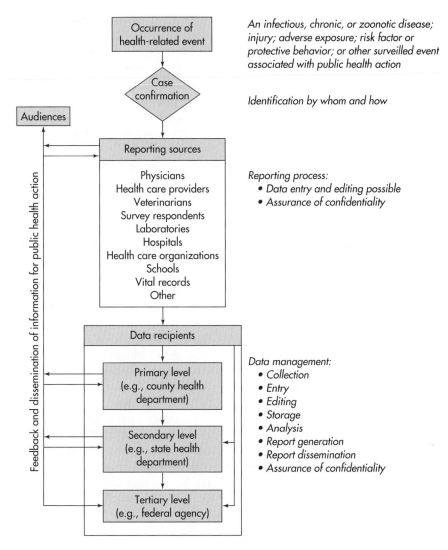

**FIGURE 11-13** United States surveillance system flow chart. (From Centers for Disease Control and Prevention [CDC]: Updated guidelines for evaluating surveillance systems, *MMWR* 50[No. RR-13]:1-35, 2001, p. 8.)

Public health surveillance activities date back more than three centuries. In the United States these activities were formalized by Congress in 1878 when Congress authorized the U.S. Marine Hospital Service (the forerunner of today's Public Health Service) to collect morbidity reports from U.S. consuls overseas (CDC, 1998). Consistent with the development of epidemiology, public health surveillance was traditionally limited to the monitoring of infectious diseases. Today public health surveillance systems monitor a variety of issues, including the incidence and prevalence of infectious and noninfectious diseases; the impact associated with these conditions; health risk behaviors in the overall population; components of population growth; and health services, resources, and policy trends. There is a wide range of public health surveillance data collection systems in the United States. Some of them can be found at the CDC's website.

On a national level, the CDC is the major agency responsible for public health surveillance. It maintains a national morbidity reporting system that collects, compiles, and publishes demographic, clinical, and laboratory data on many infectious and chronic diseases and conditions from each state. Each state has a department or departments responsible for morbidity reporting to the CDC. In Tennessee, the fourteen health department regions across the state weekly electronically transmit the incidence of reportable diseases in their areas to the Communicable and Environmental Disease Services section of the Tennessee Department of Health. At the state level, these statistics are analyzed and discussed at a weekly surveillance meeting and are then transmitted electronically to CDC. Figure 11-13 shows the reporting relationships between local, state, and federal agencies. These relationships extend internationally. The CDC provides an annual summary of disease reports from states to the World Health Organization (WHO) and promptly notifies WHO of any reported cases of the internationally quarantinable diseases (CDC, 1996).

Because reporting can be mandated only at the state level, reporting to CDC by the states is *voluntary*. State health departments maintain a morbidity reporting system based on regulations adopted by the state board of health. The state board of health derives its authority to issue regulations from acts of the state legislature.

The Council of State and Territorial Epidemiologists is now the CDC's primary collaborator for determining what diseases and conditions are nationally reported. "A notifiable disease is one for which regular, frequent, and timely information on individual cases is considered necessary for the prevention and control of the disease" (CDC, 1994, p. 800). As of January 1, 1998, 52 infectious diseases were notifiable nationally. A listing of notifiable diseases and conditions is provided in Box 11-3.

## INFECTIOUS DISEASE: A NEGLECTED PUBLIC HEALTH MANDATE

Deaths from infectious disease decreased markedly in the United States during most of the twentieth century. However, between 1980 and 1992 the death from infectious diseases increased 58%. This increase includes only those for whom the primary cause of death was infectious disease (Figure 11-14). The sharp increase in 1918 and 1919 was caused by the influenza epidemic pandemic, which killed more than 20 million people worldwide and over 500,000 in the United States (CDC, 1998).

Emerging infectious diseases are posing a major threat in the United States and worldwide. Box 11-4 defines the term and presents reasons for why they are occurring. In 1994, the CDC launched the first phase of a nationwide effort to revitalize the nation's capacity to protect the public from infectious disease. The document, *Preventing Emerging Infectious Diseases: A Strategy for the 21st Century*, describes the agency's plans for the next 5 years. It can be downloaded from CDC's website at *http://www.cdc.gov/*. Box 11-5 lists emerging infectious disease issues.

## A Global Perspective

The world is facing a global crisis in infectious disease prevention and control. Annually almost half of the 50 million deaths worldwide are directly related to an infectious or parasitic disease; among children, 4.1 million deaths are related to respiratory infections, 3 million are related to diarrheal disease and TB, and 1 million each are related to malaria and measles. Additionally, almost half of the population of the world is exposed to malaria to some degree, over one third of the world's population is now infected with M. *tuberculosis*, more than 2 billion people are infected with the hepatitis B virus, and more than 16 million adults and 1 million children have acquired HIV infection since the start of the HIV/AIDS epidemic (WHO, 1995, pp. 192-195).

To address the magnitude of global infectious diseases, the International 1997 Dahlem Conference on Disease Eradication established four criteria for a disease to be considered eradicable: (1) humans must be critical to maintaining transmission, (2) accurate diagnostic tests must be available, (3) an effective intervention must be available,

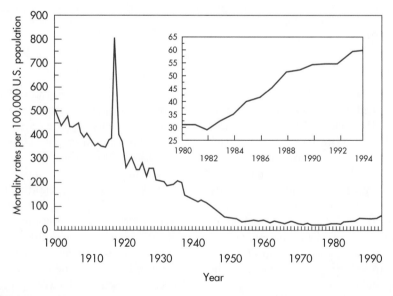

**FIGURE 11-14** Trends in deaths caused by infectious diseases in the United States, 1900-1994. (From Centers for Disease Control and Prevention (CDC): *Preventing emerging infectious diseases. A strategy for the 21st century,* Atlanta, 1998, CDC, p.1.)

and (4) it must be possible to interrupt transmission for a prolonged period in a large geographic area (Orenstein, Strebel, Papania, et al., 2000, p. 1521). In addition, there must be political and societal support in the countries where the efforts are occurring. In countries where people worry about enough to eat on a daily basis, it is not difficult to understand why they do not place disease eradication at a high priority. Much work went toward eliminating yellow fever, yaws, malaria, and smallpox, but epidemiologists finally learned that only smallpox met the four criteria that made eradication possible. The last case in the world occurred in 1977 in Somalia (Chin, 2000).

However, success in reducing the frequency of other diseases has been noteworthy (Aylward, Hennessey, Zagaria, et al., 2000, p. 1515). The annual incidence of polio has fallen by more than 90% worldwide, from an estimated 350,000 cases when an eradication effort was launched in 1988 to slightly more than 7000 reported in 1999. It has been totally eradicated from 3 of the 6 regions of the WHO, and it remained endemic in only 30 countries at the end of 2000. WHO has a goal of global eradication by 2050. There was a

97% reduction in cases of guinea worm worldwide, and measles has been all but eliminated in the United States and Europe.

Appendix 11-3 presents epidemiological information about select common communicable diseases. Chapter 13 addresses the epidemiology of commonly acquired sexually transmitted diseases, including AIDS.

## Universal Precautions: An Essential But Not Sufficient Control Measure

Preventing and controlling infectious disease requires that persons at risk for transmitting or acquiring infections change their behaviors. Behavioral aspects of infectious disease control are a leading factor in allowing these diseases to spread. Persons at risk include health care providers as well as clients. It is well documented that lack of adherence to infection control procedures, such as handwashing, has

**BOX 11-4**

*What Are Emerging Infectious Diseases and Why Are They Emerging?*

As defined in the 1992 Institute of Medicine report, emerging infectious diseases include diseases whose incidence in humans has increased within the past two decades or threatens to increase in the near future. Modern demographic and environmental conditions that favor the spread of infectious diseases include:

- Global travel.
- Globalization of the food supply and centralized processing of food.
- Population growth and increased urbanization and crowding.
- Population movements due to civil wars, famines, and other man-made or natural disasters.
- Irrigation, deforestation, and reforestation projects that alter the habitats of disease-carrying insects and animals.
- Human behaviors, such as intravenous drug use and risky sexual behavior.
- Increased use of antimicrobial agents and pesticides, hastening the development of resistance.
- Increased human contact with tropical rain forests and other wilderness habitats that are reservoirs for insects and animals that harbor unknown infectious agents.

From Centers for Disease Control and Prevention (CDC): *Preventing emerging infectious diseases. A strategy for the 21st century,* Atlanta, October 1998, CDC, p. 3; Institute of Medicine (IOM): *Emerging infections: microbial threats to health in the United States,* Washington, DC, 1994, National Academy Press.

**BOX 11-5**

*Emerging Infectious Disease Issues*

- *Antimicrobial Resistance:* Many drug choices for the treatment of common infections are becoming increasingly limited, expensive, and in some cases, nonexistent.
- *Foodborne and Waterborne Diseases:* Changes in how food is processed and distributed have resulted in multistate outbreaks. New waterborne pathogens are unaffected by routine disinfection.
- *Vectorborne and Zoonotic Diseases:* Many emerging diseases are acquired from animals or are transmitted by arthropods.
- *Diseases Transmitted Through Blood Transfusion/Products:* Because blood is a human tissue it is a natural vehicle for transmission of organisms such as HIV and hepatitis C.
- *Chronic Diseases Caused by Infectious Agents:* Several chronic diseases once thought caused by lifestyle or the environment are caused or intensified by infectious agents.
- *Vaccine Development and Use:* Numerous childhood diseases have been eliminated by vaccination; new vaccines are currently under development for some diseases.
- *Diseases of People with Impaired Host Defenses:* The numbers of people with HIV, organ transplants, and chemotherapy has increased dramatically.
- *Diseases of Pregnant Women and Newborns:* Pregnant women with infections often endanger their fetuses. Some racial and ethnic minorities experience high rates of maternal infection.
- *Diseases of Travelers, Immigrants, and Refugees:* People who cross international borders may be at increased risk for contracting infectious disease; this aggregate is increasing.

From Centers for Disease Control and Prevention (CDC): *Preventing emerging infectious diseases. A strategy for the 21st century,* Atlanta, October 1998, CDC.

caused infectious disease among health care workers and clients.

Adherence to universal precautions is essential. This method of infection control was developed by the CDC in the mid-1980s to highlight the need to maintain safeguards for protecting workers who are at risk of exposure to blood-borne pathogens, such as the human immunodeficiency (HIV) and hepatitis B (HBV) viruses, and other potentially infectious materials (CDC, 1987). The importance of maintaining universal precautions was reinforced in 1992 when the Occupational Safety and Health Administration's (OSHA) regulation of bloodborne pathogens was passed (OSHA, 1992).

Based on CDC's universal precautions recommendation, OSHA's bloodborne pathogens standard *requires* that all employers and employees "assume that *all* human blood and specified human body fluids are infectious for HIV, HBV, and other bloodborne pathogens. Where differentiation of types of body fluids is difficult or impossible, *all* body fluids *are* to be considered as potentially *infectious*" (OSHA, 1992). All clinical sites should have a copy of OSHA's *Bloodborne Pathogens Standards*, which reinforces the need to use sound infection control techniques in the clinical setting, such as handwashing, use of protective equipment, and proper care of needles.

Implementation of universal precautions does not eliminate the need for other category or disease-specific isolation precautions such as those for infectious diarrhea or pulmonary TB. Special precautions are strongly recommended for oral examinations and treatments in the dental setting and during phlebotomy. In addition to universal precautions, detailed precautions have been developed for procedures and/or settings in which prolonged or intensive exposures to blood occur, such as invasive procedures, dentistry, autopsies or morticians' services, dialysis, and the clinical laboratory.

## TB: The Need for Constant Attention

With the development of anti-TB medication in the 1940s, there was hope that the disease would soon be eradicated. There was a steady decline in the incidence of TB in the United States from 1953 though 1984. However, from 1985 through 1992, the number of cases increased by 20%. The major reason for this increase was the collapse of TB public health systems in the United States, which then fostered a new outbreak of the disease, including new drug-resistant strains (Institute of Medicine [IOM], 2000, p. 1). The HIV/AIDS epidemic, immigration from countries where TB is common, and transmission of TB in congregate settings such as prisons also contributed to the increase.

The resurgence of cases cost the city of New York as much as $1 billion and stimulated more public health funding for the identification and treatment of persons with TB. Since 1993, the number of reported cases of TB has again

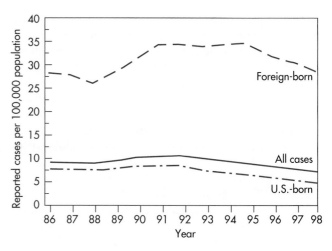

**FIGURE 11-15** Tuberculosis case rates by origin: United States, 1986-1998. (From Centers for Disease Control and Prevention [CDC]: *Core curriculum on tuberculosis. What the clinician should know,* Atlanta, 2000b, CDC, p. 18.)

 **BOX 11-6**

## *Persons at Higher Risk for Developing TB Disease Once Infected*

- HIV infected
- Recently infected
- Persons with certain medical conditions
- Persons who inject illicit drugs
- History of inadequately treated TB

From Centers for Disease Control and Prevention (CDC): *Core curriculum on tuberculosis. What the clinician should know,* Atlanta, 2000b, CDC, p. 20.

declined. In 1998, a total of 18,261 cases (6.8 per 100,000 population) were reported (CDC, 2000b, p. 16).

The proportion of TB cases among foreign-born people has increased significantly, from 27% in 1992 to 42% in 1998 (CDC, 1999b). The TB rate for foreign-born persons has remained at least four to six times higher than that for U.S.-born persons. Figure 11-15 graphically depicts this difference.

Figure 11-16 depicts the fact that racial and ethnic minorities and the elderly are disproportionately infected with TB. Compared with non-Hispanic whites, Asians are almost 16 times more likely to have TB; African Americans 8 times more likely; and Hispanics, Native Americans, and Alaskan Natives 5 times more likely (CDC, 1999b). There is some evidence that socioeconomic factors account for at least some of those disparities (Cantwell, McKenna, McCray, et al., 1998, p. 1016). Box 11-6 lists persons at higher risk of developing TB disease once they are infected.

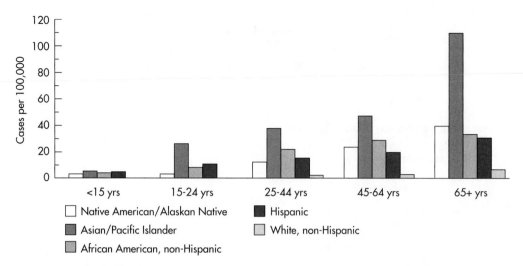

**FIGURE 11-16** TB case rates by age group and race/ethnicity, United States, 1999. (From Centers for Disease Control and Prevention [CDC]: *Core curriculum on tuberculosis. What the clinician should know,* Atlanta, 2000b, CDC. Retrieved from the internet October 2, 2000. *http://www.cdc.gov/nchstp/tb/pubs/slidesets/surv/surv/1999/18.gif*)

Resistance to anti-TB drugs remains a public health problem, although the proportion and number of multidrug-resistant TB (MDR TB) cases is decreasing. The decrease in MDR TB and TB is laudable; however, the lessons of the late 1980s should not be forgotten: epidemiologists cannot cease being vigilant. TB remains a leading cause of death worldwide, and many people in the United States carry latent infections. Without continual prevention and casefinding, the trends could again move sharply upward.

## UTILIZING THE EPIDEMIOLOGICAL PROCESS WITH CHRONIC DISEASE

Historically, the focus of the epidemiologist was infectious diseases because they were the primary health problems of the nineteenth century. In 1878 national morbidity data on cholera, smallpox, plague, and yellow fever were collected by the U.S. Marine Hospitals to institute quarantine measures to prevent the introduction and spread of these diseases into the United States.

Today, those four infectious diseases are almost unknown in this country. Antibiotics, good nutrition, safe water, and vaccines, among other variables, have changed the leading causes of death to chronic diseases. This category of disease is defined as "those illnesses that are prolonged, do not resolve spontaneously, and are rarely cured completely" (Marks, 1998, p. 6). They are responsible for 7 of 10 deaths in the United States; medical costs for people with chronic illnesses total more than 60% of total medical care expenditures (CDC, 1999c, p. vii). Four chronic diseases, cardiovascular disease, cancer, chronic obstructive pulmonary disease, and diabetes account for almost 72% of all of the deaths in this country. Figure 11-17 depicts the top 10 causes of death and shows how chronic illness fits into the total picture of deaths for all causes. The problems of chronic illness in the United States are emerging as problems that threaten to overwhelm a health care system that was designed primarily to meet the often different needs of acute-care clients (Marks, 1998, p. 7). It is crucial that epidemiologists focus their skills on this area of concern.

Currently, data about the prevalence of selected chronic conditions are collected regularly by the National Center for Health Statistics by means of the National Health Interview Survey. In this survey, a condition is considered chronic if (1) the condition is described by the respondent as having been first noticed more than 3 months before the week of the interview, or (2) it is one of the conditions always classified as chronic regardless of time of onset. Examples of conditions always viewed as chronic are ulcers, emphysema, diabetes, arthritis, neoplasms, all congenital anomalies, and psychoses and other mental disorders (National Center for Health Statistics, 1996). The National Health Interview Survey also examines the concepts of impairment and disability related to chronic disease and conditions. These concepts are discussed in Chapter 18.

People of any age can evidence chronic conditions; these conditions are not synonymous with old age. Aging is the normal process of biological, psychological, and sociological change over time. However, because aging involves a gradual lessening in levels of efficiency and functioning in the various body systems, elderly people are more likely than young people to have chronic conditions. They also are likely to have more of them.

Chronic conditions cause significant stress for families, individuals, and society. Roughly 41 million Americans had some degree of activity limitation in 1995, of which

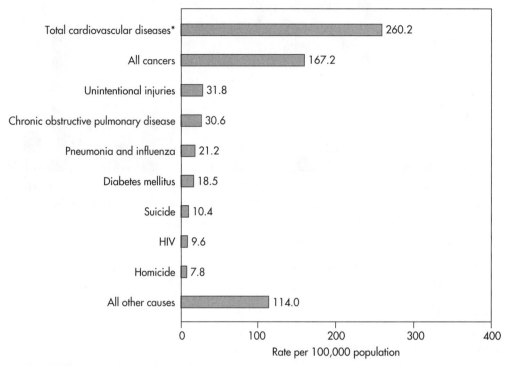

All data are age adjusted to 1970 total U.S. population.
*The total cardiovascular disease death rate includes the rate of death due to ischemic heart disease
(131.0 per 100,000) and the rate of death due to stroke (42.0 per 100,000).

**FIGURE 11-17** Most common causes of death, United States, 1996. (From Centers for Disease Control and Prevention [CDC]: *Chronic diseases and their risk factors: the nation's leading causes of death,* Atlanta, 1999c, CDC, p.3.)

12 million were unable to carry out a major life activity. Collectively, chronic conditions account for three of every four deaths in the United States (The Institute for Health and Aging, 1996, pp. 4, 8).

The risks and burdens associated with chronic conditions vary by age, race, the nature of the condition, and socioeconomic status. Chapters 16 through 20 discuss these variations. However, it is important to remember that many chronic conditions found in later life have their roots in childhood or young adulthood and continue throughout the life span. Because life expectancy is increasing for people with chronic conditions, as well as for the general population, a major concern is emerging about the nation's ability to provide for chronic care services for all who need them. The emphasis in health care spending must be on preventing chronic conditions in childhood and young adulthood.

## Levels of Prevention for Chronic Disease

The primary goal of epidemiology is to control and prevent disease. Although chronic illnesses are among the most prevalent and costly of all diseases, they also are among the most preventable. To a certain degree, the major chronic disease killers—cardiovascular disease, cancer, diabetes, and chronic obstructive pulmonary disease—are related to what people do or do not do as they live each day. Three risk fac-

tors in particular, tobacco use, lack of physical activity, and poor nutrition, are major contributors to the leading killers. Primary prevention of these problems via education and community policies and practices is essential; however, changing behaviors is difficult. Epidemiologists need to focus research on the most effective means of helping people change their behaviors.

Detection and treatment of chronic conditions (secondary prevention) are often possible. For many conditions such as diabetes, hypertension, breast cancer, and glaucoma, large-scale national programs for early detection represent an economical approach to secondary prevention. Early diagnosis plays a significant role in the control of chronic disease and conditions.

A major secondary prevention effort relative to chronic illness occurred in the United States when the National Health Survey was authorized and conducted in 1956 to secure information about health conditions in the general population. This survey was enacted under the National Health Survey Act, which was proposed in 1955 by the U.S. Department of Health, Education, and Welfare. Under this act, the Surgeon General of the Public Health Service was authorized to conduct a survey to produce uniform national statistics on disease, injury, impairment, disability, and related topics.

In 1972 a new survey mechanism initiated by USDHEW, the National Health and Nutrition Examination Survey (NHANES), began. Persons 1 to 74 years of age were examined, with emphasis on their nutritional status. Statistical data were collected on health records, fertility patterns, morbidity, and mortality. Today NHANES is the primary source of nationwide data on illnesses, disabilities, and physiological measurements.

Tertiary prevention activities also should be part of the care of people who have chronic conditions. Tertiary prevention involves rehabilitation, with the ultimate goal being cure or full restoration of the client's level of functioning. For some chronic conditions, this may be impossible; hence, the ideal goal must be replaced by more limited objectives such as maximizing remaining functional potential or minimizing further deterioration. Another option would be to learn to live within the limitations that the chronic disease has imposed. A more detailed discussion of the concept of rehabilitation is presented in Chapter 18.

## Approaches to the Study of Chronic Conditions

Two basic approaches to the study of chronic conditions are retrospective and prospective studies.

*Retrospective studies* look at people who are diagnosed as having a disease and compare them with those who do not have disease. The persons who do not have the disease are called *controls*. The controls come from the same general population segment as the individuals who have the condition and have the same characteristics as the study group except for the disease condition. A retrospective study examines factors in the person's past experience. One of the disadvantages of retrospective studies is that detailed information may not be available or accurate. The greatest problem, however, is finding a control group that is alike in all respects except for the condition under study. The advantages of this type of study are cost and the number of subjects needed. Retrospective studies are relatively inexpensive and require a small sampling size because cases are identified at the onset.

*Prospective studies* start with a group of people, a *cohort,* all presumed to be free from a condition but who differ in their exposure to a supposedly harmful factor. This cohort is followed over a period to discover differences in the rate at which disease develops in relation to exposure to the harmful factor. A major advantage of this type of study is that the cohort is chosen for study before the disease develops. The cohort is therefore not influenced by knowledge that disease exists, as in retrospective studies.

Prospective studies allow calculation of incidence rates among those exposed and those not exposed. Thus absolute difference in incidence rates and the true relative risk can be measured. The major disadvantage is that a prospective study is a long, expensive project. A large cohort must be used, especially if the disease has low incidence. Also, the larger the number of factors to be studied, the larger the cohort must be. The loss of people from the cohort as a result of death, lack of interest, or job mobility is a major problem when a study lasts over an extended period. Changes in diagnostic criteria, administrative problems, loss of staff or funding, and the high cost of record keeping can all contribute to make this a study that should not be undertaken without careful planning.

Retrospective and prospective studies assist in identifying causes of disease and effective disease control mechanisms. It is not intended that this brief description of retrospective and prospective studies will prepare community health nurses to do them. The purpose is to familiarize readers with the basic concepts involved in the study of chronic conditions.

## Screening as a Method for Detection and Control of Chronic and Infectious Conditions

One major activity at the primary and secondary levels of prevention of illness is screening. The purpose of screening is to either detect individuals with risk factors for disease or to identify those with early or asymptomatic disease.

There are two types of screening programs: the *single screening test,* in which only one condition is being identified, such as giving a group of prisoners a TB skin test, and the *multiphasic screening test,* in which a battery of tests is used at one time to detect several disease conditions. Doing height and weight measurements, audiometry, and vision screening of all persons at a county fair is an example of multiphasic screening.

Screening tests do not provide a conclusive diagnosis of a disease but rather are used to identify asymptomatic individuals who may unknowingly have a problem. Anyone who shows evidence of symptoms of a disease through a screening program should have further medical diagnostic testing. This is essential because early diagnosis and treatment are the primary goals of a screening program. Early diagnosis and treatment are particularly beneficial for conditions such as hypertension and cancer for which treatment measures are available to prevent progression of the condition.

Advantages of screening programs are that often they are relatively inexpensive; take little time; need few professionals to administer them; provide opportunity for prevention, early diagnosis, and treatment; and present statistics on the prevalence of disease when there is adequate follow-up. Major disadvantages of screening programs are that people tend to substitute them for medical examination; findings of screening programs are presumptive and further testing should be done to confirm a diagnosis; screening programs often do not reach vulnerable groups of people; and conditions may be missed during screening, resulting in persons receiving a false impression of their health status.

The following principles are seen as essential to good screening practices (Wallace, 1998, p. 907-908):

1. The condition sought should be an important health problem (affect a significant percentage of people).
2. There should be an accepted treatment for clients with recognized disease.
3. Facilities for diagnosis and treatment should be available.
4. There should be a recognizable latent or early symptomatic stage.
5. There should be a suitable test or examination that is able to detect the disease earlier than without screening.
6. The test should be acceptable to the population.
7. The natural history of the condition, including development from latent to declared disease, should be adequately understood.
8. The cost of casefinding (including diagnosis and treatment) should be economically balanced in relation to possible expenditure for medical care as a whole.
9. Casefinding should be thought of as a continuing process and not a "once and for all" project.

Although screening can be one method for early discovery of asymptomatic disease, it should be used judiciously and discriminately. Screening results need to be thoroughly evaluated, and the conditions found must be treated. An especially valuable reference for evaluating the effectiveness of screening tests and procedures is the *Guide to Clinical Preventive Services* (1996) by the U.S. Preventive Services Task Force.

## BIOLOGICAL/CHEMICAL WARFARE: AN EPIDEMIOLOGICAL CHALLENGE

Many contemporary challenges for epidemiologists exist. One of them is **biological/chemical warfare and terrorism,** defined as the deliberate use of biological/chemical agents to harm civilian populations (Lillibridge, Bell, Roman, 1999, p. 463). The use of biological weapons for war is well known in history. In the sixth century the Assyrians poisoned the wells of their enemies with rye ergot. In this country, during the French and Indian War, the English gave "gifts" of blankets infected with smallpox to Native Americans who were loyal to the French. Because the Native Americans had no immunity, many of them died.

Events and threats of terrorism (e.g., anthrax) have increased in the last decade from countries hostile to Western democracies. The former Soviet Union had an extensive program to develop these weapons and now that it has been dismantled, there is fear that scientists with extensive backgrounds in the field have gone to other countries in search of a livelihood. Libya, Iraq, Iran, and Syria have been noted as "aggressively seeking nuclear, biological, and chemical weapons" (Eitzen, Pavlin, Cieslak, et al., 1998, p. 9). Biological and chemical weapons are characterized by being readily available, cheap, very small and thus easy to carry about, and difficult to detect. Further, they would destroy people but not the infrastructure of a country. Table 11-11 lists clinical characteristics of some critical biological agents.

The CDC has been designated by the USDHHS to coordinate and lead the overall planning effort to upgrade national public health capabilities at local, state, and federal levels to respond to this threat. Initial detection of a covert act of bioterrorism is likely to be made by public health workers at the local level and thus, the first component of CDC's bioterrorism preparedness plan is surveillance. Box 11-7 lists epidemiological clues that may indicate a covert bioterrorist attack. Surveillance is the foundation because it is only when the clustering of events is recognized that the conclusion that a deliberate act has been made to cause them can be reached.

The other components of CDC's bioterrorism preparedness and response include rapid laboratory detection, epidemiological investigation and implementation of control measures, communication, and readiness assessment. Likely the local health departments of the readers of this text are involved in some manner with CDC's plan. Their website (*http://www.bt.cdc.gov*) provides details of the plan and ways in which healthcare workers can become involved.

## SUMMARY

The epidemiological process helps community health nurses to identify the health status of the community in which they are working and to prevent infectious and chronic diseases. This process places emphasis on analyzing the needs of aggregates rather than the needs of individual clients. Like the nursing process, it is a scientific, systematic problem-solving approach to the study of health needs.

Several key concepts are inherent in the understanding and utilization of the epidemiological process. These are study of aggregates at risk, natural life history of the disease, levels of prevention, host-agent-environment relationships, multiple causation of disease, and person-place-time relationships. These concepts provide a foundation for understanding the dynamics of disease transmission and occurrence and aggregate-focused preventive interventions. In addition to these concepts, a community health nurse must understand biostatistics to effectively use the epidemiological process.

By applying the concepts and methods of epidemiology, community health nurses play a vital role in the prevention of disease, injuries, and social problems in a community. Through their contacts in a variety of settings, they are in a key position to do casefinding, eliminate barriers to the control of disease, and promote health through teaching and counseling.

**TABLE 11-11**

## Clinical Characteristics of Critical Biological Agents

| DISEASE | SIGNS AND SYMPTOMS | PHYSICAL EXAMINATION | CLINICAL TESTS | KEY DIFFERENTIAL DIAGNOSIS | INCUBATION PERIOD | DURATION OF ILLNESS | CASE FATALITY | US EPIDEMIOLOGY |
|---|---|---|---|---|---|---|---|---|
| Inhalational anthrax | Fever, malaise, cough, mild chest discomfort; possible short recovery phase then onset of dyspnea, diaphoresis, stridor, cyanosis, shock; death 24-36 hours after onset of severe symptoms; hemorrhagic meningitis in up to 50% | Nonspecific physical findings | Serology, Gram stain, culture, polymerase chain reaction (PCR); CXR-widened mediastinum | Hantavirus pulmonary syndrome (HPS), dissecting aortic aneurysm (no fever) | 1-6 days [up to 45 days] | 3-5 days | ~100% if untreated | None |
| Pneumonic plague | High fever, chills, headache, hemoptysis, and toxemia; rapid progression to dyspnea, stridor, and cyanosis; death from respiratory failure, shock, and bleeding | Rales, hemoptysis, purpura | Gram stain, culture, serum immunoassay for capsular antigen, PCR, immunonhistochemical stains (IHC) | HPS, TB, community acquired pneumonia (CAP), meningococcemia rickettsioses | 2-3 days | 1-6 days | Usually fatal unless treated in 12-24 hr | 2-3 cases/yr mainly in SW US |
| Tularemia | Typhodial—aerosol, gastrointestinal, and intradermal challenge; fever, headache, malaise, chest discomfort, anorexia, nonproductive cough; pneumonia in 30-80%. Oculoglandular from inoculation of conjunctiva with periorbital edema | No adenopathy with typhodial illness | Serology, culture, PCR, IHC; CXR-pneumonia, mediastinal lymphadenopathy, or pleural effusion | Atypical CAP, Q fever, Brucellosis | 1-10 days [average 3-5 days] | >2 wks | 10-35% if untreated | 150 cases/yr transmitted by ticks/deer flies or contact with infected animals |
| Smallpox | Fever, back pain, vomiting, malaise, headache, rigors; papules 2-3 days later, progressing to pustular vesicles; abundant on face and extremities initially | Papules, pustules, or scabs of similar stage, many on face/extremities, palms/soles | Guarnieri bodies on Giemsa or modified silver stain, virions on electron microscopy, PCR, viral isolation, IHC | Varicella, vaccinia, monkeypox, cowpox, disseminated herpes zoster | 7-17 days [average 12 days] | 4 wks | Up to 30%; higher in flat-type or hemorrhagic disease | None |

From United States Army Medical Research Institute of Infectious Disease: *Biological warfare and terrorism: medical issues and response, student material booklet,* Fort Detrick, Md, 2000, USAMRIID, p. 15.

*Continued*

**TABLE 11-11**

*Clinical Characteristics of Critical Biological Agents*

| DISEASE | SIGNS AND SYMPTOMS | PHYSICAL EXAMINATION | CLINICAL TESTS | KEY DIFFERENTIAL DIAGNOSIS | INCUBATION PERIOD | DURATION OF ILLNESS | CASE FATALITY | US EPIDEMIOLOGY |
|---|---|---|---|---|---|---|---|---|
| Botulism | Ptosis, blurred vision, diplopia, generalized weakness, dizziness, dysarthia, dysphonia, dysphagia, followed by symmetrical descending flaccid paralysis and respiratory failure | No fever, client alert, postural hypotension, pupils unreactive, normal sensation, variable muscle weakness | Serology, toxin assays/anaerobic cultures of blood/stool; electromyography studies | Guillain-Barré, myasthenis gravis, tick paralysis, Mg++ intoxication, organophosphate poisoning, polio | 1-5 days | Death 24-72 hr or respiratory support for months | High mortality without respiratory support | 30 cases/yr; food intoxication, wound infections, or honey ingestion (infants) |
| Filoviruses (Maburg, Ebola) | Fever, severe headache, malaise, myalgia, maculopapular rash day 5; progression to pharyngitis, hematemesis, melana, uncontrolled bleeding; shock/death days 6-9 | Petechia, ecchymosis, conjunctivitis, uncontrolled bleeding | Serology, PCR, IHC, electrom microscopy (EM); elevated liver enzymes, thrombocytopenia | Meningococcemia, malaria, typhus, leptospirosis, borreliosis, thrombotic thrombocytopenic purpura (TTP), rickettsiosis, hemolystic uremic syndrome (HUS), arenaviruses | 2-19 days [average 4-10 days] | days to weeks | >80% | None |
| Arenaviruses (Lassa, Junin, Sabia, Machupa, Guanarito) | Fever, malaise, myalgia, headache, N/V, pharyngitis, cough, retrosternal pain, bleeding, tremors of tongue and hands (Junin), shock, aseptic meningitis, coma, hearing loss in some | Conjunctivitis, petechia, ecchymosis, flushing over head and upper torso | Serology, viral isolation, PCR, IHC; leukopenia, thrombocytopenia, proteinuria | Leptospirosis, meningococcemia, malaria, typhus, borreliosis, rickettsiosis, TTP, HUS, filoviruses | 5-21 days Lassa; 7-16 days Sabia, Junin, Machupa, Guanarito | 7-15 days | 15-30% | None |

From United States Army Medical Research Institute of Infectious Disease: *Biological warfare and terrorism: medical issues and response, student material booklet,* Fort Detrick, Md, 2000, US-AMRIID, p. 15.

**BOX 11-7**

*Epidemiological Clues that May Signal a Biological or Chemical Terrorist Attack*

1. Large numbers of ill persons with a similar disease or syndrome
2. Large numbers of cases of unexplained diseases or deaths
3. Unusual illness in a population (e.g., renal disease in a large population may suggest exposure to a toxic agent such as mercury)
4. Higher morbidity and mortality in association with a common disease or syndrome or failure of such clients to respond to usual therapy
5. Single case of disease caused by an uncommon agent (smallpox, viral hemorrhagic fever, pulmonary anthrax)
6. Several unusual or unexplained diseases coexisting in the same client without any other explanation
7. Disease with an usual geographic or seasonal distribution (e.g., tularemia in a nonendemic area, influenza in the summer)
8. Illness that is unusual or atypical for a given population or age group (e.g., outbreak of measles in adults)
9. Unusual disease presentation (e.g., pulmonary instead of cutaneous anthrax)
10. Similar genetic type among agents isolated from distinct sources at different times or locations
11. Unusual, atypical, genetically engineered, or antiquated strain of an agent (or antibiotic resistance pattern)
12. Stable endemic disease with an unexplained increase (e.g., tularemia, plague)
13. Simultaneous clusters of similar illness in noncontiguous areas, domestic or foreign
14. Atypical disease transmission through aerosols, food, or water, which suggests deliberate sabotage
15. Ill persons who seek treatment at about the same time (point source with compressed epidemic curve)
16. No illness in persons who are not exposed to common ventilation systems (have separate closed ventilation systems) when illness is seen in persons in close proximity who have a common ventilation system
17. Unusual pattern of death or illness among animals (which may be unexplained or attributed to an agent of bioterrorism) that precedes or accompanies illness or death in humans

From United States Army Medical Research Institute of Infectious Diseases: *Biological warfare and terrorism: medical issues and response, student material booklet*, Fort Detrick, Md, 2000, USAMRIID, p. 13.

## CRITICAL THINKING
*exercise*

It is Friday afternoon at 4:45 PM and you, as the supervisor, are the only nurse remaining at the local health department on a hot summer day. Within 15 minutes, you receive two calls. The first one is from a mother saying that she, her husband, and two young children had tacos at the popular San Francisco Taco Company the evening before and that now they are all vomiting. She states, "I just know we had poisoned food from that place." Moments later there is a call from an irate man saying that he ate at the San Francisco Taco Company for lunch that day and now is "deathly ill." He tells you to "close that place down. This is the second time this month this has happened to me."

1. Do you believe that you have a serious foodborne outbreak occurring?
2. Is this a problem that can wait until Monday to be investigated?
3. What should your response be to the two calls?

## REFERENCES

Ali AR, Smales ORC, Aslam M: Surma and lead poisoning, *Br Med J* 2:915-916, 1978.

Atkinson W, Furphy L, Gantt J, et al., editors: *Epidemiology and prevention of vaccine-preventable diseases*, Atlanta, 1995, Centers for Disease Control and Prevention.

Aylward B, Hennessey KA, Zagaria N, et al.: When is a disease eradicable? 100 years of lessons learned, *Am J Public Health* 90:1515-1520, 2000.

Bates B: *Bargaining for life*, Philadelphia, 1992, University of Pennsylvania Press.

Cantwell MF, McKenna MT, McCray E, et al.: Tuberculosis and race/ethnicity in the United States. Impact of socioeconomic status, *Am J Respir Crit Care Med* 157:1016-1020, 1998.

Centers for Disease Control (CDC): Recommendations for prevention of HIV transmission in health care settings, *MMWR* 36(Suppl S-2), August 21, 1987.

Centers for Disease Control and Prevention (CDC): National notifiable disease reporting, 1994, *MMWR* 43:800, 1994.

Centers for Disease Control and Prevention (CDC): Notifiable disease surveillance and notifiable disease statistics-United States, June 1946 and June 1996, *MMWR* 25(45):531-537, 1996.

Centers for Disease Control and Prevention (CDC): *Preventing emerging infectious diseases. A strategy for the 21st century*, Atlanta, October 1998, CDC.

Centers for Disease Control and Prevention (CDC): Summary of notifiable diseases, United States 1998, *MMWR* 47(53) 1999a, iv.

Centers for Disease Control and Prevention (CDC): *Reported tuberculosis in the United States, 1998*, August 1999b, CDC.

Centers for Disease Control and Prevention (CDC): *Chronic diseases and their risk factors. The nation's leading causes of death*, Atlanta, 1999c, CDC.

Centers for Disease Control and Prevention (CDC): *FoodNet 1999 Surveillance Results, Preliminary Report*, Atlanta, March 2000a, CDC.

Centers for Disease Control and Prevention (CDC): *Core curriculum on tuberculosis. What every clinician should know*, Atlanta, 2000b, CDC.

Centers for Disease Control and Prevention (CDC): Updated guidelines for evaluating surveillance systems, *MMWR* 50(No. RR-13):1-35, 2001.

Centers for Disease Control, Training and Laboratory Program Office: *Principles of epidemiology: agent, host, environment* (self-study course 3030-G, manual 1), Atlanta, 1987a, CDC, pp. 12-30.

Chin J, editor: *Control of communicable diseases manual*, ed 17, Washington, DC, 2000, American Public Health Association.

Communicable Disease Center: *Food-borne disease investigation: analysis of field data*, Atlanta, 1964, US Public Health Service.

Dubos RJ: *Mirage of health: utopias, progress, and biological change*, Rutgers, NJ, 1959, Rutgers University Press.

Eitzen E, Pavlin J, Cieslak T, et al., editors: *Medical management of biological casualties handbook*, Fort Detrick, Md, 1998, US Army Medical Research Institute of Infectious Diseases.

Friedman GE: *Primer of epidemiology*, New York, 1974, McGraw-Hill.

Gordis L: *Epidemiology*, Philadelphia, 1996, Saunders.

Grimes DE: *Infectious diseases*, St Louis, 1991, Mosby.

The Institute for Health and Aging, University of California, San Francisco: *Chronic care in America: a 21st century challenge*, Princeton, NJ, 1996, The Robert Wood Johnson Foundation.

Institute of Medicine (IOM): *Emerging infections: microbial threats to health in the United States*, Washington, DC, 1994, National Academy Press.

Institute of Medicine (IOM): *Ending neglect: the elimination of tuberculosis in the United States*, Washington, DC, 2000, National Academy Press.

Jekel JF, Elmore JG, Katz DL: *Epidemiology, biostatistics, and preventive medicine*, Philadelphia, 1996, Saunders.

Johnson NE: *Health profiles of Michigan populations of color*, Lansing, Mich, 1995, Michigan Department of Public Health.

Jones TF, Craig AS, Valway SE, et al.: Transmission of tuberculosis in a jail, *Ann Intern Med* 131:557-563, 1999.

Jones TF, Moore W, Craig A, et al.: Hidden threats: lead poisoning from unusual sources, *Pediatrics* 104:1223-1225, 1999.

Krieger N: Epidemiology and the web of causation: has anyone seen the spider? *Soc Sci Med* 39:887,1994.

Last JM, editor: *Maxcy-Rosenau public health and preventive medicine*, ed 12, Norwalk, Conn, 1986, Appleton-Century-Crofts.

Last JM: *A dictionary of epidemiology*, ed 3, New York, 1995, Oxford University Press.

Leavell HR, Clark EG: *Preventive medicine for the doctor in his community: an epidemiological approach*, New York, 1965, McGraw-Hill.

Lillibridge SR, Bell AJ, Roman SJ: Centers for disease control and prevention bioterrorism preparedness and response, *Am J Infect Control* 27:463-464, 1999.

MacMahon B, Pugh T: *Epidemiology principles and methods*, Boston, 1970, Little, Brown.

Marks JS: Looking back offers perspectives for meeting challenges that lie ahead, *Chronic Diseases Notes and Reports* 11:2-9, 1998, Centers for Disease Control and Prevention.

McGinnis MJ, Foege WH: Actual causes of death in the United States, *JAMA* 270:2207-2212, 1993.

National Center for Health Statistics: *Health, United States, 1995*, Hyattsville, Md, 1996, Public Health Service.

National Center for Health Statistics (NHCS): *Health, United States, 2000, with adolescent health chartbook*, Hyattsville, Md, 2000, NHCS.

Occupational Safety and Health Administration (OSHA): *Occupational exposure to bloodborne pathogens*, Washington, DC, 1992, OSHA.

Orenstein WA, Strebel PM, Papania M, et al.: Measles eradication: is it in our future? *Am J Public Health* 90:1521-1525, 2000.

Robey B: Two hundred years and counting: the 1990 census, *Pop Bull* 44(1), Washington, DC, 1989, Population Reference Bureau.

Rodriquez-Garcia R, Akhter M: Human rights: the foundation of public health practice, *Am J Public Health* 90:693-694, 2000.

Rothman SM: *Living in the shadow of death; tuberculosis and the social experience of illness in America*, New York, 1994, Basic.

Ryan F: *The forgotten plague. How the battle against tuberculosis was won and lost*, Boston, 1993, Little, Brown and Company.

Spargo J: *The bitter cry of the children*, New York, 1906, Macmillan.

Strawbridge WJ, Walhagen MI, Shema SJ: New NHLBI clinical guidelines for obesity and overweight: will they promote health? *Am J Public Health* 90:340-343, 2000.

Susser I, Stein Z: Culture, sexuality, and women's agency in the prevention of HIV/AIDS in Southern Africa, *Am J Public Health* 90:1042-1048, 2000.

Susser M, Susser E: Choosing a future for epidemiology: I. Eras and paradigms, *Am J Public Health* 86:668-673, 1996a.

Susser M, Susser E: Choosing a future for epidemiology: II. From black box to Chinese boxes and eco-epidemiology, *Am J Public Health* 86:674-677, 1996b.

Surgeon General of the United States: *Healthy People: the Surgeon General's report on health promotion and disease prevention*, vol II, Washington, DC, 1979, US Government Printing Office.

Tierney L, McPhee S, Papadakis M: *Current medical diagnosis and treatment*, ed 36, Stamford, Conn, 1997, Appleton & Lange.

US Army Medical Research Institute of Infectious Diseases: *Biological warfare and terrorism: medical issues and response*, student material booklet, Fort Detrick, Md, 2000, USAMRIID.

US Department of Health and Human Services (USDHHS): *Healthy People 2000: national health promotion and disease prevention objectives, full report with commentary*, Washington, DC, 1991, US Government Printing Office.

US Department of Health and Human Services (USDHHS): *Healthy People 2010: with understanding and improving health and objectives for improving health* (in 2 volumes), ed 2, Washington, DC, 2000, US Government Printing Office.

US Preventive Services Task Force: *Guide to clinical preventive services*, Baltimore, 1996, Williams and Wilkins.

Wallace BR: Screening for early and asymptomatic conditions. In RB Wallace, editor: *Maxcy-Rosenau-Last Public Health and Preventive Medicine* (pp. 907-908), 1998, Stamford, Conn, Appleton & Lange.

World Health Organization (WHO): Health status, *World Health Statistical Q* 48:189-199, 1995.

## SELECTED BIBLIOGRAPHY

Anderson ET, McFarlane J: *Community as partner*, ed 3, Philadelphia, 2000, Lippincott.

Centers for Disease Control and Prevention (CDC): Biological and chemical terrorism: strategic plan for preparedness and response, recommendations of the CDC strategic planning workgroups, *MMWR Morbid Mortal Weekly Rep* 49(RR-4):1-14, 2000, CDC.

Centers for Disease Control and Prevention (CDC): State-specific prevalence of selected health behaviors, by race and ethnicity—Behavioral Risk Factor Surveillance System, 1997, *MMWR Morbid Mortal Weekly Rep* 49 (SS-2):1-60, 2000, CDC.

Centers for Disease Control and Prevention (CDC): Surveillance for foodborne-disease outbreaks—United States, 1993-1997, *MMWR Morbid Mortal Weekly Rep* 49(SS-1): 1-62, 2000.

Centers for Disease Control and Prevention (CDC):Youth risk behavior surveillance—United States, 1999, *MMWR Morbid Mortal Weekly Rep* 49(SS-5): 1-94, 2000.

Gordis L: *Epidemiology*, ed 2, Philadelphia, 2000, Saunders.

MacMahon B, Trichopoulos D: *Epidemiology: principles and methods*, Boston, 1996, Little, Brown and Company.

Raczynski JM, DiClemente RJ, editors: *Handbook of health promotion and disease prevention*, New York, 1999, Kluwer Academic/Plenum Publishers.

Thornton TN, Craft CA, Dahlberg LL, et al.: *Best practices of youth violence prevention, a source book of community action*, Atlanta, 2000, CDC, National Center for Injury Prevention and Control.

US Department of Health and Human Services (USDHHS):*Tracking Healthy People 2010*, Washington, DC, 2000, US Government Printing Office.

Valantis B: *Epidemiology in health care*, ed3, Stamford, Conn, 1999, Appleton & Lange.

Verbrugge LM, Patrick DL: Seven chronic conditions: their impact on U.S. adult's activity levels and use of medical services, *Am J Public Health* 85:173-182, 1995.

# Gastroenteritis Questionnaire

Fill in the blank or circle **Yes/No/Don't Know** to complete questionnaire.

Interviewer _____ (Initials)                    Date of Interview _____/_____/_____

| | |
|---|---|
| Patient's Name (last, first): | DOB: |
| Parent's Name (if child): | Pt's phone #: |
| Occupation: | |
| Name and Address of Employer, daycare, or school | |
| Home Address:                    City: | State & Zip: |
| Age:                    Sex: | Race: (Circle) Caucasian/African American/Asian/Other |

| SYMPTOM HISTORY | | What was the first symptom? |
|---|---|---|
| Nausea        Y  N  DK       Chills        Y  N  DK | | Date of onset: (mo/day/yr) |
| Vomiting     Y  N  DK       Headache   Y  N  DK | | Time of onset: (military) |
| Diarrhea     Y  N  DK       Backache   Y  N  DK | | Date of onset of diarrhea: |
| Blood in stool  Y  N  DK    Muscle aches  Y  N  DK | | Time of onset of diarrhea: |
| Cramps       Y  N  DK       Fatigue       Y  N  DK | | Duration of diarrhea: (days) |
| Constipation  Y  N  DK      Other _____ | | Date of recovery: |
| Fever          Y  N  DK      _____ | | Time of recovery: |
| Temp _____ | | Comments: |

Please check **Yes/No/Don't Know** and complete blank spaces as requested.

1. Have you been seen by a physician?
   Yes    No    Don't Know
   If yes, name of physician _____
                    Address _____
                  City/State _____
                     Phone (____)_____

2. Was a stool culture done?
   Yes    No    Don't Know
   Date of culture: _____/_____/_____
   Stool culture results: _____    Lab: _____    Date: _____/_____/_____

# APPENDIX 11-1

# Gastroenteritis Questionnaire (cont'd)

3. Were you hospitalized?

   Yes    No    Don't Know

   If yes, give name of hospital: _____ How long? _____ days

4. Did you travel anywhere in the week before your illness?

   Yes    No    Don't Know

   If yes, give place(s) that you traveled to: _____

   _____ When: _____/_____/_____ to _____/_____/_____

   If airline travel, what airline? _____ Flight No. _____

5. Did you come into contact with any animals, or did you visit a farm with animals during the week before you became ill?

   Yes    No    Don't Know

   If yes, when? _____ Where? _____

   What kind of animal? _____

6. Did you go swimming in the week before you became ill?

   Yes    No    Don't Know

   If yes, where? _____ When? _____

7. Did you participate in group gatherings, parties, field trips, or other group activities in the week before your illness?

   Yes    No    Don't Know

   If yes, list activities: _____

   Where? _____ When? _____

8. Do you know anyone else who has been ill with diarrhea during the past week?

   Yes    No    Don't Know

   If yes, who (relationship and name)? _____

9. Did you have contact with young children in a day-care setting during the past week?

   Yes    No    Don't Know

   If yes, when: _____/_____/_____ to _____/_____/_____ and where: _____

   Phone: _____

10. Where did you shop for groceries eaten during the week before your illness?

    _____      _____

    _____      _____

# Foodborne Outbreak Investigation Associated with a Japanese Steak House

## CHATTANOOGA-HAMILTON COUNTY HEALTH DEPARTMENT

## SUMMARY

A foodborne investigation was conducted July 6-11, 2000, following food/restaurant complaints from two people who developed similar symptoms after eating together at a Japanese steak house on July 5, 2000. A total of 12 people who had eaten at the restaurant on the evening of July 5, 2000, were identified and interviewed. Six of the twelve interviewed met the case definition of foodborne illness. Symptoms reported included nausea/vomiting, diarrhea, abdominal cramps, fever/chills, fatigue, and headache.

## INTRODUCTION

The nurse epidemiologist at the Chattanooga-Hamilton County Health Department received two food/restaurant complaints on July 6, 2000, from two different families who had both consumed meals from the same restaurant on the same night. The two families were not acquaintances before dining together on the evening of July 5.

Environmental Services staff members were notified of the reports, as was Dr. Valerie Boaz, the Health Officer of the Health Department. Because the restaurant did not open for business until 4 PM, the environmentalist went out at that time on July 7, 2000, to perform the inspection.

The nurse epidemiologist and Chest Clinic Nurse Manager began the task of interviewing the family members who had made the initial complaints. The manager of the restaurant was contacted to provide names of other people who had also eaten there that same evening. These additional people were also interviewed by phone. Some of them also met the case definition of a foodborne illness. During the interviews, those who reported having symptoms of diarrhea were strongly encouraged to provide a stool specimen or to come in for a rectal swab for the purpose of being able to identify the causative agent.

The Tennessee Department of Health was also notified on July 6 by phone that a foodborne investigation was in process.

## METHODS

The case definition for foodborne illness in this investigation was the following: Any person who ate at the Japanese steak house on July 5, 2000, who developed nausea and/or vomiting and/or diarrhea within 30 minutes to 72 hours after eating. Diarrhea was further defined as loose, watery stools occurring more than twice within an 8-hour period.

The Gastroenteritis Questionnaire in Appendix 11-1 was used in conducting phone interviews and obtaining the needed information. Attack rates for those interviewed were calculated, as was the relative risks of the various food items eaten.

## RESULTS

A total of 12 questionnaires were administered.
Six (50%) of the people interviewed met the case definition of a foodborne illness.
Four (67%) of the ill cases were women.
Two (33%) of the ill cases were men.

Ages of the ill group ranged from 13 years of age to 56 years of age with the median age of 35 years. Of the ill group:

3 (50%) experienced nausea and/or vomiting
5 (83%) experienced diarrhea
4 (67%) experienced abdominal cramps
4 (67%) experienced fatigue
2 (33%) experienced fever/chills
2 (33%) experienced headache

The incubation period varied from 1 to 12.5 hours with a median of 5 hours. The duration of illness varied from 7 to 24 hours with a mean of 15 hours. No one required hospitalization or a physician's visit for treatment. Symptoms resolved rapidly, within 24 hours, with much improvement within just a few hours. The attack rate calculations and the relative risks indicate a suspicion of the steak and shrimp served that particular evening.

Courtesy Virginia Young, BSN, RN, Nurse Epidemiologist, Chattanooga-Hamilton County Health Department.

# Foodborne Outbreak Investigation Associated with a Japanese Steak House (cont'd)

The result of the restaurant inspection was a score of 85 out of a possible 100. Violations included the following:

- No thermometer in refrigerator
- Food uncovered in the walk-in refrigerator
- Ice scoop handle buried in ice
- Dirty wiping cloths in sink
- Bottom of reach-in refrigerator dirty
- Tables in back dirty
- Floors dirty
- Food splashed on walls
- Dish soap stored on cart with food

Samples of chicken, beef, shrimp, salad, and salad dressing were sent to the State Public Health Laboratory in Knoxville but were not tested because these foods were only available in raw form. Testing is carried out only on cooked food.

## DISCUSSION

The causative agent was suspected to be either *Staphylococcus aureus* or *Bacillus cereus* because of the short incubation time and also the short duration of the symptoms. Both of these organisms have the capability of causing nausea, vomiting, diarrhea, and abdominal cramps.

No clinical specimens were obtained primarily because the ill people were mildly ill for the most part and their recovery time was so short that they did not see the need to submit stool specimens for tests, even for our epidemiologic purposes.

Food samples were obtained by the environmentalist and sent to the Knoxville State Laboratory. The State Laboratory did not test the food samples because they were raw, not cooked. They chose not to test the salad sample either. Cooked food could not be obtained from the evening of July 5 for the following reasons: the restaurant discards all left-

over food each evening, and food is prepared on site at the customer's table. No food handlers were found to be an obvious source of contaminating the food.

## RECOMMENDATIONS

The Chattanooga-Hamilton County Health Department recommended the following guidelines to the managers of the restaurant to improve the sanitation practices at this facility:

1. Employees should practice good personal hygiene by washing their hands frequently.
2. Cross-contamination must be prevented. Utensils that have been used to handle raw meats must be washed, rinsed, and sanitized before they are used to handle cooked meats.
3. All raw meats must reach the following internal cooking temperatures before being served: chicken, 165° F; beef, 145° F; pork, 150° F; and shrimp, 146° F.

An inservice program was given to reinforce the above recommendations.

## ACKNOWLEDGEMENTS

Thank you to all the people who contributed to this investigation. Investigations are a team effort and cannot be done by a single person alone. A special thanks goes to the management of the Japanese steak house for their cooperation and assistance in this investigation. Appreciation also goes to Angela Pierce, RN, Chest Clinic Supervisor, for conducting most of the interviews and also to Bonnie Deakins, the environmentalist, for doing the restaurant inspection and also the tedious task of collecting food samples. Acknowledgement is also due Jim Parks, Tammy Burke, and Dr. Boaz for their input and management of the investigation process.

From Virginia Young, BSN, RN, Nurse Epidemiologist, Chattanooga-Hamilton County Health Department. Used with permission.

# Common Communicable Diseases

| DISEASE | ETIOLOGICAL AGENT | PRIMARY RESERVOIR | INCUBATION PERIOD | MODE OF TRANSMISSION | PERIOD OF COMMUNICABILITY | SYMPTOMS | TREATMENT |
|---|---|---|---|---|---|---|---|
| Hepatitis A (infectious) | Virus | Humans | 15-50 days (30 days average) | Person-to-person by fecal-oral route | Maximum infectivity during the incubation period and continuing for a few days after onset of jaundice; no carrier state | Abrupt and "flu-like" with loss of appetite, nausea and vomiting, abdominal discomfort, jaundice, dark brown urine, light brown stool (may be asymptomatic) | No specific treatment (bedrest, increased fluids, no alcoholic beverages, no fried or fatty foods) |
| Hepatitis B (serum) | Virus | Humans | 2 weeks-9 months (60-90 day average) | Percutaneous or permucosal exposure to infected body fluids (blood, saliva, semen, and vaginal fluids) | Weeks before onset of symptoms and infective for entire clinical course; carrier state can exist | Onset is gradual with symptoms similar to those of hepatitis A | Same as hepatitis A |
| Rubella (German measles) | Virus | Humans | 14-21 days | Usually person-to-person (direct contact or droplet spread) | At least 4 days before rash and at least 4 days after onset of rash; very contagious | Mild febrile illness with a macular rash (adults may experience more serious illness); rash on scalp, body, and limbs; usually lasts 1-3 days | No specific treatment (bedrest, increase fluids) |
| Measles | Virus | Humans | 7-21 days (10 days average) | Usually person-to-person (direct contact or droplet spread) | At least 4 days before rash and at least 4 days after onset of rash; very contagious | Resembles a bad cold with eyes and nose running, red blotchy rash beginning usually on face (often behind ears) and then becoming generalized, cough, Koplik spots, more severe symptoms than in rubella; lasts about 4 days | No specific treatment (bedrest increase fluids, place in darkened room if eyes hurt) |

Data from Chin J: *Control of communicable diseases manual*, ed 17, Washington, D.C., 2000, American Public Health Association; Last JM: *A dictionary of epidemiology*, ed 3, New York, 1995, Oxford University Press. Tierney L, McPhee S, Papadakis M: *Current medical diagnosis and treatment*, ed 36, Stamford, Conn, 1997, Appleton & Lange.
*Continued*

# Common Communicable Diseases (cont'd)

| DISEASE | ETIOLOGICAL AGENT | PRIMARY RESERVOIR | INCUBATION PERIOD | MODE OF TRANSMISSION | PERIOD OF COMMUNICABILITY | SYMPTOMS | TREATMENT |
|---|---|---|---|---|---|---|---|
| Mumps | Virus | Humans | 14-26 days (18 days average) | Person-to-person (direct contact with saliva or droplet spread) | At least 6 days before parotitis and up to 9 days after; very infective about 2 days before symptoms | Pain and swelling in one or both parotid glands, fever, pain on opening and shutting mouth (may need to use a straw to drink) | No specific treatment (bedrest, increase fluids) |
| Chickenpox | Virus | Humans | 12-21 days (14 days average) | Person-to-person (direct contact; droplet or airborne spread) | 2 days before vesicles and 6 days after vesicles appear; very contagious | Sudden onset; maculopapular rash that becomes vesicular and leaves a crusty scalp; generalized rash, itchy | No specific treatment (topical applications for itching, bedrest, encourage fluids, dress in loose clothing and caution person not to become overheated) |
| Pink eye | Multiple agents | Humans | 24-72 hours | Person-to-person by direct contact, also through contaminated clothing, fomites | Entire course of disease, until redness and discharge have disappeared | Lacrimation, eye irritation, and redness of lids; photophobia and mucopurulent discharge | Treatment dependent on causative agent |
| Ringworm | Fungi | Humans | 4-14 days (variable) | Direct skin-to-skin or indirect contact from items such as chairs, barber clippers | As long as lesions are present | Scalp: scaly patches of temporary baldness, crusty lesions, hair may become brittle Body: flat, spreading ring-shaped lesions that are red on the periphery and vesicular or pustular in center Feet: "athlete's foot" characterized by scaling or cracking of the skin between the toes, itching | Topical fungicide: oral medication as prescribed |

| Disease | Agent | Reservoir | Incubation period | Mode of transmission | Period of communicability | Symptoms | Treatment |
|---|---|---|---|---|---|---|---|
| Scabies | Mite (*Sarcoptes scabiei*) | Humans | 2-6 weeks for initial infestation; 1-4 days for reinfection | Direct skin-to-skin contact; transfer may occur from clothing | As long as condition is present—until mites and eggs are destroyed by treatment | Papular or vesicular; may show evidence of "burrows" on skin like grayish-white threads; lesions prominent around webs of fingers, wrists, elbows, belt line; intense itching | Kwell lotion |
| Pediculosis | Louse | Humans | 2 weeks (8-10 days average) | Direct person-to-person or indirect contact with infected personal belongings | As long as eggs or lice are alive | Scalp: itching; swollen lymph nodes; can often see nits or lice in hair. Pubic: itching; swollen glands | Kwell lotion or shampoo |
| Giardiasis | *Giardia lamblia*, a flagellate protozoan | Humans | 5-25 days or longer (7-10 days average) | Ingestion of cysts in fecally contaminated water or food; person-to-person by hand-to-mouth transfer of cysts from feces | Entire period of infection | Chronic diarrhea, steatorrhea, abdominal cramps, bloating, frequent loose and pale greasy stools, fatigue, weight loss | Atabrine is drug of choice; metronidazole (Flagyl) is also effective; furazolidone pediatric suspension for young children and infants; enteric precautions should be used |
| Salmonellosis | Numerous serotypes of salmonella (bacterial); *S. typhimurium* is the most common | Humans and domestic and wild animals, including poultry, swine, cattle, rodents, and pets (e.g., dogs, cats, turtles, chickens) | 6-72 hours (12-36 hours average) | Ingestion of organisms in food contaminated by feces; person-to-person by fecal-oral route | Entire period of infection, sometimes over 1 year; antibiotics can prolong this period | Acute enterocolitis, with sudden onset of headache, abdominal pain, diarrhea, nausea, and sometimes vomiting; dehydration; fever nearly always present; anorexia and loose bowels persist for days | Rehydration and electrolyte replacement with oral glucose-electrolyte solution; antibiotics (ampicillin or amoxicillin) for infants under 2 months, the elderly, and the debilitated, or clients with prolonged symptoms (antibiotics may prolong carrier state) |

*Continued*

# Common Communicable Diseases (cont'd)

| DISEASE | ETIOLOGICAL AGENT | PRIMARY RESERVOIR | INCUBATION PERIOD | MODE OF TRANSMISSION | PERIOD OF COMMUNICABILITY | SYMPTOMS | TREATMENT |
|---|---|---|---|---|---|---|---|
| Shigellosis | Shigella (Group A, *S. dysenteriae*; Group B, *S. flexneri*; Group C, *S. boydii*; Group D, *S. sonnei*); bacterial | Humans | 1-7 days (1-3 days average) | Person-to-person by fecal-oral route | During acute infection and until infectious agent is no longer present (usually within 4 weeks) | Diarrhea accompanied by fever, nausea, and sometimes toxemia, vomiting, cramps, and tenesmus; blood, mucus, pus in stool | Fluid and electrolyte replacement; antimotility agents contraindicated; antibiotic therapy (e.g., ampicillin, tetracyclines), based on antibiogram of isolated strain, for clients with severe symptoms |
| Tuberculosis | *Mycobacterium tuberculosis* and *M. africanum* primarily from humans, and *M. bovis* primarily from cattle | Humans | From infection to demonstrable primary lesion 4-12 weeks; risk after infection may persist for a lifetime as a latent infection | Person-to-person (airborne droplet); ingestion of unpasteurized milk or dairy products | As long as sputum is positive for tubercular bacilli; children with primary tuberculosis are generally not infectious | Imperceptible onset of cough that progressively worsens and is associated with production of mucopurulent sputum Hemoptysis, chills, myalgia, sweating, anorexia, weight loss, or low-grade fever that persists over weeks to months may occur | Drug therapy with a combination of antimicrobial drugs (e.g., isoniazid, rifampin, and pyrazinamide) Rest/maintain adequate fluid and caloric intake |
| Impetigo | Bacteria (often *streptococci* or *staphylococci*) | Humans | Variable, but commonly 4-10 days | Person-to-person contact with lesions or secretions and mildly infectious through fomites | As long as purulent lesions continue | Draining, crusty skin lesions that may resemble ringworm or dry scales; often accompanied by fever, malaise, headache, and loss of appetite | Antibiotics such as penicillin and erythromycin and antibiotic creams and lotions |

# 12

# Theoretical Models for Health Education and Health Promotion

*Joan Uhl Pierce*
*Maureen Nalle*

## OBJECTIVES

*Upon completion of this chapter, the reader should be able to:*

1. Describe the historic and contemporary roles of the community health nurse related to health education.
2. Identify the *Healthy People 2010* objectives for health education and health promotion.
3. Define health education and health promotion.
4. Discuss the theoretical foundations for health education and health promotion.
5. Describe the essential steps in the community health education process.
6. Define the three levels of evaluation involved in health education interventions.
7. Identify key resources for implementing community health education programs.

## KEY TERMS

Diffusion of Innovations (DI)
Formative evaluation
Health Belief Model (HBM)
Health education
Health education process
Health literacy
Health promotion

Illness behavior
Impact evaluation
Multidimensional Health Locus of Control Assessment (MHLCA)
Outcome evaluation
Pender's Health Promotion Model
PRECEDE-PROCEED

Preventive behavior
Process evaluation
Readiness to learn
Sick role behavior
Social Cognitive Theory (SCT)
Theory of Reasoned Action (TRA)

---

Health education is deeply rooted in nursing practice and historically has been an integral component of community health nursing. Among all health disciplines, nurses have long been recognized as consistently providing health education. The role of the nurse as a health educator has its foundations in Florence Nightingale, an early promoter of the nurse as a health missioner and teacher. In the context of community health, Lillian Wald and the Henry Street Settlement nurses used home instruction to improve the health of new mothers, children, and invalids and prepared families to care for their ill members (see Chapter 1). Both of these nursing pioneers encouraged health education to promote healthy lifestyles (Morgan, Marsh, 1998).

Lina Rogers, a Henry Street Settlement nurse and author of the first school nursing text, focused on using health education concepts in her practice. Rogers taught personal hygiene to school age children and their families to promote wellness and reduce the spread of disease. Through federal *Maternal and Child Health Grants* during the 1920s and 1930s, funds were made available to hire community health nurses to teach family life education, child care, and nutrition. The grants also allocated monies for community-wide preventive health teaching. Indeed, education for the public about health risks and lifestyle changes contributed significantly to improved health of the public during the twentieth century (Rothstein, 2001).

As early as 1918, the *National League for Nursing Education* recognized the need to prepare nurses to meet the teaching demands of the profession (Campbell, 1999; National League for Nursing Education, 1918). Since that time, the role of the nurse in health education has been incorporated throughout nursing curricula. The health education role is included in the American Nurses Association's (ANA) *Standards of Community Health Nursing Practice* (American Nurses Association [ANA, 1986]) and *Scope and Standards of Public Health Nursing Practice* (ANA, 1999). Nursing's commitment to health education and health promotion also is evident in the ANA's *Social Policy Statement* (1995), which highlights practices that "mobilize healthy patterns of living, foster personal and family development, and support self-defined goals of individuals, families, and communities" (p. 11).

Health education roles for nurses are incorporated in state *Nurse Practice Acts*. The nurse's mandate for health education is incorporated into the *Patient's Bill of Rights*, which discusses client teaching as a basis for informed decision making and preparation for self-care. The Joint Commission on Accreditation of Healthcare Organizations (JCAHO) also has identified educational standards as a priority area for health care facilities (JCAHO, 2000).

## HEALTH EDUCATION AND HEALTH PROMOTION

Health promotion and health education are so integrally linked it is difficult to discuss one without the other. **Health promotion** encompasses a variety of mechanisms and implementation strategies, which include fostering self-care, risk factor detection, health enhancement, and health maintenance (Joint Commission on Health Education Terminology [JCHET], 1991). Strategies for health promotion include activities designed to improve personal and public health. "The task of health promotion is both to understand health behavior and to transform knowledge about behavior into useful strategies for health enhancement" (Glanz, Lewis, Rimer, 1997a, p. 20). Health promotion strategies have been described as:

Those related to individual lifestyle—personal choices made in a social context that can have a powerful influence over one's health prospects. These priorities include physical activity and fitness, nutrition, tobacco, alcohol and other drugs, family planning, mental health and mental disorders, and violent and abusive behavior. Education and community-based programs can address lifestyle in a crosscutting fashion (U.S. Department of Health and Human Services [USDHHS], 1991, p. 6).

Numerous factors influence the need for health promotion. Social and political factors, such as escalating health care costs, increased incidence of chronic disease, and issues surrounding access to resources have moved the U.S. away from a focus on acute care toward a focus on health promotion and preventive health care. Health promotion provides a framework for changing the health behaviors and lifestyles of individuals, groups, and communities and moving them toward an optimal state of health.

Health education is an essential component of health promotion. **Health education** is defined as "the continuum of learning which enables people, as individuals, and as members of social structures, to voluntarily make decisions, modify behaviors, and change social conditions in ways that are health enhancing" (JCHET, 1991, p. 257). Although the emphasis of health education is on primary prevention, focusing on health promotion and disease prevention, all levels of prevention may be addressed. Nurses in the community use health education across the life span to help clients prepare for normative life events, develop lifestyle patterns that foster optimal health, prevent disease and chronic health problems, and address rehabilitation needs.

## A Contemporary Look at Health Education and Health Promotion

Health care in the U.S. historically has been based primarily on a medical model that focused on treatment of disease and a narrow definition of health as the absence of disease. The World Health Organization's (WHO) (1978) holistic concept of health (see Chapter 11) incorporated efforts to support healthy lifestyles, promote well-being, and build healthy public policy (Raphael, 1998). This broader, more holistic view of health was accompanied by expanded efforts in both personal and public health promotion.

In the early 1970s the U.S. Congress passed the *Health Information and Health Promotion Act*. This was a turning point in health care and initiated an era that emphasized health promotion as a significant and important public health intervention. In that same decade *Healthy People*, the first Surgeon General's Report on health promotion and disease prevention, was published and the Healthy People Initiative began (see Chapter 4). *Healthy People* cited evidence-based data that were used to establish national health objectives. These objectives targeted specific populations and incorporated health education and health promotion activities. *Healthy People* focused on primary prevention and moved away from a medical, "treatment model" of health care. Health promotion became an accepted intervention through its inclusion in health policy and related health practice. On the federal level, the *Office of Disease Prevention and Health Promotion* (ODPHP) was established.

*Healthy People* linked causes of mortality in the United States with behavioral factors such as smoking, diet, and sedentary lifestyle. With growing recognition of the complex interaction between social, economic, and political factors that influence health, efforts began to be focused on the context in which individual health behavior occurs. With an increasingly diverse population, it became evident that health behavior must be understood in terms of the social and cultural context in which it occurs. Specific strategies need to be developed that address the needs of minority and ethnic groups and communities (Thompson, Gifford, Thorpe, 2000).

"The central concern of health promotion and health education is health behavior" (Glanz, Lewis, Rimer, 1997b, p. 9). Kasl and Cobb (1966) identified three categories of health behavior: **preventive behavior** of an individual who perceives himself to be healthy (asymptomatic) and seeks to prevent or detect illness; **illness behavior** of an individual who perceives himself to be ill and seeks a remedy; and **sick role behavior** in which the individual considers himself to be ill and seeks treatment.

Personal values, attitudes, beliefs, and perceptions have an effect on health behavior patterns. More expansive definitions of health behavior incorporate the actions of individuals, groups, and communities, and the determinants and consequences of those actions such as enhanced quality of life, improved coping skills, social change, and policy development (Glanz, Lewis, Rimer, 1997b). Consequently, health promotion and health education models and interventions are being designed not only to influence individual behavior but also to address the health of communities (Ottoson, Green, 2001).

The inclusion of health care disciplines, organizations, systems, and practitioners who collaborate in the utilization of health promotion models is an essential ingredient to provide health education programs that increase health awareness and knowledge, affect attitudes and motivation, and ultimately change health behavior. *Healthy People 2010* has incorporated an interdisciplinary approach to health care and continued the nation's primary prevention agenda through health education and health promotion activities.

## HEALTHY PEOPLE 2010: HEALTH EDUCATION AND HEALTH PROMOTION

The Healthy People Initiative established goals for the nation's health, highlighting the importance of effective education and community-based strategies in achieving widespread adoption of more healthful lifestyles and practices (Philips, Chambers, Whiting, et al., 2001). The Initiative's documents have consistently incorporated health education and health promotion strategies.

A personal responsibility for health behavior is implicit in the concept of health promotion: lifestyle practices and self-care actions that influence health status and quality of life as well as cost of health care (Acton, Malathum, 2000). This orientation toward self-responsibility creates a mindset that facilitates the adaptation of an active orientation to health behavior (Gleit, 1998). Many of the national health objectives relate to learning new behaviors and skills and changing lifestyles, with a focus on primary prevention in the areas of diet, exercise, and other health behaviors.

*Healthy People 2010* objectives consistently provide direction for both individual and community health education programs (Box 12-1). These objectives focus on the quality,

### BOX 12-1
### *Educational and Community-Based Activities*

**School Setting**

1. Increase high school completion.
2. Increase the proportion of middle, junior high, and senior high schools that provide comprehensive school health education to prevent health problems in the following areas: unintentional injury; violence; suicide; tobacco use and addiction; alcohol or other drug use; unintended pregnancy; HIV/AIDS and other STD infections; unhealthy dietary patterns; inadequate physical activity; and environmental health.
3. Increase the proportion of college and university students who receive information from their institution on each of the six priority health-risk behavior areas.
4. Increase the proportion of the nation's elementary, middle, junior high, and senior high schools that have a nurse-to-student ratio of at least 1:750.

**Worksite Setting**

5. Increase the proportion of worksites that offer a comprehensive employee health promotion program to their employees.
6. Increase the proportion of employees who participate in employer-sponsored health promotion activities.

**Health Care Setting**

7. Increase the proportion of health care organizations that provide client and family education.
8. Increase the proportion of clients who report that they are satisfied with the client education they receive from their health care organization.
9. Increase the proportion of hospitals and managed care organizations that provide community disease prevention and health promotion activities that address the priority health needs identified by their community.

**Community Setting and Select Populations**

10. Increase the proportion of Tribal and local health service areas or jurisdictions that have established a community health promotion program that addresses multiple *Healthy People 2010* focus areas.
11. Increase the proportion of local health departments that have established culturally appropriate and linguistically competent community health promotion and disease prevention programs for racial and ethnic minority populations.
12. Increase the proportion of older adults who have participated during the preceding year in at least one organized health promotion activity.

Source: United States Department of Health and Human Services (USDHHS): *Healthy People 2010, conference edition*, Washington, DC, 2000, US Government Printing Office, pp. 7-12 to 7-25.

availability, and effectiveness of community-based educational programs designed to prevent disease and improve health and quality of life for targeted populations in diverse settings such as schools, worksites, and health departments. National health objectives address behavioral risk factors associated with chronic diseases such as hypertension, diabetes, arthritis, and asthma, which contribute significantly to morbidity and mortality in the United States.

Graham (1998) suggests that achievement of *Healthy People 2010* objectives depends to a large degree on a knowledgeable and concerned public. With this in mind, Ottoson and Green (2001) stress that health education strategies that target communities and population groups are integral to this effort.

## HEALTH BEHAVIOR THEORIES AND MODELS

It is essential that community health professionals understand human behavior in order to change risk behaviors and promote health (DiClemente, Raczynski, 1999). Theories of health behavior help explain why people engage in health-promoting behaviors. With foundations in such disciplines as sociology, psychology, and other social and behavioral sciences, many health behavior theories and models have focused on processes that address those behaviors relating to health. Many of these theories have been incorporated into health education methods to provide a blueprint for sound and organized program planning and evaluation.

"A theory is a set of interrelated concepts, definitions, and propositions that present a systematic view of events or situations by specifying relations among variables in order to explain or predict the events or situations" (Glanz, Rimer, 1997, p. 11). Theory reflects ways of knowing and understanding that may be tested in various ways. Numerous theories and models provide a blueprint for planning, implementing, and evaluating health education programs and activities. The most effective way to contribute to the recognition and increased utilization of effective health promotion and disease prevention programs is through the use of "theoretically driven, methodologically sound, evidence-based research" that includes a rigorous evaluation method (DiClemente, Raczynski, 1999, p. 6). Theories guide this type of research.

Theories and models of health behavior help us understand the nature of targeted behaviors and guide health education and health promotion strategies (Glanz, Rimer, 1997). Models, and the theoretical concepts that support these models, are recognized as providing an orderly way to prepare for the assessment, analysis, planning, implementation, and evaluation of health education programs that focus on reducing risk behaviors of individuals, groups, and populations. Health education and health promotion programs that are most likely to succeed are those based on a clear understanding of the targeted health behavior.

Two of the most widely used theories reflected in models for health education programs for health promotion and disease prevention are Bandura's *Social Learning Theory* (1977) and *Social Cognitive Theory* (1986) and Ajzen and Fishbein's *Theory of Reasoned Action* (1980). Models have been derived from these theories that provide direction for nursing action and intervention.

## Social Cognitive Theory

It is important to differentiate between the theories that drive and guide models for utilization by educators and researchers and the models themselves that have evolved and been based on those theories. Bandura's Social Learning Theory and later his **Social Cognitive Theory** (SCT) are perhaps the basis for all models used today.

SCT was developed on the premise that behavior be examined in the context of the environment and the personal factors that influence it. The theory assumes that people and their environments interact continuously (Glanz, Rimer, 1997). This approach to understanding what initiates behavioral changes is identified as *reciprocal determinism*, in that when a behavior is manifest it is prompted by the individual's need or desire (personal factors) in addition to being acceptable in an environment that accommodates, allows, or approves of that behavior. These phenomena interact and are dependent on each other; therefore the behavior is reinforced and is established as part of the repertoire of the individual.

The focus of SCT is on the interpersonal level. A basic premise of the theory is that people learn not only through their own experiences but also by observing the actions of others (Glanz, Rimer, 1997). The theory synthesizes a number of constructs that help us understand health behavior (Table 12-1). It highlights the dynamic relationship between behaviors and the continuing interactions between person and the environment (reciprocal determinism). Multiple factors influence a person's behaviors, including the environment, the person's need to know about what to do and how to do it (behavioral capability), outcome expectations, and a person's confidence in his or her ability to take health action (self-efficacy). A basic premise of the theory is that people can be influenced by modeling behaviors (observational learning) and through positive reinforcement and their own experiences.

Health educators and community health nurses focus on changing unhealthful behavior in the best interest of an individual, group, aggregate, or population. Change is a key factor in all of this and changing a behavior is extremely complex in that it entails modifying beliefs, attitudes, knowledge, motivation, and the social and cultural dynamics that enter into willingness to change. The SCT provides a more intricate way of understanding the capabilities of individuals who are about to learn and behave in a variety of ways. These learning capabilities include *forethought capability* (an expectation about what might happen in a situa-

**TABLE 12-1**

*Social Learning Theory or Social Cognitive Theory*

| CONCEPT | DEFINITION | APPLICATION |
|---------|------------|-------------|
| Reciprocal Determinism | Behavior changes result from interaction between person and environment; change is bidirectional | Involve the individual and relevant others; work to change the environment, if warranted |
| Behavioral Capability | Knowledge and skills to influence behavior | Provide information and training about action |
| Expectations | Beliefs about likely results of action | Incorporate information about likely results of action in advice |
| Self-Efficacy | Confidence in ability to take action and persist in action | Point out strengths; use persuasion and encouragement; approach behavior change in small steps |
| Observational Learning | Beliefs based on observing others like self and/or visible physical results | Point out others' experience, physical changes; identify role models to emulate |
| Reinforcement | Responses to a person's behavior that increase or decrease the chances of recurrence | Provide incentives, rewards, praise; encourage self-reward; decrease possibility of negative responses that deter positive changes |

Source: Glanz K, Rimer BK: *Theory at a glance. A guide for health promotion practice,* Washington, DC, 1997, National Institutes of Health/National Cancer Institute, p. 23.

tion), *vicarious capability* (acquiring knowledge through observing others), *self-regulatory capability* (setting of personal goals and self-evaluation), and *self-reflective capability* (reflecting on learning and previous actions).

Bandura (1977) further suggested that the "outcome expectations" of any given attempt to learn, adapt, or change is critical to the behavior being manifest. The expectation of a behavior being worth the effort to acquire and to be maintained is essential for persons to change their behavior. These expectations are acquired through direct experiences, vicarious experiences, judgments and opinions of others, and a synthesis of knowledge available.

The relevance and importance of SCT in guiding the planning and evaluation of programs for health promotion and disease prevention is evident. The SCT focuses on examining what influences behavior change. The goals of health promotion programs are aimed at behavioral change and at understanding what would be most effective to affect the behavior of individuals, groups, and aggregates.

### Theory of Reasoned Action

Ajzen and Fishbein (1980) developed the Theory of Reasoned Action (TRA) to examine the complex set of explanations that address individuals' behaviors and behavioral patterns. This theory proposes a category of external variables (Figure 12-1) that consists of things like demographics, attitudes toward people and institutions, and individual personality traits and their effects on the beliefs and motivation of individuals.

The theory is a complex model that is fundamental to the study of attitudes and behaviors and predicting behavior from intention. It emphasizes that behavioral intention is directly influenced by attitudes toward performing the behavior and subjective norms. Subjective norms are derived from evaluating how important individuals in the environment view performing a behavior (Glanz, Lewis, Rimer, 1997b). Behavior is a result of an individual's motivation to comply or not comply with these norms.

The TRA links values and beliefs to behavior, addresses the effects of external variables on personality traits and behavior, and proposes that when these beliefs and external variables are analyzed, behavior can be predicted. Simply stated, the theory prompts health professionals to think about how a client's behavior, related perceptions, beliefs, and expected outcomes influence health behavior and how this attitude component is influenced by peer norms or pressure (Doyle, Ward, 2001).

### Diffusion of Innovations

When considering how to influence behavior change, it is helpful to understand and predict the expected adoption of a new idea and/or behavior. Decades of work and study by Everett Rogers provide a community health nurse health educator with a sound basis upon which the expectation of the adoption of a new innovation may be predicted. Roger's Diffusion of Innovations (DI) is a paradigm that is used to explain how new ideas and information are spread and incorporated into a belief system and result in an adopted behavior.

Diffusion may be used to explain a spontaneous or an unplanned spread of a new idea. Rogers (1983) uses the word "diffusion" to include both the planned and the spontaneous spread of new ideas. "Diffusion is the process by which an *innovation* is *communicated* through certain

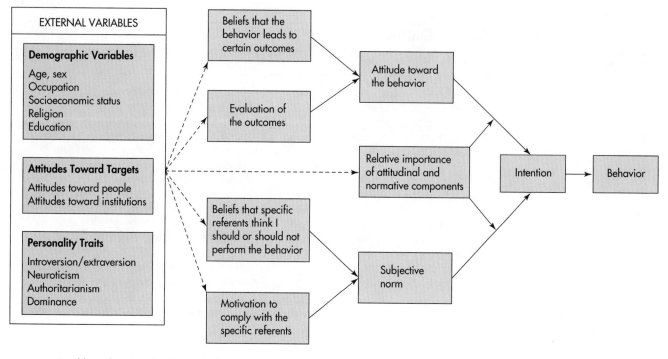

----► Possible explanations for observed relations between external variables and behavior

──────► Stable theoretical relations linking beliefs to behavior

**FIGURE 12-1** Indirect effects of external variables on behavior. (From Ajzen I, Fishbein M: *Understanding attitudes and predicting social behavior,* Englewood Cliffs, NJ, 1980, Prentice-Hall, Inc., p. 84.)

*channels* over *time* among the members of a *social system*" (Rogers, 1983, p. 5). According to Rogers, an innovation is viewed as "…an idea, practice, or object that is perceived as new" (Rogers, 1983, p. 11). The diffusion process is one that is concerned with new ideas and the adoption of the innovation. This type of communication is a "…two-way process of convergence" as opposed to a "…one-way linear act" (Rogers, 1983, p. 5). The DI theory focuses on the community level and "addresses how new ideas, products and social practices spread within a society or from one society to another" (Glanz, Rimer, 1997, p. 40). Key concepts addressed in the DI theory and their applications are given in Table 12-2. The theory suggests that the rate of adoption of an innovation is influenced by the characteristics of an innovation, including the relative advantage, compatibility, complexity, trialability, and observability of an innovation.

Diffusion researchers have been particularly interested in the rate of adoption of an innovation over time. A diffusion curve has resulted that provides a baseline to predict the percentage of those who adopt an innovation over time. The rate of adoption of an innovation also is influenced by the characteristics of the adopter as well as the characteristics of the innovation. Figure 12-2 portrays the adoption of an innovation by five adopter categories: innovators, early adopters, early majority, late majority, and laggers. These categories assist program planners in predicting the *rate of*

*adoption* for an innovation. These adopter categories provide a distribution that is S-shaped over time and depicts the influence of the "increasing rate of knowledge and adoption or rejection of the innovation in the system" (Rogers, 1983, p. 269).

As Figure 12-2 depicts, the S-shaped curve "takes off" by representing a few early adopters and then gradually increasing adopters toward a plateau that represents the *saturation point* of adoption of the innovation at a later time. This saturation point may be construed as the time when the innovation changes from being an innovation to an acceptable behavior within the social structure of the adopters.

Both DI and SCT address similar ideas. Both theories view the phenomenon of change as a result of things such as communication of all types (e.g., personal exchanges or multimedia blitzes) and by observation of peers. Bandura and Rogers focus on understanding the effects of information on behavior. Network links that accommodate information exchanges also are identified by both as being the "…main explanation of how individuals alter their behavior" (Rogers, 1983, p. 305). It is not difficult to acknowledge these constructs today knowing the huge impact of television and information technology, especially the internet, on health behavior and the significant influence of peers in influencing health behaviors.

**TABLE 12-2**

*Diffusion of Innovations Theory*

| CONCEPT | DEFINITION | APPLICATION |
|---------|-----------|-------------|
| Relative Advantage | The degree to which an innovation is seen as better than the idea, practice, program, or product it replaces | Point out unique beneifts: monetary value, convenience, time saving, prestige, etc. |
| Compatibility | How consistent the innovation is with values, habits, experience, and needs of potential adopters | Tailor innovation for the intended audience's values, norms, or situation |
| Complexity | How difficult the innovation is to understand and/or use | Create program/idea/product to be uncomplicated, easy to use and understand |
| Trialability | Extent to which the innovation can be experimented with before a commitment to adopt is required | Provide opportunities to try on a limited basis, e.g., free samples, introductory sessions, money-back guarantee |
| Observability | Extent to which the innovation provides tangible or visible results | Assure visibility of results: feedback or publicity |

Source: Glanz K, Rimer BK: *Theory at a glance. A guide for health promotion practice,* Washington, DC, 1997, National Institutes of Health/National Cancer Institute, p. 28.

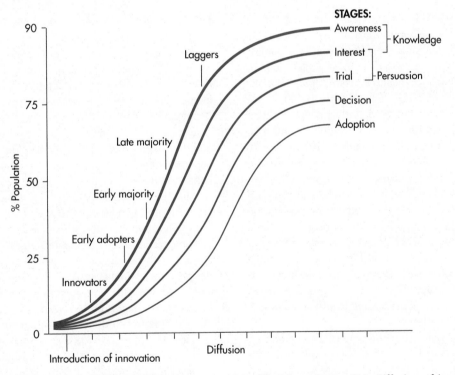

**FIGURE 12-2** Adoptions of Innovations Curve. (Modified from Rogers EM: *Diffusion of innovations,* ed 3, New York, 1983, Free Press.)

In addition to the theories discussed, it is important for the nurse to become familiar with the conceptual/theoretical models that have been used and shown to be successful in facilitating change among individuals, groups, aggregates, and populations.

## Theoretical Models

Many health behavior and health promotion models exist. Other models often used in nursing include the Health Belief Model, PRECEDE-PROCEED, Pender's Health Promotion Model, and the Multidimensional Health Locus of

**TABLE 12-3**

## *Health Belief Model*

| CONCEPT | DEFINITION | APPLICATION |
|---|---|---|
| Perceived Susceptibility | One's opinion of chances of getting a condition | Define population(s) at risk, risk levels<br>Personalize risk based on a person's features or behavior<br>Heighten perceived susceptibility if too low |
| Perceived Severity | One's opinion of how serious a condition and its sequelae are | Specify consequences of the risk and the condition |
| Perceived Benefits | One's opinion of the efficacy of the advised action to reduce risk or seriousness of impact | Define action to take:<br>how, where, when; clarify the positive effects to be expected |
| Perceived Barriers | One's opinion of the tangible and psychologic costs of the advised action | Identify and reduce barriers through reassurance, incentives, assistance |
| Cues to Action | Strategies to activate "readiness" | Provide how-to information, promote awareness, reminders |
| Self-Efficacy | Confidence in one's ability to take action | Provide training, guidance in performing action |

Source: Glanz K, Rimer BK: *Theory at a glance. A guide for health promotion practice*, Washington, DC, 1997, National Institutes of Health/National Cancer Institute, p. 19

Control. One of the best-known models is the Health Belief Model, which was the prototype for other models including PRECEDE-PROCEED. All of these models and instruments are discussed and have been tested and used in planning, implementing, and evaluating health education programs.

HEALTH BELIEF MODEL. The **Health Belief Model (HBM)** was one of the first models that adapted theory from the behavioral sciences to health problems and it remains widely used today (Glanz, Lewis, Rimer, 1997b; Strecher, Rosenstock, 1997). The model initially was created in the 1950s by Rosenstock (1960, 1966, 1974) following the initial study devised by researchers in the U. S. Public Health Service, which served as an explanatory model to explain the widespread failure of people to participate in programs to prevent or detect disease (Strecher, Rosenstock, 1997). The HBM is known as "...a single model with components that interact to explain health behavior" (Kohler, Grimley, Reynolds, 1999) and is an attempt to explain the use of preventive health services such as childhood immunizations.

Over the past 50 years, the HBM has been continuously refined and modified to help identify and explain the behavior of those who accessed the health care system to prevent illness. It was originally a disease-oriented model that looked at why some people take specific actions to prevent a disease or condition and some who do not. More recently, the HBM has been adapted for a much broader use to explain a variety of health behaviors and to design interventions that would improve client access to preventive measures (Harrison, Mullen, Green, 1992; Janz, Becker, 1984; Mirotznik, Feldman, Stein, 1995; Reynolds, West, Aiken, 1990). Table 12-3 defines the concepts in the model and addresses their application. Figure 12-3 illustrates the links between individual perceptions, modifying factors, and likelihood of action and behavioral change in the model.

The premise for the conceptual base of the model is that an individual's *perceived susceptibility* and *perceived severity* of disease determine a *perceived threat* that will increase the *likelihood of the preventive action* or participation in a health intervention that will decrease or lessen that perceived threat. Acknowledgment of both perceived susceptibility and perceived severity must exist before a perceived threat becomes sufficient to motivate a readiness for action and behavior change.

*Modifying factors* such as social milieu, culture, economic bracket, age, gender, level of understanding, education, knowledge, and overall readiness for action can affect a person's perceived susceptibility and perceived seriousness of a given health problem. These modifying factors also affect the perceived benefits and barriers to health action. For example, adolescents often have low perceived susceptibility in relation to health problems and this can lead to not taking appropriate health action (e.g., teen smoking).

*Cues to action* provide suggestions on how to trigger health action. *Perceived benefits* to action are weighed minus *perceived barriers* and estimate the likelihood of a desired behavioral change. Cues to action include public and media information, health education, environmental events, and body changes such as the discovery of disease symptoms. Cues to action may help motivate clients to take preventive health measures and in fact the community health nurse is often the source of such cues.

The HBM encompasses some of the conceptual, personal characteristics, and subsequent interventions that influence readiness to take health action. The following example illustrates application of the HBM.

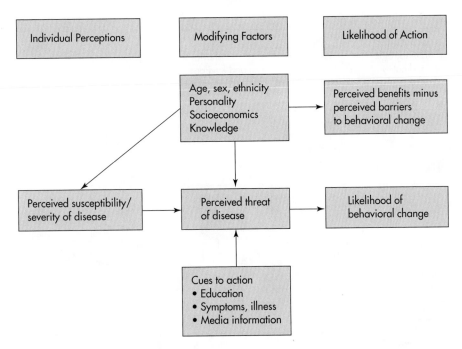

**FIGURE 12-3** The Health Belief Model. (From Strecher VJ, Rosenstock IM: The Health Belief Model. In Glanz K, Lewis FM, Rimer BK, editors: *Health behavior and health education: theory, research, and practice,* ed 2, San Francisco, 1997, Josey-Bass, p. 48.)

**CASE Scenario** A young woman is asked about her belief of the perceived susceptibility she has to contracting a sexually transmitted disease (STD). It is necessary to add to her perceived susceptibility the perceived degree of severity she attaches to STDs. Modifying factors such as age, gender, sexual activity, knowledge, culture, socioeconomic level, and educational level are identified and examined as to their effect on how susceptible she perceives herself to contracting an STD and how seriously she views and understands STDs to be. Modifying factors also require analyses to determine which factors are perceived as benefits and barriers to behavioral change.

The HBM is useful to the nurse in explaining health promoting behaviors that are triggered by an interest in preventing disease. The use of the model helps identify important factors that influence behavioral change. The most promising application of the HBM is for helping develop messages that are likely to persuade individuals to make healthy decisions. It is an effective model for nurses to use in disease prevention actions planned for clients. Many models have emerged that reflect the basic underpinnings of the HBM.

**PRECEDE-PROCEED.** The *PRECEDE Model* was originally conceived and presented by Green, Kreuter, Deeds, et al. (1980) as a model to guide the health education process. The PRECEDE acronym stands for Predisposing, Reinforcing, and Enabling Causes in Educational Diagnosis and Evaluation. It wasn't until the model was used over time and its usefulness determined that Green and Kreuter (1999) proposed the PROCEED part of the model to sup-

port health education program planning efforts. The PROCEED acronym stands for *Policy, Regulatory and Organizational Constructs in Educational and Environmental Development.* The **PRECEDE-PROCEED** model has nine phases (Figure 12-4). The model incorporates community assessment through: social diagnosis (Phase 1), epidemiological diagnosis (Phase 2), and behavioral and environmental diagnosis (Phase 3). These three phases highlight the multidimensional nature of community health problems (see Chapter 12) and the multiple causation of disease (see Chapter 11).

*Phase 1—Social Diagnosis* addresses the collection and analysis of objective and subjective data related to the quality of life of the target population. Quality of life indicators include, but are not limited to, social indicators such as absenteeism, achievement, alienation, comfort, crime, crowding, discrimination, ethics, happiness, hostility, illegitimacy, performance, riots, self-esteem, voters, unemployment, and welfare. Both assets and needs are identified during this phase. Assets mapping helps communities identify their assets including people, associations, and institutions.

Indicators that bear on the quality of life of individuals who comprise the target population may be obtained through national data sources, state and county records, and through general and cultural informants who belong to and represent the target population. Following the analysis of these data, a quality of life diagnosis can be formulated to guide the planning, implementation, and evaluation of a relevant health education program aimed at health promotion and/or disease prevention.

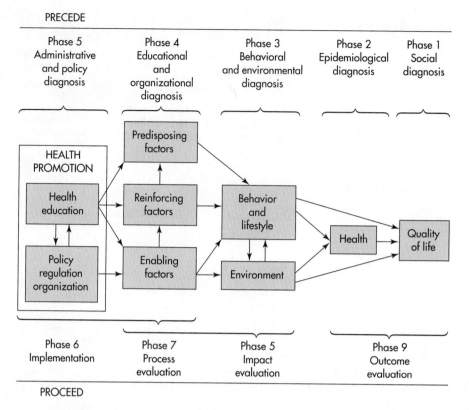

**FIGURE 12-4** PRECEDE-PROCEED. (From Green LW, Kreuter MW: *Health promotion planning: an educational and ecological approach,* ed 3, Mountain View, Calif, 1999, Mayfield, p. 35.)

*Phase 2—Epidemiological Diagnosis* addresses the assessment of the health of the target population. This assessment and diagnosis is concerned with pinpointing important health problems of the target population. Chapter 11 discusses in-depth epidemiological assessment. Of paramount importance to this assessment is to determine which health problems are important to quality of life and which behavioral and environmental factors contribute to the occurrence of those health problems. The community health nurse is particularly interested in the relationship between health (includes the epidemiological assessment data) and social problems (included in the social assessment data).

The epidemiological diagnosis may be formulated from the data obtained from vital indicators of health and the vital indicator dimensions of health. Vital indicators include, but are not limited to disability, discomfort, fertility, fitness, morbidity, mortality, and physiologic risk factors. Vital indicators include data that are available for such things as the distribution, duration, incidence prevalence, intensity, functional level, longevity dimensions of health, and disparities in health among the target population. It is through the two areas of the health assessment (vital indicators and vital indicator dimensions) that analyses will manifest the epidemiological diagnosis for the target population.

*Phase 3—Behavioral and Environmental Diagnosis* examines behavioral and environmental risk factors related to potential or actual health problems in the targeted population and

makes behavioral links to the goals or problems identified in the epidemiological and social diagnoses phases. "Behavioral factors are those behaviors or lifestyles of the individual at risk that contribute to the occurrence and severity of the health problem" (Gielen, McDonald, 1997, p. 366). Behavioral factors might include (but are not limited to) compliance, coping, consumption patterns, self-care, preventive actions, and utilization of resources, whereas the behavioral dimensions for assessment include things such as frequency of behavior, persistence, promptness, quality, range, and other dimensions as appropriate for the group or aggregate and the program planned for them. Green and Kreuter (1991) identified five steps to develop a behavioral diagnosis:

1. Separating behavioral and nonbehavioral causes of the health problem.
2. Developing an inventory of behaviors.
3. Rating behaviors according to their importance.
4. Rating behaviors according to their changeability.
5. Choosing behavioral targets.

Environmental indicators include things such as the economics/affordability, physical environment, biological environment, social environment, access, and services. Environmental diagnosis represents an analysis of the environment and factors that could be causally linked to behavior, health, and quality of life.

*Phase 4—Educational and Organizational Diagnosis* consists of the Predisposing, Reinforcing, and Enabling (the

Individual
Characteristics
and Experiences

Behavior-Specific
Cognitions
and Affect

Behavioral
Outcome

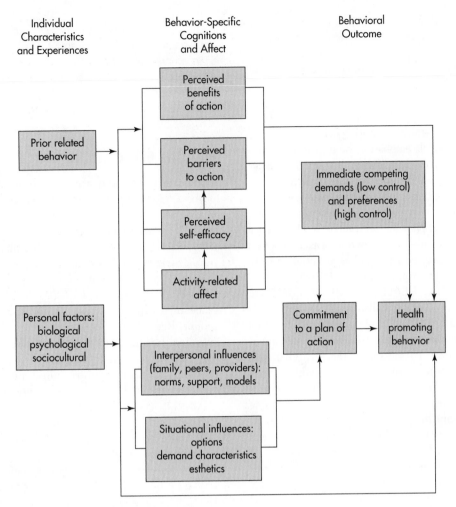

**FIGURE 12-5** Pender's Health Promotion Model. (From Pender NJ: *Health promotion in nursing practice,* ed 3, Stamford, Conn, 1996, Appleton & Lange, p. 67.)

PRE of PRECEDE) factors affecting individual or collective behaviors. The predisposing factors are those antecedents to behavior that provide the rationale or motivation for the behavior; the enabling factors are the antecedents to behavior that enable a motivation to be realized; and the reinforcing factors are those subsequent to a behavior that provide the continuing reward or incentive for the behavior and contribute to its persistence or repetition (Green, Kreuter, 1991). During this phase emphasis is placed on identifying variables that will promote health action.

*Phase 5—Administrative and Policy Diagnoses* is the last phase of the PRECEDE part of the model and involves selecting intervention strategies to address the health problem in question. During this phase, necessary planning for facilitating implementation is addressed. This involves establishing objectives, policies, and the coordination of organizational and community resources.

*Phases 6 to 9—PROCEED* involves the implementation and evaluation of the health education program. Evaluation occurs from three perspectives: process, impact, and outcome. These forms of evaluation are discussed later in this chapter.

The PRECEDE-PROCEED model has been found to be useful in addressing various community issues (Green, Kreuter, 1999). The model helps health planners, in collaboration with consumers, organize assessment data and program planning processes. Community health nurses use the model as a guide to assess, plan, implement, and evaluate successful health promotion programs.

**PENDER'S HEALTH PROMOTION MODEL.** Pender's **Health Promotion Model** was developed by a nurse and reflects a nursing-specific approach to health promotion. This model, in contrast to the HBM, examines health-promoting behaviors that are wellness oriented rather than disease focused.

Pender's *Behavior-Specific Cognitions and Affect* components of the model are considered the major motivational determinants of behavioral outcome. The behavior-specific influences found within Pender's model (Figure 12-5) are perceived benefits of action; perceived barriers to action; perceived self-efficacy; activity-related effect or negative and positive feeling states about a behavior; interpersonal influences from family, peers, providers, and norms; and situational influences that are perceptions of options available, demand characteristics, and esthetic features of environment (Pender, 1996).

Pender (1996) suggests that the biological, psychological, and sociocultural characteristics and prior related behaviors influence health behaviors through behavior-specific cognitive and affective processes. The action outcome is designated by Pender as the health-promoting behavior.

Health behavior models emphasize the importance of assessing more than cognitive understanding or knowledge when determining learner readiness. Often underlying psychosocial factors are the key variables that influence why people do or do not engage in positive health action. For example, it is known that peer pressure (an interpersonal influence in Pender's model) influences health action or lack of action among adolescents. Thus, peer counselors are often used to promote healthy lifestyle activities among adolescents.

MULTIDIMENSIONAL HEALTH LOCUS OF CONTROL ASSESSMENT. Wallston and Wallston (1978, 1984) attempt to clarify the beliefs of clients concerning personal control of their own health status. The **Multidimensional Health Locus of Control Assessment (MHLCA)** instrument assesses perceptions of an individual's health control (Wallston, Wallston, Devellis, 1978). This instrument is designed to determine the way in which different people view certain important health-related issues. The information available to the nurse following completion of the MHLCA instrument analysis provides an indication of the extent to which clients believe they can influence health status through personal behaviors. If clients believe they have *little* control over their own health, these beliefs may need to be changed. Another approach is to use behavior change strategies that have been shown to be successful with persons low in internal control but high in external control; for example, the use of peer pressure groups for weight control. However, if clients score high on beliefs concerning personal control of health, they exhibit an important prerequisite for active participation in self-care.

*Stop and Think About It*

Your agency is concerned about the increased incidence of STDs among the young adult population in your community. Which theory or model do you think is most applicable to community health nursing practice? Why? Describe how you would use the theory or model to address the issue of concern.

## HEALTH EDUCATION PROCESS

Community focused health education, designed to extend beyond traditional health care settings, is fundamental to health promotion and quality of life (USDHHS, 2000, pp. 7-3) Health education activities are designed to identify and address individual, political, social, and economic determinants of health that impede or facilitate clients' movement toward a healthy lifestyle. As addressed in *Healthy People 2010*, health education takes place in diverse settings with individuals, families, and groups. Regardless of the environment in which community health nurses practice, the health education process can be used to establish partnerships with their clients, providing education and counseling to promote self-management of health status (Clark, Gong, Schork, et al., 1997).

The **health education process** has been defined as "the continuum of learning that enables people, as individuals and members of social structures, to voluntarily make decisions, modify behaviors, and change social considerations in ways that are health enhancing" (Aspen Reference Group, 1997, p. 7). The process utilizes a comprehensive lifespan approach to understand the development of health behaviors, awareness of health risks, and appropriate strategies for promoting health behavior and risk reduction for each age group.

The health education process follows a systematic, organized framework similar to the nursing process (Table 12-4) and is individualized to meet the learning needs of clients.

**TABLE 12-4**

*Relationship of Teaching Process to Nursing Process*

| ASSESSMENT | DIAGNOSIS | GOALS | INTERVENTION | EVALUATION |
|---|---|---|---|---|
| *Nursing Process* | | | | |
| General screening questions to detect client's need to learn | One of problem statements may be a need to learn or a nursing diagnosis | Learning goals are a subset of goals | Teaching intervention may be delivered with other intervention | Evaluating whether nursing care outcome was met |
| *Teaching Process* | | | | |
| Refined assessment of need and readiness to learn | Learning diagnosis | Setting of learning goals | Teaching | Evaluating learning |

From: Redman BK: *The practice of patient education*, ed 9, St Louis, 2001, Mosby, p. 5.

Each of the steps contributes to the overall success of the process to facilitate client learning and promote positive health behaviors (Boyd, 1998). Teaching clients to make their own health decision is a significant contribution to assuming accountability for health (Gleit, 1998). Health education models (described previously in this chapter) also facilitate a systematic approach to the development of health education interventions for specific target groups (Kline, 1999).

The teaching-learning process is summarized in Figure 12-6, and a discussion of the steps of this process follows. This dynamic process involves working collaboratively with clients in determining learning needs and strategies to meet these needs. Integral to this process is community involvement in program planning, implementation, and evaluation to achieve social and behavioral outcomes and enhance program maintenance (Frankish, Lovato, Shannon, 1999). Program planning concepts are addressed in Chapter 15.

## Assessment

A comprehensive, holistic assessment of the learner, the environment, and available resources is important to establish appropriate learning objectives and effective interventions and to ensure optimal learning outcomes. Primary community health nursing responsibilities during assessment include (1) developing a trusting and therapeutic relationship, (2) collecting data on multiple parameters of health, and (3) using a variety of data collection methods. *Data collection methods* vary according to feasibility and the client population (individuals, targeted populations, communities, resources allocated, time constraints, and other factors). These methods include, but are not limited to, literature review, interview, questionnaires, surveys, and analysis of existing databases and census data.

*Focus groups* are a good tool for identifying needs of a specific population. Such groups allow participants to openly explore their health issues and identify common concerns or barriers to learning or behavior change (Gettleman, Winkleby, 2000).

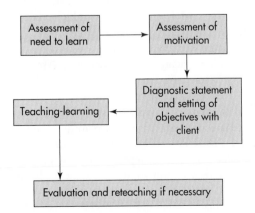

**FIGURE 12-6** The Teaching-Learning Process. (From Redman BK: *The practice of patient education,* ed 9, St Louis, 2001, Mosby, p. 4.)

A priority task during assessment is to gather data about the client's learning needs. This data includes information on health status, health values, developmental characteristics, and prior learning experiences in relation to health (Whitman, 1998). Accurate assessment of the client's **readiness to learn** or to take health action is important. Validation of learner readiness and willingness to engage in behavioral change is crucial to developing learning objectives and teaching plans (Gleit, 1998).

Readiness is a complex, multidimensional phenomenon involving the interaction between variables such as the client's perception of health and illness, family patterns of health care, availability of resources, and client priorities and motivation. It can be influenced by illness, crises, fear, physiologic demands, and concern for other family members (Whitman, 1998). Although many clients are aware of their health education and health promotion needs, they are not ready to act on them. The models previously discussed in this chapter help identify why the learner is not ready to take action.

The nurse needs to understand that client awareness of a need does not always indicate readiness to act on the need (*awareness versus readiness*). An example of awareness versus readiness is seen in a young mother who is aware of the need to obtain immunizations for her preschool children. The community health nurse has spoken to the mother on numerous occasions about immunization schedules, where immunizations can be obtained, and the importance of these immunizations in preventing communicable disease. However, the young mother has not obtained the necessary immunizations for her children. Barriers such as cost, transportation, and clinic hours that conflict with the mother's work hours have kept her from acting on this need.

### *Stop and Think About It*

Think of a personal health care need that you are aware of but are not ready to act on at this time. What is keeping you from acting on this need? Do you think that clients have similar reasons for not being able to act on health care needs? What are some of the reasons that clients may be aware of a need but not ready to act on it?

Self-assessment inventories, interviews, and checklists facilitate identification of learning needs. In addition, learner motivation and evidence of information-seeking behavior also should be assessed. The client's level of knowledge, language skills, and reading ability should be assessed to determine not what can be learned, but rather, the strategies the nurse should use to help clients learn (Whitman, 1998). Additionally, the role of the social and cultural influences on health must be assessed to assist in planning health education programs that are culturally sensitive and relevant (Frankish, Lovato, Shannon, 1999).

It is important to assess the learning environment for factors that facilitate or impede learning, including the physical and psychosocial context of health teaching (Graham,

1998). External factors such as health education program fees, location, and teaching materials may influence learner participation as well as behavioral outcomes. Other important environmental characteristics to assess are resources such as time, space, personnel, financial support, and technical assistance that support educational interventions.

## Analysis

Analysis is a cognitive process that involves categorization of assessment data, identification of health education diagnoses, and prioritizing learning needs. In this phase, the focus is on learning about the behaviors and environmental influences that need to be changed, as well as the possible barriers to achieving the desired health behavior (Glanz, Rimer, 1997). When working with populations and communities, the analysis process yields (1) a description of the learning needs, (2) specific target groups who are affected, (3) an understanding of contributing factors, and (4) identification of interventions that would prevent or eliminate the health problem (Kline, 1999). For each potential area of group intervention, the influence of predisposing, enabling, and reinforcing factors (see PRECEDE-PROCEED model in this chapter) must be analyzed to determine which factors, if modified, will result in improved health (Butler, 1994).

An important outcome of this process is the *health education diagnosis*. Based on interpretation of data about the client's health status and learning needs, the educational diagnosis provides direction related to what the client needs to learn and what the nurse needs to teach. Diagnoses may reflect actual or potential health problems related to lack of knowledge or skill or a diagnosis related to wellness enhancement for an individual, group, or community (Whitman, 1998).

Health education diagnoses may encompass risk behaviors, health-promoting behaviors, self-management skills, or disease prevention activities (Bartholomew, Parcel, Kok, et al., 2001). Multiple diagnoses may be drawn for an individual, family, or group. For example, *lack of knowledge* or awareness of preventive safety measures may influence childhood injury rates in a given community. Other possible diagnoses related to childhood injury rates might be *inadequate parenting skills* and *potential for injury related to environmental hazards*.

During the analysis phase, health education priorities are determined based on the importance of the health issue, resources and time available, and potential for change as a result of health education (Doyle, Ward, 2001). When several health-related behaviors or concerns are identified, more extensive analysis may be needed to clarify target areas for intervention. The impact of multiple factors on health and quality of life will help establish health education priorities, but these must be determined in collaboration with the client. When the health problems and behaviors of the target group, as well as modifying variables have been estab-

lished, planning for health education interventions can be initiated (Kline, 1999).

## Planning

Individual, family, and community involvement is important in all stages of health education planning to promote ownership and participation and ensure socially and culturally appropriate health education (Thompson, Gifford, Thorpe, 2000). The learning/educational diagnosis established between the client and nurse is used as a foundation for planning for health education activities.

Planning begins with establishing mutually determined goals and objectives for the learning experience. *Goals* are broad statements of expected end products of the educational intervention, generally stated as short-term or long-term outcomes, depending on client needs and time available (Boyd, 1998). *Learning objectives* identify the behavioral outcomes of the health education process. Written from the perspective of the learner, learning objectives must be stated in realistic, specific, measurable terms that clearly identify *who* will do *what* and in *what time frame*, as well as *how it will be measured* (Boyd, 1998). The following is an example of a learning objective: *At the end of the teaching session each member of the class will be able to state one community resource for family planning information.*

Learning objectives will address a specific *domain of learning*: cognitive, affective, or psychomotor. Objectives in the *cognitive domain* relate to changes in health knowledge or awareness and are frequently the focus of health education planning and intervention. Objectives in the *affective domain* address attitudes and beliefs that influence health behavior, while *psychomotor domain* objectives focus on specific behaviors and skills (diet, exercise) essential to healthy lifestyles (Butler, 1994). Once learning objectives are determined, interventions are tailored to achieve a specific health behavior. Although there is no foolproof combination to ensure educational effectiveness, interventions should consider the characteristics of the client and level of change desired (Kline, 1999). Interventions that are sensitive to language, literacy needs, values, and culture are more likely to be successful (Gettleman, Winkleby, 2000).

Critical components of planning encompass selecting and sequencing content, identifying health education resources (e.g., American Heart Association, American Lung Association), selecting teaching methods, and selecting a method of evaluation. A review of the literature is often beneficial in identifying effective strategies for a particular group and specific health issue. A planning model such as PRECEDE-PROCEED (Green, Kreuter, 1999) may facilitate the identification of appropriate strategies to address behavioral and environmental influences on health when working with populations and communities.

Effective health teaching is based on several important principles. First, the content should reflect specificity and simplicity, providing "needed" versus "nice-to-know" information. Content should be organized from the simple to the more complex, building on ideas over time. Because the first, third, and last fourth of content is retained best, repetition and reinforcement is beneficial to most learners (Boyd, 1998).

A variety of teaching formats may be used, depending on the content and the target audience. Box 12-2 highlights some teaching methods for individuals and groups. Additional strategies include games, films and videotapes, case presentations, debate, structured controversy, media clips, discussing a problem of local interest, and the use of newspaper or magazine articles to stimulate discussion.

Materials selected must serve a purpose, be appropriate to learner needs and abilities, and be suitable to achieving the stated objectives. All materials should be previewed and evaluated before use. Other considerations in planning teaching methods relate to the availability of financial and personnel resources and access to materials. Are there qual-

ified personnel to teach the content? What is already developed? Is there a national or school-based curriculum? In developing health education content, materials available through volunteer health agencies such as the American Heart Association, American Lung Association, American Diabetes Association, Alzheimer's Association, or Arthritis Foundation are valuable resources. The nurse may elect to develop educational materials for a specific target group if this would better meet their learning needs. An increasing selection of health education materials is also available on the internet (discussed later in this chapter).

Timing needs to be considered in planning. For example, an acute episode of illness may present "teachable moments" for new information about a disease process, while newly diagnosed clients may not be ready or motivated to learn. Teachable moments present an opportunity to initiate health education and behavior change (Campbell, 1999). However, stress, financial concerns, and other family

---

 **BOX 12-2**

## *Individual and Group Teaching Methods*

### Cognitive

**DISCUSSION (ONE-ON-ONE OR GROUP)**
May involve nurse and client or nurse with several clients
Promotes active participation and focuses on topics of interest to client
Allows peer support
Enhances application and analysis of new information

**LECTURE**
Is a more formal method of instruction because it is controlled by teacher
Helps learner acquire new knowledge and gain comprehension

**QUESTION-AND-ANSWER SESSION**
Is designed specifically to address client's concerns
Assists client in applying knowledge

**ROLE PLAY, DISCOVERY**
Allows client to actively apply knowledge in controlled situation
Promotes synthesis of information and problem solving

**INDEPENDENT PROJECT (COMPUTER-ASSISTED INSTRUCTION), FIELD EXPERIENCE**
Allows client to assume responsibility for completing learning activities at own pace
Promotes analysis, synthesis, and evaluation of new information and skills

### Affective
**ROLE PLAY**
Allows expression of values, feelings, and attitudes

**DISCUSSION (GROUP)**
Allows client to acquire support from others in group
Permits client to learn from other experiences
Promotes responding, valuing, and organization

**DISCUSSION (ONE-ON-ONE)**
Allows discussion of personal, sensitive topics of interest or concern

### Psychomotor
**DEMONSTRATION**
Provides presentation of procedures or skills by nurse
Permits client to incorporate modeling of nurse's behavior
Allows nurse to control questioning during demonstration

**PRACTICE**
Gives client opportunity to perform skills using equipment
Provides repetition

**RETURN DEMONSTRATION**
Permits client to perform skill as nurse observes
Is excellent source of feedback and reinforcement

**INDEPENDENT PROJECTS, GAMES**
Require teaching method that promotes adaptation and origination of pyschomotor learning
Permit learner to use new skills

From Potter PA, Perry AG: *Basic nursing: theory and practice*, ed 4, St Louis, 1999, Mosby, p. 258.

crises often present real barriers to effective learning, and every effort should be made to negotiate a more appropriate time for the health education.

## Implementation

The implementation phase of the teaching process involves carrying out activities related to the accomplishment of the health education plan, goals, and objectives. In addition to specific nursing interventions with the client, these activities may include indirect professional responsibilities such as the selection of resources, marketing to promote the program, procurement of equipment and facilities, as well as budget and resource decisions (Butler, 1994).

In implementing a health education or health promotion activity the nurse needs to realize that simply supplying information does little to promote behavior change. Involving individuals, families, and communities in implementation activities gives them a sense of ownership, which tends to increase compliance with the learning plan and facilitates achievement of behavioral objectives. Participant involvement also helps ensure self-empowerment through improved skills and motivation to modify personal behavior and can stimulate community action related to public health concerns (Gettleman, Winkleby, 2000).

Preliminary aspects of implementation focus on establishing administrative support and securing the necessary resources; later activities relate to carrying out learning activities and keeping them focused on the defined outcomes (Kline, 1999). Putting together a detailed curriculum plan, including specific learning materials, is another important component of health education implementation (Doyle, Ward, 2001). Because modifications in the health education process are expected during the implementation phase, it is important to establish mechanisms for monitoring program progress.

## Evaluation

Evaluation is an ongoing, cyclic process. It provides the basis for strengthening the health education process, and lays the foundation for further program development. In evaluating health education and health promotion programs, it is important to determine both their short- and long-term effectiveness on health behavior. Evaluation is accomplished at different levels throughout the health education process.

**Impact evaluation** is based on established behavioral objectives for the health education program and provides a measure of change in health knowledge, attitudes, and behavior in the client or target group (Kline, 1999). With impact evaluation, the short-term, immediate effects of health education can be evaluated (Doyle, Ward, 2001).

**Process evaluation** is conducted during the development and implementation phases of the health education process to assess the quality of the program and appropriateness of implementation activities (Kline, 1999). The nurse would be interested in the overall teaching process

and what could be done to make the teaching session more effective, including such aspects as appropriateness of teaching strategies, intended effects, and client or group participation responses.

**Outcome evaluation** looks at the achievement of learning objectives over time such as long-term effects on morbidity, mortality, and quality-of-life measures (Doyle, Ward, 2001) or ability to carry out a medical procedure, activity of daily living, or a developmental task. Difficulties in evaluating health trends over extended periods arise because of the complexity of these programs and their costs in terms of time and resources (Kline, 1999).

**Formative evaluation** is used during the presentation to detect a need for immediate modification(s). An example of the use of formative evaluation would be the nurse noting that participants looked confused. In response to this feedback, one action in response might be to go back and restate material that had been presented.

The types of evaluation used will depend on the purpose of the evaluation—demonstrating program effectiveness, an increase in health knowledge, or a change in health behavior. Both qualitative (e.g., focus groups, interviews, observation) and quantitative (e.g., measurement scales, pretest and posttest) evaluation methods may be appropriate, depending on the focus of the evaluation. A literature review often provides direction for specific appropriate evaluation methods and techniques.

## LITERACY AND HEALTH

**Health literacy** is defined as "the capability of individuals to obtain, interpret, and understand basic health information and services as well as the competence and motivation to use such information and services in ways that enhance their health" (Kiefer, 2001, p. 2). Health literacy limitations may range from an inability to read prescription bottles and appointment slips to misunderstanding a provider's directions for care (Baker, Parker, Williams, et al., 1997). In practice, the impact of these limitations is reflected in higher incidence of medication errors, adverse drug events, and poor compliance with health provider recommendations. Other literacy problems in relation to health care include a lack of understanding of abbreviations, medical jargon, increasingly complex health care information, or instructions given for care (Davis, Meldrum, Tippy, et al., 1996).

Many adults in the United States also experience difficulty in assuming responsibility for their health (Root, Stableford, 1999), and illiteracy contributes to this. With a tendency to delay seeking needed services, those with low levels of literacy also incur greater costs for health care. In 1998, the toll for more frequent doctors visits and longer hospital stays reached an estimated $35 billion to $73 billion (Friedland, 1998).

It is estimated that more than 40 million Americans are functionally illiterate, having less than fifth grade reading skills, and an additional 50 million are marginally literate (Kiefer, 2001). Among groups with low literacy skills, many live in poverty, many are unemployed or on public assistance, and many have physical or mental health problems that keep them from work or school. Beyond the economic and social costs, illiteracy represents a serious public health problem in terms of access to service, resource utilization, and compliance problems. People who are illiterate often have difficulty acquiring health knowledge and skills and frequently lack knowledge about effective health behaviors.

The elderly, as a result of limitations with vision and hearing, share similar characteristics to low literacy groups. Many Medicare enrollees age 60 and older lack basic skills required to choose insurance coverage and make informed health care decisions and need special consideration in relation to health literacy (Gazmararian, Baker, Williams, et al., 1999; Williams, Parker, Baker, et al., 1995).

## Literacy Assessment

Community health professionals will need to assess the functional literacy level of clients as well as the reading level of educational materials in order to provide effective health education. Low educational attainment and poor literacy skills may limit comprehension of basic health educational materials (Gettleman, Winkleby, 2000). For teaching to be effective, an assessment should be made of the client's reading level and ability to comprehend the elements of the proposed program. It is also important for the nurse educator to communicate ideas and techniques at the level of the learner and to be aware of the appropriateness of the teaching materials. One cannot equate level of education with literacy level because self-report of grades completed is not always consistent with actual reading level (Wilson, 1995).

Specific screening tools such as the *Rapid Assessment of Adult Literacy in Medicine* (REALM) (Davis, Long, Jackson, et al., 1993) and the *Short Test of Functional Health Literacy in Adults* (Parker, Baker, Williams, et al., 1995) are easy to administer and provide a more definitive approach to health literacy assessment. Less formal approaches such as one-on-one interactions and use of non–health-related materials also may be used to determine clients' reading ability and comprehension skills (Kiefer, 2001). Readability formulas, based on the difficulty of vocabulary in the text and the average length of sentences, provide an estimate of the grade level of the content (Root, Stableford, 1999). These formulas are relatively easy to use and available as a component of most word processing packages used today.

## Health Education Strategies

Teaching strategies useful in working with low literacy clients are given in Box 12-3. When working with low literacy clients, selection of strategies for teaching should take into consideration the participants' reading level and their ability to understand the content to be presented.

**BOX 12-3**
*Teaching Low-Literacy Clients*

Teaching strategies useful in promoting self-care for low-literacy clients include the following:

### Less Is More
Determine what is essential information and define the "bottom line" in terms of skills and behaviors necessary. THINK SURVIVAL. Teach the smallest amount possible to do the job. Use of a teaching checklist is beneficial for structure and consistency.

### Making the Point
In teaching, use the simplest terms possible, avoiding medical jargon. Make sure common terms are understood. Always illustrate or demonstrate important skills. Drawings, teaching aids, or simple medical equipment are often helpful.

### Test Comprehension
The easiest method for testing comprehension is to ask for a return demonstration of important skills or behaviors. Ask the client to state to you what he/she has learned in his/her own language. In many cases, there will be a need for repetition or alternate instructions.

### Review
Allow some time between teaching and review so that clients can practice their new skills and knowledge. Encourage the use of teaching aids such as handouts, booklets, or brochure.

Modified from Doak C, Doak L, Root J: *Teaching patients with low literacy skills,* ed 2, Philadelphia, 1996, JB Lippincott.

Reading levels are frequently a concern with written materials, both in terms of what the reading level is and what it should be for the intended audience (Bartholomew, Parcel, Kok, et al., 2001). Research has demonstrated a gap between consumer reading comprehension and the reading level of commonly used health education materials. While the national reading comprehension level is estimated at or below the eighth grade level, the majority of health information available through the government, health agencies, and industry sources requires a reading level of tenth grade or higher (Davis, Crouch, Wills, et al., 1990; Hartman, McCarthy, Park, et al., 1994).

Audiovisual aids are an important component of effective teaching. However, these alone are not sufficient to ensure learning because they usually do not require participation or return demonstration (Doak, Doak, Root, 1996). It is also critical to remember that not all teaching materials will produce the same results for everyone and teaching plans should be individualized. Depending on the complexity of language and content area, methods of delivering health messages, such as pamphlets, brochures, posters, and newsprint, may require adaptation for use by low literacy groups. However, merely changing words does not guarantee increased comprehension of health content. Effective health messages must be presented in an appealing and simple format, using culturally appropriate language with supportive illustrations to deliver "need-to-know" information (Root, Stableford, 1999). In assisting people with low health literacy, various strategies, including one-on-one teaching, group assistance, visual tools, and reading programs, have been shown to be useful interventions (Kiefer, 2001). The tasks of the health care provider in teaching low-literacy clients includes:

- Focusing on working around barriers to help them perform a minimum set of instructions or behaviors
- Allowing them to achieve a reasonable level of competency for self-management of health care problems
- Helping them process the message and decide to make the necessary behavioral change

It is important to remember that the goal of self-help cannot become a reality unless the client is able to understand what they are supposed to do (Doak, Doak, Root, 1996). The nurse needs to assure that the client understands the health care information presented.

## HEALTH EDUCATION IN COMMUNITY HEALTH SETTINGS

Community health education parallels the health education process for an individual client/group but targets a larger population. Health education in the community is generally directed at health problems that are identified as a community priority by the local public health department or other community agency responsible for community health planning. Planning community health programs is part of the community assessment and planning process (see Chapters 14 and 15). *Healthy People 2010* addressed educational and community-based programs in a variety of settings (see Box 12-1).

Many community health sites lend themselves for community health education. Since the inception of health education, schools have been a focal point for efforts to reduce health-risk behaviors and improve the health status of youth (Butler, 1994). Based on their potential to reach a large number of children, schools are a logical site for interventions that help youth develop skills, change health behaviors, and empower them to take responsibility for their own health (USDHHS, 2000, p. 7-5). Some of the most effective health education efforts for youth incorporate peer support, which is an inherent benefit of school-based programs (Perry, 1999; Wren, Janz, Caravano, et al., 1997). Although most schools require health education, teacher competence and comfort in relation to controversial or sensitive topics is often a barrier to school health education (Sanderson, 2000). Topics for school health education and the role of the school nurse in education are discussed in Chapter 20.

Worksite health education is beneficial to managers, employees, and the community. These programs provide an opportunity to support health while reducing health care costs, increasing worker productivity, and decreasing absenteeism (USDHHS, 2000, p. 7-5). Based on employee risk appraisal and environmental assessments, interventions in the workplace may target behavior change, the development of policies to facilitate a healthy and safer workplace, and environmental support to maintain behavioral changes (Campbell, 1999). Although the role of occupational and environmental health nurses is clearly focused on health education and health promotion (see Chapters 6 and 21), policies and resources for health teaching may be lacking in certain work environments, thus limiting the extent to which preventive health measures are implemented and supported.

The value of health education also is being emphasized by many health care organizations. While the quantity and quality is frequently affected by policies and administrative support in different settings, the importance of health teaching is reflected in role expectations, job descriptions, and inclusion in mission and philosophy statements (Graham, 1998). Organization administrators are now required to meet JCAHO standards by providing the necessary support and resources for patient teaching. In addition, an external incentive to clinicians and administrators concerning the value of health education is also required by JCAHO (Patterson, Garcia, Simmons, 2000).

## HEALTH EDUCATION RESOURCES AND TECHNOLOGY

Multiple channels of communication deliver and influence health messages. Enhanced health communication channels include print media, radio, television, audiovisual, internet, and computer-based programs. The impact of multimedia on health has been positive and negative, varying according to age and individual ability to discriminate and evaluate content.

The mass media has an ability to reach large numbers of people and is increasingly used in the development and delivery of health messages (Abrams, Emmon, Linnan, 1997). The media can be a powerful and influential tool that influences health decisions and health behavior change and delivers significant health education messages. Media advertising of health education activities includes, but is not limited to, such opportunities as promoting program participation, highlighting individual and organizational efforts, and reporting on health activities (Helvie, 1998). Another advantage of the mass media in health education is its potential to modify the social environment and social policy in order to support and reinforce desired changes (Flay, Burton, 1990). Nurses are using the media as channels for health advocacy as well as for disseminating health information to multiple community groups.

The internet represents a tremendous health care resource and increased access to health information for health care providers, educators, and consumers. Multiple websites producing health-related information targeted to various consumers include massive accesses to information and health education.

When using the internet, it is important for health care professionals and consumers to determine that the source of information found is reliable. The nurse needs to consider which applications the internet might provide to assist educating individuals, groups, and communities. It also is important for professionals to consider how the use of the internet may benefit reaching the goals of health education and health promotion and help meet the objectives of *Healthy People 2010*.

Numerous opportunities exist to use technology to keep current and to develop teaching materials related to health promotion. With the rapid expansion of health-related websites, evaluation of content for timeliness, accuracy, and source of information is essential. A sample evaluation format is available through the Centers for Disease Control and Prevention (CDC) website (*http://www.cdc.gov*). Government-sponsored websites and publications are excellent sources of health information and are readily accessible through many government agencies discussed throughout this text. Also, health education materials may be accessed through the websites of voluntary health organizations such as the American Heart Association, American Cancer Society, American Diabetes Association, and the American Lung Association. Many professional organizations and publications related to health education and health promotion are now available on-line.

## THE FUTURE OF HEALTH EDUCATION

Current health care trends suggest the need for cost-effective approaches that emphasize health promotion and disease prevention programs (Murray, Zentner, Samiezade-Yazd, 2001). The community health nurse has tremendous potential for improving the health and well-being of individuals, families, and communities through interventions that "confront and challenge people to change what they believe and how they behave in order to preserve or regain their health" (Bruhn, 2001, p. vii).

Educators and service personnel are examining ways to strengthen health promotion interventions for the community. Hills and Lindsey (1994) proposed a health promotion framework with a more holistic, preventive approach to nursing education. They described this framework as a "philosophy change to a humanistic, phenomenologic, and critical social orientation that considers the changing health needs of our society" (p. 159). This change encompasses not merely a relabeling of previous content, but of adopting a new curriculum to address inequities, create service-education collaboration, and encourage community participation in health. Service-education partnerships have been able to demonstrate community-based health education/ health promotion interventions that are cost effective and

accessible for vulnerable groups, such as homeless populations, who are at increased risk of health-damaging behaviors (Schaffer, Mather, Gustafson, 2000).

At a time when health care decisions are driven by cost containment measures, health promotion interventions and health education can help improve quality of life and decrease health care costs. Nursing interventions, traditionally focused on providing information to help people engage in health promoting behaviors, must expand to reflect and address the influence of the sociopolitical and cultural environment on health choices. From this perspective, nurses may be viewed as "pacesetters" and advocates for health promotion with the potential to ensure maximal health for all citizens (Morgan, Marsh, 1998). In the words of C. Everett Koop, the former Surgeon General of the United States, "An informed and aroused public can change the health of each of us."

## SUMMARY

Health education has traditionally been an important part of the role of the community health nurse. Health promotion and disease prevention are integral components of the nursing care for individuals, families, aggregates, and communities in multiple practice settings. Similar to the nursing process, theoretical models for the health education process outline a systematic approach to the identification of learning needs, educational diagnoses, planning and implementing health education, and evaluating the health outcomes of these interventions. Health education theories and models provide direction for interventions related to changes in health attitudes, beliefs, knowledge, and skills and provide a foundation upon which the nurse can tailor this process to meet the specific needs of targeted community groups.

In light of national trends focused on changing lifestyle factors that contribute significantly to disease and chronic illness, all nurses have a significant role in health education and health promotion efforts. Community-based health care provides expanded opportunities for health education in schools, worksites, and health care organizations. The effectiveness of health education with health promotion programs is greatly enhanced within a framework addressing multiple levels of influence related to individual behaviors, social norms, community variables, and public policy.

## CRITICAL THINKING
*exercise*

The community health nurse is planning a health education program for a rural community population. A significant number of residents have not completed high school, and there is a high rate of unemployment. Using the PRECEDE-PROCEED health assessment and planning model, and considering the needs of rural populations, identify factors that might contribute to poor health status in this community. Discuss whom you might contact to obtain specific information about community health needs.

## REFERENCES

Abrams D, Emmon K, Linnan L: Health behavior and health education: the past, present, and future. In Glanz K, Lewis FM, Rimer B, editors: *Health behavior and health education: theory, research, and practice*, ed 2, San Francisco, 1997, Josey-Bass.

Acton G, Malathum P: Basic need status and health-promoting self-care behavior in adults, *West J Nurs Res* (22)7:796-811, 2000.

Ajzen I, Fishbein M: *Understanding attitudes and predicting social behavior*, Englewood Cliffs, NJ, 1980, Prentice-Hall, Inc.

American Nurses Association (ANA): *Standards of community health nursing practice*, Washington, DC, 1986, ANA.

American Nurses Association (ANA): *Social policy statement*, Washington, DC, 1995, ANA.

American Nurses Association (ANA): *Scope and standards of public health nursing practice*, Washington, DC, 1999, ANA.

Aspen Reference Group: *Community health education and promotion: a guide to program design and evaluation*, Gaithersburg, Md, 1997, Aspen.

Baker D, Parker R, Williams M, et al.: The relationship of patient reading ability to self-reported health and use of health services, *Am J Public Health* 87(6):1027-1030, 1997.

Bandura A: *Social learning theory*, Englewood Cliffs, NJ, 1977, Prentice Hall.

Bandura A: *Social foundations of thought and action. A social cognitive theory*, Englewood Cliffs, NJ, 1986, Prentice Hall.

Bartholomew LK, Parcel G, Kok G, et al.: *Intervention mapping: designing theory-and evidence-based health promotion programs*, Mountain View, Calif, 2001, Mayfield.

Boyd M: The teaching process. In Boyd M, Graham B, Gleit C, et al., editors: *Health teaching in nursing practice. A professional model*, Stamford, Conn, 1998, Appleton & Lange.

Bruhn J: Forward, *Fam Community Health* 23(4):vii, 2001.

Butler T: *Principles of health education and health promotion*, Englewood, Colo, 1994, Morton Publishing.

Campbell K: Adult education: helping adults begin the process of learning. *AAOHN J* 47(1):31-40, 1999.

Clark N, Gong M, Schork M, et al.: A scale for assessing health care providers' teaching and communication behavior regarding asthma, *Health Educ Behavior* 24(2):245-256, 1997.

Davis TC, Crouch MA, Wills G, et al.: The gap between patient reading comprehension and the readability of patient education materials, *J Fam Practice* 31:533-538, 1990.

Davis TC, Long SW, Jackson RH, et al.: Rapid estimate of adult literacy in medicine: a shortened screening instrument, *Fam Med* 25:391-395, 1993.

Davis TC, Meldrum H, Tippy P, et al.: How poor literacy leads to poor health care, *Patient Care* 30(16):94-103, 1996.

DiClemente R, Raczynski J: The importance of health promotion and disease prevention. In Raczynski J, DiClemente R: *Handbook of health promotion and disease prevention*, New York, 1999, Kluwer Academic/Plenum Publishers.

Doak C, Doak L, Root J: *Teaching patients with low literacy skills*, ed 2, Philadelphia, 1996, JB Lippincott.

Doyle E, Ward S: *The process of community health education and health promotion*, Mountain View, Calif, 2001, Mayfield.

Flay B, Burton D: Effective mass communication strategies for health campaigns. In Atkins C, Wallach L, editors: *Mass communication and public health*, Newbury Park, Calif, 1990, Sage.

Frankish CJ, Lovato C, Shannon W: Models, theories, and principles of health promotion with multicultural populations. In Huff R, Kline M, editors: *Promoting health in multicultural populations: a handbook for practitioners*, Thousand Oaks, Calif, 1999, Sage.

Friedland RB: *Understanding health literacy: new estimates of the costs of inadequate health literacy.* Presented at the Pfizer Conference on Health Literacy, "Promoting Health Literacy: A Call to Action." Washington, DC, October 7-8, 1998.

Gazmararian JA, Baker DW, Williams MV, et al.: Health literacy among Medicare enrollees in a managed care organization, *JAMA* 281:545-551, 1999.

Gettleman L, Winkleby M: Using focus groups to develop a heart disease prevention program for ethnically diverse, low-income women, *J Community Health* 25(6):439-453, 2000.

Gielen AC, McDonald EM: The PRECEDE-PROCEED planning model. In Glanz K, Lewis FM, Rimer BK, editors: *Health behavior and health education: theory, research and practice*, ed 2, San Francisco, 1997, Josey-Bass.

Glanz K, Lewis FM, Rimer BK: Linking theory, research, and practice. In Glanz K, Lewis FM, Rimer BK, editors: *Health behavior and health education: theory, research, and practice*, ed 2, San Francisco, 1997a, Josey-Bass.

Glanz K, Lewis FM, Rimer BK: The scope of health promotion and health education. In Glanz K, Lewis FM, Rimer BK, editors: *Health behavior and health education: theory, research, and practice*, ed 2, San Francisco, 1997b, Josey-Bass.

Glanz K, Rimer BK: *Theory at a glance. A guide for health promotion practice*, Washington, DC, 1997, National Institutes of Health/National Cancer Institute.

Gleit C: Theories of learning. In Boyd M, Graham B, Gleit C, et al., editors: *Health teaching in nursing practice. A professional model*, Stamford, Conn, 1998, Appleton & Lange.

Graham B: The environment. In Boyd M, Graham B, Gleit C, et al., editors: *Health teaching in nursing practice. A professional model*, Stamford, Conn, 1998, Appleton & Lange.

Green LW, Kreuter MW: *Health promotion planning: an educational and environmental approach*, ed 2, Mountain View, Calif, 1991, Mayfield.

Green LW, Kreuter MW: *Health promotion planning: an educational and ecological approach*, ed 3, Mountain View, Calif, 1999, Mayfield.

Green LW, Kreuter MW, Deeds SG, et al.: *Health education planning: A diagnostic approach*, Palo Alto, Calif, 1980, Mayfield.

Harrison JA, Mullen PA, Green LW: A meta-analysis of studies of the health belief model with adults, *Health Educ Research: Theory and Practice* 7:107-116, 1992.

Hartman TJ, McCarthy PR, Park RJ, et al.: Evaluation of the literacy level of participants in an urban expanded food and nutrition education program, *J Nutr Educ* 26(1):37-41, 1994.

Helvie C: *Advanced practice nursing in the community*, Thousand Oaks, Calif, 1998, Sage.

Hills M, Lindsey E: Health promotion: a viable curriculum framework for nursing education, *Nurs Outlook* 42:158-162, 1994.

Janz NK, Becker MH: The health belief model: a decade later, *Health Educ Q* 11:1-47, 1984.

Joint Commission for Accreditation of Healthcare Organizations (JCAHO): *Joint Commission for Accreditation of Healthcare Organizations Standards*, Washington, DC, 2000, JACHO.

Joint Commission on Health Education Terminology (JCHET): Report of the 1990 Joint Commission on Health Education terminology, *J Sch Health* 61:257-264, 1991.

Kasl SV, Cobb S: Health behavior, illness behavior, and sick-role behaviors, *Arch Environ Health* 12:246-266, 1966.

Kiefer KM: *Health literacy: responding to the need for help*, Washington, DC, 2001, Center for Medicare Education.

Kline M: Planning health promotion and disease prevention programs in multicultural populations. In Huff R, Kline M, editors: *Promoting health in multicultural populations: a handbook for practitioners*, Thousand Oaks, Calif, 1999, Sage, pp. 73-100.

Kohler CL, Grimley D, Reynolds K: Theoretical approaches guiding the development and implementation of health promotion programs. In Raczynski JM, DiClemente RJ, editors: *Handbook of health promotion and disease prevention*, New York, 1999, Kluwer Academic/Plenum Publishers.

Mirotznik J, Feldman L, Stein R: The health belief model and adherence with a community center-based, supervised coronary heart disease exercise program, *J Community Health* 20:233-247, 1995.

Morgan I, Marsh M: Historic and future health promotion contexts for nursing, *Image: J Nurs Sch* 30(4):379-383, 1998.

Murray RB, Zentner JP, Samiezade-Yazd C: Sociocultural influences on the person and family. In Murray RB, Zentner JP, editors: *Health promotion strategies through the lifespan*, ed 7, Upper Saddle River, NJ, 2001, Prentice Hall.

National League for Nursing Education (NLNE): *Standard curriculum for schools of nursing*, Baltimore, 1918, Waverly.

Ottoson J, Green L: Public health education and health promotion. In Novick L, Mays G, editors: *Public health administration: principles for population-based management*, Gaithersburg, Md, 2001, Aspen.

Parker RM, Baker DW, Williams MV, et al.: The test of functional health literacy in adults: a new instrument for measuring a patients' literacy skills, *J Gen Int Med* 10:537-541, 1995.

Patterson C, Garcia C, Simmons R: National trends and developments in patient education: new challenges for health education, *Health Promotion Practice* 1(4):323-326, 2000.

Pender NJ: *Health promotion in nursing practice*, ed 3, Stamford, Conn, 1996, Appleton & Lange.

Perry C: *Creating health behavior change: how to develop community-wide programs for youth*, Thousand Oaks, Calif, 1999, Sage.

Philips B, Chambers D, Whiting L, et al.: Ethical issues in community-based cancer control: considerations in designing interventions, *Fam Community Health* 23(4):62-74, 2001.

Potter PA, Perry AG: *Basic nursing: theory and practice*, ed 4, St Louis, 1999, Mosby.

Raphael D: Emerging concepts of health and health promotion, *J Sch Health* 68(7):297-299, 1998.

Redman BK: *The practice of patient education*, ed 9, St Louis, 2001, Mosby.

Reynolds KD, West SG, Aiken LS: Increasing the use of mammography: a pilot program, *Health Educ Q* 17:429-441, 1990.

Rogers EM: *Diffusion of innovations*, ed 3, New York, 1983, Free Press.

Root J, Stableford S: Easy to read consumer communications: a missing link in Medicaid managed care, *J Health Politics Policy Law* 24(1):1-26, 1999.

Rosenstock IM: What research in motivation suggests for public health, *Am J Public Health* 50:295-301, 1960.

Rosenstock IM: Why people use health services, *Milbank Mem Fund Q* 44:94-124, 1966.

Rosenstock IM: Historical origins of the Health Belief Model, *Health Educ Monographs* 2:328-335, 1974.

Rothstein W: Trends in mortality in the twentieth century. In Lee P, Estes C, editors: *The nation's health*, ed 6, Boston, 2001, Jones & Bartlett.

Sanderson C: The effectiveness of a sexuality education newsletter in influencing teenagers' knowledge and attitudes about sexual involvement and drug use, *J Adolescent Research* 15(6):674-681, 2000.

Schaffer M, Mather S, Gustafson V: Service learning: a strategy for conducting a health needs assessment of the homeless, *J Health Care Poor Underserved* 11(4):385-399, 2000.

Strecher VJ, Rosenstock IM: The Health Belief Model. In Glanz K, Lewis FM, Rimer BK, editors: *Health education and health behavior: theory, research, and practice*, ed 2, San Francisco, 1997, Josey-Bass.

Thompson S, Gifford S, Thorpe L: The social and cultural context of risk and prevention: food and physical activity in an urban aboriginal community, *Health Educ Behavior* 27(6):725-743, 2000.

US Department of Health and Human Services (USDHHS): *Healthy People 2000, full report with commentary*, Washington, DC, 1991, US Government Printing Office.

US Department of Health and Human Services (USDHHS): *Healthy People 2010: conference edition*, Washington, DC, 2000, US Government Printing Office.

Wallston BS, Wallston KA: Locus of control and health: a review of the literature, *Health Educ Monographs* 6(2):107-117, 1978.

Wallston BS, Wallston KA: Social psychological models of health behavior: an examination and integration. In Baum A, Taylor S, Singer J, editors: *Handbook of psychology and health*, vol 4, Hillsdale, NJ, 1984, Erlbaum.

Wallston KA, Wallston BS, Devellis R: Development of the multidimensional health locus of control (MHLC) scales, *Health Educ Monographs* 6(2):160-170, 1978.

Whitman N: Developmental characteristics. In Boyd M, Graham B, Gleit C, et al.: *Health teaching in nursing practice. A professional model*, Stamford, Conn, 1998, Appleton & Lange, pp. 135-155.

Williams MV, Parker RM, Baker DW, et al.: Inadequate functional health literacy among patients at two public hospitals, *JAMA* 274:1677-1682, 1995.

Wilson FL: Monitoring patients' ability to read and comprehend: a first step in patient education, *Nurs Connections* 8(4):17-25, 1995.

World Health Organization (WHO): *Report of the International Conference on Primary Health Care*, held in Alma Alta, USSR, Geneva, Switzerland, 1978, WHO.

Wren PA, Janz N, Caravano K, et al.: Preventing the spread of AIDS in youth: principles of practice from 11 diverse projects, *J Adolesc Health* 21:309-317, 1997.

## SELECTED BIBLIOGRAPHY

Association of State and Territorial Directors of Nursing: *Public health nursing: a partner for healthy populations*, Washington, DC, 2000, American Nurses Publishing.

Bracht N, editor: *Health promotion at the community level: new advances*, Thousand Oaks, Calif, 1999, Sage.

Bruhn J: Ethical issues in intervention outcomes, *Fam Community Health* 23(4):24-35, 2001.

Edelman CL, Mandle CL, editors: *Health promotion throughout the lifespan*, ed 4, St Louis, 1998, Mosby.

Green LW: Health education's contributions to public health in the twentieth century: a glimpse through health promotion's rear-view mirror. In Fielding JE, editor, Lave LB, Starfield B, associate editors: *Annual Review of Public Health*, vol 20, Palo Alto, Calif, 1999, Annual Reviews.

Kulbok PA, Baldwin JH, Cox CL, et al.: Advancing discourse on health promotion: beyond mainstream thinking, *Advances in Nurs Science* 14(4):80-84, 1997.

McKenzie JF, Smeltzer JL: *Planning, implementing, and evaluating health promotion programs: a primer*, ed 3, Needham Heights, Mass, 2001, Allyn & Bacon.

Minnesota Department of Health (MDH): *Public health interventions: examples from public health nursing*, Minneapolis, 1997, MDH.

Mondragon D, Brandon J: Two major ethical issues in health education and promotion: assessing stage of change and cancer screening, *Fam Community Health* 23(4):50-61, 2001.

National Center for Education Statistics: *Adult literacy in America: a first look at the results of the National Adult Literacy Survey*, ed 2, Washington, DC, 1993, US Department of Education.

US Department of Health and Human Services, Public Health Services, National Institutes of Health, Office of Cancer Communications, National Cancer Institute: *Making health communications work*, NIH Pub No 92-1493, Washington, DC, April 1992, USDHHS.

# Aggregate-Focused Contemporary Community Health Issues

*Ella M. Brooks*

## OBJECTIVES

*Upon completion of this chapter, the reader should be able to:*

1. Discuss select aggregate-focused contemporary community health issues.
2. Discuss health risks of minorities and disadvantaged populations.
3. Apply roles of the community health nurse in addressing select aggregate-focused contemporary health problems.

4. Apply the levels of prevention when intervening to resolve select contemporary community health problems.
5. Understand health risks associated with selected contemporary community health issues.
6. Discuss community-focused interventions for addressing selected contemporary community health issues.

## KEY TERMS

Community empowerment
Cultural competence
Cultural diversity
Cultural sensitivity
Excess deaths
Health disparities

Health risk behaviors
Minority health
Poverty
Primary prevention
Process of addiction

Secondary prevention
Stages of addiction
Substance abuse
Tertiary prevention
Violent and abusive behavior

---

*Individual health is closely linked to community health—the health of the community and environment in which individuals live, work, and play [and] every community in every State and territory determines the overall health status of the Nation (USDHHS, 2000a, p. 3).*

---

Numerous health issues face the nation. The vision for Healthy People 2010 is *Healthy People in Healthy Communities* because "over the years, it has become clear that individual health is closely linked to community health" (USDHHS, 2000a, p. 3). Although some health issues may be more salient in one community and less in another, most communities are affected by contemporary health issues. Geographically, health issues vary and community health nurses must keep abreast of health concerns in their respective communities. Because of the ease of geographic mobility and spread of disease, no community can ever live in ignorance, thinking, "This will not happen here, and I don't need to know about this." It is imperative that community health nurses be aware of contemporary community health issues throughout the nation and the world.

Frequently contemporary health problems are multifaceted and individuals are caught in a web of social problems. Figure 13-1 illustrates the web of social problems that influence the development of many health problems. These social problems can increase the risk for disease occurrence and make it more difficult to plan and implement effective interventions to address contemporary health issues.

*Healthy People 2010* has two major goals: to increase the quality and years of life and to eliminate health disparities (USDHHS, 2000a, p. 2). To achieve these goals, our nation

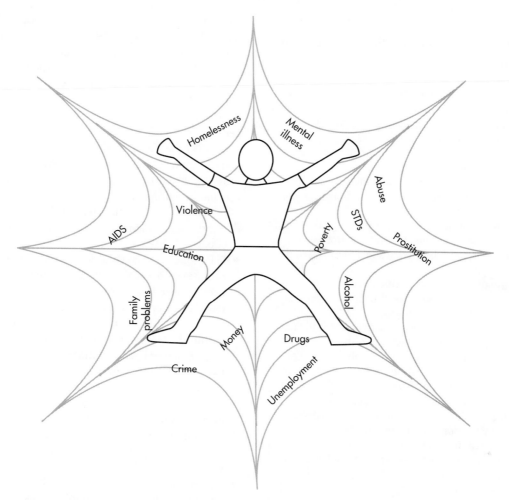

**FIGURE 13-1** Aggregates experiencing a web of social problems that influence the development of many health problems. (Modified from Massaro J, Pepper B: The relationship of addiction to crime, health and other social problems. In Crowe AH, Reeves RR: *Treatment for alcohol and other drug abuse: opportunities for coordination*, DHHS Pub No (SMA)94-2075, Rockville, Md, 1994, US Government Printing Office, p. 14.)

must implement community interventions that address health-related threats to individuals across the life span, health risks for disadvantaged populations, and specific issues involving population groups at risk for poor health. Contemporary community health issues must be analyzed to determine the web of variables influencing the occurrence of these problems and to develop appropriate interventions to solve them.

Chapters 16 through 22 discuss the health profiles of specific developmental age groups and aggregates at risk among these groups. This chapter focuses on "universal" contemporary health issues that reach across developmental stages throughout the life span and affect multiple aggregates. Using *Healthy People 2010* goals and objectives, the needs of select populations are addressed. Specifically, these select populations include minorities, those with low income, abusers of alcohol and drugs, the homeless, those at risk for sexually transmitted diseases and human immunodeficiency

virus/acquired immunodeficiency syndrome (HIV/AIDS), and those who are affected by violence. Issues entangled in the web of these problems create challenges and opportunities for community health nurses.

A comprehensive, multifaceted intervention approach is needed to address the web of problems experienced by aggregates at risk in contemporary society. As community health nurses deal with these aggregates, they must be prepared to assess and intervene both collaboratively and individually to meet the multifaceted needs. The role of the nurse in primary, secondary, and tertiary prevention of these issues is discussed, with emphasis on primary prevention.

## MINORITY HEALTH

**Minority health** has been a major focus over the past decade. This focus continues as the nation has entered into the new century. Race and ethnicity are important variables to con-

### BOX 13-1

## Guidelines for Reporting Federal Data on Race and Hispanic Origin

**American Indian or Alaska Native.** A person having origins in any of the original peoples of North and South America (including Central America) and who maintains tribal affiliation or community attachment.

**Asian**. A person having origins in any of the original peoples of the Far East, Southeast Asia, or the Indian subcontinent including, for example, Cambodia, China, India, Japan, Korea, Malaysia, Pakistan, the Philippine Islands, Thailand, and Vietnam.

**Black or African American**. A person having origins in any of the black racial groups of Africa. Terms such as "Haitian" or "Negro" can be used in addition to "Black or African American."

**Native Hawaiian or Other Pacific Islander**. A person having origins in any of the original peoples of Hawaii, Guam, Samoa, or other Pacific Islands.

**White**. A person having origins in any of the original peoples of Europe, the Middle East, or North Africa.

**Hispanic or Latino.** A person of Cuban, Mexican, Puerto Rican, South or Central American, or other Spanish culture or origin, regardless of race. The term "Spanish origin" can be used in addition to "Hispanic or Latino." Persons of Hispanic origin may be of any race and persons in the various race groups may be of any origin.

**Combined Race and Ethnicity.** Individuals who identify with more than one race may report each. For example, an individual whose mother is Asian and father is Black or African American may report both Asian and Black or African American.

Modified from US Department of Health and Human Services (USDHHS): *Tracking Healthy People 2010*, Washington, DC, 2000b, US Government Printing Office, pp. A-13-14.

sider when addressing contemporary community health issues. "Race and ethnicity are important determinants of health patterns in the United States" (Sondik, Lucas, Madans, et al., 2000, p. 1709). The Office of Minority Health (OMH), a subdivision of the U.S. Department of Health and Human Services (USDHHS), was established to analyze these health patterns and to develop, coordinate, and monitor national strategies to improve minority health. This office has made minority health a public concern and was the impetus for addressing minority health disparities in the *Healthy People* initiatives.

The size of U.S. minority populations has increased dramatically over the past few decades. As a result, the U.S. has become more culturally diverse. This diversity has been reflected in the population census reports over time. In 1976, the federal government began to classify individuals into the following racial groups: black, white, Asian or Pacific Islander, and American Indian or Alaskan Native. His-

panics were classified as "other" populations (National Center for Health Statistics, 1996, p. 108). At that time, Hispanics were first classified separately in the 1980 population reports. "The increasing diversity of the population has necessitated modification of the way race data are collected" (USDHHS, 2000b, p. A-6). As a result, additional changes have been made in classifications for gathering population census data.

In 1997 the OMB developed new standards for collecting and maintaining data on race and ethnicity. These standards were developed to provide a common language that more accurately reflects the increasing diversity of populations (Wallman, Evinger, Schechter, 2000). Under the new standards, the following major changes were made (USDHHS, 2000b, pp. A-13-A-14):

- "Hispanic" is now considered ethnicity and *is no longer classified as a racial group*. The category "Hispanic" has been replaced by "Hispanic or Latino." This can also include black or white races. For example, "Puerto Rican," "Mexican," and "Cuban" may be reported separately within the "Hispanic or Latino" group.
- The "Asian or Pacific Islander" category was divided into two separate categories: "Asian" and "Native Hawaiian or Other Pacific Islander."
- The former "Black" category is replaced by "Black or African American."
- Central and South American Indians, formerly not included in the "American Indian" category, are now included.
- In the case of multiracial backgrounds, people are encouraged to report more than one race.

Box 13-1 presents the guidelines for reporting data on race and ethnicity. These guidelines were used for the 2000 census data collection.

Although the descriptions in Box 13-1 seem clear and easy to follow, the 1997 guidelines provide the basis to "blend" these categories because, as surveys are being conducted, persons who identify with more than one race have the option to check multiple race categories. "Many Americans have multiple ethnic and racial identities" (Henderson, 2000, p. 12). Because of this, the standards were changed to allow individuals who have parents from different races to report more than one race in the data gathering process (Wallman, Evinger, Schechter, 2000). *Healthy People 2010* uses population estimates from the U.S. Census Bureau. *The 1997 changes will make it more difficult to trend and compare current minority health data with data that were collected before the 1997 standards were instituted* (Burhansstipanov, Satter, 2000; Sondik, Lucas, Madans, et al., 2000; Waters, 2000). However, these changes have the potential for helping the nation track the health needs of subpopulations under major racial categories.

Minority populations continue to grow rapidly. Figure 13-2 depicts the U.S. population by race and by growth of population since 1980. This demonstrates the dramatic increase in

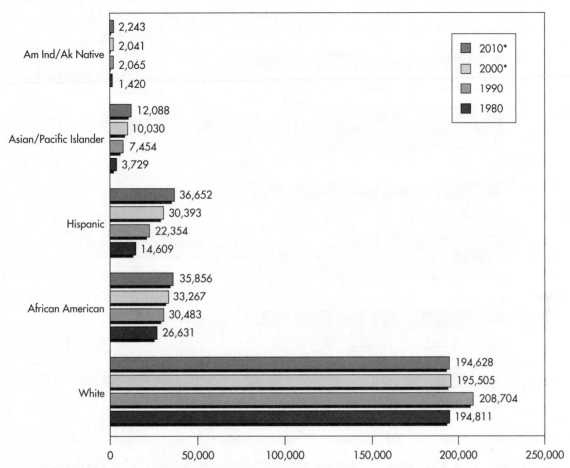

**FIGURE 13-2** U.S. total population (number in thousands) with 2000* and 2010* population projections. (Modified from US Census Bureau: *Statistical abstract of the United States, 1999*, Washington, DC, 1999, US Government Printing Office.)

the minority population groups since 1980. Hispanics and Asian-Pacific Islanders continue to be the fastest growing groups (Henderson, 2000).

### *Stop and Think About It*

Why is it beneficial for community health nurses to understand how race and ethnicity data are categorized? What are the characteristics of population groups in your community? How does having knowledge about the demographic characteristics of population groups in a community help community health nurses plan more effective community-focused interventions?

### Minority Populations and Health Disparities

**Health disparities** continue to exist among minority populations. For example, the infant death rate among African Americans is double that of whites; Hispanics have higher rates of blood pressure than non-Hispanic whites; Native Americans and Alaskan Natives have an infant death rate almost double the rate for whites; new cases of hepatitis and tuberculosis are much higher among Asians and Pacific Is-

landers in the United States than the number of cases for whites; and Native Americans and Alaskan Natives have a much higher death rate from accidents and suicides than their white counterparts (USDHHS, 2000a, p. 12). To address this disparity, one of the two major *Healthy People 2010* goals is to "eliminate health disparities among segments of the population, including differences that occur by gender, race or ethnicity, education or income, disability, geographic location or sexual orientation" (USDHHS, 2000a, p. 11). Current genetic and biological information regarding the characteristics of health problems associated with minority groups does not account for the health disparities that exist among these same groups. Hence, "these disparities are believed to be the result of complex interactions among genetic variations, environmental factors and specific health behaviors" (USDHHS, 2000a, p. 12).

A survey by the Commonwealth Fund found that minority groups overall were more likely to experience more stress and violence, eat unhealthy diets, fail to exercise, live in substandard housing, have difficulty accessing health assistance, and have incomplete education (Commonwealth Fund,

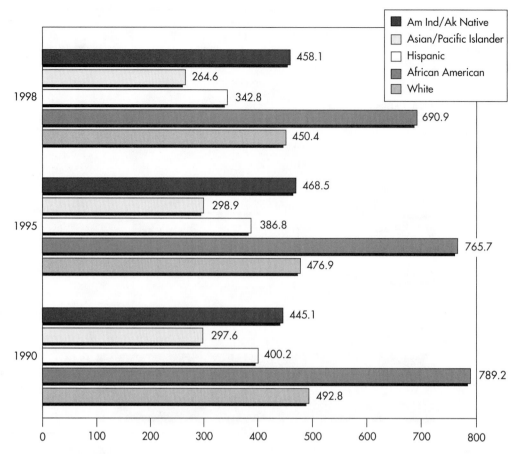

**FIGURE 13-3** Death rates per 100,000 population for all causes by race, all ages, age adjusted, 1990-1998. (Modified from National Center for Health Statistics: *Health, United States, 2000, with adolescent health chartbook,* Hyattsville, Md, 2000, National Center for Health Statistics.)

1995). These problems all contribute to a poorer quality of life. The gap between minority and majority health is most dramatic when mortality is measured in "excess deaths."

## Minority Populations and Excess Deaths

Excess deaths are defined as deaths that would not have occurred if minorities had the same age and sex-specific death rate as the majority population (OMH—Resource Center, 1989, p. 1). The majority of minority excess deaths fall into the categories of heart disease, cancer, diabetes, infant mortality, homicide, HIV/AIDS, and injuries (USDHHS, 2000a). Even when the socioeconomic effects (e.g., poverty, education) are accounted for, health and survival disparities still exist. This was supported in a national longitudinal study involving 530,000 subjects (Sorlie, Backlund, Keller, 1995), which reported significantly higher mortality in African Americans than whites after adjusting for socioeconomic effects. An understanding of the extent and causes of mortality variations between the minority and majority populations provides a foundation for targeting services and designing interventions to reduce these disparities (Blane, 1995).

Figure 13-3 depicts the death rates by race in the United States and displays the disparity in deaths between whites

and minorities. Deaths among minorities exceed those among whites in all age groups except those 15 to 19 and those 85 and over. The life expectancy has been consistently lower in the minority populations than the white majority.

## Nursing and Health of Minority Populations

As discussed in Chapter 1, Lillian Wald and the Henry Street Settlement nurses worked to improve the health of immigrants in the United States (Wald, 1915). This concern with the health of minority populations has continued into contemporary community health nursing practice. Nursing organizations across the nation are working with diverse minority populations to improve their health outcomes.

## Nurses' Commitments to Health of Minority Populations

The American Nurses Association (ANA) made a legislative commitment to encourage unified efforts of health care providers and educators to meet the health care needs of minority groups (ANA, 1995, p. 23). According to this legislative commitment, "ANA will lobby for expansion of health care programs to ensure quality health care for all populations . . . [and ANA] will pursue educational funding for health care workers to increase the number of ethnically and culturally competent professionals" (ANA, 1995, p. 23). ANA's commitment to minorities includes programming to target minority health and the education and development of culturally competent health care providers. It is also designed to strengthen "public health nursing's capacity for population health services" (ANA, 2000, p. 21).

## Nurses and Cultural Competence

Chapters 7 and 9 elaborate on the concepts of **cultural sensitivity** and culturally competent care. **Cultural competence** is an essential component in providing effective health services for diverse populations (USDHHS, 2000c). To provide competent care to culturally diverse minority populations, nurses must have an understanding of the health needs of the minority population being considered. They must also "possess specific knowledge and information about the particular cultural groups they are working with" (Randall-David, 1994, p. 3).

The ANA's (1996b) *Position Statement on Cultural Diversity* provides an operational definition for cultural diversity to guide nurses in their practice with minority groups. "**Cultural diversity** refers to the differences between people based on a shared ideology and valued set of beliefs, norms, customs, and meanings evidenced in a way of life" (ANA, 1996b, p. 90). In practice, it is important for nurses to be *culturally sensitive*, meaning that nurses must be sensitive to the values, beliefs, traditions, and health practices of various cultures that may affect nursing interventions. As previously discussed in Chapter 9, nurses must be able to understand both the language and cultural beliefs and practices of the population that they are working with in order to make a difference in positive health outcomes (Chweadyk, 2000).

## Community Empowerment

Using the health education strategy to mobilize communities to make decisions regarding their own health care needs and solutions (as discussed in Chapters 3 and 12), **community empowerment** is one intervention that can help reduce the disparities in the health status of minority populations. "Empowering people about health issues" is a required activity of all public health nurses (ANA, 2000, p. 13). "Health education can empower [mobilize] individuals to take control of their lives, empower communities to influence public policies, and raise awareness among health service providers about their crucial health promotion role" (McDermott, 1995). Mobilizing communities means getting individuals and aggregates involved and enthused about taking responsibility for their own health destiny. There is no doubt that community involvement is crucial to reducing health disparities. As budgets are cut, government and private agencies "are increasingly turning their support to community empowerment initiatives" (Eisen, 1994). Community health nurses must be involved in developing initiatives in their respective communities (ANA, 2000).

## Facilitating Community Empowerment

Effective community health nurses facilitate community empowerment when they work with minority populations. To effectively facilitate empowerment, community health nurses must demonstrate competence—by incorporating variances in cultural behaviors, beliefs and values—during the assessment, planning, and implementation phases of empowerment programs (USDHHS, 2000c). It is important that health intervention programs be specific to group needs because many health-promoting behaviors are group specific (Marin, Burhansstipanov, Connell, et al., 1995). For example, in developing a cancer prevention program for an African American minority group one must consider that "perceptions and beliefs are known to play an integral part in cancer prevention" (Underwood, 1994, p. 20). Many African Americans recognize the severity of cancer but "tend to believe that little can be done to prevent it" (Underwood, 1994, p. 20). For a prevention program to effectively mobilize the targeted aggregate, these beliefs must be *incorporated* in planning the interventions. Box 13-2 provides some key considerations for delivering culturally competent care to a targeted minority population.

Community health nurses can be instrumental in getting health education materials and programs to minority aggregates, ensuring that these materials are culturally sensitive, improving accessibility to services, and serving as advocates for minority health and research. Strategies for reaching minority aggregates are discussed in Chapter 15.

**BOX 13-2**

*Key Considerations for Providing Culturally Competent Care to a Target Minority Population*

- Identify the culture.
- Describe its demographics, health beliefs, health practices, health attitudes, and values.
- Describe its communication patterns, religious beliefs, rituals, and symbols.
- Identify one's own personal culture, health values, health beliefs and practices, rituals, and symbols that affect communication with targeted population.
- Identify cultural differences between oneself and the targeted population.
- Determine whether personal cultural values and beliefs or an understanding of the targeted population's values is guiding communication and health planning with the targeted population.
- Establish collaborative relationships with key community leaders.
- Involve the client in all aspects of the planning process.
- Develop health planning and intervention strategies based on the targeted population's values, needs, and characteristics.

Although minority populations have increased and continue to increase, they make up a small percentage of the registered nurse population and professional school enrollments (Eisen, 1994; Waters, 1996). The National Coalition of Ethnic Minority Nurses has advanced an agenda to increase the number of minority nurses and to develop more nurse minority scientists (Ericksen, 2000). Minority nurses will find a "dynamic field of opportunity" (Marquand, 2000, p. 23). There is a particular need for minority nurses to provide mental health services. In response to this need, "the American Nurses Association's Ethnic Minority Fellowship Program offers funding to attract more minority nurses to the [mental health] specialty" (Marquand, 2000, p. 23). Nurses at all levels can encourage minorities to become health care professionals and ultimately leaders and advocates for their communities. One community intervention could be to target select minority populations in local private and public schools and health systems and work with career counselors to deliver culturally specific and community-specific career opportunity programs. It is advantageous to seek out minority professionals to participate in these programs to enhance cultural competence.

Because lifestyles vary according to culture, lifestyle assessments are a key component in meeting health care needs of the culturally diverse (Pender, 1996, pp. 132-135). Prevention efforts that are not culturally sensitive will be ineffective because they will not be understood by targeted individuals, groups, and populations (Bayer, 1994, p. 895). A health promotion program with characteristics appropriate to a targeted Hispanic or Latino population may not necessarily be appropriate to the needs of another community group such as a Native American population in the same community. Health education programs must be culturally congruent. A lack of cultural sensitivity will impede or inhibit implementing health promotion interventions.

Chapter 7 provides characteristics about specific cultures that may influence health practices and should be taken into consideration during health programming. However, a culturally competent practitioner "understands that diversity *within* cultures is as important as diversity *between* cultures" (Randall-David, 1994, p. 3). Working with key community leaders helps practitioners identify this diversity and develop cultural competence (see Chapter 14). Grossman (1994, p. 62) described seven steps to help nurses develop cultural competence:
1. Know yourself.
2. Keep an open mind.
3. Respect differences in people.
4. Be willing to learn.
5. Learn to communicate effectively.
6. Don't judge.
7. Be resourceful and creative.

Chapter 9 provides guidelines for establishing a therapeutic relationship with clients of other cultures. Two key factors to consider when working with aggregates are "involving community members in every step of the process and networking with community-based organizations that already have good working relationships with the target population" (Randall-David, 1994, p. 23).

### Transcultural Resources

Numerous nursing research studies and publications have addressed transcultural issues. The Transcultural Nursing Society is an international organization that addresses cultural care and diversity in nursing. The nurse can also obtain current information on local, state, and federal minority health programs, resources, publications, and statistics by calling the Office of Minority Health's Resource Center at 1-800-444-MHRC.

## POVERTY

Income is the most common measure of socioeconomic status and provides a basis for formulating health policy (USDHHS, 2000b). Low socioeconomic status is the basis of many health problems experienced by Americans and minority groups. "In general, population groups that suffer the worst health status are also those that have the highest poverty rates and the least education" (USDHHS, 2000a, p. 12). Income is the most common measure of socioeconomic status and is used as the basis for health policy formulation. In determining poverty status, income is adjusted for family size and inflation that allows for making comparisons among groups over time (USDHHS, 2000b).

**Poverty** status measures family income relative to family size by using the poverty thresholds that are developed by the U.S. Census Bureau. These thresholds vary by family size and composition and are updated annually. (USDHHS, 2000b, p. A-18). Table 13-1 gives information on the 1998 poverty thresholds by size of family unit with number of related children under 18 years of age. If the family's income is less than that threshold shown in the table, then that family is considered impoverished. For example, for a family unit of four, with no related children under 18 years of age, the poverty threshold for this family is $16,813 (USDHHS, 2000b, p. A-19). As discussed in Chapter 4, much legislation throughout the years has focused on the issues of poverty and health. One of the three overall goals of *Healthy People 2010* focuses on eliminating social and economic disparities in health over the next decade (USDHHS, 2000b). A major role for community health nurses in the future will be the political advocate role. The health of every disadvantaged group must be safeguarded during all state and federal legislative sessions.

### Poverty and Health Risk Factors

Poverty coexists with many risk factors that influence health. Studies have shown that socioeconomic status is a determinant of illness, death, and other health outcomes (Cubbin, LeClere, Smith, 2000). Poor academic achievement, cognitive and developmental delays, decreased pro-

**TABLE 13-1**

*Poverty Thresholds in 1998, Income by Size of Family and Number of Related Children Under 18 Years*

| | NUMBER OF RELATED CHILDREN UNDER 18 YEARS AND FAMILY INCOME (POVERTY THRESHOLD) | | | | | | | | |
|---|---|---|---|---|---|---|---|---|---|
| SIZE OF FAMILY UNIT | NONE | 1 | 2 | 3 | 4 | 5 | 6 | 7 | 8 |
| One person | | | | | | | | | |
| Under 65 years | $8,480 | | | | | | | | |
| 65 years and older | 7,818 | | | | | | | | |
| Two persons | | | | | | | | | |
| Householder under 65 years | 10,915 | 11,235 | | | | | | | |
| Householder 65 years and older | 9,853 | 11,193 | | | | | | | |
| Three persons | 12,750 | 13,120 | 13,133 | | | | | | |
| Four persons | 16,813 | 17,088 | 16,530 | 16,588 | | | | | |
| Five persons | 20,275 | 20,570 | 19,940 | 19,453 | 19,155 | | | | |
| Six persons | 23,320 | 23,413 | 22,930 | 22,468 | 21,780 | 21,373 | | | |
| Seven persons | 26,833 | 27,000 | 26,423 | 26,020 | 25,270 | 24,395 | 23,435 | | |
| Eight persons | 30,010 | 30,275 | 29,730 | 29,253 | 28,575 | 27,715 | 26,820 | 26,593 | |
| Nine persons or more | 36,100 | 36,275 | 35,793 | 35,388 | 34,723 | 33,808 | 32,980 | 32,775 | 31,513 |

Modified from US Department of Health and Human Services (USDHHS): *Tracking Healthy People 2010*, Washington, DC, 2000b, US Government Printing Office, p. A-19.

ductivity in adulthood, high infant mortality, inadequate housing, unaffordable and inaccessible health care, poor nutrition, decreased mental well-being, and unemployment are some of the poverty risks that influence a community's health status (Benjamin, 1996; Garbarino, 1996; Grimes, 1996; Hartmann, Spalter-Roth, Chu, 1996). Increasingly the importance of the interrelationships between environmental, socioeconomic forces, and the health status of aggregates is being recognized (Mackenbach, Kunst, Groenhof, et al., 2000). Forces such as the economy of the nation, state, and local community; the availability of affordable health care services; and health policies greatly affect health programming and outcome.

A dynamic relationship also exists between low socioeconomic status and health risks such as lifestyle behaviors including smoking, drug use, exercise, and diet (Link, 1996). Death rates of people below the poverty level are much higher than those persons who are above the poverty level (USDHHS, 2000b). This is consistent with the fact that health risks increase significantly in lower-income families. Low income has been identified as the key factor in contributing to almost all of the chronic illnesses in the United States (USDHHS, 2000a). Additionally, low income has been a factor contributing to a higher incidence of adverse birth outcomes in infants of low-income mothers (Turner, Newschaffer, Cocroft, et al., 2000). Chapter 16 elaborates on health risks of children living in poverty.

Clearly community efforts are needed in this country to increase educational and socioeconomic opportunities that would decrease risks of mortality in the less fortunate. Changes in income and educational attainment can positively influence the health status of populations. This was illustrated in a longitudinal study that, after adjusting for various socioeconomic and demographic factors, demonstrated a decrease in mortality in both men and women under 65 years of age as income and educational level increased (Sorlie, Backlund, Keller, 1995). Hence community efforts to encourage education to help decrease socioeconomic disparities and ultimately develop healthy communities must be continually reiterated.

Like minority Americans, Americans with low income have difficulty affording and gaining access to health care and preventive services. Lack of appropriate health care places individuals at high risk for the development of acute and chronic illnesses. To reduce health disparities among low-income Americans, national, state, and community efforts are needed to increase access to health care and decrease the number of people living in poverty.

## Where Is Poverty?

Poverty spans all ages, exists in rural America as well as inner city America, and exists in white populations as well as minority populations (CDF, 2000). Poverty exists at some level in every geographic community. Young families and one-parent families are particularly at risk for poverty. Single-mother families are more likely to experience poverty than almost any other family (CDF, 2000).

Although minority groups experience a disproportionate amount of poverty, the majority of Americans living in poverty are white and reside in rural or suburban areas. Additionally, the majority of poor families with children work. "Seventy-four percent of poor children live in working families who cannot make enough to escape poverty" (CDF, 2000, p. xi).

Historically, community health nurses have served low-income families. At the Henry Street Settlement, Lillian Wald saw and responded to the health care needs of the poor in the community. Concerns such as poor nutrition and sanitation, poor infant health, child labor, lack of recreational facilities, school absences caused by sickness, and lack of access to appropriate health services became areas addressed by the Henry Street nurses. At the Frontier Nursing Service, Mary Breckenridge worked with poor, rural Appalachian families to promote health.

Today's community health nurses provide numerous services to low-income populations. Nurses need to be sensitive to the needs and concerns of these populations and be familiar with community resources that can assist them. Examples of resources that can assist low-income families and children are Medicaid, Temporary Assistance to Needy Families, WIC, and Food Stamps. Other resources are shared throughout the text.

*Stop and Think About It*

How many families do you know or have you worked with who are at poverty level? How have you determined them to be at poverty level? What interventions are needed for these families to rise above poverty level?

## Poverty and Nursing Interventions

Working with low-income populations provides many challenges and opportunities for community health nurses. Managed-care models, neighborhood health clinics, and community-based nursing centers are some ways of meeting the challenges of providing effective, culturally sensitive care to these aggregates (Craig, 1996; McCreary, 1996; Murphy, 1995). Community health nurses need to be innovative in developing interventions to promote health and create ways to "link people to needed health services and assure the provision of health care when otherwise unavailable" (ANA, 2000, p. 17). They need to become politically active and work with communities in holding elected officials accountable for protecting poor families. Currently, "states have more than $2.5 billion in unspent Temporary Assistance for Needy Families (TANF) funds and more than $3 billion in unspent Children's Health Insurance Program (CHIP) funds" (CDF, 2000, p. xxv).

How can nurses intervene? As budgets are cut, financial resources become more and more difficult to obtain, and as responsibility for developing solutions shifts from federal programs to states and local communities, health care providers and local community leaders must become resourceful and creative in developing interventions to solve many of the problems associated with poverty. Certainly one cannot expect to eliminate poverty and poverty-related health risks in one step or by a one-provider approach. However, it is possible for nurses to identify at-risk aggregates (e.g., teen parents) that can be targeted for preventive interventions. Nurses can develop collaborative interventions and make great strides toward improving health and reducing the risk of people living in poverty.

Interventions cannot be developed before risks and problems are defined in communities. One way for nurses to identify health risks and problems is to conduct an assessment of needs within a local community (Chapter 14 elaborates on how to conduct a community health assessment). Box 13-3 is an example of risk identification at a local community level. In this example, the nurses identified a high-risk aggregate and targeted this population for preventive interventions. Efforts such as these are needed to expand the limited resources available for health programming in local communities.

Interventions vary from one community to another based on each respective community's risks and needs. The most effective interventions for aggregate health are those that are population based, that mobilize populations to be enthusiastic about taking personal responsibility for their future health, and that shape the overall health of the community (Eisen, 1994; Woodson, 1996). Interventions that involve collaborative efforts (e.g., health care agencies and key community leaders) are thought to have higher outcomes than

### BOX 13-3

## An Example of Risk Identification at a Community Level: School-Based Tuberculin Testing

A review of tuberculosis surveillance data from a program of school-based tuberculin testing demonstrates the natural evolution of targeted populations. In the 7 years encompassed by this study, the prevalence of tuberculin reactivity ranged from 4.3% to 6.1% in the Amarillo public school populations which were tested. The initial screening was a sampling of all students in the school district. In subsequent years' screening, the targeted populations were increasingly refined to eliminate lower-risk populations. Children enrolled in "English as a Second Language" (ESL) classes were found to have an 8.5% tuberculosis infection rate. The purpose of this study was to alert nurses that culturally sensitive approaches are needed for successful future testing.

From Denison AV, Shum SY: The evolution of targeted populations in a school-based tuberculin testing program, *Image J Nurs Sch* 27(4):263-266, 1995.

noncollaborative interventions (Marin, Burhansstipanov, Connell, et al., 1995).

Historically community health nurses have demonstrated their impact on population-based approaches (ANA, 2000). Collaborating with community agencies and mobilizing partnerships are essential activities for public health nurses (ANA, 2000). Clearly the most ideal interventions are those that focus on primary prevention, including health promotion and specific protection. It costs less to prevent than to cure.

As nurses address the health risks of populations in communities, it is helpful to keep in mind the various roles of community health nurses in addressing the health needs of populations. Some examples of key community health nursing roles that may be implemented with the impoverished in a community are that of *health planner*, *casefinder*, *advocate*, *teacher*, and *clinic nurse*. Some typical situations in which these roles emerge are as follows:

* *Health planner:* Collaborate with local community health agencies and educational systems to determine population-specific health needs. Box 13-4 provides an example of a community-specific collaborative effort to complete a needs assessment that benefited all involved partners. Collaborative relationships are also being developed to plan innovative health programs. For example, commu-

nity health nurses in Texas developed a community partnership to plan a health program designed to reduce infant mortality. Volunteer mothers in the community were used for outreach to teach Hispanic women at risk about the importance of early prenatal care in reducing the incidence of low-birth-weight babies. "Since the beginning of the program in 1989, not one low-birth-weight baby has been born to a woman followed by a volunteer mother" (McFarlane, 1996, p. 880). Chapter 15 elaborates on this example and illustrates the health planning role with aggregates at risk.

* *Advocate:* Meet with local health agency personnel to promote development of a mobile health unit to access low-income populations at risk in the community or work with legislators to develop outreach programs to increase enrollment of eligible people in health assistance programs.

* *Casefinder:* Conduct a community assessment to identify at-risk aggregates, such as a population living in a potentially toxic environment or outreach to get high-risk mothers in for early prenatal care.

* *Teacher:* Apply teaching and learning principles to educate a group of single teen mothers about parenting skills that foster healthy child development. Keep in mind that "effective health education interventions should be tailored to a specific population" (Freudenberg, Eng, Flay, et al., 1995, p. 297). For example, peer education strategies are often very effective with teen mothers.

* *Clinic nurse:* Focus on all three levels of prevention and use many community health nursing roles in addressing the needs of the less fortunate. For example, as a *casefinder*, identify risks (such as nutritional deficiencies, violence, STDs) among the clinic clientele; as a *researcher*, document trends (such as nutritional deficits, abuse, STD incidence and prevalence) within the clinic population; and as a *counselor*, develop "culturally sensitive," population-specific interventions (e.g., community nutritional education programs to reduce hypertension, a support group for grandparents who are parenting young children, or a survivors' grief support group for families that have experienced violence).

---

### BOX 13-4

### *An Example of a Community-Specific Collaborative Effort to Determine Population-Specific Needs*

Health care reform can provide opportunities for collaboration between universities and the public at large. An advanced community nursing class within a post-RN program at a university combined resources with a nearby rural community to complete a community health and social needs assessment. The partners in the project included the local hospital, health unit, and the university; funding was secured from the Regional Center for Health Promotion and Community Studies, and the two health agency partners also made a financial donation. Community liaisons, who were both registered nurses and residents of the community, were instrumental in completing tasks and activities related to the project. The students were taught the various data collection methods and participated in class assignments refining the necessary skills required for the actual assessment. This project benefited the community by providing baseline health status and social needs data in an era of dramatic health care reform while simultaneously affording undergraduate nursing students the opportunity to apply theory to practice.

From Kulig JC, Wilde IW: Collaboration between communities and universities: completion of a community needs assessment, *Public Health Nurs* 13(2):112-119, 1996.

## HOMELESSNESS

Homeless persons are becoming more and more common in communities across the United States, and the number of Americans who are homeless is increasing dramatically. Factors that have contributed to homelessness include the lack of affordable housing, employment or income that is less than a living wage, domestic violence, mental illness, disability, and drug and alcohol use (Wright, 2000). Other factors that influence homelessness were identified in a major national qualitative study in which the researcher interviewed 777 homeless parents with 2,049 homeless children (Nunez, 1999). The researcher found race, low educational level, poor employability, and dependence on welfare as the major themes that emerged from the findings (Nunez, 1999). Like other contemporary health-related problems, few communities are exempt from homeless populations. Community health nurses must be astute in identifying and meeting the needs of the homeless in their respective communities.

Over the past two decades, the number of homeless persons has dramatically increased with more than 400,000 families in homeless shelters throughout the United States at one point in time (Nunez, 1999). An accurate estimate is almost impossible to obtain because definitions of homelessness vary, sampling and survey methods differ (Link, Susser, Stueve, et al., 1994), and the number of people homeless at any given time differs greatly from the number of people who have ever experienced homelessness in their lifetimes. Regardless of the precise number of homeless persons, it cannot be disputed that the number is continuing to increase for a variety of reasons.

Young families are the fastest-growing group of homeless people in the United States. The typical homeless family today is a single parent with two or three children whose average age is 5 (Nunez, 1999). This is not unlike findings from studies earlier in the past decade that found one-parent families, usually headed by women, represented the majority of all homeless families nationwide (Burg, 1994; Mihaly, 1991; Norton, Ridenour, 1995; Wagner, Menke, Ciccone, 1995).

Homelessness may have a lifelong impact on children that adversely affects them in adulthood. This impact was demonstrated in a Los Angeles County study of 1563 homeless adults, in which the majority reported growing up in poor socioeconomic conditions and over half had experienced some type of housing disruption as children that ranged from subsidized housing, eviction, crowded living conditions, and homelessness (Koegel, Melamid, Burnam, 1995, p. 1647). It is necessary to intervene early to prevent the cycle of homelessness in ongoing generations and to promote the health of children so that they will be healthy, contributing individuals as they move into adulthood.

## Health Problems Among the Homeless

Homeless adults have a high prevalence of social, physical, and chronic problems that may have their roots in a homeless childhood. Homeless children have numerous health problems that may contribute to chronic problems in adulthood. Studies have noted that homeless children have incomplete immunizations or immunization delays, putting them at increased risk of serious and disabling communicable disease. Wagner, Menke, and Ciccone (1995) studied the health of 76 rural homeless families, which included 125 children ranging from 1 month to 12 years of age, and identified several health risks including allergies, bronchitis, incomplete immunizations, and developmental risks. Eighty-five of the children in this study were under 6 years of age, and over half (52%) were found to have develop-

mental delays (based on Denver Developmental Screening Tests), including 20 children who completely failed fine motor testing.

Findings from the study of homeless children in Los Angeles were consistent with findings in the Ohio study by Wagner, Menke, and Ciccone (1995). Zima, Wells, and Freeman (1994) supported findings from other studies that noted homeless children were more likely to be academically delayed and have depressive and social disorders than those not homeless. Another study revealed that homeless children had various chronic physical disorders including asthma, anemia, and malnutrition, and that skin ailments, ear infections, eye disorders, dental problems, upper respiratory infections, and gastrointestinal problems were also common (Berne, Dato, Mason, et al., 1990, p. 8). The mental health of homeless children in this study was profoundly affected. Developmental delays, depression, anxiety, suicidal ideation, sleep problems, shyness, withdrawal, and aggression were evident. The homeless often feel devalued and lose their sense of self-identity (Boydell, Goering, Morrell-Bellai, 2000). Homeless children often do not have regular schooling, lack stable familial support systems, and lack friends. This can be personally and developmentally devastating, which leaves them vulnerable to a variety of health, social, and behavioral problems as they mature to adulthood.

Many lifestyle factors involved in being homeless present barriers for homeless individuals to attain or maintain good health (Smith, 1999). Both adults and children who are homeless often find it difficult to obtain health care services. Inaccessibility of health care is a major risk factor with homelessness (Smith, 1999). Riemer, Van-Cleve, and Galbraith (1995) identified some common barriers that impede preventive health care for homeless children. These barriers included difficulties in selecting and obtaining health care providers, resource variables such as waiting time for obtaining care and during appointments, attitudes of health care professionals, and transportation costs. Most homeless people do not have health insurance, and the cost of health care services is often prohibitive. The challenge for community health nurses is to find ways to reach out to the homeless populations in their communities. Outreach services are often essential for the homeless.

There is no doubt that homeless children are at risk for health, developmental, and social problems that may extend into adulthood. It is important for community health nurses to assess the childhood experiences of homeless adults, as well as assessing the homeless children themselves when intervening with homeless populations. Homeless adults who were homeless as children may have unidentified health and developmental problems that began in childhood.

## The Homeless and Their Environment

Persons who are homeless are exposed to the elements (Figure 13-4) and experience overcrowding and unsanitary con-

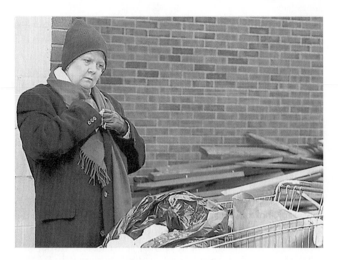

**FIGURE 13-4** Homelessness is often the cause and effect of multiple social and chronic health problems. (Copyright CLG Photographics, Inc.)

ditions. Homelessness is often a cause and effect of multiple social and chronic health problems. It is not surprising that homeless people have a high prevalence of severe and chronic mental disorders and substance abuse; a high risk of becoming victims of rape and violence; an increased incidence of physical problems, such as hypertension and trauma; an increased susceptibility to infectious disease conditions, including tuberculosis, influenza, scabies, lice, and pneumonia; and a variety of nutritional deficiencies.

Murray (1996), from interviews with 150 homeless men who were part of a day treatment program for mentally ill and chemically dependent persons, described two major fears of homeless men: fear of violence and fear of being unable to meet basic needs. A third of the men had suffered some kind of violent assault such as beating (most common), knifing, robbing, or shooting. As a result, the majority feared violence and were fearful of being unable to protect themselves. The homeless also cited frustration with shelter staff and negative reactions of other people. These data reflect the need for nurses to holistically address, and be sensitive to, the needs of the homeless without passing judgment in order to competently intervene. Nurses who work with the homeless visit them in a variety of places, including homeless shelters, shacks, benches in a park, and under bridges.

## Homelessness and Legislation

On a national level, the *Stewart B. McKinney Homeless Assistance Act* (Public Law 100-77) provides assistance to protect and improve the lives and safety of the homeless with special emphasis on the elderly, handicapped persons, and families with children. The Act authorized emergency food and shelter, supportive housing, programs for primary health care, substance abuse services, community mental

health care, adult education, education for children and youth, job training, and studies of homelessness. Further information about this Act can be found in Chapter 4.

## Homelessness and Isolation

Homeless people are often isolated from the mainstream of society. Families find themselves without the necessary support or resources to cope with even minor problems and difficulties. Kinzel's (1991) research with the homeless found that a recurring theme among people who are homeless was the need to interact with a caring person. "The feeling that no one cares, a lack of self-worth, and a sense of limited control over their lives may lead to depression, hopelessness, and finally illness. The extent and effectiveness of health-seeking behaviors among this group are limited because of decreased trust, decreased motivation for self-care, and isolation from social and health care systems" (Kinzel, 1991, p. 189).

Reports over time continue to show that approximately one third of homeless people have serious mental health and substance abuse problems that have interfered with their own ability to seek health care and provide shelter for themselves (Caton, Hasin, Shrout, et al., 2000; Smith, 1999). In response to this, five large multisite demonstration projects known as the *Center for Mental Health Services* (CMHS), funded by the Stewart B. McKinney Homeless Assistance Act, began in 1990 and targeted the homeless mentally ill in five sites: Boston, Baltimore, San Diego, and two projects in New York (USDHHS, 1994c).

The CMHS projects involved a total of 896 homeless adults who were between 36 and 40 years old and had mental illnesses such as nonaffective psychotic disorder, schizophrenia, and depression. The majority (67%) were single, about 33% were high school dropouts, about 25% were veterans, over 50% had alcohol or drug abuse problems, and less than 33% had any income benefits (USDHHS, 1994c, pp. i-ii). Within this CMHS multisite population, 75% were homeless for 1 year or more, 30% for 10 or more years, and 22% before age 18 (USDHHS, 1994c, pp. i-ii). The interim key findings from these longitudinal projects that have implications for the development of community health outreach services are as follows (USDHHS, 1994c, pp. ii-iii):

1. Homeless people with severe mental illnesses will use accessible, relevant community health services.
2. Appropriate services decrease homelessness.
3. Advocacy helps increase access to entitlement income.
4. Formerly homeless persons with severe mental illnesses are an important resource.
5. Substance abuse is a major factor in homelessness among persons with severe mental illness.
6. Housing stability, appropriate mental health treatment, and increased income lead to an improved quality of life.

In addition to the key findings, the CMHS interim report (USDHHS, 1994c, p. iii) identified five policy implications that need to be considered when providing for the health needs of the homeless:

1. Service systems must be integrated at all levels to remove barriers and promote efficient services.
2. Substance abuse treatment must be an integral part of comprehensive services for persons with severe mental illnesses to prevent recurrent homelessness.
3. A range of housing options is required to respond to the needs and preferences of the homeless.
4. Preventive health care and health education are critical components in health planning for the homeless, because many are at risk for acute and chronic illnesses.
5. Longer-term follow-up studies should focus on how to sustain early gains.

From the CMHS key findings, including policy implications, there is no doubt that interventions with the homeless must be *community-based, population-specific,* and designed to meet the needs of the particular homeless populations in communities throughout the country. Despite the recognized need of outreach programs to access the homeless "there are virtually no health insurance programs that support the efforts of outreach workers" (Wells, 1996). Because of this, there is a tremendous need to develop methods to enhance the primary care, mental health, and substance abuse resources available to the homeless.

## Nursing Interventions with the Homeless

Community health nurses provide health care to people who are homeless in traditional settings such as health departments, outpatient clinics, and homeless shelters. Consistent with the changing health care delivery system, community health nurses from traditional and other settings are also demonstrating that innovative community-based approaches to caring for the homeless are effective. Community health nurses are establishing community-based centers and clinics targeting the homeless (McNeal, 1996; Scholler-Jaquish, 1996; Simandl, 1996), providing health promotion and protection activities such as tuberculosis treatment and control in homeless shelters (Kitazawa, 1995; May, Evans, 1994; Mayo, White, Oates, et al., 1996), and taking care to the "streets" with on-the-spot mobile units (Berne, Dato, Mason, et al., 1990). Lillian Wald's Henry Street Settlement House in New York provides supportive, 24-hour care to homeless families. In Lexington, Kentucky, nurses are addressing the health needs of the homeless through the "Hope Center," a nurse-managed clinic (Ossege, Berry, 1994, p. 22). Wells (1996) emphasized the need for outreach programs to be mobile and to meet the homeless wherever they are, which means going beyond clinics and offices to parks, bridges, and shelters.

Berne, Dato, Mason, et al. (1990) described a model program that used comprehensive pediatric mobile units to access children living in homeless shelters and hotels in New York City. A major component of the program included public health nurses on-site at homeless centers to casefind

and do initial client assessments and nurse practitioners to diagnose and treat health problems. Clients were referred to community resources such as WIC, the department of social services, and community mental health services. A primary focus in working with the homeless is to mobilize their skills and capacities to become self-sufficient and to break the homeless cycle by building hope and self-esteem that fosters personal responsibility. Specific self-esteem enhancement interventions are discussed in Chapter 18. These type of interventions assist clients to increase their personal judgment of self-worth (McCloskey, Bulechek, 2000, p. 580).

Nurses can provide the "caring" aspect that people who are homeless covet in service provision. A nursing study with homeless veterans found high levels of depression were linked to low levels of self-esteem, hope, and self-efficacy (Tollett, Thomas, 1996). Through the use of a nursing theory–based intervention, Tollett and Thomas were able to "care" for the veterans and make significant changes in their level of hope (1996, p. 87). Specifically, Tollett and Thomas (1996) used small-group therapy sessions to assist veterans in identifying reasons for hope, personal strengths, and areas in which they felt pride. The researchers believed that a personal feeling of having hope was an essential first step before the homeless veterans could learn to be self-sufficient. It is vital to intervene whenever possible to increase self-sufficiency and decrease the risk of intergenerational homelessness.

Like other contemporary problems, the most ideal intervention is primary prevention. Prevention should be inherent in every facet of health programming for the homeless. A primary long-term outcome goal should always be directed toward providing the homeless with tools to become self-motivated and self-sufficient in maintaining their own health and shelter. Prevention is the most cost-effective way to address homelessness and the focus should be on ameliorating the causes of homelessness (Smith, 1999). Nurses can help link people who are homeless to community resources and provide the "caring" aspects of health care. Community health nurses carry out a significant role with the homeless. Through mobilizing partnerships (ANA, 2000) and community planning and political activism (Smith, 1999), community health nurses help many homeless persons and families achieve self-sufficiency. It is evident that the most efficient interventions are those that are community and population specific. Collaborative efforts between a multidisciplinary health care team and the homeless assists communities in developing population-specific interventions. "No single service system can adequately address the many service needs of people recovering from homelessness and mental illnesses" (Wells, 1996, p. 8).

## SUBSTANCE ABUSE

**Substance abuse** undermines health and is a serious problem in the United States. Each year millions of Americans abuse alcohol and other drugs. "On any given day, more than 700,000 people in the United States receive alcoholism treatment in either inpatient or outpatient settings" (Fuller, Hiller-Sturmhofel, 1999). Substance abuse is associated with many of the problems in the United States and contributes significantly to violence, injury, HIV infection, child and spousal abuse, motor vehicle crashes, teen pregnancy, school failure, low worker productivity, and homelessness (USDHHS, 2000a, pp. 32-33). The economic costs from substance abuse problems are in the billions of dollars annually. The psychological, familial, and social damage that accompanies substance abuse is devastating. A rising concern is the increased substance abuse among children. The younger the age of initiation to substance use, the more predictive it is of later problems with the same substances (Kosterman, Hawkins, Guo, et al., 2000). "The younger a person becomes a habitual user of illicit drugs, the stronger the addiction becomes and the more difficult it is to stop use" (USDHHS, 2000a, p. 33). The *Monitoring the Future Project* discussed in Chapter 16 provides data annually on the range of substance abuse among American youth. Smoking is discussed extensively in Chapter 17.

*Healthy People 2010* has a separate priority area for substance abuse (alcohol and other drugs), with numerous national health objectives. Both government and private organizations are working to combat substance abuse in the nation. *Healthy People 2010* has specific indicators that focus on reduction of substance use among adolescents and binge drinking among adults. Binge drinking has been associated with young adults and has been a particular problem on college campuses nationwide over the past few years. Binge drinking is defined as the "consumption of large-enough amounts of alcohol in short-enough periods of time to put the drinker and others at risk. Each year binge drinking causes numerous student deaths, thousands more injuries and a host of other problems" (Wechsler, 2000). College campuses have vast opportunities for student nurses to engage in health promotion activities, particularly primary and secondary prevention. These health promotion activities facilitate empowerment, which can reduce substance abuse among college students.

Two federal government agencies assist local communities in developing effective programs for addressing substance abuse. The National Clearinghouse on Alcohol and Drug Abuse offers information, educational materials, and referral sources. The National Institute on Alcohol Abuse and Alcoholism strives to increase knowledge and promote effective strategies to deal with the health problems associated with alcoholism. It sponsors research and educational programs including youth alcohol awareness programs, education on alcohol and pregnancy, and national drunk driving awareness.

## Health Risks of Alcoholism

Alcoholism contributes to numerous health problems, and differences exist among ethnic groups. For example, Native Americans have significantly higher rates of alcoholism and alcohol-related problems than their white counterparts (USDHHS, 1999). The effects of alcohol create health risks for all populations, although the incidences may vary among various cultural groups. (USDHHS, 1999). Long-term drinking can lead to heart disease, cancer, liver disease, and pancreatitis (USDHHS, 2000a). Alcohol is a contributing factor in causes of death, including accidents, suicides, and homicides. Nearly half of all traffic deaths are alcohol related. Studies show that careless handling of smoking materials by intoxicated persons is dangerous and contributes substantially to burn injuries, death, and property damage.

Alcohol abuse is a serious health problem. The effects of alcohol abuse are devastating to the health of communities (Emblad, 1995, p. 4). The psychosocial consequences of alcoholism are immense. Such consequences include disruption of family life, loss of on-the-job productivity and financial prosperity, lowered self-esteem, and devastating emotional effects for friends and coworkers. The families of alcoholics are victims of alcoholism themselves. Self-help groups such as Alcoholics Anonymous, Children of Alcoholics, and counseling services are available for alcoholics and their families. The National Council on Alcoholism is a voluntary organization that offers information and referral services. Many employers have employee assistance programs that help employees obtain help with their drinking problems. Because of the cultural variations in substance abuse, models for treatment must be culturally competent in order to develop effective solutions to the problem (USDHHS, 1999).

## Fetal Alcohol Syndrome

Fetal alcohol syndrome (FAS) is a major public health concern that is completely preventable (Shah, Hoffman, Shinault, et al., 1998). FAS consists of a variety of health problems with infants that have been linked to exposure to alcohol in utero. The adverse effects of alcohol on fetal development have been and continue to be a health concern. "An estimated 30,000 children are born each year with disabilities from prenatal alcohol exposure" (USDHHS, 2000d, p. 1). The infants of mothers who consume alcohol suffer retarded growth, low birth weight, facial dysmorphology, mental retardation, developmental delays, behavioral disorders, microcephaly, language, and sensory and perceptual disabilities (USDHHS, 2000d). Studies have shown that both chronic drinking and binge drinking affect pregnancy outcomes.

The public is becoming increasingly aware of conditions such as FAS, but education about this problem is an important element in a FAS prevention program. Women of childbearing years, especially pregnant women, need to know the effects of drinking during pregnancy. Increased programs to help pregnant women prevent FAS by eliminating alcohol and substance use during pregnancy are needed to decrease the health risks to the mother, the fetus, and the infant. Primary prevention through education can completely irradicate FAS and its long-term consequences to children.

## Health Risks of Illegal Drugs

Drug use is a serious health concern among adults as well as children. Millions of Americans use illicit drugs each year. More and more youth are experimenting with illicit drugs, including marijuana, cocaine, crack, heroin, acid, inhalants, and methamphetamines (USDHHS, 2000a, p. 33). According to Friend (1996), some of the reasons for the increased use of drugs by teens included failure to recognize harmful effects of drugs, peer pressure, unhappy homelife, curiosity, and a reglamorization of drug use by the movie industry. Clearly drug prevention programs must target adolescents and young adults before addiction cycles are established. Drug use is linked to other concerns such as death, violent crime, transmission of HIV, and physical, behavioral, and developmental problems in infants of drug-addicted mothers.

Drug use is a direct or contributing factor in thousands of deaths each year in the United States. Accidental overdose is the most common cause of these deaths. Alcohol, heroin, cocaine, crack, marijuana, stimulants, and tranquilizers are commonly ingested in overdoses (Leland, 1996; Schoemer, 1996). There is a disproportionate number of drug deaths among minorities.

Violent crimes are linked to drug use and the drug trade. Often crimes are committed in an effort to procure drugs when addicted persons do not have the cash resources to maintain their addiction (Needle, Mills, 1994). Research has shown that there is a relationship between drug use and crime, and more than 50% of the individuals in correctional facilities have alcohol and other drug abuse problems (Massaro, Pepper, 1994, p. 11). More than half of the men and women booked for crimes in many of the nation's larger cities have tested positive for illicit drugs at the time of their arrest (Massaro, Pepper, 1994, p. 13).

Illicit drug use is related to the transmission of HIV. HIV is prevalent among intravenous drug users. Substance abuse

---

### BOX 13-5

*Family and Environmental Factors Contributing to Alcohol and Drug Addiction*

*Family Factors*

- **Parent and sibling drug use.** Parental and sibling alcoholism and use of illicit drugs increases the risk of alcoholism and drug abuse in offspring. Attitudes and early drinking behaviors appear to be shaped more by parents and relatives than by peers (Hawkins, Lishner, Jenson, et al., 1987; Knott, 1986).
- **Poor and inconsistent family practices.** Children from families with lax supervision, excessively severe or inconsistent disciplinary practices, and low communication and involvement between parents and children are at high risk for later delinquency and drug use (Hawkins, Lishner, Jenson, et al., 1987). Lack of acceptance, closeness, warmth, and praise for good behavior also are family characteristics associated with adolescent substance abuse (Jaynes, Rugg, 1988).
- **Family conflict.** Children raised in families with high rates of conflict appear at risk for both delinquency and illicit drug use. It is the conflict, rather than the actual family structure (e.g., "broken home" or single-parent family), that predicts delinquency and drug use (Hawkins, Lishner, Jenson, et al., 1987).
- **Family social and economic deprivation.** Social isolation, poverty, poor living conditions, and low-status occupations are circumstances that appear to elevate the risk of delinquency and drug use (Hawkins, Lishner, Jenson, et al., 1987).

*School-Related Factors*

- **School failure.** School failure is a predictor of delinquency and drug use. Truancy, placement in special

classes, and early dropout from school are factors associated with drug abuse (Hawkins, Lishner, Jenson et al., 1987).
- **Low degree of commitment to education and attachment to school.** This factor is sometimes called *school bonding*. Low commitment to school is related to drug use. Drug users are more likely than nonusers to be absent from school, to cut classes, and to perform poorly. Dropouts tend to have patterns of greater drug use (Hawkins, Lishner, Jenson, et al., 1987).

*Behavioral and Attitudinal Factors*

- **Early antisocial behavior.** Conduct problems in early elementary grades have been associated with continued delinquency and use of drugs in adolescence. Early delinquent behavior appears to predict early initiation of the use of illicit drugs; and early initiation of drug use increases the risk for regular use and the probability of involvement in crime (Hawkins, Lishner, Jenson et al., 1987).
- **Attitudes and beliefs.** Alienation from the dominant values of society, low religiosity, and rebelliousness are related to drug use. Adolescents who are problem drinkers tend to value independence and autonomy, be more tolerant of deviance, and place more importance on the positive than on the negative functions of drinking. They also tend to have lower expectations of achievement. Individuals with positive attitudes toward drug use are more likely to become substance users. Perceiving substance use as normal and widespread behavior is correlated with

Modified from Crowe AH, Reeves RR: *Treatment for alcohol and other drug abuse: opportunities for coordination,* DHHS Pub No (SMA)94-2075, Rockville, Md, 1994, US Government Printing Office, p. 27.

has many other adverse health consequences. Some of these consequences include malnutrition, low-birth-weight and premature infants, accidental injuries and death, infectious diseases, and mental disorders. The devastating effects of illegal drugs hit hardest among some of the most vulnerable population groups in our country: the poor, women and children, minorities, and those infected with HIV. Drug abuse has killed hundreds of thousands of young adults who will never have the opportunity to contribute their skills to society.

## Who Becomes Addicted?

In the largest global study on cocaine use ever undertaken by the World Health Organization (WHO) it was reported that drug abuse has no boundaries. The study concluded "that there is no average cocaine user, there is an enormous variety in the types of people who use cocaine" for a variety of reasons, and cocaine users often use other drugs as well (Cocaine use, 1995, p. 25). This means that drug abuse transcends boundaries of race, culture, religion, communi-

ties, economics, and age. No community is exempt from substance users, and community health nurses have a tremendous responsibility to identify populations at risk for substance abuse. Community health nurses can then intervene before addiction occurs.

No one begins to use drugs and alcohol with the intention of becoming addicted (Crowe, Reeves, 1994, p. 2). However, all too frequently what began as an experience to satisfy curiosity leads to a point of no return where addiction has occurred. The process of addiction progresses from experimental, social use to dependency and addiction (Crowe, Reeves, 1994, p. 1). Substance abuse is multifaceted, and numerous views have been espoused in relation to causes of substance addiction (Crowe, Reeves, 1994, p. 25). Family and environmental factors have been thought to contribute to addiction (Box 13-5). Additionally, other factors such as genetics, altered brain chemistry, personality traits, social learning, and self-medication also have been thought to be possible risk indicators in addiction (Crowe, Reeves, 1994, p. 29).

### BOX 13-5

## *Family and Environmental Factors Contributing to Alcohol and Drug Addiction—cont'd*

engaging in substance use. The initiation into use of any substance is preceded by values favorable to its use (Hawkins, Lishner, Jenson, et al., 1987; Knott, 1986; Schinke, Botvin, Orlandi, 1991).

### *Environmental Factors*

- **Neighborhood attachment and community disorganization.** Disorganized communities, such as those with high population density, high neighborhood crime rates, and lack of informal social controls, have less ability to limit drug use among adolescents (Hawkins, Lishner, Jenson, et al., 1987).
- **Peer factors.** Drug behavior and drug-related attitudes of peers are among the most potent predictors of drug involvement. Adolescents tend to increase use of drugs because of the influence of friends, and they also tend to choose friends who reinforce their own drug norms and behaviors (Hawkins, Lishner, Jenson, et al., 1987). Adolescents who are problem drinkers usually do not feel their peer group and their parents are compatible, are more easily influenced by peers than by parents, and feel more pressure from peers for drinking and drug use (Knott, 1986).
- **Mobility.** Transitions (such as from elementary to middle school and from junior high to senior high school) and residential mobility are associated with high rates of drug initiation and frequency of use (Hawkins, Lishner, Jenson, et al., 1987).

### *Constitutional and Personality Factors*

- **Constitutional factors.** These factors are often present from birth or early childhood and are thought to have

neurological or physiological origins. Attention and cognitive deficits, such as low verbal ability and poor language and problem-solving skills, have been associated with delinquent behavior. There also is evidence of a constitutional predisposition toward alcoholism, suggesting that genetic factors may play a role in this area (Hawkins, Lishner, Jenson, et al., 1987).
- **Personality factors.** Alienation, low motivation, sensation-seeking, willingness to take risks, and need for stimulation are associated with drug and alcohol use (Hawkins, Lishner, Jenson, et al., 1987). Other characteristics associated with substance use include low self-esteem and self-confidence, need for social approval, high anxiety, low assertiveness, rebelliousness, low personal control, and low self-efficacy (Schinke, Botvin, Orlandi, 1991).

### *Physical and Sexual Abuse*

- This area of investigation is relatively new. However, some studies have found a high correlation between physical and/or sexual abuse and drug use and/or other deviant behavior. It is postulated that child maltreatment leads adolescents to become disengaged from conventional norms and behaviors and to initiate patterns of deviant behaviors (Dembo, Williams, Wish et al., 1988). There also appears to be a high correlation between parents' abuse of drugs and alcohol and abuse and neglect of their children. These emotional wounds, in turn, increase the likelihood that youth will use substances to compensate for unmet emotional needs (Nowinski, 1990).

**TABLE 13-2**
*The Process of Addiction*

| STAGE | FREQUENCY OF USE | SOURCES | REASONS FOR USE | EFFECTS | BEHAVIORAL INDICATORS |
|---|---|---|---|---|---|
| 1. Experimental and Social | Occasional, perhaps a few times monthly; usually on weekends when at parties or with friends. May use when alone. | Friends/peers primarily. Youth may use parent's alcohol. | To satisfy curiosity. To acquiesce to peer pressure. To obtain social acceptance. To defy parental limits. To take a risk or seek a thrill. To appear grown up. To relieve boredom. To produce pleasurable feelings. To diminish inhibitions in social situations. | At this stage the person will experience euphoria and return to a normal state after using. A small amount may cause intoxication. Feelings sought include: Fun, excitement. Thrill. Belonging. Control. | Little noticeable change. Some may lie about use or whereabouts. Some may experience moderate hangovers. Occasionally there is evidence of use, such as a beer can or marijuana joint. |
| 2. Abuse | Regular, may use several times per week. May begin using during the day. May be using alone rather than with friends. | Friends; begins buying enough to be prepared. May sell drugs to keep a supply for personal use. May begin stealing to have money to buy drugs/alcohol. | To manipulate emotions. To experience the pleasure the substances produce. To cope with stress and uncomfortable feelings such as pain, guilt, anxiety, and sadness. To overcome feelings of inadequacy. Persons who progress to this stage of drug/alcohol involvement often experience depression or other uncomfortable feelings when not using. Substances are used to stay high or at least maintain normal feelings. | Euphoria is the desired feeling; may return to a normal state following use or may experience pain, depression, and general discomfort. Intoxication begins to occur regularly. Feelings sought include: Pleasure. Relief from negative feelings, such as boredom and anxiety. Stress reduction. May begin to feel some guilt, fear, and shame. May have suicidal ideations/attempts. Tries to control use but is unsuccessful. Feels shame and guilt. More of a substance is needed to produce the same effect. | School or work performance and attendance may decline. Mood swings. Changes in personality. Lying and conning. Change in friendships—will have drug-using friends. Decrease in extracurricular activities. Begins adopting drug culture appearance (clothing, grooming, hairstyles, jewelry). Conflict with family members may be exacerbated. Behavior may be more rebellious. All interest is focused on procuring and using drugs/alcohol. |
| 3. Dependency/ Addiction | Daily use, continuous. | Will use any means necessary to obtain and secure needed drugs/alcohol. Will take serious risks. Will often engage in criminal behavior such as shoplifting and burglary. | Drugs/alcohol are needed to avoid pain and depression. Many wish to escape the realities of daily living. Use is out of control. | Person's normal state is pain or discomfort. Drugs/alcohol help person feel normal; when the effects wear off, the person again feels pain. Unlikely to experience euphoria at this stage. May experience suicidal thoughts or attempts. Often feel guilt, shame, and remorse. May experience blackouts. May experience changing emotions such as depression, aggression, irritation, and apathy. | Physical deterioration includes weight loss, health problems. Appearance is poor. May experience memory loss, flashbacks, paranoia, volatile mood swings, and other mental problems. Likely to drop out of or be expelled from school or lose jobs. May be absent from home much of the time. Possible overdoses. Lack of concern about being caught— focused only on procuring and using drugs/alcohol. |

Data from Beschner, 1986; Institute of Medicine, 1990; Jaynes, Rugg, 1988; Macdonald, 1989; Nowinski, 1990. Modified from Crowe AH, Reeves RR: *Treatment for alcohol and other drug abuse: opportunities for coordination,* DHHS Pub No (SMA) 94-2075, Rockville, Md, 1994, US Government Printing Office, pp. 2-4.

## The Process of Addiction

The process of addiction generally occurs in three stages of addiction: experimenting, abuse, and addiction. The first stage involves experimental and social use of alcohol and/or drugs. During this stage drugs or alcohol are used intermittently, and there are periods of abstinence (Crowe, Reeves, 1994, p. 2). Table 13-2 on the process of addiction identifies reasons for drug and alcohol use, the frequency and the effects of use, and the sources of alcohol and drugs.

The second stage in the addiction process is characterized by abuse of alcohol and drugs. The amount and frequency of substance used is increased with frequent intoxication. In this stage some negative consequences start to appear (note the behavior indicators listed in Table 13-2). Users are considered dependent when they stop taking the drugs and experience some physical and psychological distress with drug withdrawal (Crowe, Reeves, 1994, p. 3).

The third stage of the addiction process is that of addiction. With addiction users have no self-control over using the substance. There is a compulsive need to maintain the addiction, and to do so, criminal activity, including prostitution, is not uncommon (Crowe, Reeves, 1994, pp. 3-4). The consequences of alcohol and drug use during this stage are profoundly negative.

## Substance Abuse and the Role of the Community Health Nurse

Figure 13-5 diagrams the process of addiction through its various stages. As substance users progress through the stages of addiction, various personal, social, and psychological problems occur. When drug users undergo recovery, community health nurses must keep in mind that recovery is not an *end*; instead, recovery is a *process* that is ongoing. Therefore preventive efforts must also include tertiary prevention interventions that focus on how to prevent intermittent relapses. Understanding the process helps health care providers casefind and develop primary, secondary, and tertiary preventive programs and interventions.

Assessment is the first stage of any treatment or intervention process. The community health nurse's role with populations who are substance abusers begins with a comprehensive assessment. Special attention should be placed on assessing for this problem among pregnant women. A comprehensive assessment is essential to design appropriate interventions for appropriate problems (Crowe, Reeves, 1994). Often drug users are caught up in a web of personal, social, and cultural problems (see Figure 13-1) and require services from multiple community resources. Therefore a comprehensive assessment must be multifaceted and holistic, with interagency collaboration. Figure 13-6 depicts a holistic approach, which involves a collaborative network of care in treatment and relapse prevention.

Crowe and Reeves (1994) described five key objectives in conducting a comprehensive substance abuse assessment:
- Identify drug abusers and those at risk for drug abuse.
- Assess the full spectrum of problems and risks that may need interventions.
- Plan appropriate interventions.
- Involve appropriate family or significant others in the intervention process.
- Evaluate effectiveness of interventions that have been implemented (p. 48).

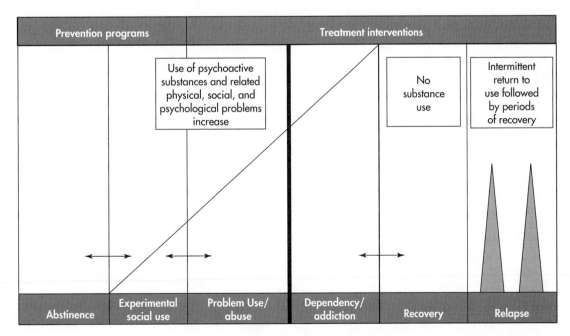

**FIGURE 13-5** The process of addiction. (From Crowe AH, Reeves RR: *Treatment for alcohol and other drug abuse: opportunities for coordination*, DHHS Pub No (SMA)94-2075, Rockville, Md, 1994, US Government Printing Office, p. 5. Data from Doweiko, 1990, Institute of Medicine, 1990.)

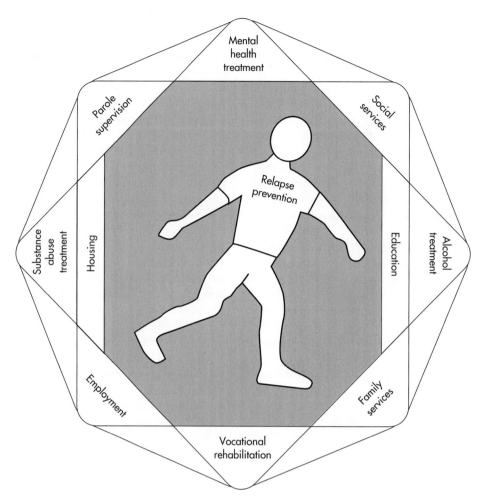

**FIGURE 13-6** Substance abuse populations in a collaborative network of care. (From Massaro J, Pepper B: The relationship of addiction to crime, health, and other social problems. In Crowe AH, Reeves RR: *Treatment for alcohol and other drug abuse: opportunities for coordination*, DHHS Pub No (SMA)94-2075, Rockville, Md, 1994, US Government Printing Office, p. 21.)

**BOX 13-6**

*Key Considerations in Screening for Alcohol and Drug Abuse*

- Screening should be conducted on persons recognized to be at risk, in a variety of settings, by a range of professionals.
- There should be collaboration among agencies and professionals on screening processes, techniques, and instruments.
- All instruments and processes should be sensitive to racial, cultural, socioeconomic, and gender-related concerns.
- Initial screening procedures should be brief.
- Information should be gathered from various sources.

From Crowe AH, Reeves RR: *Treatment for alcohol and other drug abuse: opportunities for coordination*, DHHS Pub No (SMA)94-2075, Rockville, Md, 1994, US Government Printing Office, p. 53.

Box 13-6 provides key factors to consider when screening for alcohol and drug abuse. Screening procedures assist health care providers in identifying clients who need a comprehensive substance abuse assessment.

Identifying risk factors is an essential element in a comprehensive assessment. Box 13-7 describes areas of assessment and questions to ask to aid in determining substance abuse and risk factors for substance abuse. Most agencies have an assessment protocol that guides the nurse in data collection. Every health history should include questions about substance use, including the use of alcohol and illegal and prescription drugs. Community health nurses should be alert to signs of substance abuse. The answer to questions in the comprehensive assessment can help nurses recognize substance abuse signs. Nurses can also use these questions as a guide when working with other community personnel and families to teach them about early signs and symptoms of substance abuse.

BOX 13-7

## Comprehensive Substance Abuse Assessment: Areas of Assessment Through Client and Collateral Interviews

- **Drug history and current patterns of use.** When did alcohol or other drug use begin? What types of alcohol or other drugs does the individual currently use? Does the person use over-the-counter medications, prescription drugs, tobacco, and caffeine? How frequently are the substances used and in what quantity?
- **Substance abuse treatment history.** Has the individual ever received treatment for substance abuse? If so, what type of treatment (inpatient, outpatient, methadone maintenance, 12-step programs, etc.)? Were these treatment experiences considered successful or unsuccessful and why? Has the person been sober and experienced relapse, or has he or she never attained recovery?
- **Medical history and current status.** What symptoms are currently reported by the client? Are there indicators of infectious and/or sexually transmitted diseases? Has the individual been tested for HIV and other infectious diseases? Are there indicators of risk for HIV or other diseases for which testing should be done? What kind of health care has been received in the past? The causes and effects of various illnesses and traumas should be explored.
- **Mental status and mental health history.** Is the individual orientated to person, place, and time? Does he or she have the ability to concentrate on the interview process? Are there indicators of impaired cognitive abilities? What is the appropriateness of responses during the interview? Is the person's affect (emotional response) appropriate for the situation? Are there indicators from collateral sources of inappropriate behavior or responses by the person? Is there evidence of extreme mood states, suicidal potential, or possibility of violence? Is the individual able to control impulses? Have there been previous psychological or psychiatric evaluations or treatment?
- **Personal status.** What are this person's critical life events? Who constitutes his or her peer group? Does the individual indicate psychosocial problems that might lead to substance abuse? Does the person demonstrate appropriate social, interpersonal, self-management, and stress management skills? What is the individual's level of self-esteem? What are the person's leisure time interests? What are his or her socioeconomic level and housing and neighborhood situation?

- **Family history and current relationships.** Who does the individual consider his or her family to be; is it a traditional or nontraditional family constellation? What role does the individual play within the family? Are there indicators of a history of physical or sexual abuse or neglect? Do other family members have a history of substance abuse, health problems or chronic illnesses, psychiatric disorders, or criminal behavior? What is the family's cultural, racial, and socioeconomic background? What are the strengths of the family and are they invested in helping the individual? Have there been foster family or other out-of-home placements?
- **Positive support systems.** Does the person have hobbies, interests, and talents? Who are his or her positive peers or family members?
- **Crime or delinquency.** Have there been previous arrests and/or involvement in the criminal or juvenile justice system? Has the person been involved in criminal or delinquent activity but not been apprehended? Is there evidence of gang involvement? Is the person currently under the supervision of the justice system? What is the person's attitude about criminal or delinquent behavior?
- **Education.** How much formal education has the person completed? What is the individual's functional educational level? Is there evidence of a learning disability? Has he or she received any special education services? If currently in school, what is the person's academic performance and attendance pattern?
- **Employment.** What is the individual's current employment status? What employment training has been received? What jobs have been held in the past and why has the person left these jobs? If currently employed, are there problems with performance or attendance?
- **Readiness for treatment.** Does the client accept or deny a need for treatment? Are there other barriers to treatment?
- **Resources and responsibilities.** What is the individual's socioeconomic status? Is the person receiving services from other agencies, or might he or she be eligible for services?

Data from Doweiko, 1990; McLellan, Dembo, 1992; Tarter, Ott, Mezzich, 1991.
From Crowe AH, Reeves RR: *Treatment for alcohol and other drug abuse: opportunities for coordination,* DHHS Pub No (SMA)94-2075, Rockville, Md, 1994, US Government Printing Office, p. 55.

To develop appropriate interventions, community health nurses must be aware of the social supports and resources that are available and needed in their respective communities. Local communities often have substance abuse hotlines, resources, and support groups. The nurse's knowledge about community resources, payment systems, and the referral process (see Chapter 10) can assist the drug abuse population in obtaining treatment services. The intervention plan should identify interventions needed to decrease drug involvement and address related psychosocial and financial problems. Interventions may include such things as preventive and primary care, testing for infectious diseases (e.g., AIDS, TB), counseling, support group intervention, periodic drug screening, and relapse prevention (Crowe, Reeves, 1994, p. 56). Engendering motivation for clients to change their substance-using behaviors is key to successful interventions.

Under revised treatment protocols, new emphasis is given on *motivation for change* because studies have shown that motivation is a strong predictor of whether an individual's substance use will change or remain the same (USDHHS, 2000e). Motivational approaches emphasize treating the client as an individual and shifting control from the clinician to the client. This type of intervention actively involves the substance abusers and has been shown to have positive outcomes (USDHHS, 2000e). Box 13-8 shows strategies for motivating a client to change substance-using behavior.

The community health nurse can carry out health education activities, actively participate in the treatment program, offer support to the client, remain nonjudgmental, and refer the client to appropriate community resources. Other nursing roles include that of researcher regarding

such issues as the most effective treatment modalities and reasons for the upward trends in substance abuse. As an advocate, the community health nurse may have an active role in developing policies and advocating for services at the local, state, and federal levels.

## SEXUALLY TRANSMITTED DISEASES

Historically, sexually transmitted diseases (STDs) have been a major community health problem. STDs are common in the United States, with an estimated 15 million new cases reported each year (USDHHS, 2000a). A conservative estimate of the cost of STDs is $17 billion annually. STDs and their impact can be prevented through responsible and protected sexual behavior. One of the leading health indicators for *Healthy People 2010* is to foster responsible sexual behavior. Abstinence is the only method of complete protection, but condoms, if used correctly, can prevent STDs and unintended pregnancies (USDHHS, 2000a, p. 34).

Because of the current epidemic of HIV/AIDS and its devastating effects, STDs and HIV/AIDS are discussed in two separate categories. However, there is often a reciprocal connection in which "STDs and HIV infection are often linked not only by common underlying risk behaviors but also by biological mechanisms" (USDHHS, 1995, p. 116). Because of this reciprocal connection, prevention and treatment efforts for STDs or HIV/AIDS cannot be addressed to the exclusion of the other without considering the dynamics of disease transmission (e.g., underlying health risk behaviors).

The following section addresses STDs and HIV/AIDS in separate categories, discusses health risks related to both STDs and HIV/AIDS, and presents nursing's role in prevention and treatment of STDs and HIV/AIDS. The epidemiological control measures for STDs and other infectious diseases are examined in Chapter 11.

Control and prevention of STDs has been, and continues to be, a high priority in public health programming. It is estimated that millions of new cases occur each year, and a large percentage of these cases occur among adolescents and young adults. A *Healthy People 2010* objective specifically aims to "reduce the proportion of adolescents and young adults with *Chlamydia trachomatis* infections (USDHHS, 2000b, p. B25-3).

New methods for screening, determining the epidemiology of the disease process, diagnoses, and treatments are emerging. Today some STDs are becoming drug resistant and very difficult to treat. The emergence of HIV in the 1980s as a major STD has brought about a heightened awareness and mass campaign to prevent STDs. However, because of the overwhelming focus on AIDS, other STDs have been considered as a neglected public health priority, thereby increasing their prevalence (Yankauer, 1994, p. 1895). Neglecting

### BOX 13-8

## *Strategies for Motivating a Client to Change Substance Using Behavior*

- Focus on the client's strengths instead of the weaknesses.
- Respect the client's autonomy and decisions.
- Make treatment individualized and client centered.
- Do not depersonalize the client by using labels like "addict" or "alcoholic."
- Develop a therapeutic partnership.
- Use empathy, not authority or power.
- Focus on early interventions.
- Extend motivational approaches into nontraditional settings.
- Focus on less intensive treatments.
- Recognize that substance abuse disorders exist along a continuum.
- Recognize that many clients have more than one substance use disorder.
- Recognize that some clients may have other coexisting disorders that affect all stages of the change process.
- Accept new treatment goals, which involve interim, incremental, and even temporary steps toward ultimate goals.
- Integrate substance abuse treatment with other disciplines.

From US Department of Health and Human Services (USDHHS): *Enhancing motivation for change in substance abuse treatment*, Pub No SMA 00-3460, Washington, DC, 2000e, US Government Printing Office, p. xvii.

STD control increases the risk of HIV transmission. "It is known that the STDs that cause ulcerative lesions such as syphilis, chancroid, or genital herpes increase the risk of HIV transmission" (Newmann, Nishimoto, 1996, p. 20). Behavioral risk factors such as intravenous drug use and unprotected sex place individuals at risk for development of STDs and HIV. Hence HIV prevention efforts must also include STD prevention (USDHHS, 2000h).

STDs affect all people, regardless of gender, race, or socioeconomic status. However, the incidence of STDs is higher in young people than ever before and is continuing to increase in youth and women, with the highest incidence among persons between ages 15 and 25 years (Cohen, Spear, Scribner, et al., 2000; USDHHS, 2000f). Overall the incidence is disproportionately higher for the poor and minority groups, and African Americans and Hispanics have higher rates of STDs than whites (USDHHS, 2000a).

Early in 1996 the Centers for Disease Control and Prevention (CDC) identified six prominent nationally notifiable STDs that have the highest incidence and prevalence: AIDS, chancroid, chlamydia, gonorrhea, pediatric HIV infection (not notifiable in all states, however), and syphilis (CDC, 1996). Appendix 13-1 provides information about the most commonly acquired STDs. The CDC plays a major role in national disease surveillance and works collaboratively with local, state, and territorial health departments and health care providers in maintaining a national disease reporting system. (Chapter 11 elaborates on the CDC's role in public health surveillance.) The primary responsibility for monitoring and controlling STDs rests on surveillance by state and local health departments. However, the surveillance activities by these organizations would be incomplete without the assistance of other health care providers and services (USDHHS, 1995, p. 116). Most local health departments have STD clinics that provide diagnostic and treatment services at no cost to the individual.

Recently there has been both an increase in abstinence and the use of condoms among sexually active young people (USDHHS, 2000a). However, the estimated 15 million new cases of STDs annually indicates that there is a long road ahead to noticeably decrease the incidence and prevalence of STDs. *Healthy People 2010* fosters responsible sexual behavior that specifically includes behavioral objectives to increase the proportion of adolescents who abstain from sexual intercourse or use condoms if currently sexually active. Another national objective is to increase the proportion of sexually active persons who use condoms (USDHHS, 2000a). Achievement of these objectives could dramatically decrease the incidence and prevalence of STDs. Clearly decreasing STDs can only occur if changes in sexual behaviors are made. "Preventing the spread of STDs requires that persons at risk for transmitting or acquiring infections change their behaviors" (CDC, 1998a, p. 3).There is compelling worldwide evidence that indicates that the presence of other STDs increases the chances for both transmitting and acquiring HIV (USDHHS, 2000a).

## HIV/AIDS

HIV and AIDS were first diagnosed in the early 1980s and are now epidemic worldwide. Nearly 700,000 cases of AIDS have been reported since the epidemic began in the 1980s (USDHHS, 2000a). It is estimated that 800,000 to 900,000 people are infected with HIV. The estimated lifetime health care costs associated with HIV is $155,000 per person. Over one-half of the people infected with HIV are under age 25, and the majority are infected through sexual behavior (USDHHS, 2000a).

AIDS cases are reported to the CDC based on a uniform case definition and a case report form. The number of persons living with AIDS increased in all groups between 1992 and 1997 as a result of the 1993 expanded AIDS definition. In 1993 the definition was revised to include severe immunosuppression, based on CD4 T-lymphocyte cell counts and an expanded set of HIV-associated illnesses (USDHHS, 2000h). These changes in the AIDS definition, the long incubation period between HIV infection and symptoms, and the variation in state HIV surveillance and reporting have made it difficult to accurately predict the number of AIDS cases. These factors have made it difficult to uniformly gather surveillance data (CDC, 1998b). AIDS surveillance trends have also been affected by the incidence of HIV infection and revised guidelines for reporting HIV infection (CDC, 1999). However, as with STDs, surveillance and reporting for HIV/AIDS are the responsibility of state and local health departments.

HIV is the leading cause of death for African-American men between ages 25 to 44 years (USDHHS, 2000a). The highest overall number of deaths has been among minorities (USDHHS, 2000f). The human and economic costs of the AIDS epidemic are astronomic and beyond estimation. AIDS initially appeared in gay men, and many people still think that it is a disease of this aggregate. Even though men who have sex with men continue to account for the largest proportion of cases, other segments of the population such as substance users; those who are homeless, incarcerated, or mentally ill; and runaway youths (USDHHS, 2000f) are affected. Clearly, HIV is not limited to one segment of the population and the number of AIDS cases resulting from heterosexual transmission continues to drastically rise. As a result, women are increasingly developing AIDS. AIDS cases are currently increasing faster among women than among men (Lauby, Smith, Stark, et al., 2000). Figure 13-7 shows AIDS cases in the United States at time of diagnosis, according to race for persons 13 years of age and over diagnosed through December 1999. Note the dramatic increase in 1993 for all races and the decline in 1994. The increase reflects the 1993 revisions in the AIDS case definition rather than a drastic increase in the incidence of AIDS.

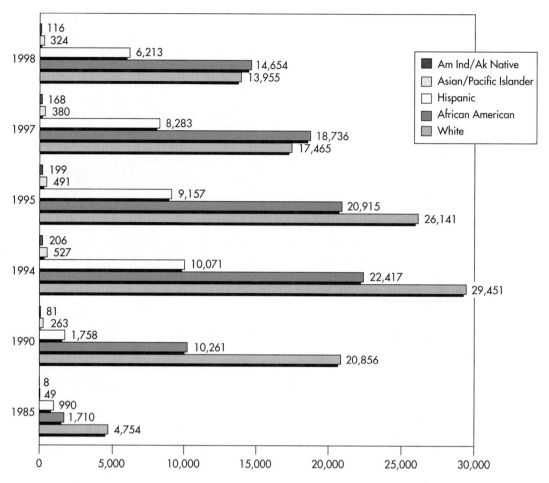

**FIGURE 13-7** AIDS cases per 100,000 population in the United States at time of diagnosis over age 13, by race and selected years, 1985-1998. (Modified from National Center for Health Statistics: *Health, United States, 2000, with adolescent health chartbook*, Hyattsville, Md, 2000, National Center for Health Statistics.)

## Health Risks Related to STDs and HIV/AIDS

Health risks related to STDs and HIV/AIDS are addressed in two categories. The first discusses health behaviors that increase the risk of acquiring STDs and HIV/AIDS. The second category addresses opportunistic infections that increase the risk of AIDS and AIDS mortality.

HEALTH RISK BEHAVIORS. Numerous health risk behaviors place individuals in danger of developing STDs and HIV/AIDS. The Healthy People 2010 objectives focus on changing behaviors that minimize transmitting and acquiring STDs and HIV/AIDS with heavy emphasis on adolescents and young adults (USDHHS, 2000a).

Progress was made toward *Healthy People 2000* HIV infection objectives. However, objectives were not achieved as noted in the high incidence of STDs. Therefore *Healthy People 2010* objectives focus on strategies for reducing the risk behaviors for acquiring STDs and HIV through changing personal behaviors. A few of these strategies include abstinence from sexual intercourse, use of condoms if currently

sexually active, and increasing prime time advertising messages that promote responsible sexual behavior.

Almost 4 million of the estimated 15 million new cases of STDs reported each year occur in adolescents. A national youth risk behavior study in 1994 revealed some startling information regarding unhealthy adolescent behaviors. It was found that approximately one of three 14- to 15-year-old youths had engaged in sexual intercourse; almost four of five had had intercourse by ages 18 to 21; and 12.1% of the 18- to 21-year-old males who participated in the study had reported having their first sexual intercourse by age 12 (Adams, Schoenborn, Moss, et al., 1995). Although the number of adolescents having sexual intercourse has increased, there has also been an increase in the number of adolescents using condoms (USDHHS, 2000a). Clearly STD and HIV prevention efforts must target young adolescents so that they can begin to develop healthy behaviors at an early age to minimize the risk of STDs and HIV. Box 13-9 lists unhealthy behaviors that increase the risk of acquiring STDs and HIV/AIDS.

Even though progress has been made in reducing risk behaviors in communities throughout the United States, there are still populations who have not grasped the serious and potentially fatal consequences of engaging in high-risk sexual activities. In a study involving knowledge and behavioral issues with 175 HIV-positive subjects, Sowell, Seals, and Cooper (1996) identified 10 reasons the HIV-infected participants gave for engaging in unprotected sex. These reasons are displayed in Box 13-10.

Sowell, Seals, and Cooper (1996) found that "being drunk or high" was the most frequently cited reason for engaging in unsafe sexual behavior. This study has tremendous implications for primary prevention. Preventive interventions must be multifaceted and include education about all facets of disease transmission, including various reasons for engaging in unhealthy sexual activities.

Sowell, Seals, and Cooper's (1996) study suggests that in addition to educating persons about the disease process and risk factors, discussing responsible sexual behavior and the building of trusting intimate relationships is essential. Knowledge alone will not prevent the spread of HIV. Sowell, Seals, and Cooper's study does reflect, however, that there is still a lack of knowledge about HIV and how it is spread. It is imperative that populations fully understand the nature of HIV and the manners in which it may be spread. Education must also increase awareness that the exchange of body fluids between HIV-infected persons "may result in reinfection with HIV or exposure to other harmful pathogens that can cause morbidity" (Sowell, Seals, Cooper, 1996). It is crucial that HIV-infected persons understand that it is not "safe" to engage in unprotected sex regardless of the circumstances (see the Teaching Tips in Box 13-11).

**OPPORTUNISTIC INFECTIONS AMONG HIV POPULATIONS.** It is important to remember that "HIV is an asymptomatic disease and the host is infectious for many years" (Hitchcock, 1996, p. 83). For this reason many individuals can be infected with HIV before the host carrier is personally aware of being HIV infected. The time between being infected with HIV and developing AIDS varies, and the first realization that the host is infected often occurs with the manifestation of an opportunistic infection. There are numerous opportunistic infections. The CD4 T-lymphocyte counts are used to guide clinicians in placing HIV-infected persons on prophylaxis that protects them against opportunistic infections and delays the development of AIDS (USDHHS, 2000h; CDC, 1998b).

A great deal of progress has been made in the treatment of HIV/AIDS. Research has shown that opportunistic infections in HIV-infected persons significantly increase the risk of developing additional opportunistic infections (Finkelstein, Williams, Molenberghs, et al., 1996). Findings from this research also provided support that the risk of developing opportunistic infections can be predicted (and used to begin AIDS prophylaxis that is consistent with CDC 1993 revised recommendations) by monitoring the

## BOX 13-9

### *Risk Behaviors for STDs and HIV/AIDS*

- Engaging in unprotected anal, vaginal, or oral sexual activities (both receptive and insertive)
- Having sex with a person known to be HIV-positive
- Sharing, or having sex with persons who share drug needles, syringes, or other injection equipment that has been used by others
- Having multiple sex partners
- Having sex in exchange for drugs, money, or other inducements
- Using alcohol and drugs with sexual activity
- Having a history of STDs, especially genital lesions (e.g., syphilis, chancroid, herpes), and engaging in sexual activity

Modified from CDC: *HIV counseling, testing, and referral: standards and guidelines,* Atlanta, 1994a, CDC, p. 7.

## BOX 13-10

### *Reasons for Engaging in Unprotected Sex*

- Was drunk or high on alcohol/drugs
- Did not have condom available
- Was turned on and didn't want to stop
- Did not know at the time that it was risky
- Did not know reason why
- Knew risk but chose to take it
- Safer sex was not satisfying
- Does not like condoms
- Was not comfortable asking partner
- Both partners HIV-positive and monogamous

From Sowell RL, Seals BF, Cooper JA: HIV transmission knowledge and risk behaviors of persons with HIV infection, *AIDS Patient Care and STDs* 10(2):111-115, 1996, p. 115.

CD4 T-lymphocyte cell counts in HIV-infected persons (USDHHS, 2000h). Clearly, with HIV-infected populations, attention must focus on promoting healthy behaviors and lifestyles that would decrease transmission to uninfected persons, decrease the risk of developing opportunistic infections, and prolong the time before the development of AIDS (USDHHS, 2000f).

Acquiring opportunistic infections increases the progression of HIV and the onset of AIDS (CDC, 1998b). People who are HIV infected are at high risk for developing active tuberculosis (TB), particularly in settings where cough-inducing procedures (sputum induction and aerosolized pentamidine treatments) are being performed. Persons with HIV have a more rapid conversion to active TB than those who are not HIV infected and have a higher probability of contracting TB on exposure because of the risk factors (CDC, 2000).

### What Does It Mean to Practice "Safer Sex"?

The term "safer sex" refers to the practice of protecting yourself against sexually transmitted diseases (STDs), sometimes referred to as venereal disease (VD). There are at least 50 different kinds of these diseases; some of them are even life threatening. You can catch an STD by having sex with someone who is infected.

### What If I Have Sex Without Actually Having Intercourse?

You can still get an STD without having vaginal intercourse or penetration. STDs are spread by having vaginal, oral, or anal sex with an infected person. STD-causing germs can pass from one person to another through body fluids such as semen, vaginal fluid, saliva, and blood; genital warts and herpes are STDs that are spread by direct contact with a wart or blister.

### No One I Dated Looks to Me as If They Could Have an STD. They Look Really Healthy.

You can't tell if a person has an STD just by appearance. In fact, some people with STDs have no signs at all and may not even know they are infected. Still, some signs to look for in your partner are a heavy discharge, rash, sore, or redness near your partner's sex organs. If you see any of these, don't have sex or be sure to use a condom.

### How Can I Tell If I Might Have an STD?

You may have an STD if you experience burning or pain when urinating; sores, bumps, or blisters near the genitals or mouth; swelling around the genitals; fever, chills, night sweats, or swollen glands; or tiredness, vomiting, diarrhea, or sore muscles. In addition, you may have an unusual discharge or smell from the vagina; burning and itching around the vagina; pain in the lower abdomen; vaginal pain during sex; or vaginal bleeding between periods. *But don't forget: you may not have any warning signs at all. Regular medical checkups are essential to your health . . . If you have sex with more than one partner, routine cultures and blood tests may be needed.*

### I Think I Have an STD! What Should I Do?

Get help right away. If you don't, you may pass the STD to your partner or, if you're pregnant, to your baby. In fact, without treatment an STD may make it impossible for you to have a baby at all. You also may develop brain damage, blindness, cancer, heart disease, or arthritis. In some cases you can even die. So go to a doctor or clinic right away.

If your health care provider determines that you do have an STD, tell your partner or partners to get tested, too. Take all of your medication; don't stop just because all your symptoms go away. Do not have sex until you have received full treatment. The disease could still be present in your body. Finally, keep all your appointments, and always use a condom and spermicide when you have sex.

### What Are the Signs of STDs?

There are many different kinds of STDs, and some of them have similar symptoms. You should never attempt to make a diagnosis on your own. The nurse can give you a list with general descriptions of a few of the most common sexually transmitted diseases.

### How Can I Reduce My Chances of Contracting an STD?

Remember, the more sexual partners you have, the greater your risk. Naturally, the best way to reduce your risk is by not having sex or by having sex with one mutually faithful, uninfected partner, or by using a latex condom and spermicide with nonoxynol-9 during sex. Some STDs may be avoided by placing spermicide in the vagina before having sex, because it kills sperm and some STD germs. It helps to urinate and wash after sex (but do not douche, because douching may actually force germs higher up into the body). Avoid having sex with someone who uses intravenous drugs or engages in anal sex. Do not engage in oral, anal, or vaginal sex with an infected person. If you think you may be at risk for AIDS or an STD, seek medical help immediately. Use a new condom each time you have sexual intercourse.

### What If the Condom Breaks? What Should We Do?

If a condom breaks, do not douche. Insert more spermicide into the vagina right away. Men should wash their genitals immediately. Go to a doctor or clinic for an STD examination as soon as possible.

From *Mosby's patient teaching guides,* St Louis, 1995, Mosby, p. 221.

TB has a strong epidemiological link with AIDS and is prevalent among the HIV/AIDS population, although surveillance data are limited by incomplete reporting of HIV status for persons with TB (CDC, 1998c). Therefore the prevalence may actually be higher than has been reported (CDC, 2000). Because of the increased incidence and prevalence of TB among AIDS populations, community health nurses must always consider the possibility of TB, be-

come vigilant in assessing for comorbidity (Grimes, Grimes, 1995, p. 166), and increase TB surveillance along with HIV surveillance (Sbarbaro, 1996, p. 33). This means that any person who is HIV positive should be considered high risk and be automatically tested for TB (CDC, 2000).

There is still no cure for AIDS, but antiretroviral therapy has dramatically improved the health of people living with HIV/AIDS (USDHHS, 2000f). A cure or vaccine for AIDS does not seem to be on the near horizon. Although progress has been made "in vaccine development and in understanding the complexities of viral-host immune response, the prospect of widely available biomedical preventive measures are still in development stages" (USDHHS, 2000h, p. 43). Vaccine development is uncertain and has been impeded because of the long incubation period of AIDS, as well as the enormous costs for vaccine development (Koopman, Little, 1995). Clearly the emphasis with AIDS needs to be on prevention of the disease. The war against AIDS must continue, and all possible avenues of prevention and cure must be considered.

## The Nursing Role and STDs

The American Nurses Association (ANA) has made a commitment to support all efforts of disease prevention (ANA, 1995, p. 20). Community health nurses have a unique opportunity to help decrease incidence, prevalence, and complications of STDs through primary, secondary, and tertiary prevention activities. Nurses have access to populations across the life span and have the opportunity to be involved in community education programs that address preventive interventions for all age groups.

The National Institute of Nursing Research's (NINR) commitment to AIDS is reflected in its research priorities. NINR has awarded grants to promote research in nursing care of persons with AIDS and continues to fund nursing research in relation to HIV/AIDS. Nursing research is playing an active part in finding a solution to the AIDS epidemic.

To provide competent care, nurses need to be aware of their own attitudes about STDs when working with clients. People with STDs, and especially people with AIDS, are well aware of the prejudices that have surrounded the disease. One study found that nurses' attitudes toward persons with AIDS were significantly different according to the mode in which AIDS was acquired (Cole, Slocumb, 1993). Clients who acquired AIDS through blood transfusions were thought of as innocent victims and were viewed more favorably than those who acquired the disease through homosexual contact or use of drug needles (Cole, Slocumb, 1993, p. 116). A goal for all community health nurses should be that clients will never feel that they lack support from their nurses. Nurses have unique skills to help fight this terrible disease and must make every effort to prevent its spread.

## Primary, Secondary, and Tertiary Preventive Nursing Interventions

A continuum of preventive services is essential to address problems associated with AIDS and other STDs. The key goal when addressing STDs and HIV/AIDS control is primary prevention. The most successful outcomes will come from comprehensive and collaborative efforts that are community specific. These efforts must address the needs of communities and aggregates and involve clients and a range of community organizations and providers (e.g., health care agencies, nurses, physicians, volunteers, and educators) in providing preventive and treatment services. This means developing community outreach programs that access at-risk populations where they are.

STD/HIV/AIDS education is a vital component at all levels of prevention. Nurses are working with local community and school leaders to provide STD/HIV/AIDS awareness education to community members, parents, teachers, school children, adolescents, college students, homeless shelters, family planning clinics, and other community-based clinics such as emergency rooms and 24-hour emergency agencies. Nurses need to assume a major role in educating people about STDs/HIV/AIDS by providing competent nursing care and linking clients with appropriate community resources. Education is an important asset. Lack of knowledge about STDs/HIV/AIDS can lead to risk-taking behaviors, delays in seeking testing and treatment, exclusion from clinical drug trials, and higher mortality rates. Nurses working with persons who have STDs/AIDS must be able to deal with personal biases to be competent therapeutic agents. Education is a vital component at all levels of prevention.

Standards and guidelines exist for STDs and HIV that must be adhered to in working with STD populations (CDC, 1999). CDC guidelines for prevention and control of STDs and HIV emphasize four main areas: (1) education to reduce risk or transmission; (2) detection of asymptomatic and symptomatic infected persons; (3) effective diagnosis and treatment of infected persons; and (4) evaluation, treatment, and counseling of sex partners of those who have an STD (CDC, 1993, p. 3). Table 13-3 addresses these guidelines and provides examples of select nursing interventions, categorized as primary, secondary, and tertiary prevention. Confidentiality is extremely important with STD populations.

PRIMARY PREVENTION. Primary prevention focuses on active prevention of contracting STDs/HIV. Primary prevention of STDs/HIV is carried out by identifying those at risk for transmitting and acquiring STDs and working with them to change their risky behaviors. Preventive efforts should be population specific and tailored to the particular risks that have been identified in the assessment of that population. For example, it has been found among some ethnic and socioeconomic groups that mass media educational efforts do not adequately address the educational needs of these groups (Calvillo, 1992), who would benefit from a more focused educational experience that particularly addresses the clients' needs.

Prevention messages must be developmentally appropriate. For example, it is important to understand that sexual inquisitiveness is normal in adolescents because they are beginning to establish their own sexual identities. Therefore prevention messages that take into consideration sexual inquisitiveness must target the young so that they can develop safe and healthy habits at an early age instead of engaging in risky behavior that may lead to acquiring STDs.

**TABLE 13-3**

*Nursing Application of Primary, Secondary, and Tertiary Levels of Prevention for STDs and HIV/AIDS*

| PREVENTION LEVEL | PRIMARY PREVENTION | SECONDARY PREVENTION | TERTIARY PREVENTION |
|---|---|---|---|
| AREAS TO FOCUS OBJECTIVES | PROMOTE HEALTHY BEHAVIORS ADVOCATE SPECIFIC PROTECTION | EARLY DIAGNOSIS PROMPT TREATMENT | REHABILITATION PREVENT RELAPSE |
| Examples of nursing interventions | • Conduct risk assessments to identify populations at risk for acquiring STDs<br>• Develop community education programs:<br>  • STD/AIDS awareness<br>  • Involve community residents and agencies such as teachers, parents, health care agencies, community centers, etc.<br>• Provide "safe sex" education such as the proper use of condoms and advocate abstinence and monogamy in high-risk groups<br>• Teach adolescents about risks of acquiring STDs in sexual experimentation associated with alcohol and drug use<br>• Educate groups of parents and teachers on how to recognize risk behaviors (such as alcohol and drug abuse) in their children or students | • Conduct risk assessment to casefind, identify STD-exposed partners, and refer individuals to appropriate community agency for diagnosis and treatment<br>• Conduct TB screening in HIV-infected and refer for prompt treatment<br>• Educate STD/HIV-infected populations that abstaining from sexual activity is the most effective way to prevent disease transmission; additionally educate regarding use of protective methods that prevent exchange of body fluids<br>• Refer drug and alcohol abusers for treatment<br>• Work with HIV populations to eliminate risk behaviors (such as sharing drug syringes and needles) that would spread the disease | • Case manage STD/HIV-infected persons to prevent disease complications<br>• Conduct periodic risk assessments in infected populations to casefind and prevent disease reinfection and development of opportunistic infections<br>• Work with support agencies to keep alcohol and drug populations in treatment to prevent abuse relapse<br>• Provide supportive nursing care, such as adequate nutrition, to improve quality of life and delay progression of HIV infection to AIDS |

The predominant theme in primary prevention should be that *abstinence* is the only sure method of preventing and acquiring an STD. Other methods, such as using condoms, decrease risks of transmitting and acquiring STDs but do not insure absolute safety. Latex condoms provide a strong protection against HIV if properly used. The CDC recommends that prevention messages on the effectiveness and proper use of condoms should be clear and tailored to the population (CDC, 1993, p. 5). It is imperative for the nurse to adequately instruct clients on how to use condoms properly.

In primary prevention of STDs, the concern is with promoting healthy behaviors and avoiding or changing risky behaviors, such as unprotected sex or drug and alcohol use. Nursing activities focus on health promotion and specific prevention of STDs.

SECONDARY PREVENTION. Secondary prevention focuses on early diagnosis and treatment of STDs and those who are infected with HIV. Secondary prevention stresses early and immediate management of infections, promotion of the practice of healthy habits to prevent transmission of the disease to others, and prevention of opportunistic infections. For example, if partners are HIV positive, the message

must include that it is not "safe" to engage in unprotected sex regardless of the circumstances because of the risk of reinfection or the potential of being infected with other STDs or opportunistic infections.

Secondary prevention also includes finding those who have been exposed to STDs and notifying partners of STD-infected persons of the need for diagnosis and treatment. Referral for treatment can be by client referral, in which the infected person notifies the partner(s), or by provider referral, in which the provider (e.g., physician) refers the infected person to the local health department for contact follow-up on partners for early treatment (CDC, 1993, p. 7). Regardless of the type of contact follow-up done, health care providers do report actual cases of STDs and AIDS to the official local reporting agency (see Chapter 11).

Early intervention is intervening before there are symptoms (CDC, 1993, p. 11). Early intervention links people to appropriate community resources for treatment and support. If the population includes drug users, particularly IV drug users, then secondary prevention and treatment is concerned with getting this population into drug treatment programs and preventing the sharing of equipment.

Many community health agencies are developing innovative needle exchange programming to prevent the spread of infection.

Collaborative efforts are needed to effectively address the complexity of STD transmission. It is not sufficient to only diagnose and treat the disease. An effective control program must include identifying contributing behaviors (e.g., alcohol and drugs) that enhance the risk for reinfection and transmission. This can be done through risk assessment to determine individualized risks and also by developing an intervention plan that appropriately targets the risk behaviors in aggregates (USDHHS, 2000a).

TERTIARY PREVENTION. **Tertiary prevention** for STDs and HIV is concerned with rehabilitation. Nursing activities focus on preventing reinfection, preventing complications from STDs, preventing opportunistic infections to delay HIV progression to AIDS, and providing supportive nursing care. Treatment for STDs or HIV should not be done without assessing other areas of risks, such as IV drug use, that may contribute to reinfection or transmission. Like other contemporary problems a web of cofactors must often be addressed to have successful outcomes. In tertiary prevention the ideal is to prevent unhealthy behaviors that would increase the risk of STD transmission, or reinfection, and progression of HIV infection to AIDS.

Although there is no cure for AIDS, much has been done to delay the progression of HIV infection to AIDS by various drugs that delay development of AIDS. Again, tertiary prevention involves comprehensive and collaborative activities. Tertiary prevention in HIV populations is concerned with strengthening the immune system. This includes pharmacologic drug management as well as promoting healthy behaviors. CDC provides recommended guidelines for pharmacologic management of HIV opportunistic infections and for STDs (CDC, 1993, 1995; USDHHS, 2000h).

# VIOLENT AND ABUSIVE BEHAVIOR

Violent behavior refers to behaviors that intentionally inflict injury to self (as in suicide) and to others (Rosenberg, O'Carroll, Powell, 1992). More than two million people are injured by violent assaults each year (USDHHS, 1995, p. 60). Violent and abusive behavior poses enormous threats, with considerable physical costs and emotional consequences, to the health and safety of communities, workplaces, and schools.

When costs are examined in monetary expenditures the amount is staggering. Medical expenses, lost earnings, and the financing of public programs dealing with violent crime are estimated to cost $105 billion annually. When pain, suffering, and reduced quality of life are added to this, the cost is estimated at $450 billion annually, with violent crime accounting for $426 billion and property crime the other $24 billion (Miller, Cohen, Wiersema, 1996). Every effort must be made to eliminate violence.

Why violence is so widespread, often occurring in families where bonds are strongest, is difficult to understand. Hanrahan, Campbell, and Ulrich (1993) have summarized various explanations for violence in our society (Box 13-12). Different cultures have varying interpretations about what constitutes violence, and the nurse must consider others' views of violence from economic, kinship, and territoriality perspectives, as well as the influence of spiritual, moral, psychological, and metaphysical issues (Hanrahan, Campbell, Ulrich, 1993, p. 30).

Violent and abusive behavior was a major priority area in the *Healthy People 2000* document. The national objectives were directed toward reducing morbidity and mortality associated with violence, including homicides, suicides, and domestic partner and child assault (USDHHS, 1991). The following section discusses homicide and suicide, addresses domestic violence with a focus on violence against women, and discusses nursing interventions for violent and abusive behaviors.

## Homicide and Suicide

Because no other crime is monitored accurately or precisely, homicide is a reliable indicator of all other violent crimes (USDHHS, 2000a). *Healthy People 2010* has set objectives to reduce homicides. Many factors that contribute to injuries are also factors that have been found to be closely associated with violent and abusive behavior (USDHHS, 2000a). There has been a trend of increasing violence among children and adolescents. Recently, violence in the schools has been brought to the forefront of awareness, and increased school safety awareness programs throughout the country are being initiated.

Violent behavior is a complex issue involving a web of cofactors and no single solution. Violence on television and movies is a normal portrayal that provides lasting impressions to the viewers and is thought to be a major contributor to the increasing episodes of violent behavior (Hamilton, 2000). Like other contemporary problems, violent behavior cannot be addressed as a separate entity without examining the societal and socioeconomic cofactors often associated with the violence. For example, alcohol, substance abuse, poverty, drug trafficking, socioeconomic status, adolescent criminal activity, easily accessible weapons, and victims of family violence are some factors that are known to contribute to violent behavior and place aggregates at risk for homicides (Stephenson, 1992, p. 43; USDHHS, 1995, p. 60). Many of the cofactors that increase the risk for homicide also place individuals at risk for suicide. Specifically it has been found that suicide results from an interaction of many cofactors and usually involves a history of psychosocial problems and mental illness that often do not surface until after the suicide has occurred (CDC, 1994b).

As a result of the *Healthy People 2000* initiatives, some progress toward reducing the suicide rate as been made in the last decade (USDHHS, 2000g). In the overall population,

## BOX 13-12

### Summaries of Explanations of Violence

#### Biological

Aggression is an innate characteristic that is either an instinctual drive (the instinctivist school of thought) or neurologically based (neurophysiological theories). The latter examines how brain functioning and/or hormones influence degrees of aggressive tendencies and/or violent behaviors. Research evidence links increased testosterone levels to increases in aggression, but the studies do not indicate a causal relationship and factors such as mood, sampling difficulties, and environment must be considered as intervening characteristics.

#### Role of Alcohol

Research indicates that alcohol seems to facilitate aggression because of the negative affect it has on conscious cognitive processing, yet violence occurs as frequently *without* the presence of alcohol. Alcohol is often used as an excuse or a justification for violence.

#### Psychoanalytical Viewpoint

This position, espoused by Freud and followers, states that violence results from ego weaknesses and the internal need to discharge hostility. Frustration is the stimulus that leads to the expression of aggression. Catharsis or the expression of the aggression results in a decrease of subsequent aggressive behaviors.

#### Social-learning Theory

Aggression and violence are learned responses and may be considered adaptive or destructive, depending on the situation. The family, television, and environmental conditions serve as models for children to learn how to be aggressive and/or violent.

#### Cultural Attitudes Fostering Violence

Tacit acceptance of violence as a means to resolve conflict. War and weapons are justified as protection. In everyday language, we jokingly threaten to "kill" people or "beat them up." We accept physical punishment as a way to discipline children under "certain circumstances." Pornographic depictions of women are legal and deemed as erotica.

#### Power and Violence

Violence or its threat is often used as a method of persuasion, as in rape or incest. Fear of being a victim of violence keeps people, primarily women, in positions of submission.

#### Poverty

Being poor is a condition of oppression, and aggression and violence are methods of expressing such oppression. Poverty needs to be considered as a circumstance in which violence occurs rather than as factor causing such behaviors.

#### Subculture of Violence

There is a theme of violence that permeates the lifestyle values of the individuals who are part of this "cultural group." Violence is a fairly typical method of resolving conflict.

From Hanrahan P, Campbell J, Ulrich Y: Theories of violence. In Campbell J, Humphreys J, editors: *Nursing care of survivors of family violence,* St Louis, 1993, Mosby, p. 6.

---

the number of suicides has remained stable over the last decade. However, suicide is a leading cause of death among 13- to 19-year-old adolescents, and many teens seriously consider suicide without completing suicide (USDHHS, 2000g, p. 38). Some of the factors thought to contribute to suicidal ideation include the following (USDHHS, 2000g, p. 38):

- Depression
- Feelings of hopelessness and worthlessness
- Preoccupation with death
- Impulsive, aggressive, or antisocial behavior
- Family influences
- Family disruption
- History of violence and family disruption
- Rapid sociocultural change
- Substance abuse or dependence
- Severe stress in school, family, or social life

*Healthy People 2010* identifies a reduction in the rate of suicide attempts by adolescents as a critical adolescent objective (USDHHS, 2000g, p. 38). Clearly, this is a health problem in which community nurses can play an active role

through primary and secondary prevention. These factors should be assessed in health promotion activities with adolescents who are high risk for suicide. Homicide is also increasing among adolescents.

In 1997, homicide was the leading cause of death for children aged 5 to 14 years (USDHHS, 2000a). The number of homicides occurring annually demonstrates regression from the *Healthy People 2000* objective for reducing homicides. Many factors, such as unemployment, high school dropout, lack of education, low income, and substance abuse, are closely associated with violent and abusive behavior (USDHHS 2000a, 2000g). Men are more often the victims and perpetrators of homicides, and homicide rates are significantly increased among young African-American men (USDHHS, 2000a).

### The Role of the Nurse with Homicide and Suicide

Community health nurses play an important role in primary prevention of violent and aggressive behavior. Nurses have

**BOX 13-13**

*Questions to Determine the Extent of Violence and Resources Addressing Violence in the Community*

How safe do you feel in the community?

Are the schools in the community safe? What is the incidence of truancy and dropout?

Is there any indication of gang activity?

What is the incidence of stolen property, auto vehicle theft, and breaking and entering homes?

Are the community parks safe? For what are the parks used? Who uses them?

Is there a homeless population in the community?

What is the number of single-parent families?

What is the average socioeconomic status?

What is the poverty rate?

What is the unemployment rate?

What is the illiteracy rate?

Is there evidence of drug dealing? At what ages?

What are the alcohol use, abuse, and/or addiction rates in the community?

What are the number of driving arrests related to intoxication?

What are the drug use, abuse, and/or addiction rates?

What is the incidence of adolescent violence?

What are the homicide and/or attempted homicide statistics?

What are the suicide and/or attempted suicide statistics?

What is the incidence of adolescent suicide and/or attempted suicide?

Is there suicide education that spans all ages?

Is there a high incidence of domestic violence in the community?

What is the incidence of child abuse?

Is there a shelter for domestic abuse victims?

What support groups are active? What peer support groups are needed?

What crisis intervention exists (for suicide, drugs, alcohol, STDs, AIDS, victims of violence, families/friends of suicide/homicide victims)?

What, if any, are the crisis hotline telephone numbers?

Where are the centers?

What referral agencies are available?

Are there community partnerships to deal with violence?

How many worksites have employee assistance programs?

How many worksites have developed policies to address alcohol, drugs, and violence?

How does the media address the issue of violence in the community?

---

opportunities to intervene with populations across the life span. They develop collaborative relationships with other health care providers for the purpose of developing comprehensive health programming that targets aggregates at risk for suicide and homicide. Because of the complexity of violent and aggressive behavior, social cofactors must be considered when developing multifaceted community interventions to eliminate violent and abusive behavior in the communities (USDHHS, 2000a).

Community health nurses are involved in community risk assessment, determining populations at risk for violence and suicide, and developing and implementing interventions to decrease violence in the community (see Chapters 14 and 15 for assessing and planning interventions with communities and aggregates at risk). Solutions to eliminate violence are complex and require multidisciplinary and multifaceted approaches. Like other contemporary problems, the most effective intervention is prevention. Interventions to prevent violent behavior that leads to homicide and suicide must include long-range planning that begins at home; is supported in the schools and communities; and involves state, local, media, religious, and cultural organizations (Wolman, 1995, p. xix). Chapter 16 presents a range of preventive interventions to reduce youth suicide and violence.

Working collaboratively with other disciplines and agencies to identify those at risk and to intervene effectively through prevention is crucial. To be effective it is important

to mobilize partnerships with community resources in developing prevention programs (ANA, 2000). This requires community health nurses to be knowledgeable about the resources available in the community. Knowledge of community resources is necessary for any intervention with community populations, and community health nurses must be able to identify which resources exist and which are needed and have a strong network with community agencies to develop preventive and treatment measures.

Recognizing populations that are prone to violent behavior is essential. Multiple social, economic, and psychological factors, such as unemployment and societal attitudes about violence and drug abuse, place aggregates at risk for homicides. Like other social problems, this one does not exist in isolation, and there is no single indicator. However, certain characteristics are known to contribute to homicide and suicide. These characteristics are part of a larger web of crime cofactors and are a point from which to begin a risk assessment. A few questions nurses might ask to ascertain the extent and cofactors of violence that may be existing in their communities are listed in Box 13-13.

Answers to these questions can provide a starting point for understanding the potential web of violence in respective communities and can provide a base for developing preventive interventions. This would include such things as public awareness campaigns, supporting law enforcement in arrest, supporting stringent legal sanctions for perpetrators

**TABLE 13-4**

*Nursing Application of Primary, Secondary, and Tertiary Levels of Prevention for Violent and Abusive Behavior*

| PREVENTION LEVEL | PRIMARY PREVENTION | SECONDARY PREVENTION | TERTIARY PREVENTION |
|---|---|---|---|
| GOAL | STOP VIOLENCE | STOP VIOLENCE | STOP VIOLENCE |
| Examples of nursing interventions | • Conduct risk assessment to identify populations at risk for violent behavior<br>• Develop community public awareness programs to alert public of indicators of criminal activity<br>• Involve community members such as teachers, parents, health care agencies, and community centers in prevention<br>• Educate aggregates (e.g., parents, teachers, adolescents) on how to recognize signs of suicidal ideation<br>• Collaborate with community leaders to destroy the base of violence, suicide, and homicide, and provide awareness of domestic abuse shelters and other options for protection<br>• Advocate policy development that limits access to drugs and weapons | • Research the number of suicide attempts in the population, crime statistics, domestic abuse police calls, drug/alcohol-related arrests, and injuries related to violent behavior<br>• Refer victims of violence to support groups and shelters<br>• Support enforcement of legal sanctions for perpetrators<br>• Casefind by screening select populations for depression and refer for counseling/treatment<br>• Work with affected populations to eliminate risk behaviors (such as drug and alcohol abuse)<br>• Facilitate development of peer support groups | • Conduct follow-up risk assessments for relapse<br>• Coordinate follow-up therapy of victims of violence to prevent recurrence and to break the cycle of abuse<br>• Collaborate with community providers to establish community support groups for helping perpetrators stop violent behavior<br>• Advocate enforcement of stringent legal sanctions for perpetrators<br>• Collaborate with support agencies to ensure ongoing treatment for victims and perpetrators<br>• Advocate for development of shelters for victims |

and treatment for the chemically addicted, treating injured victims, advocating for shelter, and advocating for strong protective and treatment policy development.

Community health nurses can intervene at the primary, secondary, and tertiary levels of prevention. The roles of the community health nurse may vary with various interventions. Every aspect of prevention and intervention should have an overall goal to *stop violence*. Table 13-4 shows examples of various nursing interventions and nursing roles involved in eliminating violent behavior.

## Domestic Violence

Domestic violence awareness has increased over the past decade. As a result, many myths concerning domestic abuse have been dispelled, and it has become clear that domestic violence occurs in every community. Domestic violence occurs in every race at all socioeconomic levels, all educational levels, all ages, in both men and women, among the employed and unemployed and celebrities and noncelebrities. In other words, no populations are unaffected by domestic violence. Every reader of this textbook will undoubtedly

have heard of, or personally known, someone within his or her community who has been a victim of domestic violence. Domestic violence has serious ramifications for the individual, family, and community. It can result in physical and emotional injury, death, temporary or permanent separation of families, and financial hardship. Intrafamilial violence is more prevalent than is often recognized. Domestic violence has no boundaries and crosses the life span.

Although domestic violence has been prevalent for some time, in recent years more stringent laws have been passed that enable protective action before behaviors escalate into physical injury and death. For example, in the early 1990s antistalking legislation was passed that gives the police power to arrest individuals for this behavior, and currently almost all states and the District of Columbia have passed antistalking legislation (U.S. Department of Justice, 1996b). In 1994 Congress passed the Violence Against Women Act, which has resulted in national campaigns for violence against women. As a result, every state has established a state organization of Violence Against Women. A national hotline (1-800-799-SAFE) has been established, and many states have developed toll-free hotlines as well (U.S. Department of Justice, 1996a).

Domestic violence laws vary from state to state in the types of acts (e.g., stalking, assaults, threats) they cover. How each state defines domestic violence determines what constitutes a crime (Stark, Flitcraft, 1996, p. 160; U.S. Department of Justice, 1996b). A study conducted by the National Institute of Justice (NIJ) and CDC interviewed 8000 women and 8000 men about their experiences with rape, physical assault, and stalking (NIJ, 1998). Some of the key findings from this study include the following:

- Physical assault is widespread, and 52% of the women in the study said they were physically assaulted as a child or adult by an adult perpetrator.
- 1.9% of the women experienced assault within 12 months of the interview.
- Findings supported an estimate that 1.9 million women are assaulted annually.
- 18% of the women said they experienced a completed or attempted rape at some time in their life and 0.3% said they had experienced completed or attempted rape within 12 months of the interview.
- These findings suggest that interventions should focus on rapes perpetrated against children and adolescents.
- There were racial and ethnic differences in the reported incidences of rape and physical assault. Native American/Alaskan Native women were most likely to report rape and physical assault victimization. Hispanic women were less likely to report rape victimization than non-Hispanic women.
- Women experience significantly more partner violence than men and said they were raped and/or physically assaulted by a current or former spouse, cohabiting partner, or date in their lifetime.
- 1.5% of surveyed women and 0.9% of surveyed men said they were raped in the previous 12 months of the interview.
- Violence against women is primarily partner violence.
- Women are more likely than men to be injured during an assault.
- Stalking is more prevalent than previously thought (NIJ 1998, p. 2).

The findings from this study are being used as a basis to develop more effective programming to prevent and treat domestic violence.

Both men and women are victims of domestic violence, but women are the most frequently and seriously injured victims. Both men and women are stalkers and have been stalked (Brownstein, 2000). Studies suggest that at least 2 million women are physically battered each year by intimate partners, including husbands, former husbands, boyfriends, and lovers, including gay or lesbian partners (Crowell, Burgess, 1996, p. 1). The findings from a national crime victimization survey provided some poignant facts

**BOX 13-14**

*Victims of Domestic Violence: Select Facts from a National Crime Victimization Survey*

- Women are attacked about six times more often by offenders with whom they had an intimate relationship than are male violence victims.
- Nearly 30% of all female homicide victims are known to have been killed by their husbands, former husbands, or boyfriends.
- In contrast, just over 3% of male homicide victims are known to have been killed by their wives, former wives, or girlfriends.
- Husbands, former husbands, boyfriends, and ex-boyfriends committed more than 1 million violent acts against women.
- Family members or other people that the victim knew committed more than 2.7 million violent crimes against women.
- Husbands, former husbands, boyfriends, and ex-boyfriends committed 26% of rapes and sexual assaults.
- About 45% of all violent attacks against female victims 12 years old and older by multiple offenders involve offenders they know.
- The rate of intimate-offender attacks on women separated from their husbands was about three times higher than that of divorced women and about 25 times higher than that of married women.
- Women of all races are equally vulnerable to attacks by intimates.
- Female victims of violence are more likely to be injured when attacked by someone they know than female victims of violence who are attacked by strangers.

Modified from US Department of Justice: *Domestic violence awareness: stop the cycle of violence,* Pub No USGPO: 1996-405-033/54261, Washington, DC, 1996a, US Government Printing Office, p. 5.

about victims of domestic violence. These facts are shown in Box 13-14.

As mentioned previously, no segment of the population is free of battered women. Battered women come from all walks of life. However, some characteristics of domestic violence victims that have been observed with consistency include an early exposure to violence as a child, economic dependence on one's partner, lack of awareness of alternatives, poor self-image, and inadequate support systems. Often friends and relatives of the battered woman find it easier to ignore the situation or even sanction the abuse than get involved. Between 21% and 30% of all women in the United States are estimated to have been beaten by a partner at least once, and more than 1 million women each year seek help for injuries caused by battering (Alpert, 1999). This help is often sought out at emergency rooms where fewer questions may be asked and anonymity may be maintained.

When a victim of domestic abuse presents to the emergency room or clinic, nurses are often the first contact the victim has following the assault. Because of the complexity of the abuse cycle, nurses must be sensitive to the fear experienced by these victims when questioning and intervening. This is especially critical in cases of rape, where nurses are dealing with emotional trauma and may also be gathering forensic evidence that will be used if legal charges are filed against the perpetrator (Crowell, Burgess, 1996, p. 109). Domestic violence involves battering (such as pushing, slapping, punching, kicking, knifing, shooting, and throwing objects) and verbal and emotional abuse. Most battering relationships "pass through phases marked by increasing fear, isolation, and control, often accompanied by increasingly complex psychological and psychosocial adaptations" (Stark, Flitcraft, 1996, p. 205).

Within these phases there is often a time of remorse; the perpetrator may feel guilty and remorseful following an episode of abuse, and things may calm down for a time. However, it does not take much to trigger a new episode. In fact, the abuse cycle is very likely to occur again, and it may become more severe. A violent relationship can easily go on to become a violent system that ultimately leads to death. Nurses must be perceptive and prepared to comprehensively assess, intervene, and refer appropriately when victims seek care.

Domestic violence is different from other forms of violence in that the victim is in close relationship to the perpetrator, and the perpetrator has continued access to the victim (Stark, Flitcraft, 1996, p. 161). Domestic violence is often difficult to identify. Travis (1996) has described three predominant indicators to distinguish domestic violence from other forms of violence: (1) The victim often knows the perpetrator, and often there have been repeated offenses that have progressively become more violent; (2) the victim often lives in a state of terror and powerlessness as the perpetrator exerts physical, psychological, and emotional control over the victim; (3) and the violence is often known to the community, where there have been fragmented indicators of abuse in medical records, police records, and school and work records that reflect patterns of absence or visible signs of battering, yet the community has looked the other way and ignored the indicators (Travis, 1996, pp. 24-25). When the violence is finally noted, it is often severe and in some cases deadly. It is crucial for community health nurses to be aware of these characteristics to intervene in an efficacious manner.

The battered victim may be kept from contact with others who could provide help. The victim may be depressed and may frequently mention minor somatic complaints when seen by health care personnel. She may or may not show obvious signs of physical injury. Many women who have experienced battering are unrecognized during health care visits (Davidson, 1996, p. 13). Domestic violence is difficult to deal with because of emotional ties between the individuals involved (NIJ, 1996, p. 28).

Shelters and safe homes for battered women exist in many communities throughout the country. As mentioned earlier, there is a national hotline (1-800-799-SAFE) with daily 24-hour coverage by people who respond to requests for information, discuss options, and provide shelter referrals. Individuals who call the hotline can get an immediate crisis intervention referral to agencies in their local communities, including domestic abuse shelters and emergency services. The National Coalition against Domestic Violence in Washington, D.C. (202-638-6388) is an excellent source of information and referral. In response to the Violence Against Women Act, the NIJ is carrying out extensive research on this problem, and new data and information will be forthcoming in the next few years.

## The Role of the Nurse with Domestic Violence

The American Nurses Association has developed a strong position statement on violence against women. The position document defines violence against women as "behavior intended to inflict harm and includes slapping, kicking, choking, punching, pushing, use of objects as weapons, forced sexual activity, and injury or death from a weapon" (ANA, 1996a, p. 203). ANA has made an active commitment to eliminate all forms of domestic violence "through the legislative, regulatory, and health care arena" (ANA, 1995).

Because nurses have the unique opportunity to interact with clients individually as well as in groups, it is important to complete thorough interviews with victims or potential victims to more effectively intervene and identify the most appropriate referrals. Humphreys (1993) believes that every family should be assessed for family violence. Table 13-5 lists the indicators of potential or actual wife abuse from history. Table 13-6 gives the indicators of wife abuse from physical examination. Indicators for child abuse are identified in Chapter 16.

Davey and Davey (1996) encourage nurses to interview clients when screening for abuse because the victims are more likely to disclose personal information during an interview with a nurse than when responding to a written form. Box 13-15 provides teaching tips for domestic violence and Box 13-16 gives a list of guidelines to use when interviewing victims about domestic violence. Community health nurses can use these guides to assess women at risk. Assessment data are used as a basis for developing nursing interventions, including referral to community resources as indicated. Identifying women at risk is essential for intervention at both primary and secondary levels of prevention (Davidson, 1996, p. 13).

An important role of the community health nurse is casefinding. The community health nurse is in a unique position to see the family at home and may be the first to ob-

**TABLE 13-5**

## Indicators of Potential or Actual Wife Abuse from History

| AREA OF ASSESSMENT | AT-RISK RESPONSES* |
|---|---|
| ### Primary Concern/Reason for Visit | |
| | Unwarranted delay between time of injury and seeking treatment |
| | Inappropriate spouse reactions (lack of concern, overconcern, threatening demeanor, reluctance to leave wife, etc.) |
| | Vague information about cause of injury or problem; discrepancy between physical findings and verbal description of cause; obviously incongruous cause of injury given |
| | Minimizing serious injury |
| | Seeking emergency room treatment for vague stress-related symptoms and minor injuries |
| | Suicide attempt; history of previous attempts |
| ### Family Health History | |
| Family of origin | Traditional values about women's role taught |
| | Spouse abuse or child abuse (may not be significant for wife but should be noted) |
| Children | Children abused |
| | Physical punishment used routinely and severely with children |
| | Children are hostile toward or fearful of father |
| | Father perceives children as an additional burden |
| | Father demands unquestioning obedience from children |
| Partner | Alcohol or drug abuse |
| | Holds machismo values |
| | Experience with violence outside of home, including violence against women in previous relationships |
| | Low self-esteem; lack of power in workplace or other arenas outside of home |
| | Uses force or coercion in sexual activities |
| | Unemployment or underemployment |
| | Extreme jealousy of female friendships, work, and children, as well as other men; jealousy frequently unfounded |
| | Stressors such as death in family, moving, change of jobs, trouble at work |
| | Abused as a child or witnessed father abusing mother |
| Household | Poverty |
| | Conflicts solved by aggression or violence |
| | Isolated from neighbors, relatives; few friends; lack of support systems |
| ### Past Health History | |
| | Fractures and trauma injuries |
| | Depression, anxiety symptoms, substance abuse |
| | Injuries while pregnant |
| | Spontaneous abortions |
| | Psychophysiological complaints |
| | Previous suicide attempts |
| Nutrition | Evidence of overeating or anorexia as reactions to stress |
| | Sudden changes in weight |
| Personal/social | Low self-esteem; evaluates self poorly in relation to others and ideal self, has trouble listing strengths, makes negative comments about self frequently, doubts own abilities |
| | Expresses feelings of being trapped, powerlessness, that the situation is hopeless, that it is futile to make future plans |
| | Chronic fatigue, apathy |
| | Feels responsible for spouse's behavior |
| | Holds traditional values about the home, a wife's prescribed role, the husband's prerogatives, strong commitment to marriage |
| | External locus of control orientation, feels no control over situation, believes fate or other forces determine events |

From Campbell J, McKenna LS, Torres S et al.: Nursing care of abused women. In Campbell J, Humphreys J, editors: *Nursing care of survivors of family violence,* St Louis, 1993, Mosby, pp. 255-256.

*At-risk responses are derived from clinical experience and review of the literature.

*Continued*

**TABLE 13-5**

*Indicators of Potential or Actual Wife Abuse from History—cont'd*

| AREA OF ASSESSMENT | AT-RISK RESPONSES* |
|---|---|
| Personal/social— cont'd | Major decisions in household made by spouse, indicates far less power than he has in relationship, activities controlled by spouse, money controlled by spouse |
|  | Few support systems, few supportive friends, little outside home activity, outside relationships have been discouraged by spouse or curtailed by self to deal with violent situation |
|  | Physical aggression in courtship |
| Sleep | Sleep disturbances, insomnia, sleeping more than 10 to 12 hours per day |
| Elimination | Chronic constipation, diarrhea, or elimination disturbances related to stress |
| Illness | Frequent psychophysiological illnesses |
|  | Treatment for mental illness |
|  | Use of tranquilizers and/or mood elevators and/or antidepressants |
| Operations/ hospitalizations | Hospitalizations for trauma injuries |
|  | Suicide attempts |
|  | Hospitalization for depression |
|  | Refusals of hospitalization when suggested by physician |
| Personal safety | Handgun(s) in home |
|  | History of frequent accidents |
|  | Does not take safety precautions |
| Health care utilization | No regular provider |
|  | Indicates mistrust of health care system |
| Review of systems | Headaches, undiagnosed gastrointestinal symptoms, palpitations, other possible psychophysiological complaints |
|  | Sexual difficulties, feels husband is "rough" in sexual activities, lack of sexual desire, pain with intercourse |
|  | Joint pain and/or other areas of tenderness, especially at the extremities |
|  | Chronic pain |
|  | Pelvic inflammatory disease |

serve an abusive relationship. The nurse must be comfortable in exploring possible abuse issues with clients. This may involve examining personal attitudes and beliefs related to domestic abuse (Dickson, Tutty, 1996). Community health nurses, like other health care providers, are legally responsible for reporting abuse, and it is imperative that nurses do not allow personal issues and biases to interfere with their professional responsibility to clients. It is essential for nurses to look not only for obvious signs of abuse but also for less obvious signs (Gerard, 2000). Early intervention is necessary to break the cycle of abuse and prevent the escalation of violence. The nurse can help clients look at their situation and seek alternatives to their current lifestyle. This usually involves examining available community resources and agencies for both immediate and long-term assistance. A collaborative approach is necessary for assessment, intervention, and prevention of domestic violence.

Referrals for counseling, shelters for battered women and their children, self-help programs, job training, and financial assistance are a few of the community services available to help domestic violence victims. Community health nurses

provide supportive assistance when the client is using these community services. Community health nurses also facilitate, through referral, coordination, and managed-care roles, comprehensive ongoing care that is coordinated with other community groups and agencies. Nurses also refer clients to safe houses and serve as client advocates. They work to decrease barriers to the access of care.

Increasingly, community health nurses are providing valuable services in shelters for battered women and children. Nurses complete health assessments, make referrals to community resources, provide health counseling, conduct group health education sessions, and provide consultation to the shelter staff relative to the health aspects of operating a group home. Community health nurses' knowledge of the community and health issues make them valuable members of a domestic violence team.

In sheltered group settings community health nurses are active members of an interdisciplinary team and provide a unique perspective to the delivery of comprehensive health care. Their focus on preventive, as well as curative, services enhances the care provided to this population group. Be-

**TABLE 13-6**

## Indicators of Wife Abuse from Physical Examination

| AREA OF ASSESSMENT | AT-RISK FINDINGS |
|---|---|
| General appearance | Increased anxiety in presence of spouse |
| | Watching spouse for approval of answers to questions |
| | Signs of fatigue |
| | Inappropriate or anxious nonverbal behavior |
| | Nonverbal communication suggesting shame about body |
| | Flinches when touched |
| | Poor grooming, inappropriate attire |
| Vital statistics | Overweight or underweight |
| | Hypertension |
| Skin | Bruises, welts, edema, or scars, especially on breasts, upper arms, abdomen, chest, face, and genitalia |
| | Burns |
| Head | Subdural hematoma |
| | Clumps of hair missing |
| Eyes | Swelling |
| | Subconjunctival hemorrhage |
| Genital/urinary | Edema, bruises, tenderness, external bleeding |
| Rectal | Bruising, bleeding, edema, irritation |
| Musculoskeletal | Fractures, especially of facial bones, spiral fractures of radius or ulna, ribs |
| | Shoulder dislocation |
| | Limited motion of an extremity |
| | Old fractures in various stages of healing |
| Abdomen | Abdominal injuries in pregnant women |
| | Intraabdominal injury |
| Neurological | Hyperactive reflex responses |
| | Ear or eye problems secondary to injury |
| | Areas of numbness from old injuries |
| | Tremors |
| Mental status examination | Anxiety, fear |
| | Depression |
| | Suicidal ideation |
| | Low self-esteem |
| | Memory loss |
| | Difficulty concentrating |

From Campbell J, McKenna LS, Torres S, et al.: Nursing care of abused women. In Campbell J, Humphreys J, editors: *Nursing care of survivors of family violence*, St Louis, 1993, Mosby, p. 257.

cause of the complex dynamics related to family violence, confidentiality in regard to the location of shelters for battered victims is maintained by health professionals in many communities. Crisis hotlines help clients access services from these shelters. Nurses have been working to strengthen services for victims of domestic violence across the nation.

The Nursing Network on Violence Against Women (NNVAW) was founded in 1985 during the first National Nursing Conference on Violence Against Women held at the University of Massachusetts at Amherst. The ultimate goal of NNVAW is to provide a nursing presence in the struggle to end violence in women's lives. A book written specifically for nurses on family violence is *Nursing Care of Survivors of Family Violence* (1993) by Campbell and Humphreys. The book is an excellent practical resource for clinicians, researchers, and teachers. The authors stress that preventive interventions at both the family and community level are essential to reduce future domestic violence.

Nursing activities developed by the Iowa Intervention Project to intervene in abuse protection are listed in Box 13-17. As research continues, more publications will become available, and as researcher roles are implemented, community health nurses will make a contribution to nursing's knowledge base for preventing and intervening in violent and abusive behavior.

## BOX 13-15
### Domestic Violence Guide*

I. Identify Signs and Signals:
  A. Physical (any injuries if pregnant, hair missing, edema, limited motion)
  B. Emotional (feels depressed, suicidal, or responsible for abuse and for meeting partner's needs)
  C. Behavioral (hypervigilant, quiet in partner's presence, victimizes others)
  D. Social (isolated from friends and family, few financial or other resources)
II. When Domestic Violence Is Suspected:
  A. Assess the existence of violence and presence of danger
  B. Educate about domestic violence and choices
  C. Assist in the development and practice of a safety plan
  D. Encourage short- and long-term counseling
III. Assess the Abuser for Increasing Threat:
  A. Threatens homicide or suicide
  B. Acutely depressed or feeling hopeless
  C. Brings gun or other weapon into home
  D. Obsessive about partner or family
  E. Increases frequency or roughness of battering
  F. Uses drugs or alcohol
  G. Hurts or kills family pets
  H. Rages or fights with other people
IV. Identify Options:
  A. Seek legal advice
  B. Get protective order
  C. Have abuser arrested

D. Leave
E. Stay
F. Develop safety plan
V. Establish a Client-Centered Safety Plan:
  A. Determine the effects of violence on the client's children, how to predict imminent danger, how to physically leave situation
  B. Hide money, important papers, cards, numbers, clothing, medication for quick, easy access
  C. Hide extra keys for house and give extra set to trusted person
  D. Set up "code" with family and friends so they'll know when to call police
  E. Hide phone number for local shelter, establish contact with social worker
  F. Reestablish contact with estranged family and friends
  G. Identify places of sanctuary
  H. Make current plan more detailed than last "escape" attempt
VI. Organizing Framework for the Clinician:
  A. Develop protocol for handling domestic violence, put in Policies and Procedures manual
  B. Offer educational sessions for staff
  C. Post phone numbers for local domestic violence shelters in prominent place
  D. Compile a list of therapists and social workers who specialize in treating victims on an outpatient basis
  E. Contact attorney general to learn status of laws about reporting abuse in your state

From Davey PA, Davey DB: Domestic violence: a clinical view, *Home Health Focus* 2(10):78-79, 1996.
*This document is for use by clinicians only and is not to be left in the home.

## BOX 13-16
### Guidelines for Interviewing Clients About Domestic Violence

Remember that your client is a survivor.
Talk unhurriedly in a private environment.
Maintain confidentiality.
Use active listening skills.
Maintain eye contact without staring.
Show empathetic concern, not horror.
Don't offer simplistic solutions.
Don't use demonstrative sympathy or anger.

Don't ask "why" questions.
Believe your client; don't disregard or minimize the situation.
Don't make judgments.
Acknowledge injustice.
Give supportive messages.
Respect your client's right of self-determination.
Record without judgments what has been said and observed.

From Davey PA, Davey DB: Domestic violence: a clinical view, *Home Health Focus* 2(10):78-79, 1996.

● **BOX 13-17**

## NIC Nursing Intervention: Abuse Protection Support

*Definition*

Identification of high-risk, dependent relationships and actions to prevent further infliction of physical or emotional harm

*Nursing Activities*

Identify adult(s) with a history of unhappy childhoods associated with abuse, rejection, excessive criticism, or feelings of being worthless and unloved as children

Identify adult(s) who have difficulty trusting others or feel disliked by others

Identify whether individual feels that asking for help is an indication of personal incompetence

Identify level of social isolation present in family situation

Determine whether family needs periodic relief from care responsibilities

Identify whether adult at risk has close friends or family available to help with children when needed

Determine relationship between husband and wife

Determine whether adults are able to take over for each other when one is too tense, tired, or angry to deal with a dependent family member

Determine whether child/dependent adult is viewed differently by an adult based on gender, appearance, or behavior

Identify crisis situations that may trigger abuse, such as poverty, unemployment, divorce, or death of a loved one

Monitor for signs of neglect in high-risk families

Observe a sick or injured child/dependent adult for signs of abuse

Listen to the explanation on how the illness or injury happened

Identify when the explanation of the cause of the injury is inconsistent among those involved

Encourage admission of child/dependent adult for further observation and investigation as appropriate

Record times and duration of visits during hospitalization

Monitor parent-child interactions and record observations as appropriate

Monitor for underreactions or overreactions on the part of an adult

Monitor child/dependent adult for extreme compliance, such as passive submission to hospital procedures

Monitor child for role reversal, such as comforting the parent, or overactive or aggressive behavior

Listen attentively to adult who begins to talk about own problems

Listen to a pregnant woman's feelings about pregnancy and expectations about the unborn child

Monitor new parent's reactions to infant, observing for feelings of disgust, fear, or unrealistic expectations

Monitor for a parent who holds newborn at arm's length, handles newborn awkwardly, or asks for excessive assistance

Monitor for repeated visits to a clinic, emergency room, or physician's office for minor problems

Monitor for a progressive deterioration in the physical and emotional care provided to a child/dependent adult in the family

Monitor child for signs of failure to thrive, depression, apathy, developmental delay, or malnutrition

Determine expectations adult has for child to determine whether expected behaviors are realistic

Instruct parents on realistic expectations of child, based on developmental level

Establish rapport with families who have a history of abuse for long-term evaluation and support

Help families identify coping strategies for stressful situations

Instruct adult family members on signs of abuse

Refer adult(s) at risk to appropriate specialists

Inform the physician of observations indicative of abuse

Report any situations in which abuse is suspected to the proper authorities

Refer adult(s) to shelters for abused spouses as appropriate

Refer parents to Parents Anonymous for group support as appropriate

From McCloskey JC, Bulecheck GM, editors: *Nursing interventions classification (NIC)*, ed 3, St Louis, 2000, Mosby, pp. 107-108.

## SUMMARY

Aggregate-focused contemporary community health issues are multifaceted and complex. Community health nurses have an important role in assessing populations at risk, identifying health problems, and developing interventions to promote the health of the community. This chapter addressed the issues involving select population groups at risk and discussed the community health nurse's role in primary, secondary, and tertiary prevention of contemporary health issues. Particular emphasis was given to primary prevention and developing community-based interventions.

As responsibility for meeting the needs of disadvantaged populations shifts from the federal government to state and local communities, the need for comprehensive community-based programming is a priority. In community-based programming, interventions are tailored specifically to the needs of communities. Examples of such interventions include the use of peer counselors and the use of culturally relevant health education materials.

Community-based programming requires a holistic approach that addresses the multifaceted web of contemporary health problems (poverty, homelessness, substance addiction, STDs, HIV/AIDS, violence, and abusive behavior). Many of the problems do not exist in isolation but are part of a larger web of social, economic, and other related health issues. Because community health nurses have access to the populations at risk and knowledge of the resources in their respective communities, they play an important role when they use the nursing process in intervening with aggregates to assist and diagnose contemporary health issues and to implement and evaluate effective interventions.

## CRITICAL THINKING
*exercise*

Read the following scenario (Berne, Dato, Mason, Rafferty, 1990, p. 11) and then write a paragraph describing your feelings and the course of action you would take in the next week. Do you believe that this situation could ever happen to you or someone that you know?

### Imagine You Are Homeless . . .

Imagine you are a 33-year-old woman with three children. Your apartment burned down 6 months ago. You and your children had been living with your sister in her cramped apartment until she had another baby, and now there simply is not enough room for everyone.

You sleep in your car at night. During the day, you walk the streets with your children trying to find an apartment you can afford. Finally, you go to the department of social services to try to find shelter for the night and are told that your children may have to be placed in foster care if a place cannot be found for all of you. Knowing that the foster care system in this city is unreliable and sometimes unsafe, you agree to spend the first night in an overcrowded warehouse-type shelter, where you end up sleeping on the floor.

You and your children have no privacy here. Many of the children and adults have colds, and you hear that tuberculosis has been an increasing problem among the homeless. When the opportunity arises, you agree to move into one of the single-room occupancy hotels that the city is using to house homeless families "temporarily." That temporary shelter becomes your home for 13 months.

The temporary shelter consists of one 10 ft × 10 ft room. You have no kitchen, no refrigerator, no stove or cooking facilities. There is one bed for you and your three children.

You pull the mattress off the bed at night to make room for all of you to sleep and then pull the sheets off the bed in the day to eat on the floor.

You use running water to keep your baby's milk cool and you do the dishes in the tub where you bathe and store things.

There is no place for your children to play, no place to sit, no place to do homework. When they try to play in the hall, they are approached by drug dealers and sometimes even pimps.

This is what life is like for you and your children. Imagine the gradual dissipation of your own and your children's self-esteem and the isolation and depression that eventually overwhelm you. Imagine having a future without space, without privacy, without hope.

---

*Ella M. Brooks acknowledges the work from previous editions of this text in the development of this chapter.*

## REFERENCES

Adams PF, Schoenborn CA, Moss AJ, et al.: Health risk behaviors among our nations youth: United States, 1992, National Center for Health Statistics, Vital Health Statistics 10(192), 1995.

Alpert EJ, editor: Partner violence: how to recognize and treat victims of abuse: a guide for physicians and other health care professionals, ed 3, Waltham, Mass, 1999, Massachusetts Medical Society.

American Nurses Association (ANA): Legislative and regulatory initiatives for the 104th Congress, American Nurses Association: Department of Governmental Affairs, 1995, ANA.

American Nurses Association (ANA): American Nurses Association position statement on physical violence against women, Washington, DC, 1996a, ANA.

American Nurses Association (ANA): American Nurses Association position statement on cultural diversity in nursing practice, Washington, DC, 1996b, ANA.

American Nurses Association (ANA): Public health nursing: a partner for health populations, Washington, DC, 2000, ANA.

Bayer R: AIDS prevention and cultural sensitivity: are they compatible? Am J Public Health 84(6):895-897, 1994.

Benjamin R: Feeling poorly: the troubling verdict on poverty and health care in America, National Forum 76(3):39-42, 1996.

Berne AS, Dato C, Mason DJ, et al.: A nursing model for addressing the health needs of homeless families, Image J Nurs Sch 22(1):8-13, 1990.

Beschner G: Understanding teenage drug use. In Beschner G, Friedman AS, editors: Teen drug use, Lexington, Mass, 1986, D.C. Heath.

Blane D: Social determinants of health—socioeconomic status, social class, and ethnicity, Am J Public Health 85(7):903-905, 1995 (editorial).

Boydell K, Goering, P, Morrell-Bellai TL: Narratives of identity: representation of self in people who are homeless, Qualitative Health Research 10(1):26-38, 2000.

Brownstein A: In the campus shadows, women who are stalkers as well as being stalked, The Chronicle of Higher Education XLCII(15): A40-A2, December 8, 2000.

Burg M: Health problems of sheltered homeless women and their dependent children, Health Soc Work 19(2):125-131, 1994.

Burhansstipanov L, Satter DE: Office management and budget racial categories and implications for American Indians and Alaskan Natives, Am J Public Health 90(11):1720-1723, 2000.

Calvillo ER: AIDS knowledge and attitudes among Latinos. In Western Institute of Nursing: Communicating nursing research, silver threads: 25 years of excellence, vol 25, Boulder, Colo, 1992, The Institute.

Campbell JC, Humphreys JC: Nursing care of survivors of family violence, St Louis, 1993, Mosby.

Campbell J, McKenna LS, Torres S, et al.: Nursing care of abused women. In Campbell J, Humphreys J, editors: *Nursing care of survivors of family violence*, St Louis, 1993, Mosby.

Caton CL, Hasin D, Shrout E, et al.: Risk factors for homelessness among indigent urban adults with no history of psychotic illness: a case—control study, *Am J Public Health* 90(2): 258-263, 2000.

Centers for Disease Control and Prevention (CDC): 1989 sexually transmitted diseases treatment guidelines, *MMWR Morbid Mortal Wkly Rep* 38(No. S-8):4-40, 1989.

Centers for Disease Control and Prevention (CDC): 1993 sexually transmitted diseases treatment guidelines, *MMWR Morbid Mortal Wkly Rep* 42(No. RR-14):1-102, 1993.

Centers for Disease Control and Prevention (CDC): *HIV counseling, testing, and referral: standards and guidelines*, Atlanta, 1994a, CDC.

Centers for Disease Control and Prevention (CDC): Programs for the prevention of suicide among adolescents and young adults, *MMWR Morbid Mortal Wkly Rep* 43(RR-6):3-18, April 22, 1994b.

Centers for Disease Control and Prevention (CDC): USPHS/IDSA guidelines for the prevention of opportunistic infections in persons infected with human immunodeficiency virus: a summary, *MMWR Morbid Mortal Wkly Rep* 44(RR-8), 1995.

Centers for Disease Control and Prevention (CDC): Changes in notifiable diseases data presentation, *MMWR Morbid Mortal Wkly Rep* 45(2):41-42, January 19, 1996.

Centers for Disease Control and Prevention (CDC): 1998 guidelines for treatment of sexually transmitted diseases, *MMWR Morbid Mortal Wkly Rep* 44(RR-1):1-116, 1998a.

Centers for Disease Control and Prevention (CDC): *HIV/AIDS surveillance report* 10(2):1-43, 1998b.

Centers for Disease Control and Prevention (CDC): Prevention and treatment of tuberculosis among patients infected with human immunodeficiency virus: principles of therapy and revised recommendations, *MMWR Morbid Mortal Wkly Rep* 47(RR-20), 1998c.

Centers for Disease Control and Prevention (CDC): Guidelines for national human immunodeficiency virus case surveillance, including monitoring for human immunodeficiency virus infection and acquired immunodeficiency syndrome, *MMWR Morbid Mortal Wkly Rep* 48(RR13):1-28, 1999.

Centers for Disease Control and Prevention (CDC): *Core curriculum on tuberculosis*, ed 4, Atlanta, 2000, CDC.

Children's Defense Fund (CDF): *The state of America's children yearbook 2000*, Washington, DC, 2000, CDF.

Chweadyk P: Speaking of cultural competence, *Minority Nurse* (Spring 2000):28-31.

Cocaine use: the largest global study ever undertaken, *World Health* 4(July-August):25, 1995.

Cohen D, Spear S, Scribner R, et al.: "Broken windows" and the risk for gonorrhea, *Am J Public Health* 90(2):230-236, 2000.

Cole F, Slocumb E: Nurses' attitudes toward patients with AIDS, *J Adv Nurs* 83:112-117, 1993.

Commonwealth Fund: *National comparative survey of minority health care*, New York, 1995, Commonwealth Fund.

Craig C: Making the most of the nurse-managed clinic, *Nurs Health Care* 17(3):124-126, 1996.

Crowe AH, Reeves RR: *Treatment for alcohol and other drug abuse: opportunities for coordination*, DHHS Pub No (SMA)94-2075, Rockville, Md, 1994, US Government Printing Office.

Crowell NA, Burgess AW: *Understanding violence against women*, Washington, DC, 1996, National Academy Press.

Cubbin C, LeClere FB, Smith GS: Socioeconomic status and the occurrence of fatal and nonfatal injury in the United States, *Am J Public Health* 90(1):70-77, 2000.

Davey PA, Davey DB: Domestic violence: a clinical view, *Home Health Focus* 2(10):78-79, 1996.

Davidson L: Preventing injuries from violence toward women, *Am J Public Health* 86(1):12-14, 1996 (editorial).

Dembo R, Williams L, Wish ED, et al.: The relationship between physical and sexual abuse and illicit drug use: a replication among a new sample of youths entering a juvenile detention center, *Int J Addict* 23(11):1102-1123, 1988.

Denison AV, Shum SY: The evolution of targeted populations in a school-based tuberculin testing program, *Image J Nurs Sch* 27(4):263-266, 1995.

Dickson F, Tutty LM: The role of public health nurses in responding to abused women, *Public Health Nurs* 13(4):263-268, 1996.

Doweiko HE: *Concepts of chemical dependency*, Pacific Grove, Calif, 1990, Brooks/Cole.

Eisen A: Survey of neighborhood-based, comprehensive community empowerment initiatives, *Health Educ Q* 21(2):235-252, 1994.

Emblad J: Dispelling the myths, *World Health* 4:4(July-August), 1995.

Ericksen AB: An umbrella of advocacy, *Minority Nurse* (Fall):16-18, 2000.

Finkelstein DM, Williams PL, Molenberghs G, et al.: Patterns of opportunistic infections in patients with HIV infection, *J Acquir Immune Defic Syndr Hum Retrovirol* 12:38-45, 1996.

Freudenberg N, Eng E, Flay B, et al.: Strengthening individual and community capacity to prevent disease and promote health: in search of relevant theories and principles, *Health Educ Q* 22(3):290-306, 1995.

Friend T: Cover story: today's youth just don't see the dangers, *USA Today*, August 21, 1996, A1, A2.

Fuller RK, Hiller-Sturmhofel: Alcoholism treatment in the United States, *Alcohol Research and Health* 23(2):69-77, 1999.

Garbarino J: Children and poverty in America, *National Forum* 76(3):28-31,42, 1996.

Gerard M: Domestic violence: how to screen and intervene, *RN* 63(12):52-56, 2000.

Grimes D, Grimes M: Tuberculosis: what nurses need to know to help control the epidemic, *Nurs Outlook* 43(4):164-173, 1995.

Grimes ML: Forum on education and academics, middle-class morality: Postures toward the poor, *National Forum* 76(3):3-4, 1996.

Grossman D: Enhancing your cultural competence, *Am J Nurs* 94:58-62, 1994.

Hamilton JT: The market for television violence, *National Forum* 80(4):15-18, 2000.

Hanrahan P, Campbell J, Ulrich Y: Theories of violence. In Campbell J, Humphreys J, editors: *Nursing care of survivors of family violence*, St Louis, 1993, Mosby.

Hartmann H, Spalter-Roth R, Chu J: Poverty alleviation and single-mother families, *National Forum* 76(3):24-27, 1996.

Hawkins JD, Lishner DM, Jenson JM, et al.: Delinquents and drugs: what the evidence suggests about prevention and treatment programming. In Brown BS, Mills AR, editors: *Youth at high risk for substance abuse*, Rockville, Md, 1987, National Institute on Drug Abuse.

Henderson G: Race in America, *National Forum* 80(2):12-15, 2000.

Hitchcock PJ: Adolescents and sexually transmitted diseases, *AIDS Patient Care* 10(2):79-86, 1996.

Humphreys J: Children of battered women. In Campbell J, Humphreys J, editors: *Nursing care of survivors of family violence*, St Louis, 1993, Mosby.

Institute of Medicine (IOM): *Treating drug problems* (vol 1), Washington, DC, 1990, National Academy Press.

Jaynes JH, Rugg CA: *Adolescents, alcohol and drugs*, Springfield, Ill, 1988, Charles Thomas.

Kinzel D: Self-identified health concerns of two homeless groups, *West J Nurs Res* 13(2):181-194, 1991.

Kitazawa S: Tuberculosis health education needs in homeless shelters, *Public Health Nurs* 12(6):409-416, 1995.

Knott DH: *Alcohol problems: diagnosis and treatment*, New York, 1986, Pergamon Press.

Koegel P, Melamid E, Burnam A: Childhood risk factors for homelessness among homeless adults, *Am J Public Health* 85(12):1642-1649, 1995.

Koopman JS, Little RJ: Assessing HIV vaccine effects, *Am J Epidemiol* 142(10):1113-1119, 1995.

Kosterman R, Hawkins JD, Guo J, et al.: The dynamics of alcohol and marijuana initiation: patterns and predictors of first use in adolescence, *Am J Public Health* 90(3):360-266, 2000.

Kulig JC, Wilde IW: Collaboration between communities and universities: completion of a community needs assessment, *Public Health Nurs* 13(2):112-119, 1996.

Lauby JL, Smith P, Stark M, et al.: A community-level HIV prevention intervention for inner-city women: results of the women and infants demonstration projects, *Am J Public Health* 90(2):216-222, 2000.

Leland J: The fear of heroin is shooting up: kids on dope are still rare, but parents are right to be scared, *Newsweek*, pp 55-56, Aug 26, 1996.

Link B: Understanding sociodemographic differences in health—the role of fundamental social causes, *Am J Public Health* 86(4):471-473, 1996 (editorial).

Link B, Susser E, Stueve A, et al.: Lifetime and five-year prevalence of homelessness in the United States, *Am J Public Health* 84(12):1907-1912, 1994.

Macdonald DI: *Drugs, drinking and adolescents*, St Louis, 1989, Mosby.

Mackenbach JP, Kunst AE, Groenhof F, et al.: Socioeconomic inequalities in mortality among women and men: an international study, *Am J Public Health* 89(12):1800-1806, 2000.

Marin G, Burhansstipanov L, Connell CM, et al.: A research agenda for health education among underserved populations, *Health Educ Q* 22(3):346-363, 1995.

Marquand B: Nursing the human spirit, *Minority Nurse* (Fall):19-23, 2000.

Massaro J, Pepper B: The relationship of addiction to crime, health, and other social problems. In Crowe AH, Reeves RR, editors: *Treatment for alcohol and other drug abuse: opportunities for coordination*, DHHS Pub No (SMA)94-2075, Rockville, Md, 1994, US Government Printing Office.

May K, Evans G: Health education for homeless populations, *J Community Health Nurs* 11(4):229-237, 1994.

Mayo K, White S, Oates SK, et al.: Community collaboration: prevention and control of tuberculosis in a homeless shelter, *Public Health Nurs* 13(2):120-127, 1996.

McCloskey JC, Bulechek GM, editors: *Nursing interventions classification (NIC)*, ed 3, St Louis, 2000, Mosby, pp. 107-108.

McCreary M: Collaboration among communities: NLN's new center for collaborating organizations and community groups introduces exciting plan for health care futures, *NLN Update* 2(2):3, 5, 1996.

McDermott S: The health promotion needs of older people, *Prof Nurse* 10(8):530-533, 1995.

McFarlane J: De Madres a Madras: an access model for primary care, *Am J Public Health* 86:879-880, 1996.

McLellan T, Dembo R: *Screening and assessment of alcohol and other drug (AOD)–abusing adolescents* (Treatment Improvement Protocol 3), Rockville, Md, 1992, Center for Substance Abuse Treatment.

McNeal G: Mobile health care for those at risk, *Nursing and Health Care: Perspectives on Community* 17(3):134-140, 1996.

Mihaly LK: *Homeless families: failed policies and young victims*, Washington, DC, 1991, Children's Defense Fund.

Miller TR, Cohen MA, Wiersema B: *Victim costs and consequences: a new look*, National Institute of Justice research report, Pub No NIJ 155282, Washington, DC, February 1996, US Department of Justice.

*Mosby's patient teaching guides*, St Louis, 1995, Mosby.

Murphy B, editor: *Nursing centers: the time is now*, New York, 1995, National League for Nursing.

Murray RB: Stressors and coping strategies of homeless men, *J Psychosoc Nurs* 34(8):16-22, 1996.

National Center for Health Statistics: *Health, United States, 1995, Chartbook*, Pub No (PHS) 96-1232, Hyattsville, Md, 1996, US Government Printing Office.

National Center for Health Statistics: *Health, United States, 2000, with adolescent health chartbook*, Hyattsville, Md, 2000, National Center for Health Statistics.

National Institute of Justice (NIJ): *The criminalization of domestic violence: promises and limits*, Rockville, Md, 1996, US Department of Justice.

National Institute of Justice (NIJ): *Prevalence, incidence, consequences of violence against women: findings from the national violence against women survey*, Washington, DC, 1998, US Government Printing Office.

Needle RH, Mills AR: *Drug procurement practices of the out-of-treatment chronic drug abuser*, NIH Pub No 94-3820, Rockville, Md, 1994, National Institutes of Health.

Newmann RE, Nishimoto PW: 1996 Human Immunodeficiency Virus Update for the primary care provider, *Nurse Pract Forum* 7(1):16-22, 1996.

Norton D, Ridenour N: Homeless women and children: the challenge of health promotion, *Nurse Pract Forum* 6(1):29-33, 1995.

Nowinski J: *Substance abuse in adolescents and young adults: a guide to treatment*, New York, 1990, Norton.

Nunez R: A snapshot of family homelessness across America, *Political Science Q* 114(2):289-307, 1999.

Office of Minority Health—Resource Center (OMH-RC): Cancer hits some minorities hard. In *Cancer and minorities: closing the gap*, Washington, DC, 1989, Department of Health and Human Resources.

Ossege J, Berry R: Nurse managed care for the homeless in Lexington, Ky, *Nurse* 43(4):22, 1994.

Pender N: *Assessment of health, health beliefs, and health behaviors. Health promotion in nursing practice*, ed 3, 1996, Appleton & Lange.

Randall-David E: *Culturally competent HIV counseling and education*, McLean, Va, 1994, The Maternal and Child Health Clearinghouse.

Riemer J, Van-Cleve L, Galbraith M: Barriers to well child care for homeless children under age 13, *Public Health Nurs* 12(1):61-66, 1995.

Rosenberg ML, O'Carroll PW, Powell KE: Let's be clear, violence is a public health problem, *JAMA* 267(22):3071-3072, 1992.

Sbarbaro J: TB control is indeed an exercise in vigilance, *Public Health Rep* III:32-33, 1996.

Schinke SP, Botvin GJ, Orlandi MA: *Substance abuse in children and adolescents: evaluation and intervention*, Newbury Park, Calif, 1991, Sage.

Schoemer K: Rockers, models and the new allure of heroin, *Newsweek*, pp. 50-54, August 26, 1996.

Scholler-Jaquish A: Walk-in health clinic for the homeless, *Nurs Health Care* 17(3):119-123, 1996.

Shah S, Hoffman R, Shinault R, et al.: Screening for pregnancy and contraceptive use among women admitted to a Denver detoxification center, *Public Health Reports* 113(4):336-340, 1998.

Simandl G: Nursing students working with the homeless, *Nurse Educ* 21(2):18-22, 1996.

Smith SP: Homelessness as a lifestyle: a risk factor, *Home Health Care Management & Practice* 11(4):38-44, 1999.

Sondik EJ, Lucas JW, Madans JH, et al.: Race/Ethnicity and the 2000 census: implications for public health, *Am J Public Health* 90(11):1709-1713, 2000.

Sorlie P, Backlund E, Keller J: U.S. mortality by economic demographics and social characteristics: the national longitudinal study, *Am J Public Health* 85(7):949-956, 1995.

Sowell RL, Seals BF, Cooper JA: HIV transmission knowledge and risk behaviors of persons with HIV infection, *AIDS Patient Care and STDs* 10(2):111-115, 1996.

Stark E, Flitcraft A: *Women at risk: domestic violence and women's health*, Thousand Oaks, Calif, 1996, Sage.

Stephenson GM: *Preparedness for crime, the psychology of criminal justice*, Cambridge, Mass, 1992, Blackwell.

Tarter RE, Ott PJ, Mezzich AC: Psychometric assessment. In Frances RJ, Miller SI, editors: *Clinical textbook of addictive disorders*, New York, 1991, Guilford Press.

Tollett JH, Thomas SP: A theory-based nursing intervention to instill hope in homeless veterans, *Adv Nurs Sci* 18(2):76-90, 1996.

Travis J: Violence against women: reflections on NIJ's research agenda, *National Institute of Justice Journal* 2(230):21-25, 1996.

Turner BJ, Newschaffer CJ, Cocroft J, et al.: Improved birth outcomes among HIV-infected women with enhanced medicaid prenatal care, *Am J Public Health* 90(1):85-91, 2000.

Underwood SM: Issues and challenges in cancer nursing research: increasing the participation and involvement of African-Americans in cancer programs and trials. In American Cancer Society, editor: *Nursing Research and Underserved Populations*, 1994, The Society.

US Census Bureau: *Statistical abstract of the United States, 1999*, Washington, DC, 1999, US Government Printing Office.

US Department of Health and Human Services (USDHHS): *Healthy People 2000: national health promotion and disease prevention objectives, full report, with commentary*, Washington, DC, 1991, US Government Printing Office.

US Department of Health and Human Services (USDHHS): *HIV counseling, testing and referral standards and guidelines*, Public Health Service, Washington, DC, 1994a, US Government Printing Office.

US Department of Health and Human Services (USDHHS): *HIV infection and AIDS: are you at risk?* Public Health Service, Washington, DC, 1994b, US Government Printing Office.

US Department of Health and Human Services (USDHHS): *Making a difference: interim status report of the McKinney Demonstration Program for homeless adults with serious mental illness*, Rockville, Md, 1994c, Center for Mental Health Services, Substance Abuse and Mental Health Services Administration.

US Department of Health and Human Services (USDHHS): *Healthy People 2000: midcourse review and 1995 revisions*, Washington, DC, 1995, US Government Printing Office.

US Department of Health and Human Services (USDHHS): *Cultural issues in substance abuse treatment*, Pub No SMA 99-3278, Public Health Service, Washington, DC, 1999, US Government Printing Office.

US Department of Health and Human Services (USDHHS): *Healthy People 2010: Understanding and improving health*, ed 2, Washington, DC, 2000a, US Government Printing Office.

US Department of Health and Human Services (USDHHS): *Tracking Healthy People 2010*, Washington, DC, 2000b, US Government Printing Office.

US Department of Health and Human Services (USDHHS): *Cultural competence standards*, Washington, DC, 2000c, US Government Printing Office.

US Department of Health and Human Services (USDHHS): *Diagnosis prevention and treatment of fetal alcohol syndrome*, Washington, DC, 2000d, US Government Printing Office.

US Department of Health and Human Services (USDHHS): *Enhancing motivation for change in substance abuse treatment*, Pub No SMA 00-3460, Washington, DC, 2000e, US Government Printing Office.

US Department of Health and Human Services (USDHHS): *The AIDS epidemic and the Ryan White CARE Act: past progress, future challenges*, Washington, DC, 2000f, US Government Printing Office.

US Department of Health and Human Services (USDHHS): *Health, United States, 2000, with Adolescent Health Chartbook*, Pub No 00-1232, Washington, DC, 2000g, US Government Printing Office.

US Department of Health and Human Services (USDHHS): *A guide to the clinical care of women with HIV*, Washington, DC, 2000h, US Government Printing Office.

US Department of Justice: *Domestic violence awareness: stop the cycle of violence*, Pub No USGPO: 1996-405-033/54261, Washington, DC, 1996a, US Government Printing Office.

US Department of Justice: *Domestic violence, stalking, and antistalking legislation*, Pub No 1996-405-037/40024, Washington, DC, 1996b, US Government Printing Office.

Venereal Disease Action Coalition: *Sexually transmitted diseases: a community information and resource guide*, Detroit, 1983, United Community Services of Metropolitan Detroit.

Wagner JD, Menke EM, Ciccone JK: What is known about the health of rural homeless families? *Public Health Nurs* 12(6):400-408, 1995.

Wald L: *The house on Henry Street*, New York, 1915, Holt.

Wallman KK, Evinger S, Schechter S: Measuring our nation's diversity: developing a common language for data on race and ethnicity, *Am J Public Health* 90(11):1704-1708, 2000.

Waters CM: Professional development in nursing research—a culturally diverse postdoctoral experience, *Image J Nurs Sch* 28(1):47-50, 1996.

Waters CM: Immigration, intermarriage, and the challenges of measuring racial/ethnic identities, *Am J Public Health* 90(11):1735-1737, 2000.

Wechsler H: Binge drinking: should we attack the name of the problem?, *The Chronicle Review*, pp B12-B3, October 20, 2000.

Wells SM: Recovering from homelessness and serious mental illness, *Access: Information from the National Resource Center on Homelessness and Mental Illness* 8(2):1,3-4,8, 1996.

Wolman B: Foreword. In Adler LL, Denmark FL, editors: *Violence and the prevention of violence*, Westport, Conn, 1995, Praeger.

Woodson RL: Welfare reform, *National Forum* 79(3):15-19, 1996.

Wright T: Resisting homelessness: global, national, and local solutions, *Contemp Sociology* 29(1):27-43, 2000.

Yankauer A: Sexually transmitted diseases: a neglected public health priority, *Am J Public Health* 84(12):1894-1897, 1994.

Zima B, Wells K, Freeman H: Emotional and behavioral problems and severe academic delays among sheltered children in Los Angeles County, *Am J Public Health* 84(2):260-264, 1994.

## SELECTED BIBLIOGRAPHY

Campbell JC: Violence against women: where policy needs to go, *Nurs Policy Forum* 1(6):10-17, 1995.

Centers for Disease Control and Prevention (CDC):HIV/AIDS prevention research project. *Compendium of HIV prevention interventions with evidence of effectiveness*, Atlanta, November 1999, CDC.

Centers for Disease Control and Prevention (CDC): Building duty systems for monitoring and responding to violence against women: recommendations from a workshop, *MMWR Morbid Mortal Wkly Rep* 49(RR-11):1-16, 2001.

Coker A, Smith P, McKeown R, et al.: Frequency and correlates of intimate partner violence by type: physical, sexual, and psychological battering, *Am J Public Health* 90(4):523-526, 2000.

Cubbin C, Pickle L, Fingerhut L: Social context and geographic patterns of homicide among U.S. black and white males, *Am J Public Health* 90(4):579-587, 2000.

Cull V: Exposure to violence and self-care practices of adolescents, *Fam Community Health* 19(1):31-41, 1996.

Dalaker J, Proctor BD: *Poverty in the United States: 1999*, US Census Bureau, Current Population Reports, Series P60-210, Washington, DC, 2000, US Government Printing Office.

Dickson F, Tutty LM: The role of public health nurses in responding to abused women, *Public Health Nurs* 13(4):263-268, 1996.

Killion C: Special health care needs of homeless pregnant women, *Adv Nurs Sci* 18(2):44-46, 1995.

Lloyd SA: Intimate violence, *National Forum* 80(4):19-22, 2000.

McFarlane J, Parker B, Soeken K: Abuse during pregnancy: frequency, severity, perpetrator, and risk factors of homicide, *Public Health Nurs* 12(5):284-289, 1996.

Miller RB, Boyle JS: "You don't ask for trouble": women who do sex and drugs, *Fam Community Health* 19(3):35-48, 1996.

Pollack W: The Columbine syndrome: boys and the fear of violence, *National Forum* 80(4):39-42, 2000.

Rouse BA, editor: *Substance abuse and mental health statistics sourcebook*, DHHS Pub No (SMA)95-3064, Washington, DC, 1996, US Government Printing Office.

Schafran LH: Topics for our times: rape is a major public health issue, *Am J Public Health* 86(1):15-17, 1996.

Sharpe KE: Addicted to the drug war, *The Chronicle Review*, pp B14-B15, October 6, 2000.

Talashek ML, Gerace LM, Starr KL: The substance abuse pandemic, determinants to guide interventions, *Public Health Nurs* 11(2):131-139, 1994.

Whalen M: *Counseling to end violence against women*, Thousand Oaks, Calif, 1996, Sage.

# Commonly Acquired Sexually Transmitted Diseases

| DISEASE | USUAL SYMPTOMS | DIAGNOSIS | POSSIBLE COMPLICATIONS | TREATMENT | SPECIAL CONSIDERATIONS |
|---|---|---|---|---|---|
| *Gonorrhea*[a] *(clap, dose, drip)* Cause: *Neisseria gonorrhoeae* bacterium | Appear in 2-10 days or up to 30 days *Women:* 80% have no symptoms; may have puslike vaginal discharge; lower abdominal pain; painful urination *Men:* Thick, milky discharge from penis and/or painful urination; 10-20% have no symptoms *Men and women:* Sore throat, pain and mucus when defecating; often no anal symptoms | *Women:* Culture from vagina, cervix, throat and/or rectum *Men:* Smear or culture from penis, rectum, and/or throat | *Women:* Pelvic inflammatory disease (10-20% of cases) (see PID on the next page) *Men:* Narrowing of urethra; sterility; swelling of testicles *Men and women:* Arthritis, blood infections, dermatitis, meningitis, and endocarditis *Newborns:* Eye, nose, lung, and/or rectal infections | Ceftriaxone plus doxycycline or tetracycline or spectinomycin Ceftriaxone | 3-10 days after treatment and again in 4-6 weeks a culture test should be done (to show cure) |

Data from Venereal Disease Action Coalition: *Sexually transmitted diseases: a community information and resource guide,* Detroit, 1983, United Community Services of Metropolitan Detroit, pp. 9-11.; Centers for Disease Control: 1989 sexually transmitted diseases treatment guidelines, *MMWR Morbid Mortal Wkly Rep* 38(No. S-8):4-40, 1989; Centers for Disease Control and Prevention (CDC): 1993 sexually transmitted diseases treatment guidelines, *MMWR Morbid Mortal Wkly Rep* 42(No. RR-14):3-59, 1993; Centers for Disease Control and Prevention (CDC): 1998 guidelines for treatment of sexually transmitted diseases, *MMWR Morbid Mortal Wkly Rep* 47(No. RR-1), 1998a.

Symbols indicate that a particular STD also may be contracted in the following ways:

[a]Infants: while in birth canal of an infected mother.

[b]Increased risk through use of the intrauterine device (IUD) as a method of contraception.

[c]Fluid from chancre coming in contact with cuts in the skin; infants: while in infected mother's womb.

[d]Sharing wet towels with an infected person.

[e]Change in pH balance of vagina from pregnancy, diabetes, birth control pills, antibiotics, stress, douching.

[f]Puncture of skin with contaminated needle; using toothbrush, razor, etc., of an infected person.

[g]May be spread by fingers from one hairy area to another; or by sharing linen or clothing of an infected person.

[h]Close physical contact (sexual or nonsexual).

*Continued*

## APPENDIX 13-1

# Commonly Acquired Sexually Transmitted Diseases (cont'd)

| DISEASE | USUAL SYMPTOMS | DIAGNOSIS | POSSIBLE COMPLICATIONS | TREATMENT | SPECIAL CONSIDERATIONS |
|---------|----------------|-----------|------------------------|-----------|------------------------|
| *Nongonococcal Urethritis/Cervicitis[a] (NGU, NGC)*<br><br>Common cause:<br>*Chlamydia trachomatis*<br>Other causes:<br>*Ureaplasma urealyticum, Trichomonas vaginalis, Candida albicans,* and *herpes simplex virus* | Appear in 1-3 weeks<br>*Women (NGC):* Usually have no symptoms; may have frequent uncomfortable urination; vaginal discharge<br>*Men (NGU):* Mild-to-moderate discomfort on urination; thin, clear, or white morning discharge from penis | *Women:* No highly definitive diagnostic tool is currently available for chlamydial infection; culture (to rule out gonorrhea) and a vaginal smear (to rule out trichomonas and yeast)<br>*Men:* Culture (to rule out gonorrhea) and a smear | *Women:* Pelvic inflammatory disease (see PID below), cervical dysplasia (currently under study), ectopic pregnancy, and infertility<br>*Men:* Prostatitis, epididymitis<br>*Newborns:* Eye infections, pneumonia | Doxycycline or azithromycin (erythromycin for pregnant women) | |
| *Pelvic Inflammatory Disease (PID)[b]*<br><br>*Affects only women*<br>Usual causes: *Neisseria gonorrhoeae, Chlamydia trachomatis,* enteric bacteria | Onset of symptoms varies; abnormal vaginal discharge; severe pain and tenderness in lower abdominal/pelvic area; painful intercourse and/or menstruation; irregular bleeding; chills and fever; nausea, vomiting | History, culture, and examination to rule out other problems (ectopic pregnancy, appendicitis, etc.); pelvic ultrasound; laparoscopy | Sterility; chronic abdominal pain; chronic infection (of the fallopian tubes, uterus and/or ovaries); ectopic pregnancy, death | *Inpatient:* Cefoxitin IV in combination with doxycycline or clindamycin and gentamicin IV<br>*Ambulatory:* Cefoxitin IM in combination with ceftriaxone and doxycycline or tetracycline; bed rest and no sex for at least 2 weeks | Usually the result of untreated gonorrhea or chlamydial infection<br>Scarring of fallopian tubes may increase risk of future ectopic pregnancies<br>IUD, if present, should be removed and replaced by another form of birth control<br>Careful medical follow-up is essential |
| *Human Papillomavirus Infection/Condylomata Acuminata (HPV, genital/venereal warts)*<br><br>Cause: Human papillomavirus | Appear in 1-6 months; firm, flesh-colored or grayish-white warts on vulva, anus, lower vagina, penis, scrotum, mouth, throat; lesions on cervix usually not visible to the naked eye; itching | Clinical examination and Pap smear of colposcopy for lesions on cervix | Blockage of vaginal, rectal, or throat openings; cervical dysplasia; cancer (currently under study) | Cryotherapy with liquid nitrogen or cryoprobe; podophyllin benzoin (contraindicated in pregnancy) or trichloroacetic acid; electrocautery | Warts and invisible lesions are highly contagious; both will continue to multiply until completely removed |

| DISEASE | USUAL SYMPTOMS | DIAGNOSIS | POSSIBLE COMPLICATIONS | TREATMENT | SPECIAL CONSIDERATIONS |
|---|---|---|---|---|---|
| *Herpes, Genital or Oral (cold sores; fever blisters on mouth)* Causes: herpes simplex virus I (HSV I; oral); herpes simplex virus II (HSV II; genital) | May occur immediately or as late as 1 year after contact or not at all; some people exhibit few or no symptoms Itching, tingling sensation followed by painful blister-like lesions that appear in clusters at the site of infection (i.e., lips, nose, inner and outer vaginal lips, clitoris, rectum, thighs, buttocks); blisters dry up and disappear generally leaving no scar tissue HSV II symptoms in women may include increased vaginal discharge, painful intercourse and urination; painless lesions on cervix may go undetected *Primary episodes:* HSV II—some experience fever, body aches, flulike symptoms, swollen lymph nodes near infected areas *Recurrent episodes:* HSV I and HSV II—generally lessen in frequency and severity over time | Culture from sore, clinical examination or Tzanck smear Definitive diagnosis only possible when lesions are present | *Oral:* Autoinoculation to skin or eyes *Genital:* Possible increased risk of cervical cancer; disturbance of bladder or bowel functioning (neuralgia); meningitis (nonfatal) *Newborns:* Blindness, brain damage, and/or death to baby passing through birth canal of mother with active lesions | No known cure at present The following may be helpful in reducing symptoms and/or recurrences: oral acyclovir; stress reduction techniques (yoga, meditation, etc.); keeping sores dry/clean; healthy diet and exercise; inpatient therapy in severe cases; acyclovir IV | HSV I can be found genitally and HSV II can be found orally due to oral-genital sex or autoinoculation Recurrent attacks are unpredictable but often appear at times of high stress, when fatigued, after vigorous intercourse, around menstruation, at time of other illnesses; research is inconclusive regarding whether herpes is occasionally contagious when there are no active lesions Many experience difficult but not insurmountable, adjustments in self-image and sexual behavior *Women:* Should have Pap smears twice yearly and if pregnant, inform their health care provider (of their herpes); cesarean delivery is indicated if mother has active lesions at the time of delivery; cervical lesions may go undetected because *they are not painful* |

*Continued*

**APPENDIX 13-1**

# Commonly Acquired Sexually Transmitted Diseases (cont'd)

| DISEASE | USUAL SYMPTOMS | DIAGNOSIS | POSSIBLE COMPLICATIONS | TREATMENT | SPECIAL CONSIDERATIONS |
|---|---|---|---|---|---|
| **Syphilis[c]** (*syph, lues, pox, bad blood*) Cause: *Treponema pallidum* (spirochete bacterium) | First stage—(appears in 10-90 days, average 3 weeks): painless sores (chancres) where bacteria entered body (genitals, rectum, lips, breasts, etc.) Second stage—(1 week to 6 months after stage 1): rash; flulike symptoms; mouth sores; genital/anal sores (condylomata lata); inflamed eyes; patchy balding Latent stage—(10-20 years after stage 2): None Final stage—See possible complications | Blood test; clinical examination | *Adult:* Blindness, deafness (usually reversible); brain damage; paralysis, heart disease, death *Newborns:* Damage to skin, bones, eyes, teeth, and/or liver; death | Penicillin (tetracycline or doxycycline for penicillin-allergic clients; doxycycline used in nonpregnant clients only) | Many women will not notice chancre because it is painless and may be deep inside vagina Complications can be prevented if treated at first or second stage Return for blood test 1 month after treatment and once every 3 months for 1 year |
| **Vulvovaginitis** Causes: *Trichomonas vaginalis* (protozoa)[d]; *Candida albicans* (fungus)[e]; *Gardnerella/Haemophilus vaginalis* (bacteria)[f] | A. *Trichomoniasis* (Trich, TV, A, B, C Vaginitis) appear in 1-6 weeks *Women:* Thin, foamy yellow-green or gray vaginal discharge with foul odor; burning, redness, itching and/or frequent urination | *Women:* Vaginal smear; microscopic identification; urinalysis; culture (to rule out gonorrhea); clinical examination *Men:* Hard to diagnose | A. None | A. Metronidazole (Flagyl) | A. All partners should be treated even if they have no symptoms Cautions about metronidazole: very high doses have been shown to cause cancer in laboratory animals Should not be taken by pregnant or breastfeeding women |

| DISEASE | USUAL SYMPTOMS | DIAGNOSIS | POSSIBLE COMPLICATIONS | TREATMENT | SPECIAL CONSIDERATIONS |
|---|---|---|---|---|---|
| *Vulvovaginitis—cont'd* | *Men:* Usually no symptoms. May have slight, clear morning discharge from penis; itching after urination | | | | Alcohol should be avoided when taking Flagyl because it may cause severe headaches and nausea |
| | B. Candida infections (yeast, monilia); onset of symptoms varies | | B. *Newborns:* Mouth and throat infections | B. Miconazole nitrate, clotrimazole, butaconazole, or teraconazole intravaginally | A, B, and C. Recurrent infections are common and can be prevented: tub bathing during menstruation, loose clothing and cotton panties; also avoid use of bubble bath, deodorant tampons, scented soaps, vaginal sprays, and douches (because these may irritate the vagina and/or change the pH balance) |
| | *Women:* Thick, white, cottage cheeselike, foul-smelling discharge that adheres to the vaginal walls; intense itching and irritation of genitals | | C. None | C. Metronidazole (Flagyl) or clindamycin (effective in 50-60% of cases) | |
| | *Men:* usually no symptoms; dermatitis on penis | | | | |
| | C. *Gardnerella infections;* onset of symptoms varies | | | | |
| | *Women:* Thin, foul-smelling, yellow-gray discharge; may have some vaginal burning | | | | |
| *Hepatitis B* Cause: hepatitis B virus | Appear in 1-6 months, but often no clear symptoms | Blood tests; clinical examination | Chronic hepatitis; chronic acute hepatitis; cirrhosis; liver cancer; death | Supportive and symptomatic care; bed rest; lots of fluids; a light, healthy diet and no alcohol; no specific drug therapy (antiretroviral agents about 40% effective) | Often confused with flu or a bad cold and thus not treated early Recovery usually 2-3 months |

*Continued*

# APPENDIX 13-1

## Commonly Acquired Sexually Transmitted Diseases (cont'd)

| DISEASE | USUAL SYMPTOMS | DIAGNOSIS | POSSIBLE COMPLICATIONS | TREATMENT | SPECIAL CONSIDERATIONS |
|---------|----------------|-----------|------------------------|-----------|------------------------|
| *Hepatitis B—cont'd* | General flulike symptoms; liver deterioration marked by darkened urine, lightened stool, yellowed eyes and skin, skin eruptions, enlarged and tender liver | | | | Will not recur once cured<br>Hepatitis B vaccine will provide immunity |
| *Pediculosis Pubis[g] (crabs, cooties, lice)*<br>Cause: *Phthirus pubis* (crab louse) | Appear in 4-5 weeks<br>Intense itching in hairy areas (usually begins in pubic hair) | Clinical examination; self-examination may reveal blood spots on underwear, eggs or nits | None | Lindane (Kwell) cream, lotion, or shampoo (not recommended for pregnant or breastfeeding women); pyrethrins and piperonyl butoxide applications | Common soap will not kill crabs<br>All clothes and linen must be washed in hot water or dry-cleaned or removed from human contact for 1-2 weeks |
| *Scabies[h] (the itch)*<br>Cause: *Sarcoptes scabiei* (parasite mite) | Appear in 4-6 weeks<br>Severe itching and raised reddish tracts; may appear anywhere on body and are caused by the mite burrowing under the skin | Clinical examination; microscopic observation | Secondary bacterial infection (from scratching) | Lindane (Kwell) cream, lotion, or shampoo (not recommended for pregnant or breastfeeding women) or crotamiton (Eurox) cream or lotion | Common soap will not kill the mites<br>All clothing and linen much be washed in hot water or dry-cleaned or removed from human contact for 1-2 weeks |

# 14

# Community Assessment and Diagnosis

*Susan Clemen-Stone*

---

## OBJECTIVES

*Upon completion of this chapter, the reader should be able to:*

1. Describe the relevance of community analysis activities to community health nursing practice.
2. Discuss the importance of developing partnerships when assessing a community.
3. Discuss the application of the nursing process to community-oriented practice.
4. Identify parameters for assessing a community's level of functioning.
5. Summarize methods for assessing a community's health status.
6. Explain the relevance of public health statistics to community health nursing practice.
7. Summarize international, federal, state, and local sources for obtaining community data.
8. Formulate guidelines for implementing community analysis activities in the practice setting.

---

## KEY TERMS

Coalition
Community analysis
Community assessment guide
Community dynamics
Community education strategies
Community-focused nursing functions

Community forums
Community health profile
Community partnership
Community survey
Focus group interviews
Grass-roots movement

Key informants
Participant observation
Secondary data
Walking tours
Windshield surveys

---

*Communities of concern will change the world.*

JIM MANN (2001)

Chapter 2 explored the American Nurses Association's (ANA) and the American Public Health Association's (APHA) definitions of community health nursing practice, which state that the dominant responsibility of nurses in community health is to the community or the population as a whole (ANA, 1999; APHA, 1996). Recently private foundations, governmental related agencies, and nursing organizations confirmed the importance of focusing on the health of the community (ANA, 1999; Institute of Medicine, 1997; National League for Nursing [NLN], 1993; Pew Health Professions Commission, 1995; U.S. Department of Health and Human Services [USDHHS], 2000). These organizations' visions for the future emphasize a consumer-driven, community-based health care system and the need for changes in the educa-

tion of health professionals. They advocate that health professionals be educated to address health promotion and disease prevention needs at population and community levels, as well as at the personal care level (NLN, 1993). This emphasis is consistent with the *Healthy People 2010* initiative (USDHHS, 2000) that challenges communities to develop local health plans to reduce morbidity and premature mortality through health promotion and disease prevention activities. Communities of concern will succeed in doing so.

Health promotion and disease prevention action at the community level requires the implementation of community analysis strategies that allow health providers to work with community residents in identifying a unique community profile. To establish this profile, community health nurses must "see," "smell," and "hear" the community and describe its people, its environment, its health status, and its health resources. Further, they must work with the community to systematically analyze all facets of community dynamics (described in Chapter 3) for the purpose of

**449**

identifying appropriate community- and population-focused health promoting interventions.

"Community analysis is the process of assessing and defining needs, possible barriers, opportunities and resources involved in initiating community health action programs" (Rissel, Bracht, 1999, p. 59). This process involves a variety of assessment and diagnostic activities that aid the community in setting priorities for health planning. This chapter focuses on examining these activities.

## WHY ASSESS THE COMMUNITY

It is essential for the community health nurse to have an understanding of community dynamics because health action occurs in the community. Every community has *patterns* of functioning or community dynamics that either contribute to or detract from its state of health. The community health nurse must recognize these patterns to anticipate community responses to health promotion and disease prevention activities and to facilitate community health planning efforts. Without this knowledge it is difficult to effect change.

Knowledge of community dynamics is obtained through systematic community assessment. Community assessment helps the nurse and other health care professionals identify cultural differences in relation to consumer interests, strengths, concerns, and motivations. This assessment also assists health care professionals in analyzing processes through which community beliefs, values, and attitudes are transmitted. Having this information allows health professionals to individualize community program planning.

It is important for the community health nurse to recognize that, as the traditions and health experiences in each community vary, the type of programs designed to meet consumer needs also should vary. Programs appropriate for one community, or for a population within a community, may be ineffective in meeting the needs of other communities and populations.

Calvillo (1992) substantiated the importance of individualizing health programs for specific populations in a community through her research on acquired immunodeficiency syndrome (AIDS). She examined AIDS knowledge and attitudes among Latina women in Los Angeles compared to a national sample of Hispanic women in the United States. The Los Angeles sample had lower educational and income levels. These respondents were less knowledgeable about AIDS and held more erroneous misconceptions about the transmission of AIDS than their national counterparts. Calvillo (1992) also found that "women in the Los Angeles sample who were more acculturated had significantly higher knowledge scores, fewer erroneous beliefs and greater knowledge of preventive measures" (p. 415). These facts suggested to Calvillo that socioeconomic status, differing levels of acculturation, and ethnicity all affect health programming and that *targeted* educational efforts are needed to meet the needs

of diverse subgroups within communities. Other researchers (DiClemente, Wingood, Vermund, et al., 1999; Magilvy, Brown, Moritz, 1999; Marin, Burhansstipanov, Connell et al., 1995; Winkleby, Flora, Kraemer, 1994) also have found that community health interventions must take into consideration the unique demographic, socioeconomic, and cultural characteristics of community residents and need to be tailored for differing subgroups to produce *sustained* health behavior change.

Studies such as those conducted by Calvillo reinforce the need to study the characteristics of the community in which one is working. They demonstrate that assumptions cannot be made about community response to health promotion and disease prevention interventions. Such studies also point out the relevance of identifying factors that facilitate or inhibit health behavior change and the need for collaborative consumer and health provider relationships.

## COMMUNITY HEALTH ASSESSMENT: A PARTNERSHIP PROCESS

Within any community setting, concerned citizens and professionals from many disciplines are interested in community assessment activities designed to identify unmet needs and community assets. Because it would be impossible for any one group to handle all the health care needs of a community, efforts by many should be promoted and supported. Developing effective partnerships with clients and other health providers is the key to successful health planning in the future. "Public health, in a reformed health care system, will forge partnerships between communities and all levels of government. Communities and public health agencies—together—will keep the public healthy by assessing the community's health needs fully, developing the best policies to meet those needs, and assuring that all of us have access to high quality health and medical services and the highest attainable level of individual and community health" (APHA, 1993, unnumbered foreword).

Public health leaders across the nation endorse the importance of forging community health partnerships (ANA, 1999; Association of State and Territorial Directors of Nursing [ASTDN], 1998; Berkowitz, 2000; Bracht, Kingsbury, Rissel, 1999; Children's Defense Fund [CDF], 1996; Flynn, Ray, Rider, 1994; Institute of Medicine [IOM], 1996; Kreuter, 1992; McFarlane, 1996; Oberle, Baker, Magenheim, 1994). Frequently cited benefits of such partnerships are displayed in Box 14-1. Partnerships are being established to develop local *Healthy People 2010* objectives, to strengthen a community's capacity to respond to health problems, and to revitalize communities. They also are being used to improve access to health care, advocate for underserved populations, increase public awareness about the consequences of unhealthy lifestyles, and establish culturally relevant and age-appropriate health interventions.

## BOX 14-1

### *Selected Potential Benefits of Community Partnerships*

- Raise the public's consciousness concerning health status indicators, available community resources, gaps in service delivery, and health behavior interventions
- Promote a shared vision regarding health goals and outcomes
- Encourage individuals and organizations to use their skills and resources in collective health action
- Activate citizens to participate in health decision making
- Promote a community-wide focus on "health for all"
- Help health care providers focus on priority concerns of community residents
- Demonstrate respect for cultural diversity and the needs of differing community subgroups
- Expand community health action resources
- Promote commitment to community health improvement efforts
- Facilitate development and implementation of culturally sensitive health interventions

## *Teaching* TIPS BOX 14-2

### *Strategies for Educating the Community About Health Issues*

- Elicit the community's perspective of health issues through focus group discussions or community surveys.
- Use the community partnership approach to share community assessment data with culturally diverse segments of the population.
- Conduct a health fair that provides information on major health problems across the age continuum and health promotion activities to prevent these problems.
- Write a health column for the local newspaper or newsletters sent home from schools, churches, and other community organizations.
- Use the mass media (e.g., radio or television) to inform the public about significant community health issues.
- Sponsor special events around national health celebration days (e.g., smoking cessation and healthy heart activities during Healthy Heart month or on the Great American Smoke-out day).
- Sponsor a community health awareness symposium.
- Place health information on bulletin boards in local gathering places (e.g., grocery stores, laundromats, churches, or community centers).
- Have a health booth at local community events (e.g., ethnic festivals, county fairs, powwows).

A **community partnership** is a union of people that is focused on collective action for a common endeavor or goal (see Chapter 3). Phrases including *coalition, grass-roots movement, leadership boards, networks, consortia,* and *citizen panels* reflect the movement to have people actively participate in community health action efforts. The differences in terminology relate to how partnerships are organized and citizen participation is facilitated (Bracht, Kingsbury, Rissel, 1999). For example, the term **coalition** is used when *formal* community structures (existing organizations and groups) are linked together to address a pressing community issue such as violence. On the other hand, a **grass-roots move-ment** uses *informal* structures such as church groups or parents of disabled children to mobilize community residents for health action (Bracht, Kingsbury, Rissel, 1999).

Successful community partnerships promote an active participatory process that encourages individuals and organizations to use their skills and resources in collective action for health. The community partnership process can promote understanding of community health problems and local ownership of health promotion activities and programs. Building active community participation in health activities can be challenging at times. However, it is absolutely crucial to engage the community in health action. No community agency can address by itself health problems such as violence, homelessness, and infant mortality. Educating the community about such health issues can promote community interest in the issues. Box 14-2 delineates community education strategies that practitioners have found useful in helping community residents identify community

needs. **Community education strategies** are educational interventions focused on reaching the community as a whole or an aggregate in the community. As mentioned previously, an aggregate, or a population group, has classically been defined as a group of individuals who have in common one or more personal or environmental characteristics (William, 1977).

### *Stop and Think About It*

You are a nurse employed by Family Hospice and Home Care. A pastor from an inner city church came to you expressing concern about the number of children in his parish who had experienced the loss of a significant other as a result of violence, illness, or injury. He asked your agency to assist him in helping these children and their families deal with death and dying and in preventing violence in the community. Who else in your community might be dealing with similar concerns? Who might you partner with to address this need?

## THE NURSE'S ROLE IN COMMUNITY ASSESSMENT

Community health nursing staff as well as administrators participate in community assessment and development activities to identify a community's health status. Although nursing administrators have the primary responsibility for establishing mechanisms that facilitate community health assessment activities, staff nurses play a pivotal role in identifying community needs on a daily basis. While working with clients in the community setting, staff nurses assess the characteristics of their work environment (neighborhood, census tract, or district) and the health status of aggregates or population groups (e.g., the homeless, elderly residents in a senior citizens' housing project, pregnant teenagers, or Asian refugees) within these work regions. This assessment process aids staff in identifying barriers to service delivery and in determining ways to mobilize community resources to reduce these barriers.

The public health nursing stories in Box 14-3 illustrate the advantage of staff nurse involvement in community health assessment activities. The data collected from the two adolescents described in these stories assisted the nurses in realizing that community efforts were needed to ensure positive pregnancy outcomes for teenagers in their communities. This type of knowledge facilitates community development activities and the planning of relevant programs and services for populations at risk. Community health nurses at all levels of practice are actively participating in program planning, implementation, and evaluation activities.

"Public (community) health nurses have great opportunities for community development because of their knowledge of and positions in the community" (Clarke, Beddome, Whyte, 1993, p. 309). Their daily contact with families and individuals provide significant linkages with the community as a whole, which allows them to gain knowledge and trust of the community (Conley, 1995). "This trust provides the public (community) health nurse with ready access to client populations that are difficult to engage, to agencies, and to health care providers" (Conley, 1995, p. 3). Having access to underserved populations and key community leaders permits community health nurses to gain a qualitative perspective about a community's health status. This type of perspective is not achieved when only statistical health status indicators are analyzed. Qualitative data are needed to identify *determinants* of health and disease (Conley, 1995).

In addition to assessing their work environments, community health nurses participate in comprehensive community health status assessment activities. Public health agencies have the responsibility to "regularly and systematically collect, assemble, analyze, and make available information on the health of the community, including statistics on health status, community health needs, and epidemiological and other studies of health problems" (IOM, 1988, p. 9). Community partnerships are being formed to fulfill this function. As an active member of these partnerships, community health nurses use various data collection methods, such as key informant and focus group interviews, to examine the characteristics of the communities in which they work. These and other data collection approaches are described in a later section of this chapter.

The community health nurse's primary purpose in assessing a community's health status is to identify strengths, assets, and needs in relation to preventive health practices. When needs are identified, community health nurses work with consumers and other health care professionals to improve disease prevention and health promotion practices. "Only programs that systematically work to promote health and to prevent disease and injury on a community-wide basis can keep people from getting sick. It has always been the mandate of public health to prevent, rather than merely treat, our health problems" (APHA, 1993, p. 1).

## DIAGNOSING COMMUNITY ASSETS AND UNMET PREVENTIVE HEALTH NEEDS

When participating in community analysis activities, the community health nurse uses the nursing process as described in Chapter 9 but shifts emphasis from the family as client and partner to the community as client and partner. Data are collected from multiple sources (*assessing*) and *analyzed* to formulate community-focused *nursing diagnoses*. Community-focused nursing diagnoses about existing health needs, community dynamics that either positively or negatively influence health action, and gaps in the existing health care delivery system are generated for the purpose of facilitating community organization and health planning efforts. Nursing diagnoses about community strengths and assets also are made because

**BOX 14-3**

*Assessment Function*

**Michigan's Public Health Nurses Tell Their Stories. . .**

The public health nursing staff at a local health department kept encountering teens in the community who not only were pregnant but also were living in community environments that were unhealthy for them and their unborn children.

For example, in one case, a 15-year-old female who was 4 months pregnant was living at a local shelter with a man in his 20s. In another situation, a 16-year-old female who was 8 months pregnant was living with older friends in unsanitary conditions. Both of these adolescents had difficulty maintaining prenatal care appointments because of lack of permanent and stable living arrangements and lifestyles. As a result, the nursing staff began working with the community to develop a transitional living program for pregnant and parenting teens.

Modified from Nurse Administrators Forum: *Promoting healthy Michigan communities: the role of public health nursing in health reform,* Lansing, Mich, 1994, Michigan Department of Public Health, p. 9.

it is through its strengths and assets that a community is able to build its future (Kretzmann, McKnight, 1993).

"A nursing diagnosis is a clinical judgment about an individual, family, or community response to actual or potential health problems/life processes…which…provides the basis for selection of nursing interventions to achieve outcomes for which the nurse is accountable" (North American Nursing Diagnosis Association [NANDA], 1999, p. 149). Although most nursing diagnoses classification systems focus primarily on the individual as a unit of analysis rather than the family or community (refer to Chapter 9, nursing classification section), there are beginning efforts to formulate community-focused nursing diagnoses. The NANDA classification system includes two such diagnoses. These are *Potential for Enhanced Community Coping and Ineffective Community Coping* (NANDA, 1999, pp. 76-77). These diagnoses examine the problem-solving abilities of a community. Other examples of community-focused nursing diagnoses are identified in the following lists. These examples examine functional health patterns in a community, based on Gordon's (1987) functional patterns. These diagnoses were developed by Kriegler and Harton (1992) in consultation with Gordon. Gordon's functional health patterns were discussed in Chapter 9.

- Potential dysfunction in health-perception–health management pattern: knowledge deficit of risk factors of heart disease related to lack of comprehensive educational programs.
- Potential dysfunction of coping-stress tolerance pattern: underutilization of community support groups related to knowledge deficit of existing resources (Kriegler, Harton, 1992, p. 233).

Gordon (2000) contends that "a useful nursing diagnosis statement consists of terms describing (1) the problem or condition and (2) the primary etiological or related factor(s) contributing to the problem or conditions that is the focus of nursing treatment" (p. xi). Consistent with epidemiological concepts presented in Chapter 11, Muecke (1984) proposed that a community-focused nursing diagnosis identify the population at risk when examining the problem or condition of concern. This is based on the belief that "community health nursing integrates the epidemiological approach with the nursing process to make fundamental decisions about care at the level of the population as a whole" (Muecke, 1984, p. 27). The epidemiological model aids the practitioner in estimating risk among populations as well as identifying direct and indirect factors contributing to problems or conditions. Examples of community-focused nursing diagnoses grounded in knowledge of epidemiology follow:

- In 2001, children in census tracts 10 and 11 are still at risk for lead poisoning. This risk is related to living in poorly repaired homes built before 1950 and inadequately enforced housing regulations.

- Teenagers in Green Oak Township are at risk for unwanted pregnancies. This risk is related to the fact that health care resources in the township refuse to provide teenagers birth control without parental consent.
- Senior citizens in Manchester County are at risk for social isolation. This isolation is related to a lack of recreational activities in the county and affordable public transportation.

Community-focused nursing diagnoses are derived from a synthesis of community assessment data, nursing knowledge, and epidemiological concepts, especially the concept of risk in populations (discussed in Chapter 11). These types of nursing diagnoses describe situations that can be influenced by nursing intervention. Note the sample nursing diagnoses just shared. These diagnoses reflect several aggregates at risk in the community (e.g., children, teenagers, and the elderly) and pertinent functional nursing roles. For example, community health nurses are often in a key position to prevent or diagnose lead poisoning among children. Because many families are unaware of the dangers of this condition and its causes (etiology), community health nurses frequently plan and implement health education programs designed to inform the public about lead poisoning. They also carry out lead poisoning surveillance activities by assessing the environment during home visits and when traveling through their districts. If community health nurses identify that a significant number of homes in their work regions are old and in poor condition, they also may implement screening programs to identify children with lead poisoning.

Once nursing diagnoses are established, the community health nurse uses the principles of health planning (see Chapter 15) and the nursing process to plan, implement, and evaluate interventions to resolve unmet community need. Refer again to the nursing diagnosis previously identified that addresses social isolation among seniors in Manchester County. Box 14-4 presents how the community health nurse might use the nursing process to *initially* plan interventions for addressing this isolation. A range of **community-focused nursing functions** categorized by the phases of the nursing process is presented in Box 14-5. These functions were identified by community health nursing leaders across the nation and are discussed throughout the text.

Community health nurses frequently develop partnerships when planning community-focused interventions because they know that active participation by consumers and other professionals promotes long-term support and involvement. Using the partnership model to intervene at the community level is elaborated on in Chapters 2, 3, and 15. The partnership model focuses on building on community strengths and assets to resolve unmet needs. "Each community boasts a unique combination of assets upon which to build its future," including individuals, associations, and institutions (Kretzmann, McKnight, 1993, p. 6).

**BOX 14-4**

*Manchester County: Initial Care Plan for Addressing Social Isolation Among Seniors*

### Assessment Data

- Over 15% of the population in Manchester County was 65 years of age or older in 2001, which is significantly higher than the state (12.6%) and the U.S. (12.7%) rates.
- In Manchester County, over 35% of persons older than 65 were living in poverty in 2001. This percentage is significantly higher than state (15%) and national (21%) percentages.
- A record audit of nursing charts revealed that 40% of the senior clients served by nurses at the county health department expressed feelings of social isolation. Major causes for this were identified as a lack of transportation or inadequate financial resources to participate in social activities.
- Over 25% of the seniors in Manchester County seen by the Area Council on Aging have no cars.
- Currently there is no affordable public transportation for seniors in Manchester County.
- Focus group data collected by the Health Improvement Planning Coalition revealed that seniors are concerned about their limited recreational opportunities.

### Nursing Diagnosis

Senior citizens in Manchester County are at risk for social isolation. This isolation is related to the lack of low-cost recreational activities in the county, the low economic status of many senior residents, and the lack of low-cost public transportation.

### Expected Client (Community) Outcomes

- Community risk control: social isolation of seniors.
- Community develops enhanced coping strategies: active planning by the community in relation to senior citizen concerns.

### Nursing Interventions

- Use the media (local newspaper) to inform the public about significant community health issues, including the concerns of senior residents.
- Collaborate with local church leaders in developing an action plan for addressing senior citizens' concerns.
- Mobilize senior citizen groups for health action.
- Advocate for senior citizens during county commissioner meetings, especially in relation to a need for a neighborhood senior center in Manchester County.

### Evaluation Criteria

- The five churches in Manchester County donate space in their facilities for low-cost recreational activities for aging residents and are providing volunteers to organize these activities.
- The local chapter of the American Red Cross and the Area Council on Aging are providing transportation services for aging citizens who want to participate in recreational activities at local churches.
- Long-term plans include the county commissioners' appropriation of funds for a senior citizens' center in Manchester County.

## COMMUNITY ASSESSMENT PARAMETERS

A significant aspect of the community assessment process is the identification of what needs to be addressed during the process. Establishing assessment guidelines helps a community partnership organize data collection efforts and identify significant factors that influence a community's state of wellness.

Figure 14-1 summarizes parameters for a community health status assessment, based on the community dynamics framework discussed in Chapter 3. This assessment wheel illustrates that community wellness is a multidimensional concept, influenced by interrelated characteristics including people, the environment, and health resources. If any one of these components changes, the balance of community health is altered. For example, economic depression can reduce funding for health care services and other essential communities activities. It also can affect the physical, mental, and social health status of community residents.

In addition to delineating assessment parameters, it is important to determine questions that need to be answered during the assessment process. This helps the assessment team determine the information base and methods needed to make decisions about a community's health status. The extent of the questions to be addressed will vary, based on available resources and local health objectives. Box 14-6 displays one state's views about the *minimum* number of questions to be answered by a community health assessment.

The *Healthy People* initiative (USDHHS, 1991; USDHHS, 2000) challenged state and local health care professionals to compare community health status indicators against the benchmarks delineated in the national *Healthy People* documents (Oberle, Baker, Magenheim, 1994). To facilitate national, state, and local comparisons, a committee representing all levels of public health was convened by the Centers for Disease Control to develop a *consensus set* of health status indicators (Box 14-7). "Priority in selecting the

**BOX 14-5**

## *Community-Focused Nursing Functions*

### Assessment

1. Identifies pertinent information about community.
2. Gathers descriptive data about the community.
3. Assesses health-related learning needs of populations.
4. Participates in identifying community health states and health behaviors, including the knowledge, attitudes, and perceptions of groups regarding health and illness.
5. Collects pertinent information about community in a systematic way.
6. Aids in community health surveys.
7. Includes members of the community as partners in the assessment process.
8. Uses basic statistics and demographic methods to collect health data.
9. Collaborates with other health care providers to assess the community.
10. Consults with community leaders to describe the community.

### Analysis

11. Identifies common and recurrent health problems that have potential for illness consequences.
12. Identifies health needs of help-seeking and nonseeking populations.
13. Describes health capability of community, based on assessment.
14. Applies selected epidemiological concepts in analyzing assessment data (e.g., population-at-risk, incidence, prevalence).
15. Describes present community health problems in the perspective of time (recognizes trends).
16. Describes and analyzes resources available including patterns of utilization.
17. Analyzes data for relationships and clues to the community's health.
18. Aids/participates in analysis of community health database.
19. Forms ideas and hypotheses concerning data gathered in community assessment to derive inferences for nursing programs.
20. Includes members of the community in analyzing assessment data.

### Planning

21. Assists in developing plans to meet needs arising from gaps or deficiencies identified.
22. Develops service priorities and plans for intervention, based on analysis, community expectations, and accepted practice standards.
23. Participates in planning community health programs.
24. Determines priorities for community health care, based on information gathered during assessment.
25. Participates with community leaders in planning to meet identified health needs.

26. Participates with others in developing health plans applicable to the community at large.
27. Develops service objectives of identified community problems.
28. Uses knowledge of change process in planning community programs.
29. Plans for community-wide or age-specific screening programs.
30. Includes members of the community as partners in planning community health programs.

### Implementation

31. Mobilizes the community's collective resources to help achieve higher community health goals.
32. Functions as a health advocate for the community.
33. Serves as vital link in the communication network between all kinds of community agencies and clients.
34. Seeks opportunities to participate with other disciplines in projects to bring about changes in the availability, accessibility, and accountability of health care and related systems.
35. Sets up immunization campaigns with community leaders and public health officials.
36. Initiates and monitors disease prevention programs in the community.
37. Educates the community through media regarding health issues.
38. Organizes community groups to work on alleviating community health problems.
39. Acts as a catalyst/potentiator for community change.
40. Sets up ongoing community health education programs with community leaders and public health officials.

### Evaluation

41. Monitors health services for desired quality.
42. Continually validates appropriateness of public health programs (e.g., discusses with residents, collects more data).
43. Contributes information for use in evaluation of nursing programs.
44. Evaluates community response to nursing intervention.
45. Ensures necessary community health program evaluation data are collected accurately and systematically.
46. Analyzes results of service in relation to proportion of population served.
47. Promotes systematic evaluation of community resources.
48. Evaluates the impact of nursing activities on the health of the community as a whole.
49. Includes members of the community as partners in evaluating health programs.
50. Analyzes results of service in relation to whether community program objectives were reached.

From Anderson ET: Community focus in public health nursing: whose responsibility? *Nurs Outlook* 31:44-48, 1983, p. 46. © 1981, E. Anderson.

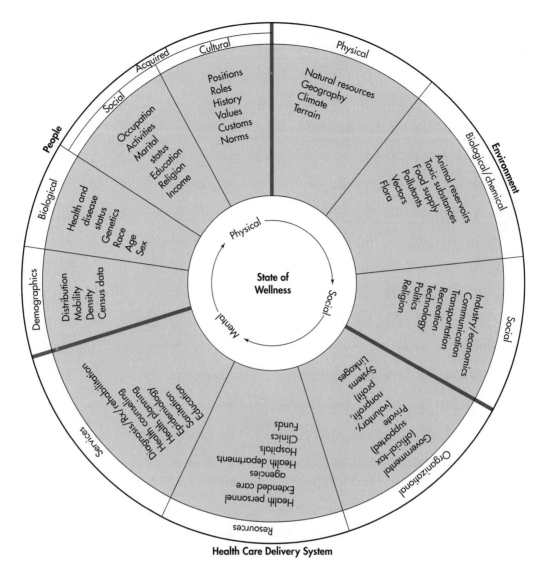

**FIGURE 14-1** The community: its people, its environment, and its health care delivery system.

 **BOX 14-6**

*Community Health Assessment*

The questions to be answered by the health assessment include, at a minimum:
1. What are the demographic, social, and economic characteristics of the community's population?
2. What is the health status?
3. What are the levels of health risk?
4. What is the utilization pattern for health services?
5. What are the key environmental/occupational health issues?
6. What are the expenditures for health care services?
7. What are the available community health resources?
8. Is the supply of health care providers (e.g., primary care practitioners) sufficient?
9. Does the population have access to health care?

From Office of Policy, Planning, and Evaluation, Michigan Department of Public Health: *List of national and state databases,* Lansing, Mich, 1995, The Office, p. 2.

indicators was given to measures for which data are readily available and that are commonly used in public health" (CDC, 1991, p. 449). These 18 indicators provide health outcome and risk parameters for persons to consider when conducting a community assessment and can facilitate interpretation of local data.

Drawing extensively from the "consensus set of indicators for community assessment and performance monitoring," the "indicators for a community health profile" (displayed in Box 14-8) also provide parameters to consider when measuring a community's health. A community health profile aids "a community to identify and focus attention on specific high-priority health issues. A community health profile is made up of indicators of sociodemographic characteristics, health status and quality of life, health risk factors, and health resources that are relevant for most communities" (IOM, 1997, p. 127). A variety of qualitative and quantitative data collection methods are used to obtain data related to community health status indicators.

**BOX 14-7**

*Consensus Set of Indicators\* for Assessing Community Health Status and Monitoring Progress Toward the Year 2000 Objectives*

*Indicators of Health Status Outcome*

1. Race/ethnicity-specific infant mortality, as measured by the rate (per 1000 live births) of deaths among infants 1 year of age

*Death Rates (Per 100,000 Population)†*

2. Motor vehicle crashes
3. Work-related injury
4. Suicide
5. Lung cancer
6. Breast cancer
7. Cardiovascular disease
8. Homicide
9. All causes

*Reported Incidence (Per 100,000 Population)*

10. Acquired immunodeficiency syndrome
11. Measles

12. Tuberculosis
13. Primary and secondary syphilis

*Indicators of Risk Factors*

14. Incidence of low birth weight, as measured by percentage of total number of live-born infants weighing 2500 g at birth
15. Births to adolescents (females age 10-17 years) as a percentage of total live births
16. Prenatal care, as measured by percentage of mothers delivering live infants who did not receive prenatal care during first trimester
17. Childhood poverty, as measured by the proportion of children 15 years of age living in families at or below the poverty level
18. Proportion of persons living in counties exceeding U.S. Environmental Protection Agency standards for air quality during previous year

From Centers for Disease Control and Prevention (CDC): Consensus set of health status indicators for the general assessment of community health status—United States, *MMWR* 40(27):449-451, 1991, p. 450.
\*Position or number of the indicator does not imply priority.
†Age-adjusted to the 1940 standard population.

**BOX 14-8**

*Proposed Indicators for a Community Health Profile*

*Sociodemographic Characteristics*

1. Distribution of the population by age and race/ethnicity
2. Number and proportion of persons in groups such as migrants, homeless, or the non-English speaking, for whom access to community services and resources may be a concern
3. Number and proportion of persons aged 25 and older with less than a high school education
4. Ratio of the number of students graduating from high school to the number of students who entered ninth grade 3 years previously
5. Median household income
6. Proportion of children less than 15 years of age living in families at or below the poverty level
7. Unemployment rate
8. Number and proportion of single-parent families
9. Number and proportion of persons without health insurance

*Health Status*

10. Infant mortality rate by race/ethnicity
11. Numbers of deaths or age-adjusted death rates for motor vehicle crashes, work-related injuries, suicide, homicide, lung cancer, breast cancer, cardiovascular diseases, and all causes, by age, race, and gender as appropriate
12. Reported incidence of AIDS, measles, tuberculosis, and primary and secondary syphilis, by age, race, and gender as appropriate
13. Births to adolescents (ages 10-17) as a proportion of total live births
14. Number and rate of confirmed abuse and neglect cases among children

*Health Risk Factors*

15. Proportion of 2-year-old children who have received all age-appropriate vaccines, as recommended by the Advisory Committee on Immunization Practices
16. Proportion of adults aged 65 and older who have ever been immunized for pneumococcal pneumonia; proportion who have been immunized in the past 12 months for influenza
17. Proportion of the population who smoke, by age, race, and gender as appropriate
18. Proportion of the population aged 18 and older who are obese
19. Number and type of U.S. Environmental Protection Agency air quality standards not met
20. Proportion of assessed rivers, lakes, and estuaries that support beneficial uses (e.g., fishing and swimming approved)

*Health Care Resource Consumption*

21. Per capita health care spending for Medicare beneficiaries (the Medicare adjusted average per capita cost [AAPCC])

*Functional Status*

22. Proportion of adults reporting that their general health is good to excellent
23. During the past 30 days, average number of days for which adults report that their physical or mental health was not good

*Quality of Life*

24. Proportion of adults satisfied with the health care system in the community
25. Proportion of persons satisfied with the quality of life in the community

From Institute of Medicine: *Improving health in the community*, Washington, DC, 1997, National Academy Press, pp. 129-130.

## METHODS FOR ASSESSING A COMMUNITY'S HEALTH STATUS

No one assessment method is sufficient for obtaining a comprehensive view of how a community is functioning. With the increasing recognition that effective community health assessment efforts must address factors that influence health and disease occurrence (e.g., environmental influences and lifestyle patterns), as well as health status outcomes and risk indicators, the need to use multiple methods for data collection becomes quite evident.

Regardless of the method used to obtain community information, community analysis efforts should be structured. Structure can be obtained in various ways, including developing specific goals and expected outcomes for the process, establishing focused questions for community interviews, and using survey tools and assessment guides. Focusing data collection efforts helps to ensure that sufficient data for establishing community diagnoses are collected. Both primary and secondary community data are examined to identify appropriate community diagnoses.

### Conduct Windshield and Walking Tours

As mentioned in Chapter 3, two important methods for obtaining primary community data quickly are windshield surveys and walking tours. **Windshield surveys** (Figure 14-2) are driving tours of a geographic area at varying times for the purpose of observing and recording information about community characteristics (Sharpe, Greaney, Lee, et al., 2000). When these tours are done on foot, they are labeled **walking tours.**

Windshield surveys and walking tours can help community assessment teams examine a variety of community characteristics, including such things as existing community resources, the safety or walkability of the environment (Pollack, 1999), the type of social interactions, and community values through observations of community symbols (Sharpe, Greaney, Lee, et al., 2000). For example, community values are often reflected in the way families build their

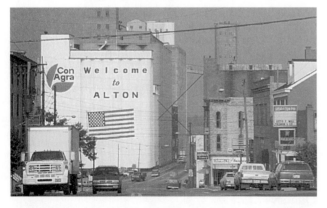

**FIGURE 14-2** Direct observation of a community provides the nurse with valuable assessment data.

homes, messages on bulletin boards, and graffiti on buildings (Wilson, Mitrano, 1996). Appendix 14-1 provides parameters to examine during windshield and walking tours.

### Use Assessment Guides

Use of a community assessment guide is one way to obtain focused information about community dynamics. A **community assessment guide** is a formal, structured instrument that provides a focus for collecting and organizing community data around essential assessment components.

Reference citations for several community assessment guides that assist the practitioner in obtaining community data were presented in Chapter 3. The assessment guide in Appendix 14-2 is systematically organized around the components of a community and community dynamics. This guide is based on concepts derived from epidemiology and sociology. It helps the practitioner examine data related to the person, place, and time variables analyzed in the epidemiology chapter and community systems data identified by Sander (1966) in his classic work on the community (refer to Chapter 3). This guide aids the practitioner in doing a comprehensive community assessment over an extended period.

To use a community assessment guide effectively, an assessment team must have an understanding of community dynamics and community health concepts that describe the qualitative and quantitative aspects of community assessment. Having a theoretical understanding of community concepts helps the practitioner focus on significant clues about community functioning and critical assessment parameters.

### Analyze Secondary Data

In any community secondary data are available that help the community assessment team identify community strengths, assets, and needs. **Secondary data** are data that have already been collected and have frequently been analyzed. Examples of secondary data usually available for most communities are census data; health status data, including vital statistics and leading causes of mortality and morbidity; resources information that describes health, welfare, and other social services in the community; and historical information that addresses the economic, political, educational, and social community trends over time. Where to obtain these types of data is addressed in a later section of this chapter. Frequently used health status statistics were presented in Chapter 11.

Secondary data can help the community assessment team identify aggregates at risk; predict health needs of individuals, families, and populations; determine priorities when needs are greater than resources; support the need for additional funding for community health services; and understand community dynamics. The following case scenario illustrates how knowledge of census data and statistics related to program attendance helped one community health nurse identify an aggregate at risk (single-parent, working mothers) and potential health educational interests.

**Scenario**    One community health nurse was concerned because parents in one of the schools she serviced were not participating in a program designed to promote child safety. When this nurse looked at census tract data, she found that 64% of the households in her district were headed by single-parent, working mothers who had marginal incomes. This information suggested to the nurse that to reach these women she would have to plan activities around the mothers' work schedules. It also pointed out to her that she was dealing with families who were at risk for financial, social, and psychological crises. These data stimulated the nurse to design health programs that were relevant to mothers' and children's needs.

One program, *How to Meet Your Social Needs While Caring for Small Children,* was particularly well received. This program was planned because the nurse on several home visits heard mothers complain about the lack of time for leisure activities. The expressed concerns of these mothers, coupled with knowledge obtained from census tract data, led the nurse to believe that other mothers in the area had the same concern. Her nursing diagnosis was supported and resulted in a meaningful health program that was well attended. Because this one program was so well received, an ongoing activity and discussion group for these mothers was established, with equally positive results. The processes this nurse used to develop her mothers' group and to maintain it are presented in Chapter 23.

Secondary data often provide the basis for decision making in the face of uncertainty. Take, for example, the community health nurse who has several requests for the establishment of a well-baby clinic in various locations. If only one clinic can be funded, this nurse may use secondary statistical data to document a need for a clinic in a specific location. The concentration of preschool children in a given area and the level of childhood immunization protection can all be obtained from secondary data sources. These data may provide information about where the greatest need exists and can be used to substantiate a decision a nurse might make about clinic location.

It is important for health care professionals to analyze a range of available health or health-related data, such as demographic, morbidity, and mortality statistics, to assess community assets, strengths, and needs. Comparing local, state, and national data is equally important. Analyzing data related to the national consensus health status indicators identified previously in this chapter or *Healthy People 2010* data can facilitate these comparisons.

Examining trends over time is essential. These analyses help a community assessment team to more effectively make decisions about a community's health status and needed health action. For example, if a community's death rate for breast cancer is significantly higher than state and national rates over a 5-year period, this community should seriously consider developing a breast cancer prevention program. However, if this situation was noted only in 1 given year, the community would want to establish an effective monitoring system to determine whether this was an isolated occurrence or the beginning of a trend.

GRAPHIC PRESENTATION OF DATA. Graphic presentation of secondary and primary data is an efficient way to show large numbers of observations at one time. Numerical figures are more easily remembered when presented graphically because data are organized and relationships are demonstrated. Tables, graphs, and charts are some of the instruments used to present statistical information symbolically. Guidelines for presenting data in this form include the following:

* Illustrate only the amount of data that is visually appealing.
* Number a table, graph, or chart if more than one is used.
* Title each table, graph, or chart, including in the title information identifying *what, where,* and *when.*
* Define unclear terms and/or abbreviations in the footnote.
* Label both the horizontal and vertical axes of the graphic presentation.
* Identify the source of the data at the bottom of the chart, including author, title of publication, publisher, date of publication, and reference page number.

When these guidelines are used, a table would look like the example presented in Table 14-1.

Graphic presentation of data has popular appeal and is frequently used to portray quickly a large number of facts. Graphs, charts, and tables can be misused or misunderstood, however, especially if one attempts to relate data that are unrelated. Also, attempting to present too many facts in one table defeats the purpose for using data display methods. When this is done, it confuses rather than clarifies the event being illustrated. Available data on a community should be used in the most effective way possible to get across the significance of a community's health problems.

## Carry Out Surveys

Surveys are conducted in community health nursing practice when existing health and health-related data are inadequate to substantiate a need for the development of a particular health program. For example, standard sources of data may show that suicide is one of the leading causes of death for older adolescents. This information is significant in that it focuses attention on a major health problem of this developmental age group. It is not sufficient, however, to identify health action needed in a particular community for reducing adolescent suicide. Other types of information must be collected before initiating a local health program. Data about things such as adolescent use of available mental health resources, attitudes of professionals and consumers about adolescent needs, and reasons for teenage sui-

**TABLE 14-1**

*Distribution of Reported AIDS Cases by Exposure Category, Age, and Sex in the United States, Cumulative Totals Through June 2000*

| Horizontal Axes | | | | |
|---|---|---|---|---|
| | PERCENTAGE OF AIDS CASES | | | |
| EXPOSURE CATEGORY (RISK GROUP) | MEN* (N = 620,189) | WOMEN* (N = 124,911) | CHILDREN <13 YR (N = 8,804) | TOTAL (N = 753,907†) |
| *Vertical Axes* | | | | |
| Male homosexual contact with HIV | 56% | — | — | 47% |
| IV drug users (IVDU) | 22% | 42% | — | 25% |
| Male homosexual and IVDU | 8% | — | — | 6% |
| Heterosexual contact with HIV | 4% | 40% | — | 10% |
| Transfusion recipient‡ | 1% | 3% | 3% | 1% |
| Mother with HIV | — | — | 91% | 1% |
| Hemophiliac | 1% | — | 4% | 1% |
| Undetermined§ | 8% | 15% | 2% | 9% |
| Total | 100% | 100% | 100% | 100% |

Modified from Centers for Disease Control and Prevention: *HIV/AIDS surveillance report, midyear edition* 12(1):1-41, 2000, p. 12.
*Includes adults and adolescents.
†Includes 3 persons whose sex is unknown and persons known to be infected with human immunodeficiency virus type 2 (HIV-2).
‡Thirty-nine adults/adolescents and 2 children developed AIDS after receiving blood screened negative for HIV antibody. Thirteen additional adults developed AIDS after receiving tissue, organs, or artificial insemination from HIV-infected donors. Four of the 13 received tissue, organs, or artificial insemination from a donor who was negative for HIV antibody at the time of donation.
§Includes 151 persons who acquired HIV infection perinatally but were diagnosed with AIDS after age 13. These 151 persons are tabulated under the adult/adolescent, not pediatric, exposure category.

cide must be ascertained before health planning can be effective. A survey is frequently conducted to obtain this type of information.

A community survey is a systematic study "that focuses on obtaining information regarding the activities, beliefs, preferences, and attitudes of people via direct questioning of a sample of respondents" (Polit, Hungler, 1997, p. 469). A variety of self-reported data can be obtained from a survey including information about a specific segment of the population or the health care system and the health status of the entire community. Several methods can be used to survey community residents. Face-to-face interviews (Figure 14-3), telephone interviews, or mailed written questionnaires are a few examples of ways to complete a community survey.

The scope of a survey varies, depending on the purpose and the financial and workforce resources available. While a survey can provide essential data for health programming, it is important to clearly define the reason for a survey, because this process can be costly and time-consuming.

Survey research is well suited for obtaining information on a wide range of topics and many segments of the population (Polit, Hungler, 1997). Surveys should be used to obtain data that are not available from other sources. For example, accurate data can generally be obtained about vital events (births, deaths, or marriages), but morbidity data are often incomplete. Surveys are frequently used to obtain in-

formation about health-related phenomena that are usually underreported, such as alcoholism, mental disorders and child abuse, and health care access issues.

Data obtained from a survey provide the foundation for a more intensive investigation of health needs in a community. Frequently, information obtained through the survey method tends to be relatively superficial (Polit, Hungler, 1997). Other assessment methods such as focus group and key informant interviews are used to obtain more in-depth information about a community's health status.

## Conduct Focus Group Interviews

Conducting focus group interviews is another approach for obtaining information about health needs, assets, and strengths from a community's perspective. The focus group or *group interview* (Morgan, 1998) "is a qualitative approach to learning about population subgroups with respect to conscious, semiconscious and unconscious psychological and sociocultural characteristics and processes" (Basch, 1987, p. 411). The focus group method is useful for obtaining culturally relevant and community-specific assessment data. It assists practitioners in obtaining data about peoples' perceived needs and priorities, community attitudes and beliefs about issues, and community preferences regarding health programming (Gonzalez, Gonzalez, Freeman, et al., 1991; Morgan, 1998).

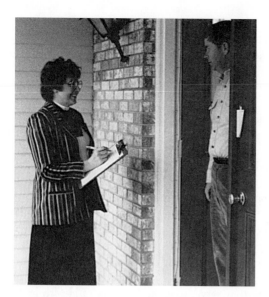

**FIGURE 14-3** House-to-house surveys assist health care professionals in obtaining a comprehensive understanding of their local communities. A well-planned survey can provide data about such things as resource utilization patterns, social concerns, and specific health needs of a subgroup within the community. The public health professional pictured was a member of an epidemiological team that was conducting a city-wide family health study. Higher-than-average infant deaths prompted the local health department to initiate this study. The results of the survey helped the health department to target its maternal-child health (MCH) efforts on high-risk groups. Because of its low infant mortality rate, this local community no longer qualified for special state MCH funds 5 years after the survey was completed. (Courtesy Henry Parks.)

The standard focus group format is similar to the processes used with any small groups (Basch, 1987; Gearhart-Pucci, Haglund, 1992; Krueger, 1994; Morgan, 1998). The leader or moderator uses a variety of leadership interventions to establish the focus groups, to promote a supportive group atmosphere and to accomplish specific goals. These interventions are discussed in Chapter 23 and include such things as finding an appropriate setting, creating a nonthreatening group climate, facilitating group process, and addressing cultural factors that influence group process and outcomes. For example, Strickland (1999) found, when working with two Native American tribes in Washington state, that communication patterns and tribal traditions were important elements to consider when conducting focus groups cross-culturally. Strickland allowed for additional time (2 to 4 hours versus the normal 1 to 3 hours) for the focus group interview. This time was used for traditional cultural activities including time to get acquainted, for the prayer songs, and gift giving.

Like other small groups, a focus group usually lasts no more than 1 to 3 hours. A focus group differs from many small groups in that the participants are usually homogenous with respect to characteristics such as age, sex, and so-

cial variables. Focus group interviews are structured around a specific set of questions designed to identify community needs and strengths. This structure is established to learn about and assist the community as a whole, rather than individual group participants (Basch, 1987).

A diversity of views is needed to detect patterns and trends in relation to critical health problems, priorities for health programming, and strategies for addressing concerns of multiple aggregates at risk. When using a focus group approach, diversity is achieved by controlling the size of the group and conducting a *series* of group interviews or by interviewing multiple groups with similar participants. The size of the focus group should be small enough to allow all participants to share their insights yet large enough to promote diversity of perceptions. Usually a focus group is composed of six to eight participants (Morgan, 1998). The selection of these participants is based on the purpose of the focus group and the type of information needed.

## Stop and Think About It

Data obtained from a mailed survey to community residents identified that access to health care continues to be a major issue in your community. Your agency has decided to conduct focus groups to identify specific barriers to access of health care. Considering agency resources and the demographic characteristics of your community, including such things as age structure, cultural diversity, and socioeconomic status and educational levels across census tracts, what type of participants would you want to involve in the focus group process? How many focus groups would you conduct? Where would you want to hold your focus group sessions? Who would you contact in your community to assist you in recruiting focus group participants?

## Conduct Community Forums

The community forum approach to data collection is similar to the focus group approach in that it is a qualitative method designed to obtain grass-roots opinions. Both approaches place people in natural, real-life situations that can increase the possibility of spontaneous, candid expression of views. Both approaches also can provide speedy results and cost relatively little (Krueger, 1994).

Although community forums may contain some of the characteristics of a focus group, there are significant differences. Community forums are open meetings for all members of the community (Balacki, 1988). This is in contrast to the homogenous, structured focus group. Focus groups are structured to promote public opinion representation from a variety of at-risk groups. The open approach of a community forum may not attract this type of representation. Also Balacki (1988) questions the assumption that the neediest within a community will attend an open formal gathering and be a vocal element. Even though community forums do provide a naturalistic environment for discussion, many people find it difficult to express their views in a large group setting.

Community forums, commonly called *town hall meetings*, have been used across the nation to elicit public opinion about health care issues (Group takes pulse of public via town hall meetings, 1992; Harris, 1993; Lauter, 1993; Ross, 1993; Toner, 1994; Town meetings air reform issues, 1993). Technology is facilitating citizen participation in a variety of political, consumer, and health care issues. Presidents Clinton and Bush Sr. and other politicians have used telecommunication to bring their health care reform messages to residents in local communities. Many communities air their significant political and decision-making meetings (e.g., city council and school boards) on local cable television channels (Snider, 1994). "Electronic town hall meetings" are the wave of the future (Snider, 1994).

Like other group intervention strategies, a successful community forum requires careful planning and organization. Chapter 23 discusses factors that nurses take into consideration when planning a group experience for client action. In relation to a community forum, the literature consistently highlights the need for a concerted mass media saturation before a forum, strong leadership that can focus participants on forum objectives, and a method for recording consumer input (Balacki, 1988; Group takes pulse of public via town hall meetings, 1992; Warheit, Bell, Schwab, 1974).

Town hall meetings are a creative strategy that actively engages the community in dialogue about community needs and interests (Randall-David, 1994). They can assist practitioners in identifying perceived unmet need as well as factors that inhibit or promote health action. Although community forums may not provide representative views from all segments of the population, they can provide direction for more focused community group experiences.

## Conduct Research

Research to document the effectiveness of nursing services and to identify cause-and-effect relationships is critically needed in the community health nursing setting. Funders of health care services are demanding concrete data that support the need for nursing personnel, the need for certain health programs, and the value of specific community health interventions.

Clinical research can help the health care professional document community needs as well as interventions that effectively address these needs (Magilvy, Brown, Moritz, 1999). A study conducted by Street Health, a community-based nursing organization in Toronto that operates clinics for women and men who are homeless or underhoused, illustrates the importance of clinical research (Crowe, Hardill, 1993). Recognizing that they lacked quantitative data to document both the health problems of their homeless clients and barriers to services—structural and attitudinal—the Street Health nurses established a survey research project to

obtain the data needed to strengthen their lobby efforts for homeless people.

The Street Health survey showed that homeless women and men had health problems similar to the general population but that the prevalence of many health problems, such as emphysema, chronic bronchitis, and epilepsy, was significantly greater in the homeless population than in the general public. It also showed that life circumstance had a tremendous impact on homeless persons' abilities to cope with these problems and that a number of barriers were preventing the homeless from receiving appropriate and/or compassionate care (Crowe, Hardill, 1993).

Based on their survey results, Street Health staff developed over 40 recommendations that targeted various community health agencies and educational institutions. For example, Street Health recommended that emergency room personnel receive sensitivity training about the community they serve, that the Ministry of Health prohibit all publicly funded health care institutions from refusing care to individuals who do not have their health card, and that Toronto's metro police develop a standing order to address the problem of discriminatory treatment of and violence toward homeless people (Crowe, Hardill, 1993). The Street Health nurses used these research findings to advocate for health services needed by their clients.

Research utilization is a critical component of professional nursing practice. It is imperative that the community health nurse be familiar with research in the field and integrate research findings into clinical nursing practice. The *Annual Review of Nursing Research* is a unique nursing research reference that helps practitioners provide evidenced-based nursing interventions. This reference has been published every year since 1983 and provides a synthesis of nursing research in selected areas by experts in the field. A number of areas that have been addressed in the *Review* would be of interest to community health nurses. *The Handbook of Clinical Nursing Research* (Hinshaw, Feetham, Shaver, 1999) also provides a synthesis of nursing research that can facilitate research utilization in the practice setting. "Not all nurses need to conduct research, but all should use it to guide their practice" (Lusk, 1993, p. 153).

## Contact Key Community Informants

Contact with key community persons, or *informants,* can help community health nurses understand factors influencing health behavior and identify those with whom they might work to enhance their effectiveness. Key informants are individuals well versed in a phenomenon of interest and who are willing to share their knowledge and insight with the researcher. Key informants frequently are interviewed when need assessments are conducted (Polit, Hungler, 1997).

Examples of key informants are directors of housing projects, clergy, professionals in other health care agencies, local politicians, owners of long-established businesses, and unofficial community spokespersons. These individuals can help the nurse gain knowledge about the power relationships within a local area, community values and attitudes, and environmental factors that enhance or detract from a community's state of health. Unofficial spokespersons often provide the most candid opinion of how the consumer views health and the health care delivery system. Clergy, agency clients, and cultural organizations, such as International Neighbors or the Polish club, can frequently assist a community health nurse in identifying these unofficial spokespersons.

A community health nurse should use every opportunity available to relate to community people. The opportunities are limitless and require only motivation on the part of the nurse and supervisory support to take advantage of them. Spontaneous dialogue with community residents aids community health nurses in gaining community trust and creating a positive professional image. The ability to relate to others in the community, such as school principals, physicians, administrators in mental health agencies, secretaries, and clergy, is essential if one wants to diagnose community assets, strengths, and needs accurately.

### Observe, Listen, and Analyze

Data about a community can be obtained daily by observing, listening, and analyzing. What the environment looks like when the nurse drives in the district, how families are dressed when they are seen in the clinic setting, and who relates to whom during community meetings all provide the community health nurse with clues about a community's state of health.

**Participant observation** during significant community events such as community health and political meetings, social gatherings, religious ceremonies, and special celebrations is an important process for community health nurses. This process can assist the health care provider in learning about people's behavior and practices and their differences and similarities. During this process the nurse might notice how business is conducted, how decisions are made, who attends community events, health concerns of community residents, and differences in attitudes about service usage (Gonzalez, Gonzalez, Freeman, et al., 1991; Randall-David, 1989). Participant observations help the community health nurse identify significant cultural differences in the community and health concerns that need to be addressed. They also assist the nurse in identifying key informants.

Community health nurses who are population oriented and community focused take time to analyze their community observations. They are alert to environmental conditions that adversely affect the state of a community's health. If, when driving through the district, a nurse finds children playing in the streets and sees no recreational facilities, she or he would raise questions about the need for safe play areas. An astute nurse can promote positive environmental change as illustrated in the following case scenario.

**CASE Scenario**  One community health nurse was able to promote environmental changes in her district because she identified that the parents in the area were genuinely concerned about the welfare of their children. Rat-infested vacant lots in the neighborhood presented a serious threat to the children who played in them. This nurse, with the assistance of a minister, was able to mobilize parents' energies so that the garbage from these lots was removed and rats were killed. Maintaining the lots as suitable play areas became a major community project.

A community health nurse who views the community as the unit of service is more likely to meet the needs of individual families than the nurse who focuses only on family health care needs. Family problems are interrelated with community problems and often cannot be resolved until changes occur within community systems or the environment. The preceding case situation reflects this view.

## SOURCES OF COMMUNITY DATA

A community health nurse can contact numerous international, federal, state, and local agencies and individuals to obtain community health status data. Although some were mentioned previously in this chapter, they are summarized here to give a composite picture of the multiple sources of data one can use when diagnosing community needs.

### International Sources

The United Nations is the major source of worldwide health and health-related data. Most countries report demographic statistics and health data to this organization, which then compiles the data into two major documents. The *Demographic Year Book* is a comprehensive collection of international demographic statistics. The *World Health Statistics Annual* is a yearly publication of information on vital statistics and causes of death (National Center for Health Statistics, 1999). These documents permit the United States to compare its health status with other developed nations. They also help local communities with high immigration rates identify among immigrants' health problems that are not normally experienced in the United States. Chapter 11 identifies some of these problems.

### National Sources

The federal agency specifically established for the collection and dissemination of health data is the Public Health Services' National Center for Health Statistics. This center conducts the National Health Survey, which provides valuable information on the health and illness status of U.S. residents (see Chapter 11). In addition, it provides official information on vital statistics and data about the supply and use of health resources (Office of the Federal Register, 2000).

**TABLE 14-2**

*Ongoing National Health Data Collection Systems and Health Surveys*

| SYSTEM/SURVEY | PURPOSE | LEAD AGENCY |
|---|---|---|
| *Data Collection Systems* | | |
| National Vital Statistics System | Collect and publish data on births, deaths, marriages, and divorces in the United States | National Center for Health Statistics |
| National Notifiable Diseases Surveillance System | Provide weekly provisional information on the occurrence of notifiable diseases | Epidemiology Program Office of CDC |
| AIDS surveillance | Epidemiological surveillance of AIDS | National Center for Infectious Diseases |
| Abortion surveillance | Epidemiological surveillance of abortions | National Center for Chronic Disease Prevention and Health Promotion |
| National Traumatic Occupational Fatalities Surveillance System | Monitor occupational fatalities | National Institute for Occupational Safety and Health |
| Estimates of National Health Expenditures | Compile annually estimates of health expenditures by type of expenditure and source of funding | Office of the Actuary, Health Care Financing Administration |
| Surveillance, Epidemiology, and End Results Program | Provide data on all residents diagnosed with cancer during the year and current follow-up information on all previously diagnosed clients | Eleven population-based registries throughout the nation and Puerto Rico under contract of the National Cancer Institute |
| Behavioral Risk Factor Surveillance System | Monitor key health risk behaviors (e.g., alcohol use, smoking behaviors, and AIDS attitude and knowledge awareness) in the U.S. population | State health departments in cooperation with CDC |
| *Health Surveys* | | |
| National Survey of Family Growth | Provide national data on the demographic and social factors associated with childbearing, adoption, and maternal and child health | National Center for Health Statistics |
| National Health Interview Survey | Identify annually changes in illnesses, injuries, impairments, chronic conditions, and utilization of health resources | National Center for Health Statistics |
| National Health and Nutrition Examination Survey | Estimate through health interviews and examination the national prevalence and reasons for secular trends of select diseases and risk factors and contribute to an epidemiological understanding of these diseases (e.g., cardiovascular, respiratory, arthritis, hearing, and diabetes) | National Center for Health Statistics |
| National Home and Hospice Care Survey | Provide annual information about the demographic and health characteristics of home health and hospice clients and characteristics of agencies serving these clients | National Center for Health Statistics |
| National Household Surveys on Drug Abuse | Monitor trends in use of marijuana, cigarettes, alcohol, and cocaine among persons 12 years of age and older | Substance Abuse and Mental Health Services Administration, Office of Applied Studies |
| Monitoring the Future Study | Epidemiological annual survey of drug use and related attitudes among college and high school seniors and eighth and tenth graders | University of Michigan's Institute for Social Research under contract of the National Institute of Drug Abuse |
| Annual Survey of Occupational Injuries and Illnesses | Collect annual statistics on occupational injuries and illnesses | Bureau of Labor Statistics of Department of Labor |

From National Center for Health Statistics: *Health, United States, 1999 with health and aging chart book,* Hyattsville, Md, 1999, US Government Printing Office, pp. 326-359; Michigan Department of Community Health: *Health risk behaviors: results from Michigan Behavioral Risk Factor Survey,* Lansing, Mich, 2000, Michigan Department of Community Health.

The U.S. Public Health Service also publishes two documents that provide extensive resource information related to our nation's major health issues. Its *Starting Points for Creating a Healthy Community* document delineates resources that assist communities in establishing "Healthy Cities and Communities" programs, and identifies national, state, and local agencies that provide information related to the priority areas in the *Healthy People* initiative. Its *Federal Health Information Centers and Clearinghouses* document lists almost 300 centers or organizations that serve as a resource for health information and provides both website information and telephone numbers (National Health Information Center [NHIC], 1999).

Several other federal and national agencies will supply health data on request. The Substance Abuse and Mental Health Services Administration, the National Institutes of Health, the Bureau of the Census, the Alan Guttmacher Institute, and the Public Health Foundation are a few examples of such agencies. The *United States Government Manual*, which can be purchased from the Superintendent of Documents, U.S. Government Printing Office, Washington, D.C., is a valuable reference for identifying other government agencies that disseminate health data. This manual is updated regularly and describes the purposes and programs of most federal agencies. The *Health, United States* document, a report on the health status of the nation, is also updated regularly and contains information on both federal and private agencies that provide health information.

Selected ongoing national health data collection systems and health surveys are displayed in Table 14-2. Select websites for governmental and public health resources are presented in Tables 14-3 and 14-4. The national health data collection systems regularly publish major reports on trends. These reports can be obtained in most professional libraries or from the federal agency that assumes responsibility for ongoing data collection.

The Bureau of the Census is another important source of population data. Census data include the size, distribution, structure, and change of populations in the United States. These data demonstrate patterns over time and provide general characteristics of a community's total population. Knowing the age structure in a community assists health care professionals located there in predicting the types of health problems and health care services needed. This knowledge, as well as census data about the economic status, housing conditions, and household composition in an area, assists community health nurses in predicting aggregates at risk in segments of the population. The previously discussed case situation about the needs of a high concentration of single working mothers in a nurse's district illustrates the importance of using census tract data.

Population or disease/condition-specific organizations on all three levels of governments are significant sources of community data. Examples of such organizations are the

**TABLE 14-3**

*Select Public Health Resources on the Web*

| ORGANIZATION | INTERNET ADDRESS |
| --- | --- |
| Agency for Healthcare Research and Quality (formerly AHCPR) | *http://www.ahcpr.gov/* |
| Agency for Toxic Substance and Disease Registry (ATSDR) | *http://www.atsdr.cdc.gov/* |
| Association of State and Territorial Health Officials | *http://www.astho.org/* |
| Centers for Disease Control and Prevention (CDC) | *http://www.cdc.gov/* |
| CDC's Public Health Images Library | *http://phil.cdc.gov/phil/* |
| Consumer Product Safety Commission (CPSC) | *http://www.cpsc.gov/* |
| Department of Health and Human Services (DHHS) | *http://www.dhhs.gov/* |
| Environmental Protection Agency (EPA) | *http://www.epa.gov/* |
| Food and Drug Administration (FDA) | *http://www.fda.gov/* |
| Health Care Financing Administration (HCFA) (Centers for Medicare and Medicaid Services [CMS]) | *http://www.hcfa.gov/* |
| Health Resources and Services Administration (HRSA) | *http://www.hrsa.dhhs.gov/* |
| National Center for Complementary and Alternative Medicine (NCCAM) | *http://altmed.od.nih.gov/* |
| National Center for Health Statistics (NCHS) | *http://www.cdc.gov/nchs/* |
| National Institutes of Health (NIH) | *http://www.nih.gov/* |
| Occupational Safety and Health Administration (OSHA) | *http://www.osha.gov/* |
| Pan American Health Organization (PAHO) | *http://www.paho.org/* |
| State and Local Government on the Net | *http://www.piperinfo.com/state/index.cfm* |
| Substance Abuse and Mental Health Services Administration (SAMHSA) | *http://www.samhsa.gov/* |
| The Office of Disease Prevention and Health Promotion (ODPHP) | *http://odphp.osophs.dhhs.gov/* |
| Thomas | *http://thomas.loc.gov/* |
| U.S. Bureau of the Census | *http://www.census.gov/* |
| World Health Organization (WHO) | *http://www.who.int/* |

**TABLE 14-4**

*Select Center for Disease Control and Prevention Websites*

| DIVISION | INTERNET ADDRESS |
|---|---|
| Centers for Disease Control and Prevention (CDC) | *http://www.cdc.gov* |
| CDC National AIDS Clearinghouse (CDC National Prevention Information Network) | *http://www.cdcnpin.org* |
| CDC National Center for HIV, STD, and TB Prevention Services (NCPS) | *http://www.cdc.gov/nchstp/od/nchstp.html* |
| CDC National Center for Infectious Diseases (NCID) | *http://www.cdc.gov/ncidod* |
| CDC National Institute for Occupational Safety and Health (NIOSH) | *http://www.cdc.gov/niosh/homepage.html* |
| CDC National Center for Injury Prevention and Control (NCIPC) | *http://www.cdc.gov/ncipc/ncipchm.htm* |
| CDC National Center for Health Statistics (NCHS) | *http://www.cdc.gov/nchs* |
| CDC Wonder (Healthy People Initiatives) | *http://wonder.cdc.gov* |
| CDC Bioterrorism | *http://www.bt.cdc.gov* |

American Association of Retired Persons (AARP), the Children's Defense Fund (CDF), National Council on Disability, American Cancer Society, American Diabetes Association, Mothers and Students Against Drunk Drivers (MADD and SADD), and National Coalition Against Domestic Violence. These organizations provide significant demographic, health status and health risk data, as well as information about community resources and major service delivery issues. Many of them provide information that helps a community assessment team compare local health data with national and state trends. For example, the Public Policy Institute of the AARP has published on a yearly basis since 1991 the document titled *Reforming the Health Care Systems: State Profiles.* This document provides a profile for each state that addresses health care information as well as demographic and health status data.

Legislators and public officials on all three levels of government are also valuable resources. They often are willing to assist health care professionals in analyzing social and health care legislation. Laws and ordinances related to community health reflect the values and priorities of a community, the state, and the federal government. Every health care professional should be familiar with legislation that influences the health of his or her community.

### State Sources

State health departments are a major source of health data. Vital statistics, morbidity data, health workforce, and resource information usually are collected and disseminated by this agency. Frequently this agency has health information clearinghouses and hot lines that quickly provide health information to interested providers and consumers. State health departments often have an extensive listing of health promotion and disease prevention resources.

Legislators and the population or disease/condition-specific organizations previously identified are also valuable information resources on the state level. The Department of Education, the Bureau of Mental Health, and the Office of Services to the Aging are some of the state agencies that supply health and health-related information. Obtaining a

state directory of health and social service agencies will help each reader determine which agencies in his or her state furnish information about specific health needs in local communities. These directories often can be obtained from local health councils or at local libraries.

### Local Sources

On the local level, some key sources for obtaining community data are the chamber of commerce, city planner's office, health department, county extension office, intermediate school district, libraries, health and welfare professionals, hospital records, clergy, community leaders, and consumers. In addition to providing data about major health problems, health, education, and social service agencies can share significant information about service utilization patterns. The city planner's office can provide population mobility data that can assist health providers in predicting service needs. Community residents provide important qualitative data about perceived community needs, the traditions of the community, and informal information resources.

Most cities and counties have directories that provide information on the major health and welfare resources in their community. These directories are often published by local health departments or United Way organizations. Experienced practitioners are valuable resources for new practitioners who are interested in learning about formal community services. Experienced practitioners are also very knowledgeable about informal community resources.

## SYNTHESIZE ALL AVAILABLE DATA

Once community data are assembled, they should be organized in a meaningful way so that patterns and trends can be ascertained. Many techniques can be used to synthesize community data. Charts, figures, and tables are often used for this purpose. Graphic presentation of population distributions, morbidity data, or vital statistics for several decades can be very effective in pinpointing significant community problems. Growth or lack of growth in a community, for instance, can be identified when population distributions are graphically visualized. Growth or lack of growth in a community is important to address because these situations can affect the availability of health and social service resources.

Comparing community rates with state and national rates is essential. This comparison can highlight specific health problems and community strengths and can help a community to determine priorities for program planning. For example, if a community's infant and maternal mortality rates are much higher than state and national rates, a community would examine carefully its maternal-child health programming. On the other hand, a community may find when making these comparisons, that its maternal-child health statistics are far superior to those of other areas. This in turn could demonstrate to the community the value of maintaining adequate health programs for these two age groups in the population.

Analysis of data often supports the need for further data collection. This is illustrated in the following case scenario:

**CASE Scenario** The health department became aware of a maternal-infant health problem in one census tract of a large urban area. This census tract was a residential rental area with basement efficiency apartments renting for $640 or higher per month. The population was 75% students and young working people, referred to as the "yuppies." Of the remaining 25%, 20% were elderly second-generation immigrant merchants, and 5% were young families living in the city housing project. The area had a high reported incidence of mugging, purse snatching, and apartment thefts, with rumors of drug manufacturing, pushing, and usage.

Few referrals were made to the health agencies in the area; casefinding was negligible; and records of nursing services showed few home visits to individuals in this district. The explanation given for this situation was that the majority of the population in this census tract was either at school or working and, therefore, inaccessible to agency personnel during the working day. Evening office hours were scheduled by private physicians and several health clinics in the area.

The health department became particularly concerned about the lack of referrals from this census tract when they analyzed the infant and maternal mortality (death) rates for the entire county. It was discovered that only in this census tract did these rates significantly vary from national statistics.

Infant and maternal mortality rates for the specified census tract were:
23.4 infant deaths per 1000 live births
5.2 maternal deaths per 1000 live births

Infant and maternal mortality rates in the United States during the same time period were:
7.1 infant deaths per 1000 live births
3.1 maternal deaths per 1000 live births

It was obvious from these vital statistics that something had to be done to improve the health status of mothers and children in this area. However, more specific data were needed to determine causes of death, health status of area residents, and use of health care services, as well as related health problems, including socioeconomic difficulties, drug use, and attitudes about the "establishment." Personnel from a drug clinic and the student organization at a local college assisted the health department in collecting the data they needed. Lack of transportation, extremely limited incomes, lack of knowledge, inadequate nutrition, and resistance to normal channels of health care were some of the major problems identified. The establishment of a neighborhood health clinic, staffed mostly by college students and area residents, produced positive results. Data analysis at the end of 3 years reflected a significant decrease in both the infant and maternal mortality rates for this area.

This scenario dramatically illustrates the importance of synthesizing data once they are compiled. Community diagnostic activities are carried out so that appropriate decisions about health planning can be made. When data analysis is lacking, significant health issues can be missed.

## TIPS FOR IMPLEMENTING COMMUNITY ANALYSIS ACTIVITIES

Community assessment and diagnostic activities are exciting and challenging. It should be apparent, however, that they cannot be left to chance. To effectively implement these activities, time for planning, assessing, and analyzing must be set aside. Equally important is the need to always keep the framework of the "community" in clear perspective when providing nursing care.

### BOX 14-9
*Selected Community-Focused Orientation Activities*

- Analyze census tract and vital statistics data to learn about population characteristics in your district.
- Attend case conferences and community meetings (PTA, social service council, citizen group activities) with an experienced employee.
- Conduct a windshield survey of your clinical area (Figure 14-3).
- Attend a board of health meeting or other policy-focused meetings to identify the values and attitudes of leaders in policy-making positions.
- Identify the locations of health and social service resources, recreational facilities, local churches, school systems, and shopping areas.
- Shop in your district to determine cost of essentials such as food and clothing.
- Make field visits with personnel from other departments in your agency (environmental health, mental health or nutrition)
- Observe in clinic settings (well-baby, STD, adult screening, or prenatal).

Presented in Box 14-9 are suggestions for maintaining a focus on the community when newly involved in community activities. Peers and supervisory personnel in the clinical setting can assist a newly employed practitioner to identify appropriate community activities. These individuals can help the new practitioner obtain community health status information or insight about significant community traditions. Community residents are also key resources that should be contacted when learning about the community.

## SUMMARY

Meeting the health needs of at-risk aggregates or populations is a major community health nursing function. A nurse must know the community before this responsibility can be effectively carried out. A variety of strategies are used to assess the health status, the health capability, and the health action potential of the nurse's community. Data are analyzed, as well as collected, so that target groups for nursing service can be identified. Use of the nursing process facilitates implementation of these activities. Developing community partnerships also facilitates this process. Interdisciplinary collaboration and consumer participation is critical during the community assessment process because no one person alone can appropriately diagnose community needs.

Exploring the community, its organization, and its activities is extremely rewarding. This exploration provides a clearer picture of community health action and a foundation for health planning activities designed to improve the health status of high-risk groups. It further helps the community health nurse to assist individual families more effectively. Often family health problems cannot be resolved until changes occur in community systems.

## CRITICAL THINKING
*exercise*

You are a community health nurse who works for a local health department that was directed by the city commissioners to develop short- and long-range plans to combat local community violence. The agency's violence task force, of which you are a member, recognizes that it has insufficient data to make decisions about specific community interventions. Thus the committee's first goal is to assess community perceptions regarding this problem and to collect and analyze quantitative data relative to the nature of the problem. Taking into consideration that several types of violence (e.g., child and elder abuse, domestic violence, homicide, and intentional and unintentional injury) occur in a community, identify the key informants who could assist your task force in obtaining the community's perspective about the problem. Additionally, discuss the kinds of quantitative data you would need to document the extent of violence in your community and where and how you might obtain these data. Further, discuss how community attitudes about violence could facilitate or inhibit your data collection process.

## REFERENCES

American Nurses Association (ANA) Quad Council of Public Health Nursing Organizations: *Scope and standards of public health nursing practice,* Washington, DC, 1999, ANA.

American Public Health Association (APHA): *Public health in a reformed health care system: a vision for the future,* Washington, DC, 1993, APHA.

American Public Health Association (APHA), Public Health Nursing Section: *The definition and role of public health nursing: a statement of APHA public health nursing section,* Washington, DC, 1996, APHA.

Anderson ET: Community focus in public health nursing: whose responsibility? *Nurs Outlook* 31:44-48, 1983.

Anderson ET, McFarlane J: *Community as partner: theory and practice in nursing,* ed 3, Philadelphia, 2000, JB Lippincott.

Association of State and Territorial Directors of Nursing (ASTDN): *Public health nursing: a partner for progress. A document which links nursing, public health core functions and essential services,* Washington, DC, 1998, ASTDN.

Balacki MF: Assessing mental health needs in the rural community: a critique of assessment approaches, *Issues Ment Health Nurs* 9:299-315, 1988.

Basch C: Focus group interview: an underutilized research technique for improving theory and practice in health education, *Health Educ Q* 14:411-448, 1987, Winter.

Berkowitz B: Collaboration for health improvement: models for state, community, and academic partnerships, *J Public Health Manage Prac* 6:1-6, 67-72, 2000.

Bracht N, Kingsbury L, Rissel C: A five-stage community organization model for health promotion: empowerment and partnership strategies. In Bracht N, editor: *Health promotion at the community level,* ed 2: *New advances,* Thousand Oaks, Calif, 1999, Sage, pp. 83-104.

Calvillo ER: AIDS knowledge and attitudes among Latinas. In Western Institute of Nursing: *Communicating nursing research, silver threads: 25 years of nursing excellence,* vol 25, Boulder, Colo, 1992, The Institute, p. 415.

Centers for Disease Control and Prevention (CDC): Consensus set of health status indicators for the general assessment of community health status—United States, *MMWR* 40 (27):449-451, 1991.

Centers for Disease Control and Prevention (CDC): *HIV/AIDS surveillance report,* midyear edition 12(1):1-41, 2000.

Children's Defense Fund (CDF): *The state of America's children yearbook 1996,* Washington, DC, 1996, CDF.

Clarke HF, Beddome G, Whyte NB: Public health nurses' vision of their future reflects changing paradigms, *Image: J Nurs Sch* 25:305-310, 1993.

Conley E: Public health nursing within core public health functions: "back to the future," *J Public Health Manage Pract* 1:1-8, 1995.

Crowe C, Hardill K: Nursing research and political change: the Street Health Report, *Can Nurse* 88:21-24, 1993.

DiClemente R, Wingood G, Vermund S, et al.: Prevention of HIV/AIDS. In Raczynski J, DiClemente R, editors: *Handbook of health promotion and disease prevention,* New York, 1999, Kluwer Academic.

Flynn BC, Ray DW, Rider MS: Empowering communities: action research through Healthy Cities, *Health Educ* 21:395-405, 1994.

Gearhart-Pucci L, Haglund BJA: Focus groups: a tool for developing better health education materials and approaches for smoking intervention, *Health Promotion Int* 7:11-15, 1992.

Gonzalez U, Gonzalez J, Freeman U, et al.: *Health promotion in diverse cultural communities*, Palo Alto, Calif, 1991, Health Promotion Resource Center, Stanford Center for Research in Disease Prevention.

Gordon M: *Nursing diagnosis: process and application*, ed 2, New York, 1987, McGraw-Hill.

Gordon M: *Manual of nursing diagnosis*, ed 9, St Louis, 2000 Mosby.

Group takes pulse of public via town hall meetings, *Public Relations J* 48:5, 1992.

Harris HR: A heavy dose of questions for Clinton's health care plan, *The Washington Post* 116:DCI(Col 1), October 21, 1993

Hinshaw AS, Feetham, SL, Shaver JL, editors: *Handbook of clinical nursing research*, Thousand Oaks, Calif, 1999, Sage

Institute of Medicine (IOM): *The future of public health*, Washington, DC, 1988, National Academy Press.

Institute of Medicine (IOM): *Healthy communities: new partnership for the future of public health*, Washington, DC, 1996, National Academy Press.

Institute of Medicine (IOM): *Improving health in the community*, Washington, DC, 1997, National Academy Press.

Kretzmann J, McKnight J: *Building communities from the inside out*, Chicago, 1993, ACTA Publications.

Kreuter MW: PATCH: its origin, basic concepts, and links to contemporary public health policy, *J Health Educ* 23:135-139, 1992.

Kriegler N, Harton M: Community health assessment tool: a patterns approach to data collection and diagnosis, *J Community Health Nurs* 9(4):229-234, 1992.

Krueger RA: *Focus groups: a practical guide for applied research*, ed 2, Thousand Oaks, Calif, 1994, Sage.

Lauter D: Town hall health hearing presents few cures, *Los Angeles Times* 112:A21 (col 1), March 13, 1993.

Lusk SL: Linking practice and research, *AAOHN J* 41:153-157, 1993.

Magilvy JK, Brown NJ, Moritz P: Community-focused interventions and outcomes strategies. In Hindshaw AS, Feetham SL, Shaver JL, editors: *Handbook of clinical nursing research*, Thousand Oaks, Calif, 1999, Sage, pp. 125-143.

Mann J: Communities of concern will change our world, *Futurist* 35(3):68-69, 2001.

Marin G, Burhansstipanov L, Connell C, et al.: A research agenda for health education among underserved populations, *Health Educ Q* 22:346-363, 1995.

McFarlane J: De Madras a Madres: an access model for primary care, *Am J Public Health* 86:879-880, 1996.

Michigan Department of Community Health: *Health risk behaviors: results from Michigan Behavioral Risk Factor Survey*, Lansing, Mich, 2000, Michigan Department of Community Health.

Morgan P: *The focus group guidebook: focus group kit*, Thousand Oaks, Calif, 1998, Sage.

Muecke M: Community health diagnosis in nursing, *Public Health Nurs* 1(1):23-35, 1984.

National Center for Health Statistics: *Health, United States, 1999 with health and aging chartbook*, Hyattsville, Md, 1999, US Government Printing Office.

National Health Information Center (NHIC) (1999): *Federal health information centers and clearinghouse*, Washington, DC, 1999, Office of Disease Prevention and Health Promotion.

National League for Nursing (NLN): *A vision for nursing education*, New York, 1993, NLN.

North American Nursing Diagnosis Association (NANDA): *Nursing diagnoses: Definitions and classifications, 1999-2000*, Philadelphia, 1999, NANDA.

Nurse Administrators Forum: *Promoting healthy Michigan communities: the role of public health nursing in health reform*, Lansing, Mich, 1994, Michigan Department of Public Health.

Oberle MW, Baker EL, Magenheim MJ: Healthy People 2000 and community health planning, *Annu Rev Public Health* 15:259-275, 1994.

Office of the Federal Register: *United States government manual, 2000/2001*, Washington, DC, 2000, The Office.

Office of Policy, Planning, and Evaluation, Michigan Department of Public Health: *List of national and state databases*, Lansing, Mich, 1995, The Office.

Pew Health Professions Commission: *Critical challenges: revitalizing the health professions for the twenty-first century*, San Francisco, 1995, UCSF Center for the Health Professions.

Polit D, Hungler B: *Essentials of nursing research: methods, appraisal and utilization*, Philadelphia, 1997, Lippincott.

Pollack PB: *Liveable communities! An evolution guide*, Washington, DC, 1999, AARP Public Policy Institute.

Randall-David E: *Strategies for working with culturally diverse communities and clients*, Bethesda, Md, 1989, The Association for the Care of Children's Health.

Randall-David E: *Culturally competent HIV counseling and education*, McLean, Va, 1994, The Maternal and Child Health Clearinghouse.

Rissel C, Bracht N: Assessing community needs, resources, and readiness: Building on strengths. In Bracht N, editor: *Health promotion at the community level: new advances*, ed 2, Thousand Oaks, Calif, 1999, Sage, pp. 59-7l.

Ross M. Health plan takes heat at GOP meetings, *Los Angeles Times* 113:A20 (col 1), December 5, 1993.

Sander IT: *The community: an introduction to a social system*, ed 2, New York, 1966, Ronald Press.

Sharpe P, Greaney M, Lee P, et al.: Assets-oriented community assessment, *Public Health Reports* 115(2,3):205-211, 2000.

Snider JH: Democracy on-line: tomorrow's electronic electorate, *The Futurist* 28(5):15-19, 1994.

Strickland CJ: Conducting focus groups cross-culturally: experiences with Pacific Northwest Indian people, *Public Health Nurs* 16(3):190-197, 1999.

Toner R: Wanting health care help, voters tell of apprehension, *The New York Times* 143(Sec 1):1 (col 2), April 3, 1994.

Town meetings air reform issues, *Employee Benefit Plan Review* 47:12, 1993.

US Department of Health and Human Services (USDHHS): *Healthy People 2000: national health promotion and disease prevention objectives, full report, with commentary*, Washington, DC, 1991, US Government Printing Office.

US Department of Health and Human Services (USDHHS): *Healthy people 2010 (conference edition, volume 1)*, Washington, DC, 2000, US Government Printing Office.

Warheit GJ, Bell RA, Schwab JJ: *Planning for change: needs assessment approaches*, Rockville, Md, 1974, National Institute of Mental Health.

William CA: Community health nursing: What is it? *Nurs Outlook* 24:250-254, 1977.

Wilson K, Mitrano T: *An assets-based approach to neighborhood and community development*, Columbia, SC, 1996, University of South Carolina, Institute for Families in Society.

Winkleby MA, Flora JA, Kraemer HC: A community-based heart disease intervention: predictors of change, *Am J Public Health* 84:767-771, 1994.

## SELECTED BIBLIOGRAPHY

Bloom Y, Figgs L, Baker E, et al.: Data uses, benefits, and barriers for the behavioral risk factor surveillance system: a qualitative study of users, *J Public Health Management Practice* 6(1):78-86, 2000.

Cote-Arsenault D, Morrison-Beedy P: Practical advice for planning and conducting focus groups, *Nurs Res* 48(5):280-283, 1999.

Courtney R, Ballard E, Fauver S et al.: The partnership model: working with individuals, families, and communities toward a new vision of health, *Public Health Nurs* 113:177-186, 1996.

Doerr B, Wantuch C: Cudahy High School survey and focus groups: assessment of the needs of a teen population. A community-campus collaboration, *Public Health Nurs* 17(1):11-15, 2000.

Eisen A: Survey of neighborhood-based, comprehensive community empowerment initiatives, *Health Educ Q* 21:235-252, 1994.

Finnegan L, Ervin NE: An epidemiological approach to community assessment, *Public Health Nurs* 6:147-151, 1989.

Freudenberg N, Lee J, Germain LM: Reaching low-income women at risk of AIDS: a case history of a drop-in center for women in the South Bronx, New York City, *Health Educ Res* 9:119-132, 1994.

Goeppinger J: Health promotion for rural populations: partnership interventions, *Fam Community Health* 16:1-10, 1993.

Hagopian A, House P, Dyck S, et al.: The use of community surveys for health planning: The experience of 56 northwest rural communities, *J Rural Health* 16(1):81-90, 2000.

Hamilton P: Community nursing diagnosis, *Adv Nurs Sci* 5(3):21-36, 1983.

Hornberger C, Cobb A: A rural vision of a healthy community, *Public Health Nurs* 15(5):363-369, 1998.

Keppel K, Pearcy J: Healthy People 2000: an assessment based on the health status indicators for the United States and each state, *Healthy People 2000 Statistical Notes*, 19, 1-31, 2000.

Labonte R: Health promotion and empowerment: reflections on professional practice, *Health Educ Q* 21:253-268, 1994.

Norris T, Pittman M: The healthy communities movement and the coalition for healthier cities and communities, *Public Health Rep* 115(2):118-124, 2000.

Polivka B, Lovell M, Smith B: A qualitative assessment of inner city elementary school children's perceptions of their neighborhood, *Public Health Nurs* 15(3):171-179, 1998.

Poulton B: Use involvement in identifying health needs and shaping and evaluating services: is it being realized? *J Adv Nurs* 30(6):1284-1296, 1999.

Schultz PR: When client means more than one: extending the foundational concept of person *Adv Nurs Sci* 10:71-86, 1987.

Stanley S, Stein D: Health Watch 2000: community health assessment in south central Ohio, *J Community Health Nurs* 15(4):225-236, 1998.

Stevens PE: Focus groups: collecting aggregate-level data to understand community health phenomena, *Public Health Nurs* 13:170-176, 1996.

United States Department of Health and Human Services (USDHHS): *Healthy People 2010: understanding and improving health*, ed 2, Washington, DC, 2000, US Government Printing Office.

# Learning About the Community on Foot

| | OBSERVATIONS | DATA |
|---|---|---|
| **I. Community Core**<br>**1. History**—What can you glean by looking (e.g., old, established neighborhoods; new subdivisions)? Ask people willing to talk: How long have you lived here? Has the area changed? As you talk, ask if there is an "old timer" who knows the history of the area. | | |
| **2. Demographics**—What sort of people do you see? Young? Old? Homeless? Alone? Families? What race do you see? Is the population homogeneous? | | |
| **3. Ethnicity**—Do you note indicators of different ethnic groups (e.g., restaurants, festivals)? What signs do you see of different cultural groups? | | |
| **4. Values and Beliefs**—Are there churches, mosques, temples? Does it appear homogeneous? Are the lawns cared for? With flowers? Gardens? Signs of art? Culture? Heritage? Historical markers? | | |
| **II. Subsystems**<br>**1. Physical environment**—How does the community look? What do you note about air quality, flora, housing, zoning, space, green areas, animals, people, human-made structures, natural beauty, water, climate? Can you find or develop a map of the area? What is the size (e.g., square miles, blocks)? | | |

Note: Supplement your impressions with information from the census, police records, school statistics, chamber of commerce data, health department reports, etc., to confirm or refute your conclusions. Tables, graphs, and maps are helpful and will aid in your analysis.
From Anderson ET, McFarlane JM: *Community as partner: theory and practice in nursing,* ed 3, Philadelphia, 2000, JB Lippincott, pp. 168-170.

*Continued*

# Learning About the Community on Foot (cont'd)

| | OBSERVATIONS | DATA |
|---|---|---|
| **2. Health and Social Services**— Evidence of acute or chronic conditions? Shelters? "Traditional" healers (e.g., curanderos, herbalists)? Are there clinics, hospitals, practitioners' offices, public health service, home health agencies, emergency centers, nursing homes, social service facilities, mental health services? Are there resources outside the community but accessible to its members? | | |
| **3. Economy**—Is it a "thriving" community, or does it feel "seedy"? Are there industry, stores, places for employment? Where do people shop? Are there signs that food stamps are used/accepted? What is the unemployment rate? | | |
| **4. Transportation and Safety**—How do people get around? What type of private and public transportation is available? Do you see buses, bicycles, taxis? Are there sidewalks, bike trails? Is getting around in the community possible for persons with disabilities? What type of protective services are there (e.g., fire, police, sanitation)? Is air quality monitored? What are the types of crimes committed? Do people feel safe? | | |
| **5. Politics and Government**—Are there signs of political activity (e.g., posters, meetings)? What party affiliation predominates? What is the governmental jurisdiction of the community (e.g., elected mayor, city council with single member districts)? Are people involved in decision making in their local governmental unit? | | |

Note: Supplement your impressions with information from the census, police records, school statistics, chamber of commerce data, health department reports, etc., to confirm or refute your conclusions. Tables, graphs, and maps are helpful and will aid in your analysis.
From Anderson ET, McFarlane JM: *Community as partner: theory and practice in nursing,* ed 3, Philadelphia, 2000, JB Lippincott, pp. 168-170.

# Learning About the Community on Foot (cont'd)

| | OBSERVATIONS | DATA |
|---|---|---|
| **6. Communication**—Are there "common areas" where people gather? What newspapers do you see in the stands? Do people have televisions and radios? What do they watch/listen to? What are the formal and informal means of communication? | | |
| **7. Education**—Are there schools in the area? How do they look? Are there libraries? Is there a local board of education? How does it function? What is the reputation of the school(s)? What are major educational issues? What are the dropout rates? Are there extracurricular activities available? Are they used? Is there a school health service? A school nurse? | | |
| **8. Recreation**—What do children play? What are the major forms of recreation? Who participates? What facilities for recreation do you see? | | |
| *III. Perceptions*<br>**1. The Residents**—How do people feel about the community? What do they identify as its strengths? Problems? Ask several people from different groups (e.g., old, young, field workers, factory workers, professional, minister, housewife) and keep track of who gives what answer. | | |
| **2. Your Perceptions**—General statements about the "health" of this community. What are its strengths? What problems or potential problems can you identify? | | |

# Community Assessment Guide

| COMMUNITY _____ DATE _____<br>CHECK (√) APPROPRIATE COLUMN* | STRENGTH | POTENTIAL NEED | PROBLEM | DESCRIPTION/COMMENTS |
|---|---|---|---|---|
| I. *People*<br>A. Vital and demographic statistics<br>   1. Population density | | | | |
| 2. Population composition<br>   a. Sex ratio | | | | |
| b. Age distribution | | | | |
| c. Race distribution | | | | |
| d. Ethnic origin | | | | |
| 3. Population characteristics<br>   a. Mobility | | | | |
| b. Socioeconomic status | | | | |
| c. Level of unemployment | | | | |
| d. Educational level | | | | |
| e. Marriage rate | | | | |
| f. Divorce rate | | | | |
| g. Dependency ratio | | | | |
| h. Fertility rate | | | | |
| i. Head of household | | | | |
| 4. Mortality characteristics<br>   a. Crude death rate | | | | |
| b. Infant mortality rate | | | | |
| c. Maternal mortality rate | | | | |
| d. Age-specific death rate | | | | |
| e. Leading causes of death | | | | |
| 5. Morbidity characteristics<br>   a. Incidence rate (specific diseases) | | | | |
| b. Prevalence rate (specific diseases) | | | | |

*Place check in only one column—strength, potential need, or problem.
*Note*: The material presented in Chapters 3, 4, 5, 11, 14, and 15 and the cultural assessment tool in Chapter 7 are especially helpful to the nurse when using this assessment tool. The nurse initially collects available data and then adds to this assessment on an ongoing basis.

# Community Assessment Guide (cont'd)

| CHECK (√) APPROPRIATE COLUMN* | STRENGTH | POTENTIAL NEED | PROBLEM | DESCRIPTION/COMMENTS |
|---|---|---|---|---|
| B. History of community (e.g., founding, cultural groups) | | | | |
| C. Values, attitudes, and norms | | | | |
| D. Individual and family living practices | | | | |
|   1. Types of families | | | | |
|   2. Number of children per family | | | | |
|   3. Leisure activities | | | | |
| II. *Environmental*<br>A. Physical<br>  1. Natural resources | | | | |
|   2. Geography, climate, terrain | | | | |
|   3. Roads/transportation | | | | |
|   4. Boundaries | | | | |
|   5. Housing (types available by percent, condition, percent rented, percent owned) | | | | |
|   6. Other major structures | | | | |
| B. Biologic and chemical<br>  1. Water supply | | | | |
|   2. Air (color, odor, particulates) | | | | |
|   3. Food supply (sources, preparation) | | | | |
|   4. Pollutants, toxic substances, animal reservoirs, or vectors | | | | |
|   5. Flora and fauna | | | | |
|   6. Is this a predominantly urban, suburban, or rural community? (How is land used?) | | | | |
| III. *Systems*<br>A. Health<br>  1. Preventive health care practices and facilities (list) | | | | |
|   2. Treatment health care facilities (e.g., acute care, medical, and surgical hospitals) (list) | | | | |

*Continued*

# Community Assessment Guide (cont'd)

| CHECK (√) APPROPRIATE COLUMN* | STRENGTH | POTENTIAL NEED | PROBLEM | DESCRIPTION/COMMENTS |
|---|---|---|---|---|
| 3. Rehabilitation health care facilities (e.g., alcoholism) (list) | | | | |
| 4. Long-term health care facilities (e.g., nursing homes) (list) | | | | |
| 5. Respite care services for special population groups (list) | | | | |
| 6. Hospice care services (list) | | | | |
| 7. Catastrophic health care facilities and services (list) | | | | |
| 8. Special health services for population groups (what and how provided) <br> a. Preschool | | | | |
| b. School age | | | | |
| c. Adult or young adult | | | | |
| d. Occupational health | | | | |
| e. Adults and children with disabling conditions | | | | |
| 9. Voluntary health care resources | | | | |
| 10. Sanitation services | | | | |
| 11. Health work force (population ratios) | | | | |
| 12. Health education activities | | | | |
| 13. Methods of health care financing (approximate percent) <br> a. Private pay | | | | |
| b. Health insurance | | | | |
| c. HMO | | | | |
| d. Medicaid/Medicare | | | | |
| e. Worker's Compensation | | | | |
| f. Uninsured | | | | |
| g. Underinsured | | | | |

# Community Assessment Guide (cont'd)

| CHECK (√) APPROPRIATE COLUMN* | STRENGTH | POTENTIAL NEED | PROBLEM | DESCRIPTION/COMMENTS |
|---|---|---|---|---|
| 14. Prevalent diseases and conditions (list) | | | | |
| 15. Linkages with other systems | | | | |
| 16. Health care resource overall availability | | | | |
| 17. Health care resource overall use | | | | |
| B. Welfare<br>  1. Official (public) welfare resources<br>    a. General (list; e.g., Department of Social Services) | | | | |
|     b. Safety and protection (list; e.g., fire department) | | | | |
|   2. Voluntary welfare resources (list) | | | | |
|   3. Transportation resources (public and private) | | | | |
|   4. Facilities to meet needs (e.g., shopping areas, public housing) | | | | |
|   5. Special services for population groups (list) | | | | |
|   6. Resource accessibility | | | | |
|   7. Resource use | | | | |
| C. Education<br>  1. Public educational facilities (list) | | | | |
|   2. Private educational facilities (list) | | | | |
|   3. Libraries (list) | | | | |
|   4. Educational services for special populations<br>    a. Pregnant teens | | | | |
|     b. Adults | | | | |
|     c. Developmentally disabled children and adults | | | | |
|     d. Other | | | | |
|   5. Resource accessibility | | | | |
|   6. Resource use | | | | |

*Continued*

# Community Assessment Guide (cont'd)

| CHECK (√) APPROPRIATE COLUMN* | STRENGTH | POTENTIAL NEED | PROBLEM | DESCRIPTION/COMMENTS |
|---|---|---|---|---|
| D. Economic<br>  1. Major industry and business (list) | | | | |
|   2. Banks, savings and loans, credit unions (list) | | | | |
|   3. Major occupations (list) | | | | |
|   4. General socioeconomic status of population | | | | |
|   5. Median income | | | | |
|   6. Percentage of population below poverty level | | | | |
|   7. Percentage of population who are retired | | | | |
| E. Government and leadership<br>  1. Elected official leadership (list with title) | | | | |
|   2. Nonofficial leadership (list with title affiliations) | | | | |
|   3. City offices (location, hours, services) | | | | |
|   4. Accessibility to constituents | | | | |
|   5. Support of community resources | | | | |
| F. Recreation<br>  1. Public facilities (list) | | | | |
|   2. Private facilities (list) | | | | |
|   3. Recreational activities frequently used (list) | | | | |
|   4. Leisure activities frequently used (list) | | | | |
|   5. Coordination with educational recreation facilities and programs | | | | |
|   6. Programs for special population groups<br>   a. Elderly | | | | |
|    b. People who are disabled | | | | |
|    c. Others | | | | |

# Community Assessment Guide (cont'd)

| CHECK (√) APPROPRIATE COLUMN* | STRENGTH | POTENTIAL NEED | PROBLEM | DESCRIPTION/COMMENTS |
|---|---|---|---|---|
| 7. Resource accessibility | | | | |
| 8. Resource use | | | | |
| G. Religion<br>1. Facilities by denomination (list) | | | | |
| 2. Religious leaders (list) | | | | |
| 3. Community programs and services | | | | |
| 4. Resource accessibility | | | | |
| 5. Resource use | | | | |
| IV. *Community dynamics* (describe) | | | | |
| A. Communication (diagram and describe)<br>1. Vertical (community to larger society) | | | | |
| 2. Horizontal (community to itself) | | | | |
| 3. Specific resources (e.g., television, radio, newspapers) | | | | |
| V. *Major sources of community data* | | | | |
| A. Government (list; e.g., local health department, city planning office) | | | | |
| B. Private (list; e.g., chamber of commerce; key informants) | | | | |

*Continued*

## QUESTIONS FOR THE COMMUNITY HEALTH NURSE

1. In general, are resources readily available and accessible?
2. What does the community see as its major strengths and needs?
3. How self-sufficient is the community in meeting its perceived needs?
4. What does the community health nurse see as the community's major strengths and needs?
5. How does the community's health status indicators compare to state and national indicators?

6. Are there established health coalitions to address community needs?
7. Health care
   a. How does the community view and use the health care system? (Specify cultural barriers.)
   b. What does the community see as its health care needs?
   c. What are the goals and major activities of the health system?
   d. How self-sufficient is the community in meeting its health needs?

# Community Assessment Guide (cont'd)

| DATE | GOALS | ACTIVITIES TO IMPLEMENT |
|------|-------|-------------------------|
| **COMMUNITY HEALTH CARE GOALS AND ACTIVITIES TO IMPLEMENT THEM** | | |
| | | |

Assessor _____ Date _____

Assessor _____ Date _____

Assessor _____ Date _____

# 15

# Community Organization and Health Planning for Aggregates at Risk

*Susan Clemen-Stone*

## OBJECTIVES

*Upon completion of this chapter, the reader should be able to:*

1. Discuss the concepts of community organization and health planning.
2. Distinguish between comprehensive health planning and health program planning.
3. Understand the relationships among the concepts inherent in epidemiology, demography, community organization, and health planning.
4. Trace the development of comprehensive health planning activities and legislation in the United States and discuss trends that influenced this development.
5. Analyze the steps of the health program planning process.
6. Describe how to work with communities as partners to solve contemporary health problems.
7. Discuss the use of health planning concepts in community health nursing practice.
8. Discuss barriers to health planning.

## KEY TERMS

Assessment Protocol for Excellence in Public Health (APEX/PH)
Asset assessment
Basic Priority Rating System
Block grant
Categorical grants
CDC's framework for program evaluation

Community Health Improvement Process (CHIP)
Comprehensive health planning
Formative evaluation
Health program planning
Health resource inventory
Outcomes
Partnership process

Planned Approach to Community Health (PATCH)
PEARL factors
Planning
Policy development
PRECEDE/PROCEED Model
Program efficiency
Resource assessment
Summative evaluation

---

*Predetermine the objectives you want to accomplish.*
*Think big, act big, and set out to accomplish big results.*

MARK VICTOR HANSEN

Chapter 3 describes how the community is the client for the community health nurse and discusses the importance of identifying aggregates at risk within the community. Classically aggregates, or populations, have been defined as groups of persons who have one or more shared personal or environmental characteristics (Williams, 1977). Some of these characteristics may put these persons

at risk for morbidity, mortality, and/or social problems. For example, persons who are exposed to family violence are at risk for injury and death. A distinguishing feature of the community health nursing practice area is a focus on interventions that protect and promote the health of aggregates at risk and communities. This chapter describes how nurses put that concept into practice.

Examples of aggregate-focused problems that contemporary community health nurses frequently encounter include AIDS, crack-addicted neonates, family violence, child abuse, and drug and alcohol abuse. In addition, too many people face limited family incomes, lack of access to health

**481**

care, hunger, and homelessness. These are awesome problems that require interventions different from those developed by nurses working with individual clients and family members. Community health nurses use community-based health planning processes to address these problems. They are involved in policy decisions that address the environmental, social, and behavioral variables making an impact on the health of families, populations or aggregates, and communities.

Lillian Wald, the founder of modern community health nursing, was a role model for policy advocacy behavior (see Chapter 1). She described how nurses helped make the community a positive environment that facilitates the self-actualization of individuals through the life span. In describing how nurses from the Henry Street Settlement House functioned, she wrote that the nurses are "enlisted in the crusade against disease and for the promotion of right living, beginning even before life itself is brought forth, through infancy, into school life, on through adolescence.... The nurse is being socialized, made part of a community plan for the communal health. Her contribution to human welfare, unified and harmonized with those powers which aim at care and prevention, rather than at police power and punishment, forms part of the great policy of bringing human beings to a higher level" (Wald, 1915, p. 60). Wald noted early in her career that working with political leaders to change the social and physical environment was as important as helping individuals modify their health behaviors. This activist changed child labor laws, helped build playgrounds, and established school nursing, all examples of how political and social structures influence the health of communities, aggregates, families, and individuals.

Community organizations using health planning processes facilitate work with communities as partners, assisting and motivating aggregates to bring about changes. These changes are designed to solve health problems and to create environments that prevent health problems from developing. Using this approach to deal with health concerns means that community health nurses shift from a one-to-one reactive model of care to a multidisciplinary, proactive, community-focused model that involves the community in problem identification and resolution. The nation's health agenda, *Healthy People 2010* (U.S. Department of Health and Human Services [USDHHS], 2000a) emphasizes the need for aggregate and community-based comprehensive health planning, guided by a multidisciplinary and lay partnership model for health.

## DEFINING HEALTH PLANNING

Health planning is an ongoing process whereby information about the nation, a state, or a local community is systematically collected and *used* to structure a health improvement plan that facilitates client empowerment for health action. "Planning is a systematic method of trying to attain explicit objectives for the future through the efficient and appropri-

ate use of resources, available now and in the future" (Green, 1999, p. 3).

The health planning process is a scientific problem-solving approach that helps a community evaluate and bring about specific changes for the purpose of improving the health status of the community. In community health practice, this approach is used on a community-wide level to develop "healthy public policy" that supports health promotion and disease prevention efforts (Green, 1999; Kickbusch, Draper, O'Neill, 1990). "Such policies are articulated not only in laws and regulations that govern the behavior of individuals but also in practice guidelines for health care providers, educational requirements for health professionals, and reimbursement schemes for health care" (Scherl, Noren, Osterweis, 1992, p. 3).

Community-wide planning helps provide a framework for the development of population-focused interventions and the coordination of client and provider health action efforts. For example, the *Healthy People 2010* documents, which have been developed at all levels of government, provide direction for targeting interventions for aggregates at risk as well as resources to resolve priority health problems.

Community-wide health planning is known as *comprehensive health planning* or *policy planning*. In the community setting, planning also occurs at the organizational level to develop strategies for thriving in a competitive environment (*strategic* and *visionary planning*) and to develop health programs and services (*health program planning* or *operational planning*). This chapter expands discussion on comprehensive health planning and health program planning.

## COMPREHENSIVE HEALTH PLANNING: HISTORICAL AND CURRENT PERSPECTIVES

Comprehensive health planning began as a *voluntary movement* in the early 1930s with the establishment of area-wide hospital planning councils. These councils were formed to raise and allocate money for hospital construction and modernization. Their membership included lay persons involved in philanthropic and civic affairs and professionals such as hospital administrators (National Academy of Sciences, 1980, p. 13).

Formalized government involvement in health planning became evident in the mid-1930s. At that time, a provision of the Social Security Act of 1935 provided aid to states for maternal child health and disease control service programming with the stipulation that states develop plans on how to use this aid (Bergwall, Reeves, Woodside, 1973). Since that time, most federal legislation that provides aid to states for the development of health services or the construction of health facilities has commonly required state planning activities. A classic example of this was the Hill-Burton Act. This legislation authorized grants to states for statewide planning for hospitals and public health centers and construction grants for health facilities. An annual updated state plan was required to maintain Hill-Burton funding. The Heart Disease, Cancer, and Stroke Amendments of 1965, known as The Regional Medical Program, also had planning requirements. It involved professionals in health planning for regional centers for treatment of heart disease, cancer, and stroke.

Initially, comprehensive health planning was primarily reactive. Only after a health problem affected a large number of people was there an attempt to solve it. However, beginning with some of President Johnson's "Great Society" programs in the 1960s, the emphasis in health planning became more comprehensive, with the recognition that all components of the community influenced the health status of the community. Consistent with this belief, consumer participation in the planning process was stressed. The National Commission on Community Health Services (1966) summarized these beliefs in its classic report, *Health Is a Community Affair.*

Action planning for health should be community wide in area, continuous in nature, comprehensive in scope, all-inclusive in design, coordinative in function, and adequately staffed. . . . The Community Action Studies Project (CASP) analysis especially emphasizes the relationship of one aspect of community health to another, and the interrelatedness of health with the total social, educational, and economic enterprise. Action-planning should be all-inclusive in design—a partnership between private, voluntary, and governmental sectors representing all elements of the community, including consumers as well as providers of services, civic leaders, and, importantly, health professionals (pp. 168-169).

Based on these beliefs, two types of legislation designed to improve the health status of communities emerged— community development and health planning legislation.

## Community Development Legislation

Through the Economic Opportunity Act of 1964, the federal government supported broad community development initiatives to make a comprehensive attack on poverty. These initiatives had a "healthy cities" focus. They established community action agencies that worked to revitalize distressed communities and to help people in these communities obtain needed education, social services, and housing. Some of them focused on improving the physical environment. Although the Office of Economic Opportunity eventually disbanded, local community action agencies continue to operate (General Accounting Office [GAO], 1995b, p. 7).

Private sector efforts, especially private foundation support, also have advanced community revitalization programs since the early 1960s. At least 2500 private nonprofit Community Development Corporations around the country focus their efforts on improving distressed geographical areas (GAO, 1995b). However, many of them do not offer comprehensive services. It is the hope of planners that the Empowerment Zones and Enterprise Communities Program, adopted in 1992 under the Omnibus Budget Reconciliation Act, will continue to promote comprehensive community revitalization efforts (GAO, 1995b). Currently

the Healthy Communities Initiatives are seen as powerful models for community improvement and revitalization (Clark, 2000; Minkler, 2000; Sharpe, Greaney, Lee, et al., 2000; Wallerstein, 2000).

## Health Planning Legislation

Comprehensive health service planning efforts ran parallel to the community revitalization efforts. The Comprehensive Health Planning and Public Health Service Amendment of 1966 was passed to enable states and communities to plan for better use of health resources. Because this legislation was not effective, other legislative action was developed in the mid-1970s (Reeves, Coile, 1989).

The National Health Planning and Resources Development Act of 1974 consolidated several health planning and development programs. This act was passed to facilitate the development of a national health planning policy and to augment state and local health planning. The goals of this act were improved accessibility of health care services, curtailment of rising costs, and monitoring of the quality of care being provided. The National Health Planning and Resources Development Act emphasized the need for strong local planning and control over the development of services. Additionally, it mandated consumer and third-party payer participation in the planning process.

The antiregulatory philosophy of the Reagan administration advanced the belief that the control of health planning and service development should occur at the local level. The Omnibus Budget Reconciliation Act (OBRA) of 1981 ended the federal mandate for planning under the National Health Planning and Resources Development Act. It also consolidated federal programs and reorganized how federal expenditures were allocated to the states under its *block grant* provision. OBRA created 9 block grants by consolidating more than 50 categorical grant programs and 3 existing block grants; 4 of the 9 block grants were for health, 3 were for social services, 1 was for education, and 1 was for community development (GAO, 1995a, p. 27). The four areas of health covered by block grants were maternal and child health; preventive health and health services; alcohol, drug abuse, and mental health; and primary care.

A **block grant** is a funding mechanism through which the federal government supports state and local health programs. In contrast to **categorical grants,** which specifically designate how the funds are to be spent, the block grant provides a lump sum of money to states and allows states to determine how these monies will be spent. This type of federal aid is designed to provide states greater discretion in the use of federal funds. However, state flexibility was reduced over time as funding constraints were added to the block grants (GAO, 1995a).

By the end of the 1980s it became evident that the focus on cost containment was affecting health planning activities at state and local levels. The Committee for the Study of the Future of Public Health (Institute of Medicine [IOM], 1988) identified that "increases in public health spending were not keeping pace with the growing need for assessment, policy development, and assurance activities demanded by the range of immediate and impending crises and ongoing problems in public health" (p. 80). Once again, health planning was becoming primarily reactive, responding to the issue of the moment rather than benefiting from careful assessment processes (IOM, 1988). The IOM Committee challenged the nation to strengthen essential public health activities to improve the health and well-being of the American people.

## COMPREHENSIVE HEALTH PLANNING: THE 1990s AND BEYOND

The 1990s produced dramatic changes in health planning activities and legislation. Experience with the abolishment of the national health planning framework, created under the National Health Planning and Resources Development Act, showed that the "free market" of business had neither controlled costs nor had it adequately addressed the health problems of the American people (Reeves, Coile, 1989). Major debates about the most effective and cost-efficient way to meet the health needs of all occurred at every level of government and among professional and lay advocacy groups during the 1990s. These debates continue.

The health planning experiences in the 1980s also showed that some form of external oversight and guidance for health planning was essential. During this time, the type and degree of health planning activities at state and local levels became very diverse. Coalitions, appointed state and local health committees, and health task forces increasingly emerged to provide a needed structure for community health planning efforts (Reeves, Coile, 1989).

Health planning experiences during the 1980s and early 1990s highlighted the need to reexamine the nation's health planning efforts. Many of the visions of the 1960s National Commission on Community Health Services are reemerging as central themes in health planning. Currently the concepts of comprehensive community health status assessment and action, professional and consumer partnerships for health, and community revitalization are being emphasized. Importantly, planning efforts are focusing on the significant influence that environmental factors have on health. In contrast to the 1960s' emphasis on how changes in health services delivery will resolve community problems, the current health planning focus is on identifying *community health assets* (Doyle, Ward, 2001; Kretzmann, McKnight, 1993; McKenzie, Smeltzer, 2001) and *needs* (Altschuld, Witkin, 2000). Health planning efforts also are focused on mobilizing the community for health action.

As discussed in Chapter 2, many international and national movements have reoriented health planning and policy toward prevention during the past decade. "Two phrases that capture the essence of a new vision for health care in the 1990s [were] *promoting health* and *preventing disease...*

A significant catalyst for action has been *Healthy People 2000: National Health Promotion and Disease Prevention Objectives*" (Scherl, Noren, Osterweis, 1992, p. 1). The Healthy People Initiative continues to stimulate health action across the nation (USDHHS, 2000a).

## HEALTHY PEOPLE INITIATIVE PROMOTES HEALTH PLANNING

The Healthy People Initiative, the nation's vision for improving the health status of all citizens, has provided an impetus for government agencies, private organizations and businesses, and local communities to strengthen their community development and health planning efforts. This mandate created a framework for monitoring the nation's changing health status and for guiding public health policy at all levels of government (Stoto, 1992; USDHHS, 2000a). "*Healthy People 2010* outlines a comprehensive, nationwide health promotion and disease prevention agenda" (USDHHS, 2000a, p. 1).

The *Healthy People 2010* initiative challenges states and local communities to develop their own *Healthy People 2010* objectives and action plans to address these objectives. It is expected that these governmental units will carry out the core public health functions—assessment, policy development, and assurance (IOM, 1988)—to promote healthy community living (see Chapter 4).

The *Healthy People 2010* objectives help local communities advance comprehensive community and aggregate-focused health planning efforts. These objectives assist local agencies to increase awareness and understanding of how problems and activities at the local level reflect national and state community health problems. They also aid local agencies in formulating a clear vision about local community needs, in advocating for budget or resource prioritization, and in building partnerships for health action (Oberle, Baker, Magenheim, 1994; USDHHS, 2000a).

## COMMUNITY DIAGNOSIS

To facilitate the development of *Healthy People 2010* plans, states and local communities complete a population-based community health status assessment. Understanding the concepts presented in Chapter 14 relative to community diagnosis, along with the epidemiological variables of person, place, and time, is essential to answer the key questions that health planners must ask as they assess health planning needs. *Person* involves the "who" of community diagnosis. The cultural, ethnic, psychosocial, spiritual, and biological characteristics of the person variable must be considered when health services are planned. These characteristics influence how persons define health and illness and use health services. For example, when a population narrowly defines health as the absence of disease, the population may respond more favorably to curative health services than preventive health services.

*Place* describes the setting where services are planned, which may be rural, urban, inner city, or suburbia. When the characteristics of place are examined, the availability, accessibility, and cost of present services should be analyzed. Size is also a factor that needs to be considered. A community with 1000 residents will have different needs than a community with a population of 1 million. The cost to deliver health services, the kinds of personnel and financial resources that are available, the scope of the program, and the complexity involved in planning and implementing services are some factors that vary among populations of different sizes (McKenzie, Smeltzer, 2001).

*Time* in relation to urgency also needs to be considered during the health planning process. If the problem under consideration, for example, is an emergency such as influenza among aging citizens, immediate action must be taken. Other health problems such as accident prevention may not require immediate action but can necessitate action over time.

It is also important to determine the appropriate time to initiate the health program under consideration. Analyzing community values and attitudes, availability of resources, and cost-benefit factors aids the health planner in determining the appropriate time to begin health-planning intervention.

Examining a community's developmental history is another significant factor to examine when considering timing. An older, inner-city ethnic community might have more established values and attitudes about health and illness than a newer community such as a prospering subdivision. Analyzing how values and attitudes have evolved over time in an older community assists the health planner in identifying key community leaders. Community leaders should be actively engaged in developing interventions that would be acceptable to community residents. The Community Health Improvement Process provides a framework for involving community leaders and residents in diagnosing community needs and planning, implementing, and evaluating intervention to meet these needs.

## Framework for Community Health Improvement

A recent IOM report (Durch, Bailey, Stoto, 1997) has provided a framework that can be used to guide local communities as they develop, implement, and evaluate Healthy People community improvement action plans. This framework, the **Community Health Improvement Process** or **CHIP**, is presented in Figure 15-1. CHIP is a tool used "for developing a shared vision and supporting a planned and integrated approach to improve community health" (Durch, Bailey, Stoto, 1997, p. 5).

The community health improvement process encourages local public health agencies and community groups to form a community health coalition for the purpose of promoting health improvement action. A CHIP involves two princi-

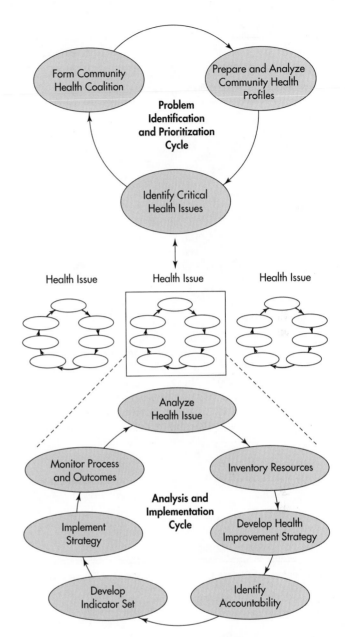

**FIGURE 15-1** The community health improvement process (CHIP). (From Durch JS, Bailey LA, Stoto MA, editors: *Improving health in the community: a role for performance monitoring,* Washington, DC, 1997, National Academy Press, p. 79.)

pal interacting cycles (see Figure 15-1). The first cycle focuses on problem identification and prioritization. The second cycle is designed to analyze pressing community health issues, promote the development of intervention strategies to address these issues, and monitor the implementation process and outcomes (Durch, Bailey, Stoto, 1997). An important step of CHIP is the development of indicators sets to help link interventions with outcomes (see Figure 15-1). This, in turn, aids a community improvement team or community coalition in monitoring performance and outcomes.

**TABLE 15-1**

*Criteria for Health Planning Priority Setting*

| CRITERIA | POTENTIAL EVALUATION PARAMETERS |
|----------|--------------------------------|
| Size of problem | Percentage of population with health problem |
| | Population to be considered (entire population or a target group) |
| Seriousness of the problem | *Urgency*—emergent nature of problem; importance relative to the public (epidemic/endemic, community's perception of problem) |
| | *Severity*—premature mortality; years of potential life lost; disability; community beliefs about seriousness of the health problem |
| | *Economic loss*—to the community (city/county/state); to the individual |
| | *Involvement of others*—potential impact on populations (measles) or impact on family groups (child abuse, homicide) |
| Estimated effectiveness of interventions | Is there an acceptable preventive/treatment intervention? |
| | Does the intervention improve the likelihood of favorable health outcomes? |
| | What is the potential adverse effect(s) of the interventions (e.g., screening tests)? |
| | What proportion of the target population can be reached by the intervention? |

From Centers for Disease Control and Prevention (CDC): *A guide for establishing public health priorities,* Atlanta, undated, CDC, p. 4; Pickett GE, Hanlon JJ: *Public health administration and practice,* ed 9, St Louis, 1990, Mosby, pp. 226-227.

**TABLE 15-2**

*Criteria for Scoring Size of a Health Problem*

| PERCENT OF POPULATION WITH HEALTH PROBLEM | "SIZE OF PROBLEM" RATING |
|-------------------------------------------|--------------------------|
| 25% or more | 9 or 10 |
| 10% through 24.9% | 7 or 8 |
| 1% through 9.9% | 5 or 6 |
| 0.1% through 0.9% | 3 or 4 |
| 0.01% through 0.09% | 1 or 2 |
| Less than 0.01% (1/10,000) | 0 |

From Centers for Disease Control and Prevention (CDC): *A guide for establishing public health priorities,* Atlanta, undated, CDC, p. 3.

Examples of indicator sets were presented in Chapter 14 (see Boxes 14-7 and 14-8).

The document, *Tracking Healthy People 2010,* will greatly enhance the nation's and local communities' abilities to monitor progress in achieving the *Healthy People 2010* objectives (USDHHS, 2000b). This document identifies a measure or indicator for each of the *Healthy People 2010* objectives for assessing progress toward or away from goal achievement.

## Setting Priorities for Health Planning

Throughout the nation, local communities are using *Healthy People 2010* plans to establish priorities for the effective and efficient use of scarce health resources. This has become an especially difficult task because communities are facing an increasing range of pressing problems that require community-based interventions (Centers for Disease Control and Prevention [CDC], undated).

A review of the literature reveals that a common set of criteria is frequently used for setting health planning priorities. This set of criteria is labeled either the Hanlon Method or the **Basic Priority Rating System** (CDC, undated; Pickett, Hanlon, 1990). These criteria and potential evaluation parameters for each are presented in Table 15-1. Following is the formula for establishing a numerical score when these criteria are used (CDC, undated; Pickett, Hanlon, 1990):

$$\text{Basic Priority Rating} = (A + 2B) \times C$$
$$A = \text{size of the problem}$$
$$B = \text{seriousness of the problem}$$
$$C = \text{estimated effectiveness of interventions}$$

This formula reflects that the *seriousness of the problem* and the *effectiveness of interventions* receive a higher priority than the size of the problem.

Tables 15-2, 15-3, and 15-4 provide examples of how to obtain a numerical rating when using the Basic Priority Rating (BPR) formula. How to rank problems based on the

**TABLE 15-3**

*Criteria for Scoring Seriousness of a Health Problem*

| HOW SERIOUS | "SERIOUSNESS" RATING |
|-------------|----------------------|
| Very serious (e.g., very high death rate; premature mortality; great impact on others; etc.) | 9 or 10 |
| Serious | 6, 7, or 8 |
| Moderately serious | 3, 4, or 5 |
| Not serious | 0, 1, or 2 |

From Centers for Disease Control and Prevention (CDC): *A guide for establishing public health priorities,* Atlanta, undated, CDC, p. 5.

BPR system is illustrated in Table 15-5. The ranking varies from one community to another, based on community characteristics. One community may rank a health problem a number 1, while a neighboring community may rank the same problem a number 5. These rankings are based on both quantitative data and qualitative perceptions of the problem. For example, a local community may rank motor vehicle accidents among its youth higher than another community, if the rate of mortality from motor vehicle accidents among people 15 to 24 years has significantly increased over the past year. The local community's ranking might be influenced by the community's emotional reactions to the premature death of its youth, as well as by statistical data (cause-specific and age-specific mortality rates).

After rating the size and seriousness of the problem and intervention effectiveness, a group of factors commonly known as the PEARL factors are examined. These factors—*propriety, economics, acceptability, resources,* and *legality*—do not relate directly to the health problem but significantly influence a community health agency's ability to address the problem (CDC, undated). The questions addressed by the PEARL factors are presented in Table 15-6. "Yes-or-no" scoring is used with the PEARL factors. Health problems that receive a *no* answer to any of the PEARL questions are either dropped from consideration for the present or receive further investigation to determine if the PEARL factor can be corrected (CDC, undated).

The PEARL factors help a community health coalition examine the nature of the problem as well as the adequacy

**TABLE 15-4**

*Criteria for Scoring Effectiveness of Intervention*

| EFFECTIVENESS OF INTERVENTIONS | "EFFECTIVENESS" RATING |
|---|---|
| Very effective (80%-100% effective) (e.g., vaccine) | 9 or 10 |
| Relatively effective (60%-80% effective) | 7 or 8 |
| Effective (40%-80% effective) (e.g., laser treatment for diabetic retinopathy to prevent blindness) | 5 or 6 |
| Moderately effective (20%-40% effective) | 3 or 4 |
| Relatively ineffective (5%-20% effective) (e.g., smoking cessation interventions) | 1 or 2 |
| Almost entirely ineffective (less than 5% effective) | 0 |

From Centers for Disease Control and Prevention (CDC): *A guide for establishing public health priorities,* Atlanta, undated, CDC, p. 6.

**TABLE 15-6**

*PEARL Component of Priority Setting*

| PEARL FACTORS | QUESTIONS CONSIDERED* |
|---|---|
| **P** = Propriety | Is the problem one that falls within the agency's overall scope of operation? |
| **E** = Economic feasibility | Does it make economic sense to address the problem? Are there economic consequences if the problem is not addressed? |
| **A** = Acceptability | Will the community and/or target population accept a program to address the problem? |
| **R** = Resources | Are, or should, resources be available to address the problem? |
| **L** = Legality | Do current laws allow the problem to be addressed? |

From Centers for Disease Control and Prevention (CDC): *A guide for establishing public health priorities,* Atlanta, undated, CDC, p. 5.
*Health problems that receive a *no* answer to any of the PEARL questions are either dropped from consideration for the present or receive further investigation to determine if the PEARL factor can be corrected.

**TABLE 15-5**

*Problem Ranking Using the Basic Priority Rating (BPR)*

| HEALTH PROBLEM | COMPONENTS | | | BPR SCORE | |
|---|---|---|---|---|---|
| | A | B | C | (A + 2B) × C | RANK |
| Access to preventive care | 6 | 9 | 7 | 168.00 | 4 |
| Teen pregnancy | 5 | 9 | 2 | 46.00 | 6 |
| Uninsured | 6 | 8 | 9 | 198.00 | 2 |
| Ground water protection | 9 | 9 | 9 | 243.00 | 1 |
| Sexually transmitted diseases | 7 | 8 | 6 | 138.00 | 5 |
| Motor vehicle accidents | 6 | 9 | 8 | 192.00 | 3 |

From Centers for Disease Control and Prevention (CDC): *A guide for establishing public health priorities,* Atlanta, undated, CDC, p. 7.

of resources and the community's interest in addressing the problem in question. Green and Kreuter (1999) stress that when prioritizing health needs, it is important to examine the "changeability" of the health issue, as perceived by community residents and health professionals working in collaboration with these residents. Some health issues may be highly important, based on the nature of the problem. However, if the community will not accept a program to "change" the situation, resources should be directed at more "changeable" health situations. Changeable situations are determined in partnership with community residents.

## THE COMMUNITY HEALTH NURSE AND HEALTH PLANNING

Nurses have played a significant role in promoting action for health. It was a nurse, in cooperation with a local community, who started the Healthy Cities initiative (see Chapter 3) in the United States (Flynn, Ray, Rider, 1994). Nurses are assuming leadership roles at all levels of government in carrying out the core public health functions of assessment, policy development, and assurance (ASTDN, 1998; Berkowitz, 1995, 2000; Conley, 1995). Nurses also are assuming leadership roles in the new emerging health care structures, where they advocate for quality client services (Keller, Strohschein, Lia-Hoagberg, et al., 1998; Storfjell, Mitchell, Daly, 1997).

The community health nurse is particularly well qualified to work with community citizens in carrying out population-based health planning. Each day the nurse sees the needs of aggregates at risk within the community through home visits, clinics, classes, schools, and other nursing activities. She or he is able to obtain a composite picture of the health needs of an aggregate such as lack of prenatal care, family planning services, or public transportation. The nurse's continual, comprehensive contact with the community makes her or him knowledgeable about available resources, gaps in service provision, and unhealthy environmental conditions.

Nurses usually see only the "tip of the iceberg" when diagnosing problems common to families in their caseloads. What has been assessed, however, can become the basis for an epidemiological investigation of community needs. Epidemiological studies examine groups of families in an agency's geographical area. They frequently involve investigation of needs in census tracts or specific political boundaries such as cities, towns, or counties. "Public health nurses provide a critical linkage between epidemiological data and clinical understanding of health and illness as it is experienced in peoples' lives" (American Public Health Association [APHA], 1996, p. 3). This linkage assists planners in validating community needs, strengths, and capacity.

Nurses also provide a critical linkage between providers and consumers. They articulate community needs to health planners and policy makers and advocate for essential health policies and programs (American Nurses Associa-

tion [ANA], 1999; APHA, 1996). Additionally, nurses plan, implement, and evaluate population-focused health services (ANA, 1999; Diekemper, SmithBattle, Drake, 1999; Keller, Strohschein, Lia-Hoagberg, et al., 1998). Examples of health planning interventions commonly implemented by community health nurses are the planning and implementation of health screenings at the worksite or health fairs in schools, shopping malls, and other settings, and the development of clinic services for the uninsured and other underserved populations. Health planning opportunities are abundant in the community setting.

## PROGRAM PLANNING FOR HEALTH*

Program planning for aggregates at risk involves the same steps used in the individual and family-centered nursing process: assessing, analyzing, planning, implementing, and evaluating (Table 15-7). Basic concepts of epidemiology, biostatistics, and demography (see Chapter 11) and management principles (see Chapter 24) are used to refine decision-making and diagnostic skills and to expand intervention options during the program planning process.

The emphasis in the program planning model is on the health of aggregates at risk and the community as a whole, and problems, solutions, and interventions are defined on this level. In contrast, the clinical practice model focuses on the individual as the unit of service. During the program planning process, the community and aggregates at risk are viewed as the client and a vehicle for social action (McKenzie, Smeltzer, 2001).

Another distinguishing feature of community and aggregate-based program planning is its focus on the prevention of existing health problems in the population being served, as well as on the promotion of health and well-being. The goals are to have "healthy people in a healthy world" and to "make prevention a way of life, not just an idea" (CDC, 1995, pp. 1, 5). Community planning strategies that assist consumers and health professionals to achieve these goals are addressed in this chapter and Chapters 16 through 23.

### Trends Affecting Health Program Planning

Having an understanding of the demographic, epidemiological, and health care delivery trends in the United States helps community residents identify priority health needs and plan programs that meet these needs. Prevailing attitudes, as well as these trends, influence both the services needed and the organization of these services. Box 15-1 pre-

---

*Christine DeGregorio, PhD, while a University of Rochester doctoral student in political science, first wrote the phases and steps of the community planning process as outlined here. Much of the content and many of the illustrations in this section reflect her thinking and creativity. It is used with her permission.

**TABLE 15-7**

*Comparison of the Nursing, Epidemiology, and Health Care Planning Processes*

| NURSING PROCESS | EPIDEMIOLOGICAL PROCESS | HEALTH PLANNING PROCESS |
|---|---|---|
| Assessing<br>Data collection to determine nature of client problems | I. Determine the nature, extent, and scope of the problem<br>　A. Natural life history of condition<br>　B. Determinants influencing condition<br>　　1. Primary data (essential agent)<br>　　　a. Parasite, bacterium, or virus<br>　　　b. Nutrition<br>　　　c. Psychosocial factor<br>　　2. Contributory data<br>　　　a. Agent<br>　　　b. Host<br>　　　c. Environment<br>　C. Distribution patterns<br>　　1. Person<br>　　2. Place<br>　　3. Time<br>　D. Condition frequencies<br>　　1. Prevalence<br>　　2. Incidence<br>　　3. Other biostatistical measurements | Preplanning<br>Assessment<br>Data collection to determine needs of populations and the community as a whole<br>Assessment of resources |
| Analyzing | II. Formulate tentative hypothesis(es) | Development of problem statement, goals, expected outcomes |
| Formulation of nursing diagnoses or hypotheses | III. Collect and analyze further data to test hypothesis(es) | Policy development |
| Planning | IV. Plan for control | Plan strategies to achieve expected outcomes |
| Implementing | V. Implement control plan | Implementation |
| Evaluating | VI. Evaluate control plan | Evaluation |
| Revising or terminating | VII. Make appropriate report | |
| | VIII. Conduct research | |

sents examples of trends that are influencing health planning efforts. An examination of these trends makes it clear that the health care delivery system and local communities are dealing with unprecedented demands that require creative health planning and programming.

## THE PROGRAM PLANNING PROCESS

After identifying priority health needs, local health agency improvement teams will initiate the health planning process, in partnership with the community, to address community needs and gaps in service delivery. As illustrated in Table 15-7, the program planning process is orderly and logical. It is a tool that helps those using it to organize large amounts of community data that describe community assets, strengths, and problems, as well as health planning solutions. For purposes of discussion, the program planning process is divided into five phases: *preplanning, assessment, policy development, implementation,* and *evaluation.* Each of

these phases will be separately described, but in reality they are overlapping and inseparable. For example, in practice, evaluative activities may occur during any phase of the process or goals may be altered when resource implications of different alternatives are discussed, with the realization that original goals were too ambitious or overly cautious (Green, 1999).

### The Preplanning Phase

The preplanning phase builds a foundation for the rest of the process. Before proceeding with health planning efforts, it is crucial that planners test their ideas and validate that what they perceive as a problem is also seen by others as a problem severe enough to warrant changes. "Validation amounts to double checking, or making sure that an identified need is the real need" (McKenzie, Smeltzer, 2001).

"Planning an effective program is more difficult than implementing it. Planning, implementing, and evaluating programs are all interrelated, but good planning skills are

**BOX 15-1**

*Examples of Trends Affecting Health Care Planning*

*Epidemiological Trends*

- *Conditions of aging* such as cardiovascular disease or cognitive impairments are placing increased demands on the health care system.
- *Diseases of lifestyle and behavior* such as substance abuse, homelessness, and domestic violence are major threats to health and require comprehensive health action.
- *Technology-related reduction in premature mortality* also has produced social, legal, and ethical dilemmas.
- *Current emerging and resurgent infectious diseases* are producing immeasurable human suffering and health care costs.
- *Environmental factors* that predispose to and/or cause disease are increasing and are causing a heavy demand on health care resources.
- *A recognition that prevention of disease* is much more complex than once thought. Scientific advances have helped health care professionals recognize that genetic predisposition interacts with multiple environmental factors to produce or prevent disease.
- *Health disparities among different segments* of the population are presenting a range of health improvement challenges.

*Demographic Trends*

- *The graying of American society* will increase the demand for health services well into the twenty-first century.

- *Increasing consumer involvement* is impacting the demand for service and influencing the nature of consumer professional relationships.
- *Growing ethnic diversity* among the young and the old in America increases the need to bridge the cultural gap between traditional and nontraditional intervention strategies.
- *Significant changes in the family structure* influence both client needs and service delivery strategies.

*Health Care Delivery Trends—Pew Commission*

- *A system* more managed with better integration of services and financing.
- *A system* more accountable to those who purchase and use health services.
- *A system* more aware of and responsive to the needs of enrolled populations.
- *A system* able to use fewer resources more effectively.
- *A system* more innovative and diverse in how it provides for health.
- *A system* less focused on treatment and more concerned with education, prevention, and care management.
- *A system* more oriented to improving the health of the entire population.
- *A system* more reliant on outcome data and evidence.

From Pew Health Professions Commission: *Critical challenges: revitalizing the health professions for the twenty-first century*, San Francisco, 1995, UCSF Center for the Health Professions, pp. 9-10; Pew Health Professions Commission: *Recreating health professional practice for a new century: the fourth report of the Pew Health Professions Commission*, San Francisco, 1998, UCSF Center for the Health Professions; Brownson RC, Kreuter MW: Future trends affecting public health: challenges and opportunities, *J Public Health Management Practice* 3(2):49-60, 1997.

prerequisite to programs worthy of evaluation" (Brekson, Harvey, Lancaster, 1998, p. 145). The planning organization and environment needs to be "tested" to ascertain whether sufficient resources and commitment are available to devote to the work required to bring about the change.

The preplanning phase has six steps: (1) obtaining community and consumer support and participation, (2) development of a broadly defined problem statement, (3) development of a goal statement, (4) delineation of a timetable that accounts for the phases of the process, (5) assessment of resources for the task that needs to be accomplished, and (6) planning for data collection strategies to be used. Each of these steps helps build a framework needed for future planning activities.

OBTAINING COMMUNITY SUPPORT AND PARTICIPATION. Encouraging people to be involved in decision making that affects their quality of life helps ensure that programs will effectively address the health issues of concern. Environmental as well as individual client changes are often needed to reduce premature morbidity and mortality in a community.

Community support and participation are needed to make environmental changes. For example, teenagers can be taught the importance of wearing seat belts, driving the posted speed limits, and not drinking while driving. However, this behavior is enhanced by making environmental changes that increase road safety, such as decreasing hidden curves or installing adequate shoulders on the road.

A variety of models to promote community participation have been tested. Phrases including *community participation, community organization, community empowerment,* and *empowerment education* reflect the movement to have people "buy into" the changes needed for healthy living. Community organization activities are designed to stimulate conditions for change and to mobilize citizens and communities for health action. A major goal during this process is to facilitate community empowerment. As discussed in Chapters 2 and 3, to be empowered means that one (community, family, or individual) has the knowledge, skills, and capacity for effective and self-determined action (Courtney, 1995, p. 370; Courtney, Ballard, Fauver, et al., 1996, p. 180).

It is well supported that a partnership relationship that focuses on community assets and active client participation in the health planning process is needed to strengthen a community's capacity for self-care (ANA, 1999; ASTDN, 1998; Berkowitz, 2000; Bracht, 1999; Durch, Bailey, Stoto, 1997; Flynn, 1998). As stated previously, "a *partnership process* is the negotiated sharing of power between health professionals and individual family and/or community partners. These partners agree to be involved as active participants in the process of mutually determining goals and actions that promote health and well-being. The ultimate goal of the partnership process is to enhance the capacity of individual, family, and community partners to act more effectively on their own behalf" (Courtney, Ballard, Fauver, et al., 1996, p. 180). Active client participation, mutual goal-setting, and community capacity building are key goals during the health planning process. Although all clients may not wish to engage in a partnership relationship, it is important for the health care professional to develop a therapeutic relationship with clients, which strengthens clients' self-care capabilities.

"Mobilizing community partnerships and action to identify and solve health problems" (CDC, 1995) is viewed as an essential public health service. The process of facilitating community empowerment through a partnership relationship can occur in various ways. Schlaff (1991), in a prize-winning idea for a Secretary's Award for Innovation in Health Promotion and Disease Prevention, described an ideal scenario in one city: a health center worked with the neighborhood council to deal with health problems. The council was an elected body of residents and activists representing the community. The health center director reported directly to the council, and working with them were lay community health workers who reflected the ethnic and cultural diversity of the community. Community health workers carried out health education in homes, and local people assisted planners in accurately defining problems that needed correction. The program combined the use of community organization activities, efforts to form organizational structures involving members of the community, and the use of lay health workers who lived in the community where they worked.

Another illustration of facilitating community empowerment to change both the health behavior of individuals and their collective health is the Abbotsford Community Nursing Center in Philadelphia. The Center is located in a tenant-managed public housing development and delivers primary health services ranging from prenatal to geriatric care. Need for the services offered was in part based on a resident-administered survey that defined the major health issues in the community. Residents have control of the 12-member board that makes final decisions about program design, hiring of personnel, and policy. Residents of the project are hired to be the outreach workers, drivers, security personnel, and receptionists. Use of these resources puts money directly back into the community being served and also brings information about the community to the Center. The outreach workers visit households in the development on a regular basis, provide information on health education and prevention issues, and follow up on missed appointments and concerns such as prenatal and postnatal difficulties. The Center is *community driven*, which means that the residents have control both over the resources and ownership in the results of the program (Resources for Human Development, Inc., and the Abbottsford Homes Tenant Management Corporation, undated). This behavior illustrates well the first step of program planning: obtaining community and consumer support and participation.

## Stop and Think About It

You are a public health nurse working for a county health department in an urban community. Your town newspaper recently highlighted a local hospital's annual report that addressed the increasing prevalence of childhood asthma and challenged community residents to address this problem. With whom might you network or partner to determine the causes of asthma in your community? Where might you go to obtain more information about the extent of this problem in your community?

**DEVELOPMENT OF A PROBLEM STATEMENT.** A problem is a condition that is sufficiently distressing that change to bring relief is desired or sought. An example of a broadly defined problem statement from which policy development could begin might be the following: "Deaths from motor vehicle accidents for people 15 to 24 years of age in Jones County have substantially increased over the past year." This statement has a broad, yet clear, focus. All involved in the planning process would know that the concern is increased motor vehicle accidents for a certain age group in a specific area in a given year. The identification of a community problem is often the initial stimulus for developing a health action partnership.

**DEVELOPMENT OF A GOAL STATEMENT.** A goal is a general statement of intent or purpose that provides guidance for the activities that are to take place to address the identified problem. A goal emanating from the above problem statement might be, "Jones County citizens will work toward reducing the rate of fatalities from motor vehicle accidents among people 15 to 24 years of age by 10% in 3 years."

**DELINEATION OF A TIMETABLE.** To develop a realistic timetable that accounts for the remaining phases of the process, planners must have a general idea of what they plan to accomplish in the months ahead. After a specific goal is delineated, a health planning team or coalition conducts a preliminary discussion about what needs to be done to achieve the stated goal, and how the team can facilitate community participation for action. This discussion focuses on examining the nature of the tasks to be accomplished and what is feasible for community agencies and citizens to

**TABLE 15-8**

*Timetable for Jones County Health Department's Motor Vehicle Accident Project*

| | TIME IN MONTHS | | | | | | | | | | | |
|---|---|---|---|---|---|---|---|---|---|---|---|---|
| **PHASES** | **DEC** | **JAN** | **FEB** | **MAR** | **APR** | **MAY** | **JUNE** | **JULY** | **AUG** | **SEPT** | **OCT** | **NOV** |
| Preplanning | ___ | ___ | | | | | | | | | | |
| Assessment | | ___ | ___ | ___ | ___ | | | | | | | |
| Policy development | | | | ___ | ___ | ___ | ___ | ___ | | | | |
| Implementation | | | | | | | ___ | ___ | ___ | ___ | | |
| Evaluation | | | | | | | | | ___ | ___ | ___ | ___ |

do together, considering other priorities. Table 15-8 presents a sample health planning timetable. As discussed earlier, this table illustrates how the phases overlap and build on one another.

ASSESSMENT OF RESOURCES. Resources are needed to effectively carry out the planning process. A **resource assessment** is completed to determine whether current resources are adequate to accomplish program planning goals. "Resources include all the people and things needed to carry out the desired program" (McKenzie, Smeltzer, 2001, p. 219). Resources can be both internal (part of the organization) and external to an organization. Examples of resources include money, enthusiasm for the planning goals, community commitment, space in which to work, time, staff competencies, and experienced workers who have popularity, esteem, charisma, and commitment to the planning project. If resources are inadequate, planning goals may need to be altered, or strategies for obtaining sufficient resources will need to be developed.

One of the most valuable health planning resources is a committee that works toward the goal and that has power and authority to make decisions. To be viable, the committee must have tasks assigned to it that are crucial to the goal. The committee also must have an audience that expects results. Health planning committee members should be chosen on the basis of their interpersonal skills, their knowledge of the planning process and the community, and their commitment to the goals. Not every committee member will likely have all of these ingredients for successful planning. However, these ingredients must be present in some degree if successful planning is to take place.

An example of how community leaders (resources) are organized to deal with health problems is the collaborative Healthy Cities Indiana project that involves an academic setting, a professional organization, and six Indiana cities (Flynn, 1996; Flynn, Rider, Bailey, 1992). Healthy Cities Indiana is a community development approach to health promotion that involves a public-private partnership in developing healthier cities. Citizens participate in examining problems and solutions to enhance community capacity for health action. Community leadership development that supports health promotion is fundamental. Central to the

process is the local healthy city committee that represents the community. Its members come from various sectors of the community, including arts and culture, business, dentistry, education, employment, environment, finance, health and medical care, local government, media, parks, and other areas such as religion and transportation. The Healthy Cities Indiana program emphasizes experiential learning with these leaders, teaching what people want and need rather than setting goals for them. Emphasis is on strengthening a community's capacity to deal with its own perceived needs.

DEVELOPING DATA COLLECTION STRATEGIES. A plan needs to be developed so that the community health improvement team can assess the problem of concern. When developing this plan, the health improvement team focuses on *what* data are needed, from *whom* they need input, *how* they should obtain data, *who* will be responsible for collecting the data, and *when* the data collection process will be completed. For example, the Jones County Health Department planning team would want active participation from at least parents, students, teachers, legislators, police officers, and health providers when they examine vehicle fatalities among managers.

The plan for data collection should be written in sufficient detail so that all involved parties are clear about what needs to be accomplished. A worksheet such as the one presented in Table 15-9 facilitates the planning process.

At the conclusion of the preplanning phase, the planning team should have a good grasp of the problem, should be aware of the power and authority they have from the involved community, should know their strengths and limitations, and should have delineated the time frame for the process. The team is then ready to move to the next phase of the planning process: *assessment*.

## The Assessment Phase

In population-based planning, community health nurses "evaluate health trends and risk factors of population groups and help determine priorities for targeted interventions" (APHA, 1996, p. 3). Examining risk factors as well as health trends broadens the health planner's perspective and reflects a recognition that health problems are influenced by

**TABLE 15-9**

*Jones County Health Department Motor Vehicle Accident Project: Worksheet for Planning Data Collection Strategies*

*Goal:* Reduce the rate of motor vehicle accidents among 15- to 24-year-old youth in Jones County.
*Rationale for Goal:* The rate of fatal motor vehicle accidents among 15- to 24-year-old youth has increased 5% in the past year.

| TYPE OF DATA | DATA SOURCE | COLLECTION METHOD | TIME FOR COMPLETION | RESPONSIBILITY OF |
|---|---|---|---|---|
| *Data Collection Plan for Organizational Assessment* | | | | |
| Characteristics of accident victims | Clients | Personal interview | April 30, 2002 | Staff CHN |
| Epidemiological data | Accident reports and interview data | Review of reports | April 30, 2002 | Planning committee |
| | | | | |
| | | | | |
| *Data Collection Plan for Community Assessment* | | | | |
| Causes of accidents | Law enforcement officers | Mail survey | April 30, 2002 | Planning committee |
| Content covered in driver education courses | Driver education staff | Telephone interview | April 30, 2002 | Planning committee |
| | | | | |
| | | | | |
| | | | | |

multiple interrelated factors. Identifying the multiple forces that influence illness aids communities in developing appropriate interventions. "The ultimate aim of a [community] health plan is to improve levels of health rather than health services—although the latter may, of course, be an important means to that end" (Green, 1992, p. 167). A variety of interventions are used to improve the health of populations (Keller, Strohschein, Lia-Hoagberg, 1998; McKenzie, Smeltzer, 2001).

In population-based planning, three steps in the assessment phase of the health care planning process are completed. These are (1) conducting a needs and an asset assessment, (2) setting priorities upon which the planning committee can focus, and (3) specifying outcomes to which organizational and community resources can be applied. Each of these steps helps planners become more specific as they progress through the planning process.

CONDUCTING A NEEDS AND AN ASSET ASSESSMENT. During the program planning process, health planners build upon community data obtained during the community health status assessment process and use epidemiological concepts to identify the specific nature of the problem being addressed. When examining the nature and extent of the problem, health improvement teams discern trends over a specified period of years and cite the problem's significance, implications, and comparisons with norms or other standards.

Assessing a population's need relative to a circumscribed health problem (e.g., motor vehicle accidents, domestic violence, or teenage pregnancy) is a complex matter that goes beyond defining the population at risk. Needs are relative, and they are based on values, cultures, history, and the experiences of the individual, the family, and the community. Human needs are not easily identified but are diffuse and related. For example, motor vehicle deaths may be related to poor roads that are the result of a low-level tax base for road repairs, which is due to high unemployment. Human needs often change because the forces that influence need often change. A need today may not be a need next year.

Translating assessed needs into community programs and interventions is greatly influenced by the availability of human and financial resources in addition to the availability of technology. Thus an asset assessment that delineates population strengths, such as concerned citizen groups, service organizations, and social institutions is completed. Community assets are tapped throughout the program planning process to strengthen planning efforts.

A key component of an asset assessment is a **health resource inventory**. A health resource inventory identifies the type of services community agencies are providing in relation to the specified health problems. This inventory also examines service utilization patterns and barriers and perceived community need. Major goals for completing this inventory are to prevent duplication of services, identify potential partnerships for action, and determine effective strategies for increasing service utilization.

Box 15-2 presents a sample needs assessment tool designed to collect data about motor vehicle accidents in Jones County. It can be used as an assessment guide to collect data about other health needs in a community. How

and where health planners obtain data for a needs assessment is presented in Chapter 14.

**ASSET-FOCUSED AND NEED-BASED ASSESSMENT PROCESSES.** As discussed in Chapter 3, two frequently used processes for asset-oriented and need-based community assessments and community capacity building are the **Assessment Protocol for Excellence in Public Health (APEX/PH)** and **Planned Approach to Community Health (PATCH).** Both of these processes are designed to increase a community's capacity to plan, implement, and evaluate comprehensive, community-based health promotion or disease prevention programs. Both also promote citizen participation throughout the process and encourage assessment of community resources as well as needs.

The basic elements of APEX/PH and PATCH are presented in Chapter 3. Essentially, these models help a community assess and prioritize health needs; inventory community resources; and develop, implement, and evaluate community-wide interventions. It is anticipated that a community's capacity for health promotion will be strengthened when either of these models are used.

Another widely used model for community health assessment is Green and Kreuter's (1999) **PRECEDE/PROCEED Model.** This model is presented in depth in Chapter 12. Basically it provides an organizing framework for needs assessment as well as program planning. From a needs assessment perspective, it guides a community assessment team in examining variables that influence the community's quality of life (see Chapter 12). Data obtained during the assessment phase (PRECEDE) are used to plan, implement, and evaluate (PROCEED phase) programs for populations at risk.

The Community Health Improvement Process (CHIP), discussed previously in this chapter (see Figure 15-1), also provides a framework for asset and need assessments as well as population-focused planning and development activities. CHIP can help a community "take a comprehensive approach to maintaining and improving health, assessing its health needs, determining its resources and assets to promoting health, developing and implementing a strategy for action, and establishing where responsibility should lie for specific results" (Durch, Bailey, Stoto, 1997, p. 77). CHIP promotes community problem solving and active citizen involvement in the health planning process.

**SETTING PRIORITIES.** During this step in the assessment process, community health improvement teams make decisions about priorities for a *program* focus. To determine this focus, health planners examine the factors influencing problem occurrence, as well as gaps in existing services. Based on this exploration, a target population is identified and the nature of the problem is specifically defined. Using the motor vehicle mortality problem in Jones County among youth ages 15 to 24 years as an example, possible target groups could be all youth in the 15- to 24-year-old age span, or high school students ages 15 through 18, or young adults ages 18 through 24. Jones County program developers determined

---

● **BOX 15-2**

## A Sample Needs Assessment Tool: Motor Vehicle Accidents in Jones County

1. Community assessment of factors influencing fatalities from motor vehicle accidents
   a. Mortality data
   b. Morbidity data (incidence and prevalence) trends in recent years
   c. Demographic characteristics associated with mortality and morbidity (at-risk aggregates) in the defined community
   d. Local factors, such as road conditions, thought to influence trends
   e. Lifestyle of population groups
      (1) Environmental characteristics promoting health or illness
      (2) Economic base of population, income, and occupation
      (3) Lifestyle behaviors, such as drinking patterns, that influence health status
   f. Local perception of needs, problems, or priorities
2. Community resources
   a. Health services, strengths, and limitations
   b. Population coverage
   c. Usage rates for health services and barriers to use
3. Extent of knowledge related to the problem under consideration
   a. Magnitude of the problem in other populations: national and state data
   b. Etiological factors (*results* of case-control and cohort studies or theories)
   c. Physiological, sociological, and psychological processes related to pathology
   d. Inferences for *primary* prevention and early detection of problems
   e. Treatment potential
      (1) Inferences for therapeutic strategies at the individual, family, or aggregate level
      (2) Inferences for *secondary* and *tertiary* prevention (inferences regarding treatment potential are based on *results* of clinical trials and other types of evaluative studies or theories)

that priority should be placed on addressing the problem among high school students because the majority of fatal accidents were occurring among this age group. It was further established that addressing drinking and driving should be the program emphasis because all deaths among high school students were associated with excessive alcohol intake.

Analysis of health statistics aids planners in making decisions about priorities for a program focus. Criteria similar to those previously discussed in this chapter also are used to guide decision making regarding priorities. Green (1999) cautions planners to be aware of the danger of "paralysis by analysis" syndrome, in which no action is taken until all data are available. One of the objectives of the program may be to focus on data collection if gaps in data are identified and the problem is considered a major health concern.

Whatever method is used by the planning committee to set priorities, the priority chosen will affect the timing and the amount of resources allocated to that priority. Human as well as financial resources are important to consider when establishing resource needs. With the rapidly changing nature of practice in health care organizations, *staff competencies* are a critical factor to assess as well.

SPECIFY OUTCOMES. The last step in this assessment phase is to specify outcomes to which organizational and community resources can be applied over a specified period of time. Outcomes are specific, concrete, measurable statements that need to be accomplished in order to eventually reach a broad goal. They are intended to guide the operations of the agency to reach the goal.

Outcomes focus on the what and when. They specify *results*, not strategies for getting results. For example, outcomes that help reach the goal of reducing the rate of fatalities from motor vehicle accidents might be (1) lower the motor vehicle fatality rate for youth ages 15 to 18 years in Jones County by 3% in the next year; (2) ensure enforcement of the provisions of the Zero Tolerance Bill (no alcohol at school activities) during the 2001-2002 school year; (3) limit teenage access to alcohol by 2002; and (4) develop and implement an ongoing alcohol awareness educational program during 2001-2002. These outcomes are designed to provide direction for achieving the goal of the program, "Jones County Citizens will work toward reducing the rate of fatalities from motor vehicle accidents among people 15 to 24 years of age by 10% in 3 years."

When establishing outcomes, it is important to take into consideration what can be accomplished feasibly in a specified time frame. Ideally, Jones County would like to reduce fatal motor vehicle accidents among their youth by 5% immediately. However, this is not realistic considering the nature of the problem, the characteristics of the target population, and the resources needed to affect change. Multiple factors influence the motor vehicle accident fatality rate, especially among youth. Teenagers and young adults are known to engage in behaviors (e.g., drinking while driving, driving without a seat belt, and speeding) that place them at high risk for fatal driving accidents. Comprehensive programming is needed to address all of these factors, which can require extensive resources and time.

At the conclusion of the three steps of the assessment phase, planners will know the details of the problem under consideration. They also will know the resources available within the organization and the community that can help deal with the problem. When this information is known, health planners concentrate on the third step in the planning process, *policy development*.

## The Policy Development Phase

Policy development involves the determination of strategies to achieve the expected outcomes that emerge as the result of the assessment done in phase two of the planning process. These strategies include methods for allocating resources such as money, personnel, and equipment and interventions directed toward prevention. The strategies also clarify relationships that affect rights, status, and resources.

During the policy development phase, planners pay attention to social and political parameters: Where are the greatest resources? Where is there resistance to the expected outcomes? What methods or strategies could best achieve the expected outcomes? How can the community be mobilized for health action? Will one of the strategies be a modification of what already exists or will it be a new innovative approach? Will the strategies to meet the expected outcomes involve contracts with other organizations and/or support for these organizations so that they can better meet the expected outcome? Answers to questions like these will result in an allocation of resources; the identification of responsibilities; and finally, the establishment of an action plan that has tasks, responsibilities, interventions, and a time frame clearly delineated.

Policy development is frequently a process of negotiation among the different groups involved in the planning process: consumers, service providers, decision makers, and resource persons. Further, during the policy development phase planners must anticipate expected changes in services, legislation, and general trends, and then must foresee what impact these changes will have on the local community. A balance must be achieved that will most effectively use community resources to meet the needs perceived by ordinary citizens, as well as needs perceived by professionals with expertise.

It is easier to discuss the policy development phase of the planning process by dividing it into four steps: (1) assess various strategies to achieve expected outcomes; (2) match tasks with resources; (3) negotiate new organizational liaisons as needed; and finally, (4) establish contracts as needed. The result is an action plan.

GENERATE STRATEGIES TO ACHIEVE EXPECTED OUTCOMES. Generating alternatives to meet the expected outcomes written in phase two is one of the most exhilarating steps in the process. It is a time to be creative and innovative, to exercise a flair for originality.

Various ways to generate strategies can be effective in reaching desired outcomes. Reviewing the literature that addresses successful and unsuccessful strategies related to the health problem of concern is one. Talking with communities and/or advocacy groups that are dealing with similar problems is another. *Brainstorming*—throwing caution to the wind and citing any idea that comes to mind—or conducting a *think tank* with people affected by the health problem are two other approaches for generating community-based interventions.

One of the most exciting aspects of this phase of the health planning process is the development of client inter-

ventions that will reach the target population. In community health practice, a major challenge is to develop interventions that reach underserved populations. Freudenberg, Eng, Flay, et al. (1995) have proposed principles to consider when planners mobilize communities for the purpose of addressing the needs of the underserved. These guidelines are presented in Box 15-3 and reinforce many of the concepts presented throughout this chapter. Another major challenge for professionals when planning community education interventions is to provide culturally appropriate educational messages. Guidelines for presenting culturally relevant educational messages are presented in Box 15-4. The Centers for Disease Control and Prevention (CDC)

## BOX 15-3
### *Principles for Building Individual and Community Capacity*

- Effective health education interventions should be tailored to a specific population within a particular setting.
- Effective interventions involve the participants in planning, implementation, and evaluation.
- Effective interventions integrate efforts aimed at changing individuals, social and physical environments, communities, and policies.
- Effective interventions link participants' concerns about health to broader life concerns and to a vision of a better society.
- Effective interventions use existing resources within the environment.
- Effective interventions build on the strengths found among participants and their communities.
- Effective interventions advocate for the resources and policy changes needed to achieve the desired health objectives.
- Effective interventions prepare participants to become leaders.
- Effective interventions support the diffusion of innovation to a wider population.
- Effective interventions seek to institutionalize successful components and to replicate them in other settings.

From Freudenberg N, Eng E, Flay B, et al.: Strengthening individual and community capacity to prevent disease and promote health: in search of relevant theories and principles, *Health Educ Q* 22:290-306, 1995, pp. 297-298.

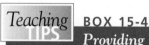

**BOX 15-4**
## *Providing Culturally Appropriate Community Educational Messages*

- Learn about the learning style of the members in the community. Most audiences relate more when they hear, see, and then do.
- Use many different strategies for educating culturally diverse communities.
- Limit the use of lectures and workshops.
- Employ strategies that exist in the community when making group presentations, such as the "call and response" method used in the African-American community. With this strategy, the leader/teacher/preacher states a message in an emphatic way and the audience calls back a response.
- Use a *format* that actively engages the community, such as games, dance, street theater, videos, and storytelling.
- Use existing community educational strategies (e.g., church newsletters, announcements at street fairs or tribal gatherings, and neighborhood flyers).
- Identify language (e.g., street vocabulary or vernacular) that is most appropriate to use and rules for communicating.
- Limit the use of brochures, because most people remember only 10% of what they read.
- For imparting the message, choose a *messenger* who is respected by the targeted segment(s) of the community (e.g., spiritual leaders, healers, influential opinion leaders, gang leaders, sports figures, and tenant association leaders).
- Design a *message* that is simple, uncomplicated, and "do-able," that is consistent with the cultural values of the community and encourages community members to take charge.
- Offer education in settings that are familiar, safe, clean, and easily accessible (e.g., natural gathering places such as community centers, playgrounds, soup kitchens, and malls).

Modified from Randall-David E: *Culturally competent HIV counseling and education,* McLean, Va, 1994, Maternal and Child Health Clearing House, pp. 24-26.

has a division of health communications that can assist local communities with health communication planning and implementation that effectively reaches local community groups (Parvanta, Freimuth, 2000).

Examples of community-based *interventions* used to prevent disease and promote health are peer modeling and education, use of lay health advisors, coalition building for advocacy, educating policy makers and members of community leadership groups (e.g., Tribal Councils and City Councils), participating in community events (e.g., health fairs and pow-wows), and using an education format that actively engages the community (e.g., distribution of useful items with imprinted messages such as T-shirts and use of videos, plays, art, or music) (Freudenberg, Eng, Flay, et al., 1995; Marin, Burhansstipanov, Connell, et al., 1995; Randall-David, 1994).

MATCH TASKS WITH RESOURCES. After strategies have been chosen for each expected outcome, resources need to be assigned to make certain that the task or strategy is accomplished. This results in an action plan specifying the work activities needed to achieve the expected outcome. It includes what is to be done, who is responsible, and by what date each step should be completed. It should be possible to accomplish action steps in 1 to 12 months. Each expected outcome may have many action steps. For example, if one expected outcome is "To limit teenager access to alcohol by 2002," the action plan that matches strategies with resources to achieve this outcome might look like the one presented in Table 15-10.

Step two of the policy development phase results in an action plan that delineates specific action steps with responsible individuals, along with a realistic time frame. This type of plan facilitates the completion of necessary health planning activities.

ESTABLISH ORGANIZATIONAL LIAISONS AND CONTRACTS. These steps help planners complete action steps. For example, if Ms. Alexander is responsible for a monthly newspaper article focused on alcohol awareness issues, she will need to have a firm commitment from the editor that the paper will print the article. This may involve a visit by administrative personnel in the health department to the editorial director of the newspaper and a written or verbal

agreement that such a plan is feasible. Several activities may also be needed if support from law enforcement agencies is desired. For example, it may be necessary for the community health coalition to take steps to encourage legal agencies to enforce state and local regulations. The community health coalition might partner with citizen organizations and businesses to strengthen its policy advocacy efforts designed to obtain support for regulation enforcement.

Table 15-11, showing the planning sequence, summarizes the differences between goals, plans, outcomes, and action steps, as well as the following parameters of each of these: functions, leadership, database, time span, and accountability. Having an awareness of these differences is important, because each level of planning must be completed to ensure effective and efficient community health planning.

## The Implementation Phase

The fourth phase of the health care planning process is implementation. All the work of the other phases finally leads to achievement of concrete outcomes in the real world. Implementation is, to a great extent, a political process that requires that those seeking to bring about change be very aware of the various forces present in the community. Will these forces help the changes take place or can they be mobilized to provide support for the changes? This phase calls for trust, rapport, and patience to work out new and different relationships and to respond to the unanticipated ramifications of the change.

In short, implementation is carrying out the plan. It involves organizing, delegating, and managing work so that the action steps prepared in the last phase are completed and outcomes are accomplished within the specified time. These are the questions that planners need to answer in the implementation phase: What is to be done? How will it be done? Who will do it? What are the deadlines for each step? Who will monitor progress? How and when will the solution be evaluated?

A timeline flowchart delineating operational activities to be accomplished to achieve program goals is used throughout the implementation phase. This flowchart visually displays the major program activities and a time frame in which each activity is to take place. One of the first timeline

---

**TABLE 15-10**

## *Jones County Health Department: One Action Plan for the Motor Vehicle Accident Project*

*Expected Outcome:* To limit teenager access to alcohol by 2002.

| ACTION STEPS | DATE | PERSON RESPONSIBLE |
|---|---|---|
| Get support of the 15 Jones County PTAs | March 15, 2001 | Eigsti |
| Get support of all law enforcement agencies | March 15, 2001 | Clemen and Jones |
| Put one article each month of the year in the "Jones County Chronicle" | Monthly | Alexander |
| Get support of grocery association | August 1, 2001 | McGuire |

**TABLE 15-11**

*The Planning Sequence*

| PLANNING LEVEL | FUNCTION | PRIMARY LEADERSHIP | DATABASE | TIME SPAN | ACCOUNTABILITY |
|---|---|---|---|---|---|
| Goals | To provide broad purpose and general direction for the organization | Board | Ideology, values, role, mission | Infinite | Everyone |
| Plans | To provide definitive direction and a plan for the organization | Chief executive Planning chairperson Planning committee Adopted by board | Operational Societal (issues and trends) Opinions of community leaders, key internal lay and staff leaders | 2-3 years | President, planning chairperson, executive director |
| Outcomes | To provide measurable specification of attainable outcomes within operational goals | Unit executives Unit boards and committees | Operational Clients Community Opinions of key internal lay and staff leaders of operating units | 1 year | Executive director, specific staff |
| Action steps | To provide specification of steps to be taken and activities to be conducted to achieve outcomes; persons responsible; completion dates | Unit Executives Staff | Operational Available resources | 1-12 months | Individual staff |

Developed by Christine DeGregorio, PhD, while a doctoral student in political science, University of Rochester, Rochester, NY.

flowcharts to be formalized was the Gantt chart (Timmreck, 1995). Usually only a simple Gantt chart (Figure 15-2) is used at the program planning level in community health practice.

On a simple timeline flowchart, only major activities of a project rather than a breakdown of the elements of activities are identified. For example, "train staff" on Figure 15-2 is a major activity. Elements of this activity, such as needs assessment of staff, development of training materials, and implementation and evaluation of training, are not displayed. The projected completion time for each major activity is indicated on the chart by a solid line or arrow. The original Gantt chart reflected projected starting time and desired completion time but did not indicate what actually occurred during the specified time frame. Some agencies modify the Gantt chart to include this type of information.

A timeline flowchart helps program directors avoid planning too many tasks for the same time period or tackling less urgent tasks until all essential tasks have been completed. It is important to monitor the implementation plan to make certain that the correct sequence of activities needed to achieve program goals and expected outcomes is being carried out. This monitoring enables the organization to identify successful and unsuccessful strategies and organi-

zational issues related to program implementation. While monitoring the implementation phase, the emphasis among planners is on the next phase of the health planning process—*evaluation*.

## The Evaluation Phase

The fifth phase of the health care planning process, *evaluation*, is best seen as a continuous feedback process. It looks back on actions to determine their efficiency in order to make decisions regarding future actions. Figure 15-3 illustrates the feedback nature of the evaluation process.

Evaluation is an objective critical assessment of the degree to which entire services or their component parts (e.g., effectiveness and efficiency of a specific intervention or completion of activities within a specified time frame) fulfill stated goals (St. Leger, Schnieden, Walsworth-Bell, 1992, p. 1). Evaluation occurs throughout the health planning process *(formative evaluation)* to document progress in carrying out program activities within the designated time frame and to monitor achievement of intermediate outcomes. Evaluation also occurs as the program ends *(summative evaluation)* to assess program impact or outcome and efficiency. When program impact is evaluated, the relationship between program interventions and outcomes as

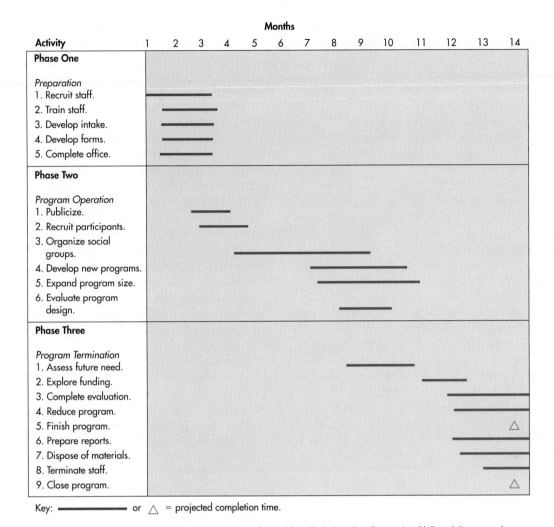

**FIGURE 15-2** Modified Gantt chart. (Developed by Christine De Gregorio, PhD, while a graduate student in political science, University of Rochester, Rochester, NY.)

well as actual program outcomes are examined (Timmreck, 1995). "**Program efficiency** is used to ascertain if the same outcomes could have been achieved in a more effective manner at a lower cost" (Timmreck, 1995, p. 182).

The classic program evaluation framework examines program effectiveness and efficiency from three perspectives (Donabedian, 1982): *structure* (environment in which program operates), *process* (how well program activities are planned and services are delivered), and *outcomes* (program impact and efficiency). Chapters 12 and 25 examine these concepts more extensively. In the evolving managed care environment, emphasis is on both program impact (outcomes) and efficiency.

The evaluation phase has three steps: documenting progress, comparing achievements against a performance standard, and preparing for needed modifications. If any one of these steps is ignored, the evaluation process will be incomplete.

**DOCUMENT PROGRESS.** Keeping accurate and complete records of successes and problems in the process is a

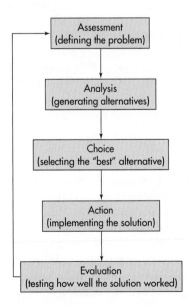

**FIGURE 15-3** Summary of the planning process. (Developed by Christine De Gregorio, PhD, while a graduate student in political science, University of Rochester, Rochester, NY.)

key activity to a productive evaluation. Examples of the type of questions asked to document progress are identified below:

1. Are problems clearly defined?
2. Are the problems documented?
3. Are the solutions appropriate?
4. Do the solutions have many associated risks?
5. Is the envisioned scope of change satisfactory?
6. What impact will the change have on rights, resources, and structures?
7. Are the risks worth the gains?
8. Are the objectives feasible?
9. Are outcomes being achieved within the specified time frame?
10. Is the evaluation plan appropriate?

With the information obtained by asking these questions, planners can move to the next step in the evaluation phase.

**COMPARE ACHIEVEMENTS AGAINST A PERFORMANCE STANDARD.** Performance standards are based on the expected outcomes that were written in the assessment phase of the process. For each action step written to reach each expected outcome, criteria or indicators should be established before implementation. "An indicator is an objective, measurable, well-defined variable relating to the structure, process, or outcome of care" (Joint Commission on Accreditation of Healthcare Organizations [JCAHO], 1990, p. 29). For example, if the expected outcome is "to reduce teenager access to alcohol by 2002," and one of the action steps is to get support of the 15 Jones County Parent Teacher Associations (PTAs), standards to evaluate this action step might be:

1. High achievement—support of all 15 PTAs
2. Adequate achievement—support of 10 PTAs
3. Inadequate progress—support from fewer than 10 PTAs

Indicators for evaluation should be established before implementing action steps. In addition, ways to determine whether the indicators were met should be developed. The method to obtain data about PTA support might involve a verbal report from the coordinating PTA group. This method would be delineated on an action plan as follows:

1. Source of data: verbal report from coordinating PTA group
2. Time: March 2001
3. Responsibility: Mary Cox, CHN

Developing performance indicators that address structure, process, and outcome dimensions of evaluation is challenging in the community setting. Many aggregates at risk, such as the homeless and those dealing with domestic violence, have multiple and complex needs, and only a comprehensive health programming approach is adequate to address the needs experienced by these groups. This type of programming is difficult to evaluate because the range of variables that need to be addressed is extensive and "numerous personal and societal factors outside the clinicians'

control may impact the final outcomes for individual clients" (Bureau of Primary Health Care, USDHHS, 1996, p. ii). When planners develop performance standards for comprehensive programming, they *selectively* evaluate those outcomes they are able to influence.

Table 15-12 displays key questions planners might ask to evaluate whether providers are addressing program outcomes for the homeless. These questions examine how well the system (structure and process standards) functions on behalf of homeless people, as well as the impact that interventions have on individual clients (outcome standards). For each of the desired outcomes (e.g., increased level of functioning or improved access to services), performance indicators are developed. For example, if the expected outcome is "to increase the level of functioning of homeless school-age children during the 2001-2002 academic year," a performance indicator that addresses school attendance would be appropriate because school attendance is a major standard used to assess a child's level of functioning. To measure school attendance, planners might use the following indicators:

- High achievement—less than 5 school days missed (the national average number of days missed per school-age child is 3.8 days.)
- Adequate achievement—less than 8 school days missed
- Inadequate progress—more than 8 school days missed

In this era of cost containment, the importance of objectively measuring program impact and efficiency cannot be overemphasized. Program funders expect health care providers to demonstrate an ability to produce quality, cost-effective outcomes (Bureau of Primary Health Care, USDHHS, 1996).

All five phases of the planning process—preplanning, assessment, policy development, implementation, and evaluation—are interrelated and are, in reality, not carried out separately in the manner that they have been presented. When the basic elements included in each phase are followed, planners have a much greater likelihood of success than when they are passed over. The health care planning process is a valuable tool for professionals who wish to bring about change to solve a difficult problem.

**PREPARE FOR NEEDED MODIFICATION.** The information obtained in the final step of the evaluation phase is used by planners to make decisions about the changes that need to be made in the objectives and associated action plans. Questions such as the following need to be asked about the planning process:

1. Have any key informants or stakeholders been left out of the community planning process—citizens, professionals, leaders?
2. Was an adequate decision-making process used?
3. Have responsibilities and tasks been allocated appropriately?
4. Has there been negative feedback or a destructive impact (lost trust or commitment or heightened resistance) thus far?

**TABLE 15-12**

*Measuring Client-Level and System-Level Outcomes Key Questions for Health Care for the Homeless Providers*

| | SELECTED HEALTH CONDITIONS | | | |
|---|---|---|---|---|
| **OUTCOMES** | **VIOLENCE AGAINST WOMEN (ADULTS)** | **OTITIS MEDIA (PEDIATRICS)** | **MENTAL ILLNESS** | **SUBSTANCE ABUSE** |
| *Client-Level Outcomes* | | | | |
| **Involvement in treatment** | Are women involved in counseling? | Are children receiving antibiotics? | Are clients engaged in treatment? | Are clients engaged in treatment? |
| **Improved health status** | Is victimization reduced? Is self-esteem improved? | Do children have fewer recurring infections? Is hearing loss reduced? | Are psychiatric symptoms reduced? Is physical health addressed? | Are co-morbid physical and psychiatric symptoms reduced? |
| **Improved level of functioning** | Are physical, psychiatric, and social functioning improved? | Are children missing fewer days of school? | Are physical, psychiatric, and social functioning improved? | Are physical, psychiatric, and social functioning improved? |
| **Disease self-management** | Can women avoid risks? Are they involved in self-help groups? | Do children and their parents understand risks and how to avoid them? | Are clients able to manage their symptoms? Are they involved in self-help groups? | Are clients able to reduce their usage? Are they involved in self-help groups? |
| **Improved quality of life** | Do women have safe housing? Do they have a support network? Do they have income or work? | Do children have safe housing? Do they have family support? Are they in school? | Are clients housed? Do they have a support network? Do they have income or work? | Are clients housed? Do they have a support network? Do they have income or work? |
| **Client choice** | Do women feel they have treatment options? | Do parents (and older children) feel they have treatment options? | Do clients feel they have treatment options? | Do clients feel they have treatment options? |
| **Client satisfaction** | Are women satisfied with the services they receive? | Are parents (and older children) satisfied with the services they receive? | Are clients satisfied with the services they receive? | Are clients satisfied with the services they receive? |
| *System-Level Outcomes* | | | | |
| **Access** | Do providers screen for violence? Do they conduct outreach? | Do clients receive care for acute symptoms within 24 hours? | Are appointment times convenient? Is crisis care available? | Are detox and residential services available? |
| **Comprehensive services** | Are appropriate options available that are attractive to clients? | Are appropriate options available to meet the child's needs? | Are appropriate options available that are attractive to clients? | Are appropriate options available that are attractive to clients? |
| **Continuity of care** | Is a referral network available? Are referrals successful? | Do providers offer follow-up care? Do they make specialty referrals? | Do providers offer follow-up care? Do they make specialty referrals? | Do providers offer follow-up care? Do they make specialty referrals? |
| **Systems integration** | Do other providers (e.g., housing, employment) make services available to clients? | Are other key systems (e.g., education) involved in the child's care? | Do other providers (e.g., housing, employment) make services available to clients? | Do other providers (e.g., housing, employment) make services available to clients? |

From Bureau of Primary Health Care, USDHHS: *The working group on homeless health outcomes, meeting proceedings,* Rockville, Md, June 1996, The Bureau, pp. 14-15.

*Continued*

**TABLE 15-12**

*Measuring Client-Level and System-Level Outcomes Key Questions for Health Care for the Homeless Providers—cont'd*

| | SELECTED HEALTH CONDITIONS | | | |
|---|---|---|---|---|
| **OUTCOMES** | **VIOLENCE AGAINST WOMEN (ADULTS)** | **OTITIS MEDIA (PEDIATRICS)** | **MENTAL ILLNESS** | **SUBSTANCE ABUSE** |
| **Cost-effectiveness** | Are emergency room visits and repeat episodes reduced? | Are surgical procedures and emergency room visits reduced? | Are emergency room visits and inpatient care reduced? | Are emergency room visits and inpatient care reduced? |
| **Prevention** | Is educational material available? Do providers screen for gun possession? | Is educational material available for parents and clients? | Is educational material available? Are risk factors addressed? | Is educational material available? Are risk factors addressed? |
| **Client involvement** | Do clients participate in treatment decisions? | Do parents (and older children) participate in treatment decisions? | Do clients participate in treatment decisions? | Do clients participate in treatment decisions? |

From Bureau of Primary Health Care, USDHHS: *The working group on homeless health outcomes, meeting proceedings,* Rockville, Md, June 1996, The Bureau, pp. 14-15.

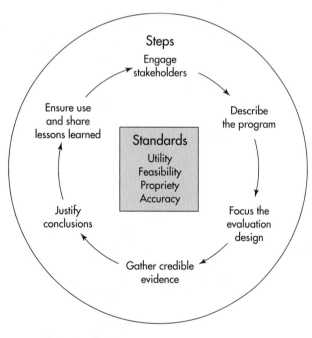

FIGURE 15-4 Framework for program evaluation. (From Centers for Disease Control and Prevention [CDC]: Framework for program evaluation in public health, *MMWR* 48[RR-11]: 1-46, 1999, p. 4.)

5. What positive community responses (improved cooperation, trust, problem solving, heightened commitment, or greater resources) have occurred thus far?
6. Are resources adequate to achieve desired outcomes?
7. Are program goals, objectives, and performance indicators appropriate?

FRAMEWORK FOR PROGRAM EVALUATION. Figure 15-4 presents a framework for program evaluation developed by a Centers for Disease Control and Prevention (CDC) work

 **BOX 15-5**

*CDC's Program Evaluation Standards*

> *Utility standards* ensure that information needs of evaluation users are satisfied.
> *Feasibility standards* ensure that the evaluation is viable and pragmatic.
> *Propriety standards* ensure that the evaluation is ethical.
> *Accuracy standards* ensure that evaluation produces findings that are considered correct.

From Centers for Disease Control and Prevention (CDC): Framework for program evaluation in public health, *MMWR* 48(RR-11):1-40, 1999, pp. 27,29.

group that included evaluation experts, health care professionals and other interested individuals. CDC's **framework for program evaluation** provides a comprehensive approach for developing and implementing program evaluation activities and highlights evaluation activities discussed previously.

The CDC framework (CDC, 1999) for program evaluation involves six steps: stakeholders are engaged in the evaluation process; the program is described in detail so there is a clear understanding of mission, goals, objectives, and stage of program development; the evaluation design is focused; appropriate measures or indicators are developed and credible evidence is gathered to support program outcomes; conclusions are supported by comparing evidence against acceptable standards; and evaluation results are disseminated. In the center of the framework is a set of evaluation standards that helps evaluators prioritize evaluation options. These standards are organized into four groups (Box 15-5).

The CDC framework for program evaluation helps program planners structure evaluation activities while tailoring these activities to local needs. For example, the stakeholders, program design and evaluation process will vary, based on individual community needs and assets. The advantage of the framework is the structure it provides for organizing evaluation activities. An in-depth discussion of this framework is presented in a *Morbidity and Mortality Weekly Report* (CDC, 1999).

## SUMMARY

Health planning for populations at risk is a major function of the community health nurse. In any community setting there are aggregates at risk for specific health problems. The community health nurse uses a variety of intervention strategies to meet the needs of these at-risk populations. This chapter focuses on the health planning and program planning processes.

Health planning occurs at all levels of government and within national, state, and local private organizations. Health planning occurs at a community-wide level (com-

*prehensive health planning)* to identify the health status of the community and to promote the development of healthy public policy. Health planning also occurs at the operational level (*program planning*) in an organization to develop health programs, services, and interventions. Both types of planning are essential for addressing the health needs of the community and aggregates within the community. The *Healthy People Initiative* provides direction for all types of health planning.

During the health planning process, emphasis is placed on mobilizing the community for health action. Partnership building facilitates the achievement of this goal and supports a community in effective and self-determined action. Innovation in practice is needed to address the complex needs of populations at risk.

Community health nurses actively participate on health planning teams and provide unique contributions during the health planning process. Involvement in health planning activities can be exciting and rewarding.

## A view from the field

### MADRES A MADRES: A COMMUNITY PARTNERSHIP FOR HEALTH

*Joan Mahon, MS, RN; Judith McFarlane, RN, PhD; and Katherine Golden, BSN, RN*

**ABSTRACT** To increase the number of Hispanic women who begin early prenatal care, a community partnership for health was initiated among the general public, businesses, 14 volunteer mothers, and one community health nurse. Volunteer mothers living in the targeted community were taught how to identify Hispanic women at risk for not starting early prenatal care and how to provide social support and community resource information within a culturally acceptable milieu. At the end of the first year of the partnership, over 2000 women at risk for not starting early prenatal care had been contacted by the volunteer mothers.

As a single teenage mother, I felt alone and frightened when I was pregnant. I asked myself what I was going to do, how I would manage, where I could go for help, and who would help me. Women in my community need information and support during pregnancy.
— *19-year-old single parent and volunteer mother in de Madres a Madres*

### A National Disgrace

Almost 40,000 infants die each year before their first birthday due to low birth weight. The cost of intensive care, special education, and social services for these infants and their families can average $400,000 over the children's life. In comparison, the cost of routine prenatal care is $400 (American Public Health Association, 1989a). The Surgeon General's goal for the nation was that by 1990, 90% of all pregnant women would begin prenatal care within the first three months of pregnancy (USDHHS, 1980). Based on the 1978-1986 rate of progress, however, the nation will not meet this goal until the year 2094, 100 years after the target date (Children's Defense Fund, 1989). As reported by the American Public Health Association (1989b), maternal and infant health has clearly suffered and markedly declined in recent years, as chronicled by 12 key indicators, including prenatal care, rates of low birth weight, and infant mortality.

### A Widening Minority Gap

Compounding the problem are major disparities between the maternal and infant health of white and minority Americans (USDHHS, 1989). Between 1984 and 1985 there was no improvement in the proportion of infants

From Mahon J, McFarlane J, Golden K: Madres a madres: a community partnership for health, *Publ Health Nurs* 8(1):15-19. ©1991 Blackwell Scientific Publications, Inc. Reprinted by permission of Blackwell Scientific Publications, Inc.
Address correspondence to Judith McFarlane, RN, Professor and Director, de Madres a Madres: A Community Partnership for Health, Texas Woman's University, College of Nursing, 1130 M.C. Anderson Boulevard, Houston, TX 77030.
Joan Mahon is the clinical nurse associate with de Madres a Madres and Katherine Golden is research associate. Both are at Texas Woman's University. This program was aided by grant CHE-255 from the Texas Gulf Coast Chapter, March of Dimes Birth Defects Foundation.

*Continued*

*A view from the field*

with low birth weight. Among African-American and nonwhite infants, the frequency of low birth weight increased (Children's Defense Fund, 1989).

Low birth weight, infant mortality, and pregnancy complications are clearly associated with inadequate prenatal care. To improve access to prenatal care, the National Institute of Medicine (1988) set forth a seminal document detailing demographic risk factors associated with insufficient prenatal care, barriers to the use of prenatal care, and recommendations to improve the use of prenatal care. The report profiled Hispanic women as substantially less likely than non-Hispanic white mothers to begin prenatal care early, and three times as likely to obtain late or no care. Moreover, Hispanic mothers as a group are more likely than non-Hispanic African-American mothers to begin prenatal care late or not at all. Clearly, when compared with non-Hispanic white and African-American women, Hispanic women are at far greater risk to not receiving early prenatal care; many receive no prenatal care. In addition to minority status, age is a major indicator, with teenagers and mothers over age 40 years being at highest risk of receiving late or no prenatal care. Women with less than a high school education are also at increased risk. Finally, poverty was cited as one of the most important correlates of insufficient prenatal care.

In Houston, the fourth largest city in the nation, the minority health gap is widening. According to the latest figures from the City of Houston Health Department (1988), 68.6% of pregnant women initiate prenatal care during the first trimester; for Hispanic women the figure falls to 60.4%. Stated another way, 40% of the Hispanic women in Houston do not receive early prenatal care. The 1989-1990 Texas State Health Plan designated access to prenatal and maternity care for low-income pregnant women in Texas as the top priority issue. Texas accounts for 8% of all births nationally. Nearly 1 in every 12 infants in this country who died in 1985 was a Texas resident (Texas Department of Health, 1988). Improving birth outcomes in the state would have a major impact on meeting the Surgeon General's goals for the nation.

### Culturally Relevant Social Support and Information to Facilitate Early Prenatal Care

With the Hispanic woman at high risk for not receiving early prenatal care, innovative approaches to provide access to care are essential. Barriers were well defined and verified by the National Institute of Medicine (1988) as sociodemographic (age, education, parity),

system access (transportation, clinic availability, insurance), and cultural-personal (fear, stress, depression, denial). To mitigate barriers to prenatal care, de Madres a Madres: A Community Partnership for Health was initiated in a Hispanic community. (De Madres a Madres means "from mothers to mothers.")

The program is a collaborative effort among the general public, businesses, and volunteer mothers to identify Hispanic women at risk for not starting early prenatal care. Other objectives are to provide social support and information on community resources within a culturally acceptable framework. The value of social support in promoting a healthy pregnancy is well supported in the literature (American Nurses Association, 1987; Gray, 1987; Nuckolls, Cassel, Kaplan, 1972; Norbeck, Tilden, 1983; Omer et al., 1987). The use of lay volunteers and paraprofessionals to offer education and support services in the home setting to pregnant women is also widely reported in the literature (National Institute of Medicine, 1988; Heins, Nance, Ferguson, 1987; Olds, Henderson, Tatelbaum, et al., 1986). The conceptual basis for the program was drawn directly from a community as client model (Anderson, McFarlane, 1988). An analysis of each community system was completed to yield community strengths and portals for intervention as well as identify community leaders and levers for change. Community as client information was used to strategize planning, implementation, and evaluation of the de Madres a Madres program.

The pregnant women in all cited studies received intensive social support by volunteers or lay professionals after they initiated prenatal care in a clinic setting, which for most was in the second or third trimester. No program has been reported to date that offers targeted support and information to high-risk women before they enter the health care system. De Madres a Madres proposed culturally relevant social support and community resource information to identified at-risk women before they entered the system. The premise was that culturally relevant social support coupled with community resource information would enable pregnant women to transcend barriers to early prenatal care.

The program will be evaluated by the number of women who begin early prenatal care before as compared with after implementation of the program. The percentage of pregnant women who obtain early prenatal care at the neighborhood health clinic, located within the target community and the only provider of public prenatal care, will be evaluated for the two years of the program

*A view
from the field*

and compared with a two-year period before the program was initiated. Additional variables include the number of at-risk women visited by the volunteer mothers and the number of health and social service referrals completed by the volunteer mothers. Finally, structured interviews of at-risk women who are assisted by the volunteer mothers will be used to evaluate the program. Requirements for the volunteer mothers include residence in the community, at least 18 years of age, and completion of an eight-hour training program offered by the community health nurse. Community awareness, involvement, commitment, and ownership are the essential program elements.

## Community Awareness and Recruitment of Volunteer Mothers

Begun in 1989 and funded by a two-year community service grant from the local chapter of the March of Dimes, de Madres a Madres employed one master's-prepared community health nurse (CHN). Based on the fact that Houston's Hispanic women are the least likely to obtain early prenatal care, an inner-city Hispanic community was selected by the March of Dimes for program implementation. This community has a population of 13,555, of which 34% are women of childbearing age. Median family income is $12,782, and 19% of the households receive public assistance. The CHN completed a community assessment that identified 31 key community leaders.

The 31 community leaders, many of whom were Hispanic, included school principals, the clergy, civic leaders, attorneys, social service administrators, a state representative, health care providers, elected city council representatives, school board members, and law enforcement officers. Most were visited individually several times. The objectives and purpose of the program were explained during each visit. Each community leader was asked for names of potential volunteer mothers. (Because most community leaders were men, sharing the names of women yielded an endorsement for the program from the male hierarchy.)

Simultaneously, the CHN made formal presentations about the program at scheduled community functions, including school meetings, civic association gatherings, church functions, and crime-prevention meetings. At least 100 people attended most formal meetings and learned about de Madres a Madres. In addition, informal presentations were made by the community health nurse at community health fairs, school-sponsored fiestas, and church-supported bazaars and social events.

The CHN assimilated herself into community activities, and on a typical day might begin by visiting with a cluster of women at the local bakery to learn of their concerns during pregnancy and perceived barriers to care. The next stop might be a discussion with the school nurse regarding how the de Madres a Madres program could be integrated into the nurse's regularly scheduled group meeting with pregnant teens. Then on to churches in the area to meet with lay groups of volunteer women interested in outreach and community service. The evening might consist of making a formal presentation on the program at a neighborhood meeting to prevent crime, followed by informal chats with women interested in becoming volunteer mothers.

The community assessment and establishment of trust between the CHN and residents was the lengthiest phase of the program. It was quickly learned that, although most of the 13,000 residents were considered of Hispanic ethnicity, the residents segregated themselves by nation of birth. For example, second-generation Mexican-Americans would not associate with the newly immigrated Mexicans, and neither group would mingle with Guatemalans, El Salvadorans, or Nicaraguans. Values, beliefs, and health practices were nationality specific. It was necessary to recruit volunteer mothers from each group. In addition to nation of origin, immigration status differed widely and was a definite barrier to prenatal care. Women in the amnesty program were at highest risk of not receiving prenatal care and, like teen mothers, required special efforts on the part of the volunteer mothers and CHN.

## Community Commitment and Involvement

At the end of nine months, 14 volunteer mothers had completed the eight-hour training session with the CHN. They ranged in age from 19 to 65 years, had experienced roles from teenage mother to grandmother, and, because of their positions in the community, came into daily contact with women at risk for not starting early prenatal care. The women met in small groups for two hours and were guided through information on the importance of early prenatal care, how to identify women at risk for not starting early care, resources for pregnant women, and effective supportive communication skills. The mothers learned and shared their perceptions of the many barriers to obtaining care during pregnancy. Information was provided on how effective listening and social support can decrease isolation and enable pregnant women to obtain resources and early prenatal care. The volunteer mothers

*Continued*

*A view from the field*

learned how to be advocates for healthy pregnancies. The following is an outline of the curriculum:

A. Role as advocate
  1. Overview of de Madres a Madres: A Community Partnership for Health
  2. Importance of volunteer neighborhood mothers
  3. Volunteer role in the home and the community
B. Resources in the community
  1. Health, food, job training, education, financial aid, transportation, housing
C. Communication/support techniques
  1. Development of trust; use of empathy; verbal skills relating to trust and empathy
  2. Nonverbal skills relating to trust and empathy; use of touch
D. Effective supportive communication skills
  1. Techniques for effective communication; barriers to communication; ways of facilitating communication
E. Aspects of quality prenatal care
  1. Places to receive prenatal care; probable cost; what the visit will entail; outcome of good prenatal care; maternal complications from lack of prenatal care; ambivalence about pregnancy and fears of prenatal care
F. Health resources (detailed description)
  1. Agencies offering prenatal care; eligibility requirements; how agencies coordinate care
G. Low-birth-weight infants, known causes
  1. Prenatal care
  2. Nutrition
  3. Substance abuse
  4. Stress (battering)
H. Family dynamics, interpersonal relationships
  1. Supportive family relationships
  2. Spousal abuse
I. Importance of social support, effects of stress on pregnancy
  1. Methods to decrease stress and increase problem solving skills
  2. Effective listening; decreasing isolation; guiding to proper resources; role modeling
  3. Increasing mother's self-worth

Strategies for presenting the curriculum varied. Some of the content was taught during a visit to the local hospital's intensive care unit for low-birth-weight infants. Other sessions focused on role playing and group sharing of experiences. Guest speakers discussed how to obtain health and social services programs for pregnant women.

Volunteers who completed the training program were given a tote bag with the program name and logo. They proudly carried the bag daily and turned queries about the logo into discussion sessions about the program with colleagues at work as well as the general public.

A great deal of camaraderie developed among the volunteer mothers, who established a strong social support network for each other. Such group support was essential for the successful coping of these volunteers as they assisted women in dire circumstances. The mothers met regularly with the CHN to discuss their experiences and plans for community events and receive additional and updated information. They also met informally as a group and began to establish an organizational infrastructure with leadership positions.

Because these mothers were of the same culture and spoke the same language as women in their community, information was offered in a culturally acceptable milieu. Methods of providing the information varied. One mother invited women into her home to discuss concerns and community resources for a healthy pregnancy. Others visited women in their homes. Several of them were present at the food pantry in the community where they offered social support and community resource information with 75 to 100 women weekly. Many of the women who frequented the pantry were undocumented residents and unaware of how to obtain care for their pregnancy without fear of reprisal.

Although the fact of pregnancy is frequently obvious, exact status was not solicited. The basic premise of de Madres a Madres is primary prevention. If at-risk women are offered culturally relevant information, they will be able to use it when a pregnancy is confirmed. It also was assumed that mothers would share the information with family and friends, creating a ripple effect of information throughout the community. The volunteer mothers were taught that information is empowering and contact is success. The at-risk women would choose when and how to use the information.

The volunteer mothers planned and implemented several community-wide events to share information, including a de Madres a Madres party for all women in the community and an information booth at community functions. A brochure that included community resources and a video about the program were developed for use by the volunteers. A small purse mirror with community resource numbers was given to all mothers visited by the volunteers.

*A view from the field*

## MADRES A MADRES: A COMMUNITY PARTNERSHIP FOR HEALTH—cont'd

### A Community Partnership for Health

Community ownership follows community awareness, involvement, and commitment. To facilitate community ownership, the second year of the de Madres a Madres program will focus on strengthening involvement of the business community, including financial support for the program. The CHN will assist the community in exploring sources for continuation funding, including the United Way and Hispanic Chamber of Commerce. A community advisory board will be formed, with representatives from business, community leaders, and volunteer mothers. A task of the board will be to assume future direction and support mechanisms for the program.

After the first year of the program, more than 2000 at-risk women had received information from a volunteer mother. The type of woman seen daily is exemplified by Olivia.

Olivia, age 21, was five months pregnant and a recent immigrant to Houston. She did not speak English and had not begun prenatal care. After seeing a notice about a de Madres a Madres event, she walked the one mile to the neighborhood elementary school where the program was being held. At the event, Olivia learned about community resources including the location of the prenatal clinic and health and social service agencies. A volunteer mother arranged to visit her the next day. During the home visit, Olivia stated that she was in need of basic food staples for her family, and that her husband was physically abusive. The volunteer mother offered information about the shelter for battered women, location of neighborhood food pantries, and eligibility requirements for specific health and social services. After contact with the volunteer mother, Olivia initiated prenatal care, enrolled in the Women, Infants, and Children (WIC) program, and received weekly food staples from the neighborhood pantry.

Maternal and child health is essential for a healthy and prosperous community. De Madres a Madres developed a community support network to form a partnership of the general public, businesses, and volunteer mothers to protect and promote the health of pregnant women. When a volunteer mother with two children who works full time was asked why she donated her time, her reply was quick and sure, "Why would I not help these women? This community is my home. I care about these women."

### REFERENCES

American Nurses Association: *Access to prenatal care: key to preventing low birthweight,* Kansas City, Mo, 1987, ANA.

American Public Health Association: *The nation's health* [editorial], Washington, DC, 1989a, APHA.

American Public Health Association (APHA): *Monitoring children's health: key indicators,* Washington, DC, 1989b, APHA.

Anderson E, McFarlane J: *Community as client. Application of the nursing process,* Philadelphia, 1988, JB Lippincott.

Children's Defense Fund (CDF): *The health of American's children. Maternal and child health data book,* New York, 1989, CDF.

City of Houston Health Department: *The health of Houston 1984-1986,* Houston, 1988, City of Houston Health Department.

Gray L: A descriptive study on perceived social support among clients assessed by public health nurses. Unpublished thesis, Houston, 1987, Texas Woman's University.

Heins HC, Nance NW, Ferguson JE: Social support in improving perinatal outcome: the resource mothers program, *Obstet Gynecol* 70:263-266, 1987.

National Institute of Medicine: *Prenatal care: reaching mothers, reaching infants,* Washington, DC, 1988, National Academy Press.

Norbeck JS, Tilden VP: Life stress, social support, and emotional disequilibrium in complications of pregnancy: a prospective multivariate study, *J Health Soc Beh* 24:30-46, 1983.

Nuckolls KB, Cassel J, Kaplan BH: Psychosocial asserts, life crises, and the prognosis of pregnancy, *Am J Epidemiol* 95:431-441, 1972.

Olds DL, Henderson CR, Tatelbaum R, et al.: Improving the delivery of prenatal care and outcomes of pregnancy: a randomized trial of nurse home visitation, *Pediatrics* 77:16-28, 1986.

Omer H, Elizur V, Barnea T, et al.: Psychological variables and premature labour: a possible solution for some methodological problems, *J Psychosomatic Res* 30:559-565, 1987.

Texas Department of Health: *1989-90 Texas state health plan,* Texas Statewide Health Coordinating Council, Austin, 1988, Texas Department of Health.

US Department of Health and Human Services (USDHHS): *Promoting health/preventing disease: objectives for the nation,* Washington, DC, 1980, Government Printing Office.

US Department of Health and Human Services (USDHHS): *Health, United States, 1988,* Washington, DC, 1989, Government Printing Office.

## CRITICAL THINKING
*exercise*

"A View From the Field" describes de Madres a Madres, a community partnership for health, and how community health nurses used the health care planning process to begin solving the problem of lack of prenatal care in an aggregate at risk. "Since the beginning of the program in 1989, not one low-birthweight baby has been born to a woman followed by a volunteer mother" (McFarlane, 1996, p. 880). Analyze how the concepts of community empowerment and education were used in the program. What changes would you make to increase community involvement in the program?

## REFERENCES

Altschuld JW, Witkin BR: *From needs assessment to action: transforming needs into solution strategies,* Thousand Oaks, Calif, 2000, Sage.

American Nurses Association (ANA), Quad Council of Public Health Nursing Organizations: *Scope and standards of public health nursing practice,* Washington, DC, 1999, ANA.

American Public Health Association (APHA), Public Health Nursing Section: *The definition and role of public health nursing: a statement of APHA Public Health Nursing Section,* Washington, DC, 1996, APHA.

Association of State and Territorial Directors of Nursing (ASTDN): *Public health nursing: a partner for progress. A document which links nursing, public health core functions, and essential services,* Washington, DC, 1998, ASTDN.

Bergwall DF, Reeves PN, Woodside NB: *Introduction to health planning,* Washington, DC, 1973, Information Resources Press.

Berkowitz B: Health system reform: a blueprint for the future of public health, *J Public Health Management Pract* 1:1-6, 1995.

Berkowitz B: Collaboration for health improvement: models for state, community, and academic partnerships, *J Public Health Management Practice* 6(1):67-72, 2000.

Bracht N, editor: *Health promotion at the community level: new advance,* ed 2, Thousand Oaks, Calif, 1999, Sage.

Brekson DJ, Harvey JR, Lancaster RB: *Community health education: settings, roles, and skills for the 21ˢᵗ century,* ed 4, Gaithersburg, Md, 1998, Aspen.

Brownson RC, Kreuter MW: Future trends affecting public health: challenges and opportunities, *J Public Health Management Practice* 3(2):49-60, 1997.

Bureau of Primary Health Care, USDHHS: *The working group on homeless health outcomes, meeting proceedings,* Rockville, Md, June 1996, The Bureau.

Centers for Disease Control and Prevention (CDC): *A guide for establishing public health priorities,* Atlanta, undated, CDC.

Centers for Disease Control and Prevention (CDC): *CDC vision: healthy people in a healthy world through prevention,* Atlanta, 1995, CDC.

Centers for Disease Control and Prevention (CDC): Framework for program evaluation in public health, *MMWR Morbid Mortal Wkly Rep* 48(RR-11):1-46, 1999.

Clark DC: The city government's role in community health improvement, *Public Health Reports* 115(2,3):216-221, 2000.

Conley E: Public health nursing within core public health functions: "back to the future," *J Public Health Management Pract* 1:1-8, 1995.

Courtney R: Community partnership primary care: a new paradigm for primary care, *Public Health Nurs* 12:366-373, 1995.

Courtney R, Ballard E, Fauver S, et al.: The partnership model: working with individuals, families, and communities toward a new vision of health, *Public Health Nurs* 13:177-186, 1996.

Diekemper M, SmithBattle L, Drake MA: Bringing the population into focus: a natural development in community health nursing practice, Part 1, *Public Health Nurs* 16(1):3-10, 1999.

Donabedian A: *Exploration in quality assessment and monitoring,* vol 2, Ann Arbor, Mich, 1982, Health Administration Press.

Doyle E, Ward S: *The process of community health education and promotion,* Mountain View, Calif, 2001, Mayfield.

Durch JS, Bailey LA, Stoto MA, editors: *Improving health in the community: a role for performance monitoring,* Washington, DC, 1997, National Academy Press.

Flynn BC: Healthy Cities: toward worldwide health promotion, *Annu Rev Public Health* 17:229-309, 1996.

Flynn BC: Communicating with the public: community-based nursing practice, *Public Health Nurs* 15(3):165-170, 1998.

Flynn BC, Ray DW, Rider MS: Empowering communities: action research through Healthy Cities, *Health Ed* 21:395-405, 1994.

Flynn BC, Rider MS, Bailey WW: Developing community leadership in healthy cities: the Indiana model, *Nurs Outlook* 40(3):121-126, 1992.

Freudenberg N, Eng E, Flay B, et al.: Strengthening individual and community capacity to prevent disease and promote health: in search of relevant theories and principles, *Health Educ Q* 22:290-306, 1995.

General Accounting Office (GAO): *Block grants: characteristics, experience, and lessons learned,* Washington, DC, 1995a, GAO.

General Accounting Office (GAO): *Community development: comprehensive approaches address multiple needs but are challenging to implement,* Washington, DC, 1995b, GAO.

Green A: *An introduction to health planning in developing countries,* New York, 1992, Oxford University Press.

Green A: *An introduction to health planning in developing countries,* ed 2, Oxford, NY, 1999, Oxford University Press.

Green LW, Kreuter MW: *Health promotion planning: an educational and ecological approach,* ed 3, Mountain View, Calif, 1999, Mayfield.

Institute of Medicine (IOM): *The future of public health,* Washington, DC, 1988, National Academy Press.

Joint Commission on Accreditation of Healthcare Organizations (JCAHO): *Quality assurance in home care and hospice organizations,* Oakbrook Terrace, Ill, 1990, JCAHO.

Keller LO, Strohschein S, Lia-Hoagberg B, et al.: Population-based public health nursing interventions: a model from practice, *Public Health Nurs* 15(3):207-215, 1998.

Kickbusch I, Draper R, O'Neill M: Healthy public policy: a strategy to implement the Health for All philosophy at various governmental levels. In Evers W, Farrant W, Trojan A, editors: *Healthy public policy at the local level,* Boulder, Colo, 1990, Westview Press.

Kretzmann JP, McKnight JL: *Building communities from the inside out: a path toward finding and mobilizing a community's assets,* Chicago, 1993, ACTA Publications.

Mahon J, McFarlane J, Golden K: De Madres a Madres: a community partnership for health, *Public Health Nurs* 8(1):15-19, 1991.

Marin G, Burhansstipanov L, Connell C, et al.: A research agenda for health education among underserved populations, *Health Educ Q* 22:346-363, 1995.

McFarlane J: De Madres a Madres: an access model for primary care, *Am J Public Health* 86:879-880, 1996.

McKenzie JF, Smeltzer JL: *Planning, implementing, and evaluating health promotion programs: a primer,* ed 3, Boston, 2001, Allyn and Bacon.

Minkler M: Using participatory action research to build healthy communities, *Public Health Reports* 115(2,3):191-197, 2000.

National Academy of Sciences, Institute of Medicine: *Health planning in the United States: issues in guidelines development,* Washington, DC, 1980, The National Academy.

National Commission on Community Health Services: *Health is a community affair,* Cambridge, Mass, 1966, Harvard University Press.

Oberle MW, Baker EL, Magenheim MJ: Healthy People 2000 and community health planning, *Annu Rev Public Health* 15:259-275, 1994.

Parvanta C, Freimuth V: Health communication of the Centers for Disease Central and Prevention, *Am J Health Behav* 24(1):18-25, 2000.

Pew Health Professions Commission: *Critical challenges: revitalizing the health professions for the twenty-first century,* San Francisco, 1995, UCSF Center for the Health Professions.

Pew Health Professions Commission: *Recreating health professional practice for a new century. The fourth report of the Pew Health Professions Commission,* San Francisco, 1998, UCSF Center for the Health Professions.

Pickett GE, Hanlon JJ: *Public health administration and practice,* ed 9, St Louis, 1990, Mosby.

Randall-David E: *Culturally competent HIV counseling and education,* McLean, Va, 1994, Maternal and Child Health Clearing House.

Reeves PN, Coile RC: *Introduction to health planning,* ed 4, Arlington, Va, 1989, Information Resources Press.

Resources for Human Development, Inc., Abbotsford Homes Tenant Management Corporation: *Project abstract,* Philadelphia, undated, The Corporation.

Scherl D, Noren J, Osterweis M: *Promoting health and preventing disease,* Washington, DC, 1992, Association of Academic Health Centers.

Schlaff AL: Boston's Codman Square community partnership for health promotion, *Public Health Reports* 106(2):186-191, 1991.

Sharpe PA, Greaney ML, Lee PR, et al.: Assets-oriented community assessment, *Public Health Reports* 115(2,3):205-211, 2000.

St. Leger AS, Schnieden H, Walsworth-Bell JP: *Evaluating health services' effectiveness: a guide for health professionals, service managers and policy makers,* Philadelphia, 1992, Open University Press.

Storfjell JL, Mitchell R, Daly G: Nurse-managed healthcare: New York's Community Nursing Organization, *JONA* 27(10):21-28, 1997.

Stoto MA: Public health assessment in the 1990s, *Annu Rev Publ Health* 13:59-78, 1992.

Timmreck T: *Planning, program development, and evaluation: a handbook for health promotion, aging, and health services,* Boston, 1995, Jones & Bartlett.

US Department of Health and Human Services (USDHHS): *Healthy People 2010, conference edition, 2 volumes,* Washington, DC, 2000a, USDHHS.

US Department of Health and Human Services (USDHHS): *Tracking Healthy People 2010,* Washington, DC, 2000b, US Government Printing Office.

Wald L: *The house on Henry Street,* New York, 1915, Henry Holt.

Wallerstein N: A participatory evaluation model for healthier communities: developing indicators for New Mexico, *Public Health Report* 115(2,3):199-204, 2000.

Williams CA: Community health nursing: what is it? *Nurs Outlook* 24:250-254, 1977.

## SELECTED BIBLIOGRAPHY

American Public Health Association (APHA): *APHA advocate's handbook,* Washington, DC, 1999, APHA.

Braden S: *Evaluating nursing interventions: a theory-driven approach,* Thousand Oaks, Calif, 1998, Sage.

Breckon DJ: *Managing health promotion programs: leadership skills for the 21st century,* Gaithersburg, Md, 1998, Aspen.

Cornish E: Outlook 2001: recent forecasts from *The Futurist Magazine* for 2001 and beyond, *The Futurist* 34(6):29-40, 2000.

Eisen A: Survey of neighborhood-based, comprehensive community empowerment initiatives, *Health Educ Q* 21:235-252, 1994.

Fetterman D, Kaftarian SJ, Wandersman A: *Empowerment evaluation: knowledge and tools for self-assessment and accountability,* Thousand Oaks, Calif, 1996, Sage.

Green LW, Ottoson JM: *Community and population health,* ed 8, Boston, 1999, McGraw-Hill.

Kelly ED, Becker B: *Community planning: an introduction to the comprehensive plan,* Washington, DC, 2000, Island Press.

Kreuter MW, Lezin NA, Kreuter MW, et al.: *Community health promotion ideas that work: a field-book for practitioners,* Sudbury, Mass, 1998, Jones and Bartlett.

Minkler M, editor: *Community organizing and community building for health,* New Brunswick, NJ, 1998, Rutgers University Press.

Rothschild ML: Ethical considerations in support of the marketing of public health issues, *Am J Health Behav* 24(1):26-35, 2000.

Smith W: Social marketing: an evolving definition, *Am J Health Behav* 24(1):11-17, 2000.

Wates N: *The community planning handbook,* London, 2000, Earthscan Publications.

Wilcox R, Knapp A: Building communities that create health, *Public Health Reports* 115(2,3):139-143, 2000.

# 16

# Care of Infants, Children, Adolescents, and Their Families

*Susan Clemen-Stone*

## OBJECTIVES

*Upon completion of this chapter, the reader should be able to:*

1. Discuss the significance of the infant and maternal mortality trends in the United States.
2. Describe select *Healthy People 2010* maternal, infant, and child health objectives.
3. Articulate major maternal and infant health risks and factors associated with these risks.
4. Discuss demographic characteristics and major health risks of children and adolescents.
5. Analyze factors associated with the major health risks of children and adolescents.

6. Analyze health promotion needs of families with infants and children and community health nursing anticipatory guidance interventions in relation to those needs.
7. Discuss community-based services and community health nursing interventions designed to address the health risks of mothers and children.
8. Discuss significant legislation that has influenced maternal and child health service delivery.

## KEY TERMS

Acute conditions
Anticipatory guidance
Child maltreatment
Children's Health Insurance Program (CHIP)
Congenital anomalies
Developmental disabilities
Failure to thrive (FTT)
Fetal alcohol syndrome (FAS)
*Healthy People 2010* maternal and child health (MCH) objectives

Homicide
Individuals with Disabilities Education Act (IDEA)
Lead poisoning
Maternal and child health programming
Maternal mortality
Morbidity
National Family Planning Program
Neonatal period
Postneonatal period

Postpartum depression (PPD)
Sexually transmitted diseases (STDs)
Substance abuse
Sudden infant death syndrome (SIDS)
Suicide cluster
Teenage pregnancy
Unintended pregnancy
Vaccine preventable infectious diseases (VPDs)
Youth violence

---

*Stand for Children: Leave No Child Behind*

CHILDREN'S DEFENSE FUND

On June 1, 1996, parents, grandparents, religious and civic community leaders, advocates for children, and concerned citizens converged upon Washington, D.C., to take a "stand for all children" (Children's Defense Fund [CDF], 1996). This national mobilization effort was a day of spiritual, family, and community re-

newal and personal commitment to children. At the Lincoln Memorial, masses of people from communities nationwide stood united in their commitment to help all children (Figure 16-1) have a healthy start, a head start, a fair start, a safe start, and a moral start (CDF, 1996). This national day for children was a day for speaking out against violence, child abuse and neglect, poverty, disparities in health care and health status, and political and socioeconomic forces that contribute to family and community stress and crisis. It was a day for sharing the fact that it is no longer acceptable for even one child to suffer from life's hardships.

The 1990s marked an era of experimentation and national effort to promote healthy family and child growth and development (Knitzer, Page, 1996). National campaign efforts, such as the Stand for All Children's March just described and the 1997 Presidents' Summit for America's Future in Philadelphia, which was designed to rekindle the spirit of volunteerism, promoted the need for strong *community action* on behalf of all children. Significant federal and state funds were used to develop special initiatives, addressing the needs of families and children. Emphasis was on increasing efforts to promote the well-being of children at the earliest years, ages birth to 3, and to lay a solid foundation for school and other life experiences. The importance of all children having a stable relationship with at least one adult, a safe environment, adequate health care, and marketable skills also was stressed (Abu-Nasr, 1997).

Although concerted attempts were made throughout the twentieth century to improve the health status of all children in our nation, as well as worldwide, these efforts have fallen short of their goals. There are still over 9 million children in the United States who have been left behind. These high-risk children have four or more family disadvantages that place them at risk of experiencing poor outcomes (O'Hare, Ritualo, 2000). "Almost one-third of American children are living in a one-parent household, 28% live with parent(s) without steady full-time employment, and for more than one in five, the family income is below the poverty line" (O'Hare, Ritualo, 2000 p. 29).

"With our feet still fresh on the sand of a new century, we need to make a sacred promise to deliver to the children who will be born into our world the health and nutrition, the education and protection, that is their birth right" (UNICEF, 2001a, p. 4). Globally, over 10 million children under age 5 still die each year from preventable conditions; 149 million children still suffer from malnutrition; over 100 million children are still not in primary school; and millions of children are involved in child labor, prostitution, and other illegal activities (UNICEF, 2001a, p. 3). The Global Movement for Children (GMC) and the "Say Yes for Children" campaign were launched in 2001 to address these problems and to promote the health of our children worldwide. The "Say Yes for Children" campaign proclaims "all children should be free to grow in health, peace, and dignity" (UNICEF, 2001b, p. 6). This campaign is mobilizing communities around the world to take action that eliminates stresses for children.

Strategies for promoting the well-being of infants, children, adolescents, and their families are highlighted in this chapter. Emphasis is placed on examining population and community-focused interventions needed to resolve the major health risks among children of all ages. An extensive discussion of individual child-focused interventions, designed to treat specific health problems and disease conditions, is

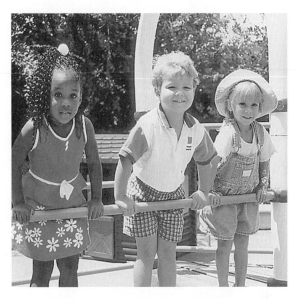

**FIGURE 16-1** All children, regardless of race, color, or creed, need positive life experiences to develop to their fullest potential. (From Wong DL, Hockenberry-Eaton M, Wilson D, et al.: *Whaley and Wong's nursing care of infants and children,* ed 6, St Louis, 1999, Mosby, p. xx.)

beyond the scope of this chapter. The reader can obtain a comprehensive understanding of these types of interventions by referring to Whaley and Wong's *Nursing Care of Infants and Children* (Wong, Hockenberry-Eaton, Wilson, et al., 1999). Select maternal issues and families' concerns related to childrearing also are addressed. Other health issues of women and men are discussed in Chapters 13 and 17.

## INFANT AND MATERNAL HEALTH: CRITICAL INDICATORS OF A NATION'S HEALTH

The importance of infant and maternal mortality rates as critical indicators of a nation's health is well documented (Federal Interagency Forum on Child and Family Statistics, 2000; Hargraves, Thomas, 1993; Maternal and Child Health Bureau, 2000; UNICEF, 2001b). These rates are used worldwide as global indicators of the health status of the population as a whole because they are closely related to socioeconomic and environmental conditions. A nation's maternal and infant mortality rates are a measure of its success in combating poverty, adverse environmental conditions such as health care access issues and water pollution, and morbidity.

Worldwide, over half a million women die each year as a result of pregnancy-related complications (UNICEF, 2001b). Maternal death rates range from approximately 520 per 100,000 live births to less than 10 per 100,000 live births, and infant death rates from 172 per 1000 live births to less than 4 per 1000 live births (Maternal and Child Health Bureau, 2000; UNICEF, 2001b; World Health Organization [WHO], 1995). As would be expected, the highest death

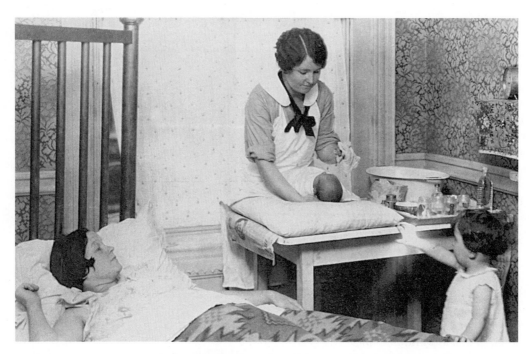

**FIGURE 16-2** A community health nurse from the Visiting Nurse Service of New York City visits a mother with a new baby at home in the early 1930s. (Courtesy Visiting Nurse Service of New York City.)

rates are in the least developed countries, such as those in Africa and Southeast Asia.

At the beginning of the century, maternal mortality rates in the United States mirrored those currently seen in developing countries. In 1935, the year when Title V of the Social Security Act was passed to improve the health of all mothers and children in the nation, the maternal mortality rate was 582 deaths per 100,000 live births, and the infant mortality rate was almost 56 deaths per 1000 live births (Maternal and Child Health Bureau, 1996). Statistics such as these motivated concerned individuals to develop community-based maternal and child health programs.

Nurses have assumed a major leadership role in maternal and child health programming since the early 1900s (Figure 16-2). Lillian Wald, the pioneer community health nurse and feminist, helped establish milk stations in 1903 at the Henry Street Settlement House in New York City to ensure the safety of milk for babies. Diarrhea caused by contaminated milk in the summer months was the cause of many deaths. The City of New York followed this example and in 1911 authorized the establishment of 15 milk stations:

A nurse is attached to each station to follow into the homes and there lay the foundation, through education, for hygienic living. A marked reduction in infant mortality has been brought about and moreover, a realization, on the part of the city, of the immeasurable social and economic value of keeping the babies alive (Wald, 1915, p. 57).

Most mothers and children in the United States are healthy, and successful efforts at preventing mortality and morbidity among these populations mean that there will be

further improvements in their health. However, the United States cannot take its maternal and child health achievements for granted. Although infant and maternal deaths have decreased significantly over the past 65 years, our nation still has serious maternal and child health issues that need to be addressed.

When the infant mortality rate for the United States is compared with the same rate in other developed countries, a striking reason is apparent why those who care about the public's health should be concerned: *this nation ranked lower than 25 other industrialized countries in 1996* (Figure 16-3). Japan and Singapore reported the lowest infant mortality rate in history in 1996. The risk of a Japanese infant dying is 48% lower than that observed in the United States (Maternal and Child Health Bureau, 2000).

The mortality disparities among American infants (Figure 16-4) are particularly distressing to the nation. The infant mortality rate for African-American infants is 2.4 times the rate for white infants. The proportional discrepancy between African-American and white rates has remained unchanged throughout the century (Maternal and Child Health Bureau, 2000). This discrepancy is noted in both neonatal and postneonatal mortality. Native Americans and Puerto Ricans also have infant mortality rates substantially higher than the United States average (United States Department of Health and Human Services [USDHHS], 2000b). These data provided the stimulus for the United States to increase its national efforts in the fight against infant mortality, with a special focus on minority infant health. Maternal, infant, and child health is one of the 28 focus areas identified in the *Healthy People 2010* initiative.

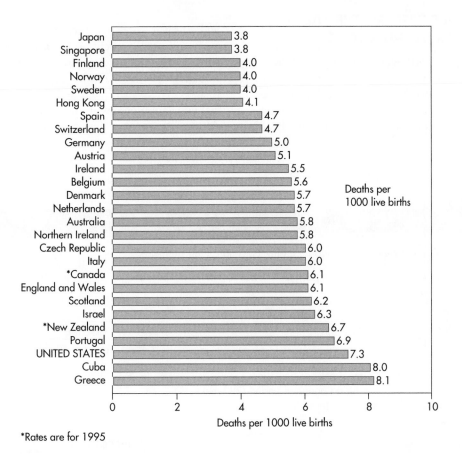

*Rates are for 1995

**FIGURE 16-3** Comparison of national infant mortality rates: 1996. (From Maternal and Child Health Bureau: *Child health USA 2000,* Washington, DC, 2000, US Government Printing Office, p. 22. Source: National Center for Health Statistics.)

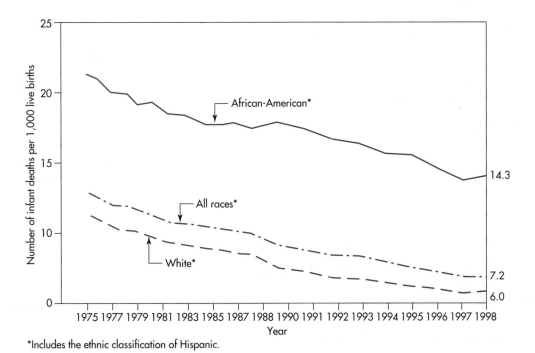

*Includes the ethnic classification of Hispanic.

**FIGURE 16-4** U.S. Infant mortality rates by race of mother: 1975-1998. (From Maternal and Child Health Bureau: *Child health USA 2000,* Washington, DC, 2000, US Government Printing Office, p. 23. Source: National Center for Health Statistics.)

### *HEALTHY PEOPLE 2010:* MATERNAL AND CHILD HEALTH OBJECTIVES

The *Healthy People 2010* maternal and child health (MCH) objectives in Box 16-1 reflect the nation's continued commitment to reduce MCH problems. These objectives build on the *Healthy People 2000* objectives and focus on children and adolescent mortality and infants' health and survival concerns, including infant mortality rates; birth outcomes; prevention of birth defects; access to preventive care; and fetal, perinatal, and other infant deaths (USDHHS, 2000b). The MCH objectives also identify factors associated with infant and maternal health risks. Special population groups are targeted, including low-income, African American, American Indian or Alaskan Native,

**BOX 16-1**
*Objectives: Maternal, Infant, and Child Health*

Goal: Improve the health and well-being of women, infants, children, and families

*Fetal, Infant, Child, and Adolescent Health*
16-1 REDUCE FETAL AND INFANT DEATHS
**Target and baseline:**

| OBJECTIVE | REDUCTION IN FETAL AND INFANT DEATHS | 1997 BASELINE | 2010 TARGET |
|---|---|---|---|
| | | *Rate per 1000 Live Births Plus Fetal Deaths* | |
| **16-1a** | Fetal deaths at 20 or more weeks of gestation | 6.8 | 4.1 |
| **16-1b** | Fetal and infant deaths during perinatal period (28 weeks of gestation to 7 days or more after birth) | 7.5 | 4.5 |

**Target and baseline:**

| OBJECTIVE | REDUCTION IN INFANT DEATHS | 1998 BASELINE | 2010 TARGET |
|---|---|---|---|
| | | *Rate per 1000 Live Births* | |
| **16-1c** | All infant deaths (within 1 year) | 7.2 | 4.5 |
| **16-1d** | Neonatal deaths (within the first 28 days of life) | 4.8 | 2.9 |
| **16-1e** | Postneonatal deaths (between 28 days and 1 year) | 2.4 | 1.2 |

**Target and baseline:**

| OBJECTIVE | REDUCTION IN INFANT DEATHS RELATED TO BIRTH DEFECTS | 1998 BASELINE | 2010 TARGET |
|---|---|---|---|
| | | *Rate per 1000 Live Births* | |
| **16-1f** | All birth defects | 1.6 | 1.1 |
| **16-1g** | Congenital heart defects | 0.53 | 0.38 |
| **16-1h** | Reduce deaths from sudden infant death syndrome (SIDS) | 0.72 | 0.25 |

16-2 REDUCE THE RATE OF CHILD DEATHS
**Target and baseline:**

| OBJECTIVE | REDUCTION IN DEATHS OF CHILDREN | 1998 BASELINE | 2010 TARGET |
|---|---|---|---|
| | | *Rate per 100,000* | |
| **16-2a** | Children aged 1 to 4 years | 34.6 | 18.6 |
| **16-2b** | Children aged 5 to 9 years | 17.7 | 12.3 |

16-3 REDUCE DEATHS OF ADOLESCENTS AND YOUNG ADULTS
**Target and baseline:**

| OBJECTIVE | REDUCTION IN DEATHS OF ADOLESCENTS AND YOUNG ADULTS | 1998 BASELINE | 2010 TARGET |
|---|---|---|---|
| | | *Rate per 100,000* | |
| **16-3a** | Adolescents aged 10 to 14 years | 22.1 | 16.8 |
| **16-3b** | Adolescents aged 15 to 19 years | 70.6 | 39.8 |
| **16-3c** | Young adults aged 20 to 24 years | 95.3 | 49.0 |

From US Department of Health and Human Services (USDHHS): *Healthy people 2010, with understanding and improving health and objectives for improving health,* ed 2, Washington, DC, 2000b, US Government Printing Office, pp. 16-12–16-50.

Native Hawaiian and other Pacific Islanders, and Hispanic or Latino groups (USDHHS, 2000b).

Progress toward achieving the nation's MCH objectives is mixed. Although infant mortality has reached record low levels, minority infant health issues have not changed. Additionally, no progress or movement in the wrong direction occurred in the areas of maternal deaths, fetal alcohol syndrome (FAS), and low-birth-weight infants (USDHHS, 2000b). However, notable gains have been made in reducing infant and fetal deaths, decreasing cesarean births (particularly repeat cesareans), and increasing women's use of health practices that help their own health and that of their infants. These health practices involve an increase in the early use of prenatal care, increased hospitalizations for

---

**BOX 16-1**

**Objectives: Maternal, Infant, and Child Health—cont'd**

*Maternal Deaths and Illnesses*

**16-4 REDUCE MATERNAL DEATHS**
**Target:** 3.3 maternal deaths per 100,000 live births
**Baseline:** 7.1 maternal deaths per 100,000 live births occurred in 1998

**16-5 REDUCE MATERNAL ILLNESS AND COMPLICATIONS DUE TO PREGNANCY**
**Target and baseline:**

| OBJECTIVE | REDUCTION IN MENTAL ILLNESS AND COMPLICATIONS | 1998 BASELINE | 2010 TARGET |
|---|---|---|---|
| | | *Per 100 Deliveries* | |
| **16-5a** | Maternal complications during hospitalized labor and delivery | 31.2 | 24 |
| **16-5b** | Ectopic pregnancies | Developmental | Developmental |
| **16-5c** | Postpartum complications, including postpartum depression | Developmental | Developmental |

*Prenatal Care*

**16-6 INCREASE THE PROPORTION OF PREGNANT WOMEN WHO RECEIVE EARLY AND ADEQUATE PRENATAL CARE**
**Target and baseline:**

| OBJECTIVE | INCREASE IN MATERNAL PRENATAL CARE | 1998 BASELINE | 2010 TARGET |
|---|---|---|---|
| | | *Percent of Live Births* | |
| **16-6a** | Care beginning in first trimester of pregnancy | 83 | 90 |
| **16-6b** | Early and adequate prenatal care | 74 | 90 |

**16-7 (DEVELOPMENTAL) INCREASE THE PROPORTION OF PREGNANT WOMEN WHO ATTEND A SERIES OF PREPARED CHILDBIRTH CLASSES**

*Obstetrical Care*

**16-8 INCREASE THE PROPORTION OF VERY LOW BIRTH WEIGHT (VLBW) INFANTS BORN AT LEVEL III HOSPITALS OR SUBSPECIALTY PERINATAL CENTERS**
**Target:** 90%
**Baseline:** 73% of VLBW infants were born at level III hospitals or subspecialty perinatal centers in 1996-1997

**16-9 REDUCE CESAREAN BIRTHS AMONG LOW-RISK (FULL TERM, SINGLETON, VERTEX PRESENTATION) WOMEN**
**Target and baseline:**

| OBJECTIVE | REDUCTION IN CESAREAN BIRTHS | 1998 BASELINE | 2010 TARGET |
|---|---|---|---|
| | | *Percent of Live Births* | |
| **16-9a** | Women giving birth for the first time | 18 | 15 |
| **16-9b** | Prior cesarean birth | 72 | 63 |

*Continued*

**BOX 16-1**

*Objectives: Maternal, Infant, and Child Health—cont'd*

## Risk Factors

**16-10 REDUCE LOW BIRTH WEIGHT (LBW) AND VERY LOW BIRTH WEIGHT (VLBW)**

**Target and baseline:**

| OBJECTIVE | REDUCTION IN LOW AND VERY LOW BIRTH WEIGHT | 1998 BASELINE | 2010 TARGET |
|---|---|---|---|
| | | *Percent* | |
| **16-10a** | Low birth weight (LBW) | 7.6 | 5.0 |
| **16-10b** | Very low birth weight (VLBW) | 1.4 | 0.9 |

**16-11 REDUCE PRETERM BIRTHS**

**Target and baseline:**

| OBJECTIVE | REDUCTION IN PRETERM BIRTHS | 1998 BASELINE | 2010 TARGET |
|---|---|---|---|
| | | *Percent* | |
| **16-11a** | Total preterm births | 11.6 | 7.6 |
| **16-11b** | Live births at 32 to 36 weeks of gestation | 9.6 | 6.4 |
| **16-11c** | Live births at less than 32 weeks of gestation | 2.0 | 1.1 |

**16-12 (DEVELOPMENTAL) INCREASE THE PROPORTION OF MOTHERS WHO ACHIEVE A RECOMMENDED WEIGHT GAIN DURING THEIR PREGNANCIES**

**16-13 INCREASE THE PERCENTAGE OF HEALTHY FULL-TERM INFANTS WHO ARE PUT DOWN TO SLEEP ON THEIR BACKS**

**Target:** 70%
**Baseline:** 35% of healthy full-term infants were put down to sleep on their backs in 1996

## Developmental Disabilities and Neural Tube Defects

**16-14 REDUCE THE OCCURRENCE OF DEVELOPMENTAL DISABILITIES**

**Target and baseline:**

| OBJECTIVE | REDUCTION OF DEVELOPMENTAL DISABILITIES IN CHILDREN | 1991-1994 BASELINE | 2010 TARGET |
|---|---|---|---|
| | | *Rate per 10,000* | |
| **16-14a** | Mental retardation | 131* | 124 |
| **16-14b** | Cerebral palsy | 32.2† | 31.5 |
| **16-14c** | Autism spectrum disorder | Developmental | Developmental |
| **16-14d** | Epilepsy | Developmental | Developmental |

*Children aged 8 years in metropolitan Atlanta, Ga, having an IQ of 70 or less.
†Children aged 8 years in metropolitan Atlanta, Ga.

**16-15 REDUCE THE OCCURRENCE OF SPINA BIFIDA AND OTHER NEURAL TUBE DEFECTS (NTDs)**

**Target:** 3 new cases per 10,000 live births
**Baseline:** 6 new cases of spina bifida or another neural tube defect (NTD) per 10,000 live births occurred in 1996

**16-16 INCREASE THE PROPORTION OF PREGNANCIES BEGUN WITH AN OPTIMUM FOLIC ACID LEVEL**

**Target and baseline:**

| OBJECTIVE | INCREASE IN PREGNANCIES BEGUN WITH OPTIMUM FOLIC ACID LEVEL | 1991-1994 BASELINE | 2010 TARGET |
|---|---|---|---|
| | | *Percent* | |
| **16-16a** | Consumption of at least 400 μg of folic acid each day from fortified foods or dietary supplements by nonpregnant women aged 15 to 44 years | 21 | 80 |
| | | *Number* | |
| **16-16b** | Median RBC folate level among nonpregnant women aged 15 to 44 years | 160 ng/ml | 220 ng/ml |

**BOX 16-1**
*Objectives: Maternal, Infant, and Child Health—cont'd*

## Prenatal Substance Exposure

**16-17 INCREASE ABSTINENCE FROM ALCOHOL, CIGARETTES, AND ILLICIT DRUGS AMONG PREGNANT WOMEN**

**Target and baseline:**

| OBJECTIVE | INCREASE IN REPORTED ABSTINENCE IN PAST MONTH FROM SUBSTANCES BY PREGNANT WOMEN* | 1996-1997 BASELINE (UNLESS NOTED) | 2010 TARGET |
|---|---|---|---|
| | | *Percent* | |
| **16-17a** | Alcohol | 86 | 94 |
| **16-17b** | Binge drinking | 99 | 100 |
| **16-17c** | Cigarette smoking† | 87 (1998) | 99 |
| **16-17d** | Illicit drugs | 98 | 100 |

*Pregnant women aged 15 to 44 years.*
†*Smoking during pregnancy for all women giving birth in 1998 in 46 states, the District of Columbia, and New York City.*

**16-18 (DEVELOPMENTAL) REDUCE THE OCCURRENCE OF FETAL ALCOHOL SYNDROME (FAS)**

## Breastfeeding, Newborn Screening, and Service Systems

**16-19 INCREASE THE PROPORTION OF MOTHERS WHO BREASTFEED THEIR BABIES**

**Target and baseline:**

| OBJECTIVE | INCREASE IN MOTHERS WHO BREASTFEED | 1998 BASELINE | 2010 TARGET |
|---|---|---|---|
| | | *Percent* | |
| **16-19a** | In early postpartum period | 64 | 75 |
| **16-19b** | At 6 months | 29 | 50 |
| **16-19c** | At 1 year | 16 | 25 |

**16-20 (DEVELOPMENTAL) ENSURE APPROPRIATE NEWBORN BLOODSPOT SCREENING, FOLLOW-UP TESTING, AND REFERRAL TO SERVICES**

| **16-20a** | Ensure that all newborns are screened at birth for conditions mandated by their state-sponsored newborn screening programs, for example, phenylketonuria and hemoglobinopathies. |
|---|---|
| **16-20b** | Ensure that follow-up diagnostic testing for screening positives is performed within an appropriate time period. |
| **16-20c** | Ensure that infants with diagnosed disorders are enrolled in appropriate service interventions within an appropriate time period. |

**16-21 (DEVELOPMENTAL) REDUCE HOSPITALIZATION FOR LIFE-THREATENING SEPSIS AMONG CHILDREN AGED 4 YEARS AND UNDER WITH SICKLING HEMOGLOBINOPATHIES**

**16-22 (DEVELOPMENTAL) INCREASE THE PROPORTION OF CHILDREN WITH SPECIAL HEALTH CARE NEEDS WHO HAVE ACCESS TO A MEDICAL HOME**

**16-23 INCREASE THE PROPORTION OF TERRITORIES AND STATES THAT HAVE SERVICE SYSTEMS FOR CHILDREN WITH SPECIAL HEALTH CARE NEEDS**

**Target:** 100%
**Baseline:** 15.7% of territories and states met Title V for service systems for children with special health care needs in fiscal year 1997

complications of pregnancy, abstinence from tobacco use during pregnancy, increased breastfeeding of newborns, and screening for fetal abnormalities and genetic disorders (USDHHS, 2000b).

National objectives for improving the health of mothers and children focus on mitigating and preventing risk factors for poor MCH outcomes. They also address modifying behaviors and lifestyles that adversely affect birth outcomes and logistical barriers to care (USDHHS, 2000b). The *Healthy People 2010* initiative challenges states and local communities to develop and implement plans to address local MCH concerns.

## MATERNAL AND INFANT HEALTH RISKS

Globally, **maternal and child health programming** is designed to address the needs of women during the childbearing years and their infants and involves preventive interventions that promote healthy lifestyle behaviors throughout the reproductive years. The goal is to improve the quality of life among all women of reproductive age and to reduce infant and maternal mortality and morbidity.

### Maternal Mortality

The World Health Organization defines **maternal mortality** as "the death of a woman while pregnant or within 42 days of termination of pregnancy irrespective of the duration and the site of the pregnancy, from any cause related to or aggravated by the pregnancy or its management" (Salter, Johnston, Henger, 1997). Although more than 99% of these deaths occur in developing countries (UNICEF, 2001a), there still were 281 maternal deaths in the United States in 1998 (Maternal and Child Health Bureau, 2000).

In the United States, over 6 million women are of reproductive age (15 to 44 years old). A typical American woman spends almost half of her lifespan at potential biological risk of pregnancy (Colley, Brantley, Larson, 2000). These women are at risk for unintended pregnancies, maternal morbidity, and maternal mortality resulting from complications that occur during pregnancy, childbirth, or the postpartum period.

**BOX 16-2**

*Factors Associated with High-Risk Pregnancy*

*Economic*
Poverty
Unemployment
Uninsured, underinsured health insurance
Poor access to prenatal care

*Cultural-Behavioral*
Low educational status
Poor health care attitudes
No care or inadequate prenatal care
Cigarette, alcohol, drug abuse
Age less than 16 or over 35 yr
Unmarried
Short interpregnancy interval
Lack of support group (husband, family, church)
Stress (physical, psychological)
African-American race

*Biological-Genetic*
Previous low-birth-weight infant
Low maternal weight at her birth
Low weight for height
Poor weight gain during pregnancy
Short stature
Poor nutrition
Inbreeding (autosomal recessive?)
Intergenerational effects
Hereditary diseases (inborn error of metabolism)

*Reproductive*
Prior cesarean section
Prior infertility
Prolonged gestation
Prolonged labor
Prior infant with cerebral palsy, mental retardation, birth trauma, congenital anomalies
Abnormal lie (breech)
Multiple gestation
Premature rupture of membranes
Infections (systemic, amniotic, extraamniotic, cervical)
Preeclampsia or eclampsia
Uterine bleeding (abruptio placenta, placenta previa)
Parity (0 or more than 5)
Uterine or cervical anomalies
Fetal disease
Abnormal fetal growth
Idiopathic premature labor
Iatrogenic prematurity
High or low levels of maternal serum $\alpha$-fetoprotein

*Medical*
Diabetes mellitus
Hypertension
Congenital heart disease
Autoimmune disease
Sickle cell anemia
TORCH infection
Intercurrent surgery or trauma
Sexually transmitted diseases

Modified from Nelson WE, Behrman RE, Kliegman RM, Algin AM, editors: *Nelson textbook of pediatrics,* Philadelphia, 1996, WB Saunders, p. 440.

The maternal mortality rate for the United States has dramatically decreased over the past century. However, this rate has not declined since 1982, nor has the disparity between African American and white women (Maternal and Child Health Bureau, 2000). The African-American maternal mortality rate is more than *three times* the rate for white women. The mother's age also is strongly associated with maternal mortality. "Regardless of race, the risk of maternal death increases for women over age 30; women 35 to 39 years old have approximately twice the risk of maternal death than those aged 20 to 24 years" (Maternal and Child Health Bureau, 2000, p. 25). Important causes of maternal mortality in the United States are ectopic pregnancies, preeclampsia and eclampsia, hemorrhage, embolism, infection, and anesthesia-related complications. Tubal scarring can result in ectopic pregnancies. The leading cause of preventable tubal scarring is pelvic inflammatory disease (PID) caused by chlamydia and gonorrhea (USDHHS, 2000b).

Factors associated with high-risk pregnancies are displayed in Box 16-2. These factors are important for nurses to consider during the prenatal period because they provide the basis for the high mortality and morbidity rates during infancy and contribute to the high maternal mortality rates. They are danger signs signaling threat to the newborn and the mother. Practitioners use these risk indicators to identify mothers and infants who have special needs and can benefit from preventive interventions.

"*Socioeconomic status is one of the most powerful risk factors for poor health outcomes*" (Hughes, Simpson, 1995, p. 88). Low socioeconomic status is associated with reduced access to health care, poor nutrition, lower education, and inadequate housing. It is also strongly linked to race, ethnicity, and unhealthy lifestyles (Hughes, Simpson, 1995).

Socially and economically deprived persons are more likely than others to have high-risk pregnancies. This is at least partially explained by the lack of adequate prenatal care, which is often unavailable to many population groups, including the inner city and rural poor, teenage mothers, and disadvantaged ethnic groups. "Risk factors for not receiving prenatal care include being less than 18 years of age, unmarried status, low educational attainment, and being in a minority group. Regardless of age, black women (Figure 16-5) are less likely to receive prenatal care than are white women" (Maternal and Child Health Bureau, 2000, p. 60). Other significant reasons for late entry into prenatal care are the mother not realizing she is pregnant, the family not having insurance or money to pay for visits, and an inability to get an appointment (Centers for Disease Control and Prevention [CDC], 2000b).

Prenatal care provides a number of benefits, including the prevention of maternal deaths; education regarding pregnancy, labor and delivery, and newborn care; the potential for linking disadvantaged women to important social services; and an increased likelihood that newborns will receive needed preventive care (Shiono, Behrman, 1995, p. 13). It also provides an avenue for preventing health problems in the newborn caused by maternal disease or health behaviors such as smoking and alcohol use. The MCH Healthy People 2010 objectives highlight a need to "increase the proportion of pregnant women who receive *early* and *adequate* prenatal care" (USDHHS, 2000b; CDC, 2001b). The goal is to have mothers enter prenatal care during the *first trimester* and to receive at least *13 prenatal* visits. Barriers that need to be addressed to achieve this goal are identified in Box 16-3.

## Maternal Morbidity

The factors associated with high-risk pregnancy identified in Box 16-2 place women of reproductive age and their infants at risk for **morbidity,** or disease, as well as mortality. The burden of disease among women in developing countries is huge. It is estimated that as many as 300 million women worldwide suffer from short- or long-term illness related to pregnancy and childbirth (UNICEF, 1996).

Morbidity related to complications of pregnancy and childbirth includes uterine prolapse, fistulae, incontinence, pain during intercourse, and infertility. Infections that result in pelvic inflammatory disease (PID) and permanent nerve

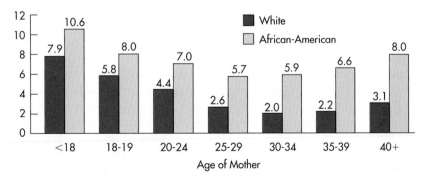

**FIGURE 16-5** Percentage of births to women with late or no prenatal care, by age and race of mother: 1998. (From Maternal and Child Health Bureau: *Child health USA 2000,* Washington, DC, 2000, US Government Printing Office, p. 60. Source: National Center for Health Statistics.)

BOX 16-3

## Barriers to Use of Prenatal Care

### I. Sociodemographic
Poverty
Residence: inner-city or rural
Minority status
Age: <18 or >39
High parity
Non–English-speaking
Unmarried
Less than high school education

### II. System-Related
Inadequacies in private insurance policies (waiting periods, coverage limitations, coinsurance and deductibles, requirements for up-front payments)
Absence of either Medicaid or private insurance coverage of maternity services
Inadequate or no maternity care providers for Medicaid-enrolled, uninsured, and other low-income women (long wait to get appointment)
Complicated, time-consuming process to enroll in Medicaid
Availability of Medicaid poorly advertised
Inadequate transportation services, long travel time to service sites, or both
Difficulty obtaining child care
Weak links between prenatal services and pregnancy testing
Inadequate coordination among such services as WIC and prenatal care
Inconvenient clinic hours, especially for working women

Long waits to see physician
Language and cultural incompatibility between providers and clients
Poor communication between clients and providers exacerbated by short interactions with providers
Negative attributes of clinics, including rude personnel, uncomfortable surroundings, and complicated registration procedures
Limited information on exactly where to get care (phone numbers and addresses)

### III. Attitudinal
Pregnancy unplanned, viewed negatively, or both
Ambivalence
Signs of pregnancy not known or recognized
Prenatal care not valued or understood
Fear of doctors, hospitals, procedures
Fear of parental discovery
Fear of deportation or problems with the Immigration and Naturalization Service
Fear that certain health habits will be discovered and criticized (smoking, eating disorders, drug or alcohol abuse)
Selected lifestyles (drug abuse, homelessness)
Inadequate social supports and personal resources
Excessive stress
Denial or apathy
Concealment

From Brown S: Drawing women into prenatal care, *Fam Plann Perspect* 21(2):75, March/April 1989. © The Alan Guttmacher Institute.

---

damage to the feet and legs as a result of obstructed labor are also significant reproductive complications (UNICEF, 1996). **Postpartum depression (PPD)** is a major concern (USDHHS, 2000b). PPD has been identified throughout history. It is estimated that between 3% and 20% of mothers suffer from this condition, with about one woman in 1000 having postpartum psychosis (Kruckman, Smith, 2001). The consequences of PPD psychosis have been highly publicized, with recent reports of mothers killing their children (Greenberg, Springen, 2001). Although PPD is widely recognized, many women delay seeking help for this condition. The Postpartum Support International has been established to provide information about PPD and support for families experiencing this condition. This center can be reached at *http://www.postpartum.net*. Community health nurses play a significant role in identifying PPD and helping mothers with this condition obtain treatment.

### Intendedness of Pregnancy

It is estimated that almost 50% of all pregnancies are unintended, either mistimed or unwanted altogether (Colley, Brantley, Larson, 2000). There are several consequences of

**unintended pregnancy.** "A woman with an unintended pregnancy is less likely to seek early prenatal care and is more likely to expose the fetus to harmful substances (such as tobacco or alcohol). The child of an unwanted conception, as distinct from a mistimed one, is especially at greater risk of being born at low birth weight, of dying in its first year of life, of being abused, and of not receiving sufficient resources for healthy development" (IOM, 1995, p. 1). An MCH year 2010 objective is to increase the proportion of pregnancies that are intended from 51% of all pregnancies to 70% of all pregnancies (USDHHS, 2000b).

Although unintended pregnancies are common among all population subgroups, the risk is higher for teenagers, women 40 years of age and older, women with lower levels of education, unmarried women, and women with low income (Colley, Brantley, Larson, 2000; USDHHS, 2000b). A major determinant of pregnancy is contraceptive use (USDHHS, 2000b). Unintended pregnancies can be the result of inconsistent or improper use of contraceptives, lack of use, or use of less effective methods (Colley, Brantley, Larson, 2000). Nonusers of contraception account for more than 50% of all unintended pregnancies (Burnhill, 1998). Some risk factors associated with nonuse are poverty, partner attitudes about contraception, client comprehension and health literacy, fear of contraceptive side effects, client's personal characteristics, lapse in use of a method, problems paying for conception, and age of mother over 30 years (Colley, Brantley, Larson, 2000). Increasing the proportion of women at risk of unintended pregnancy (and their partners) who use contraception to 100% is a critical *Healthy People 2010* goal (USDHHS, 2000b). To achieve this goal women need access to quality family planning services. Select cultural beliefs that influence contraceptive practices and postpartum care are presented in Box 16-4. Governmental funding for these services is discussed in a later section of this chapter.

## Infant Health Risks

Multiple factors influence the health status of infants before and after birth, including genetics, the health of the mother, the health behaviors of parents, and environmental conditions that affect the infant's growth and development and ability to receive adequate health care. Box 16-2 summarizes the multiple factors that impact an infant's health as well as the health of mothers.

Figure 16-6 shows the leading causes of death for children less than a year old in the United States. *Two thirds* of all infant deaths occur in the **neonatal period,** or the first 28 days of life (Maternal and Child Health Bureau, 2000). Major causes of neonatal mortality are congenital anomalies, disorders related to short gestation and low birth weight, respiratory distress syndrome, and maternal complications of pregnancy. The ranking of these causes differs by race: the primary causes of neonatal mortality for African Americans are conditions resulting from short gestation and low birth weight, while congenital anomalies are the leading causes for whites (Maternal and Child Health Bureau, 2000).

Infants most at risk during the neonatal period are low-birth-weight babies (less than 2500 g, or 5 lb 8 oz, at birth), especially very low-birth-weight babies (less than 1500 g, or 3 lb 5 oz, at birth), and those born preterm. *Low birth weight and/or preterm delivery are the major factors that fuel the proportional discrepancy between African-American and white infant mortality rates in the United States.* These factors also account for the U.S. high infant mortality ranking among industrialized countries. Countries that have a high proportion of low birth weight and preterm births have high infant mortality (Paneth, 1995). In 1998, 7.6% of all infants in the United States were born too small (Maternal and Child Health Bureau, 2000). *The percentage of newborns born at low birth weight in the United States currently rivals the incidence reported 30 years ago.* Recent increases in low-birth-weight newborns are largely attributable to the increase in multiple births among white women (Maternal and Child Health Bureau, 2000).

Congenital anomalies cause a significant number of infant deaths during both the neonatal and postneonatal periods. However, the most important cause of death during the

 **BOX 16-4**

*Some Cultural Beliefs About the Postpartum Period and Contraception*

---

### Postpartum Care

*Chinese, Mexican, Korean, and Southeast Asian women* may wish to eat only warm foods and drink hot drinks to replace blood lost and to restore the balance of hot and cold in their bodies. These women may also wish to stay warm and avoid bathing in a tub or shower, exercising, and washing their hair for 7 to 30 days after childbirth. Self-care may not be a priority; care by family members is preferred. These women may wear abdominal binders. They may prefer not to give their babies colostrum. Other family members may care for the baby.

*Haitian women* may ask to take the placenta home to bury or burn it.

*Japanese women* may request part of the umbilical cord, which they will place in a special box.

*Muslim women* follow strict religious laws concerning modesty and diet. A Muslim woman must keep her hair, body, arms to the wrist, and legs to the ankles covered at all times. She cannot be alone in the presence of a man other than her husband or a male relative. Observant Muslims will not eat pork or pork products. They are obligated to eat meat slaughtered according to Islamic law (halal meat) but will usually accept kosher meat, seafood, or a vegetarian diet if halal meat is not available.

### Contraception

Birth control is government mandated in *China*. Most Chinese women have an intrauterine device (IUD) inserted after the birth of their first child.

*Saudi Arabian women* usually do not practice birth control.

*Mexican women* are likely to choose the rhythm method because most are Catholic.

*East Indian men* are encouraged to undergo voluntary sterilization by vasectomy.

*Muslim couples* may practice contraception by mutual consent, so long as its use is not harmful to the woman. Acceptable contraceptive methods include foam, condoms, the diaphragm, and natural family planning.

---

From Lowdermilk DL, Perry SE, Bobak IM: *Maternity and women's health care,* ed 7, St Louis, 2000, Mosby, p. 615.

postneonatal period (28 days through 11 months) among all racial and ethnic groups is sudden infant death syndrome (SIDS). SIDS claims the lives of about 4000 infants annually (Anderson, Kochanek, Murphy, 1997). The rate of SIDS among African Americans is twice that of whites (USDHHS, 2000b). Unraveling the underlying reasons for ethnic variations in pregnancy outcomes is one of the great challenges to public health research (Paneth, 1995).

Many variables influence intrauterine growth and gestational duration and infant survival. "Cigarette smoking

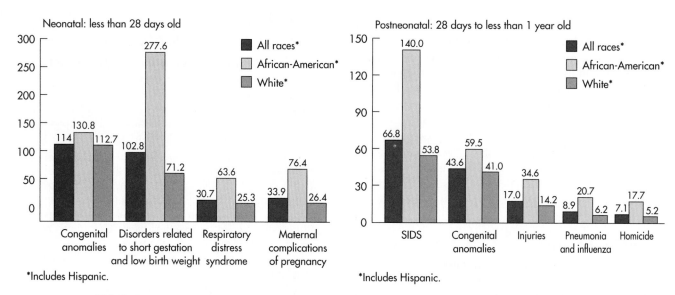

**FIGURE 16-6** Leading causes of neonatal and postneonatal mortality: 1998. (From Maternal and Child Health Bureau: *Child health USA 2000,* Washington, DC, 2000, US Government Printing Office, p. 24. Source: National Center for Health Statistics.)

during pregnancy, low maternal weight gain, and low prepregnancy weight account for nearly two-thirds of all growth-retarded infants" (Shiono, Behrman, 1995, p. 8). Use of drugs and alcohol during pregnancy, poverty, low level of educational attainment, and minority status are also factors associated with risk of low birth weight (Maternal and Child Health Bureau, 2000; USDHHS, 2000b). The impact of substance abuse during pregnancy, including **fetal alcohol syndrome (FAS),** is discussed in Chapter 13. FAS is one of the most common, preventable causes of mental retardation in the Western world.

"The lowest neonatal mortality rate occurs in infants of mothers who receive adequate prenatal care and who are 20 to 30 years of age" (Nelson, Behrman, Kliegman, Algin, 1996, p. 440). Shiono and Behrman (1995) and other health professionals (Alexander, Korenbrot, 1995; Johnson, Primas, Coe, 1994) believe that resources should be concentrated on improving the content and structure of prenatal and obstetric care, with an emphasis on addressing modifiable risks for low-birth-weight and preterm births. "The most likely known targets for prenatal interventions to prevent low birth weight rates are: (1) smoking, (2) nutrition, and (3) medical care" (Alexander, Korenbrot, 1995, p. 107).

Community-wide, well-coordinated initiatives are needed to address problems related to negative pregnancy outcomes. Because needs vary among different segments of the population, community partnerships need to be mobilized. Coalition- or constituency-building among all sectors of society is a must to enhance service delivery to mothers and children (Maternal and Child Health Bureau, 1996). From a service perspective, there is renewed interest in the importance of home visiting to reach geographically isolated and/or other disadvantaged groups (National Commission to Prevent In-

fant Mortality, 1989; Olds, Henderson, Kitzman, et al., 1999). Home visiting activities can improve many health outcomes, including increased participation in cost-effective prenatal care, decreased use of harmful substances during pregnancy, and increased involvement in healthy life-style activities (National Commission to Prevent Infant Mortality, 1989).

Problems developing before the infant reaches 1 month of age are usually related to gestational age, birth weight, and in utero problems. Problems after 1 month of age are more often related to environmental factors. Here the community health nurse plays a significant role in prevention, especially in relation to morbidity. Two health problems associated with environmental factors, failure to thrive and SIDS, are discussed in the next section. Others are discussed in a later section of this chapter.

### Stop and Think About It
Your agency is writing a grant to address the African-American infant mortality disparities in your county. What specific type of data would you want to collect to determine the nature of the problem? What community organizations might be able to help you develop culturally appropriate interventions, based on community needs?

**FAILURE TO THRIVE.** A problem associated with high-risk infants—those who are small or have other physical, familial, and psychological problems—can be their **failure to thrive (FTT).** FTT occurs when a child does not obtain and/or use sufficient calories required for growth. A child who fails to thrive deviates persistently from an established growth curve and has a weight and sometimes height that *falls below the fifth percentile* for the child's age. Three general categories of failure to thrive have been defined:

**BOX 16-5**

*Nursing Considerations to Foster Bonding Among Specific Populations*

### Women in Economically Disadvantaged Situations

Low-income mothers may have to contend with stressors that distract them from developing a relationship with their babies. Inability to pay for infant supplies or child care, chaotic home situations, and worry over eligibility for social and health care services deplete these women's psychological energy.

Nurses need to conduct nonjudgmental, individual assessments of resources and social networks to avoid inaccurate and stereotypical assumptions. Nurses can help economically disadvantaged mothers access social services, such as the Women, Infants, and Children (WIC) program and Medicaid. For mothers whose home environments provide little or no support and multiple stressors, early discharge may not be optimal. Nurses can advocate for longer hospital stays for these mothers when the hospital environment is more conducive to bonding.

Economically disadvantaged mothers, especially adolescents, are not as likely to be aware of the benefits of bonding or to be knowledgeable of normal infant behaviors. These women may not be aware of maternity care options, such as rooming-in, or may be less assertive in asking for such options. The nurse needs to be a client educator and advocate, explaining the choices and the potential benefits. The nurse should ensure a supportive, encouraging environment that will help mothers engage in positive interactions with their infants. By use of the Brazelton Neonatal Assessment Scale, the nurse can capture the mother's attention with a mother-infant interactional experience and, at the same time, increase the mother's knowledge of infant behavior. Written material can be provided after the assessment to reinforce the behavioral concepts. Examples, from sections of an individualized handout written as if from the baby, include "My Strengths: great motor maturity—I stretch my arms way up over my head" and "How you can help: swaddle my arms so I can suck on my hands" (Tedder, 1991).

### Women of Varying Ethnic and Cultural Groups

Childbearing practices and rituals of other cultures may not be congruent with standard practices associated with bonding in the Anglo-American culture. For example, Chinese families traditionally use extended family members to care for the newborn so that the mother can rest and recover, especially after a cesarean birth. Some Native American, Asian, and Hispanic women do not initiate breastfeeding until their breast milk comes in. Haitian families do not name their babies until after the confinement month. Amount of eye contact varies among cultures, too. Yup'ik Eskimo mothers almost always position their babies so that eye contact can be made.

Nurses should become knowledgeable of the childbearing beliefs and practices of diverse cultural and ethnic groups. Because individual cultural variations exist within groups, nurses need to clarify with the client and family members or friends what cultural norms the client follows. Incorrect judgments may be made about mother-infant bonding if nurses do not practice culturally sensitive care.

From Lowdermilk DL, Perry SE, Bobak IM: *Maternity and women's health care,* ed 7, St Louis, 2000, Mosby, p. 629.
Sources: Geissler EM: *Pocket guide to cultural assessment,* St Louis, 1994, Mosby; Symanski ME: Maternal-infant bonding, *J Nurs Midwifery* 37:675, 1992; Tedder JL: Using the Brazelton Neonatal Assessment Scale to facilitate the parent-infant relationship in a primary care setting, *Nurse Pract* 16(3):26, 1991.

- *Organic failure to thrive (OFTT)*, which is the result of a physical cause, such as congenital heart defects, neurological lesions, microcephaly, chronic renal failure, gastroesophageal reflux, malabsorption syndrome, endocrine dysfunction, cystic fibrosis, or acquired immunodeficiency syndrome (AIDS).

- *Nonorganic failure to thrive (NFTT)* has a definable cause that is unrelated to disease. NFTT is most often the result of psychosocial factors, such as inadequate nutritional information by the parent; deficiency in maternal care or a disturbance in maternal-child attachment; or a disturbance in the child's ability to separate from the parent, leading to food refusal to maintain attention.

- *Idiopathic failure to thrive* is unexplained by the usual organic and environmental etiologies, but it also may be classified as NFTT. Both categories of NFTT account for the majority of cases of FTT (Wong, Hockenberry-Eaton, Wilson, et al., 1999, p. 644).

Causes of failure to thrive include poverty, inadequate nutritional knowledge, health beliefs such as fad diets, family stress, feeding resistance, and insufficient breast milk (Wong, Hockenberry-Eaton, Wilson, et al., 1999). Nursing interventions vary based on the cause of FTT. Assistance to families in resolving problems that interfere with their ability to provide adequate nutrition for their children is an important element of nursing care. This assistance might involve referral to obtain funds to buy food, parent education related to child feeding techniques and food selection, stress management counseling, and education that addresses strategies for decreasing feeding resistance and attachment difficulties. Dealing with families who have a parent-child disturbance can be difficult. Wong and others (1999) discuss this care in depth. It is important for the nurse to observe infant-parent attachment when completing an infant assessment. Some factors to consider when fostering attachment or bonding among specific populations are identified in Box 16-5.

Community health nurses play an important role in preventing FTT, identifying infants at risk for FTT, and assisting families in promoting normal growth and development. It is not unusual for the community health nurse to work with parents who lack adequate resources to purchase formula or parents who lack knowledge about formula preparation. It is also not unusual for the community health nurse to work with families who are experiencing considerable stress, which can interfere with the bonding process. Bonding or attachment issues can result in parents having problems meeting an infant's basic nutritional needs.

SUDDEN INFANT DEATH SYNDROME. Another sequel to high-risk pregnancy may be **sudden infant death syndrome (SIDS).** In the United States, between 1 to 4 of every 1000 live-born infants die annually from SIDS. It is the number one cause of death in infants between the ages of 1 month and 1 year. Although SIDS was identified as early as in the writings of the New Testament, no single cause for this condition has been discovered. It is suspected that SIDS is caused by a combination of events and some type of biochemical, anatomical, or developmental defect or deficiency (Assistant Secretary for Legislation [ASL], 1997; Wong, Hockenberry-Eaton, Wilson, et al., 1999). Risk factors for SIDS are displayed in Table 16-1.

Helping parents handle grief and guilt feelings is a major role of the community health nurse in these situations. The impact of death on siblings is another area where the nurse must intervene. Increasingly, communities are setting up crisis teams to assist families who have experienced a child's death from SIDS. It is common for health departments to employ community health nurses to work with these families. These nurses facilitate family adjustment as they work through the grief process after death has come to a seemingly healthy infant. Helping families deal with their feelings about future parenting is also very important. Because the mourning process takes *at least a year* for completion of acceptance and social reorganization, nurses should call on these families periodically to evaluate their progress, or refer them to community resources such as a SIDS support group that will assist them in meeting their psychological needs (Wong, Hockenberry-Eaton, Wilson, et al., 1999).

Public health professionals have a significant preventive intervention role as well as a therapeutic role when dealing with SIDS. Since the national *Back to Sleep* education campaign was launched in 1994 to promote "Babies on Their Back to Sleep," the rate of SIDS has dropped dramatically from more than 5,000 to under 3,000 infant deaths per year (National Black Child Development Institute [NBCDI], 2000). Currently the focus is on eliminating the racial disparity in SIDS deaths. A *Resource Kit for Reducing the Risk of Sudden Infant Death Syndrome in African American Communities* is available and contains culturally relevant client materials and a leader's guide for leading group discussions in various community settings. It can be obtained from the National Institute of Child Health and Human Development (NICHD) by calling 1-800-505-CRIB or at the NICHD web site: *http://www.nichd.nih.gov.*

## TABLE 16-1

### *Epidemiology of SIDS Factors*

| FACTORS | OCCURRENCE |
|---|---|
| Incidence | 1.4:1000 live births |
| Peak age | 2 to 4 months; 95% occur by 6 months |
| Sex | Higher percentage of males affected |
| Time of death | During sleep |
| Time of year | Increased incidence in winter; peak in January |
| Racial | Greater incidence in Native Americans and African Americans, followed by whites, Asians, and Hispanics |
| Socioeconomic | Increased occurrence in lower socioeconomic class |
| Birth | Higher incidence in: |
| | Premature infants, especially infants of low birth weight |
| | Multiple births* |
| | Neonates with low Apgar scores |
| | Infants with central nervous system disturbances and respiratory disorders such as bronchopulmonary dysplasia |
| | Increasing birth order (subsequent siblings as opposed to firstborn child) |
| | Infants with a recent history of illness |
| Sleep habits | Prone position; use of soft bedding; overheating (thermal stress); possibly co-sleeping with adult |
| Feeding habits | Lower incidence in breastfed infants |
| Siblings | May have greater incidence |
| Maternal | Young age; cigarette smoking, especially during pregnancy; substance abuse (heroin, methadone, cocaine) |

From Wong DL, Hockenberry-Eaton M, Wilson D, et al.: *Whaley and Wong's nursing care of infants and children,* ed 6, St Louis, 1999, Mosby, p. 652.
*Although a rare event, simultaneous death of twins from SIDS can occur.

## DEMOGRAPHIC CHARACTERISTICS AND HEALTH PROFILES OF CHILDREN AND ADOLESCENTS

Because health risks and service needs differ by age, number of children, and other demographic characteristics, it is important for community health nurses to analyze these characteristics and mortality and morbidity rates specific to the targeted age group under consideration. This analysis helps community health nurses identify health concerns and strengths within their own community. Having this knowledge provides a foundation for allocating scarce resources for education, health, and other community services.

## Demographic Characteristics

Figure 16-7 displays the resident U.S. population by age group. Trends reflect that while the absolute number of children age 21 or younger is increasing, this age group is declining relative to other age groups in the population. It is expected that persons 65 or older will increase from 12.7% in 1999 to 17% of the population in the year 2010, whereas the child population under age 18 is expected to comprise 24% of the population. This is down from a peak of 36% at the end of the "baby boom" and 26% of the population in 1999 (Federal Interagency Forum on Child and Family Statistics, 2000). However, a significant number of children will still be residing in our nation. In 1999, there were over 85 million children through the age of 21 in the United States, representing 31.3% of the total population. Children under age 18 are expected to increase to 77.2 million in 2020, up from 70.2 million in 1999. Although the majority of children under the age of 18 (65%) were white in 1999, this ethnic group is declining relative to other ethnic groups (Federal Interagency Forum on Child and Family Statistics, 2000).

The majority of children younger than 6 (65%) and children ages 6 through 17 (78%) have mothers in the workforce. Contrary to stereotypes, the majority of poor families with children work (CDF, 2000). Although the overall number of poor children is declining, there still were 1.7 million more children living in poverty at the end of the century than in 1980 (Maternal and Child Health Bureau, 2000).

Additionally, the income gap between the rich and the poor is at a 50-year high (CDF, 2000).

Disturbingly, when comparing the U.S. child poverty rate with those in other major Western industrialized countries, the United States has made less progress in reducing poverty than other Western industrialized nations. "Other nations less wealthy than the United States have cut their child poverty rates to half, a third, or even a fifth of the U.S. poverty rate, largely through strong government action" (CDF, 2000, p. 1). The U.S. child poverty rate is significantly higher than the rate in most major Western industrialized nations. It is often two to three times higher (National Center for Children in Poverty, 2001).

In 1998, 12.8 million children under 18 years of age lived in families that had an income below the poverty level. Although the majority of children living in poverty are white, a disproportionately high percentage of African-American and Hispanic children live in poverty (Figure 16-8). Across ethnic groups, children living with unmarried mothers are particularly at risk for living in poverty. In 1998, 59.4% of children less than18 years of age in the United States lived in homes headed by a single mother. Other factors that place children at risk for experiencing poverty are low educational attainment of parents (no earned college degree) and the family wage earner having part-time or no employment (Bennett, Li, Song, Yang, 1999).

The importance of *comparing* local, state, and national health indicators is vividly illustrated when U.S. poverty rates are examined. Poverty rates for younger children living in many large cities and in specific states are higher than the national average. For example, state average poverty

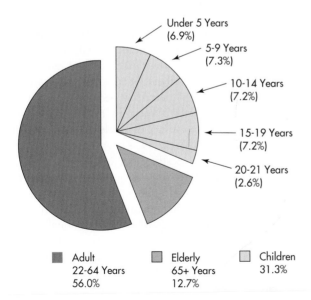

**FIGURE 16-7** U.S. resident population by age group: July 1, 1999. (From Maternal and Child Health Bureau: *Child health USA 2000*, Washington, DC, 2000, US Government Printing Office, p. 11. Source: US Bureau of the Census.)

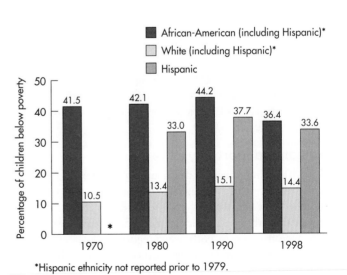

**FIGURE 16-8** Related children under 18 years of age living in families below 100% of poverty level by race/ethnicity: 1998. (From Maternal and Child Health Bureau: *Child health USA 2000*, Washington, DC, 2000, US Government Printing Office, p. 12. Source: US Bureau of the Census.)

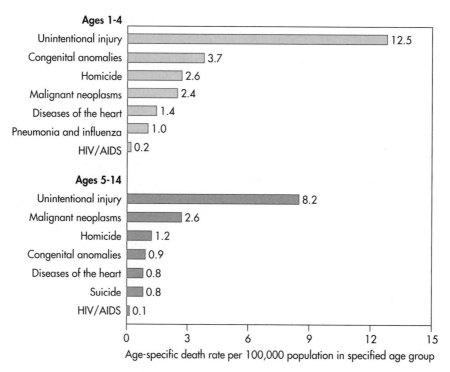

**FIGURE 16-9** Leading causes of death in children ages 1 to 4 and 5 to 14, 1998. (From Maternal and Child Health Bureau: *Child health USA 2000,* Washington, DC, 2000, US Government Printing Office, p. 32. Source: National Center for Health Statistics.)

rates for the period from 1997 to 1999 ranged from 7.6% in Maryland to 20.8% in New Mexico (Dalaker, Proctor, 2000). Although child poverty rates are highest in urban areas, poverty among young suburban children grew at a much faster pace between the 1970s and the mid-1990s than did poverty among either urban or rural young children (Bennett, Li, Song, Yang, 1999).

Chapter 13 discusses the influence of poverty on the health status of children. However, the fact that low "*socioeconomic status is one of the most powerful risk factors for poor health outcomes*" (Hughes, Simpson, 1995, p. 88) cannot be overstated. Poverty, especially in the earliest childhood years, causes lifelong damage to children's minds and bodies (UNICEF, 2001a).

### Childhood Mortality Risks

The 10 leading causes of death among children and adolescents are presented in Figures 16-9 and 16-10. As can be seen in these figures, death rates for children ages 5 to 14 are lower than those for children under 5, and compared with younger children in both age categories, adolescents have much higher mortality rates. Although overall childhood mortality rates have declined over the past several decades, disparities among racial and ethnic groups, for many causes of death, are substantial. Disparities also exist among persons with different levels of education. Individuals with less than a high school education have mortality rates at least double those persons with some college education (National Center for Health Statistics, 2000). Additionally, de-

spite declines in suicide and homicide death rates, these health problems continue to be leading causes of death among children and adolescents.

It is striking to note (see Figures 16-9 and 16-10) that the majority of childhood deaths could be prevented. It has long been documented that environmental, social, and behavioral factors greatly influence the occurrence of mortality across the life span. It was noted in our first national health plan that approximately "50 percent of our United States' deaths are due to unhealthy behavior or lifestyle; 20 percent to environmental factors; 20 percent to human biological factors; and only 10 percent to inadequacies in health care" (U.S. Department of Health, Education, and Welfare [USDHEW], 1979, p. 9).

INJURIES. Although deaths from unintentional injury have declined significantly since 1950, injuries remain the leading cause of death and disability among children and young adults. Almost 55 children and teenagers die from injuries each day (USDHHS, 2000b). Unintentional injuries claim more than *three times* as many lives among children and adolescents as the next leading cause of death (Maternal and Child Health Bureau, 2000). Motor vehicle accidents are the single largest contributing cause of unintentional-injury deaths for children of any age. Although motor vehicle mortality among teenagers has declined over the last decade, adolescents are particularly at risk for motor vehicle deaths. For adolescents aged 12 to 18 years, unintentional injury deaths increase nearly *fivefold*. Most of this increase is due to motor vehicle accidents (National Safety Council, 2000).

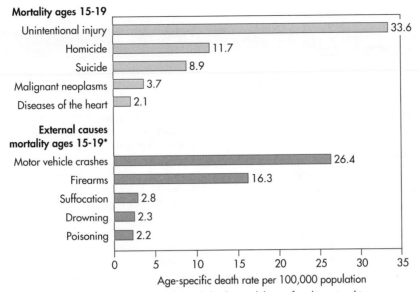

**FIGURE 16-10** Leading causes of death in adolescents ages 15 to 19: 1998. (From Maternal and Child Health Bureau: *Child health USA 2000,* Washington, DC, 2000, US Government Printing Office, p. 46. Source: National Center for Health Statistics.)

Following motor vehicle accidents, firearms, fires and related burns, and drowning are also leading causes of childhood unintentional injury deaths. Drowning fatalities are the second leading cause of injury-related death for children and adolescents aged 1 to 19 years (USDHHS, 2000b). Children ages 1 to 4 have the highest death rates from drowning, with rates over three times that for children ages 5 to 14 (Maternal and Child Health Bureau, 2000). Among children under 5, drowning occurs most frequently in swimming pools and home spas. Household fires are also a particular risk to children, with children under 5 who live in substandard housing at special risk (USDHHS, 2000b).

Firearms also cause a significant number of injury deaths among children. However, many of these deaths are intentional. In 1998, almost 47% of firearm deaths among 5- to 14-year-old children were homicides (Maternal and Child Health Bureau, 2000). In this same year, suicides and homicides accounted for over 94% of the firearm deaths among teenagers. Despite decreased homicide rates among all age groups in the United States, the decline is less dramatic among youth (USDHHS, 2000b). Additionally, our youth now have to deal with mass shootings at school that may kill or injure several children at one time.

A significant challenge for community health professionals in the next decade is to find ways to reduce fatalities from injuries. An important role of the community health nurse is to address behaviors that contribute to unintentional injuries, including safety-belt use, motorcycle helmet use, bicycle helmet use, driving while under the influence of alcohol and drugs, and riding with a driver who has been drinking. Data reflect that a significant number of adolescents engage in these risk-taking behaviors.

In 1999, over 16% of youth in grades 9 to 12 who participated in the Youth Risk Behavior Surveillance System (YRBSS) survey had rarely or never worn seat belts when riding in a motor vehicle driven by someone else; over one third (38%) of youth who rode a motorcycle had rarely or never worn a motorcycle helmet; over 85% had rarely or never worn a bicycle helmet; one third of students had ridden more than once with a driver who had been drinking alcohol; and about 13% had driven a vehicle more than once after drinking alcohol. Some risk behaviors are more common among specific gender, racial, and ethnic subgroups. For example, males are more likely than females to drive after drinking, and white students report this risk behavior more than their African-American counterparts (CDC, 2000d).

The community health nurse also can assume a major role in preventing accidents and injuries in younger school-age children through health education activities designed to prevent poisonings, fires, falls, and other causes of accidents. The Consumer Product Safety Commission (1-800-638-CPSC) provides material on consumer product safety, including product hazards, product defects, and injuries sustained in using products. This information can help the nurse plan sound educational programs. The National Child Safety Council Childwatch (1-800-222-1464) answers questions and distributes literature on safety and sponsors the Missing Kids program (publicized through milk cartons). A safety education tool can be found in Box 16-6. The National Center for Injury Prevention and Control (NCIPC) at the CDC provides extensive educational material to assist professionals and the public with injury prevention.

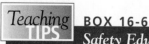

### BOX 16-6
## *Safety Education Tool*

More children die from injuries than any other cause. The good news is that most injuries can be prevented by following simple safety guidelines. Talk with your health care provider about ways to protect your child from injuries. Fill out this safety checklist.

### Safety Guidelines Checklist
Read the list below and check off each guideline that your family already follows. Work on those you don't.

### For All Ages
- Use smoke detectors in your home. Change the batteries every year and check once a month to see that they work.
- If you have a gun in your home, make sure that the gun and ammunition are locked up separately and kept out of children's reach.
- Never drive after drinking alcohol.
- Use car safety belts at all times.
- Teach your child traffic safety. Children under 9 years of age need supervision when crossing streets.
- Teach your children how and when to call **911**.
- Learn basic life-saving skills (CPR).
- Keep a bottle of ipecac at home to treat poisoning. Talk with a doctor or the local Poison Control Center before using it. Post the number of the Poison Control Center near your telephone and write it in the space on the inside front cover of this book. Also be sure to check the expiration date on the bottle of ipecac to make sure it is still good.

### Infants and Young Children
- Use a car safety seat at all times until your child weighs at least 40 pounds.
- Car seats must be properly secured in the back seat, preferable in the middle.

- Keep medicines, cleaning solutions, and other dangerous substances in childproof containers, locked up and out of reach of children.
- Use safety gates across stairways (top and bottom) and guards on windows above the first floor.
- Keep hot water heater temperatures below 120° F.
- Keep unused electrical outlets covered with plastic guards.
- Provide constant supervision for babies using a baby walker. Block the access to stairways and to objects that can fall (such as lamps) or cause burns (such as stoves).
- Keep objects and foods that can cause choking away from your child. This includes things like coins, balloons, small toy parts, hot dogs (unmashed), peanuts, and hard candies.
- Use fences that go all the way around pools and keep gates to pools locked.

### Older Children
- Use car safety belts at all times.
- Until children are tall enough so that the lap belt stays on their hips and the shoulder belt crosses their shoulder, they should use a car booster seat.
- Make sure your child wears a helmet while riding on a bicycle or motorcycle.
- Make sure your child uses protective equipment for rollerblading and skateboarding (helmet, wrist and knee pads).
- Warn your child of the dangers of using alcohol and drugs. Many driving- and sports-related injuries are caused by the use of alcohol and drugs.

### A Special Message About SIDS
Sudden Infant Death Syndrome (SIDS) is the leading cause of death for infants. Put infants to sleep on their backs to decrease the risk of SIDS.

From USDHHS: *Child health guide: put prevention into practice,* Washington, DC, 2000a, US Government Printing Office, pp. 31-33.

HOMICIDE. In 1974, **homicide** became a leading cause of death among children and young adults for the first time in the history of our nation. Between 1985 and 1991 the rate of homicide among males ages 15 to 19 increased 154%, with firearm use being a major contributor to homicide deaths. Although the homicide rates have continued to decline since 1994, current rates are still unacceptably high (CDC, 2000c). Homicide death rates in the United States are significantly higher than in many other industrialized nations (USDHHS, 2000b).

In 1998, homicide ranked third as the leading cause of deaths for children ages 1 to 4 and ages 5 to 14, and second for ages 15 to 24 (Maternal and Child Health Bureau, 2000). The death rate from homicide is the leading cause of death for African-American adolescents ages 15 to 24. The homicide rate for Hispanic and American Indians/Alaskan Natives is also much higher than the general population (USDHHS, 2000b). Children at special risk among all ethnic and minority groups are presented in Box 16-7. Identifying factors associated with violence provides the foundation for selecting and implementing appropriate preventive interventions.

Community health nurses must work in close collaboration with all agencies in the community to *prevent* homicide among youth. Comprehensive programs to prevent childhood homicide must involve many sectors of the community and multiple approaches to the problem. Activities for preventing youth violence usually employ one of three general prevention strategies: education, legal and regulatory change, and environmental modification (NCIPC, 1993, p. 11). Box 16-8 displays examples of interventions

## BOX 16-7
### Children at Risk for Violence

*Individual*
- History of early aggression
- Beliefs supportive of violence
- Social cognitive deficits

*Family*
- Poor monitoring or supervision of children
- Exposure to violence
- Parental drug/alcohol abuse
- Poor emotional attachment to parents or caregivers

*Peer/School*
- Associate with peers engaged in high-risk or problem behavior
- Low commitment to school
- Academic failure

*Neighborhood*
- Poverty and diminished economic opportunity
- High levels of transience and family disruption
- Exposure to violence

From Centers for Disease Control and Prevention (CDC): *Youth violence in the United States fact sheet,* 2000c. Retrieved from the internet Aug. 29, 2001. *http://www.cdc.gov/ncipc/dvp/yvpt/facts.htm.*

## BOX 16-8
### Activities to Prevent Youth Violence

*Education*
Adult mentoring
Conflict resolution
Training in social skills
Firearm safety
Parenting centers
Peer education
Public information and education campaigns

*Legal/Regulatory Change*
Regulate the use of and access to weapons
- Weaponless schools
- Control of concealed weapons
- Restrictive licensing
- Appropriate sale of guns
Regulate the use of and access to alcohol
- Appropriate sale of alcohol
- Prohibition or control of alcohol sales at events
- Training of servers
Other types of regulations
- Appropriate punishment in schools
- Dress codes

*Environmental Modification*
Modify the social environment
- Home visitation
- Preschool programs such as Head Start
- Therapeutic activities
- Recreational activities
- Work/academic experiences
Modify the physical environment
- Make risk areas visible
- Increase use of an area
- Limit building entrances and exits
- Create sense of ownership

From NCIPC: *The prevention of youth violence: a framework for community action,* Atlanta, 1993, CDC, p. 11.

used under each category. Community health nurses assume a significant role in planning and implementing violence control interventions in a variety of settings, including schools, clinics, churches, and other community service agencies.

**SUICIDE.** The incidence of suicide among youth has been increasing steadily for four decades. In 1998, suicide ranked *sixth* as the leading cause of death for ages 5 to 14 years and third for ages 15 to 19 years. The suicide rate nearly tripled among youth during the latter half of the twentieth century (CDC, 2001c). A major concern of health professionals is the increasing number of suicides among African-American men. Although white teens continue to have higher suicide rates than minority youth, the gap is narrowing (CDC, 2001c).

Suicide rates for both African-American and white women are significantly less than men. However, young women of all racial/ethnic groups are substantially more likely *to consider* suicide than young men. Data from the 1999 YRBSS survey reflect these differences. In 1999, about one fifth (19.3%) of all high school students had seriously considered attempting suicide, with female students (24.9%) almost twice as likely as male students (13.7%) considering suicide. Female students (18.3%) were also significantly more likely than male students (10.9%) to have made a suicide plan and to actually attempt suicide in the past 12 months (females 10.9%, males 5.7%) (CDC, 1999).

Health professionals view suicide as a problem of extreme importance in the adolescent population because it is an indicator that social, emotional, and physical stress is great. Rapidly changing societal values, population mobility, and economic pressures have presented adolescents with decision-making conflicts that result in uncertainty and stress (Figure 16-11). It is estimated that at least 90% of all persons who kill themselves have a mental or substance abuse disorder, or a combination of disorders (USDHHS, 2000b). Other risk factors include a prior suicide attempt; stressful life events; access to lethal suicide methods; family influences, including a history of violence and family disruption; and rapid sociocultural change (National Center for Health Statistics, 2000; USDHHS, 2000b).

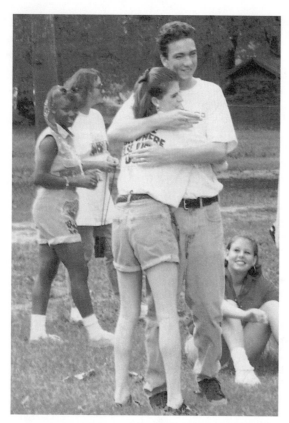

**FIGURE 16-11** Accelerated societal changes have exposed American youth to increased opportunities as well as increased stresses. American youth are exposed much earlier than their previous counterparts to such things as human sexuality concerns, pressures from peers to use alcohol and drugs, and varying lifestyles. Community health nurses are often in a favorable position to detect youth who are having difficulty coping with the demands of life. (From Wong DL, Hockenberry-Eaton M, Wilson D, et al.: *Whaley and Wong's nursing care of infants and children,* ed 6, St Louis, 1999, Mosby, p. 900.)

 **BOX 16-9**
*Youth Suicide Prevention Strategies*

- **School Gatekeeper Training**
  Directed at school staff to help them identify students at risk of suicide, refer such students for help, and respond in cases of a tragic death or other crisis in school.
- **Community Gatekeeper Training**
  Provides training for community members such as clergy, police, and recreation staff to aid them in identifying youths at risk of suicide, and referring these youth for help.
- **General Suicide Education**
  Provides students with facts about suicide, alert them to suicide warning signs, and provide them with information about how to seek help for themselves or for others.
- **Screening Program**
  Involves administration of a standardized instrument to identify high-risk youth in order to provide more thorough assessment and treatment for a smaller, targeted population.
- **Peer Support Programs**
  Designed to foster peer relationships, competency development, and social skills as a method to prevent suicide among high-risk youth.
- **Crisis Centers and Hotlines**
  Provide emergency counseling for suicidal people.
- **Means Restriction**
  Designed to restrict access to firearms, drugs, and other common means of committing suicide.
- **Intervention After a Suicide**
  Designed in part to help prevent or contain suicide clusters and to help youth effectively cope with feelings of loss that come with the sudden death or suicide of a peer.

From CDC: *Youth suicide prevention programs: a resource guide,* Atlanta, 1992, CDC, pp. ix-x.

"Suicide clusters" and the possible "contagion" effect of adolescent suicide is also a public concern. A **suicide cluster** is the occurrence of suicides or attempted suicides closer together in space and time than is considered usual for a given community. It is estimated that suicide clusters account for approximately 1% to 5% of all suicides among adolescents and young adults. In a cluster, suicides occurring later in the cluster often appear to have been influenced by earlier suicides (CDC, 1988). To combat the influence of previous suicides, persons at risk need to be identified and interviewed, personal counseling services should be provided for close friends and relatives of the victims and potentially suicidal adolescents, and the community needs to be supported in a way that minimizes sensationalism (CDC, 1994).

A comprehensive community-focused approach that emphasizes prevention and is linked as closely as possible with professional mental health resources is needed to com-

bat youth suicide (CDC, 1992). Currently a broad spectrum of youth suicide prevention programs in the United States use a variety of prevention strategies (Box 16-9). The strategies outlined in Box 16-9 focus on enhancing recognition of suicide, referral for appropriate mental health services, and promoting activities designed to address known or suspected risk factors. Most youth suicide prevention programs target adolescents despite the fact that the suicide rate among young adults 20 to 24 years of age is significantly higher than the rate among adolescents 15 to 19 years of age. Greater prevention efforts need to be targeted toward young adults (CDC, 1992, 1994).

Community health nurses, especially those functioning in the school setting, are in a key position to detect troubled youth and to work with the community in planning a comprehensive suicide prevention program. It is important to move beyond an individual-focused approach. A community-oriented approach that targets at-risk populations and uses a variety of intervention strategies is needed to address this alarming problem.

**CONGENITAL ANOMALIES.** Each year approximately 3.8 deaths per 100,000 children aged 1 to 4 years and 1.2 deaths per 100,000 children aged 5 to 14 years occur from serious **congenital anomalies** or birth defects (USDHHS, 2000b). Many factors increase the risk for congenital anomalies including genetics and a number of modifiable risk factors including poverty, poor housing, malnutrition, pregnancy at a young age, use of alcohol and cigarettes, and inadequate medical care. It has been shown that mothers in all age categories who are disadvantaged are at risk for producing an unhealthy child (Chomitz, Cheung, Lieberman, 1995; Paneth, 1995; Yoon, Rasmussen, Lynberg, et al., 2001).

The risk of having an abnormal birth increases as a mother's consumption of alcohol, illicit drugs, and tobacco increases (USDHHS, 2000b). This risk also increases among young mothers and mothers who have had inadequate health care. These mothers are more likely to have low-birth-weight babies than other mothers. Low-birth-weight infants have a high incidence of congenital malformations. These facts suggest that a preventive health program designed to reduce childhood mortality related to congenital malformations must include ways to eliminate poor environmental and social conditions, expand the use of prenatal services by young and disadvantaged mothers, and alter unhealthy behaviors (alcohol and drug consumption and smoking) that increase the risk for abnormal births. "Improving women's health before, during, and after pregnancy is the key to reducing the human and economic costs associated with infant mortality and morbidity" (Chomitz, Cheung, Lieberman, 1995, p. 132).

**MALIGNANT NEOPLASMS.** Although malignant neoplasms or cancer is rare among children, it is the chief cause of death *by disease* in youth under age 15. Common sites include the blood and bone marrow, bone, lymph nodes, brain, nervous system, kidneys, and soft tissues (American Cancer Society [ACS], 2001). Over 8000 new cases of cancer are diagnosed yearly among children ages 0 to 14 years in the United States. Leukemia accounts for one third of these new cases and one third of the deaths attributed to childhood cancer. Cancer fatality rates for children have declined 50% since 1973. Parents play a significant role in early diagnosis and treatment. Cancer in children can be detected early during regular medical or nursing checkups and by astute parents who observe unusual symptoms that persist in their children (ACS, 2001).

Cancer places a tremendous burden on families and society. The nature of this condition and the prolonged treatment needed cause pain and anguish for both the child and the family. Cancer in childhood also causes financial hardship for many families because funding for catastrophic illness is frequently not available. Health planning efforts for cancer should focus on providing early detection, treat-

ment, and supportive services; funding for research; and monies to eliminate individual financial hardships.

Community health nurses can significantly assist families in coping with childhood cancer by providing home health care services and supportive counseling and helping them obtain needed resources from community agencies. For example, the American Cancer Society supplies dressings and equipment free of charge. Other community agencies such as departments of social services provide funds for medical treatment. Helping parents establish and maintain support networks is an important role for nurses working with families who are coping with childhood cancer. Cancer support groups can often be identified by contacting local hospices, hospitals, or the American Cancer Society.

## Childhood Morbidity Risks—Acute Conditions

The incidence of acute conditions in childhood is difficult to ascertain because many acute conditions are not reportable, and many reportable acute conditions are often not reported. Additionally, acute illnesses are frequently treated at home and as a result are not brought to the attention of health professionals. Data from the National Health Surveys conducted since 1956 do provide estimated patterns of incidence over time. According to this survey, **acute conditions** are illnesses and injuries that were first noticed less then 3 months before the reference date of the interview and were serious enough to have had an impact on behavior (Adams, Hendershot, Marano, 1999, p. 1387).

The major types of childhood acute conditions for children, identified in the National Health Interview Survey, fall into five major categories. These are respiratory conditions, injuries, infective and parasitic diseases, digestive system conditions, and all other conditions. Respiratory conditions, injuries, and infective and parasitic diseases are highlighted in the following text. An extensive discussion of all acute conditions among children is beyond the scope of this book.

The average school-age child misses 4.0 days of school per year because of illness and injury. Children from families that have an income under $10,000 per year experience more acute conditions than children from families that have an income greater than $10,000 per year (U.S. Bureau of the Census, 2000).

**RESPIRATORY CONDITIONS.** Respiratory conditions, including influenza and the common cold, account for over 60% of the reported acute illnesses among school-age children. Influenza causes two thirds of the reported acute respiratory conditions. Diseases of the respiratory system are the major cause of hospitalization of younger children (see Figure 16-6). In 1998, these diseases accounted for 31% of hospital discharges of children 1 to 9 years of age. There were 3.4 million hospital discharges of children 1 to 21 years old that year. Children younger than age 18 in families with incomes less than $20,000, and African-American children regardless of income status, are at risk for hospitalization (Maternal and Child Health Bureau, 2000).

**BOX 16-10**

*Childhood Injuries: Risk Factors*

**Sex:** Preponderance of males; difference mainly due to behavioral characteristics, especially aggression
**Temperament:** Children with difficult temperament profile, especially persistence, high activity, and negative reactions to new situations (Nyman, 1987)
**Stress:** Predisposes to increased risk taking and self-destructive behavior; general lack of self-protection
**Alcohol and drug use:** Associated with higher incidence of motor vehicle injuries, drowning, homicides, and suicides
**Previous history of injury:** Associated with increased likelihood of another injury, especially if initial injury required hospitalization

*Developmental characteristics*
Mismatch between child's developmental level and skill required for activity (e.g., all-terrain vehicles)
Natural curiosity to explore environment
Desire to assert self and challenge rules
In older child, desire for peer approval and acceptance

*Cognitive characteristics (age specific)*
**Infancy:** Sensorimotor: explores environment through taste and touch
**Young child:**
Object permanence: actively searches for attractive object
Cause and effect: unaware of consequential dangers
Transductive reasoning: may fail to learn from experiences; for example, falling from a step is not perceived as same type of danger as climbing a tree
Magical and egocentric thinking: cannot comprehend danger to self or others; cannot take place of others to realize danger; if thinking something is safe, believes it to be so
**School-age child:** Transitional cognitive processes: unable to fully comprehend casual relationships; attempts dangerous acts without detailed planning regarding consequences
**Adolescent:** Formal operations: preoccupied with abstract thinking and looses sight of reality; may lead to feeling of invulnerability

*Anatomical characteristics (especially in young children)*
**Large head:** Predisposes to cranial injury
**Large spleen and liver with wide costal arch:** Predisposes to direct trauma to these organs
**Small and light body:** May be thrown easily, especially inside a moving vehicle
**Left-handedness:** Combination of environmental biases and certain neuroanatomical or biological differences may increase susceptibility to injury
**Other factors:** Poverty; family stress (i.e., maternal illness, recent environmental change), substandard alternative child care, young maternal age, low maternal education, multiple siblings

From Wong DL, Hockenberry-Eaton M, Wilson D, et al.: *Whaley and Wong's nursing care of infants and children,* ed 6, St Louis, 1999, Mosby, p. 9.

Acute respiratory conditions interfere with activities of daily living and may lead to other serious, acute and chronic conditions, such as viral pneumonia, encephalitis, and otitis media and mortality. For example, otitis media can, if untreated, result in permanent hearing loss and chronic ear infection, and respiratory syncytial virus (RSV) infection is the most common cause of bronchiolitis and pneumonia among infants. "As a group, acute respiratory diseases are one of the leading causes of death from any infectious diseases" (Chin, 2000, p. 425).

INJURIES. Injuries disproportionately strike the young and the old (Warner, Barnes, Fingerhut, 2000). Among children, injuries cause significant morbidity as well as mortality. Children experience traumatic injuries in a variety of settings including the home, at school, in cars, and all types of recreational areas.

Yearly, between 20% and 25% of all children sustain an injury that requires medical attention and/or limits their activity (NCIPC, 2000). "For every childhood death caused by injury, there are approximately 34 hospitalizations, 1000 emergency department visits, and many more visits to private physicians and school nurses, and an even larger number of injuries treated at home" (NCIPC, 1999, p. 1). Additionally, more than 2 million people call poison control centers yearly because of a poisoning incident (NCIPC, 2000).

A variety of factors place children at risk for injuries. Several risks are common to most types of injuries. Injuries occur more often in those with low socioeconomic status, especially urban African-American children and American Indian/ Alaska Natives, and males (NCIPC, 2000). Risks associated with specific types of injuries include the developmental level of the child, prevalence of threat in the environment (e.g., firearms or swimming pools), access to and use of safety measures and/or equipment, and inadequate supervision to avoid threat (e.g., young school-age child supervising a toddler near an in-ground swimming pool that lacks protective fencing) (NCIPC, 1999). Box 16-10 identifies other risks factors. It is important to consider developmental characteristics of each age group when developing safety interventions.

INFECTIVE AND PARASITIC DISEASES. Infective and parasitic diseases are of concern to all health professionals because of their contagious nature. Many of them, such as scabies, impetigo, ringworm, head lice, giardiasis, and pinworms, are still considered diseases of the poor and unclean even though this myth has been disproved. Children who experience these conditions are often socially isolated and teased by their peers.

Although the incidence of vaccine preventable infectious diseases (VPDs) among children has reached recordlow levels in the United States, indigenous (not imported) cases of all of these diseases, except for polio, continue to be reported. Additionally, despite significant progress in improving immunization rates, approximately 1 million children under the age of 2 in the United States have not been fully vaccinated (Maternal and Child Health Bureau, 2000). Figure 16-12 presents a recommended childhood

## Recommended Childhood Immunization Schedule
## United States, January-December 2001

Vaccines[1] are listed under routinely recommended ages. Bars indicate range of recommended ages for immunization. Any dose not given at the recommended age should be given as a "catch-up" immunization at any subsequent visit when indicated and feasible. Ovals indicate vaccines to be given if previously recommended doses were missed or given earlier than the recommended minimum age.

| Age ▶ Vaccines ▼ | Birth | 1 mo | 2 mos | 4 mos | 6 mos | 12 mos | 15 mos | 18 mos | 24 mos | 4-6 yrs | 11-12 yrs | 14-16 yrs |
|---|---|---|---|---|---|---|---|---|---|---|---|---|
| Hepatitis B[2] | | Hep B #1 | | | | | | | | | | |
| | | | Hep B # 2 | | | Hep B # 3 | | | | | Hep B[2] | |
| Diphtheria, Tetanus, Pertussis[3] | | | DTaP | DTaP | DTaP | | DTaP[3] | | | DTaP | Td | |
| *H. influenzae* type b[4] | | | Hib | Hib | Hib | Hib | | | | | | |
| Inactivated Polio[5] | | | IPV | IPV | | IPV[5] | | | | IPV[5] | | |
| Pneumococcal Conjugate[6] | | | PCV | PCV | PCV | PCV | | | | | | |
| Measles, Mumps, Rubella[7] | | | | | | MMR | | | | MMR[7] | MMR[7] | |
| Varicella[8] | | | | | | Var | | | | | Var[8] | |
| Hepatitis A[9] | | | | | | | | | Hep A—in selected areas[9] | | | |

Approved by the Advisory Committee on Immunization Practices (ACIP), the American Academy of Pediatrics (AAP), and the American Academy of Family Physicians (AAFP).

1. This schedule indicates the recommended ages for routine administration of currently licensed childhood vaccines, as of 11/1/00, for children through 18 years of age. Additional vaccines may be licensed and recommended during the year. Licensed combination vaccines may be used whenever any components of the combination are indicated and its other components are not contraindicated. Providers should consult the manufacturers' package inserts for detailed recommendations.

2. **Infants born to HBsAg-negative mothers** should receive the 1st dose of hepatitis B (Hep B) vaccine by age 2 months. The 2nd dose should be at least 1 month after the 1st dose. The 3rd dose should be administered at least 4 months after the 1st dose and at least 2 months after the 2nd dose, but not before 6 months of age for infants.

**Infants born to HBsAg-positive mothers** should receive hepatitis B vaccine and 0.5 mL hepatitis B immune globulin (HBIG) within 12 hours of birth at separate sites. The 2nd dose is recommended at 1-2 months of age and the 3rd dose at 6 months of age.

**Infants born to mothers whose HBsAg status is unknown** should receive hepatitis B vaccine within 12 hours of birth. Maternal blood should be drawn at the time of delivery to determine the mother's HBsAg status; if the HBsAg test is positive, the infant should receive HBIG as soon as possible (no later than 1 week of age).

**All children and adolescents** who have not been immunized against hepatitis B should begin the series during any visit. Special efforts should be made to immunize children who were born or whose parents were born in areas of the world with moderate or high endemicity of hepatitis B virus infection.

3. The 4th dose of DTaP (diphtheria and tetanus toxoids and acellular pertussis vaccine) may be administered as early as 12 months of age, provided 6 months have elapsed since the 3rd dose and the child is unlikely to return at age 15-18 months. Td (tetanus and diphtheria toxoids) is recommended at 11-12 years of age if at least 5 years have elapsed since the last dose of DTP, DTaP, or DT. Subsequent routine Td boosters are recommended every 10 years.

4. Three *Haemophilus influenzae* type b (Hib) conjugate vaccines are licensed for infant use. If PRP-OMP (PedvaxHIB® or ComVax® [Merck]) is administered at 2 and 4 months of age, a dose at 6 months is not required. Because clinical studies in infants have demonstrated that using some combination products may induce a lower immune response to the Hib vaccine component, DTaP/Hib combination products should not be used for primary immunization in infants at 2, 4, or 6 months of age, unless FDA-approved for these ages.

5. An all-IPV schedule is recommended for routine childhood polio vaccination in the United States. All children should receive four doses of IPV at 2 months, 4 months, 6-18 months, and 4-6 years of age. Oral polio vaccine (OPV) should be used only in selected circumstances. (See *MMWR* May 19, 2000/49[RR-5];1-22.)

6. The heptavalent conjugate pneumococcal vaccine (PCV) is recommended for all children 2-23 months of age. It also is recommended for certain children 24-59 months of age. (See *MMWR* Oct. 6, 2000/49[RR-9];1-35.)

7. The 2nd dose of measles, mumps, and rubella (MMR) vaccine is recommended routinely at 4-6 years of age but may be administered during any visit, provided at least 4 weeks have elapsed since receipt of the 1st dose and that both doses are administered beginning at or after 12 months of age. Those who have not previously received the 2nd dose should complete the schedule by the 11-12 year old visit.

8. Varicella (Var) vaccine is recommended at any visit on or after the first birthday for susceptible children, i.e. those who lack a reliable history of chickenpox (as judged by a health care provider) and who have not been immunized. Susceptible persons 13 years of age or older should receive 2 doses, given at least 4 weeks apart.

9. Hepatitis A (Hep A) is shaded to indicate its recommended use in selected states and/or regions, and for certain high risk groups; consult your local public health authority. (See *MMWR* Oct. 1, 1999/48[RR-12]; 1-37.)

*For additional information about the vaccines listed above, please visit the National Immunization Program Home Page at http://www.cdc.gov/nip/ or call the National Immunization Hotline at 800-232-2522 (English) or 800-232-0233 (Spanish).*

**FIGURE 16-12** Recommended childhood immunization schedule, United States, January to December 2001.

immunization schedule. An updated version of this schedule can be obtained yearly at the website listed in the footnote of Figure 16-12. CDC revises this schedule regularly as new information about vaccines is obtained. Providing parents with a written immunization schedule can help prevent confusion. Effective anticipatory guidance assists parents in determining when children should have immunizations and the value of them. The guide to contraindications and precautions to vaccinations in Appendix 16-1 helps professionals and parents to know when vaccines should be administered.

The two most common parasitic infections among children in the United States are giardiasis and pinworms (Wong, Hockenberry-Eaton, Wilson, et al., 1999). The prevalence of pinworm infections is highest in school-age children, followed by preschoolers. In some school-age populations the prevalence is near 50%. Giardiasis is the most common protozoan infection in the United States. Its prevalence may range between 1% and 30%, depending on the community and age group surveyed. Endemic giardiasis infection in the United States most commonly occurs in July to October among children under the age of 5 and adults 25 to 39 years old. It is associated with drinking contaminated surface water; swimming in bodies of fresh water, such as lakes and rivers; and having a young family member in day care (Chin, 2000).

---

*Teaching* **TIPS**
**BOX 16-11**
*Preventing Intestinal Parasitic Disease*

Always wash hands and fingernails with soap and water before eating and handling food and after toileting.
Avoid placing fingers in mouth and biting nails.
Discourage children from scratching bare anal area.
Use superabsorbent disposable diapers to prevent leakage.
Change diapers as soon as soiled and dispose of diapers in closed receptacle out of children's reach.
Do not rinse diapers in toilet.
Disinfect toilet seats and diaper-changing areas; use dilute household bleach (10% solution) or Lysol and wipe clean with paper towels.
Drink water that is specially treated, especially if camping.
Wash all raw fruits and vegetables, or food that has fallen on the floor.
Avoid growing foods in soil fertilized with human excreta.
Teach children to defecate only in a toilet, not on the ground.
Keep dogs and cats away from playgrounds or sandboxes.
Avoid swimming in pools frequented by diapered children.
Wear shoes outside.

From Wong DL, Hockenberry-Eaton M, Wilson D, et al.: *Whaley and Wong's nursing care of infants and children*, ed 6, St Louis, 1999, Mosby, p. 737.

---

The epidemiology of select common infective and parasitic diseases is presented in the Appendix of Chapter 11. The reader will find the American Public Health Association handbook, *Control of Communicable Diseases Manual*, (Chin, 2000) a valuable resource when identifying and recommending follow-up for any of these diseases. Prevention is the key to effective control of these conditions. Epidemiological investigation to determine the source of infection and to break the chain of transmission is essential. Community health nurses play a significant role in educating families and school personnel about the prevention of infective and parasitic conditions. Tips for preventing intestinal parasitic disease are found in Box 16-11.

## Childhood Morbidity Risks—Chronic Conditions

Chronic health problems during childhood are of special concern to health professionals because they can adversely affect a child's growth and development and can cause disability in later life. They can also create considerable emotional and financial stress for children and their families. "Families of children with chronic conditions share a common set of challenges: high health care costs, greater caretaking responsibilities, obstacles to adequate education, and the additional stress these issues create for the entire family" (Institute for Health and Aging, 1996, p. 26).

"Estimates of the prevalence of children with disabilities and chronic illnesses vary from 2% to 32%...Larger estimates typically include children with conditions that place few or no limitations on the child's functioning. Smaller estimates include children with conditions that place comparatively severe limitations on the child's functioning" (Ireys, Katz, 1997, p. 3). Over 4 million children and adolescents have disabilities (Kaye, 1997). High rates of activity limitations have been identified among children and youth ages 5 to 17, children and youth in families living below the poverty line, and males ages 5 to 17. Approximately half of the persons in the United States who have a disability report that their disability began either at birth to adolescence (24%) or as a young adult (27%) (Federal Interagency Forum on Child and Family Statistics, 2000).

Causes for disability among children fall under two major categories: diseases and disorders account for approximately 58% of disabling conditions, and impairment accounts for the remaining 42%. The most common *causes of disability* among children, in rank order, are asthma, mental retardation, mental disorders, diseases of the nervous system and sense organs, and speech impairments (Wenger, Kaye, LaPlante, 1996). The five most prevalent *causes of limitations* among persons under 18 years, in rank order, are asthma, learning disability and mental retardation, mental illness, speech impairments, and hearing impairments (LaPlante, Carlson, 1996). Hyperkinetic syndrome of childhood accounts for two thirds of mental illness in childhood (Kraus, Stoddard, Gilmartin, 1996).

Asthma affects more than 15 million Americans, including almost 5 million children (CDC, 1998). The CDC's National Center for Environmental Health is focusing on preventing asthma and improving the health and quality of life for persons with this disease. Asthma is a very costly disease. The estimated cost of asthma in the year 2000 was about $14.5 billion (CDC, 1998). The CDC's National Center for Environmental Health is assisting states in developing a national strategy to address this condition.

Community health nurses provide supportive assistance in a variety of ways to families whose children have chronic conditions. They assist these families in obtaining adequate health care, in making necessary adjustments in family lifestyle, and in obtaining community resources that will help them promote their child's growth and development. A major role for community health nurses who work with families who are dealing with children with disabilities is the care manager. This role in relation to persons who have disabilities is discussed in Chapter 18.

Community health nurses also assume a significant role in assisting children to accept peers who have a chronic condition. A program to help children adjust to other children with chronic disabling conditions is *Kids on the Block*. This program is a puppet presentation showing puppets in wheelchairs, with assistive devices, and with various physical and mental conditions. It stimulates discussion of children's feelings about peers who are different. Educational and health professionals can obtain more information about *Kids on the Block* by contacting 1-800-368-KIDS or *http://www.KOTB.com*.

In addition to the chronic diseases just addressed, children experience many other chronic conditions, environmental problems, and psychosocial concerns that present serious difficulties for both themselves and their families. For example, homelessness is becoming increasingly prevalent among families with children. Homelessness and other social problems including child abuse, sexually transmitted diseases, and drug abuse are discussed in Chapter 13. None of these concerns are unique to children. However, some of them are briefly highlighted in this chapter to emphasize the need for health care professionals to evaluate the influence of these problems on child growth and development. Additionally, lead poisoning and unintended teenage parenthood are addressed.

LEAD POISONING. **Lead poisoning** is one of the most common preventable *environmental* diseases of childhood in the United States. Mental retardation, learning disabilities, and other neurological handicaps are the needless results of this condition. Infants and young children are at highest risk for complications of lead toxicity because they absorb lead more readily than do adults, and their nervous systems are more susceptible to the effects of lead (CDC, 1997). Currently the blood lead level that defines childhood lead poisoning is 10 $\mu$g/dL (Landrigan, 2000). The lowest blood lead concentration associated with deficits in cognitive functioning and academic achievement requires continued exploration. A recent study by Lanphear, Dietrich, Auinger, and Cox (2000) suggests that lead may exert toxicity at concentrations lower than 5 $\mu$g/dL.

Despite recent and substantial declines in lead poisoning among children in the United States, almost 1 million American children still have elevated blood lead levels (Satcher, 2000). The risk for lead exposure remains disproportionately high for some groups, including children who are poor, non-Hispanic blacks, Mexican Americans, those living in large metropolitan areas, or those living in older housing (CDC, 2000b; USDHHS, 2000b). Young children enrolled in Medicaid are also a group at high risk for lead poisoning (Bloch, Rosenblum, Guthrie, 2000). Federal health care programs are not effectively reaching at-risk children (General Accounting Office, 1999).

Lead exposure risk is primarily determined by a child's environmental conditions (CDC, 1997). The most serious remaining sources of lead exposure for children are contaminated soil, dust, and paint (Lynch, Boatright, Moss, 2000). These sources of lead exposure continue to plague our children despite the fact that the manufacturing of residential paint with lead was eliminated in 1976 and a phase-out of leaded fuel was initiated in the 1970s (CDC, 1997).

Lead poisoning is not confined to poor children in deteriorated neighborhoods. No economic or racial subgrouping of children is exempt from the risk of adverse health effects from lead toxicity. It is estimated that 24 million U.S. dwellings, 4.4 million of which have children living in them, have deteriorated leaded paint and elevated levels of lead-contaminated house dust (CDC, 2001a). These homes are found in all types of communities.

Children from some ethnic groups (e.g., Hmong, Chinese, and Hispanic) are exposed to lead through folk remedies used to treat minor ailments. Chinese herbal medicines, Paylooah, an Asian folk medicine used for treating fever in children, and Azarcon, a Mexican folk remedy for "empacho" or chronic indigestion, have been identified as sources of lead poisoning among children (CDC, 1993a). Box 16-12 provides a description of these traditional ethnic remedies and how they are used.

Although knowledge about its etiology, pathophysiology, and epidemiology has increased significantly in the past two decades, childhood lead poisoning continues to remain a major public health problem. Federal strategies aimed at eliminating childhood lead poisoning recommend a multi-tiered approach for dealing with the problem that includes environmental management, medical follow-up based on elevated blood lead levels, universal screening of all young children, and primary preventive activities such as identification and remediation of sites of lead (CDC, 1997; President's Task Force on Environmental Health Risks and Safety Risks to Children, 2000). The most recent federal strategy (President's Task Force on Environmental Health Risks and Safety Risks to Children, 2000) aims to make

### BOX 16-12
*Ethnic Sources of Lead Exposure*

In some cultures the use of traditional ethnic remedies may contain lead and increase children's risk of lead poisoning. These remedies include:

**Azarcon** (Mexico)—For digestive problems; a bright orange powder; usual dose is ¼ to 1 teaspoon, often mixed with oil, milk, or sugar, or sometimes given as a tea; sometimes a pinch is added to a baby bottle or tortilla dough for preventive purposes

**Greta** (Mexico)—A yellow-orange powder, used in the same way as azarcon

**Paylooah** (Southeast Asia)—Used for rash or fever; an orange-red powder given as ½ teaspoon straight or in a tea

**Surma** (India)—Black powder applied to the inner lower eyelid that is used as a cosmetic to improve eyesight

**Unknown Ayurvedic** (Tibet)—Small, gray-brown balls used to improve slow development; two balls are given orally three times a day

Modified from Centers for Disease Control and Prevention (CDC): Lead poisoning associated with use of traditional ethnic remedies—California, 1991-1992, *MMWR* 42(27):521-524, 1993a; from Wong DL, Hockenberry-Eaton M, Wilson D, et al.: *Whaley and Wong's nursing care of infants and children,* ed 6, St Louis, 1999, Mosby p. 749.

### BOX 16-13
*Warning Signs of Abuse*

Physical evidence of abuse and/or neglect, including previous injuries

Conflicting stories about the "accident" or injury from the parents or others

Cause of injury blamed on sibling or other party

An injury inconsistent with the history, such as a concussion and broken arm from falling off a bed

History inconsistent with child's developmental level; such as a 6-month-old turning on the hot water

A complaint other than the one associated with signs of abuse (e.g., a chief complaint of a cold when there is evidence of first- and second-degree burns)

Inappropriate response of caregiver, such as an exaggerated or absent emotional response; refusal to sign for additional tests or agree to necessary treatment; excessive delay in seeking treatment; absence of the parents for questioning

Inappropriate response of child, such as little or no response to pain; fear of being touched; excessive or lack of separation anxiety; indiscriminate friendliness to strangers

Child's report of physical or sexual abuse

Previous reports of abuse in the family

Repeated visits to emergency facilities with injuries

From Wong DL, Hockenberry-Eaton M, Wilson D, et al.: *Whaley and Wong's nursing care of infants and children,* ed 6, St Louis, 1999, Mosby, p. 763.

---

homes lead-safe and to provide early intervention for children at highest risk, with a focus on prevention.

A comprehensive, community-wide approach is essential to prevent lead poisoning among children. This approach should focus on controlling lead exposure in high-risk areas, epidemiological investigation of environmental hazards, casefinding, early diagnosis and treatment, dissemination of educational materials to professionals and the public, and the passage of effective legal regulations. Community health nurses assume responsibility for many of these activities.

CHILD MALTREATMENT. As a result of increased reporting requirements in recent years, it is now recognized that child maltreatment is a major public health problem that affects children of all ages. **Child maltreatment** can involve physical and/or psychological abuse and neglect, emotional abuse or neglect, and sexual abuse. Examples of child maltreatment include infliction of direct harm or injury; failure to provide adequate food, clothing, shelter, and medical care; placing a child at an unreasonable risk because of the failure of an adult to intervene to eliminate that risk; and sexual exploitation (State of Michigan, 2001).

In 1998, about 903,000 children were victims of substantiated child abuse or neglect (Maternal and Child Health Bureau, 2000). *Substantiated* means that investigations by state child protective agencies confirmed that abuse or neglect occurred. A sizable proportion of these

children suffered neglect (about 56%), 23% experienced physical abuse, 12% experienced sexual abuse, 0.6 % experienced emotional abuse or neglect, and 25% other forms of maltreatment. In 1998, 1100 children died from abuse or neglect (Maternal and Child Health Bureau, 2000).

Parents of the victims are most often the perpetrator of child maltreatment. Generally younger children under 3 years of age suffer the most abuse and neglect (Maternal and Child Health Bureau, 2000). Recently greater attention is being given to the large overlap between child maltreatment and woman abuse (Edleson, 1999). Chapter 13 elaborates on this concern and other aspects of domestic violence.

Although reporting of child maltreatment has improved significantly in the last decade, this problem continues to be underreported and is often not identified (USDHHS, 1996). All health care professionals must expand their efforts to identify undetected abuse and neglect in children. The warning signs of abuse are presented in Box 16-13. Clinical manifestations of potential child maltreatment can be found in Appendix 16-2. These indicators assist nurses in identifying victims of abuse and neglect. Strategies aimed at preventing initial maltreatment or its recurrence should be focused on changing risk factors that have been demonstrated to have a major influence on child abuse. For example, strategies designed to reduce marital and financial stresses in families, such as referring families to community agencies for financial aid and counseling, are appropriately aimed at eliminating a significant risk factor.

The problems of child maltreatment are compounded for professionals who work with the school-age population because often they must deal with the lasting effects of conditions that existed during infancy and the preschool years. Longitudinal studies are beginning to report findings that indicate long-term detrimental consequences of child abuse. Children who are abused during early childhood tend to have difficulty establishing trust, have more aggressive and behavioral problems than children who have not been abused, and frequently manifest a general air of depression, unhappiness, and sadness. Children who are sexually abused initially exhibit anger, hostility, and sexual problems, but in the long term, more serious problems such as diminished self-esteem, fear, and depression emerge (Briere, Elliott, 1994; Dubowitz, 1986). In addition, data suggest that long-term effects of child maltreatment may include other problems such as juvenile delinquency, attempted suicide, substance abuse, truancy, and runaway behavior (Lindberg, Distad, 1985; Powers, Echenrode, Jaklitsch, 1990).

Many community resources are available to assist both health professionals and the public to increase their knowledge about child maltreatment and help them intervene effectively with abusive families. In 1975 the federal government established the *National Clearinghouse on Child Abuse and Neglect* (P.O. Box 1182, Washington, D.C., 20013, 1-800-394-3366) to assist communities with their educational needs regarding child abuse. This clearinghouse disseminates information and resource materials on all types of child maltreatment, responds to public inquiries, and has a computerized database that maintains updated statistics. Hotline services also are readily available to help communities and troubled families. The *National Child Abuse Hotline* (1-800-422-4453) provides information, professional counseling, and referrals for treatment. The *Parents Anonymous* National Office (909-621-6184) provides information on self-help groups for parents involved in child maltreatment. Most states have a hotline for Parents Anonymous.

**TEENAGE PARENTHOOD.** National attention is focused on unintended pregnancy (IOM, 1995), because the consequences associated with these pregnancies can burden children, parents, families, and society. Although unintended pregnancies have declined in recent years, almost 50% of all pregnancies are still unintended. Unintended pregnancies occur among women of all socioeconomic, marital status, and age groups. However, the incidence of unintended pregnancy is highest among unmarried and lower-income women and among women at either end of the age span (IOM, 1995; USDHHS, 1995). Discussion here highlights **teenage pregnancy.**

Although the birth rate for teenagers reached an all-time low in 1999 (National Center for Health Statistics, 2000), there were still 467,631 live births among teenagers that year (Maternal and Child Health Bureau, 2000). "For teenagers, the problems associated with unintended pregnancy are compounded, and the consequences are well documented. Teenaged mothers are less likely to get or stay married, less likely to complete high school or college, and more likely to live in poverty than their peers who are not mothers" (USDHHS, 2000b).

Medically, both the teenage mother and her baby are at high risk. Children born to teenage parents have a much higher neonatal, postnatal, and infant mortality rate. These babies have a higher incidence of prematurity, low birth weight, and respiratory distress. The mothers tend to have more physical problems throughout their pregnancy. Considering that adolescence is a period when marked physical changes and rapid growth occurs, it is understandable that the additional stress of pregnancy increases a teenage mother's susceptibility to health difficulties. Toxemia, hypertension, nutritional deficiencies, prolonged labor, pelvic disproportion, and cesarean sections are a few complications of pregnancy common to the teenage mother (Alan Guttmacher Institute, 1994; IOM, 1995; USDHHS, 1995).

The *Healthy People 2010* family planning objectives are aimed at reducing pregnancies among teenagers younger than 18 and unintended pregnancies among all women. The emphasis for teenagers is on reducing the incidence of sexual intercourse, increasing effective use of contraceptive methods for the purposes of preventing pregnancy and sexually transmitted diseases, and increasing the opportunities for age-appropriate sexuality education, care, and counseling (USDHHS, 2000b).

The multiplicity and complexity of needs manifested during teenage parenthood mandate close coordination among professionals from all disciplines. Pregnancy can pose serious physical and psychosocial health problems and concerns for the teenage parents, their families, and the community at large. The involved teenagers are dealing with two normative stressors, adolescence and parenthood, which may result in adverse, long-lasting psychosocial consequences if effective intervention is not available.

Population- and community-focused programming is needed to address the problems associated with teenage pregnancy. Successful pregnancy prevention programs are comprehensive in nature and provide continuity of care over several years. They also connect adolescents with peer and adult role models, include life skills education, as well as sexuality and contraceptive education and services, and provide mechanisms for buffering youth against the pressures of their environment (USDHHS, 1995).

Recently, efforts in some communities have been strengthened to prevent the negative outcomes associated with adolescent parenting. A variety of innovative approaches are being used to help teenage mothers complete their education, prevent repeat pregnancies, and encourage responsible parenting. "These approaches include alternative schools for pregnant and parenting students within the public school system, residential facilities for homeless teenage mothers on AFDC (now renamed Temporary Assistance to Needy Families), home visiting to assist teenage mothers and their families, and school-based programs that serve mothers as part of a larger effort aimed at all at-risk teenagers" (GAO, 1995, pp. 2-3). Box 16-14 displays the

### BOX 16-14

## Services to Support High School Completion Among Teenage Mothers

*Financial*
Child care
Transportation
Housing
Small scholarships

*Social*
Parenting education
Life skills classes
Counseling
Anger/stress management
Support groups
Teen fathers program
Recreational activities

*Employment/Education*
Vocational/job skills training
Job placement
Job/college fairs
Tutoring
Mentor program

*Health*
Mental health counseling
Family planning/pregnancy prevention
Child development classes
Home visits by prenatal community nurse
Substance abuse counseling
Group therapy
Health care

*Special Features*
Case management
Teen parent coordinator/advisor
Sanctions for repeat pregnancy
Summer program
Program for dropouts
In-home visits
On-site health clinic

From General Accounting Office (GAO): *Welfare to work: approaches that help teenage mothers complete high school,* Washington, DC, 1995, GAO, pp. 11-12.

range of services provided by 13 local programs that are recognized by experts as being exemplary in helping disadvantaged teenage mothers complete their high school education. A variety of approaches and services can help mothers expand life options (GAO, 1995).

Studies on the consequences of unintended pregnancies and nonmarital childbearing tend to focus on mothers and children. Fathers involved in teenage childbearing tend to be older than the mother. Males and Chew (1996) contend "what we call school age childbearing is predominantly a teen-adult phenomenon" (p. 567). It is estimated that only a minority (26%) of men involved in pregnancies among adolescent women under age 18 are that young: 35% are ages 18 to 19, and 39% are at least 20 (Alan Guttmacher Institute, 1994). Little is known about the impact of pregnancy on the fathers involved in adolescent childbearing. The limited studies that examine adolescent fathering suggest that educational and emotional problems precede rather than follow the act of fathering (Resnick, Chambliss, Blum, 1993). Community health professionals must strengthen their efforts in reaching out to fathers involved in adolescent childbearing.

**SEXUALLY TRANSMITTED DISEASES.** One alarming consequence of early initiation of sexual activity among adolescents is the high rates of **sexually transmitted diseases (STDs)** in this age category. Although STDs occur among men and women of all socioeconomic and age groups, STDs disproportionately affect the young, the poor, and minorities (USDHHS, 2000b). Almost 15 million cases of STDs occur annually, 66% of them in people under the age of 25 years (CDC, 1999; USDHHS, 2000b). Almost 4 million of the new cases of STDs occur in adolescents, and many of these adolescents are at risk for PID. Yearly more than 1 million women experience an episode of acute PID, with most cases associated with gonorrhea and chlamydia infections (CDC, 2001a). Women aged 15 to 19 years had the highest reported rates of both chlamydia and gonorrhea among women in 1998. PID can lead to infertility, tubal pregnancy, chronic pelvic pain, and other serious consequences. Over 100,000 women become infertile as a result of PID each year (USDHHS, 2000b).

Of great concern is the growing segments of young children, adolescents, and young adults affected with AIDs. As of June 2000, there were 12,669 cases of AIDs among children aged 19 and under (CDC, 2000c). Young children under the age of 13 are primarily exposed to human immunodeficiency virus (HIV) through perinatal transmission before or during birth. Adolescents are primarily exposed to HIV through receipt of blood products and high-risk behaviors, including heterosexual and male-to-male sexual contact and injecting drug use. Young adults are primarily exposed to HIV through high-risk behaviors. Among young adult men, the major exposure category associated with AIDS is male-to-male contact; among young adult women, exposure to HIV is primarily through injecting drug use or through sex with an injecting drug user. The majority of young adults are probably exposed to HIV during adolescence (Maternal and Child Health Bureau, 2000). Chapter 13 further expands on the epidemiology of AIDs.

Community health nurses working with the school-age population must realize that the occurrence of STDs is a *major* health problem in this age group. Programs that provide preventive, curative, and educative services for all children in the population served by the nurse must be planned. Use of the epidemiological process (Chapter 11) and the principles of health planning (Chapter 15) facilitate the accomplishment of such a task. For readily accessible STD information, the nurse or client may want to use the STD Hotline at 1-800-227-8922, or the AIDS Hotline at 1-800-342-AIDS. These hotlines provide information on STDs and confidential referrals for diagnosis and treatment.

"If adults are going to help teenagers avoid the outcomes of sex that are clearly negative—STDs, unintended pregnancies, abortions, and out-of-wedlock births—they must accept the reality of adolescent sexual activity and deal with it directly and honestly" (Alan Guttmacher Institute, 1994, p. 5). Teenagers encounter a host of stressors that place them at risk for pregnancy and STDs acquisition. They often lack experience in communicating with their partners about contraceptive use. They also frequently fear disclosure and avoid seeking contraceptive services to prevent others from knowing they are sexually active. Additionally, they often lack access to an appropriate source of care and must deal with numerous contradictory messages about responsible sexual behavior. Other Western democracies are much more open with adolescents about sexual relationships (Alan Guttmacher Institute, 1994). Our nation needs to learn from these countries.

SUBSTANCE ABUSE. Substance abuse among American youth is a major public health problem. **Substance abuse** involves the misuse of tobacco, alcohol, illicit drugs, prescription medication, and other substances such as glue. Data from the annual national drug survey, the *Monitoring the Future* study, indicate that substance abuse is widespread. Despite recent decline in the percentage of adolescents ages 12 to 17 reporting use of some illicit drugs in the month before the survey, the use of several drugs remained essentially unchanged in the year 2000 (Johnston, O'Malley, Bachman, 2000). Use of inhalants, LSD, "ice," Rohypnol, cigarettes, and smokeless tobacco were all down in 2000 from peak levels in the mid-1990s. Those drugs not showing a decline include amphetamines, barbiturates, tranquilizers, hallucinogens other than LSD, opiates other than heroin, and alcohol. Ecstasy use rose sharply among teens in 2000 (Johnston, O'Malley, Bachman, 2000). Marijuana is the most widely used illicit drug. Despite recent declines in smoking rates, the prevalence of smoking has increased substantially among teens since 1991.

The findings from national surveys suggest that our nation cannot afford to be lax in the attention given to the control of drug abuse among youth. Overall, drug use among high school students and young adults remains widespread. Although there are regional and population differences in the use of illicit drugs among young people, no community is free of illegal drug use by secondary and college students (Johnston, O'Malley, Bachman, 2000). "The drug problem is not an enemy which can be vanquished, as in a war. It is more a recurring and relapsing problem which must be contained to the extent possible on a long-term, ongoing basis; and, therefore, it is a problem which requires an ongoing, dynamic response from our society" (Johnston, O'Malley, Bachman, 1996, p. 29).

The dynamics associated with substance abuse, as well as the role of community health nurses in addressing this problem, are discussed in Chapter 13. For youth, drug abuse prevention programs have traditionally employed one or both of two strategies: educational or social control through policy and regulation or legislation (Goodstadt, 1989). Based on a review of pertinent research related to preventive drug intervention, Goodstadt (1989) promoted the joint development and implementation of educational and policy strategies to combat drug abuse in school settings.

Dusenbury, Falco, and Lake (1997) recently reviewed 47 nationally and currently available classroom-based drug abuse curricula that focused on primary prevention and were designed for any grade level K-12, for which samples could be obtained from program distributors. They found that "prevention curricula which give students training in social resistance skills or how to recognize influences and resist them effectively, and normative education positing that drug use is not the norm, have been shown to reduce substance use behavior. In addition, training in broader personal and social skills such as decision making, anxiety reduction, communication, and assertiveness appears to enhance program effectiveness" (Dusenbury, Falco, Lake, 1997, p. 127).

Ten of the 47 drug prevention curricula available to schools have been evaluated in rigorous research studies and have been shown to reduce substance abuse (Table 16-2). However, two curricula (Social Competence Promotion and Teenage Health Teaching Modules) need further evaluation beyond the posttest to determine the sustained effects on students' drug use. The Project Alert and DARE Curricula had variable success at reducing substance use initially but did not appear to have a long-lasting effect. Dusenbury, Falco, and Lake (1997) believe "these [two] programs may still make an important contribution to drug abuse prevention, if done within the context of ongoing and sustained prevention efforts" (p. 130). They stress that reinforcement and follow-up are critical elements of any prevention program. If a program is brief, such as the Project Alert and DARE programs, it appears that the effects diminish over time (Dusenbury, Falco, Lake, 1997).

**TABLE 16-2**

*Drug Abuse Prevention Curricula: Contact Information*

| CURRICULUM NAME | CONTACT |
|---|---|
| Alcohol Misuse Prevention Project | University of Michigan Institute for Social Research Room 2349 Ann Arbor, MI 48106-1248 734-764-8354 |
| DARE | DARE America P.O. Box 2090 Los Angeles, CA 90051-0090 800-223-DARE |
| Growing Healthy | National Center for Health Education 72 Spring Street Suite 208 New York, NY 10012-4019 800-551-3488 |
| Know Your Body | American Health Foundation 675 Third Avenue 11th Floor New York, NY 10017 212-551-2509 |
| Life Skills Training | Institute for Prevention Research Cornell University Medical 411 East 69th Street New York, NY 10021 212-746-1270 |
| Project Alert | Best Foundation 725 South Figueroa Street Suite 1615 Los Angeles, CA 90017 800-ALERT-10 |
| Project Northland | University of Minnesota Division of Epidemiology School of Public Health 1300 South Second Street Suite 300 Minneapolis, MN 55445-1015 612-624-0057 |
| Social Competence Promotion Program | Department of Psychology (M/C 285) University of Illinois at Chicago 1007 West Harrison Street Chicago, IL 60607-7137 312-413-1012 |
| STAR | Institute for Prevention Research 1540 Alcazar Street, CHP 207 Los Angeles, CA 90033 323-442-2600 |
| Teenage Health Teaching Module | Educational Development Center 55 Chapel Street Newton, MA 02158-1060 800-225-4276 |

From Dusenbury L, Falco M, Lake A: A review of the evaluation of 47 drug abuse prevention curricula available nationally, *J Sch Health* 67:127-132, 1997, p. 131.

Significant drug prevention and referral service information can be obtained from several national organizations. Alcoholics Anonymous, Cocaine Anonymous, and Narcotics Anonymous answer questions on health risks of substance abuse, provide self-help support services, and assist people in obtaining needed drug treatment services. These organizations are found in local telephone directories. The National Clearinghouse for Alcohol and Drug Information (1-800-729-6686) provides a broad range of educational materials on drug-related issues. The National Parents' Resource Institute for Drug Education (PRIDE) also disseminates lay and professional materials on substance abuse and refers families to appropriate service organizations. The National Institute on Drug Abuse hotline (1-800-662-HELP) provides general information on drug abuse and drug prevention programs and offers referrals to drug rehabilitation centers. The national plan for drug control can be obtained from the Office of National Drug Control Policy (2000). Most states and local communities also have resources that assist youth, adults, and professionals interested in obtaining drug abuse prevention and treatment information. These resources can be accessed by contacting your local health department or community mental health center.

## Stop and Think About It

You are working with teachers and students at an alternative high school to create 1- to 2-minute taped health issues announcements to be broadcast over the school's public announcement system. Taking into consideration the major causes of mortality and morbidity among adolescents and the developmental tasks of this age group, what health issues would you address? How might you creatively present these issues?

## HEALTH PROMOTION DURING INFANCY AND CHILDHOOD

All children must accomplish health promotion tasks that help them prevent mortality and morbidity, develop healthy lifestyle behaviors, and enhance future development and maturation (see Appendixes 16-3 through 16-6). Sometimes it is a struggle for children to achieve these tasks. The author of "Stuffed Rabbit" (Box 16-15) dramatically illustrates the stressful process a child goes through to develop independence during adolescence. Parents, health care professionals, and other interested individuals can help children make the growing process less stressful. They can assist children in achieving a healthy adulthood through preventive and health promoting interventions such as safety education. Because health risks and needs among children change over time, it is crucial for child caregivers to view health promotion as a longitudinal process that enhances a child's health at critical transition periods (Green, 1994). Health promotion in the newborn to 5-year-old age group is particularly important because this period provides the foundation for the physical, intellectual, and emotional health for the rest of the child's life.

Anticipatory guidance in helping parents to know what to expect of their children at different stages and when to obtain preventive health care services is one of the most *basic* and *significant* health promotion needs of parents. Through anticipatory guidance parents can gain knowledge about child growth and development and parenting activities that promote a nurturing and safe environment for their children. Anticipatory guidance is a process that involves gathering information about the child and his or her environment, establishing alliance with the parents, and providing education and guidance around development milestones and parent and child concerns (Foye, 1997). For example, a major concern of many parents is how to get quality day care services for their children. Community health nurses discuss with parents how to assess the quality of day care programs and, with some parents, where they might get financial help to pay for these services.

Appendix 16-7 presents a timeline for preventive health care. A recommended schedule for immunizations is presented in Figure 16-12, and anticipatory guidance health supervision topics for infants, children, and adolescents are presented in Appendix 16-8. Timely anticipatory guidance assists parents and children to understand developmental needs and health risks. This, in turn, helps parents and children to develop effective strategies for stress management and problem solving. For example, the community health nurse can help parents discuss sexuality issues openly and honestly with their children by helping them address their fears regarding these issues. Community health nurses also can help parents discuss concerns about common childhood needs such as dental care, adequate nutrition, and behavioral problems.

Both individual-focused and population-focused interventions are used by health care professionals to guide children and their families through the growth process. Individual-focused interventions are aimed at monitoring growth and development on a continuous basis, helping children to develop healthy lifestyle patterns, and creating a supportive family environment to enhance growth and development. The topics of anticipatory guidance presented in Appendix 16-8 assist health care providers to identify family and child strengths and health service needs. A family-centered approach to care is essential for health providers to successfully promote a child's health. Families provide the nurturing environment needed by children to successfully achieve developmental tasks across the age continuum.

From a population-focused perspective, health care providers work in partnership with communities to design health promotion programs based on community needs and national and local health objectives. Illustrative of this are the innovative cardiovascular health promotion projects developed to promote children's heart health. These programs are grounded in the belief that primary prevention is the key to successfully reduce major problems in adulthood.

The National Heart, Lung, and Blood Institute has funded several culturally relevant programs to address children's heart health. For example, the HIP HOP TO

 **BOX 16-15**

*Stuffed Rabbit*

> Stuffed rabbit
> Seven years my nocturnal security
> Now neglected worn and eyeless
> Lying in the memory-choked attic
> Stabbed by blunt dusty shafts of sunlight
> Recalling to me
> Evenings of forbidden play beneath giggle-muffling blankets
> Recalling to me the day I grew
> Too big
> Too old
> To sleep with innocence while hugging security
> I'll leave you here stuffed rabbit,
> You're dead
> But God, what a long slow funeral we're having!
>
> Gregory Smith, written at age 18

HEALTH program, designed to honor the African-American heritage, reflects children's interest in the inner city–bred phenomenon of hip-hop music. This project uses ethnic traditions and tastes in music, dancing, food, clothing, and sports to promote healthy heart eating and activity among inner-city African-American children. The PATHWAYS program is another example of a culturally relevant health promotion heart project. It uses traditional Native American games, such as "the coyote has smelly feet," an Apache version of tag, to promote an understanding of different tribal cultures and to increase physical activity among Native American children. It also helps families prepare healthy traditional tribal foods and children develop healthy nutritional habits. The 1996 special edition of the *Heart Memo* published by the National Heart, Lung, and Blood Institute, discusses both the HIP HOP TO HEALTH and the PATHWAYS programs, as well as several other heart healthy projects for children. This Heart Memo provides valuable tips for developing effective population-focused interventions for children.

## GENERAL CONCEPTS OF HEALTH PROMOTION

Health promotion needs are based on the developmental tasks and common health problems of the specific population group. For children and parenting populations, the following factors should be considered when developing a strong community-based health promotion program:

- A monitoring system to identify high-risk infants, children, and parents
- An organized community program to combat problems such as accidents, child abuse and neglect, and substance abuse
- An organized system for provision of preventive health services, such as physical examinations and immunizations

- A health education program designed to meet anticipatory guidance needs of parents and children
- A well-established procedure for follow-up care of clients with identified health needs
- Passage and revision of significant legislation, such as immunization and child abuse laws and laws addressing educational needs of special populations
- An organized process for addressing critical biopsychosocial child and parenting needs such as adequate day care services and recreational facilities.

When working with children, it is critical for all health care professionals to observe for lags in normal growth and development. Early casefinding and intervention can prevent permanent disability. A comprehensive biopsychosocial and cultural assessment should be done with every child and family when the child is not performing at the appropriate developmental age level. Intervention should be started immediately if a developmental disability is confirmed.

## Developmental Disabilities

Developmental disabilities are increasingly common among school-age children and present significant stresses to those affected. Although estimates of the number of children with developmental disabilities vary significantly, it is known that several million children and their families are dealing with this problem. A diagnosis of a disabling condition constitutes a crisis for families and may require multiple adjustments in their lifestyle. Community health nurses frequently assume a significant role in promoting physical and psychosocial well-being among families by addressing the issues related to developmental disabilities.

As with average children, the degree to which children with developmental disabilities adjust successfully as healthy individuals varies. The nature and quality of their previous and current life experiences and their physical, emotional, and cognitive status greatly influence how well children with developmental disabilities progress. Numerous variables affect the socioadaptive capacity of children with developmental disabilities. An overwhelming number of the factors are influenced by environmental conditions, which are discussed in Chapter 18.

Since the passage of Public Law 94-142, Education for All Handicapped Children Act in 1975 (renamed the **Individuals with Disabilities Education Act [IDEA]** in 1990), the number of children receiving special education services in elementary and secondary public schools has increased significantly. One in every 10 students in public schools today receives special education under IDEA (Office of Special Education Programs, 1994). Over half of all children receiving special education services in public schools are identified as having a learning disability. Almost one fourth are identified as having speech or language impairments; over one tenth are identified as having mental retardation; and almost one tenth are identified as having serious emotional disturbances (Office of Special Education Programs, 1994). Lyon

(1996) contends that "the influence of advocacy has contributed to a substantial proliferation in the number of children who have been identified with learning disabilities relative to other handicapping conditions" (p. 57).

Public Law 94-142 mandated that every school system receiving special federal educational funds must provide a "free, appropriate education for all handicapped children between the ages of six and eighteen, regardless of the type of handicap or the degree of impairment." It also provided incentive monies to extend services to children beginning at age 3 and for young adults between 18 through 21. Public Law 99-457 (the Education for All Handicapped Children Act Amendments of 1986) amended Public Law 94-142 and created a new Preschool Grant Program (currently reauthorized under P.L. 102-119). This program mandates that children, beginning at the age of 3, have the "right to education." It also created a new Handicapped Infants and Toddlers Program that provides incentive monies to enhance educational services for disabled and at-risk infants and toddlers. Provisions of this law require that each child have an Individualized Education Program (IEP) and families have an Individualized Family Service Plan (IFSP). IEPs specify measurable performance goals and indicators to assess progress toward goal achievement (Boundy, 2000).

School systems that receive IDEA funds are required to purchase whatever is needed to meet a child's educational needs. Other major mandates covered by IDEA are:
- a "child-find plan" to identify all children within the state who have special needs;
- appropriate educational opportunities in the least restrictive environment;
- due process safeguards that help parents provide input concerning their child's educational needs and challenge decisions regarding their child;
- an IEP; and
- assurance that tests and other evaluation materials do not reflect cultural or racial bias.

## COMMUNITY-BASED SERVICES FOR MOTHERS AND CHILDREN

During the past century significant federal legislation has been passed and many demonstration projects held to address the health of infants and mothers in America. The Children's Bureau was established in 1912 to improve children's health and reduce infant mortality. The Sheppard-Towner Act of 1921 created federally supported maternal and child health services at the state level. Title V of the Social Security Act of 1935 has provided grants to states for maternal and child health services and services for children with disabilities for over 65 years. The Eighty-ninth Congress, during President Johnson's time in office (1963-1968), brought huge changes in child health legislation with the establishment of the Office of Economic Opportunity and its Head Start Program, Medicaid, and the National Institutes of Child Health and Human Development. Significant current legislation continues to provide funding for maternal and child health services.

Seven major public programs help fund health services and establish programs for women and children in need. These programs are the preventive health and health services block grant; maternal and child health block grant; the Early and Periodic Screening, Diagnosis, and Treatment portion of Medicaid; the childhood immunization program; childhood lead poisoning prevention; community health centers; and migrant health centers (General Accounting Office, 1992; HRSA, 2000). Table 16-3 provides significant data related to each of these programs, which provide a broad range of health, welfare, and environmental services, such as expanded medical and social services for pregnant mothers and infants, screening services for infants and children, health care for special populations, and healthy start initiatives. In 1997, Congress created the **Children's Health Insurance Program (CHIP)** under the Balanced Budget Act, for children whose families earn too much to qualify for Medicaid but too little to afford private health insurance (CDF, 2000). A significant number of children

**TABLE 16-3**

*Programs Serving Low-Income Mothers and Children in the United States: Program Objectives and Target Population**

| PROGRAM AND AUTHORITY | PROGRAM OBJECTIVES AND TARGET POPULATION |
|---|---|
| **Community Health Centers Grant (CHC)** (Section 330, Public Health Service [PHS] Act) | This program provides preventive and primary health care services and case management of other services to medically underserved populations;[†] each CHC must demonstrate the capability to serve all age groups, and should be able to identify populations in its service area with special health care needs. |
| **Migrant Health Centers Grant (MHC)** (Section 329, PHS Act) | This program provides preventive services and management of other services to migrant and seasonal farmworkers and their families; in defining its appropriate role, each center assesses the needs of its target population. |
| **Maternal and Child Health Block Grant (M&CH)** (Title V, Social Security Act [SSA]) | This block grant program seeks to improve the health of mothers and children who do not have access to adequate health care,[‡] particularly those from low-income families: direct services include preventive and primary care for children, prenatal care and delivery services, and postpartum care, but this funding also helps to support the state service delivery infrastructure; other services must also be provided for children with special health care needs (rehabilitative services for certain categories of children under 16 who are disabled). |
| **Childhood Lead Poisoning Prevention Program (CLPPP)** (Lead Contamination Control Act, 1988) | This program provides states with resources to establish and expand programs to prevent childhood lead poisoning; program activities may include screening for lead poisoning, referral for medical treatment and environmental intervention, follow-up, and education about lead poisoning. It targets high-risk children under 6 years of age. |
| **Childhood Immunization Program (CIP)** (Section 317, PHS Act) | This program provides states with resources to establish and maintain programs to immunize children against vaccine-preventable diseases; CIP funds may be used for the planning and implementation of immunization programs, for vaccine purchase, and for assessment of immunization status. |
| **Preventive Health and Health Services Block Grant (PHHS)** (Title XIX, part A of PHS Act) | This block grant program provides states with resources for comprehensive preventive health services. Each state determines the target population to be served. |
| **Medicaid/Early and Periodic Screening, Diagnosis, and Treatment (EPSDT)** (Title XIX, SSA) | This program seeks to diagnose physical and mental problems in low-income children under 21 and to provide treatment to correct any conditions found. |

From General Accounting Office (GAO): *Federally funded health services: information on seven programs serving low-income women and children*, GAO/HRD-92-73FS, Gaithersburg, Md, May 1992, GAO, pp. 10-11.

*All seven programs are authorized to address the health care needs of women, children, or both, but each targets a slightly different population. The Abstinence Education Grant Program (HRSA, 2000) has been added to Title V (see *http://www.mhcb.hrsa.gov*).

[†]Medically underserved populations are designated by the U.S. Department of Health and Human Services (USDHHS) according to the percentage of population with income below the poverty level, percentage of population 65 years of age and over, infant mortality rate, and physicians per 1000 population.

[‡]The Maternal and Child Health Block Grant provides both grants to states and funding for set-aside programs. In this fact sheet, we are reporting only on the grants to states.

need this service because almost 12 million children are uninsured (Children's Defense Fund, 2000).

Other significant services are available for mothers and children in the community. As presented in Chapter 4, the Women, Infants, and Children Program (WIC) makes food available to at-risk pregnant and lactating women, infants, and children up to the age of 5 years. Mothers and children in need of food can also obtain food stamps through the Family Independent Agency (FIA). Additionally, federally subsidized food programs are available to children in Head Start programs, day care centers, schools, and other community agencies. A wide range of voluntary organizations in each community also provide emergency food as well as clothing, furniture, and other essentials to meet basic needs. Chapters 4 and 10 discuss these organizations and how to refer families to them.

Family planning services are important to help prevent unintended pregnancy. The **National Family Planning Program** (Title X of the Public Health Service Act) has funded family planning services for over 30 years. There are over 7000 clinic sites in the United States offering publicly funded contraceptive services (Frost, Ranjit, Manzella, 2001). Agencies providing Title X family planning services provide a broad range of contraceptive care, such as contraceptive education, medical evaluation, and screening for STDs.

A wide range of educational services also is available in the community to assist at-risk children. Some of those services provided for children with disabilities are discussed in the developmental disabilities section of this chapter and others are discussed in Chapter 18. *Healthy start* and *head start programs* are designed to promote infants and toddlers growth and development and to prepare them to succeed in school programs later in life. Families can obtain these and other services from the school system in their local communities. Community health nurses often refer at-risk children to these programs.

Numerous other services in many communities help mothers and children deal with a variety of concerns and needs. For example, mental health agencies are available to help families deal with behavioral problems and other mental health issues. Other agencies provide services at no or low cost for treatment of substance abuse and yet other organizations help children meet their recreational needs. Most health departments have resource guides that identify available maternal and child health services.

# THE ROLES OF THE COMMUNITY HEALTH NURSE

The community health nurse assumes a number of roles in providing service to mothers and children. The following section describes some of these roles.

## Advocate-Planner

Because children often cannot speak for themselves, the nurse becomes an advocate. This can involve pointing out to caregivers the safety hazards in the environment and urging necessary changes or working with managed care organizations to obtain needed services. On a broader level, the nurse is an advocate for the development of day care centers in a community and publicizes the inadequacy of health and medical care for economically disadvantaged families. An advocate must be involved in the political process to correct issues such as unemployment, lack of adequate income, overcrowding, and the cycle of poverty, which can ultimately be solved only with legislative changes. Attitudes of assertiveness, a knowledge of the political process, and a willingness to take risks are necessary tools for this role.

## Teacher

The community health nurse is frequently a teacher. This role includes demonstrating information about child care to families and involving parents in the learning process. Helping parents understand good nutrition for this age group, or the proper way to use safety seats and belts in cars, means involvement of all concerned in the process of teaching and learning and changing values and attitudes. The community health nurse is well versed in the developmental tasks of children and families. Teaching parents about these tasks is a form of anticipatory guidance and assists in task accomplishment.

## Group Worker

To meet the needs of mothers and children, the community health nurse must be attuned to opportunities for group teaching and counseling. Working with the La Leche League or Parents Anonymous, a crisis intervention program set up to help prevent damaging relationships between parents and their children, is an option. Other possibilities are numerous. One community health nurse, for example, had in his caseload area a large mobile park. Within the park he found that several families were interested in parenting classes. This staff nurse helped the parents form a weekly discussion group and the results were that isolated families received mutual supportive help in the form of babysitting, shared meals, and problem solving about how to deal with difficult parenting situations. Chapter 20 discusses group work opportunities in the school setting.

## Care Manager

Managing health care services and coordinating community resources is another significant role of the community health nurse. Often numerous services are available to families but are not well coordinated. Families can feel uncared for and torn apart when the Department of Social Services, Medicaid screening clinic, the community health nurse, the school nurse, the child guidance center, and other agencies all request the same information in detail, or when these same health professionals do not communicate with each other and plan different care goals. Community health nurses seek permission from families to coordinate their care.

Closely tied to the care manager role is the facilitating role of the nurse. Helping families and the larger community to understand their rights as people and to understand services offered in the community all facilitate the better use of these services. The nurse helps families work toward desired change. Every community has persons with ideas and skills; all that needs to be done is to give them direction and reinforcement. Milio's *9226 Kercheval: The Storefront That Did Not Burn* is the classic story of how one community health nurse helped an inner-city area establish its own day care center (Milio, 1970). This nurse found that people saw a great problem with children who were not cared for while mothers worked. She acted as a catalyst to assist in solving the problem and was a facilitator and enabler as well.

## Casefinder

Because of the nurse's proximity to infants, children, and their families, casefinding has been a strategic role for many years. At-risk children and parents are identified and followed periodically as they develop. Disabilities are lessened when treatment is begun early, and some can be prevented by primary intervention. A system needs to be established in each community to periodically screen all children for problems. The Early Periodic Screening, Diagnosis, and Treatment Program (EPSDT) of Medicaid is one schedule that can be followed.

The North American Nursing Diagnosis Association (NANDA) accepted several diagnoses that address the needs of children and families (Gordon, 2000). The defining characteristics for these diagnoses provide practitioners with useful parameters for casefinding when working with families and children under stress. Chapter 8 also provides assessment parameters to consider with families who need assistance with coping.

## Epidemiologist

Collecting data on health problems and care is an important epidemiological role. Nurses are concerned about why parents do not use available health services and what motivates those who do. They use population-focused practice models to answer these concerns and to develop targeted, aggregate-focused interventions that address the factors that impede service use (Association of State and Territorial Directors of Nursing [ASTDN], 2000). Reasons why people do and do not use health care are important elements in planning health services.

When the community health nurse visits parents after accidental poisoning incidents, the nurse can add to the epidemiological understanding of the predisposing and immediate causes of the accident and make recommendations to prevent them from occurring again. If it were the case that 75% of the families who have poisoning accidents have other health problems, there would be evidence that this kind of stress leads to poisoning accidents.

A good record system in the health agency will help nurses collect data on health problems, plan interventions, and evaluate care given. These data can provide information on changing health needs and necessary health services. A good record system will also collect data on the newborn to 5-year-old child that provide the basis for a health history on which later events in the family system can be compared and built.

## Clinic Nurse

Community health nurses have long worked in well-baby clinics where, at regular intervals, the health of children up to the age of 5 is assessed, immunizations are given, and parents have the opportunity to discuss concerns of growth and development. This role has been expanded to an assessment and treatment role. Nurses deal with physical and psychosocial problems such as delayed play, immature social behavior, and temper tantrums. With the nurse's knowledge of child development, behavior modification, and care management techniques, the roles of observer; consultant; and counselor to parents, preschool teachers, and day care workers are valuable in dealing with minor problems that can develop into major ones.

## Home Visitor

A well-known role of the nurse caring for the needs of children is that of the community health nurse who visits parents and children in their homes. Each health department sets its own priorities and standards for the care of parents and children. This ranges from the prenatal and postnatal referral of each pregnancy to the referral of only those mothers and infants at high risk. The broad background of community health nurses equips them with skills to help establish the standards as to which children and parents will be visited. In particular, families that are poor, uneducated, or headed by teenage parents often face barriers to getting the health care or social support services they need. Many experts believe that providing services in the home reduces these barriers. They also believe that home visiting for prenatal counseling or parenting education for this population group can address problems before they become irreversible or extremely costly (GAO, 1990). The following case scenarios illustrate some specific problems parents have in obtaining care for themselves and their children.

**CASE** *Scenario* Sue was 17 years old when she became pregnant. Her husband, Tom, age 18, worked as a gas station attendant. His income provided only the basic necessities of food and rent but was too high to allow them any public assistance. Sue decided to "save" money by waiting for antepartum care until near her estimated date of confinement (EDC). Upon her first antepartum visit to the doctor 1 month before delivery, she was found to be severely hypertensive and diabetic. Her infant weighed 10 lb at birth and required 1 month's hospitalization. Sue and Tom felt that they were severely criticized by the health personnel for not receiving adequate antepartum care.

*CASE*
*Scenario*   Diane and Jim Jones have four children under 5 years of age. Jim has a job-related back injury and is unemployed. The Joneses have a Medicaid card, and they use the outpatient department of a large teaching hospital in their city for medical care. They go there only when they absolutely must. The family has no car and uses the city bus line, which involves three transfers for the 4-mile trip. With four children, Mrs. Jones finds this most difficult, especially in cold weather. When she does arrive at the hospital, she must wait several hours and then sees a different physician each time so that she must repeatedly give her family's health histories. Mrs. Jones feels that "the people in that hospital don't care about or understand me and my kids."

The nurse who visits in the home, especially when both parents are present, is in a privileged position to closely and periodically assess the baby's, the parents', and the family's development. The nurse also can identify stress, help parents deal with problems of bonding, provide role modeling for bonding and parenting, give anticipatory guidance, and help reinforce positive behavior.

During home visits, the nurse aids families in using community resources as necessary. For example, when parents and a new baby with a diagnosis of spina bifida, Down syndrome, or other chronic health problems come home from the hospital, it is most often the community health nurse who introduces the family to community resources such as the Children's Special Health Care Services program for financial aid; to the physical therapy offered by the intermediate school program; or to the interdisciplinary diagnostic services of university-affiliated centers. This same nurse will likely be one of the persons to help parents as they go through the grief process related to having a baby who is less than "perfect." The nurse also can be alert to signs of stress within the family in this situation; living 24 hours a day with a help-less infant who needs additional care and problems can be an overwhelming problem for some families. Homemakers, parent's aides, and parent-support groups are useful when families are in such a situational crisis. Community health nurses are often in a pivotal position to help families help themselves in resolving parenting and child health issues.

## SUMMARY

Children are our nation's greatest resources. Decreasing infant and maternal mortality rates reflect this value, as does legislation such as Medicaid and CHIP, which provides health care for at least a segment of the maternal and child health populations. The challenge for community health nurses is to identify at-risk mothers and children who need services and then to help them obtain these services. The community health nurse assumes a variety of roles to achieve this goal.

Healthy families build healthy communities. The child's health and that of the parents is inextricably interwoven and significantly affected by environmental conditions. Community health nurses help parents provide the foundation for a child's lifelong physical, mental, and social development and to address environmental and other factors that impede development.

## CRITICAL THINKING
*exercise*

The View from the Field, "Lilly's Anger" (Dangelmaier, 1992, pp. 41-45), describes a public health nurse whose caseload was at-risk pregnant women and infants. Describe the skills the nurse used as she cared for Lilly and her baby. What resources are available in your local community to help client's like Lilly deal with their needs?

*A view*
*from the field*

### LILLY'S ANGER

I am a public health nurse providing home visits to "at risk" pregnant women and infants. The women and infants I see generally live in rural settings.

Perhaps the most challenging aspect of my work is trying to engage the client who, for a combination of reasons, is not initially receptive to help from someone perceived as an "outsider." The following situation provides insight to the challenges and complexities routinely encountered by public health nurses such as myself.

I first encountered Lilly approximately ten months ago. She was eight months pregnant and was found to have some abnormalities in her blood work at the last checkup. She needed to have an ultrasound immediately to determine if the baby was okay. The clinic was unable to reach Lilly by phone and asked me to stop by her home and urge her to get into the clinic as soon as possible for further assessment.

Lilly's need for help on the one hand, and resistance to any kind of intervention on the other hand, quickly sur-

From Dangelmaier A: Lilly's anger. In Zewekh J, Primomo J, Deal L, editors: *Opening doors: stories of public health nursing,* Olympia, Wash, 1992, Washington State Department of Health, Parent-Child Health Services, pp. 41-45.

faced in my initial contact. To begin with, she was very angry. Angry about being awakened from her sleep—I learned she worked nights in a laundry. Angry about having relinquished her first child and the pressure her parents were putting on her to do it again. Angry about her negative experiences with the Department of Social and Health Services. Angry at the prospect of the second ultrasound. "Didn't I just have one a month ago? Can things change all that much in four weeks?"

Speaking in a loud voice and in a forceful manner, Lilly had no difficulty letting me know her thoughts about her pregnancy and her generally less than desirable circumstances. Her anger and frustration were intensified by her imposing figure. Lilly is about six feet tall, large framed, has bright red hair, and is developmentally delayed. I found her presentation rather intimidating, especially in view of the dark and dreary house into which I had been invited to state my business. However, the fact that I allowed Lilly to vent seemed to be having a quieting effect. I tried as much as possible to validate her concerns, and as a result, she gradually became more open to having the second ultrasound. In fact, I actually dialed the number so she could set up the appointment. By the time I left Lilly's home, she was also indicating that she "might" be receptive to another visit. "But don't call until the late afternoon."

Driving away from Lilly's home, I reflected on what had transpired and wondered if I would ever see her again. Given the number of problems in this case, ongoing help was certainly needed, but would Lilly be open to it?

Attempts to make contact by phone got nowhere, so I decided to "drop-in" about four weeks after my first visit. My hope was that it was late enough in the day so Lilly would be up from her sleep and receptive to my visit. Apparently, my willingness to listen to her during my first visit rather than retreat during her burst of anger and frustration, earned a certain measure of respect and acceptance. Lilly invited me in and we began to explore in greater detail the concerns and issues touched on during my first contact. This conversation opened the way for me to introduce some thoughts on how she might deal with the problems at hand.

Lilly had followed through with the second ultrasound, which didn't reveal any abnormalities. However, because her blood pressure was up, she was advised to terminate her work and go on bed rest for the balance of her pregnancy— a matter of a week or so. Lilly said she had also decided to keep the baby in spite of the pressure from her parents. With her boyfriend gone, her parents antagonistic, and no apparent circle of friends, it was evident that Lilly had no adequate "support system." Lilly had none of the items she needed for

the baby, such as layette and car seat, and she was undecided whether to breastfeed or bottle feed. I was relieved and encouraged to hear that Lilly would be receptive to my help in acquiring the necessary items and in obtaining information on how to deal with her bed rest. She also had concerns about how to provide appropriate care for her newborn. Her anxiety was prompted by her complete lack of experience. Having relinquished her first child, the opportunity to learn these skills had been forfeited.

To help expand Lilly's support base, I asked if she might also be willing to see our social worker, who could provide some guidance. She said she was. In fact, at this point in our relationship, she seemed open to exploring whatever ideas and resources I felt might be helpful. The visit ended with the understanding I would return in three days, hopefully with additional information and some of the baby items she needed.

As I left Lilly's, I reflected again on all that had occurred. It was clear we had progressed in our relationship. Lilly was now actively participating in identifying her concerns and exploring resources that could meet her needs. I also thought about one of my primary objectives in this relationship: when possible, to assist Lilly in accomplishing tasks on her own rather than doing them for her. My purpose was to help Lilly gain some much needed confidence and increase her skill level. Hopefully, her trust in me and the strength of our relationship had evolved to the point where she would be comfortable rather than resistant to help. My goals were twofold: assist Lilly to feel competent in meeting the challenges of being a new mother, and help her gain the strengths, confidence and knowledge to seek appropriate help when necessary.

I was able to visit Lilly one more time before the baby was due. I provided her with some information she was interested in and was able to locate both a layette and car seat for the baby. Equally important, the visit provided the opportunity to obtain Lilly's consent for ongoing visits in the months following delivery.

Some eight months have passed since Lilly delivered a normal infant girl. The baby is happy and thriving. Monthly visits have allowed me to provide support and the chance to teach Lilly additional skills in caring for her baby. It has been interesting to observe Lilly's increasing ability to cope with problems that have arisen.

In the last few months Lilly has had to deal with being evicted from her rental home, seeing her boyfriend leave again, and continuing criticism from her parents. In spite of this, she interacts positively with the baby and provides good infant care. Lilly has also taken the initiative to find a

*continued*

*A view from the field*

full-time sitter so that she can work rather than be on welfare. She is comfortable in seeking out resources when needed, as evidenced by her participation in the WIC program, social service counseling, and the low-cost housing authority. She has demonstrated considerable growth in self-confidence and her capacity to function in general. She openly discusses the value of my visits and laughingly reflects back on our shaky beginning. We both agree that our relationship has grown. No longer is getting in touch with

Lilly a problem. In fact, she seems quite comfortable in calling me, sharing her concerns, and inviting me to "come and see baby Sarah." I will probably continue regular visits until the baby is a year old. I know that when I no longer provide visits to this family, Lilly and I will both miss the positive working relationship we have come to enjoy. It has been a growing experience for both of us.

I could have given up on Lilly after my first stressful contact. I'm glad I didn't!

## REFERENCES

Abu-Nasr D: Volunteer vision turns into reality, *The Ann Arbor News*, April 27, 1997, pp. A-1, A-11.

Adams PF, Hendershot GE, Marano MA: Current estimates from the National Health Interview Survey, 1996: National Center for Health Statistics, *Vital Health Stat* 10(200): 1387, 1999.

Alan Guttmacher Institute (AGI): *Sex and America's teenagers*, New York, 1994, AGI.

Alexander GR, Korenbrot CC: The role of prenatal care in preventing low birth weight, *The Future of Children* 5(1):103-120, 1995.

American Cancer Society (ACS): *Cancer facts and figures—2001*, Atlanta, 2001, ACS.

Anderson RN, Kochanek KD, Murphy SL: Report of the final mortality statistics, 1995, *Monthly Vital Statistics Report* 48(11, Suppl 27), 1997.

Assistant Secretary for Legislation (ASL): *Testimony on infant mortality and prenatal care by James S. Marks, M.D., M.P.H., Centers for Disease Control and Prevention*, March 13, 1997. Retrieved from the internet Sept. 20, 2001. *http://www.hhs.gov/asl/testify/t970313a.html*

Association of State and Territorial Directors of Nursing (ASTDN): *Public health nursing: a partner for healthy populations*, Washington, DC, 2000, ANA.

Bennett NG, Li J, Song Y, Yang K: *Young children in poverty: a statistical update*, New York, 1999, National Center for Children in Poverty.

Bloch AB, Rosenblum LR, Guthrie AM: Recommendations for blood lead screening of young children enrolled in Medicaid: targeting a group at high risk, *MMWR* 49(No. RR-14):1-13, 2000.

Boundy K: New regulations implementing the Individuals with Disabilities Education Act amendments of 1997—an overview (part 2), *J Poverty Law Policy* 34(112):68-83, 2000.

Briere JN, Elliott DM: Immediate and long-term impacts of child sexual abuse, *The Future of Children* 4(2):54-69, 1994.

Brown S: Drawing women into prenatal care, *Fam Plann Perspect* 21(2):73-80, 88, March/April 1989.

Burnhill MS: Contraceptive use: the U.S. perspective, *Int Gynecol Obstet* 62(Suppl 1):517-523, 1998.

Centers for Disease Control (CDC): CDC recommendations for a community plan for the prevention and containment of suicide clusters, *MMWR* 37(S-6):1-12, 1988.

Centers for Disease Control and Prevention (CDC): Youth suicide prevention programs: a resource guide, Atlanta, 1992, CDC.

Centers for Disease Control and Prevention (CDC): Lead poisoning associated with use of traditional ethnic remedies—California, 1991-1992, *MMWR* 42(27):521-524, 1993a.

Centers for Disease Control and Prevention (CDC): Standards for pediatric immunization practices, *MMWR* 42 (No RR-5):1-13, 1993b.

Centers for Disease Control and Prevention (CDC): Programs for the prevention of suicide among adolescents and young adults, *MMWR* 43(RR-6):1-7, 1994.

Centers for Disease Control and Prevention (CDC): Update: blood lead levels—United States, 1991-1994, *MMWR* 46(7):142-146, 1997.

Centers for Disease Control and Prevention (CDC): *Sexually transmitted disease surveillance, 1997*, Atlanta, 1998, CDC.

Centers for Disease Control and Prevention (CDC): *Young people at risk: HIV/AIDS among America's youth*, Washington, DC, 1999, CDC.

Centers for Disease Control and Prevention (CDC): Blood lead levels in young children—United States and selected states, 1996-1999, *MMWR* 49(50):1133-1137, 2000a.

Centers for Disease Control and Prevention (CDC): Entry into prenatal care—United States, 1989-1997, *MMWR* 49(18):393-398, 2000b.

Centers for Disease Control and Prevention (CDC): *HIV/AIDS surveillance report*, 12(1):1-41, 2000c.

Centers for Disease Control and Prevention (CDC): Youth risk behavior surveillance—United States, 1999, *MMWR* 49(SS05):1-96, 2000d.

Centers for Disease Control and Prevention (CDC): *Youth violence in the United States fact sheet*, 2000e. Retrieved from the internet Aug. 29, 2001. *http://www.cdc.gov/ncipc/dvp/yvpt/facts.htm*

Centers for Disease Control and Prevention (CDC): Fatal pediatric lead poisoning—New Hampshire, 2000, *MMWR* 50(22):457-459, 2001a.

Centers for Disease Control and Prevention (CDC): *Pelvic inflammatory disease (PID)*, May 2001b. Retrieved from the internet Sept. 5, 2001. *http://www.cdc.gov/nchstp/dstd/Fact_Sheets/FactsPID.htm*

Centers for Disease Control and Prevention (CDC): *Suicide among youth*, 2001c. Retrieved from the internet Nov. 29, 2001. *http://www.cdc.gov/communication/tips/suicide.htm*

Centers for Disease Control and Prevention (CDC): Trends in blood lead levels among children, Boston, 1994-1999, *MMWR* 50(17): 337-339, 2001d.

Children's Defense Fund (CDF): *The state of America's children yearbook 1996*, Washington, DC, 1996, CDF.

Children's Defense Fund (CDF): *The state of America's children*, Washington, DC, 2000, CDF.

Chin J: *Control of communicable diseases manual*, ed 17, Washington, DC, 2000, APHA.

Chomitz VR, Cheung LWY, Lieberman E: The role of lifestyle in preventing low birth weight, *The Future of Children* 5(1):121-138, 1995.

Colley GB, Brantley MD, Larson MK: *Family planning practices and pregnancy intention, 1997*, Atlanta, 2000, Division of Reproduction Health, National Center for Chronic Disease Prevention and Health Promotion, Centers for Disease Control and Prevention.

Dalaker J, Proctor B: *Poverty in the United States, 1999*, Current population reports, Washington, DC, 2000, US Government Printing Office.

Dangelmaier A: Lilly's anger. In Zewekh J, Primomo J, Deal L, editors: *Opening doors: stories of public health nursing*, Olympia, Wash, 1992, Washington State Department of Health, Parent-Child Health Services.

Dubowitz H: *Child maltreatment in the United States: etiology, impact and prevention*, Washington, DC, 1986, US Congress, Office of Technology Assessment.

Dusenbury L, Falco M, Lake A: A review of the evaluation of 47 drug abuse prevention curricula available nationally, *J Sch Health* 67:127-132, 1997.

Edleson JL: *The overlap between child maltreatment and woman abuse*, April 1999. Retrieved from the internet Sept. 8, 2001. *http://www.vaw.umn.edu/vawnet/overlap.htm*

Federal Interagency Forum on Child and Family Statistics: *America's children: key national indicators of well-being 2000*, Washington, DC, 2000, US Government Printing Office.

Foye HR: Anticipatory guidance. In Hoekelman RA, Friedman SB, Nelson NM, et al., editors: *Primary pediatric care*, St Louis, 1997, Mosby.

Frost J, Ranjit N, Manzella K, et al.: Family planning clinic services in the United States: patterns and trends in the late 1990s, *Fam Plann Perspect* 33(3):113-122, 2001.

General Accounting Office (GAO): *Home visiting: a promising early intervention strategy for at-risk families*, GAO/HRD-90-83, Gaithersburg, Md, July 1990, GAO.

General Accounting Office (GAO): *Federally funded health services: information on seven programs serving low-income women and children*, GAO/HRD-92-73FS, Gaithersburg, Md, May 1992, GAO.

General Accounting Office (GAO): *Welfare to work: approaches that help teenage mothers complete high school*, Washington, DC, 1995, GAO.

General Accounting Office (GAO): *Lead poisoning: federal health care programs are not effectively reaching at-risk children* (Pub No GAO/HE HS-99-18), Washington, DC, 1999, GAO.

Goodstadt MS: Substance abuse curricula vs. school drug policies, *J Sch Health* 59:246-250, 1989.

Gordon M: *Manual of nursing diagnosis*, ed 9, St Louis, 2000, Mosby.

Green M, editor: *Bright futures: guidelines for health supervision of infants, children, and adolescents*, Arlington, Va, 1994, National Center for Education in Maternal and Child Health.

Green M, Palfrey J: *Bright futures: guidelines for health supervision of infants, children, and adolescents*, ed 2, Arlington, Va, 2000, National Center for Education in Maternal and Child Health.

Greenberg SH, Springen K: The baby blues and beyond, *Newsweek* 26-29, July 2, 2001.

Hargraves M, Thomas RW: Infant mortality: its history and social construction, *Am J Preventive Medicine* 9(Suppl):17-26, 1993.

Health Resources and Services Administration (HRSA): *Understanding Title U of the Social Security Act*, Rockville, Md, 2000, Maternal and Child Health Bureau.

Hughes D, Simpson L: The role of social change in preventing low birth weight, *The Future of Children* 5(2):87-102, 1995.

Institute for Health and Aging, University of California, San Francisco: *Chronic care in America: a 21st century challenge*, Princeton, NJ, 1996, The Robert Wood Johnson Foundation.

Institute of Medicine (IOM): *The best intentions: unintended pregnancy and the well-being of children and families*, Washington, DC, 1995, National Academy of Science.

Ireys HT, Katz S: The demography of disability and chronic illness among children. In Wallace HM, Biehl RF, MacQueen JC, et al., editors: *Mosby's resource guide to children with disabilities and chronic illness*, St Louis, 1997, Mosby.

Johnson J, Primas P, Coe M: Factors that prevent women of socioeconomic status from seeking prenatal care, *J Am Acad Nurse Pract* 6(3):105-111, 1994.

Johnston LD, O'Malley PM, Bachman JG: *National survey results on drug use from the Monitoring The Future Study, 1975-1995, Vol 1*, secondary school students, Washington, DC, 1996, US Government Printing Office.

Johnston LD, O'Malley PM, Bachman JG: *Monitoring the future: national results on an adolescent drug use: overview of key findings, 2000*, (NIH Pub No 01-4923), Bethesda, Md, 2000, National Institute on Drug Abuse.

Kaye S: Education of children with disabilities, *Disability Statistics Abstract* 19:1-3, 1997.

Knitzer J, Page S: *Map and track: state initiatives for young children and families*, New York, 1996, National Center for Children in Poverty.

Kraus LE, Stoddard S, Gilmartin D: *Chartbook on disability in the United States, 1996*, Washington, DC, 1996, National Institute on Disability and Rehabilitation Research.

Kruckman L, Smith S: *An introduction to postpartum illness*, 2001. Retrieved from the internet Sept. 12, 2001. *http://www.chss.iup.edu/postpartum/preface.html*

Landrigan PJ: Pediatric lead poisoning: is there a threshold? *Public Health Reports* 115:530-531, 2000.

Lanphear BP, Dietrich K, Auinger P, Cox C: Cognitive deficits associated with blood lead concentrations $<10 \mu g/dL$ in US children and adolescents, *Public Health Reports* 115:521-529, 2000.

LaPlante M, Carlson D: *Disability in the United States: prevalence and causes, 1992*, Disability Statistics Report (7), Washington, DC, 1996, National Institute on Disability and Rehabilitation Research.

Lindberg FH, Distad LJ: Survival response to incest: adolescents in crisis, *Child Abuse and Neglect* 9:521-526, 1985.

Lowdermilk DL, Perry SE, Bobak IM: *Maternity and women's health care*, ed 7, St Louis, 2000, Mosby.

Lynch RA, Boatright DT, Moss SK: Lead-contaminated imported tamarind candy and children's blood lead levels, *Public Health Report* 115:537-543, 2000.

Lyon GR: Learning disabilities, *The Future of Children* 6(1):54-76, 1996.

Males M, Chew KSY: The ages of fathers in California adolescent births, 1993, *Am J Public Health* 86:565-568, 1996.

Maternal and Child Health Bureau: *Child health USA '95*, Washington, DC, 1996, US Government Printing Office.

Maternal and Child Health Bureau: *Child health USA 2000*, Washington, DC, 2000, US Government Printing Office.

Milio N: *9226 Kercheval: the storefront that did not burn*, Ann Arbor, 1970, University of Michigan Press.

National Black Child Development Institute (NBCDI): *Campaign's resource kit seeks to reduce incidence of SIDS in African American Communities*, Oct. 12, 2000. Retrieved from the internet Aug. 26, 2001. *http://www.hhs.gov/news/press/2000press/2000.html#Oct*

National Center for Children in Poverty: *Child poverty fact sheet*, 2001. Retrieved from the internet Sept. 28, 2001. *http://cpmcnet.columbia.edu/dept/nccp*

National Center for Health Statistics (NCHS): Births: preliminary data for 1999, *National Vital Statistics Reports* 48(14):1-20, 2000.

National Center for Injury Prevention and Control (NCIPC): *The prevention of youth violence: a framework for community action*, Atlanta, 1993, CDC.

National Center for Injury Prevention and Control (NCIPC): *Childhood injury fact sheet*, Atlanta, 1999, NCIPC.

National Center for Injury Prevention and Control (NCIPC): *Unintentional injury prevention fact sheet*, Atlanta, 2000, NCIPC

National Commission to Prevent Infant Mortality: *Home visiting: opening doors for America's pregnant women and children*, Washington, DC, 1989, The Commission.

National Safety Council: *Injury facts 2000*, Itasca, Ill, 2000, The Council.

Nelson WE, Behrman RE, Kliegman RM, Algin AM, editors: *Nelson textbook of pediatrics*, Philadelphia, 1996, WB Saunders.

Nyman G: Infant temperament, childhood accidents, and hospitalizations, *Clin Pediatr* 26(8):398-404, 1987.

Office of National Drug Control Policy: *National drug control strategy: 2000 annual report*, Washington, DC, 2000, The Office.

Office of Special Education Programs: *Implementation of the Individuals with Disabilities Education Act; sixteenth annual report to Congress*, Washington, DC, 1994, US Department of Education.

O'Hare WP, Ritualo AR: Kids count: identifying and helping America's most vulnerable, *Statistical Bulletin* 81(1):26-32, 2000.

Olds DL, Henderson CR, Kitzman HJ, et al.: Prenatal and infancy home visitation by nurses: recent findings, *The Future of Children* 9(1):44-65, 1999.

Paneth NS: The problem of low-birth weight, *The Future of Children* 5(1):19-34, 1995.

Powers JL, Echenrode J, Jaklitsch B: Maltreatment among runaway and homeless youth, *Child Abuse and Neglect* 14:87-98, 1990.

President's Task Force on Environmental Health Risks and Safety Risks to Children: *Eliminating childhood lead poisoning: a federal strategy targeting lead paint hazards*, Washington, DC, 2000, The Task Force.

Resnick MD, Chambliss SA, Blum RN: Health and risk behaviors of urban adolescent males involved with pregnancy, *Fam Soc* 366-374, 1993.

Salter C, Johnston HB, Henger N: Care for postabortion complications: saving women's lives, *Population Report*, series L10, Baltimore, 1997, Johns Hopkins.

Satcher DS: The surgeon general on the continuing tragedy of childhood lead poisoning, *Public Health Reports* 115:579-580, 2000.

Shiono PH, Behrman RE: Low birth weight: analysis and recommendations, *The Future of Children* 5(1):4-18, 1995.

State of Michigan: *Child protection law*, Lansing, Mich, 2001, Family Independence Agency.

UNICEF: *The progress of nations*, New York, 1996, UNICEF.

UNICEF: *The state of the world's children 2002*, New York, 2001a, UNICEF.

UNICEF: SOWC 2002 press kit, September 13, 2001: one week before the UN special session on children, *UNICEF says broken promises hurt the children of the 90s*, 2001b. Retrieved from the internet Sept. 14, 2001. *http://www.unicef.org/media/sowc02presskit*

US Bureau of the Census: *Statistical abstract of the United States 2000*, ed 120, Washington, DC, 2000, US Government Printing Office.

US Department of Health, Education and Welfare (USDHEW): *Healthy people: the Surgeon General's report on health promotion and disease prevention*, DHEW Pub No PHS 79-55071, Washington, DC, 1979, US Government Printing Office.

US Department of Health and Human Services (USDHHS): *Report to Congress on out-of-wedlock childbearing*, Hyattsville, Md, 1995, US Government Printing Office.

US Department of Health and Human Services (USDHHS): *Child maltreatment 1994: reports from the states to the National Center on Child Abuse and Neglect*, Washington, DC, 1996, US Government Printing Office.

US Department of Health and Human Services (USDHHS): *Child health guide: put prevention into practice*, Washington, DC, 2000a, US Government Printing Office.

US Department of Health and Human Services (USDHHS): *Healthy People 2010, with understanding and improving health and objectives for improving health, 2010,* ed 2, Washington, DC, 2000b, US Government Printing Office.

Wald L: *The house on Henry Street,* New York, 1915, Holt.

Warner M, Barnes DM, Fingerhut LA: *Injury and poisoning episodes and conditions: national health interview survey, 1997, Vital Health Stat* 10(202), 2000.

Wenger BL, Kaye S, LaPlante MP: Disabilities among children, *Disability Statistics Abstract* 15:1-4, 1996.

Winstead-Fry P, Bishop KK: Nurses and Public Law 102-119: a family-centered continuing education program, *J Contin Educ Nurs* 28(1):26-31, 1997.

Wong DL, Hockenberry-Eaton M, Wilson D, et al.: *Whaley and Wong's nursing care of infants and children,* ed 6, St Louis, 1999, Mosby.

World Health Organization (WHO): Progress towards health for all: third monitoring report: health status, *World Health Statistics Q* 48:189-199, 1995.

Yoon PW, Rasmussen SA, Lynberg MC: The national birth defects prevention study, *Public Health Report* 116:32-40, 2001.

## SELECTED BIBLIOGRAPHY

Centers for Disease Control and Prevention (CDC): Preventing pneumococcal disease among infants and young children: recommendations of the Advisory Committee on Immunization Practice, *MMWR* 49(No. RR-9), 2000.

Collins A, Carlson B: *Child care by kith and kin—supporting family, friends, and neighbors caring for children,* New York, 1998, National Center for Children in Poverty.

Gold RB, Sonfield A: Reproductive health services for adolescents under the Children's Health Insurance Program, *Fam Plann Perspect* 33(2):81-83, 2001.

Gomby DS, Culross PL, Behrman RE: Home visiting: recent program evaluations—analysis and recommendations, *The Future of Children* 9(1):4-26, 1999.

Josten L, Wedeking L, Block D, et al.: Linking high-risk, low-income, pregnant women to public health services, *J Public Health Management Practice* 3(2):27-36, 1997.

Kearney MH, York R, Deatrick JA: Effects of home visits to vulnerable young families, *J Nursing Scholarship* 32(4):369-376, 2000.

Krishnon SP, Hilbert JC, VanLeeuwen D: Domestic violence and help-seeking behaviors among rural women: results from a shelter-based study, *Fam Community Health* 24(1):28-38, 2001.

Knitzer J: *Promoting resilience: helping young children and parents affected by substance abuse, domestic violence, and depression in the context of welfare reform,* New York, 2000, National Center for Children in Poverty.

Loveland-Cherry CJ: Interventions for promoting health in adolescents. In Hindshaw AS, Feetham SL, Shaver JL: *Handbook of clinical nursing research,* Thousand Oaks, Calif, 1999, Sage.

Medoff-Cooper BS, Holditch-Davis D: Therapeutic actions and outcomes for preterm (low birth weight) infants. In Hindshaw AS, Feetham SL, Shaver JL: *Handbook of clinical nursing research,* Thousand Oaks, Calif, 1999, Sage.

Story M, Holt K, Sofka D, editors: *Bright futures in practice: nutrition,* Arlington, Va, 2000, National Center for Education in Maternal and Child Health.

US Department of Agriculture: *Nutrition and your health: dietary guidelines for Americans,* ed 5, Washington, DC, 2000, US Government Printing Office.

# Guide to Contraindications and Precautions to Vaccinations*

| TRUE CONTRAINDICATIONS AND PRECAUTIONS | NOT TRUE (VACCINES MAY BE ADMINISTERED) |
| --- | --- |
| **GENERAL FOR ALL VACCINES (DTP/DTaP, OPV, IPV, MMR, HiB, HBV)** | |
| *Contraindications* | |
| Anaphylactic reaction to a vaccine contraindicates further doses of that vaccine | Mild to moderate local reaction (soreness, redness, swelling) following a dose of an injectable antigen |
| Anaphylactic reaction to a vaccine constituent contraindicates the use of vaccines containing that substance | Mild acute illness with or without low-grade fever |
| Moderate or severe illnesses with or without a fever | Current antimicrobial therapy |
| | Convalescent phase of illnesses |
| | Prematurity (same dosage and indications as for normal, full-term infants) |
| | Recent exposure to an infectious disease |
| | History of penicillin or other nonspecific allergies or family history of such allergies |
| **DTP/DTaP** | |
| *Contraindications* | |
| Encephalopathy within 7 days of administration of previous dose of DTP | Temperature of< 40.5° C (105° F) following a previous dose of DTP |
| | Family history of convulsions§ |

From Centers for Disease Control and Prevention (CDC): Standards for pediatric immunization practice, *MMWR* 42(No RR-5):12-13, 1993b.

DTP = Diphtheria-tetanus toxoid and pertussis vaccine
DTaP = Diphtheria and tetanus toxoids and acellular pertussis
Hib = *Haemophilus influenzae* type b vaccine
HBV = Hepatitis B vaccine
IPV = Inactivated poliovirus vaccine
MMR = Measles-mumps-rubella vaccine
OPV = Oral poliovirus vaccine

*This information is based on the recommendations of the Advisory Committee on Immunization Practices (ACIP) and those of the Committee on Infectious Diseases (Red Book Committee) of the American Academy of Pediatrics (AAP) as of October 1992. Sometimes these recommendations vary from those contained in the manufacturer's package inserts. For more detailed information, providers should consult the published recommendations of the ACIP, AAP, American Association of Family Practice Physicians, and the manufacturer's package inserts.

†The events or conditions listed as precautions, although not contraindications, should be carefully reviewed. The benefits and risks of administering a specific vaccine to an individual under the circumstances should be considered. If the risks are believed to outweigh the benefits, the vaccination should be withheld; if the benefits are believed to outweigh the risks (e.g., during an outbreak or foreign travel), the vaccination should be administered. Whether and when to administer DTP to children with proven or suspected underlying neurological disorders should be decided on an individual basis. It is prudent on theoretical grounds to avoid vaccinating pregnant women. However, if immediate protection against poliomyelitis is needed, OPV, not IPV, is recommended.

‡For children with a personal or family (siblings or parents) history of convulsions, acetaminophen should be considered before DTP is administered and thereafter every 4 hours for 24 hours.

§There is a theoretical risk that the administration of multiple live-virus vaccines (OPV and MMR) within 30 days of one another if not administered on the same day will result in a suboptimal immune response. There are no data to substantiate this lack of response.

‖Persons with a history of anaphylactic reactions following egg ingestion should be vaccinated only with extreme caution. Protocols that have been developed for vaccinating such persons should be consulted (*J Pediatr* 102:196-199, 1983; *J Pediatr* 113:504-506, 1988).

¶Measles vaccination may temporarily suppress tuberculin reactivity. If testing cannot be done the day of MMR vaccination, the test should be postponed for 4 to 6 weeks.

# Guide to Contraindications and Precautions to Vaccinations* (cont'd)

| TRUE CONTRAINDICATIONS AND PRECAUTIONS | NOT TRUE (VACCINES MAY BE ADMINISTERED) |
|---|---|
| **DTP/DTaP—cont'd** ||
| *Precautions†* | Family history of sudden infant death syndrome |
| Fever of ≥40.5° C (105° F) within 48 hrs after vaccination with a prior dose of DTP | |
| Collapse or shocklike state (hypotonic-hyporesponsive episode) within 48 hrs of receiving a prior dose of DTP | Family history of an adverse event following DTP administration |
| Seizures within 3 days of receiving a prior dose of DTP‡ | |
| Persistent, inconsolable crying lasting 3 hrs within 48 hrs of receiving a prior dose of DTP | |
| **OPV§** ||
| *Contraindications* | Breastfeeding |
| Infection with HIV or a household contact with HIV | Current antimicrobial therapy |
| Known altered immunodeficiency (hematologic and solid tumors; congenital immunodeficiency; and long-term immunosuppressive therapy) | Diarrhea |
| Immunodeficient household contact | |
| *Precaution†* | |
| Pregnancy | |
| **IPV** ||
| *Contraindication* | |
| Anaphylactic reaction to neomycin or streptomycin | |
| *Precaution†* | |
| Pregnancy | |
| **MMR§** ||
| *Contraindications* | Tuberculosis or positive skin test |
| Anaphylactic reactions to egg ingestion and to neomycin‖ | Simultaneous TB skin testing¶ |
| Pregnancy | Breast-feeding |
| Known altered immunodeficiency (hematologic and solid tumors; congenital immunodeficiency; and long-term immunosuppressive therapy) | Pregnancy of mother of recipient |
| | Immunodeficient family member or household contact |
| | Infection with HIV |
| *Precaution†* | Nonanaphylactic reactions to eggs or neomycin |
| Recent (within 3 months) immune globulin administration | |
| **HiB** ||
| None identified | |
| **HBV** ||
| None identified | Pregnancy |

# Clinical Manifestations of Potential Child Maltreatment

## Physical Neglect
**SUGGESTIVE PHYSICAL FINDINGS**

Failure to thrive

Signs of malnutrition, such as thin extremities, abdominal distention, lack of subcutaneous fat

Poor personal hygiene, especially of teeth

Unclean and/or inappropriate dress

Evidence of poor health care, such as nonimmunized status, untreated infections, frequent colds

Frequent injuries from lack of supervision

**SUGGESTIVE BEHAVIORS**

Dull and inactive; excessively passive or sleepy

Self-stimulatory behaviors, such as finger-sucking or rocking

Begging or stealing food ⎫

Absenteeism from school ⎬ in older child

Drug or alcohol addiction ⎪

Vandalism or shoplifting ⎭

## Emotional Abuse and Neglect
**SUGGESTIVE PHYSICAL FINDINGS**

Failure to thrive

Feeding disorders, such as rumination

Enuresis

Sleep disorders

**SUGGESTIVE BEHAVIORS**

Self-stimulatory behaviors, such as biting, rocking, sucking

During infancy, lack of social smile and stranger anxiety

Withdrawal

Unusual fearfulness

Antisocial behavior, such as destructiveness, stealing, cruelty

Extremes of behavior, such as overcompliant and passive or aggressive and demanding

Lags in emotional and intellectual development, especially language

Suicide attempts

## Physical Abuse
**SUGGESTIVE PHYSICAL FINDINGS**

Bruises and welts

On face, lips, mouth, back, buttocks, thighs, or areas of torso

Regular patterns descriptive of object used, such as belt buckle, hand, wire hanger, chain, wooden spoon, squeeze or pinch marks

May be present in various stages of healing

Burns

On soles of feet, palms of hands, back, or buttocks

Patterns descriptive of object used, such as round cigar or cigarette burns, "glovelike" sharply demarcated areas from immersion in scalding water, rope burns on wrists or ankles from being bound, burns in the shape of an iron, radiator, or electric stove burner

Absence of "splash" marks and presence of symmetric burns

Stun gun injury—lesions circular, fairly uniform (up to 0.5 cm), and paired about 5 cm apart (Frechette and Rimsza, 1992)

Fractures and dislocations

Skull, nose, or facial structures

Injury may denote type of abuse, such as spiral fracture or dislocation from twisting of an extremity or whiplash from shaking the child

Multiple new or old fractures in various stages of healing

Lacerations and abrasions

On backs of arms, legs, torso, face, or external genitalia

Unusual symptoms, such as abdominal swelling, pain, and vomiting from punching

Descriptive marks such as from human bites or pulling the hair out

Chemical

Unexplained repeated poisoning, especially drug overdose

Unexplained sudden illness, such as hypoglycemia from insulin administration

From Wong DL, Hockenberry-Eaton M, Wilson D, et al.: *Whaley and Wong's nursing care of infants and children*, ed 6, St Louis, 1999, Mosby.

# Clinical Manifestations of Potential Child Maltreatment (cont'd)

**SUGGESTIVE BEHAVIORS**

Wary of physical contact with adults

Apparent fear of parents or going home

Lying very still while surveying environment

Inappropriate reaction to injury, such as failure to cry from pain

Lack of reaction to frightening events

Apprehensive when hearing other children cry

Indiscriminate friendliness and displays of affection

Superficial relationships

Acting-out behavior, such as aggression, to seek attention

Withdrawal behavior

## Sexual Abuse

**SUGGESTIVE PHYSICAL FINDINGS**

Bruises, bleeding, lacerations or irritation of external genitalia, anus, mouth, or throat

Torn, stained, or bloody underclothing

Pain on urination or pain, swelling, and itching of genital area

Penile discharge

Sexually transmitted disease, nonspecific vaginitis, or venereal warts

Difficulty in walking or sitting

Unusual odor in the genital area

Recurrent urinary tract infections

Presence of sperm

Pregnancy in young adolescent

**SUGGESTIVE BEHAVIORS**

Sudden emergence of sexually related problems, including excessive or public masturbation, age-inappropriate sexual play, promiscuity, or overtly seductive behavior

Withdrawn, excessive daydreaming

Preoccupied with fantasies, especially in play

Poor relationships with peers

Sudden changes, such as anxiety, loss or gain of weight, clinging behavior

In incestuous relationships, excessive anger at mother for not protecting daughter

Regressive behavior, such as bed-wetting or thumb-sucking

Sudden onset of phobias or fears, particularly fears of the dark, men, strangers, or particular settings or situations (e.g., undue fear of leaving the house or staying at the day care center or the baby-sitter's house)

Running away from home

Substance abuse, particularly of alcohol or mood-elevating drugs

Profound and rapid personality changes, especially extreme depression, hostility, and aggression (often accompanied by social withdrawal)

Rapidly declining school performance

Suicidal attempts or ideation

# Infancy* Developmental Chart

Health professionals should assess the achievements of the infant and provide guidance to the family on anticipated tasks. The effects are demonstrated by health supervision outcomes.

| ACHIEVEMENTS DURING INFANCY | TASKS FOR THE FAMILY | HEALTH SUPERVISION OUTCOMES |
| --- | --- | --- |
| Good physical health and growth<br>Regular sleep pattern<br>Self-quieting behavior<br>Sense of trust<br>Family adaptation to infant<br>Attachment between infant and parents<br>Healthy sibling interactions | Meet infant's nutritional needs<br>Establish regular eating and sleeping schedule<br>Prevent early childhood caries (baby bottle tooth decay)<br>Prevent injuries and abuse<br>Obtain appropriate immunizations<br>Promote normal development<br>Promote warm, nurturing parent-infant relationship<br>Promote responsiveness and social competence<br>Encourage vocal interactions with parents, siblings, and others<br>Encourage play with toys, siblings, parents, and others<br>Encourage safe exploration of the environment | Formation of partnership ("therapeutic alliance") between health professional and parents<br>Preparation of parents for new role<br>Optimal nutrition<br>Satisfactory growth and development<br>Injury prevention<br>Immunizations<br>Promotion of developmental potential<br>Prevention of behavioral problems<br>Promotion of family strengths<br>Enhancement of parental effectiveness |

From Green M, Palfrey J, editors: *Bright futures: guidelines for health supervision of infants, children, and adolescents,* ed 2, Arlington, Va, 2000, National Center for Education in Maternal and Child Health, p. 24.
*Infancy: under 1 year.

# Early Childhood* Developmental Chart

Health professionals should assess the achievements of the child and provide guidance to the family on anticipated tasks. The effects are demonstrated by health supervision outcomes.

| ACHIEVEMENTS DURING EARLY CHILDHOOD | TASKS FOR THE CHILD | HEALTH SUPERVISION OUTCOMES |
| --- | --- | --- |
| Regular sleeping habits<br>Independence in eating<br>Completion of toilet training<br>Ability to dress and undress<br>Ability to separate from parents<br>Progression from parallel to interactive play and sharing<br>Loving relationship and good communication with parents and siblings<br>Clear communication of needs and wishes<br>Expression of such feelings as joy, anger, sadness, and frustration<br>Self-comforting behavior<br>Self-discipline<br>Intelligible speech<br>Positive self-image<br>Demonstration of curiosity and initiative<br>Demonstration of imaginative make-believe, and dress-up play | Learn healthy eating habits<br>Practice good oral hygiene<br>Participate in physical games and play<br>Develop autonomy, independence, and assertiveness<br>Respond to limit-setting and discipline<br>Learn self-quieting behaviors and self-discipline<br>Learn appropriate self-care<br>Make friends and meet new people<br>Play with and relate well to siblings and peers<br>Learn to understand and use language to meet needs<br>Listen to stories<br>Learn how to handle conflicts without violence | Early autonomy<br>Optimal growth and development<br>Establishment of good health habits<br>Optimal nutrition<br>Injury prevention<br>Immunizations<br>School readiness<br>Promotion of developmental potential<br>Prevention of behavioral problems<br>Promotion of family strengths<br>Enhancement of parental effectiveness |

From Green M, Palfrey J, editors: *Bright futures: guidelines for health supervision of infants, children, and adolescents,* ed 2, Arlington, Va, 2000, National Center for Education in Maternal and Child Health, p. 104.
*Early childhood: 1-5 years.

# Middle Childhood* Developmental Chart

Health professionals should assess the achievements of the child and provide guidance to the family on anticipated tasks. The effects are demonstrated by health supervision outcomes.

| ACHIEVEMENTS DURING MIDDLE CHILDHOOD | TASKS FOR THE CHILD | HEALTH SUPERVISION OUTCOMES |
|---|---|---|
| Responsibility for good health | Maintain healthy eating habits | Sense of personal competence |
| Ability to play in groups | Practice good oral hygiene | Sense of self-efficacy and self-confidence |
| Development of one or more close friends | Participate in athletic programs, physical activity | Optimal growth and development |
| Identification with peer groups | Maintain appropriate weight | Active role in health supervision and promotion |
| Competence as a member of family, community, and other groups | Use vehicle safety belt | Optimal nutrition |
| Ability to express feelings | Wear protective gear for physical activities (e.g., bicycle, helmet, mouth guard, knee pads) | Good health habits |
| Belief in capacity for success | | Injury prevention |
| Understanding of right and wrong | Avoid alcohol, tobacco, and other drugs | Personal safety |
| Awareness of safety rules | Resist peer pressure to engage in risk-taking behaviors | Social competence |
| Ability to read, write, and communicate increasingly complex and creative thoughts | Control impulses | Promotion of developmental potential |
| Responsibility for homework | Resolve conflict and manage anger constructively | Prevention of behavioral problems |
| School achievement | Assume responsibility for belongings, chores, homework, and good health habits | Promotion of family strengths |
| | Play with and relate well to siblings and peers | Enhancement of parental effectiveness |
| | Communicate well with parents, teachers, and other adults | Success in school |
| | Work hard in school and develop good study habits | |

From Green M, Palfrey J, editors: *Bright futures: guidelines for health supervision of infants, children, and adolescents,* ed 2, Arlington, Va, 2000, National Center for Education in Maternal and Child Health, p. 176.
*Middle childhood: 5-11 years.

# Adolescence\* Developmental Chart

Health professionals should assess the achievements of the adolescent and provide guidance to the family on anticipated tasks. The effects are demonstrated by health supervision outcomes.

| DEVELOPMENTAL ACHIEVEMENTS | TASKS FOR THE ADOLESCENT | HEALTH SUPERVISION OUTCOMES |
|---|---|---|
| Responsibility for good health habits<br>Physical, emotional, and sexual growth and development<br>Social and conflict resolution skills<br>Good peer relationships with the same and opposite sex<br>Capacity for intimacy<br>Sexual identity and responsible sexual behavior<br>Coping skills and strategies<br>Appropriate level of autonomy<br>Personal value system<br>Progression from concrete to abstract thinking<br>Academic and career goals<br>Educational or vocational competence | Maintain good eating habits and oral hygiene<br>Engage in physical activity regularly and maintain appropriate weight<br>Use appropriate safety measures (e.g., safety belt, helmet)<br>Avoid alcohol and other drugs, tobacco, inhalants<br>Practice abstinence or safe sex<br>Engage in safe and age-appropriate experimentation<br>Manage negative peer pressure<br>Learn conflict resolution skills<br>Develop self-confidence, self-esteem, and sense of individual identity<br>Develop healthy interactions with peers, siblings, and adults<br>Learn ways to reduce risks of physical, emotional, and sexual abuse<br>Continue process of becoming more independent<br>Develop sense of community responsibility<br>Be responsible for school performance<br>Develop effective communication skills | Self-efficacy and mastery<br>Independent active role in health supervision and promotion<br>Optimal growth and development<br>Good health habits<br>Optimal nutrition<br>Reduction of high-risk behavior<br>Injury prevention<br>Promotion and developmental potential<br>Prevention of behavioral problems<br>Sense of responsibility and morality<br>Promotion of family strengths<br>Enhancement of parental effectiveness<br>Educational/vocational success |

From Green M, Palfrey J, editors: *Bright futures: guidelines for health supervision of infants, children, and adolescents,* ed 2, Arlington, Va, 2000, National Center for Education in Maternal and Child Health, p. 236.
\*Adolescence: 11-21 years.

Child Preventive Care Timeline: Recommendations of Major Authorities

**Child Preventive Care Timeline**

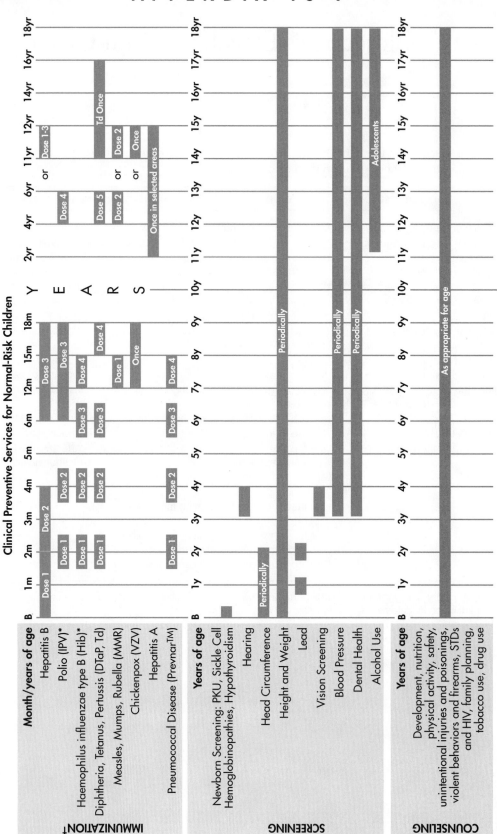

Clinical Preventive Services for Normal-Risk Children

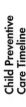

Recommended by most U.S. authorities

*Schedules may vary according to vaccine type.
†The information on immunization is based on recommendations issued by the Advisory Committee on Immunization Practices, the American Academy of Pediatrics, and the American Academy of Family Physicians.
From USDHHS: *Child health guide: put prevention into practice*, Washington, DC, 2000a, US Government Printing Office, pp. 20-21. See Figure 16-12 for a more recent immunization schedule. An immunization schedule should be obtained from the CDC on a yearly basis.

# Topics of Anticipatory Guidance

## Prenatal and Newborn

### PRENATAL VISIT

1. *Health:* pregnancy course; worries; tobacco, alcohol, drug use; hospital and pediatric office procedures
2. *Safety:* infant car seat, crib safety
3. *Nutrition:* planned feeding method
4. *Child care:* help after birth, later arrangements
5. *Family:* changes in relationships (spouse, siblings), supports, stresses, return to work

### NEWBORN VISITS

1. *Health:* jaundice, umbilical cord care, circumcision, other common problems, when to call pediatrician's office
2. *Safety:* infant car seat, smoke detector, choking, keeping tap water temperature below 120° F
3. *Nutrition:* feeding, normal weight loss, spitting, vitamin and fluoride supplements
4. *Development/behavior:* individuality, "consolability," visual and auditory responsiveness
5. *Child care:* importance of interaction, parenting books, support for primary caregiver
6. *Family:* postpartum adjustments, fatigue, "blues," special time for siblings

## First Year

### UP TO 6 MONTHS

1. *Health:* immunizations, exposure to infections
2. *Safety:* falls, aspiration of small objects or powder, entanglement in mobiles that have long strings
3. *Nutrition:* supplementing breast milk or formula, introducing solids, iron
4. *Development/behavior:* crying/colic, irregular schedules (eating, sleeping, eliminating), response to infant cues, reciprocity, interactive games, beginning eye-hand coordination
5. *Child care:* responsive and affectionate care, caregiving schedule
6. *Family:* return to work, nurturing of all family relationships (spouse and siblings)

### 6-12 MONTHS

1. *Safety:* locks for household poisons and medications; gates for stairs; ipecac; poison center telephone number; outlet safety covers; avoiding dangling cords or tablecloths; safety devices for windows/screens; toddler

car seat when infant reaches 20 pounds; avoiding toys that have small detachable pieces; supervise child in tub or near water
2. *Nutrition:* discouraging use of bottle as a pacifier or while in bed; offering cup and soft finger foods (with supervision); introducing new foods one at a time
3. *Development/behavior:* attachment, basic trust versus mistrust, stranger awareness, night waking, separation anxiety, bedtime routine, transitional object
4. *Child care:* prohibitions few but firm and consistent across caregiving settings: defining discipline as "learning" (not punishment)
5. *Family:* spacing of children

## Second Year

### 1-2 YEARS

1. *Health:* immunizations
2. *Safety:* climbing and falls common; supervising outdoor play; ensuring safety caps on medicine bottles; noting dangers of plastic bags, pan handles hanging over stove, and space heaters
3. *Nutrition:* avoiding feeding conflicts (decreased appetite is common); period of self-feeding, weaning from breast or bottle; avoiding sweet or salty snacks
4. *Development/behavior:* autonomy versus shame/doubt, ambivalence (independence/dependence), tantrums, negativism, getting into everything, night fears, readiness for toilet training, self-comforting behaviors (thumb sucking, masturbation), speech, imaginative play, no sharing in play, positive reinforcement for desired behavior
5. *Child care:* freedom to explore in safe place; day care; home a safer place to vent frustrations; needs show of affection, language stimulation through reading and conversation
6. *Family:* sibling relationships, parents modeling of nonaggressive responses to conflict (including their own conflict with their toddler)

## Preschool

### 2-5 YEARS

1. *Health:* tooth brushing, first dental visit
2. *Safety:* needs close supervision near water or street; home safety factors include padding of sharp furniture corners, fire escape plan for home, and locking up

From Foye HR: Anticipatory guidance. In Hoekelman RA, Friedman SB, Nelson NM, et al., editors: *Primary pediatric care*, St Louis, 1997, Mosby, pp. 153-154.

*continued*

# Topics of Anticipatory Guidance (cont'd)

## Preschool—cont'd

**2-5 YEARS—cont'd**

power tools; should have car lap belt at 40 pounds and bike helmet; should know (a) name, address, and telephone number, (b) not to provoke dogs, and (c) to say "no" to strangers

3. *Nutrition:* balanced diet; avoiding sweet or salty snacks; participating in conversation at meals
4. *Development/behavior:* initiative versus guilt; difficulty with impulse control and sharing; developing interest in peers; high activity level; speaking in sentences by age 3; speech mostly intelligible to stranger by age 3; reading books; curiosity about body parts; magical thinking, egocentrism
5. *Child care/preschool:* needs daily special time with parents, bedtime routine; talking about day in day care; limiting TV watching with child; reprimanding privately, answering questions factually and simply; adjusting to preschool, kindergarten readiness
6. *Family:* chores, responsibilities

## Middle Childhood

**5-10 YEARS**

1. *Health:* appropriate weight; regular exercise; somatic complaints (limb and abdominal pain, headaches); alcohol, tobacco, and drug use; sexual development; physician and child dealings (more direct)
2. *Safety:* bike helmets and street safety; car seat belts; swimming lessons; use of matches, firearms, and power tools; fire escape plan for home; saying "no" to strangers
3. *Nutrition:* balanced diet, daily breakfast, limiting sweet and salty snacks, moderate intake of fatty foods
4. *Development/behavior:* industry versus inferiority, need for successes, peer interactions, adequate sleep
5. *School:* school performance, homework, parent interest
6. *Family:* more time away but continuing need for family support, approval, affection, time together, and communication; family rules about bedtime, chores, and responsibilities; guidance in using money; parents should encourage reading; limiting TV watching and discussing

programs seen together; teaching and modeling nonviolent responses to conflict

7. *Other activities:* organized sports, religious groups, other organizations, use of spare time

## Adolescence

**DISCUSS WITH ADOLESCENT**

1. *Health:* alcohol, tobacco, and drug use, health consequences of violence, dental care, physical activity, immunizations
2. *Safety:* bike and skateboard helmet and safety, car seat belts, driving while intoxicated, water safety, hitchhiking, risk taking
3. *Nutrition:* balanced diet, appropriate weight, avoiding junk foods
4. *Sexuality:* physical changes, sex education, peer pressure for sexual activity, sense of responsibility for self and partner. OK to say no, preventing pregnancy and sexually transmitted diseases, breast and testes self-examination
5. *Development/relationships:* identity versus role confusion, family, peers, dating, independence, trying different roles, managing anger other than with verbal and physical attacks
6. *School:* academics, homework
7. *Other activities:* sports, hobbies, organizations, jobs
8. *Future plans:* school, work, relationships with others

**DISCUSS WITH PARENTS**

1. *Communication:* allowing adolescents to participate in discussion and development of family rules; needs frequent praise and affection, time together, interest in adolescent's activities
2. *Independence:* parent and child ambivalence about independence; expecting periods of estrangement; promoting self-responsibility and independence; still needs supervision
3. *Role model:* actions speak louder than words—parents provide model of responsible, reasonable, nonviolent, and compassionate behavior

# 17

# Health Promotion Concerns of Adult Men and Women

*Ella M. Brooks*

## OBJECTIVES

*Upon completion of this chapter, the reader should be able to:*

1. Discuss how achievement of developmental milestones can enhance growth in adulthood.
2. Describe common stressors experienced during adulthood and nursing interventions that assist adults in coping with these stressors.
3. Discuss nursing interventions for wellness in relation to adult roles and developmental tasks.
4. Use *Healthy People 2010* objectives to identify health risks among adults.
5. Analyze the major causes of mortality and morbidity for adult men and women.

6. Understand gender influences on health needs and behaviors.
7. Evaluate factors that increase adults' risk for mortality and morbidity.
8. Discuss the community health nurse's role in maintaining the health of adult men and women.
9. Describe aggregates at risk among adult men and women.
10. Develop primary, secondary, and tertiary interventions to promote and maintain the health of adult men and women.

## KEY TERMS

(Adult) Morbidity
(Adult) Mortality
Climacteric
Depression
Environmental tobacco smoke
Formication

Generativity
Health habits
Health promotion
Health risks
Health status statistics
Intimacy

Launching
Menopause
Osteoporosis
Quality of life
Unintentional injury
Years of healthy life

*Our understanding of the determinants of health—individual biology and behavior, physical and social environments, policies and interventions, and access to quality health care—and how they relate to one another, coupled with our understanding of how individual and community health affects the health of the Nation, is perhaps the most important key to increasing the quality and years of life and eliminating health disparities—creating healthy people in healthy communities*

(U.S. DEPARTMENT OF HEALTH AND HUMAN SERVICES [USDHHS], 2000A, PP. 20, 25).

Along with the multiple roles and responsibilities of adulthood, adults are developing as individuals and need to be concerned with their health. This chapter discusses adult aggregates at risk for high **mortality** and **morbidity**, examines health behaviors that increase mortality and morbidity risks, and discusses nursing interventions to promote health and reduce mortality and morbidity risks among adults. Other chapters present the health needs of parents of infants, children, and adolescents (Chapter 16); occupational health issues (Chapter 21); the adult with a disabling condition (Chapter 18); and older adulthood (Chapter 19). Other contemporary issues such as minority health status and trends, sexually transmitted diseases (STDs), substance abuse, and accidents and injuries are discussed in Chapter 13.

## *HEALTHY PEOPLE 2010* AND ADULT HEALTH

Adulthood is usually a time of relatively good physical and mental health when people have the opportunity to assume personal responsibility for their health behaviors. Personal choices and the social and physical environments surrounding individuals can shape health behaviors (USDHHS, 2000a). Taking personal responsibility in physical fitness and healthy eating are known to have an effect in preventing many health problems such as coronary heart disease, hypertension, stroke, diabetes, colon cancer, and obesity. Many of the leading causes of morbidity and mortality for adults are preventable through changes in lifestyle and health habits. The *Healthy People 2010* leading health indicators illuminate individual behaviors, physical factors, and social environmental factors that significantly affect the health of individuals and communities (USDHHS, 2000a, p. 24). The indicators emphasize how changes in lifestyle and health habits can positively influence quality of life.

### Health Habits/Health Risks

*Healthy People 2010* indicated that the leading causes of death generally result from a mix of environmental risk factors. These behaviors include violence and injury, dietary practices, obesity, lack of exercise, tobacco use, alcohol consumption, substance use, failure to use seatbelts, and preventive health and screening services (USDHHS, 2000a; 2000b). These behaviors contribute significantly to the five major causes of death in the United States: cancer, heart disease, stroke, unintentional injury, and chronic lung disease (USDHHS, 2000a). *Healthy People 2010* identified the leading health indicators in an effort to help everyone understand the importance of **health promotion** and disease prevention and to encourage national participation in improving health in the next decade (USDHHS, 2000a). Nurses intervene with adults at various levels of health promotion to reduce health risks and promote healthy lifestyles. Health promotion activities with adults are directed toward maximizing their health and abilities and minimizing the effects of aging (Sapp, Bliesmer, 1999). For example, a community health nurse might develop a smoking cessation program for adults in the community. A community health nurse may also identify high-risk aggregates for developing coronary heart disease and develop a worksite fitness program to help these adults address coronary heart disease risk factors such as lack of physical activity, high stress, and poor dietary habits.

Many risk factors are long-established habits that are hard to break. Such habits provide challenges for nurses to develop creative interventions and teaching strategies that are effective in helping adults reduce **health risks** and de-

**BOX 17-1**
*Educational Topics for Promoting Adult Health and Meeting Healthy People 2010 Initiatives*

- Prevention of tobacco use
- Cessation of tobacco use
- Physical activity and fitness
- Worksite injury prevention and safety
- Helmet use by bicyclists and motorcyclists
- Use of seatbelts
- Responsible driving of all types of motorized vehicles (e.g., automobiles, motorcycles, all-terrain vehicles, snowmobiles, farm and work machinery)
- Improvement of dietary behaviors and nutrition
- Prevention and reduction of elevated cholesterol levels
- Weight reduction and management
- Stress reduction and management
- Preventive health behaviors (e.g., immunizations and screening procedures)
- Prevention of alcohol use and abuse
- Cancer prevention and detection

Modified from US Department of Health and Human Services (USDHHS): *Tracking Healthy People 2010*, Washington, DC, 2000b, US Government Printing Office.

velop **health habits** and healthy behaviors. These strategies are addressed later in this chapter. Box 17-1 lists some selected educational topics for reducing risk factors among adults and achieving *Healthy People 2010* initiatives. Community health nurses can use these educational topics as a guide for developing interventions that promote the health of adults.

### The Nation's Objectives for Adult Health

The first goal of *Healthy People 2010* is to *increase quality and years of healthy life* (USDHHS, 2000a, p. 8). This is expected to be accomplished by helping people of all ages increase life expectancy and improve quality of life. **Quality of life** refers to the sense of happiness and satisfaction that people have in their lives and environment. It also reflects a personal sense of physical and mental health and an ability to react to factors in the physical and social environments. Quality of life is subjective and more difficult to measure than life expectancy, and the difference between the life expectancy and quality or **years of healthy life** reflects the average amount of time spent in less than maximal health because of acute or chronic limitations (USDHHS, 2000a, p. 10). Many of these acute and chronic limitations are preventable. *Healthy People 2010* seeks to increase life expectancy and quality of life over the next 10 years by helping people gain the knowledge, motivation, and opportunities they need to make informed decisions about their health. The goal is to assist persons to take personal responsibility for their health to prevent

**BOX 17-2**

**Health Status Goals, Risk Reduction Objectives, Services and Protection Goals**

*Health Status Goals*

Reduce coronary heart disease deaths.

Reduce stroke deaths.

Reduce diabetes and diabetes-related deaths.

Reduce the proportion of adults with high blood pressure.

Reduce the proportion of adults with high total blood cholesterol levels.

Increase the proportion of adults who have had their blood cholesterol checked within the preceding 5 years.

Reduce deaths caused by unintentional injuries.

Reduce deaths caused by motor vehicle crashes.

Reduce deaths from work-related injuries.

Reduce nonfatal injuries caused by motor vehicle crashes.

Reduce homicides.

Reduce suicides.

Increase the proportion of adults who are at a healthy weight.

Reduce the proportion of adults who are obese.

Reduce the overall cancer death rate.

Reduce the death rate from specific cancers (e.g., breast cancer, melanoma, prostate, lung, skin).

*Risk Reduction Objectives* that increase the proportion of adults who:

- are aware of the early warning signs of heart attack and stroke.
- can administer cardiopulmonary resuscitation (CPR).
- use at least one of the following protective measures that may reduce the risk of skin cancer: avoid sun between 10 AM and 4 PM, wear sun-protective clothing when exposed to sunlight, use sunscreen with a sun protective factor (SPF) of 15 or higher, and avoid artificial sources of ultraviolet light.
- had their blood pressure checked within the preceding 2 years and can state whether their blood pressure was normal or high.
- consume no more than 30% of daily calories from fat.

- engage regularly (preferably daily) in moderate physical activity for at least 30 minutes per day.
- quit smoking and/or using tobacco.
- wear helmets when operating motorcycles and bicycles.
- wear safety belts.
- apply child restraints.
- receive Pap tests and mammograms.
- participate in employer-sponsored health promotion activities.
- are taking action (e.g., losing weight, increasing physical activity, or reducing sodium intake) to control their blood pressure.
- have disabilities and report satisfaction with life.

*Services and Protection Goals* that increase the proportion of:

- health care organizations that provide client and family education.
- dentists and physicians who counsel their at-risk clients about tobacco use.
- college and university students who receive information from their institution on each of the six priority health-risk behavior areas.
- hospitals and managed care organizations that provide community disease prevention and health promotion activities that address the priority health needs identified by their community.
- local health departments that have established culturally and linguistically competent community health promotion and disease prevention programs.
- worksites that offer a comprehensive employee health promotion program to their employees.
- persons who have access to rapidly responding prehospital emergency medical services.
- persons appropriately counseled about health behaviors.
- worksites that offer nutrition or weight management classes or counseling.

Modified from USDHHS: *Tracking Healthy People 2010,* Washington, DC, 2000b, US Government Printing Office.

those limitations that decrease quality of life and life expectancy (USDHHS, 2000a, p. 10).

Numerous adult health objectives are scattered throughout the *Healthy People 2010* document. Some of the main focus areas for *Healthy People 2010* are summarized in Box 17-2. These objectives address health status measures and goals for improving health status, reducing health risk behaviors, and improving health services and protection. Because lifestyle behaviors continue to adversely influence the health of adults, many of these goals encourage changing lifestyle behaviors (e.g., smoking patterns, exercise and dietary habits) that can improve the future health of our nation.

Overweight and obesity are major contributors to many preventable health problems and causes of death. Costs for medical services and lost productivity due to overweight and obesity are in the billions of dollars annually (USDHHS, 2000a, p. 28). The prevalence of obesity has increased and the number of children, adolescents, and adults who are overweight and obese has dramatically increased over the past four decades. Currently, more than half of adults in the United States are estimated to be overweight or obese (USDHHS, 2000a, pp. 28-29). Additionally, fewer people who are overweight appear to be taking steps to control their weight through measures such as healthy eating and exercising more. For both men and women, adopting sound dietary practices and eating a healthy diet combined with regular physical activity are both important for maintaining a healthy weight (USDHHS, 2000a, p. 29). However, a significant number of people are unaware of sound dietary practices. A recent research survey showed that only about one quarter of Americans were aware of the dietary requirements for fruits and vegetables, and those who were aware of these ate more fruits and vegetables than those who were unaware (USDHHS, 1995a, p. 30). The survey also showed that nurse practitioners only routinely inquired about exercise habits in only 30% of their clients and formulated an exercise plan for only 14% of their clients (USDHHS, 1995a, p. 25). These findings suggest that health care professionals need to focus more on health promotion interventions. Exercise information should be gathered on a routine basis and nurses should be prepared to intervene in this area.

Community health nurses can play a significant role in helping the nation accomplish the *Healthy People* 2010 objectives. Nurses have the expertise to develop primary, secondary, and tertiary measures to achieve many of these objectives. Having an understanding of these objectives can assist nurses in developing individual and aggregate health interventions that address them. When developing interventions, nurses take into consideration the developmental tasks of adulthood as well as health risk factors.

## DEVELOPMENTAL TASKS OF ADULTHOOD

It has long been established that significant personality growth and development occur during adulthood (Erikson, 1963, 1982; Havighurst, 1972; Stevenson, 1977). Human beings change, learn, and pass through developmental stages that require achievement of predictable tasks. Accomplishment of these tasks provides a foundation for growth. If these tasks are not accomplished, future development can be jeopardized or altered.

Adult development is influenced by numerous variables including individual needs, interpersonal relationships (including family roles), established patterns of coping, support systems, community roles, and societal expectations. Table 17-1 illustrates the complexity of the developmental stages and tasks of adulthood. These stages are not absolute with age, and they may overlap as adults progress through the life span. As community health nurses work with and provide guidance to adults throughout the life span, it is important to remember that the developmental process and "aging is a natural experience, not a pathological process" (Eliopoulos, 2001, p. 9).

### Erikson's Intimacy, Generativity, and Ego Integrity

Erik Erikson's (1963) classic work on developmental theory stressed the importance of the psychosocial aspects of development. Erikson wrote that development was a continu-

ous process and that delays or crisis at one developmental stage could diminish successful achievement of other stages of development. His psychosocial theories address stages of development, developmental goals and tasks, psychosocial crises, and coping processes. Erikson described eight developmental stages from birth to death, three of which apply to the 18- to 65-year-old population. According to Erikson (1963, 1982) these stages are intimacy (young adult), generativity (middle adult), and ego integrity (older adult).

INTIMACY. Young adults are involved in an intense search of self. At the same time they are at the developmental stage of **intimacy** and need to begin to relate to others, become partners in friendships, and develop sexual, work, and community relationships. Young adulthood is a time for development of close personal relationships and commitment to others. Young adults may experience conflicting values, attitudes, and ideas as they sort out what life means to them and develop the ethical strength to abide by their commitments. The young adult who is successful in achieving intimacy will develop the ability to love and commit to others; unsuccessful resolution can result in isolation and self-absorption.

GENERATIVITY. As life continues into middlescence, it is expected that the middle adult will guide and care for the younger generation and assist the older one. This involves an ability to care and do for others, and when these attributes exist, the adult becomes generative in nature. **Generativity** is viewed in terms of caring and sharing, as well as procreativity, productivity, and creativity. The generative person extends herself or himself to others outside the family. One does not have to be a biological parent to be generative. Generative adults help guide others on a path to their own generativity. If this task is not reached, stagnation can occur. Stagnated adults do not demonstrate the need or inclination to care for others. Instead they are likely to be egocentric and self-absorbed.

EGO INTEGRITY. In older adulthood ego integrity is established. This is a contemplative process that involves self-assessment; evaluating where one has been; where one is going; and examining personal values, decisions, and lifestyles. One also strives to accomplish personal and civic aspirations during this stage of life and to become self-fulfilled. If life aspirations are not fulfilled, adulthood can be a time of disillusionment, disenchantment, and despair. The person who has achieved ego integrity knows and likes himself or herself and is able to accept individual strengths and weaknesses, distinguish the things over which he or she has control, and accept those things that cannot be changed. Despair is likely to occur if ego integrity is not reached.

To promote wellness and to enhance an adult's self-care capabilities, the community health nurse needs to have an understanding of the processes involved in developing intimacy, generativity, and ego integrity. Adults should be facilitated in moving toward accomplishment of these developmental tasks. Helping adults understand developmental

**TABLE 17-1**

*Developmental Tasks of the Adult (Ages 18-65): Major Goals—to Develop Intimacy, Generativity, and Ego Integrity*

| YOUNG ADULT | MIDDLESCENT | |
| | MIDDLESCENCE I | MIDDLESCENCE II |
| --- | --- | --- |
| *Age: 18-29 years* | *Age: 30-50 years* | *Age: 51-70 years\** |
| 1. Establishing autonomy from parents or parent surrogates | 1. Developing socioeconomic consolidation | 1. Maintaining flexible views in occupational, civic, political, religious, and social positions |
| 2. Choosing and preparing for an occupation | 2. Evaluating one's occupation or career in light of a personal value system | 2. Keeping current on relevant scientific, political, and cultural changes |
| 3. Developing a marital relationship or other form of companionship | 3. Helping younger persons to become integrated human beings | 3. Developing mutually supportive (interdependent) relationships with grown offspring and other members of the younger generation |
| 4. Developing and initiating parenting behaviors for use with own, and others', offspring | 4. Enhancing or redeveloping intimacy with spouse or most significant other | 4. Reevaluating and enhancing the relationship with spouse or most significant other or adjusting to his or her loss |
| 5. Developing a personal lifestyle and philosophy of life | 5. Developing a few deep friendships | 5. Helping aged parents or other relatives progress through the last stage of life |
| 6. Accepting one's role as a citizen and developing participatory citizen behaviors | 6. Helping aging persons progress through the later years of life | 6. Deriving satisfaction from increased availability of leisure time |
| | 7. Assuming responsible positions in occupational, social, and civic activities, organizations, and communities | 7. Preparing for retirement and planning another career when feasible |
| | 8. Maintaining and improving the home and other forms of property | 8. Adapting self and behavior to signals of the accelerated aging process |
| | 9. Using leisure time in satisfying and creative ways | |
| | 10. Adjusting to biological or personal system changes that occur | |

Material on middlescence from Stevenson JS: *Issues and crises during middlescence,* New York, 1977, Appleton-Century-Crofts, pp. 18, 25.
\*In her text, Stevenson assigns the age range for Middlescence II to be 50-70 years.

tasks can facilitate their achievement, promote self-esteem and personal growth, and ultimately lead to self-fulfillment.

## Adult Roles

Life for an adult is complex and changing, and adults play many interdependent roles. Some roles assumed by the adult include parent, grandparent, individual, spouse or companion, son or daughter, citizen, friend, and worker. Box 17-3 delineates the facilitation of some of these adult roles. Usually these roles are developmentally sequential or complementary. However, a person may not be ready to assume a role when it arises. Examples of role changes that people may not be prepared to make are unintended parenthood and mandatory retirement, especially if retirement is not desired. Role changes that occur abruptly may create frustration and personal crises in the adult. Nurses must assess for stressors that may precipitate adult crises and be prepared to intervene appropriately.

## SELECTED STRESSORS OF ADULTHOOD AND NURSING INTERVENTION

Adult life is usually healthy, productive, and fulfilling, but it may also include frustration, confusion, and lack of direction. Nurses can provide adults with anticipatory, supportive guidance and interact with them to promote health. Providing adults with information about community resources, preventive health practices, and developmental expectations are several ways to promote health in adults.

The life span comprises a series of life change events. Chapter 8 elaborates on experiences that signify these events. The number, duration, and type of events vary with

**BOX 17-3**

*Facilitating Role Performance Among Adults*

### Individual

Adults need to define what is personally important to them and set personal life goals. At times this can create conflict for the nurse, especially when client goals differ from the nurse's. The nurse who is sensitive and accepts the client's right of self-determination generates trust and facilitates a more collaborative working relationship. Nurses need to "individualize" care to meet client needs.

### Parent

The generative aspect of middlescence is explicit when the roles of parent and grandparent are discussed. In the role of parent the adult is expected to maintain the family physically, emotionally, and financially and assist in the socialization process. Parenting issues in the middle years often involve adolescent children and launching of adult children. It is helpful for the nurse to discuss children's developmental tasks with parents. Such discussions can assist parents in understanding what is normal (e.g., being rebellious is a part of normal adolescent behavior). The community health nurse can assist parents in achieving generational balance and understanding.

### Grandparent

Grandparenting is often part of life's middle years. Some middlescents are delighted, eagerly await grandchildren, and look forward to being involved with grandchildren—others do not. Grandparents may find that they have more time to spend with their grandchildren than they did with their own children. A grandparent can enhance the growth of younger generations. In classic writings on the family, Duvall said, "When those who are at the beginning of the journey hold hands with those who have traveled a long way and know all the turns in the road, each gains the strength needed by both" (Duvall, 1962, p. 409).

### Spouse or Companion

In adulthood time is spent in developing and redeveloping relationships with a spouse or significant other and spending time in a companionship relationship. A significant other can be anyone with whom the adult has a close, meaningful relationship. With today's many lifestyles, it is completely possible that there will be a significant other who is not a spouse. This significant other may be part of a heterosexual or homosexual relationship. Being nonjudgmental about various lifestyles is essential if the community health nurse is to help the adult achieve self-fulfillment.

### Son or Daughter

Adults are trying to maintain meaningful relationships with parents and may be experiencing role reversal with them. In these "reversed" roles some adult children become caretakers of their elderly parents. Adult children need to assist aged parents in maintaining their dignity and must refrain from dominating them, taking over their decision making, and robbing them of their independence.

It is important for the adult to deal with the eventual death of aging parents. Plans for burial arrangements and the handling of personal affairs should be considered. Health care professionals need to be comfortable in teaching and talking about death and dying. It is also crucial for adults to realize that it is normal for aging parents to talk about death. Assisting aging parents to resolve their feelings about death and articulating advanced directives can help adults in accepting their own eventual death and other grief, dying, death, and loss situations.

### Citizen/Leader

Adults are expected to take an active role in civic activities and hold local, state, and national offices. They are sought as community leaders and often serve as community volunteers. Adults are valuable resources as volunteer staff and supporters for health projects in the community. Community health nurses can assist adults in understanding the need for balancing citizen commitments with family and individual responsibilities.

### Friend

Adulthood is a time of life when developing and maintaining a few deep friendships is beneficial and rewarding. Having friends that one can count on, enjoy being with, and share activities with helps provide support and pleasure when family contacts are limited.

### Worker

The health of the worker and the role of the occupational health nurse are discussed in Chapter 21. Working is generally essential to one's economic stability and has psychological implications for the individual as well.

The young adult is in a stage of training for, and deciding on, a career. The middlescent may be at a career peak and derives much satisfaction from her or his job. This is usually the time of maximum power and influence. Americans in executive positions are often 40 to 65 years old and earn a large part of the nation's income.

---

individuals. Because of the uniqueness of individuals, a life event that is major for one person may not be considered major for another.

Unlike young children, who have parents or others to support and guide them through the experience of life change events, the adult often does not have adequate sup-

port available during times of heightened stress or may not use the help that is available because of dependency fears. Because our society emphasizes self-sufficiency during adulthood, it can be difficult for an adult to seek assistance from others. Many adults must learn that *interdependency* is a mature state.

Examples of some life change events that affect adults include the following: leaving the parental home, obtaining job education and training, pursuing a career, marriage, childbearing, child rearing, child launching, providing for an aging parent, pursuing leisure-time activities, and experiencing the death of a parent. Life change events that are more or less expected usually evoke what is termed *normative stress*. However, other life change events induce stress that goes beyond what could be considered normative and may necessitate developing new interpersonal relationships, coping mechanisms, and resources. Examples of some of these life change events are divorce or separation, loss of a child, loss of a job, development of a chronic health condition, and career changes. If these events occur in rapid succession, the adult may have difficulty adapting and may experience crisis.

An example of what can happen when major life events occur in rapid succession is seen in the Stephen Johns case scenario.

**CASE** **Scenario** In a period of less than 14 years, Mr. Johns, 32 years old, left home to enter college, completed a college education, entered a career, married, bought a house, had a child, changed jobs, moved to a new residence, became divorced, moved to another residence, changed jobs again, and experienced the death of a parent. These were all significant life events for Mr. Johns, and the rapid succession of their development left him in a depressed and disorganized state. He was overwhelmed with his life and began to question whether it had meaning. A community health nurse discussed his depression when he called the "help line" at a local health department and referred him to a mental health clinic and a psychiatric nurse practitioner. Through help from the practitioner, Mr. Johns was able to establish his life goals and take action to achieve these goals. This made him comfortable about himself as a person and gave direction and meaning to his life. He began to recognize his own strengths and to work within and accept his limitations. He began to reach out to others and saw that interdependency can be therapeutic.

Although major life events may not always be experienced this rapidly, or in this magnitude, significant stresses do occur during adulthood. While experiencing these stresses, adults are also trying to achieve a balance between their responsibilities to family and society, to develop as individuals, and to maintain health. These tasks by themselves produce stress. Thus when sudden or unexpected situational difficulties arise, such as divorce, death, or changes in job and residence, the individual is at risk for crisis.

## Helping Clients in Crisis

Crisis may be experienced at any time throughout adult life. When mobilizing coping mechanisms during times of stress, the adult has many life experiences from which to draw. However, these experiences do not necessarily prepare one to handle all situations. At each developmental stage, new or different events require different coping or adaptation strategies.

When adults are in crisis, they should be helped to look at the circumstances that precipitated the crisis and modify them to reduce future occurrences. The nurse is supportive of the client without leveling judgment and helps the client and family assess the resources and support systems they have available and make plans for the immediate future. As discussed in Chapter 8, the mastery of a crisis provides opportunities for personal growth and development.

The resources people use during crisis and time of need vary. Emotional support, encouragement, assistance with problem solving, companionship, and tangible aid have been shown to be helpful to people who are dealing with a crisis. Individuals experiencing a crisis may look for caregivers who can provide these interventions. Sometimes individuals under stress need help in identifying the need for supportive assistance.

Preventing crisis is a major goal of community health nursing practice. To achieve this goal, the community health nurse recognizes early signs and symptoms of heightened stress (see Chapter 8) and helps individuals who are experiencing these symptoms mobilize appropriate coping mechanisms that help prevent major developmental crises.

## Selected Examples of Normative Crises

As adults in contemporary society move through the life span they may experience overwhelming stress that leads to normative crises. As previously mentioned, these crises may occur at any time throughout the adult life. Selected examples of common normative crises are addressed in this section. These examples include adults dissatisfied with work, those with leisure time needs, parents who are launching their children, and adults who are caretakers of aging parents.

ADULTS DISSATISFIED WITH WORK. Job dissatisfaction is often related to other personal difficulties. Stresses at work can be compounded when an adult has home pressures to handle. This was the case with Ed Sorka.

**CASE** **Scenario** Ed Sorka was a 29-year-old husband and father of two daughters, ages 3 and 5. He became disillusioned with his job because "his boss demanded too much and gave too few rewards." Ed's wife had multiple sclerosis that was getting progressively worse. She required help with activities of daily living and found it hard to participate in social events. Ed was a devoted husband and father. All his spare time was spent with his family. He found it difficult to talk about his wife's condition or his need for leisure activities. Verbalizing stress encountered at work was much easier for him to handle. When the community health nurse helped him examine both work and home stresses, Ed discovered that he really did not want to change jobs. What he needed was time for himself and assistance at home to manage the added family responsibilities related to his wife's chronic illness. The community health nurse provided support and helped him access assistive services to lighten work at home. These assistive arrangements included homemaker services to reduce the homemaking demands on Ed's time.

The stress caused by job dissatisfaction can appear in all aspects of health and family life. When a person's job starts making him or her physically or emotionally ill and takes a toll on family life, it is time to take a serious look at the situation. The nurse can guide the family in assessing the situation, referring them to appropriate community resources, and helping them access various available community services.

ADULTS WITH LEISURE TIME NEEDS. Leisure is not an easy word to define. It means many things to many people. Leisure is antithetical to work as an economic pursuit. It is a planned activity that promotes growth and is pleasurable. Internal motivation is a key factor in planning and implementing leisure activities.

Many adults are too busy to engage in regular leisure-time activity. Leisure activities can be relaxing, rejuvenating, and refreshing. They can help provide a link between responsibilities that cannot be ignored and a need to pursue something of personal value or interest. People need time in which to enjoy themselves and relax.

Adults need leisure time. Using leisure time in satisfying and creative ways is a developmental task for adulthood. The community health nurse should encourage the adult to make a conscious effort to devote time to leisure activities. The great amount of free time that often accompanies retirement and later life will be better spent if individuals have developed leisure-time activities that are satisfying in adulthood.

Frequently the adult needs help in examining why he or she does not engage in leisure activities. Often it will be found that many adults do not know how to use the free time they have and thus they devote all their time to work or other responsibilities. One way the nurse can assist people to examine their leisure time needs is to help them identify interests they would like to develop or redevelop, as demonstrated in the following scenario.

**CASE Scenario** Sara Washington was a 40-year-old divorced woman with no children. Following hospitalization, her family physician referred her to the community health nurse for health supervision for severe hypertension. After her divorce Sara devoted herself to work. She was an interior designer who was well respected in her field; promotion came very rapidly. Most of her social involvements were work-related.

Sara's recent hospitalization scared her. When the community health nurse took a social history on her first home visit, she replied, "I know I can't keep working like I have

been, but I get bored when I don't have something to do. There is very little social life for a woman my age in this town. My peers are all married or divorced themselves. Those who are divorced are like me; they work all the time."

Community health nursing intervention helped Sara discover how much she missed contact with people on a personal level, the types of social activities she might explore, her fears about getting involved, and the middlescent's need for leisure-time activities to achieve normal growth and development. Sara had enjoyed cooking, entertaining friends, art, and drama before her divorce. Supportive encouragement by the community health nurse facilitated her involvement once again in these activities. She especially enjoyed dance lessons and found that they provided several opportunities for socializing. "You know, when one takes the time, it really isn't that difficult to find something fun to do," stated Sara during one of the nurse's home visits.

Adults who have experienced a stressful life event such as divorce may use work to reduce their tension and anxiety, overlooking leisure needs. An astute community health nurse might prevent this from happening by providing anticipatory guidance and supportive encouragement when encountering adults during times of heightened stress.

PARENTS WHO ARE LAUNCHING CHILDREN. A primary task of the parent in the middle years is launching children from the parental home. **Launching** is a normal part of growth and development and a time when the young adult becomes independent and autonomous. It can be a brief or prolonged period.

Parents who have accomplished the developmental tasks of middlescence are more likely to foster independence in their children and relinquish control than those who have not. Middlescent parents who have not faced the developmental issues of their life period find it difficult to launch their adult children. The nurse can help parents through this process by discussing launching with them and assisting parents in identifying ways to achieve satisfaction that does not involve their children. Adolescents and young adults have a greater chance of achieving healthy independence when their parents support their efforts. In successful launching, parents become less directive and recognize that young adults need time to make their own decisions and sort out what they want from life.

Launching is often a time when parents reflect on how they have raised their children. They frequently evaluate their parenting on the basis of how their children have progressed toward financial independence and whether or not they have established a stable, happy home. Many parents do not consider a child fully launched until these two tasks have been achieved.

Duvall and Miller (1985, p. 276) have discussed the family developmental tasks involved in launching as follows:

- Adapting physical facilities and resources for releasing young adults
- Meeting launching-center families' costs
- Reallocating responsibilities among grown and growing offspring and their parents
- Developing increasingly mature roles within the family
- Interacting, communicating, and appropriately expressing affection, aggression, disappointment, success, and sexuality
- Releasing and incorporating family members satisfactorily
- Establishing patterns for relating to in-laws, relatives, guests, friends, community pressures, and impinging world pressures
- Setting attainable goals, rewarding achievement, and encouraging family loyalties within a context of personal freedom

A family-centered intervention approach can help parents and children through the launching process. The needs of all family members should be addressed during this process. This is illustrated in the following scenario.

**CASE** *Scenario* John Michael, age 22, decided to live with his parents because he wanted to save money to buy a condominium. He expected to live free of charge, to have no household responsibilities in his parents' home, and to come and go as he pleased. Conflicts arose when John's parents did not agree with his plans. His parents were experiencing financial stress. They had two other children in college and had just finished spending a considerable amount of money for John's education. John was making an adequate salary and they expected him to contribute financially toward family expenses. They also felt that he should assume responsibility for some of the household chores. John became angry. He wanted the freedom of adulthood without having to assume the responsibilities that went along with this freedom.

The community health nurse was involved with John's family because Mrs. Michael was newly diagnosed with diabetes. It was during her third home visit that the nurse identified the stress between John and his parents. During the visit, John's mother was tense and tearful. Observing her distressed state, the nurse encouraged her to verbalize her feelings and afterward made arrangements to meet jointly with John and his parents. During the visit, the nurse requested that each family member share his or her perceptions of what was happening. Emphasis also was placed on identifying alternative ways to resolve the family conflict and on assisting family members to identify their needs and responsibilities.

One issue that became apparent during this conference was that John became aware of the stresses his parents were experiencing. Through this process, John learned to look

beyond himself and develop sensitivity to needs of others, including his parents. The child at launching age is able to relate, at least partially, to the needs of his or her parents, but may need some help in understanding this process.

**ADULTS WHO ARE CARETAKERS FOR AGING PARENTS.** Adults taking care of their aging parents is a role that is increasing dramatically. Although it can be rewarding and gratifying, this situation can precipitate stress and crisis (see Chapter 22). Many middlescent and even older adults are caring for older parents and at the same time working and caring for children at home. Caretaking can mean less leisure time and can provoke feelings of guilt about not doing enough. These feelings are especially prevalent when an adult may have to place a parent in a nursing home when home care is no longer feasible. The nurse can encourage families to verbalize their feelings about caretaking, assess the caretaker situation, realistically look at what they can do, and use appropriate community resources. Sometimes using community resources means that the caretaker needs to obtain services outside the home, such as adult day care services or have someone assist in the home during the day. Caregiver support can assist families in making these difficult decisions.

In addition to the developmental tasks, stresses, and crises that are occurring in adulthood, the physical nature of the human body is changing during this period. Some of these physical changes provide a challenge for adults in achieving and maintaining health.

## THE HUMAN BODY IN ADULTHOOD

Achieving health for the adult involves maintaining physical, social, and mental well-being (including successful achievement of developmental tasks). Because most adults are considered healthy, the health care needs of adults may be overlooked. Frequently adults consider themselves "too busy" or "too involved" to look after their personal health. It can be a challenge for the nurse to persuade the well adult to obtain health care and to practice preventive health practices. Having an understanding of the changes that can occur in the human body during adulthood helps the nurse address this challenge.

The human body is constantly undergoing physical and mental changes. During adulthood the person begins to develop an acute awareness of growing older and is faced with adjusting to a changing body image as physical alterations occur. This adjustment is often difficult in American society because the beauty and stamina of youth are prized. The incidence of chronic and physically disabling conditions also increases with age, and these conditions can affect how one views oneself.

Several physical changes occur in the human body during adulthood. The senses of taste and smell begin to diminish.

Vision is usually well maintained in early adulthood, but presbyopia (farsightedness) is extremely common by middlescence. Presbyopia is caused by a decreased lens elasticity that reduces the power of accommodation. It hinders the ability of the individual to view objects at close range, and glasses may be necessary for reading or close work. After age 30 the cornea begins to lose transparency and the pupil decreases in size. These changes allow less light to be admitted to the eye and result in poor illumination.

Permanent sensorineural hearing loss as a result of aging (presbycusis) accelerates during middlescence. The person experiencing presbycusis has decreased auditory acuity for higher tones and may have difficulty engaging in normal conversation, including talking over the telephone. The duration and type of noise exposure that a person encounters during earlier life influences how soon presbycusis begins. For example, the person exposed to industrial noise or the avid hunter may experience presbycusis earlier than others because of more extensive sensorineural hearing damage during youth.

Metabolic function—combining food with oxygen to create energy—decreases during adulthood. This, coupled with the fact that the person is often becoming more sedentary, can mean increased weight. The basal metabolism rate gradually decreases by middle age with a resultant need for reduction in caloric intake.

Decreasing elasticity of the blood vessels, especially the coronary arteries, predisposes the middlescent to cardiovascular disease. Many middlescents evidence the symptomatology of cardiac conditions, such as shortness of breath, chest pains, and dyspnea on exertion. Incidence of death from cardiovascular disease rises in adulthood.

In middlescence the female's ovarian estrogen production and menstruation cease. This event is called *menopause.* Menopause usually occurs between the ages of 45 and 55 years but can be earlier or later. The average age of menopause is 51 for women in the United States (Hall, 2000). Menopause is a normal transition for midlife women but is often viewed negatively. Nurses can assist women in addressing the negative aspects of menopause by helping them realize that their sexuality does not end with menopause and, after menopause, they may experience a new zest and vitality in life (Greenwood, 1996). As estrogen levels decline, women may experience a wide array of symptoms including a bizarre symptom termed *formication* (Hall, 2000). Formication is a sensation that ants are crawling all over the skin and occurs in about 20% of menopausal women (Hall, 2000). The symptoms that women experience during menopause are an interplay of psychological and physiological changes that are largely a result of decreased ovarian activity and the resultant estrogen deficiency. These symptoms generally subside after menopause. However, the symptoms may continue up to 3 years after a woman's last menstrual period (Hall, 2000). Box 17-4 lists some of the symptoms experienced by women during menopause.

**BOX 17-4**

## Common Menopausal Symptoms

- Atrophic vaginitis
- Chills
- Decreased libido
- Depression
- Dizziness
- Fatigue
- Formication
- Headaches
- Hot flashes
- Insomnia
- Irritability
- Mood swings
- Palpitations
- Poor concentration
- Short-term memory loss
- Skin changes and prickly sensations
- Sweating and night sweats
- Vaginal dryness
- Vaginitis
- Weight gain

It is important to note that a woman does not necessarily experience all of these symptoms. Some women may experience many of them and others may experience very few or pass through menopause without any symptoms. However, for some women the symptoms create significant stress and fears about one's health. For example, it is not unusual for women to fear dementia because experiencing short-term memory loss and lack of concentration during this time is common (Peters, 1996). Community health nurses have an important role in alleviating fears such as these by educating people about the normal changes with menopause. Women do not have to suffer menopausal symptoms silently. Some therapies such as hormone replacement, estrogen vaginal creams, and vaginal lubricants may be indicated (Greenwood, 1996; Hall, 2000; Hofland, Powers, 1996).

Altering behaviors, physical activity, and dietary intake may also lessen the menopausal symptoms. This includes activities such as smoking cessation and minimal alcohol intake because both may contribute to irregular bleeding and increased tension; decreasing caffeine intake because it stimulates the central nervous system, which increases tension and irritability; engaging in frequent and regular exercise, which may help reduce frequency and severity of hot flashes as well as aid in weight control; avoiding stressful situations that may increase symptoms; and being cognizant of nutritional intake such as calcium, fats, sugars, salt, and carbohydrates for weight control, as well as prevention of health problems such as osteoporosis and hypertension (Greenwood, 1996).

Once a woman passes through menopause, her childbearing capabilities cease. This often has greater psychological meaning than physical significance. To be safe, it is often recommended that a woman continue to use a reliable method of birth control for at least 1 year after she has gone 12 consecutive months without a menstrual period.

In middlescence, a man passes through a period called the *climacteric,* in which the testes decrease but do not cease testosterone production. During this time the testes may atrophy slightly, frequency of sexual activity may tend to decline, and prostate problems are common (Thompson, Wilson, 1996). A man usually goes through this period between ages 50 and 60. He may or may not experience any physical symptoms. Some symptoms such as irritability, easy frustration, depression, and change in sexual drive are sometimes evidenced. Often it is more difficult for men than women to admit to these changes or talk about them. This was profoundly described when Gail Sheehy (1996) stated, "if menopause is the silent passage [for women], male menopause is unspeakable" (p. 292). Many people are not aware that this period exists for men and are often bewildered by male behavior during the climacteric.

The human responses to menopause and the climacteric can cause stress and affect relationships. Educating adult men and women about normal life change events that occur during the menopause and climacteric can help alleviate interpersonal stresses that may negatively influence their relationships. Community health nurses have an important educative role in this area.

With menopause a woman's estrogen level drops drastically, which increases the risk for calcium loss and osteoporosis. Decalcification of the bones, a condition called *osteoporosis,* begins in middlescence. Not all older adults will develop osteoporosis, although there is a decrease in bone mass that occurs with aging (Arnaud, 1996). With osteoporosis the bones become fragile and are easily broken. Bone fractures and vertebral compression that cause back pain and other problems can occur (Greenwood, 1996). Before menopause, estrogen helps protect the bones from losing calcium (Greenwood, 1996). Estrogen replacement therapy may be advised to decrease bone loss and fracture rate associated with menopause (Arnaud, 1996; Hall, 2000). Estrogen also helps prevent heart disease (Hall, 2000; Strange, 1998). Lack of exercise, low dietary calcium intake, excess alcohol intake, and smoking are also factors that contribute to osteoporosis (Greenwood, 1996). Adequate dietary intake of calcium should begin early in young women to help increase maximum bone strength. The National Institutes of Health (NIH) has recommended that adult women ages 25 to 50 should have 1000 mg, and those over age 50 should have 1500 mg, of calcium per day (Greenwood, 1996, p. 72).

As a person ages, the amount of skeletal muscle decreases and muscle cells are replaced by adipose and connective tissue. As a result of these changes, adults have decreased muscle tone, a flabbier appearance, and decreased muscle strength. Exercise will help maintain muscle tone and strength and increase calcium absorption. The adult can engage in a variety of activities and sports, but it is advised that individuals check with a physician before beginning any vigorous exercise routine. The adult should exercise consistently, gradually increasing the amount to avoid overexertion.

An example of how an adult undergoing the physical changes of middlescence can be psychologically affected by these changes is seen in the following case scenario.

**CASE Scenario**   Marge, a 50-year-old widow and mother of three daughters, ages 24, 27, and 30, is a typical example of how many people react to body changes during middlescence. When Marge's oldest daughter celebrated her thirtieth birthday she became concerned about her own "aging" process. She sought help at a local adult screening clinic because she perceived that the physical changes she was undergoing were making her look older than her chronological age. She wanted to maintain a youthful look and stated, "I am having a hard time getting old. I fear the physical changes and the dependency associated with aging."

Marge had an established career and just recently had developed an intimate relationship with a man that could lead to marriage. She was loved and respected by her children. Friends enjoyed being with her and described her as intellectually stimulating and fun. However, Marge could focus only on her physical changes and was experiencing anxiety in relation to them.

The community health nurse who saw Marge at the adult screening clinic made arrangements to visit her at home. Marge was helped to identify her strengths and to look more realistically at the changes in her appearance. The nurse discussed normal physical and emotional change associated with middlescence. Marge gradually began to realize that if she focused on her physical appearance alone, she could jeopardize some of the other joys in her life that provided self-fulfillment.

The physical changes of the aging process can be difficult to handle, and the community health nurse works with many adults who share Marge's concerns. Some adults may seek mental health counseling to assist them in adapting to the changes and demands of adulthood, and nurses can refer clients to appropriate community resources for help. The development of generativity, intimacy, and ego integrity helps an individual adapt to physical changes associated with the aging process.

Even though physical functioning changes or decreases, mental functioning can be maintained or increased during adulthood. Cerebral capacity begins to weaken relatively slowly, unless other factors such as cerebrovascular occlusion or depression occur. General intelligence of the middlescent is often greater than at any other time of life.

## SELECTED HEALTH RISKS AMONG ADULT MEN AND WOMEN

Many diseases and conditions of adults can be prevented with changes in lifestyle and are amenable to community health nursing intervention. Figure 17-1 portrays graphically

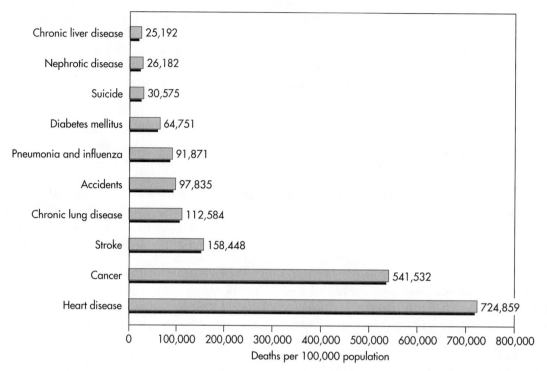

**FIGURE 17-1** Ten leading causes of death for all persons in 1998 and the total number of deaths from each cause. (Modified from National Center for Health Statistics: *Health, United States 2000, with adolescent health chartbook, United States, 2000,* DHHS Pub No 00-1232, Hyattsville, Md, 2000, National Center for Health Statistics, p. 172.)

the 10 leading causes of death for adults. Heart disease and cancer were the two leading causes in 1998. Accidents, including motor vehicle accidents, all other unintentional deaths, and adverse effects, were the third highest cause (National Center for Health Statistics, 2000). This section discusses health risks that increase morbidity and mortality among men and women in adulthood.

## Smoking and Health

One major risk factor for morbidity and mortality among adults is smoking. It was 1964 when Americans were first seriously presented with information that linked smoking and lung cancer. In that year the classic report of *Smoking and Health: Report of the Advisory Committee to the Surgeon General of the Public Health Service* (U.S. Department of Health, Education, and Welfare [USDHEW], 1964), often referred to as the *Surgeon General's Report on Smoking and Health,* was published. The report, prepared by an independent body of scientists approved by the Tobacco Institute and eight health organizations, reviewed more than 7000 studies and noted a causal relationship between cigarette smoking, lung cancer, and other serious diseases (USDHHS, 1989, p. viii). As a result, it was determined that remedial action was necessary to curtail cigarette smoking. Since that report, every Surgeon General of the United States has promoted smoking cessation and has reinforced the knowledge that smoking is one of the most significant causes of disease

and death. However, "tobacco use is pandemic [and] if the countries of the world do not act to reduce tobacco use in the next 20 to 30 years, 10 million people per year will be dying from the effect of this drug" (Satcher, 2001, p. 191).

Cigarette smoking continues to be the number one cause of preventable disease and death in the United States (USDHHS, 2000a, p. 30). According to the American Cancer Society (ACS), it is estimated that there are more than 430,000 tobacco-related deaths among adults each year (ACS, 2000, p. 28). An estimated 48 million American adult men and women are smokers and over half of all continuing smokers die prematurely from smoking (ACS, 2000). There is no safe alternative to cigarettes. All forms of tobacco use increase the risk of cancer, heart disease and chronic lung disease (ACS, 2000; Kiefe, Williams, Lewis, et al., 2001; USDHHS, 2000a). For example, spit (chew) tobacco causes cancer of the mouth, inflammation of the gums, and tooth loss (USDHHS, 2000a, p. 31). Cigar smoking causes cancer of the mouth, throat, larynx, esophagus and lungs and probably cancer of the pancreas (ACS, 2000, p. 29; USDHHS, 2000a, p. 31).

The most effective intervention for tobacco-related deaths is *prevention* by abstaining from tobacco use before a habit can be formed. The cessation of smoking and other tobacco use becomes more difficult when the habit is developed early in life because of the nicotine tolerance that is built up through years of smoking (Henningfield, Schuh,

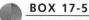

**BOX 17-5**

## *U.S. Surgeon General's Strategies to Reduce Tobacco Use by Year 2010*

### *Educational*
- Implement effective school-based prevention programs.
- Expand education to include parents.
- Focus on prevention of tobacco use.

### *Management of Nicotine Addiction*
- Advocate for universal insurance coverage for evidence-based treatment.
- Provide more intensive interventions that combine behavioral counseling and pharmacologic treatment.
- View tobacco addiction as a chronic disease with remission and relapse.

### *Regulation of Manufactured Tobacco Products*
- Regulate sale and promotion of tobacco products to protect young people from smoking initiation.
- Tighten overall advertising, sale, and promotion.
- Develop stricter warning labels on tobacco products that more accurately disclose information about the harmful effects of tobacco use.
- Develop stricter laws regulating environmental tobacco smoke (ETS) to protect nonsmokers.
- Restrict access of tobacco to minors.

### *Economic Interventions*
- Raise prices of tobacco products.
- Raise taxes on tobacco products (*Healthy People 2010* calls for state and federal taxes to average $2.00 for both cigarettes and smokeless tobacco products by 2010).

### *Comprehensive Programs*
- Implement community interventions that include schools, health agencies, city and county governments, and civic and social recreation organizations.
- Introduce countermarketing to change social norms regarding tobacco use.
- Develop policies and regulations.
- Use surveillance and evaluation processes.

### *Global Efforts*
- Collaborate with international organizations to stem pandemic of tobacco-related death and disease.

### *Elimination of Health Disparities*
- Focus research on effective interventions for various population groups.

Modified from Centers for Disease Control and Prevention (CDC): *Reducing tobacco use: a report of the Surgeon General—2000* (online service text file). USDHHS Office of Smoking and Health, 2000. Retrieved from the internet February 2, 2001. *http://www.cdc.gov/tobacco*

1996). Hence prevention efforts must target young adults before they ever begin smoking.

Studies have shown that those who quit smoking decrease their risk of cancer and other tobacco-related health problems. Some of the benefits of smoking cessation include the following (ACS, 2000, p. 29):
- living longer, regardless of age, than people who continue to smoke
- a substantially decreased risk of dying in the next 15 years compared with those who continue to smoke
- a substantially decreased risk of developing lung, throat, and other tobacco-related cancers
- a decreased risk of developing coronary heart and cardiovascular diseases

Congress has passed legislation that requires health warnings be printed on cigarette packages, cigarette advertising be banned in the broadcast media, and public awareness on the hazards of smoking be proliferated. The U.S. Public Health Service conducts research and regularly publishes reports on smoking and health. Radio and television advertisements for cigarettes are no longer allowed; programs and literature aimed at helping the smoker to stop smoking have been circulated; the rights of nonsmokers are being stressed; nonsmoking areas have been designated in many public places and on public transportation; smoking is banned on domestic airline flights and higher cigarette taxes have been levied. Many communities have adopted laws or regulations

banning smoking in public places, such as worksites, or have restricted smoking to designated areas. Despite these efforts smoking continues to be a major health risk.

Today the relationship between smoking and cardiovascular disease and lung cancer is well established (Kiefe, Williams, Lewis, et al., 2001). Smoking is a major risk factor linked to other diseases and cancers, including oral, laryngeal, esophageal, pancreatic, and urinary bladder cancer, respiratory problems, and some forms of cerebrovascular disease (Harris, 1996, p. 59). Smoking is a serious health risk in pregnancy and has been linked to retarded growth and fetal and neonatal death. Furthermore, and alarmingly, environmental tobacco smoke (including second-hand smoke) is a carcinogen for which all levels of exposure are unsafe, and it is linked to approximately 3000 lung cancer deaths each year among *nonsmokers* (ACS, 2000, pp. 29-30). Clearly, this demonstrates the need to create a smoke-free society.

A former U.S. Surgeon General, C. Everett Koop, was the first prominent public official to advocate a smoke-free society by year 2000 (Glantz, 1996, p. 156). Now a decade later, reducing tobacco use continues to be an objective of *Healthy People 2010*. The current Surgeon General continues to campaign to reduce tobacco use. In his 2000 report on tobacco use, the Surgeon General outlined strategies to make a drastic reduction in tobacco use by year 2010 (Centers for Disease Control and Prevention [CDC], 2000). These strategies are summarized in Box 17-5. Creating a

BOX 17-6
*Tobacco Focus Areas*

- Reduce tobacco use by adults: cigarette smoking, spit tobacco, cigars, other products.
- Reduce tobacco use by adolescents: tobacco products, cigarettes, spit tobacco, cigars.
- Reduce initiation of tobacco use among children and adolescents.
- Increase the average age of first use of tobacco products by adolescents and young adults.
- Increase smoking cessation attempts by adult smokers.
- Increase smoking cessation during pregnancy.
- Increase tobacco use cessation among adolescent smokers.
- Increase insurance coverage of evidence-based treatment for nicotine dependency.
- Reduce the proportion of children who are regularly exposed to tobacco smoke at home.
- Reduce the proportion of nonsmokers exposed to environmental smoke.
- Increase smoke-free and tobacco-free environments in schools, including all school facilities, property, vehicles, and school events.

- Establish laws on smoke-free indoor air that prohibit smoking or limit it to separately ventilated areas in public places and worksites.
- Reduce the illegal sales rate to minors through enforcement of laws that prohibit such sales.
- Increase the number of states and the District of Columbia that suspend or revoke state retail licenses for violations of laws prohibiting the sale of tobacco to minors.
- Eliminate tobacco advertising and promotions that influence adolescents and young adults.
- Increase adolescents' disapproval of smoking.
- Increase the number of tribes, territories, states, and the District of Columbia with comprehensive, evidence-based tobacco control programs.
- Eliminate laws that preempt stronger tobacco control laws.
- Reduce the toxicity of tobacco products by establishing a regulatory structure to monitor toxicity.
- Increase the average federal and state tax on tobacco products.

Modified from US Department of Health and Human Services (USDHHS): *Tracking Healthy People 2010*, Washington, DC, 2000b, US Government Printing Office.

smoke-free society continues to be a primary concern with community health nurses and other public health professionals. Research has shown that legislation prohibiting smoking in the workplace can have a significant effect on exposure to environmental smoke and tobacco consumption (Heloma, Jaakkola, Kahkonen, et al., 2001). Smoking prevention and smoking cessation are major goals in the *Healthy People 2010* document.

*HEALTHY PEOPLE 2010* AND SMOKING. *Healthy People 2010* highlights the significance of smoking as a major health problem. Tobacco use is one of major focus areas in the *Healthy People 2010* document (USDHHS, 2000b). Numerous objectives address tobacco use (Box 17-6). The core components of tobacco control targeted prevention, cessation, exposure to second-hand smoke, and social and environmental changes that include increased taxation for tobacco products and tighter laws regulating sales and distribution of these products (USDHHS, 2000b). Each of these areas can guide community health nurses when they develop primary, secondary, and tertiary prevention activities to decrease tobacco use and decrease the adverse effects from tobacco use. Table 17-2 provides some examples of primary, secondary, and tertiary nursing interventions designed to address smoking cessation.

SMOKING AND PREGNANCY. Smoking during pregnancy increases the risk of stillbirth, miscarriage, premature birth, and low-birth-weight infants (National Center for Health Statistics, 2000). There is evidence that heavy smoking (two or more packs per day) by pregnant women can cause serious birth defects such as mental retardation, facial anomalies, and heart defects. Infants born to women who smoked during pregnancy are more likely to die of sudden infant death syndrome (ACS, 2000). The effects of smoking endanger not only the health of the pregnant woman but also that of her fetus. Pregnant women must be taught about these risks and helped to understand the enormous responsibility they have toward the health of their unborn child. With the knowledge of these risks, it is imperative that nurses make a concerted effort to work with pregnant women to prevent and cease smoking. Nurses must work diligently to achieve the *Healthy People 2010* objective to increase smoking cessation among pregnant women. Community health nurses can intervene at all levels of prevention by educating women about the risks of smoking during pregnancy and working with them to complete smoking cessation programs.

ENVIRONMENTAL TOBACCO SMOKE. The Environmental Protection Agency (EPA) has stated that passive inhalation of smoke is a serious public health concern. This health problem is elaborated on in Chapter 6. About 3000 adult deaths each year have been attributed to nonsmokers breathing the smoke from other smokers (ACS, 2000, p. 30). Additionally, environmental tobacco smoke increases the risk of the following diseases and conditions (ACS, 2000; USDHHS, 2000a):

- heart disease
- asthma in children
- cancer

**TABLE 17-2**

*Primary, Secondary, and Tertiary Preventive Nursing Interventions to Combat Tobacco Use*

| PREVENTION LEVEL | PRIMARY PREVENTION | SECONDARY PREVENTION | TERTIARY PREVENTION |
|---|---|---|---|
| -GOAL<br>-OBJECTIVE | -SMOKE-FREE SOCIETY<br>-DON'T SMOKE/USE TOBACCO | -SMOKE-FREE SOCIETY<br>-STOP SMOKING/TOBACCO USE | -SMOKE-FREE SOCIETY<br>-AVOID RELAPSE |
| Examples of Nursing Interventions | • Develop community public awareness programs to alert public to health problems associated with dangers of tobacco use and nicotine addiction.<br>• Support state and community efforts that limit tobacco sales and restrict smoking to areas that would decrease effects of environmental tobacco smoke.<br>• Provide tobacco use prevention education that is population and developmentally specific.<br>• Advocate against products that are packaged to resemble tobacco products (e.g., bubble gum and candy), which may entice youth to experiment with tobacco use.<br>• Provide health promotion education at schools and worksites that address the value of not smoking. | • Casefind to identify smokers in a selected population and refer smokers to a smoking cessation group in community.<br>• Assess smoking-related health statistics in a select community, public areas in community, and worksites where nonsmokers are at risk for environmental tobacco smoke.<br>• Collaborate with primary health care providers in local community to routinely screen, advocate smoking cessation, and assist with cessation measures.<br>• Casefind by routinely questioning pregnant women about tobacco use and work with them to stop smoking.<br>• Assess population to identify and eliminate risk behaviors related to smoking (such as peer pressure). | • Coordinate follow-up programs to prevent former smokers from relapse.<br>• Collaborate with community providers to establish community support groups to help former tobacco users to successfully resist smoking/tobacco use.<br>• Provide follow-up and self-help materials to encourage continued smoking cessation.<br>• Assess smoking habits during routine health encounters to prevent former smokers from relapse. |

• respiratory problems (e.g., coughing, phlegm, chest discomfort)
• decreased lung function

Community health nurses must consider these risk factors when developing health promotion strategies that promote a smoke-free society.

**SMOKELESS TOBACCO.** Use of smokeless tobacco, such as snuff and chewing tobacco, is a health concern. Smokeless tobacco has been linked to various health problems such as (ACS, 2000; USDHHS, 2000a):

• cancer of the mouth, cheek, and gums
• inflammation of the gums
• tooth loss
• nicotine addiction and dependence

Teenagers as well as adults are dying of oral cancers related to smokeless tobacco. All 50 states and the District of Columbia have enacted laws prohibiting the sale of tobacco products to youth under age 18. However, enforcement varies from state to state and a *Healthy People 2010* objective calls for the enactment of stricter laws that regulate sale and distribution of tobacco products, particularly to minors.

The Comprehensive Smokeless Tobacco Education Act of 1986 (Public Law 99-252) established a program of public education to inform people of the health dangers of smokeless tobacco products. It supports educational programs, public service announcements, and research on the effects of smokeless tobacco on human health. It also regulates the advertising and labeling of smokeless tobacco products.

**TOBACCO USE AND THE COMMUNITY HEALTH NURSE.** The ultimate goal in relation to tobacco use is to create a smoke-free society. Community health nurses can significantly influence moving toward a smoke-free society because they have easy access to populations at risk in communities and health care agencies. Nurses have access to many population groups and can intervene at all levels of prevention (see Table 17-2). The most effective intervention is primary prevention. Primary prevention is accomplished through awareness and education that instills in populations the health hazards of tobacco use and motivates them to avoid using tobacco products.

Secondary prevention is accomplished through identifying those at risk, those who are using tobacco products, and those who are addicted to nicotine. Secondary interventions focus on cessation of tobacco use and breaking the addiction. "People who stop smoking tobacco, regardless of age, live longer than people who continue to smoke" (ACS, 2000, p. 29). Guiding individuals through smoking cessation groups and providing education regarding alternative activities to smoking (e.g., exercise, hobbies) are strategies that can increase life expectancy and quality of life.

Tertiary prevention focuses on helping persons remain smoke free by preventing relapse. Chapter 13 discusses the principles used in breaking the cycle of addiction, which can include nicotine addiction. Similar to other drugs, cigarette smoking tends to be a progressive addiction. People do not start out with the intention of becoming addicted to tobacco but instead addiction develops gradually (Henningfield, Schuh, 1996, p. 114). Most people are capable of quitting smoking, but the key is to prevent relapse (Miller, 1996, p. 34). Tertiary prevention is perhaps the greatest challenge because smoking cessation relapse rates tend to be high (Henningfield, Schuh, 1996; Shiffman, 1993). In some cases nicotine replacement (e.g., gum or patch) is used to aid in immediate nicotine withdrawal, although results are mixed about the effectiveness of nicotine replacements (Miller, 1996).

Tertiary prevention must focus on methods that prevent smoker relapse and help rehabilitated smokers abstain from smoking. Often smokers who have undergone smoking cessation have a single episode of relapse, which engenders feelings of weakness and failure. It affects their self-confidence and ultimately may escalate into full-blown relapse (O'Connell, Gerkovich, Cook, 1995). This should be considered when nurses develop tertiary interventions. It is important to help former smokers realize that smoking cessation is a difficult process and that relapses should not be viewed as failures. Often involvement in support groups can help former smokers recognize the struggle with smoking cessation. Community health nurses must be aware of resources in the community. The American Lung Association is one example of an excellent community resource for smoking cessation.

AMERICAN LUNG ASSOCIATION. The American Lung Association is one of the oldest private, voluntary health agencies in the United States. Its mission is to prevent and control lung disease. This association provides numerous classes and publications on smoking, smoking cessation, and lung cancer. The nurse can obtain many useful teaching tools and resources from this association, which has state affiliates all over the country and thousands of local offices.

## Gender Influences on Health

As discussed in Chapter 11, personal factors, including gender, age, race, socioeconomic status, stress, lifestyle, and health behavior, influence the epidemiology of disease occurrence and resolution. Of these factors, gender has frequently been neglected in health care practice and research. There is, however, a growing recognition that the differences in women and men produce unique health risks and needs that often require special health planning and programming. Much of the research done in the past has used male subjects. Recently the Women's Health Initiative Pro-

ject, started in 1991 by the NIH, brought about a focus on women's issues and is providing valuable data that can facilitate health planning for women. Additionally, *women's health* has emerged as a specialty focus for practitioners.

**Health status statistics** or mortality and morbidity risks of women and men differ. Although the life expectancy for persons of every age group has increased over the past century (USDHHS, 2000a, p. 8), in America women live longer than men. The life expectancy for women in the United States has been continuously higher than that of men since before 1900. Currently the life expectancy for women is 78.9 years and for men it is 72.5 years (USDHHS, 2000a, p. 9).

Socioeconomic status (SES) and lifestyle patterns have a great influence on the overall life expectancy of both men and women (Dennerstein, 1995, p.56). Genetic and biological forces also have a significant impact on certain disease-specific mortality rates according to gender and race (e.g., cancer of prostate, uterine cancer, and sickle-cell anemia).

In general, women have a higher prevalence of chronic conditions than men. For example, arthritis is more prevalent among women than men, and women experience more limitations from arthritis than men and conversely. Men have a higher incidence of heart disease than women (Kramarow, Lentzner, Rooks, et al., 1999), and the symptoms of heart disease differ between men and women. Gender differences related to selected other chronic conditions are discussed throughout this chapter.

Women also have issues that arise from their gender and roles in society such as childbirth, menstruation, and menopause. Previously seen as "diseases," these conditions are now viewed as part of the normal female physiological processes. Historically, women were treated differently and more apt to be mislabeled with a mental disorder than men (Cowan, 1996). The pain of labor, nausea in pregnancy, and menopausal changes are no longer dismissed as psychogenic. As data emerge from research on women's health issues, new light is continuously being shed on many previously mislabeled "problems" or "diseases" of women.

The Jacob Institute of Women's Health (4409 12th Street SW, Washington, D.C. 20024-2188) is an organization committed to excellence in women's health care. The Institute publishes *The Women's Health Data Book: A Profile of Women's Health in the United States*, which compiles in a single publication much of the available national data on the issues central to understanding women's health (Horton, 1995). It is highly readable and informative.

Men also have health issues that arise from their gender and their roles in society. Death rates among men from accidents, homicides, and suicides are much higher than those of women (National Center for Health Statistics, 2000). However, women are more often the victims of domestic violence than men. Violence, including domestic violence, is discussed in Chapter 13. Acquired immunodeficiency syndrome (AIDS) is a disease that at first was more prevalent among men, but its prevalence is increasing among women. AIDS is also discussed in Chapter 13.

Women and men in our culture are frequently taught that certain roles and traits are not "gender" acceptable. Nurses need to understand how gender affects the incidence and prevalence of diseases and conditions, as well as their treatments. Gender bias may exist within the caregiver or client role and may interfere with therapeutic relationships and treatments (Hawthorne, 1994, p. 79). Nurses must be aware of their own gender biases, remain sensitive to gender issues, and confront those issues as they arise.

## Cardiovascular Disease

Cardiovascular diseases (heart disease and stroke) are among the leading causes of death in the United States (see Figure 17-1). Prevention and control of heart disease and stroke is a priority area in the *Healthy People 2010* objectives. They are among the leading causes of disability and have modifiable risk factors, which include diabetes, hypertension, elevated blood cholesterol, cigarette smoking, obesity, and physical inactivity (USDHHS, 2000a).

Box 17-7 lists the major risk factors associated with heart disease and stroke. Americans are becoming increasingly aware of these risk factors. Major risk factors that cannot be changed include heredity, age, and gender (presently American men are at greater risk of experiencing a heart attack than women). Other risk factors can be alleviated through changes in behaviors, habits, and lifestyle. The more risk factors a person has, the greater the risk for heart disease (NIH, 1998).

With all cardiovascular diseases, community health nurses should fervently focus on primary prevention activities by attending to preventable and modifiable risk factors. Community health nurses promote increased awareness of cardiovascular risk factors and interventions to decrease them, encourage clients to have regular medical supervision, and inform them of available community resources. The health education activities of the nurse in this area cannot be overestimated. Box 17-8 provides some examples of nursing interventions that focus on preventing cardiovascular diseases.

### Stop and Think About It

Identify your personal cardiovascular risk factors. What personal behaviors will you change to minimize your risk profile?

HEART DISEASE. Heart disease is the number one cause of death in America (see Figure 17-1). The leading cause of death from heart disease is heart attacks. The death rate from heart attacks has been reduced over the past decade because of attention to warning signs, early intervention, and access to emergency services. In an effort to continue decreasing the heart attack death rate, increasing public awareness of emergency access services, warning signs, and persons capable of administering cardiopulmonary resuscitation (CPR) is a separate *Healthy People 2010* objective. Some warning signs of possible impending heart attack are listed in Box 17-9. Nurses can make a major contribution toward reaching this objective.

**BOX 17-7**

### Risk Factors Associated with Heart Disease and Stroke

- Age
- Diabetes
- Elevated blood cholesterol
- Excessive alcohol intake
- Excessive body weight
- Gender (male)
- Heredity
- High Blood Pressure
- Physical inactivity
- Smoking
- Stress

Modified from US Department of Health and Human Services (USDHHS): *The sixth report of the joint national committee on detection, evaluation, and treatment of high blood pressure*, NIH Pub No 94-4080, Bethesda, Md, 1997, Public Health Service.

**BOX 17-8**

### Examples of Community Health Nursing Interventions to Prevent Cardiovascular Disease in Adults

*Educate Clients About:*
- Cardiovascular risk factors
- Stroke risk factors
- Signs of heart attack and stroke
- Benefits of regular exercise
- Role of nutrition in cardiovascular disease
- Role of stress and cardiovascular disease

*Casefind By:*
- Hypertension screening
- Cholesterol screening
- Stress assessment
- Nutrition and weight assessment
- Assessing familial histories for cardiovascular diseases
- Assessing worksite populations to identify workers at risk

*Collaborate with Community Health Providers and Clients to Develop:*
- Smoking cessation groups
- Worksite exercise, smoking cessation, blood pressure, and stress management programs
- Referral resources for adults at risk
- Aggregate exercise and weight reduction programs

Smokers have a higher risk of heart attack than nonsmokers. According to the NIH, the risk of women smokers having a heart attack is two to six times that of women who are nonsmokers (NIH, 1998). It is important to promote nonsmoking and a smoke-free society. Regardless of how

### BOX 17-9

*Warning Signs of Possible Impending Heart Attack*

- Dizziness
- Heaviness, crushing, constricting, or squeezing sensation in the chest
- Indigestion
- Nausea
- Pain or numbness in jaw, neck, radiating to left arm
- Shortness of breath
- Strangling sensation
- Sweating
- Tingling sensation

### BOX 17-10

*Warning Signs of Possible Impending Stroke*

- Aphasia
- Ataxia
- Blurred vision
- Double vision
- Headache
- Loss of vision in one eye
- Numbness in one side of body
- Numbness that is transient
- Slurred speech
- Weakness in one side of body
- Weakness or numbness in one area of body (e.g., face, hand, leg)

### TABLE 17-3

*Classification of Blood Pressure for Adults Age 18 Years and Older\**

| CATEGORY | SYSTOLIC (MM HG) | DIASTOLIC (MM HG) |
|---|---|---|
| Normal† | <130 | <85 |
| High normal | 130-139 | 85-89 |
| Hypertension‡ | | |
| Stage 1 (mild) | 140-159 | 90-99 |
| Stage 2 (moderate) | 160-179 | 100-109 |
| Stage 3 (severe) | 180-209 | 110-119 |
| Stage 4 (very severe) | ≥210 | ≥120 |

From US Department of Health and Human Services (USDHHS): *The fifth report of the joint national committee on detection, evaluation, and treatment of high blood pressure,* NIH Pub No 95-1088, Bethesda, Md, 1995b, Public Health Service, p. 4.

\*Not taking antihypertensive drugs and not acutely ill. When systolic and diastolic fall into different categories, the higher category should be selected to classify the individual's blood pressure status. For instance, 160/92 mm Hg should be classified as stage 2, and 180/120 mm Hg should be classified as stage 4. Isolated systolic hypertension (ISH) is defined as SBP ≥140 mm Hg and DBP <90 mm Hg and staged appropriately (e.g., 170/85 mm Hg is defined as stage 2 ISH).

†Optimal blood pressure with respect to cardiovascular risk is SBP <120 mm Hg and DBP <80 mm Hg. However, unusually low readings should be evaluated for clinical significance.

‡Based on the average of two or more readings taken at each of two or more visits following an initial screening.

Note: In addition to classifying stages of hypertension based on average blood pressure levels, the clinician should specify presence or absence of target-organ disease and additional risk factors. For example, a client with diabetes and a blood pressure of 142/94 mm Hg plus left ventricular hypertrophy should be classified as "stage 1 hypertension with target-organ disease (left ventricular hypertrophy) and with another major risk factor (diabetes)." This specificity is important for risk classification and management.

long persons have smoked, "smoking cessation reduces the relative risk of coronary heart disease in men and women by 50%" (Judelson, 1999, p. 44).

Coronary heart disease and heart attacks are much more frequent in those who are inactive than in people who are active. Elevated serum cholesterol levels put one at risk for developing cardiovascular disease. Regular exercise can have a significant impact on reducing the risk of heart attacks and disease. Community health nurses can be instrumental in reducing the morbidity and mortality from heart attacks through interventions that focus on primary and secondary prevention. Community health nurses can educate people about the risk factors and warning signals of heart attacks, develop risk modification programs, teach families CPR, and familiarize community residents about emergency community resources. Educating adults and families regarding the importance of immediate action when a heart attack is suspected is critical to reduce the risk of mortality. For successful risk modification (e.g., activity, nutrition counseling, and

hypertension control), interventions must include awareness of personal barriers to risk modification and strategies for motivating people to change lifestyle behaviors (Biggs, Fleury, 1996). Interventions that focus on prevention and early intervention are crucial to reducing the morbidity and mortality from heart attacks.

STROKES. As previously noted in Figure 17-1, strokes rank third among all causes of death in the United States. Annually, about 600,000 Americans suffer a stroke (American Heart Association [AHA], 1997, p. 13). Strokes are a major cause of serious long-term disability that require some type of assistance to manage daily activities. Many stroke victims are disabled by paralysis and suffer resultant speech/language and memory deficits. Early signs and warnings frequently are ignored, and as a result the stroke takes a higher toll. Like heart attacks, many strokes and complications from strokes can be prevented by heeding early warning signs and seeking early treatment. Box 17-10 lists some possible warning signs of an impending stroke. Community

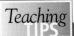

**BOX 17-11**
*Heart-Healthy Cooking*

| RECIPE INGREDIENT | SUBSTITUTION |
|---|---|
| Whole milk, light cream | Skim or 1% milk |
| Evaporated milk | Evaporated skim milk |
| 1 whole egg | 1/4 cup egg substitute or 2 egg whites |
| 1 cup butter | 1 cup margarine or 2/3 cup vegetable oil |
| Shortening | Margarine |
| Mayonnaise or salad dressing | Nonfat or light varieties |
| Cheese | Low-fat or fat-free cheese |
| Sour cream | Nonfat or low-fat sour cream or yogurt |
| 1 square unsweetened baking chocolate | 3 tbsp cocoa powder and 1 tbsp oil or margarine |
| Fat for "greasing" the pan | Nonstick cooking spray |

The way you cook is just as important as what you cook. Discuss your current cooking habits with your nurse or dietitian. Set goals for the future.

*When I Cook I Will:*

1. Trim the fat from meat before cooking it.
2. Remove the skin and fat before cooking chicken or turkey.
3. Bake, roast, grill, broil, or boil foods instead of frying.
4. Place meat on a rack to roast so the fat drips off.
5. Brown ground meat and drain off the fat before adding it to a recipe.
6. Use a nonstick pan and a small amount of cooking spray, oil, or margarine if frying.
7. Use fat-free ingredients such as wine, tomato juice, lemon juice, or bouillon to baste meats and poultry.
8. Use defatted beef or chicken broth to make gravy.
9. Cool sauces or soups in the refrigerator and skim off the fat.
10. Substitute low-fat ingredients for high-fat ingredients in recipes.
11. Add pasta, rice, dry peas, or beans to main dishes and decrease the meat.
12. Use small amounts of lean meats, herbs, or flavored seasoning (e.g., Butter Buds) to flavor vegetables, rather than fatback, saltpork, or butter.
13. Make large batches of foods and freeze meal-sized portions if you live alone. Supplement with fruit, vegetables, and breads.

From Martin KS, Larson BJ, Gorski LA, et al., editors: *Mosby's home health client teaching guides: R$_x$ for teaching,* St Louis, 1997, Mosby, p. V-A-1-9.

health nurses have an important role in health promotion by educating people about the signs of a stroke and encouraging prevention and early intervention.

Through all levels of prevention community health nurses can do much to decrease morbidity and mortality through health education activities about risk factor reduction, behavior modification, and rehabilitation services. The long-term rehabilitation needs of persons with stroke can cause great emotional and psychological distress for both client and family. When strokes occur, the community health nurse can be instrumental in helping the family work through the adaptation and rehabilitation process and assist in community resource referral, coordination, and utilization.

HYPERTENSION. Hypertension is a risk factor for heart attack and stroke. More than 50 million Americans age 6 and older have hypertension (AHA, 1997, p. 15). In 1993 high blood pressure killed almost 40,000 Americans and contributed to the deaths of thousands more (AHA, 1997). These statistics are not surprising because a large number of Americans who have high blood pressure do not know they have it; nearly three-fourths of all clients who are hypertensive are not controlling their blood pressure; a large number are on inadequate therapy; and most persons with hypertension have other risk factors for heart disease (NIH, 1997, p. 8). Table 17-3 shows the normal and abnormal blood pressure categories for adults age 18 and older.

High blood pressure is easy to detect and, through appropriate management, easy to control. Controlling high blood pressure has been shown to be one of the most effective means available for reducing mortality in the adult population. Community health nurses have a major role in prevention and control through teaching, early detection and screening activities, risk modification programs, referral for medical treatment, and facilitating clients in complying with treatment regimens. Box 17-11 provides some teaching tips for promoting cardiovascular fitness through heart-healthy cooking. Table 17-4 provides some general guidelines for hypertension screening and referral.

**TABLE 17-4**

*Recommendations for Follow-up Based on Initial Set of Blood Pressure Measurements for Adults Age 18 and Older*

| INITIAL SCREENING BLOOD PRESSURE (MM HG)* | | |
|---|---|---|
| SYSTOLIC | DIASTOLIC | FOLLOW-UP RECOMMENDED† |
| <130 | <85 | Recheck in 2 years |
| 130-139 | 85-89 | Recheck in 1 year‡ |
| 140-159 | 90-99 | Confirm within 2 months |
| 160-179 | 100-109 | Evaluate or refer to source of care within 1 month |
| 180-209 | 110-119 | Evaluate or refer to source of care within 1 week |
| ≥210 | ≥120 | Evaluate or refer to source of care immediately |

From US Department of Health and Human Services (USDHHS): *The fifth report of the joint national committee on detection, evaluation, and treatment of high blood pressure,* NIH Pub No 95-1088, Bethesda, Md, 1995b, Public Health Service, p. 6.
*If the systolic and diastolic are different, follow recommendation for the shorter time follow-up (e.g., 160/85 mm Hg should be evaluated or referred to source of care within 1 month).
†The scheduling of follow-up should be modified by reliable information about past blood pressure measurements, other cardiovascular risk factors, or target-organ disease.
‡Consider providing advice about lifestyle modifications.

**AMERICAN HEART ASSOCIATION.** The AHA is the leading voluntary, national agency actively involved in cardiovascular education, treatment, and research. The association was founded in 1924, and its mission is to reduce disability and death from cardiovascular diseases and stroke. It is actively engaged in research and has more than 2250 local affiliates in all 50 states. The AHA offers classes, publications, and numerous services to the general public. Nurses can use the association as a resource for developing health promotion activities.

## Cancer

Cancer is the leading cause of death in men and women ages 25 through 64 and is associated with a variety of risk factors. The financial costs of cancer are enormous. The National Cancer Institute estimates the yearly costs related to cancer at $107 billion (ACS, 2000, p. 3). However, dollars cannot begin to measure the toll cancer takes on human suffering and mortality. Although cancer mortality rates have not changed significantly over time, there have been changes in mortality for some age groups and for some types of cancers. Mortality could be significantly reduced by reducing risk factors. By eliminating one single risk factor, such as smoking, the cancer incidence and mortality rates could be significantly reduced. Other risk factors can also make a difference in the incidence of cancer. Community

health nurses have a key role in developing interventions to reduce these risk factors.

Cancer disproportionately strikes minority groups with "Black Americans having the highest prostate cancer incidence rates in the world" (ACS, 2000, p. 14). Varying lifestyles, including nutritional patterns among ethnic groups, screening behaviors, values and belief systems, socioeconomic status, lack of insurance, and lack of access to health services are all associated with cancer risks and may provide some explanation for the differences in health care utilization and cancer mortality among various ethnic populations (ACS, 2000, p. 16).

Gender differences also become evident when examining mortality and survival rates for many cancers. Figure 17-2 shows the 2000 estimates of new cancer cases and deaths by site and sex. It is encouraging to note that the survival rates for many cancers, with the exception of lung cancer, are increasing. Much of this is due to early detection and intervention. Although skin cancer has the highest incidence, it is amenable to prevention and treatment and does not carry a high mortality rate. Lung cancer and colon/rectum cancer carry relatively high mortality rates. Lung cancer now rivals breast cancer as the leading cause of cancer death in American women (ACS, 2000). Unfortunately, diagnostic procedures such as chest radiographs and sputum examinations usually do not reveal lung cancer until it has already spread. Cigarette smoking continues to be the most important risk factor in the development of lung cancer (ACS, 2000, p. 12). Fortunately several effective screening procedures are now available to detect breast cancer and cancers of the colon or rectum. For example, women can do regular self-examination of the breasts (Figure 17-3) and can have a physical examination and mammography. Men, age fifty and older, should have a yearly prostate-specific antigen (PSA) blood test to augment early detection of prostate cancer. Those who are at high risk for prostate cancer (e.g., African-American men or men who have a family history of prostate cancer) should have a PSA test earlier than age 50 (ACS, 2000, p. 14). Table 17-5 provides a summary of American Cancer Society (ACS) recommendations for the early detection of several types of cancer in asymptomatic people. This can be used as guide in developing health promotion strategies for cancer prevention and detection.

Community health nurses have an important educative role in teaching people about risk factors, providing nursing care, and assisting families in utilizing community resources. Using the principles of crisis intervention and grieving, as discussed in Chapter 8, the nurse can facilitate family coping and adjustment. If the need for hospice care arises, the nurse can make appropriate referrals to available resources (hospice care is discussed in Chapter 22). Many nurses are providing hospice care and are developing new hospice programs around the country. Hospice services are also provided by many home health care agencies, which provide a range of home care services.

**Cancer Cases\* by Site and Sex**

| Male | Female |
|---|---|
| Prostate 198,100 (31%) | Breast 192,200 (31%) |
| Lung and bronchus 90,700 (14%) | Lung and bronchus 78,800 (13%) |
| Colon and rectum 67,300 (10%) | Colon and rectum 68,100 (11%) |
| Urinary bladder 39,200 (6%) | Uterine corpus 38,300 (6%) |
| Non-Hodgkin's lymphoma 31,100 (5%) | Non-Hodgkins's lymphoma 25,100 (4%) |
| Melanoma of the skin 29,000 (5%) | Ovary 23,400 (4%) |
| Oral cavity 20,200 (3%) | Melanoma of the skin 22,400 (4%) |
| Kidney 18,700 (3%) | Urinary bladder 15,100 (2%) |
| Leukemia 17,700 (3%) | Pancreas 15,000 (2%) |
| Pancreas 14,200 (2%) | Thyroid 14,900 (2%) |
| All Sites 643,000 (100%) | All Sites 625,000 (100%) |

**Cancer Deaths by Site and Sex**

| Male | Female |
|---|---|
| Lung and bronchus 90,100 (31%) | Lung and bronchus 67,300 (25%) |
| Prostate 31,500 (11%) | Breast 40,200 (15%) |
| Colon and rectum 27,700 (10%) | Colon and rectum 29,000 (11%) |
| Pancreas 14,100 (5%) | Pancreas 14,800 (6%) |
| Non-Hodgkin's lymphoma 13,800 (5%) | Ovary 13,900 (5%) |
| Leukemia 12,000 (4%) | Non-Hodgkin's lymphoma 12,500 (5%) |
| Esophagus 9,500 (3%) | Leukemia 9,500 (4%) |
| Liver 8,900 (3%) | Uterine corpus 6,600 (2%) |
| Urinary bladder 8,300 (3%) | Brain 5,900 (2%) |
| Kidney 7,500 (3%) | Stomach 5,400 (2%) |
| All Sites 286,100 (100%) | All Sites 267,300 (100%) |

\*Excludes basal and squamous cell skin cancers and in situ carcinomas except urinary bladder.      ©2001, American Cancer Society, Inc., Surveillance Research

**FIGURE 17-2** Leading sites of new cancer cases and deaths—2000 estimates. (From American Cancer Society: *Cancer facts and figures—2001*, Atlanta, 2001, ACS, p. 11. Reprinted by permission of American Cancer Society.)

**NATIONAL CANCER INSTITUTE.** The National Cancer Institute is the federal government's chief source of cancer information, education, and research. The Institute has numerous publications, including pamphlets on different types of cancer and supportive care for cancer victims such as "Taking Time: Support for People with Cancer and the People Who Care about Them." "Taking Time" is an excellent resource for nurses to share with families. It covers topics including sharing the diagnosis, sharing feelings, coping within the family, assistance in obtaining equipment and/or supplies, self-image, the world outside, living each day, and resources.

By dialing 1-800-4-CANCER (1-800-638-6070 in Alaska) one can access the Cancer Information Service of the National Cancer Institute. This service provides information on community agencies and services, answers questions, and provides publications and a publication list for different types of cancer. It also provides information about active treatment centers for specific types of cancer, descriptions of clinical trials that are open for client entry, and the names of organizations and physicians involved in cancer care.

**AMERICAN CANCER SOCIETY.** The ACS is at the forefront of private sector cancer education and research in the United States. It is the largest private source of cancer research funds in the United States (ACS, 2000). The in-

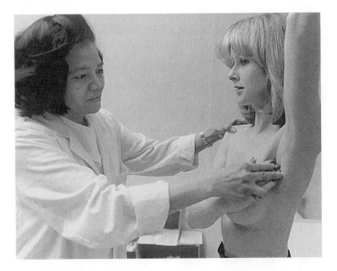

**FIGURE 17-3** Breast self-examination being taught by a health care worker. (Courtesy American Cancer Society.)

creased survival rates for many types of cancer may be a result of the support and funding of cancer research by the ACS. In 1995 ACS established the *Behavioral Health Center* that supports original behavioral and psychosocial cancer research (ACS, 2000, p. 38).

**TABLE 17-5**

*Recommendations for the Early Detection of Cancer in Asymptomatic People*

| SITE | RECOMMENDATION |
|---|---|
| Cancer-related checkup | A cancer-related checkup is recommended every 3 years for people aged 20-40 and every year for people age 40 and older. This examination should include healthy counseling, and depending on a person's age, might include examinations for cancers of thyroid, oral cavity, skin, lymph nodes, testes, and ovaries, as well as for some nonmalignant diseases. |
| Breast | Women 40 and older should have an annual mammogram, an annual clinical breast examination (CBE) by a health care professional, and should perform monthly breast self-examination. The CBE should be conducted close to the scheduled mammogram.<br>Women ages 20-39 should have a clinical breast examination by a health care professional every 3 years and should perform monthly breast self-examination. |
| Colon & Rectum | Beginning at age 50, men and women should follow *one* of the examination schedules below:<br>• A fecal occult blood test every year and a flexible sigmoidoscopy every 5 years.*<br>• A colonoscopy every 10 years.*<br>• A double-contrast barium enema every 5 to 10 years.* |
| Prostate | The ACS recommends that both the prostate-specific antigen (PSA) blood test and the digital rectal examination be offered annually, beginning at age 50, to men who have a life expectancy of at least 10 years and to younger men who are at high risk.<br>Men in high risk groups, such as those with strong familial predisposition (i.e., two or more affected first-degree relatives), or African Americans may begin at younger age (i.e., 45 years). |
| Uterus | **Cervix:** All women who are or have been sexually active or who are 18 and older should have an annual Pap test and pelvic examination. After three or more consecutive satisfactory examinations with normal findings, the Pap test may be performed less frequently. Discuss the matter with your physician.<br>**Endometrium:** Women at high risk for cancer of the uterus should have a sample endometrial tissue examined when menopause begins. |

From American Cancer Society (ACS): *Cancer facts and figures-2000,* Atlanta, 2000, ACS, p. 34. Reprinted by permission of the American Cancer Society.
*A digital rectal examination should be done at the same time as sigmoidoscopy, colonoscopy, or double-contrast barium enema. People who are at moderate or high risk for colorectal cancer should talk with a doctor about different testing schedule.

The ACS's public education programs and publications reach millions of Americans each year. The society is involved in professional education, publishes *Cancer Nursing News* (sent to about 90,000 nurses around the country), supports professorships in clinical oncology, and offers clinical oncology awards. The ACS's service and rehabilitation activities include the following resource and information services: *CanSurmount*—a short-term home visitor program for clients and their families; *Reach to Recovery*—a client visitor program that addresses the needs of women who have had breast cancer; *Man to Man*—a group program that provides information about prostate cancer and related issues; *Look Good . . . Feel Better*—a program designed to teach women cancer clients beauty techniques to help restore their appearance and self-image during chemotherapy and radiation treatments; laryngectomy rehabilitation volunteers in coordination with the International Association of Laryngectomies (IAL); ostomy rehabilitation volunteers in coordination with the United Ostomy Association; and children's camps.

## Accidents

Accidents are the leading cause of death among all persons ages 1 to 33 and are the fifth leading cause of death among people of all ages (National Safety Council, 1999, p. 10). Accidents and the term *unintentional injury* often are used interchangeably. When death occurs under "accidental" circumstances, the preferred term within the public health community is *unintentional injury* (CDC, 1996a, p. 162). Unintentional injury does not include suicides and homicides, which are separate categories that require different intervention strategies and are discussed in Chapter 13. The economic costs of fatal and nonfatal unintentional injuries are immense. In 1998 the estimated costs for unintentional injuries, including wages lost, medical, vehicle damage, fire losses, administrative, and employer costs, were more than $475 billion (National Safety Council, 1999, p. 7). However, what cannot be measured in dollars is the physical pain and suffering that results from unintentional injuries.

Table 17-6 details the leading causes of mortality among adults, including the kinds of unintentional

**TABLE 17-6**

## Leading Causes of Death and Death Rates by Age Group and Gender, 1996

| CAUSE OF DEATH BY AGE GROUP | NUMBER OF DEATHS | | | DEATH RATES* | | |
|---|---|---|---|---|---|---|
| | TOTAL | MALE | FEMALE | TOTAL | MALE | FEMALE |
| **Ages 15-24** | | | | | | |
| All Causes | 32,443 | 24,313 | 8,130 | 89.6 | 130.6 | 46.2 |
| Unintentional injuries | 13,809 | 10,273 | 3,536 | 38.1 | 55.2 | 20.1 |
| Motor-vehicle | 10,576 | 7,573 | 3,003 | 29.2 | 40.7 | 17.1 |
| Drowning | 715 | 633 | 82 | 2.0 | 3.4 | 0.5 |
| Poison (solid, liquid) | 558 | 446 | 112 | 1.5 | 2.4 | 0.6 |
| Firearms | 401 | 370 | 31 | 1.1 | 2.0 | 0.2 |
| Falls | 235 | 201 | 34 | 0.6 | 1.1 | 0.2 |
| All other unintentional injuries | 1,324 | 1,050 | 274 | 3.7 | 5.6 | 1.6 |
| Homicide and legal intervention | 6,548 | 5,655 | 893 | 18.1 | 30.4 | 5.1 |
| Suicide | 4,358 | 3,724 | 634 | 12.0 | 20.0 | 3.6 |
| Cancer | 1,632 | 955 | 677 | 4.5 | 5.1 | 3.8 |
| Heart disease | 969 | 616 | 353 | 2.7 | 3.3 | 2.0 |
| HIV | 413 | 243 | 170 | 1.1 | 1.3 | 1.0 |
| Congenital anomalies | 382 | 231 | 151 | 1.1 | 1.2 | 0.9 |
| COPD | 237 | 131 | 106 | 0.7 | 0.7 | 0.6 |
| Pneumonia and influenza | 203 | 106 | 97 | 0.6 | 0.6 | 0.6 |
| Stroke | 167 | 96 | 71 | 0.5 | 0.5 | 0.4 |
| **Ages 25-34** | | | | | | |
| All causes | 51,147 | 36,070 | 15,077 | 126.7 | 178.6 | 74.7 |
| Unintentional injuries | 12,825 | 9,658 | 3,167 | 31.8 | 47.8 | 15.7 |
| Motor-vehicle | 7,729 | 5,562 | 2,167 | 19.1 | 27.5 | 10.7 |
| Poison (solid, liquid) | 2,004 | 1,532 | 472 | 5.0 | 7.6 | 2.3 |
| Drowning | 593 | 528 | 65 | 1.5 | 2.6 | 0.3 |
| Falls | 394 | 328 | 66 | 1.0 | 1.6 | 0.3 |
| Fires, burns | 300 | 202 | 98 | 0.7 | 1.0 | 0.5 |
| All other unintentional injuries | 1,805 | 1,506 | 299 | 4.5 | 7.5 | 1.5 |
| HIV | 8,048 | 6,333 | 1,715 | 19.9 | 31.4 | 8.5 |
| Suicide | 5,861 | 4,848 | 1,013 | 14.5 | 24.0 | 5.0 |
| Homicide and legal intervention | 5,428 | 4,322 | 1,106 | 13.4 | 21.4 | 5.5 |
| Cancer | 4,845 | 2,312 | 2,533 | 12.0 | 11.5 | 12.6 |
| Heart disease | 3,350 | 2,221 | 1,129 | 8.3 | 11.0 | 5.6 |
| Stroke | 720 | 351 | 369 | 1.8 | 1.7 | 1.8 |
| Diabetes mellitus | 647 | 367 | 280 | 1.6 | 1.8 | 1.4 |
| Chronic liver disease, cirrhosis | 570 | 360 | 210 | 1.4 | 1.8 | 1.0 |
| Pneumonia and influenza | 568 | 317 | 251 | 1.4 | 1.6 | 1.2 |
| **Ages 35-44** | | | | | | |
| All causes | 96,033 | 64,304 | 31,729 | 221.3 | 298.1 | 145.4 |
| Cancer | 17,049 | 7,684 | 9,365 | 39.3 | 35.6 | 42.9 |
| Unintentional injuries | 14,267 | 10,615 | 3,652 | 32.9 | 49.2 | 16.7 |
| Motor-vehicle | 6,753 | 4,700 | 2,053 | 15.6 | 21.8 | 9.4 |
| Poison (solid, liquid) | 3,520 | 2,692 | 828 | 8.1 | 12.5 | 3.8 |
| Falls | 630 | 521 | 109 | 1.5 | 2.4 | 0.5 |
| Drowning | 586 | 495 | 91 | 1.4 | 2.3 | 0.4 |
| Fires, burns | 453 | 311 | 142 | 1.0 | 1.4 | 0.7 |
| All other unintentional injuries | 2,325 | 1,896 | 429 | 5.4 | 8.8 | 2.0 |
| HIV | 13,637 | 11,172 | 2,465 | 31.4 | 51.8 | 11.3 |
| Heart disease | 13,217 | 9,544 | 3,673 | 30.5 | 44.2 | 16.8 |

Modified from National Safety Council: *Injury facts, 1999,* Itasca, Ill, 1999, The Council, pp. 11-12.

*Deaths per 100,000 population in each group.

*Continued*

**TABLE 17-6**

*Leading Causes of Death and Death Rates by Age Group and Gender, 1996—cont'd*

| CAUSE OF DEATH BY AGE GROUP | NUMBER OF DEATHS | | | DEATH RATES* | | |
|---|---|---|---|---|---|---|
| | TOTAL | MALE | FEMALE | TOTAL | MALE | FEMALE |
| **Ages 35-44—continued** | | | | | | |
| Suicide | 6,741 | 5,300 | 1,441 | 15.5 | 24.6 | 6.6 |
| Homicide and legal intervention | 3,894 | 2,913 | 981 | 9.0 | 13.5 | 4.5 |
| Chronic liver disease, cirrhosis | 3,640 | 2,636 | 1,004 | 8.4 | 12.2 | 4.6 |
| Stroke | 2,722 | 1,445 | 1,277 | 6.3 | 6.7 | 5.9 |
| Diabetes mellitus | 1,879 | 1,139 | 740 | 4.3 | 5.3 | 3.4 |
| Pneumonia and influenza | 1,461 | 916 | 545 | 3.4 | 4.2 | 2.5 |
| **Ages 45-54** | | | | | | |
| All causes | 144,329 | 90,871 | 53,458 | 445.9 | 573.8 | 323.3 |
| Cancer | 44,627 | 22,278 | 22,349 | 137.9 | 140.7 | 135.2 |
| Heart disease | 35,034 | 25,626 | 9,408 | 108.2 | 161.8 | 56.9 |
| Unintentional injuries | 9,846 | 7,150 | 2,696 | 30.4 | 45.2 | 16.3 |
| Motor-vehicle | 4,553 | 3,104 | 1,449 | 14.1 | 19.6 | 8.8 |
| Poison (solid, liquid) | 1,714 | 1,287 | 427 | 5.3 | 8.1 | 2.6 |
| Falls | 752 | 586 | 166 | 2.3 | 3.7 | 1.0 |
| Drowning | 380 | 327 | 53 | 1.2 | 2.1 | 0.3 |
| Fires, burns | 366 | 255 | 111 | 1.1 | 1.6 | 0.7 |
| All other unintentional injuries | 2,081 | 1,591 | 490 | 6.4 | 10.0 | 3.0 |
| HIV | 6,259 | 5,321 | 938 | 19.3 | 33.6 | 5.7 |
| Stroke | 5,792 | 3,162 | 2,630 | 17.9 | 20.0 | 15.9 |
| Chronic liver disease, cirrhosis | 5,431 | 4,018 | 1,413 | 16.8 | 25.4 | 8.5 |
| Suicide | 4,837 | 3,684 | 1,153 | 14.9 | 23.3 | 7.0 |
| Diabetes mellitus | 4,258 | 2,435 | 1,823 | 13.2 | 15.4 | 11.0 |
| COPD | 2,801 | 1,413 | 1,388 | 8.7 | 8.9 | 8.4 |
| Pneumonia and influenza | 2,093 | 1,302 | 791 | 6.5 | 8.2 | 4.8 |
| **Ages 55-64** | | | | | | |
| All causes | 233,725 | 141,170 | 92,555 | 1,094.2 | 1,388.6 | 826.8 |
| Cancer | 86,828 | 47,687 | 39,141 | 406.5 | 469.1 | 349.6 |
| Heart disease | 67,335 | 46,138 | 21,197 | 315.2 | 453.8 | 189.3 |
| COPD | 10,046 | 5,302 | 4,744 | 47.0 | 52.2 | 42.4 |
| Stroke | 9,676 | 5,333 | 4,343 | 45.3 | 52.5 | 38.8 |
| Diabetes mellitus | 8,429 | 4,367 | 4,062 | 39.5 | 43.0 | 36.3 |
| Unintentional injuries | 6,871 | 4,676 | 2,195 | 32.2 | 46.0 | 19.6 |
| Motor-vehicle | 3,196 | 2,041 | 1,155 | 15.0 | 20.1 | 10.3 |
| Falls | 860 | 640 | 220 | 4.0 | 6.3 | 2.0 |
| Poison (solid, liquid) | 414 | 257 | 157 | 1.9 | 2.5 | 1.4 |
| Fires, burns | 356 | 244 | 112 | 1.7 | 2.4 | 1.0 |
| Surgical, medical complications | 320 | 161 | 159 | 1.5 | 1.6 | 1.4 |
| All other unintentional injuries | 1,725 | 1,333 | 392 | 8.1 | 13.1 | 3.5 |
| Chronic liver disease, cirrhosis | 5,312 | 3,690 | 1,622 | 24.9 | 36.3 | 14.5 |
| Pneumonia and influenza | 3,613 | 2,164 | 1,449 | 16.9 | 21.3 | 12.9 |
| Suicide | 2,925 | 2,306 | 619 | 13.7 | 22.7 | 5.5 |
| HIV | 1,794 | 1,514 | 280 | 8.4 | 14.9 | 2.5 |
| **Ages 65-74** | | | | | | |
| All causes | 473,894 | 269,173 | 204,721 | 2,538.3 | 3,233.3 | 1,979.1 |
| Cancer | 160,864 | 89,979 | 70,885 | 861.6 | 1,080.8 | 685.3 |
| Heart disease | 144,915 | 88,660 | 56,255 | 776.2 | 1,065.0 | 543.8 |
| COPD | 30,171 | 16,034 | 14,137 | 161.6 | 192.6 | 136.7 |
| Stroke | 25,306 | 12,882 | 12,424 | 135.5 | 154.7 | 120.1 |
| Diabetes mellitus | 16,553 | 7,892 | 8,661 | 88.7 | 94.8 | 83.7 |

**TABLE 17-6**

*Leading Causes of Death and Death Rates by Age Group and Gender, 1996—cont'd*

| CAUSE OF DEATH BY AGE GROUP | NUMBER OF DEATHS | | | DEATH RATES* | | |
|---|---|---|---|---|---|---|
| | TOTAL | MALE | FEMALE | TOTAL | MALE | FEMALE |
| **Ages 65-74—continued** | | | | | | |
| Pneumonia and influenza | 10,597 | 6,165 | 4,432 | 56.8 | 74.1 | 42.8 |
| Unintentional injuries | 8,780 | 5,320 | 3,460 | 47.0 | 63.9 | 33.4 |
| Motor-vehicle | 3,419 | 1,986 | 1,433 | 18.3 | 23.9 | 13.9 |
| Falls | 1,780 | 1,097 | 683 | 9.5 | 13.2 | 6.6 |
| Surgical, medical complications | 662 | 339 | 323 | 3.5 | 4.1 | 3.1 |
| Ingestion of food, object | 537 | 304 | 233 | 2.9 | 3.7 | 2.3 |
| Fires, burns | 451 | 253 | 198 | 2.4 | 3.0 | 1.9 |
| All other unintentional injuries | 1,931 | 1,341 | 590 | 10.3 | 16.1 | 5.7 |
| Chronic liver disease, cirrhosis | 5,725 | 3,443 | 2,282 | 30.7 | 41.4 | 22.1 |
| Nephritis and nephrosis | 4,633 | 2,451 | 2,182 | 24.8 | 29.4 | 21.1 |
| Septicemia | 4,058 | 2,062 | 1,996 | 21.7 | 24.8 | 19.3 |

injuries that kill people ages 15 to 74. Note that unintentional injuries are the leading causes of death until age 35, when cancer, begins to rank above accidents as leading causes of death. As persons age, diseases become more prevalent and rank higher than accidental deaths as leading causes of death. Age is a significant risk factor for developing many cardiovascular diseases, cancer, and other chronic conditions. For example, note that as people age, the death rate from falls increases; death rate from surgical and medical intervention increases; and deaths from ingestion of food/objects becomes more problematic (particularly in the 65 to 74 age groups). These have implications for designing developmentally appropriate health promotion interventions.

Gender differences also are noted when reviewing the leading causes of death for adults. For example, accidental deaths are much higher for men than for women of all age groups (see Table 17-6). This may be attributed to numerous factors such as lifestyle patterns and occupations. Men increase their risk for unintentional injury because they are more likely than women to engage in risky behaviors and work in dangerous occupations.

Community health nurses have a major educative role in primary prevention of unintentional injuries. Health promotion interventions that are developmentally specific and tailored to each community are the most effective. Like many other health problems, the most effective intervention for accidents is *prevention*. Community health nurses have the opportunity to intervene with all age groups in various settings. Schools, youth centers, fitness and sports centers, YMCA, YWCA, churches, community centers, adult health centers, adult nutrition centers, retirement centers, assisted living, and various work settings are examples of settings where health education interventions can be implemented. Part of the *Healthy People 2010*

**BOX 17-12**

*Health Promotion Topics to Prevent Unintentional Injuries*

- Child passenger safety
- Choking prevention and emergency treatment
- CPR training
- Fire safety
- Firearm safety
- Helmet use
- Local emergency medical services availability and activation
- Motor vehicle safety
- Occupational type safety (e.g., industrial and agricultural equipment, etc.)
- Pedestrian, bicycle, and motorcycle safety
- Poison prevention, control, and emergency treatment
- Prevention of falls
- Responsible and safe driving of motorized vehicles
- Safety in the home
- Seat belt use
- Snowmobile safety
- Sports safety (e.g., hiking, climbing, skiing, boating, swimming, hunting, fishing, etc.)
- Stress reduction
- Suicide prevention
- Walking/jogging safety
- Water safety
- Weather safety

agenda focuses on promoting health and safety through prevention and early intervention (Sarkis, 2000). Box 17-12 provides a list of possible health promotion topics geared toward decreasing the unintentional injury rate in this country.

## AGGREGATES AT RISK IN THE ADULT MALE AND FEMALE POPULATION

As with any age group, there are persons at special risk in the adult population who require concentrated community health nursing intervention. Throughout this text the special health needs of minorities are addressed, and minority health is discussed extensively in Chapter 13. Several groups of adults who are at risk for increased mortality and morbidity, including the homeless and those living in poverty, those who abuse drugs, those at risk for STDs, and those exposed to domestic violence, are discussed in Chapter 13. Other selected aggregates discussed here include those who suffer from depression, adults changing jobs or careers, those experiencing unemployment, adults with chronic illness, adults in marital crisis, adult gays and lesbians, and adult men and women who are incarcerated.

### Adult Men and Women Who Suffer from Depression

Depression is one of the most common diseases in the United States. It is easily treatable and the treatment of depression can be very successful and cost-effective (Ashley, Rockwell, Gladsjo, et al., 2000). Depression is often undiagnosed in older adults and the elderly. It is one of the most frequent problems seen in the elderly, and the incidence of depression increases with age (Eliopoulos, 2001). Major depression is the most common severe mental disorder in women. The onset of depression in women is most common between ages 25 and 44 and there is some evidence, such as the increased incidence of suicide attempts in young adults, that depression may be occurring at an earlier age (Horton, 1995, p. 83). Major depression and anxiety disorders have been found more frequently in children of depressed parents than in children with nondepressed parents (Faraone, Biederman, 1998).

Freud viewed depression as aggression turned inward. Depression has been described as chronic frustration stemming from environmental stresses in family, social, or work environments beyond the coping ability and resources of the client or from physiological disorders. Depression can result when stress is intensified. All persons experience times when they feel low or discouraged, but these depressed feelings are usually acute and self-limiting. Depression becomes a serious problem when it is chronic and affects the ability to cope with the events, roles, and responsibilities of daily living. Depression is often precipitated by a loss of some kind: death; separation; or loss of job, status, or health.

Some symptoms of depression include general sadness and despair, difficulty in making decisions, difficulty in carrying on a conversation, trouble concentrating, trouble sleeping, tiredness, listlessness, loss of appetite, eating binges, social regression, loss of or decreased libido, and decreased self-esteem. Persons who are depressed may be overly sensitive to what other people say or do, may be angry with others and not trust them, and may withdraw from others because of a fear of being among people.

Persons who are depressed are often not aware that they are suffering from this condition. They know that they do not feel well and often only seek medical help for minor physical problems. That is why it is so important for the community health nurse to systematically collect a complete health history (see Chapter 9) when working with adult clients. If data are collected only on the client's physical health complaints, depression can be overlooked.

Maintaining two-way communication between the client and nurse is essential. People who are depressed generally appreciate feedback on what is going on, to know that someone has listened to them, and that someone is available for support and assistance. Often the depressed client is excluded from social contacts; family, friends, and even professionals may isolate depressed clients in an attempt to protect the client from further hurt or stress. This social isolation serves to reinforce the client's feelings that no one cares.

Depressed individuals who are identified as potentially suicidal should be referred for therapeutic counseling. Some nurses are afraid to assess for suicide potential because they fear their questioning may precipitate a suicide attempt. However, suicide is not prevented by avoiding conversation about it. It is prevented by early detection and intervention to help clients get the assistance they need to deal with stresses in their daily lives.

Encountering clients who are depressed is common in community health nursing practice. At times the client is able to resolve the depressed state by using the supportive assistance of the community health nurse and significant others, such as family, friends, relatives, and lovers. At other times additional mental health counseling is necessary. However, depression will continue to exist until the individual is able to successfully mobilize coping mechanisms that enhance growth. Many chronic depressions are related to unresolved psychosocial difficulties.

The nurse can refer the client to community resources such as community mental health centers and self-help groups. Other sources of information and referral for the client and family are groups such as the Foundation for Depressive Illness (1-800-248-4344 or *http://www.depression.org*) and the National Mental Health Association (703-684-7722 or *http://nmha.org*). On the federal level, the National Institute of Mental Health (NIMH) is charged with improving the understanding, treatment, and rehabilitation of the mentally ill; preventing mental illness; and fostering the mental health of the people. NIMH is involved in prevention activities. It sponsors Project D/ART (Depression/Awareness, Recognition, and Treatment). Project D/ART is concerned with ameliorating the public health problem of depression and aims to improve the identification, assessment, treatment, and clinical management of depressive disorders through an educational program focused on the general public, primary care providers, and mental health specialists.

Project D/ART is involved with many voluntary and professional organizations and provides information and materials for the general public as well as professional audiences.

*Healthy People 2010* has a priority area that addresses mental health and mental disorders. Two objectives in this priority seek to increase mental health screening for persons seen in primary care settings and to increase the proportion of adults with mental disorders who receive treatment (USDHHS, 2000b, p. B18-8). As discussed earlier, depression is often undiagnosed and because individuals are seen for other health problems in primary settings, this provides a forum for detection and early intervention for mental disorders.

## Men and Women Changing Jobs or Careers

When changing jobs or careers, a major reorganization is required in one's life, and the stresses encountered should not be underestimated. The process can involve significant stress, particularly if changing a job or a career was not a voluntary decision (e.g., being fired or laid off), and unemployment may result. Even if the decision was a voluntary one, the individual may have doubts about the decision and may not have consensus within the family.

When some people change jobs or careers it may mean going back to school. An example of the health stresses that this could cause is seen in the McSweeney family. The family had an increased incidence of health problems when Mr. McSweeney returned to college to prepare for another career.

**CASE Scenario**  George McSweeney was a 38-year-old engineer, husband, and father of three school-age children. As a result of industrial noise, he lost 50% of his hearing. Unable to continue functioning at his job, he returned to college to prepare for another career. Financially his family had few difficulties. Although Mr. McSweeney was not eligible for workers' compensation, he received federal scholarship monies and his wife had a part-time job. The community health nurse encountered the McSweeney family after they had repeatedly taken Lisa, their 10-year-old daughter, into the emergency room for treatment of an asthmatic condition. The nurse was well received by the family because both parents were unsure of when to seek medical care for their daughter. The nurse discovered that Lisa's condition had been under good control until the family moved and she had to change schools. In addition, she found that Mr. McSweeney was having tension headaches regularly; a medical evaluation ruled out organic problems. Lisa had fewer asthma attacks and Mr. McSweeney had fewer headaches as the family began to verbalize the frustrations associated with the multiple changes they had recently experienced.

To assist the adult in dealing with change and stress, the nurse needs to assess individual and/or family perceptions of the situation. Is it viewed as a new and challenging adventure? Is it a threat to personal and economic security? Is it causing problems within the family structure?

Community health nurses should be especially sensitive to the stresses that can occur when an individual is changing jobs or careers. The nurse assesses the situation, listens to the client's concerns, and refers the client to appropriate resources (e.g., stress management, counseling services, vocational rehabilitation).

From an aggregate perspective, the number of adults experiencing the need for a job or career change is increasing. As organizations downsize and new technology emerges, the need for job or career changes is becoming a normal occurrence. The current trend in our nation reflects a need for workers to prepare for multiple careers throughout their lives. Community health nurses can assist with this process by developing support groups for those who need to make immediate changes and through preventive intervention with children and adults just starting their careers.

## Adults Experiencing Unemployment

No one is exempt from loss of employment, and this can create devastation for a family; however, some groups are more at risk for unemployment than others. The unemployment rate varies significantly by race and ethnicity and overall, unemployment is higher among African Americans than whites (U.S. Bureau of the Census, 1998).

When unemployment occurs, regardless of reason, it can be very disruptive and stressful for families involved. Family stress can mount as work responsibilities are redistributed, roles are altered, and family goals are modified. Role reversal between husband and wife may occur, and there can be increased frequency of marital disruption and role conflict. In addition to economic deprivation, unemployment can cause increased family violence, instability, and economic deprivation. Social stigma is often attached to unemployment. The unemployed family may become socially isolated and suffer altered self-esteem.

People who are unemployed often are unable to afford health care services because they lose insurance and health care benefits. Unemployment generates stress that can cause health problems. The unemployed worker may not feel well physically and have symptoms such as chest pains, shortness of breath, dizziness, dry mouth, eczema, weakness, and inability to sleep. Psychological stress among the unemployed may be evidenced by lowered self-esteem, anxiety, apathy, decreased appetite, inertia, and feelings of helplessness. The unemployed suffer from a variety of psychosomatic conditions. Family members of the unemployed can also exhibit evidence of health problems and stress related to the unemployment. Although unemployment necessitates family adjustment, change, and adaptation, the stress experienced can be minimized and positive growth can occur.

Unemployment is a major crisis physically, socially, emotionally, and financially. Community health nurses can help families understand what is happening and encourage them to use appropriate community resources. They can also work with community groups to mobilize resources for the unemployed and make referrals for crisis intervention, job training, or new employment. Community partnerships may be needed to address issues related to unemployment particularly if a community has a significantly high unemployment rate. Chapter 15 discusses mobilizing community partnerships for social and health action.

## Adults with Chronic Illness

Chronic illness is a major health problem in the American population (see Chapters 11 and 18). Illness for the individual or family is a normal part of the life cycle. Everyone expects at some point in time to have a case of the flu, a cold, or even minor surgery. Acute, nondisabling illness can often be handled by normal resources and coping mechanisms because these illnesses do not involve major lifestyle adaptation. If the illness becomes chronic, disabling, or terminal, however, the family situation can become stressful. When the adult is afflicted with a chronic health condition, major life changes may occur. These changes can involve increased health care tasks, the possibility of strained family relationships, modifications in family goals, financial stress, need for housing adaptation, and social isolation. The grieving process in relation to such conditions is discussed in Chapter 18. The individual and family may also demonstrate changes in work, school, and community experiences as a result of the illness.

The extent to which lifestyle changes occur during chronic illness varies, depending on the degree of disability encountered and the adult's perception of the event. Role reversal, changes in sexual behavior, and alterations in self-image are a few examples of the problems experienced by clients who have developed debilitating chronic illness during adulthood. The adult who is not progressing well along the developmental continuum may regress, become depressed, or become dependent when chronically ill. He or she may resist treatment or become self-absorbed and could use the illness as an escape from responsibility.

Research has shown that families who adjusted well to chronic illness viewed the illness in a positive light—that is, a greater appreciation of life for the present was developed (Hough, Lewis, Woods, 1991). Further, these families viewed themselves as competent and effective and stated that they were more sensitive and empathic about the needs of others.

Use of both the educative and problem-solving approaches to nursing intervention is essential when nurses work with families and aggregates who are dealing with a chronic condition. They need increased knowledge to realistically evaluate the changes that are occurring and that may occur. These clients also need to problem-solve to determine the most appropriate ways for them to adapt to changes, especially permanent ones. Different coping mechanisms and resources must be mobilized to reduce tension.

The possibility of death may also be a matter for the nurse to work through with chronically ill adults and their families. Families should be encouraged to articulate advance directives, express their fears and, if the client's situation warrants it, to prepare for death. Situations involving death and dying are inevitable. Yet for many Americans, death education comes late in life, and they are often not equipped to deal with it in relation to themselves or others.

When working with any chronically ill adult, the community health nurse will more than likely use the referral process. A variety of community resources, including ostomy clubs, Multiple Sclerosis Association, ACS, American Lung Association, American Heart Association, Goodwill Industries, the division of vocational rehabilitation, and the department of social services, will help clients and their families adapt to chronic illness. Chapter 22 discusses support and education for the caregiver and the client when chronic illness is present.

The community health nurse can assist the client and family by making them aware of the medical course of the client's condition, giving anticipatory guidance, and encouraging them to take an active role in health care decision making. Nurses can help the chronically ill adult accept the interdependency needed to deal successfully with his or her condition and should not make unrealistic promises of recovery or an optimistic prognosis if this is not the case. There may be no guarantee that treatment will improve the level of disability, and false hopes prevent the client from confronting and working through the crisis.

## People Who Are Experiencing Marital Crises

It is not uncommon for the community health nurse to encounter families who are experiencing some form of marital crisis such as divorce and domestic violence (discussed in Chapter 13). The divorce rate has increased dramatically in the past three decades (U.S. Bureau of the Census, 2000a), and when experienced, marital crisis is a major life stress for the adult. As a result of divorce, as well as an increase in the number of never-married parents, there has been a rise in single-parent households, which creates additional stress for many adults (U.S. Bureau of the Census, 2000b).

Marital disenchantment, separation, and divorce occur throughout adulthood. For instance, during middlescence spouses find that they have more time together, and if they are unable to reestablish intimacy or reinforce it, they may become disenchanted with their marital relationship. In addition, the sexual changes (menopause and climacteric) that occur during middlescence can also adversely affect the way in which spouses relate in the marital relationship.

Disenchantment, separation, and divorce have an impact on all family members. Adults, as well as children, need to make major changes. Experiencing feelings of uncertainty, betrayal, insecurity, failure, and loss is common during this time. As with all crises, the primary focus of the community health nurse with clients who are experiencing marital stress is on helping them achieve crisis resolution and growth. Resolution could require divorce or separation, but it also may occur through renegotiation and alteration of family patterns that are ineffective. A therapeutic approach that encourages problem solving rather than blaming can best facilitate successful resolution during this time of crisis.

From both an aggregate and family perspective, anticipatory guidance activities by community health nurses may be instrumental in preventing marital crises. Preparing young adults to handle the stresses of parenthood, or middlescent couples to deal with the conflicts during launching, may decrease the amount of stress experienced at these times. Parenting and life stress management groups are commonly found in communities throughout the country. Community health nurses frequently have an active role in establishing and conducting these groups.

## Gays and Lesbians

Gays and lesbians experience the same health problems and provider needs as that of the general population of men and women (Bell, 1999; Saulnier, Wheeler, 2000). However, gays and lesbians have health care issues that create added stress related to disclosing their sexual identity, seeking health care, and confronting attitudes from health care providers. Bias and discrimination are a reality for gays and lesbians and many "have experienced lifelong rejection from family, peers, and coworkers" (Denenberg, 1995, p. 83). Despite the fact that homosexuality was declassified as a mental illness over 20 years ago, most gays and lesbians continue to be victims of prejudice and discrimination (Carlson, 1996, p. 71; Eliason, 1996, p. 5; Hellman, 1996, p. 1094).

Deciding when or *if* they should disclose their identity to health care providers can be a highly stressful ordeal because many gays and lesbians fear that health care providers will view them negatively (Anonymous, 2000; Eliason, 1996). In traditional health care settings gay and lesbian partners are often not afforded the same recognition and partner support status as their heterosexual counterparts are granted. This adds personal stress for the client because many fear their partners may not be allowed to provide the desired emotional support. Gays and lesbians are often unable to freely express themselves in the health care setting (Hellman, 1996, p. 1095). Research has shown that many gays and lesbians, upon disclosure of their sexual identity to health care providers, have experienced reactions such as ostracism, condescension, discrimination, shock, pity, disapproval, fear, avoidance, and even rough physical handling (Eliason, 1996; Saulnier, 1999; Saulnier, Wheeler, 2000; Stevens, Hall, 1990). As a result of these types of reactions, gays and lesbians may be reluctant to seek health care, which can put them at risk for the development of health problems and disease progression by delaying early treatment (Aaron, Markovic, Danielson, 2001).

Eliason and Randall (1991) reported that lesbians were reluctant to seek care when they had health concerns because of negative past experiences and even harm. Lesbians are less likely than their heterosexual counterparts to seek regular gynecological examinations, Pap smears, breast ex-

aminations, mammograms, and other preventive services (Denenberg, 1995; Eliason, 1996). This increases their risk for development and progression of adult health problems such as cardiovascular diseases, hypertension, and cancer, which often are detected through preventive activities such as screening and Pap smears. Lesbians also have fewer pregnancies than heterosexual women, which places them at a higher risk for breast cancer. Additionally, lesbians may receive unscreened insemination or have sexual intercourse with a stranger in order to have children, which puts them at high risk for human immunodeficiency virus (HIV) (Denenberg, 1995, p. 82). Safe-sex education is as pertinent to lesbian clients as it is to heterosexual clients because they are not immune to sexually transmitted diseases (STDs) and bacterial infections.

Gay men have health needs similar to heterosexual men. Like lesbians, gay men are often reluctant to seek preventive health and treatment services for fear of discrimination and disclosure (Bell, 1999). Gay men are more likely to experience violent discrimination, such as "gay bashing," than lesbian women, which makes them more reluctant to disclose their sexual identity and to seek health care for fear of additional violence (Eliason, 1996, pp. 189-192). Gay men have higher rates of HIV/AIDS and are more apt to engage in casual sex than their lesbian counterparts, which places them at a high risk for STDs and other infections (Anonymous, 1999a; Eliason, 1996, p. 200; Mansergh, Colfax, Marks, et al., 2001). Hence safe-sex education is extremely important to this population. It also is recommended that gay men of all ages have yearly rectal examinations that screen for cancer or other infections (Eliason, 1996, p. 201).

Both gays and lesbians have higher rates of substance abuse, depression, and suicide than that of the general population (Eliason, 1996; Hall, 1993; Hellman, 1996). High-risk behaviors frequently are associated with substance abuse (Mansergh, Colfax, Marks, et al., 2001). For example, Klitzman, Pope, and Hudson (2000) found a strong relationship between abuse of the drug 3,4-methylenedioxymethamphetamine (MDMA or "Ecstasy") and unprotected anal intercourse among 169 gay and bisexual men. Clearly there is a real need for preventive and mental health treatment services for gay and lesbian adults. However, many are reluctant to seek such services because of the stigmatizing effects of receiving treatment. Many feel that they cannot be open and expressive in their treatment setting and fear further stigmatization related to their mental health (Hellman, 1996). Clearly an open environment and increased sensitivity on the part of health care providers is essential. If a provider has difficulty separating personal opinions and biases, then that provider should make an appropriate referral to someone who will provide unbiased services (Bell, 1999).

Perhaps the greatest health need for this population is for health care providers to accept gays and lesbians without prejudice and in a positive manner. Community health nurses have an opportunity to foster positive attitudes in meeting the needs of gay and lesbian adults. Clinicians need to examine their own biases and fears regarding gays and lesbians so that they do not negatively jeopardize their health care (Carlson, 1996, p. 73). No person should ever be afraid of seeking out health care providers to meet their health needs. "Health care providers need to find ways to alleviate pain and suffering, not to compound them" (Eliason, 1996, p. 187). If quality nursing care is to be given nonjudgmentally, nurses must recognize their own homophobias and identify their inaccurate knowledge base in order for all persons to receive the health care they need. Community health nurses can intervene at various levels of health promotion and prevention. Some examples of interventions include education regarding safe sexual practices that are tailored to gays and lesbians, preventive screening practices such as regular Pap smears for lesbians and anal examinations for men, suicide prevention education, screening for depression and suicide risks, and referral for treatment.

## Individuals Who Are Incarcerated

The number of individuals who are incarcerated is increasing each year. Today there are approximately 1.8 million inmates in the United States, and the population is growing at a rate of approximately 8% annually (Shinkman, 2000). The prison population spans all ages, including both men and women, and minorities are disproportionately represented. The majority of inmates are between 18 and 34 years of age, with elderly inmates being in the minority (LaMere, Smyer, Gragert, 1996). The number of women incarcerated has increased substantially. Since 1980 the number of persons in federal and state prisons more than tripled, from 329,821 persons in 1980 to a record 1,104,074 at midyear 1995 (CDC, 1996b). As the rate of crime has escalated and as more criminals are being incarcerated, the number of prison beds needed has also increased. As a result, prisons have become overcrowded. In 1995 state prisons were filled 17% to 29% above capacity, and federal prisons were 25% above capacity (Meddis, 1995, p. A3).

Incarceration and overcrowding places inmates at risk for many health problems. Demographic data reflect that incarcerated persons are primarily from lower socioeconomic backgrounds, have had problems with substance abuse, have had little health care before incarceration, and experience high rates of mental illness (Anonymous, 1999b; Petersilia, 2000). Incarcerated persons also engage in unhealthy lifestyles that increase the risk of developing illness and disease (National Institute of Justice, 1995, p. xi).

Numerous health risks and health problems exist among incarcerated populations. Many youth who are detained in juvenile corrections centers suffer from some type of physical or emotional problem (Shelton, 2000). As a result of the previous lifestyles of the inmates and the prison environment, many STDs and other communicable diseases, as well as chronic illnesses, are prevalent among incarcerated individuals. HIV/AIDS is rapidly increasing in the prison population, and HIV transmission is a serious concern (CDC, 1996c, p. 268). Many inmates who also have been IV drug users are HIV-infected before incarceration, and in some instances, incarceration may be the first time prisoners have received any health care or preventive education (Gaiter, Doll, 1996, p. 1201). Because of the diversity of the prison population, interventions must be specific to gender, cognitive, and developmental levels, and culturally sensitive (Gaiter, Doll, 1996, p. 1202). This can only be accomplished by a comprehensive understanding of risk factors (e.g., drug use, consensual as well as nonconsensual unprotected sex, alcohol use, ignorance) surrounding the HIV/AIDS-infected prison population.

The incidence and prevalence of tuberculosis (TB) in prisons also has increased significantly. The prison environment is a high-risk environment as a result of overcrowding, inadequate ventilation, and coinfection with HIV, which allows TB to easily spread among inmates. Many prisoners have latent TB, and coinfection with HIV increases the risk of developing active TB. The strongest known risk for converting latent TB to active TB is coinfection with HIV (CDC, 1996b). Because TB is spread through the air, it takes only one prisoner with active TB to infect numerous others sharing the same crowded air space (CDC, 1996b, p. 5). CDC has recommended stronger regulations to control the spread of TB in federal, state, and local prisons (CDC, 1996b).

State and local health departments have an active role in carrying out standards and practices to control TB and other health problems of the incarcerated. As a result, community health nurses are active participants in screening, intervention, and the referral process, particularly in the minimum security and community-based jail diversion program. Prison health, as it pertains to maximum security prisons such as federal and state, is a specialty in itself and beyond the scope of this book. The concern here is the incarcerated who are accessible in local county or city jails, where nurses can identify and work with at-risk groups. One of the *Healthy People 2010* objectives is to "increase the proportion of governments with community-based jail diversion programs for adults with serious mental problems" (USDHHS, 2000b, p. B18-15). The role for community health nurses in this environment primarily involves primary and secondary prevention activities that would include health education, early detection through screenings, and referrals for early intervention.

When prisoners are released, it is imperative that community support services are available for a follow-up process to control the spread of communicable disease to others, homelessness, recurring family violence, and other risk factors involved in reentry to the community (Petersilia, 2000). Community health nurses have a role in managed care that ensures ongoing care of prisoners when they are released to the community.

Nursing in prisons encompasses a wide variety of interventions that range from acute emergency care, casefinding, health education, behavioral management, treatment for STDs, psychiatric care, and substance abuse intervention to treatment for chronic illnesses such as arthritis, hypertension, and diabetes. A number of chronic illnesses and mobility problems require ongoing treatment and evaluation during incarceration. Table 17-7 presents some self-reported and physician-diagnosed illnesses of older adult inmates. Nurses must be able to work independently and meet chronic, as well as acute, health needs of the incarcerated.

As mentioned, more women have also become incarcerated. Incarcerated women have health needs that are similar to their male counterparts such as substance abuse, STDs, HIV/AIDS, TB, and mental and chronic illnesses. However, pregnancy can have societal and personal implications. Pregnant women in federal prisons may not participate in the direct care of their infants, and the birth mother has to make a choice of either placing her infant up for adoption or seeking someone who will assume guardianship responsibilities (Huft, 1992). Grandparents and other relatives often care for the children of incarcerated adults. Community health nurses frequently help these guardians access appropriate community services. Incarceration not only affects incarcerated individuals but, most powerfully, their children. Care of pregnant women involves gynecological and obstetrical care, as well as other services such as Women, Infants, and Children (WIC), and well-child care.

Care of pregnant women in prisons is complicated by stress, restrictive environments, alterations in social supports, and the displacement of the maternal role functions after birth (Huft, 1992). The environment, coupled with distorted maternal role functioning, can contribute to depression. Fogel and Martin (1992) have studied incarcerated women who are mothers and who are not mothers: both groups had high levels of depression that did not mitigate over time, but the mothers had higher levels of anxiety that remained high. Women in prisons are in need of services that would enhance their emotional and psychological health as well as their physical health.

Just as the number of individuals who are incarcerated has increased, so has the cost of prison health care. The high rate of HIV/AIDS, TB, and an increasingly aging prison population also has added to the increase in prison health costs (McDonald, 1995). To contain costs, prisons are contracting with community agencies to provide health care to the prisoners (McDonald, 1995) and are accessing telemedicine (Anonymous, 1999b).

Community health nurses and nurses in acute-care settings may be providing direct care in addition to preventive services as part of a collaborative effort to provide quality care to the incarcerated. Community placement concerns upon prison release may also be addressed by the community health nurse. Community health nurses must know the resources in the community to make appropriate referral and follow-up. They must also be knowledgeable about family dynamics and how to address changes in these dynamics as a released prisoner reenters the home environment. Like other

**TABLE 17-7**

*Percentage of Male Inmates with Lifetime History of Specific Self-Reported Physician-Diagnosed Illness*

| | AGE, Y | | |
|---|---|---|---|
| | 50-59 (*N* = 82) | >59 (*N* = 37) | OVERALL (*N* = 119) |
| Arthritis | 40.2 | 56.8 | 45.4 |
| Hypertension | 36.7 | 45.9 | 39.7 |
| Any STD | 21.5 | 21.6 | 21.6 |
| Stomach or intestinal ulcers | 18.3 | 27.0 | 21.0 |
| Prostate problems | 17.1 | 27.0 | 20.2 |
| Myocardial infarction | 17.7 | 21.6 | 19.0 |
| Emphysema | 14.6 | 27.0 | 18.5 |
| Diabetes | 10.1 | 13.5 | 11.2 |
| Asthma | 8.5 | 10.8 | 9.2 |
| Stroke | 3.8 | 16.2 | 7.8 |
| Cancer | 6.3 | 8.1 | 6.9 |
| Cirrhosis or liver disease | 4.9 | 2.7 | 4.2 |
| Injury requiring medical care | 78.5 | 73.0 | 76.7 |

From Colsher PL, Wallace RB, Loeffelholz PL, et al.: Health status of older male prisoners: a comprehensive survey, *Am J Public Health* 82(6):882, 1992.

problems that have been discussed in this chapter, providing competent care for the incarcerated will require sensitivity to issues involved with caring for the incarcerated. This will require nurses to solve personal issues and be aware of biases that may interfere with providing quality care.

**THE ROLE OF THE NURSE WITH PEOPLE WHO ARE INCARCERATED.** The American Nurses Association (ANA) has articulated several position statements for nurses working in prisons. The ANA's Council of Community Health Nurses developed the Scope and Standards of Nursing Practice in Correctional Facilities in 1985 and revised them in 1995. The purpose of these standards is to guide professional nurse practice in correctional facilities, for the general incarcerated prison population, and in specialty facilities such as those for women, juveniles, and the mentally ill. Specific ANA guidelines also exist for nurses' management and care of inmates with HIV (ANA, 1996, pp. 17-20) and TB throughout the United States (ANA, 1996, pp. 59-62).

Perhaps more than any other environment where nurses practice, the prison environment may present the greatest challenge to providing quality care. Prison nurses' personal attitudes and beliefs must be explored so they do not interfere with their role in providing the highest standard of professional care. The role of the nurse in the prison is to provide health care services that are within the scope of practice for each particular state, and the standards specifically point out that the role excludes involvement in disciplinary procedures (including execution), except for regulations that apply to nursing personnel (ANA, 1995). Primary health services in this field include using the nursing process in screening, providing direct health care services, teaching, counseling, and assisting prisoners to manage their own health care.

It has long been recognized that nurses can have role conflict when working in prisons. Alexander-Rodriguez (1983) wrote that there is a basic conflict between the goals of correctional health care and correctional institutions. A prison nurse must meet the demands of perhaps two philosophically opposite corporate cultures (Stevens, 1995, p. 8). In the public health care culture there is a prevailing belief of basic goodness, whereas in the prison system the presence of evil prevails, and as a result nurses can be polarized between the two directions (Stevens, 1995, pp. 7-8). To provide competent care in the prison environment, the prison nurse must understand the differences in values, beliefs, and norms between a corporate health care environment and a prison correctional environment. Self-awareness of issues related to caring for incarcerated populations can help allay conflict in achieving health goals and providing quality nursing care for the incarcerated.

Prisoners struggle to survive, and times of illness make them vulnerable to suffering and in need of humanistic health care (Berkman, 1995). "The biggest challenge for a nurse working in a prison, is to remain true to the humanistic philosophy of nursing and not be slowly and imperceptibly converted to the role of prison keeper. When that happens it is time to get out of prison health care" (Alexander-Rodriguez, 1983, p. 116).

Increasingly, community health nurses are expanding their services to prisoners in city and county jails. In these settings the nurse may conduct health education programs, screen for and follow-up on STDs, act as a health care resource to staff, assist prisoners in finding health care resources upon discharge, and provide supportive and problem-solving counseling. Prison systems are in need of strong primary health prevention programs, especially related to communicable disease prevention and mental health services.

## THE COMMUNITY HEALTH NURSE'S ROLE IN MAINTAINING THE HEALTH OF ADULT MEN AND WOMEN

Although community health nurses' interventions have been discussed throughout this chapter, further emphasis is needed here to highlight the significant role nurses perform in promoting the health of adults. Health is a blend of developmental, physiological, psychological, spiritual, and so-

cial factors. When one of these factors becomes out of balance, all are affected. Community health nurses take into consideration all of these factors when developing interventions to comprehensively address the needs of adult clients. Implementing comprehensive interventions requires an awareness of available resources and frequently involves collaborative and interdisciplinary teamwork.

Various approaches are often needed to plan nursing interventions that address the health needs of well adults. It is not an easy task to motivate adults to participate in health activities, especially if they consider themselves to be well. Well adults do not always recognize or act on health needs and may ignore primary prevention activities. The community health nurse implements interventions at all levels of prevention. Use of the referral process (discussed in Chapter 10) is an integral part of promoting the health of the adult. Nurses can help adults become aware of the available resources that meet their health care needs and refer them to these resources when appropriate. However, many health care resources are organized to deal with acute health care episodes rather than with preventive health care measures.

### Health Promotion Through Preventive Intervention

As discussed in earlier chapters, health promotion begins with people who are basically healthy and encourages the development of lifestyles that maintain and support health and well-being. A great deal is known about many health promotion activities such as smoking cessation, regular exercise, and dietary modifications that enhance a healthy lifestyle and risk factors that enhance disease occurrences in adulthood. However, more effective strategies are needed to assist adults in addressing these risk factors. Community-based research intervention projects, such as work-site cancer prevention that includes smoking cessation and healthy nutrition habits and prevention of functional decline (Sorensen, Thompson, Glanz, et al., 1996; Wallace, Buchner, Grothaus, et al., 1998), are emerging to address this need.

Some examples of selected health promotion activities that help healthy adult clients improve or maintain their well-being were previously displayed in Box 17-1. Other areas of health promotion, such as environmental health and occupational health and safety, are matters of legislation and enforcement as well as individual decision making. Obtaining documented data about health promotion and nursing interventions that produce successful health outcomes is critical when working toward influencing legislation and health policy. Legislative and health policy action, such as laws related to smoking in public places, are needed to comprehensively address the health needs of adult populations in the community.

Community health nurses carry out many primary prevention activities to comprehensively address the personal health needs of adults. They are particularly interested in helping the adult learn about preventable health problems and about health behaviors that can promote wellness and decrease personal health risks. A major primary prevention activity with adults is health teaching and counseling about family and personal health risk factors, accident prevention and safety, nutrition, personal hygiene, health examinations, family planning, STDs, disease transmission, and immunizations. Such health teaching, with use of resources as appropriate, may help prevent an illness or injury, dental caries, an unintended pregnancy, marital disenchantment, a suicide attempt, a case of tetanus, a case of flu, an incident of child abuse, or an STD. Health teaching activities help the adult look at health in relation to present and future functioning.

Primary prevention and health risk appraisal are major goals of health promotion but are not always easily attainable. In recent years increased emphasis has been placed on primary prevention. However, many preventive health care measures, such as yearly physical examinations, are not covered under many forms of health insurance and become out-of-pocket expenses for the client. Therefore cost is a factor that often impedes adults taking advantage of preventive services. Health screening programs can provide valuable health services to persons who otherwise would not obtain them.

The community health nurse can assess individual and family health risk factors and encourage health actions that decrease these risks. Health risk appraisal also can be handled through an automated process in which an individual's health-related behaviors and personal characteristics are compared with mortality statistics and other epidemiological data. Relating individual and group data helps individuals identify their risk of dying from a specific condition by a specified time and the amount of risk that could be eliminated by making appropriate behavioral changes in health practices. This automated approach is increasingly accessible to the general public and can have beneficial health consequences. However, the real challenge for health professionals is to help people act on personal health risks.

When counseling about health promotion activities, nurses should be sensitive and keep in mind that people bring their own beliefs, attitudes, and values to health care situations. Beliefs about individual and family susceptibility to illness, the severity of illness in terms of health and lifestyle disruption, the perceived effectiveness of diagnostic and health prevention activities, and perceived barriers to care affect the health promotion and prevention activities in which a person engages (Pender, 1996).

In addition to accident prevention, health teaching with the young adult should focus on violence prevention (see Chapter 13). Accidents, suicide, and homicide are the leading causes of death for persons 20 to 29 years of age. It is important to try to determine the nature and timing of critical precedents that place individuals at high risk for committing violent acts against themselves or others and to iden-

tify significant persons or groups in contact with high-risk individuals who could save the individual's life.

To prevent certain conditions, nurses can help adults look at their own personal health habits and risk factors. Smoking, excessive intake of alcoholic beverages, lack of sufficient rest, an inadequate diet, and other risk factors all have an impact on an adult's present and future health status.

When nurses practice from a prevention perspective, they stress the importance of medical, dental, and ophthalmological examinations for prevention, early diagnosis, and treatment of disease. Secondary preventive health measures for the adult include practicing self-examination of the breasts and testicles, yearly Pap smears, and adherence to prescribed medical and dental regimens. The adult should be assisted to see the value of monitoring and screening for conditions for which he or she has a familial or individual predisposition, such as cardiovascular accidents, diabetes, cancer, or hypertension. Practitioners can find a current preventive care timeline that summarizes adult screening procedures that should be used with adult clients and the age at which they should be done on the preventive care website (*http://www.ahcpr.gov/ppip/ppadtime.htm*). The information from this website provides parameters for discussion when the community health nurse is carrying out health counseling for ages 18 through 75 and older.

Tertiary prevention health activities that the nurse may use with the adult are related to rehabilitation activities that minimize the degree of disability of the condition. These activities are discussed in Chapter 18, where the nurse's role in rehabilitation of the disabled adult is covered. They involve interdisciplinary functioning and focus on encouraging client compliance with prescribed medical and dental regimens, as well as exploring ways to promote healthy coping behaviors.

Pender, Barkauskas, Hayman, et al. (1992, p. 108) have described three points at which a person or a group may be highly receptive to input about health promotion and disease prevention. These points are derived from a developmental and a person-environment interaction perspective that address developmental and situational stress. The three points include the following: age-specific times that are the same for most people, including menarche, parenthood, and retirement; historically specific times in the life of a society, including changes in the roles of men and women and insecurity in the labor market; and, finally, events that vary among individuals and families, including death of a partner or geographical relocation. These points can help the community health nurse develop aggregate-specific interventions aimed at reducing selected health risks.

The health risks and morbidity and mortality data for adults mandate that community health nurses continue lifelong education. Family violence, homelessness, tuberculosis, HIV/AIDS, unemployment, chronic illness—these are topics that are overwhelming in scope and that can affect practitioners themselves. Dealing with them means that nurses be well-informed; that they build in supports, both informal and formal, for the stressful times in their lives; and that political involvement at some level is crucial to ensure a basic level of health care for all.

## LEGISLATION AFFECTING ADULT HEALTH

The legislation that influences the adult also makes an impact on other age groups. The Social Security Act of 1935 and its amendments provide maternal-child health programs, which are discussed in Chapters 4 and 16. The Social Security Act also provides for Medicaid and Medicare, for which the medically indigent or terminally ill adult may qualify. The Public Health Service Act of 1944 and its amendments have helped to provide adult health care services. Health planning and environmental health legislation also have benefited adult health (see Chapter 6).

Among legislation that specifically addresses the adult population is the Occupational Safety and Health Act of 1970, which is discussed in Chapter 21. It deals with maintaining the health of the adult in the workplace and focuses on maintaining wellness. Two pieces of legislation passed in the early 1990s, The Americans with Disabilities Act and The Family and Medical Leave Act, having been positively influencing the health of adults throughout the 1990s. These acts are discussed in Chapter 4. However, the impact of welfare reform activities during the latter half of the 1990s continues to need monitoring. Community health professionals play a major role in assuring that a safety net exists to assist families to meet basic needs.

## SUMMARY

The breadth of the health issues affecting adult men and women is vast. Of all of the population groups presented in this text, adults have the greatest opportunity to improve their health status because they have monetary and physical independence. The fact that younger and older people depend on them can present burdens and challenges.

Adults who financially and emotionally support other age groups are vulnerable to unique pressures and stresses. It is often hard for them to admit that they have health problems or are experiencing stress.

The role of the nurse in helping adults achieve their developmental tasks is an important one. Understanding human development and its impact on health is essential. It is easier for adults to promote and maintain health when they know about health behaviors that enhance wellness and prevent stress. Major goals of the community health nurse when working with adults are to increase health promotion, prevent illness, and promote self-care capabilities. To accomplish these goals, nurses need a supportive work environment, engagement in the politics of health care, and a belief in lifelong learning.

## CRITICAL THINKING
*exercise*

Consider the community where you live. Identify the groups of adults at risk and their health promotion needs. Prioritize the health promotion needs and describe your reasoning. Using the three levels of prevention, outline a plan for your health promotion priority. Identify the community agencies and the resources they could provide to help address the health needs among the adult population. Describe barriers that may impede implementation of your health promotion plan. Describe factors that would facilitate implementation of your planned interventions.

*Ella Mae Brooks acknowledges the work from previous editions of this text in the development of this chapter.*

## REFERENCES

Aaron DJ, Markovic N, Danielson ME, et al.: Behavioral risk factors for disease and preventive health practices among lesbians, *Am J Public Health* 91(6):972-975, 2001.

Alexander-Rodriguez T: Prison health—a role for professional nursing, *Nurs Outlook* 31(2):115-118, 1983.

American Cancer Society (ACS): *Cancer facts and figures—2000*, Atlanta, 2000, ACS.

American Cancer Society (ACS): *Cancer facts and figures—2001*, Atlanta, 2001, ACS.

American Heart Association (AHA): *1998 heart and stroke statistical update*, Dallas, 1997, AHA.

American Nurses Association (ANA): *Scope and standards of nursing practice in correctional facilities*, Washington, DC, 1995, ANA.

American Nurses Association (ANA): American Nurses Association position statement on tuberculosis and HIV. In *Compendium of American Nurses Association position statements*, Washington, DC, 1996, ANA.

Anonymous: It can be done, *Privacy Journal* 26(2):5-6, 1999a.

Anonymous: Telemedicine reduces prison health care costs, *Corrections Forum* 8(5):59-61, 1999b.

Anonymous: Program dismantles barriers to lesbian health care, *Network News* 25(3):5, May/June 2000.

Arnaud C: Osteoporosis: using bone markers for diagnosis and monitoring, *Geriatrics* 51(4):24-30, 1996.

Ashley R, Rockwell E, Gladsjo JA, et al.: The reappearance of depression in an elderly man: what lurks behind it? *Am J Psychiatry* 157(12):1943-1947, 2000.

Bell R: ABC of sexual health: Homosexual men and women, *British Medical Journal* 318(7181):452-455, 1999.

Berkman A: Prison health: the breaking point, *Am J Public Health* 85:1616-1618, 1995.

Biggs J, Fleury J: An exploration of perceived barriers to cardiovascular risk reduction, *Cardiovasc Nurs* 30(6):41-46, November/December 1996.

Carlson K: Gay and lesbian families. In Harway M, editor: *Treating the changing family*, New York, 1996, Wiley.

Centers for Disease Control and Prevention (CDC): Mortality patterns—United States, 1993, *MMWR Morbid Mortal Wkly Rep* 45(8):161-164, March 1, 1996a.

Centers for Disease Control and Prevention (CDC): Prevention and control of tuberculosis in correctional facilities, *MMWR Morbid Mortal Wkly Rep* 45(RR-8):1-6, June 7, 1996b.

Centers for Disease Control and Prevention (CDC): HIV/AIDS education and prevention programs for adults in prisons and jails and juveniles in confinement facilities—United States, 1994, *MMWR Morbid Mortal Wkly Rep* 45(13):268-270, 1996c.

Centers for Disease Control and Prevention (CDC): *Reducing tobacco use: a report of the Surgeon General—2000* (online service text file). USDHHS Office of Smoking and Health, 2000. Retrieved from the internet February 2, 2001. *http://www.cdc.gov/tobacco*

Colsher PL, Wallace RB, Loeffelholz PL, et al.: Health status of older male prisoners: a comprehensive survey, *Am J Public Health* 82(6):881-883, 1992.

Cowan P: Women's mental health issues: reflections on past attitudes and present practices, *J Psychosoc Nurs Ment Health Serv* 34(4):20-24, 1996.

Denenberg R: Report on lesbian health, *Womens Health Issues* 5(2):81-91, 1995.

Dennerstein L: Gender, health, and ill-health, *Womens Health Issues* 5(2):53-59, 1995.

Duvall EM: *Family development,* ed 2, New York, 1962, Lippincott.

Duvall EM, Miller BC: *Marriage and family development,* ed 6, New York, 1985, Harper & Row.

Eliason MJ: *Who cares? Institutional barriers to health care for lesbian, gay, and bisexual persons,* Pub No 14-6742, New York, 1996, NLN.

Eliason MJ, Randall CE: Lesbian phobia in nursing students, *West J Nurs Res* 13(3):363-374, 1991.

Eliopoulos C: Framework for gerontological nursing. In Eliopoulos C: *Gerontological nursing,* ed 5, Philadelphia, 2001, Lippincott.

Erikson EH: *Childhood and society,* ed 2, New York, 1963, Norton.

Erikson EH: *The life cycle completed: a review,* New York, 1982, Norton.

Faraone SV, Biederman J: Depression: a family affair, *Lancet* 351:158-159, 1998.

Fogel CI, Martin SL: The mental health of incarcerated women, *West J Nurs Res* 14(1):30-47, 1992.

Gaiter J, Doll LS: Improving HIV/AIDS prevention in prisons is good public health policy, *Am J Public Health* 86(9):1201-1203, 1996 (editorial).

Glantz SA: Preventing tobacco use—the youth access trap, *Am J Public Health* 8(2):156-157, 1996 (editorial).

Greenwood S: *Menopause, naturally, preparing for the second half of life,* Volcano, Calif, 1996, Volcano Press.

Hall L: *Taking charge of menopause,* US Food and Drug Administration, Pub No (FDA) 00-1310, Rockville, Md, 2000, US Government Printing Office.

Hall M: Lesbians and alcohol: patterns and paradoxes in medical notions and lesbians' beliefs, *J Psychoactive Drugs* 25(2):109-119, 1993.

Harris JE: Cigarette smoke components and disease: cigarette smoke is more than a triad of tar, nicotine and carbon monoxide. In National Cancer Institute: *The FTC cigarette test method for determining tar, nicotine, and carbon monoxide yields of U.S. cigarettes,* NIH Pub No 96-4028, Washington, DC, 1996, NCI.

Havighurst RJ: *Developmental tasks and education,* New York, 1972, David McKay.

Hawthorne MH: Gender differences in recovery after coronary artery surgery, *Image J Nurs Sch* 26(1):75-80, 1994.

Hellman RE: Issues in the treatment of lesbian women and gay men with chronic mental illness, *Psychiatric Services* 47(10):1093-1098, 1996.

Heloma A, Jaakkola MS, Kahkonen E, et al.: Short-term impact of national smoke-free workplace legislation on passive smoking and tobacco use, *Am J Public Health* 91(9):1416-1418, 2001.

Henningfield JE, Schuh LM: Pharmacology and markers: nicotine pharmacology and addictive effects. In National Cancer Institute: *The*

FTC cigarette test method for determining tar, nicotine, and carbon monoxide yields of U.S. cigarettes, NIH Pub No 96-4028, Washington, DC, 1996, NCI.

Hofland SL, Powers J: Sexual dysfunction in menopausal woman: hormonal causes and management issues, *Geriatr Nurs* 17(4):161-165, 1996.

Horton JA, editor: *The women's health data book: a profile of women's health in the United States,* Washington, DC, 1995, The Jacob Institute of Women's Health.

Hough EE, Lewis FM, Woods NF: Family response to a mother's chronic illness: case studies of well- and poorly adjusted families, *West J Nurs Res* 13(5):568-596, 1991.

Huft AG: Psychosocial adaptation to pregnancy in prison, *J Psychosoc Nurs Ment Health Serv* 30(4):19-23, 1992.

Judelson DR: Gender gap: women and coronary heart disease, *Advance for nurse practitioners,* 7(11):43-48, 1999.

Kiefe CI, Williams OD, Lewis CE, et al.: Ten-year changes in smoking among young adults: are racial differences explained by socioeconomic factors in the CARDIA study? *Am J Public Health* 91(2):213-218, 2001.

Klitzman RL, Pope HG Jr, Hudson JI: MDMA ("Ecstasy") abuse and high-risk sexual behaviors among 169 gay and bisexual men, *Am J Psychiatry* 157(7):162-1164, 2000.

Kramarow E, Lentzner H, Rooks R, et al.: *Health and aging chartbook: health, United States, 1999.* National Center for Health Statistics, Hyattsville, Md, 1999, US Government Printing Office.

LaMere S, Smyer T, Gragert M: The aging inmate, *J Psychosoc Nurs Ment Health Serv* 34(4):25-29, 1996.

Mansergh G, Colfax GN, Marks G, et al.: The circuit party men's health survey: findings and implications for gay and bisexual men, *Am J Public Health* 91(6):1953-1958, 2001.

Martin KS, Larson BJ, Gorski LA, et al., editors: *Mosby's home health client teaching guides: Rx for teaching,* St Louis, 1997, Mosby.

McDonald DC: *Managing prison health care costs,* Washington, DC, 1995, US Department of Justice.

Meddis SV: An unprecedented level of imprisonment in USA, *USA Today,* August 10, 1995, p. A3.

Miller NH: Tips for smoking cessation, *Cardiovasc Nurs* 32(5):33-35, 1996.

National Center for Health Statistics: *Health, United States 2000, with adolescent health chartbook, United States, 2000,* DHHS Pub No 00-1232, Hyattsville, Md, 2000, National Center for Health Statistics.

National Institutes of Health (NIH): *Smoking and health: report of the advisory committee to the Surgeon General of the Public Health Service,* NIH Pub No 94-80, Bethesda, Md, 1997, Public Health Service.

National Institutes of Health (NIH): *Fact about heart disease and women: Are you at risk?* NIH Pub No 98-364, Bethesda, Md, 1998, Public Health Service.

National Institute of Justice: *Issues and practices: 1994 update, tuberculosis in correctional facilities,* Washington, DC, 1995, National Institute for Justice.

National Safety Council: *Injury facts,* 1999 ed, Itasca, Ill, 1999, National Safety Council.

O'Connell KA, Gerkovich MM, Cook MR: Reversal theory's mastery and sympathy states in smoking cessation, *Image J Nurse Sch* 27(4):311-316, 1995.

Pender N: *Health promotion in nursing practice,* ed 3, 1996, Appleton & Lange.

Pender NJ, Barkauskas VH, Hayman L, et al.: Health promotion and disease prevention: toward excellence in nursing practice and education, *Nurs Outlook* 40(3):106-113, 1992.

Peters SL: Some women on fast track feel derailed, *USA Today,* February 1, 1996, pp. 1A, 2A.

Petersilia J: When prisoners return to the community: political, economic, and social consequences, *Sentencing & Corrections: Issues for the 21st Century*, Papers from the executive sessions on sentencing and corrections, No 9, Washington, DC, 2000, US Department of Justice.

Sapp M, Bliesmer M: Promoting health through public policy and standards of care. In Stanley M, Beare PG: *Gerontological nursing: a health promotion/protection approach*, ed 2, Philadelphia, 1999, FA Davis.

Sarkis K: National health plan includes job safety goals, *Occupational Hazards* 62(4):28-30, 2000.

Satcher D: Why we need an international agreement on tobacco control, *Am J Public Health* 91(2):191-193, 2001.

Saulnier CF: Choosing a health care provider: a community survey of what is important to lesbians, *Family in Society* 80(3):254-262, 1999.

Saulnier CF, Wheeler E: Social action research: influencing providers and recipients of health and mental health care for lesbians, *Affilia* 15(3):409-433, 2000.

Sheehy G: *New passages: mapping your life across time*, New York, 1996, Ballantine Books.

Shelton D: Health status of young offenders and their families, *J Nursing Scholarship* 32(2):173-178, 2000.

Shiffman S: Smoking cessation treatment: any progress? Special section: clinical research in smoking cessation, *J Consulting Clin Psychol*, 61:718-722, 1993.

Shinkman R: Healthcare behind bars, *Modern Healthcare* 20(23):18-19, 2000.

Sorensen G, Thompson B, Glanz K, et al.: Work site-based cancer prevention: primary results from the working well trial, *Am J Public Health* 86(7):939-947, 1996.

Stevens PE, Hall JM: Abusive health care interactions experienced by lesbians: cases of institutional violence, *Response* 13(3):23-27, 1990.

Stevens R: When your clients are in jail, *Nurs Forum* 28(4):5-8, 1995.

Stevenson JS: *Issues and crises during middlescence*, New York, 1977, Appleton-Century-Crofts.

Strange CJ: *Boning up on osteoporosis*, Pub No (FDA) 97-1257, Rockville, Md, 1998, US Food and Drug Administration.

Thompson JM, Wilson SF: *Health assessment for nursing practice*, St Louis, 1996, Mosby.

US Bureau of the Census: *Population profile of the United States: 1997*, Pub No P23-194, Washington, DC, 1998, US Government Printing Office.

US Bureau of the Census: 20th century statistics, *Statistical abstract of the United States: 1999*, Washington, DC, 2000a, US Government Printing Office.

US Bureau of the Census: *Who's minding the Kids? Childcare arrangements*, Pub No P70-70, Washington, DC, 2000b, US Government Printing Office.

US Department of Health, Education and Welfare (USDHEW): *Smoking and health: report of the advisory committee to the Surgeon General of the Public Health Service*, Washington, DC, 1964, US Government Printing Office.

US Department of Health and Human Services (USDHHS): *The Surgeon General's 1989 report on reducing the health consequences of smoking: 25 years of progress*, Washington, DC, 1989, US Government Printing Office.

US Department of Health and Human Services (USDHHS): *Healthy people 2000: midcourse review and 1995 revisions*, Washington, DC, 1995a, US Government Printing Office.

US Department of Health and Human Services (USDHHS): *The fifth report of the joint national committee on detection, evaluation, and treat-*

*ment of high blood pressure*, NIH Pub No 95-1088, Bethesda, Md, 1995b, Public Health Service.

US Department of Health and Human Services (USDHHS): *The sixth report of the joint national committee on detection, evaluation, and treatment of high blood pressure*, NIH Pub No 94-4080, Bethesda, Md, 1997, Public Health Service.

US Department of Health and Human Services (USDHHS): *Healthy people 2010: understanding and improving health*, ed 2, Washington, DC, 2000a, US Government Printing Office.

US Department of Health and Human Services (USDHHS): *Tracking Healthy People 2010*, Washington, DC, 2000b, US Government Printing Office.

Wallace JI, Buchner DM, Grothaus L, et al.: Implementation of effectiveness of a community-based health promotion program for older adults, *The Journals of Gerontology* 53A(4):M301-M306, 1998.

## SELECTED BIBLIOGRAPHY

Anonymous: An arresting situation, *Nursing* 29(12):73, 1999.

Anonymous: Report highlights gay and lesbian health issues, *Nation's Health* 30(2):18, 2000.

American Public Health Association (APHA): Lesbian, gay, bisexual, and transgender health, *Am J Public Health* 91(6):841-1004, 2001.

Barbeau EM, Li Y, Sorensen G, et al.: Coverage of smoking cessation treatment by union health and welfare funds, *Am J Public Health* 91(9):1412-1415, 2001.

Breslau N, Peterson EL: Smoking cessation in young adults: age at initiation of cigarette smoking, *Am J Public Health* 86(2):214-220, 1996.

Escobedo LG, Peddicord JP: Smoking prevalence in U.S. birth cohorts: the influence of gender and education, *Am J Public Health* 86(2):231-236, 1996.

Hitchcock JM, Wilson HS: Personal risking: lesbian self-disclosure of sexual orientation to professional health care providers, *Nurs Res* 41(3):178-183, 1992.

Kearney MH: Women don't get heart attacks? *Reflections on Nursing Leadership* 26(2):18-20, 2000.

Lipp EJ, Deane D, Trimble N: Cardiovascular risks in adolescent males, *Appl Nurs Res* 9(3):102-107, 1996.

Minken MJ: Answers to your top five menopause questions, *Prevention* 53(1):89-93, 2001.

Notelovitz M, Tonnessen D: *Menopause and midlife health*, New York, 1993, St. Martin's Press.

Parascandola M: Public health then and now: cigarettes and the U.S. Public Health Service in the 1950s, *Am J Public Health* 91(2):196-205, 2001.

Peden AR, Hall LA, Rayens MK, et al.: Reducing negative thinking and depressive symptoms in college women, *J Nursing Scholarship* 32(2):145-151, 2000.

Peterson E, Schultz L, Andreski P, et al.: Are smokers with alcohol disorders less likely to quit? *Am J Public Health* 86(7):985-990, 1996.

Sherrid P: Will boomer women defy menopause? The drug industry is betting they will try, *US News & World Report* 129(10):70, 2000.

Wallace MA: Looking at depression through bifocal lenses, *Nursing* 30(9):58-61, 2000.

Zapka JG, Bigelow C, Hurley T et al.: Mammography use among sociodemographically diverse women: the accuracy of self-report, *Am J Public Health* 86(7):1016-1021, 1996.

# The Adult Who Is Disabled

*Sandra L. McGuire*

*When working with persons who are disabled, remember that first they are persons and, second, they have a disabling condition.*

SANDRA L. McGUIRE

Since early in recorded history, people have noted the disabling conditions that existed among them. Disabling conditions were recorded as early as the fourth century BC (Buscaglia, 1983, p. 152). Hippocrates, Aristotle, Galen, and others studied such conditions and sought explanations for their existence.

Primitive people often believed that only the fit should survive and many ancient societies did not treat the disabled with caring or respect (Chin, Finnocchiaro, Rosebrough, 1998; Stryker, 1977). Across the ages, attitudes toward people who are disabled have ranged from acceptance to rejection and from understanding to fear. In early times disabling conditions were sometimes viewed as a punishment for sin, and the Elizabethan Poor Law of 1601 (see Chapter 4) equated such conditions with crime. Under this law people who were disabled were often publicly punished and imprisoned (Sussman, 1966, p. 3). The classic story of the *Hunchback of Notre Dame* illustrates society's reaction to disfigurement during the eighteenth century.

In early U.S. society, people who were disabled often were kept hidden in basements or attics or placed out of the way in the back wards of hospitals (Chin, Finnocchiaro,

Rosebrough, 1998; Martin, Holt, Hicks, 1981). In the mid-to-late 1800s institutional settings for people who were mentally ill or mentally retarded began to emerge in the United States, separating them from the mainstream of society. It would not be until 1893 that the first U.S. schools for "crippled children" were opened (Chin, Finnocchiaro, Rosebrough, 1998; Mumma, 1987).

Today being disabled is no longer considered a sin or a crime. However, people who are disabled may be socially stigmatized, socially isolated, and face discrimination. People with disabilities have multiple and complex health concerns. *Healthy People 2010* is attempting to address these concerns and improve the quality of life for people who are disabled.

## HEALTHY PEOPLE 2010 AND DISABLING CONDITIONS

*Healthy People 2000* did not have a specific priority area that addressed the health needs of people with disabilities. Instead, objectives that targeted people with disabilities were integrated throughout the document. Review of these objectives showed that none of them had been met (U.S. Department of Health and Human Services [USDHHS], 2000).

Disability is a focus area in *Healthy People 2010*. National health objectives for this focus area are given in Box 18-1.

These objectives emphasize increasing the quality of life for people with disabilities by decreasing depression, unhappiness, and sadness; increasing social participation and satisfaction with life; increasing emotional support; improving access to health and wellness programs; and improving access to technology.

Disabling conditions are a serious health problem for Americans. Disabilities are disproportionately represented among minorities, the elderly, and people of lower socioeconomic status (USDHHS, 2000). It is estimated that as many as 54 million Americans, 20% of the population, are disabled (USDHHS, 2000), and millions of Americans are limited in activity because of a disabling condition. The financial costs associated with disability amount to more than $300 billion each year in the United States and the psychosocial costs are incalculable (USDHHS, 2000). The number of people who are disabled increases each year in the United States.

### Stop and Think About It

What are some of the reasons why the numbers of people who are disabled is increasing? What community resources and services could help address the needs of people with disabilities? What role could community health nurses play in providing these services?

### BOX 18-1
### Focus Area: Disability and Secondary Conditions

Goal: Promote the health of people with disabilities, prevent secondary conditions, and eliminate disparities between people with and without disabilities in the U.S. population.

- Include in the core of all relevant *Healthy People 2010* surveillance instruments a standardized set of questions that identify "people with disabilities."
- Reduce the proportion of children and adolescents with disabilities who are reported to be sad, unhappy, or depressed.
- Reduce the proportion of adults with disabilities who report feelings such as sadness, unhappiness, or depression that prevent them from being active.
- Increase the proportion of adults with disabilities who participate in social activities.
- Increase the proportion of adults with disabilities reporting sufficient emotional support.
- Increase the proportion of adults with disabilities reporting satisfaction with life.
- Reduce the number of people with disabilities in congregate care facilities, consistent with permanency planning principles.
- Eliminate disparities in employment rates between working-aged adults with and without disabilities.
- Increase the proportion of children and youth with disabilities who spend at least 80 percent of their time in regular education programs.

- Increase the proportion of health and wellness and treatment programs and facilities that provide full access for people with disabilities.
- Reduce the proportion of people with disabilities who report not having the assistive devices and technology needed.
- Reduce the proportion of people with disabilities reporting environmental barriers to participation in home, school, work, or community activities.
- Increase the number of Tribes, States, and the District of Columbia that have public health surveillance and health promotion programs for people with disabilities and caregivers.

Related objectives are found in other focus areas including: Access to Quality Health Services; Arthritis, Osteoporosis, and Chronic Back Conditions; Cancer; Diabetes; Educational and Community-Based Programs; Family Planning; Heart Disease and Stroke; Immunization and Infectious Diseases; Maternal, Infant, and Child Health; Medical Product Safety; Mental Health and Mental Disorders; Nutrition and Overweight; Occupational Safety and Health; Oral Health; Physical Activity and Fitness, Public Health Infrastructure; Respiratory Disease; Substance Abuse; Tobacco Use; and Vision and Hearing.

Source: USDHHS: *Healthy People 2010, conference edition*, Washington, DC, 2000, US Government Printing Office, pp. 6-3 to 6-26.

## CHRONIC, DISABLING, AND HANDICAPPING CONDITIONS: RELATED BUT DISTINCT PHENOMENA

Words such as *disabled* and *handicapped* often elicit negative attitudes and stereotypes and are personally devaluing. Over the years "labels" such as *impaired, crippled, disabled, handicapped,* and *handicappers* have been used with varying levels of success to describe people with disabling conditions. Such descriptors have negative connotations and do not reflect the strengths of the person being described.

Whatever descriptors are used, the "people first" philosophy is of the utmost importance. This philosophy puts the person first—before the condition. It promotes treating people with respect, enhances personal growth and independence, and facilitates more positive societal attitudes. It reflects use of appropriate language, such as "The person who is disabled," instead of saying "The disabled person." Putting the person first is not just a matter of semantics; it is a matter of value and belief. The distinctions between chronic, disabling, and handicapping conditions are explained.

### Chronic Conditions

**Chronic conditions** were defined in Chapter 11 as "those illnesses that are prolonged, do not resolve spontaneously, and are rarely cured completely" (Marks, 1998, p. 6). They are responsible for 7 of 10 deaths, and medical costs for people with chronic illnesses total more than 60% of health care expenditures in the United States (Centers for Disease Control and Prevention [CDC], 1999). Chapter 16 looks at chronic conditions with children, and Chapter 17 looks at these conditions with adults. Box 18-2 outlines some common risk factors for chronic conditions.

### BOX 18-2

### *Common Risk Factors for Chronic Conditions*

Many chronic conditions share common risk factors, all of which can be partially or totally controlled including the following:

- Smoking
- Poor nutrition
- Sedentary lifestyle
- Alcohol and substance abuse
- Inadequate access to preventive health services (e.g., prenatal care, immunizations)
- Unprotected sexual intercourse

Developing strategies and actions plans to address these risk factors can have a profound effect on increasing the quality of life and years of healthy life.

From NCCDPHP: *CDC/NCCDPHP: turning research findings into effective community programs,* Atlanta, 1996, CDC; USDHHS: *Healthy People 2010, conference edition,* Washington, DC, 2000, US Government Printing Office.

Four chronic diseases—cardiovascular disease, cancer, chronic obstructive pulmonary disease (COPD), and diabetes—greatly diminish the quality of life for millions of Americans and account for about 75% of U.S. deaths each year. Other chronic conditions are arthritis; asthma; orthopedic impairments; cerebral palsy; epilepsy; mental retardation; mental illness; muscular dystrophy; multiple sclerosis; hearing and vision impairments; spinal cord injury; drug addiction; alcoholism; and perceptual handicaps such as dyslexia, brain dysfunction, and developmental aphasia.

Chronic conditions are a lifelong reality that creates a demand for new self-care practices (Eliopoulos, 1997). Research exploring the experience of people living with chronic conditions has shown recurring themes: maintaining hope, restructuring, reshaping or reconstituting self, regaining control, redefining health, managing, self-transcendence, and empowering potential as important to everyday life and adaptation to the condition (Thorne, Paterson, 1998).

*Although the prevalence of chronic conditions increases with age, they occur across the life span.* For example, traumatic injuries to the spinal cord occur most often to young men between the ages of 16 and 30 (Stucki, 1995, p. 10), and hearing, vision, and speech impairments are common in children and young adults. With advances in knowledge, science, and technology the number of people living with chronic conditions will continue to increase.

*Not all chronic conditions are disabling.* People can have a condition for a lifetime and not consider themselves disabled. Chronic conditions become disabling when they cause functional limitations, or "impairments," and adversely affect an individual's ability to carry out one or more *major life activity.* Major life activities include communication, ambulation, self-care, education, vocational training, employment, and transportation.

### Disabling Conditions

There is no consensus on a definition for the term **disability.** Historically, the definition of disability has been based on the medical model and emphasized functional limitations associated with the disability (Moore, Feist-Price, 1999). Within this model, disability refers to physical or psychological dysfunction that results in functional limitations. In its classic report, *Disability in America: Toward a National Agenda for Prevention,* the Institute of Medicine (IOM) recommended that a conceptual framework, standard measures of disability, and a national disability surveillance system be developed (Pope, Tarlov, 1991, pp. 102-103, 273, 275).

Our society's way of viewing disability is changing. Individuals and groups such as *Disabled Peoples International* favor definitions that define disability in terms of barriers in the environment rather than in terms of deficits in the individual (Richardson, 1997). Nurses need to be careful not to define people with disabilities by their limitations. Box 18-3 gives some definitions of disability.

### BOX 18-3
## *Some Definitions of Disability*

The *World Health Organization* (1981, p. 8) has defined a disability as any restriction or lack of ability to perform an activity in the manner, or within the range, considered normal for a human being.

The *National Institute on Disability and Rehabilitation Research (NIDRR)* has defined disability as a limitation in activity caused by a chronic condition or impairment. (Using this definition, a child under age 5 with a disability is one who is unable to participate in play activities; a child age 5 to 17 with a disability is one who needs to attend a special school or is limited or unable to attend school; and an adult with a disability is one who cannot work or do housework, is limited in the amount or kind of work or housework, or is limited in other activities) (Max, Rice, Trupin, 1996).

The *Americans with Disabilities Act* defined a disability as a physical or mental impairment that substantially limits one or more of an individual's major life activities. Included under this definition are individuals who have a record of an impairment or are regarded as having such an impairment.

A definition favored by disability rights advocates defines disability as "the loss or limitation of opportunities that prevents people who have impairments from taking part in the normal life of the community on an equal level with others due to physical and social barriers" (Finkelstein, French, 1993, p. 28).

According to the IOM (Pope, Tarlov, 1991, p. 3), health professionals should look at the risks for developing a disability or secondary condition related to the disability, assess how quality of life is affected by disabling conditions, and work toward improving it. The IOM also recommended conducting longitudinal studies that assist in determining the causes and rates of transition between pathology, impairment, functional limitation, and disability and that priorities be established for disability prevention. A model of disability that shows the interaction of the disabling process, quality of life, and risk factors is given in Figure 18-1.

Frequently a *secondary condition* will develop in relation to an existing disabling condition (e.g., pressure ulcers in a person with quadriplegia). Other common secondary conditions include contractures, phlebitis, cardiopulmonary conditions, and depression. *Healthy People 2010* addresses the need to limit secondary conditions. Nursing interventions play an important role in keeping these conditions from occurring.

Various personal, societal, and environmental variables influence the progression of a condition from pathology to disability, affect the degree of limitation a person experiences and the occurrence of secondary conditions, and have an impact on adaptation to the disability (Pope, Tarlov, 1991, p. 10). Interestingly, people with similar underlying

pathologies can have varying degrees of limitation (Lafata, Koch, Weissert, 1994, p. 1813). For example, a person with cerebral palsy may evidence functional abilities ranging from independence to total dependence. Figure 18-2 illustrates some functional limitations of adults with disabilities. Conditions such as developmental disabilities, birth defects, mental retardation, mental illness, emphysema, heart disease, orthopedic conditions, and arthritis are often disabling.

More than one third of people with disabilities have two or more disabling conditions (Trupin, Rice, 1995, p. 1). The risk of having multiple disabling conditions increases with age. Overall only 40% of people with disabling conditions rate their health as fair or poor (Trupin, Rice, 1995, p. 2). However, people with multiple disabling conditions have poorer health and use more medical services than those with only one condition (Trupin, Rice, 1995, p. 1).

LEVELS OF DISABILITY. The level of disability experienced by a person is generally looked at in terms of functional limitations. Functional limitations adversely affect an individual's ability to carry out one or more major life activity. Figure 18-3 presents the percentage of people experiencing limitation of major activity as a result of a disability by age. Functional limitations are determined by combining the results of the health history, clinical evaluation, assessment of client and family perception of the situation, and measurement of ability to carry out **activities of daily living (ADLs)** and **instrumental activities of daily living (IADLs).** ADLs include self-care activities necessary to survive such as eating, dressing, bathing, ambulating, and toileting. IADLs include activities such as performing housework, managing finances, cooking/meal preparation, doing laundry, shopping, running errands, taking medicine without help, and using the telephone. The level of disability caused by a handicapping condition determines client needs, and intervention strategies. General levels of disability are given in Box 18-4.

## Handicapping Conditions

**Handicap** refers not so much to an individual but to a social state—a status assigned to the person with impairment or disability by societal expectations and interactions (Patrick, 1994, p. 1724). Society creates handicaps—a disability becomes a handicap by societal definition. A handicap involves societal devaluation. An example of this is the public's attitude toward disfiguring impairments; these impairments often cause no functional limitation but impose a disability by affecting social acceptance and interaction (Pope, Tarlov, 1991, pp. 9-10, 91).

According to the World Health Organization (WHO) (1981, p. 8) a disease or condition becomes a handicap, according to the following schema:

Disease/condition → impairment → disability → handicap

Progression from one stage to another is not always linear or unidirectional. Individuals with handicapping conditions

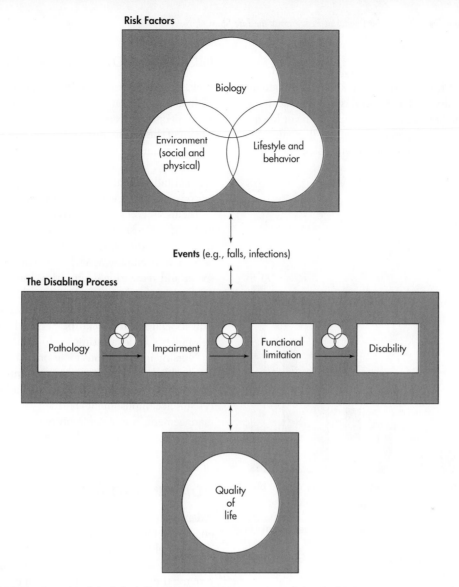

**FIGURE 18-1** Model of disability showing the interaction of the disabling process, quality of life, and risk factors. The potential for additional risk factors is shown between the stages of the model (e.g., falls, infections). (Reprinted with permission from Pope AM, Tarlov AR, editors: *Disability in America: toward a national agenda for prevention*, Washington, DC, 1991, National Academy Press, pp. 9, 85. © 1991 by the National Academy of Sciences. Courtesy of the National Academy Press, Washington, DC).

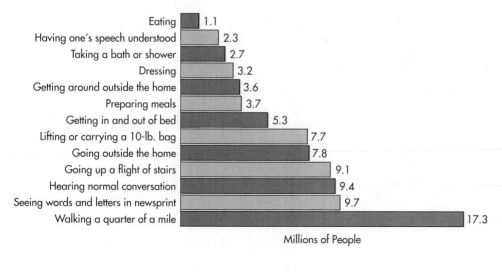

**FIGURE 18-2** Some functional limitations of adults with disabilities. (From US Department of Commerce: *Statistical abstract of the United States 1995,* ed 115, Washington, DC, 1995, US Government Printing Office, p. 138.)

have complex social, emotional, physical, educational, and financial needs that involve redefining family and community roles, relationships, and responsibilities. A handicap significantly limits one or more of an individuals' major life activities and results in functional limitations that affect an individual's ability to fulfill normal societal roles.

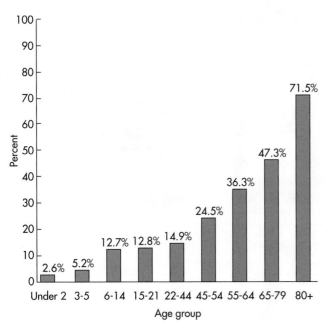

**FIGURE 18-3** Disability status of people by age. (From US Department of Commerce: *Statistical abstract of the United States: 1999*, ed 119, Washington, DC, 1999, US Government Printing Office, p. 151).

## INCLUSIVE COMMUNITY ACTIVITIES

Inclusive community activities help include the person with a disability into the *mainstream* of community life. Many people who are disabled already function in the mainstream of the community and are difficult to distinguish from other community members. For others, special efforts need to be taken for this integration to occur (e.g., persons who are mentally retarded, persons with spinal cord injury, and persons who are severely physically handicapped).

Inclusive community activities help people live as normal a life as possible. They involve assisting people in participating in the same activities as other community members such as employment, home maintenance, school, and social and recreational activities. Inclusive activities focus on maximizing the strengths of people who are disabled, enhancing their quality of life, and reducing their social isolation. Social isolation can be personally devaluing and developmentally devastating.

Nursing interventions focus on assisting individuals who are disabled in becoming integrated into the mainstream of community life and living as normal a life as possible. Successful accomplishment of such outcomes requires care management, use of community resources, and recognition that people who are disabled are entitled to the same rights and respect as everyone else.

## ADAPTING TO A DISABILITY

Adapting to a disability is a complex process and is influenced by individual, family, and societal variables. How these variables interact with each other determines how well the individual and family adapts. Limiting disability and improving the quality of life are goals of the adaptation process. Box 18-5 lists variables affecting adaptation to a disability. These variables are discussed in the following sections.

 **BOX 18-4**

*Levels of Disability*

*Level I:* Partial disability characterized by slight limitation in one or more of the major life activities; able to take part in school, competitive employment, and self-care

*Level II:* Partial disability characterized by moderate limitation in one or more of the major life activities; generally able to attend school, work regularly or part-time (but the employment may need to be modified); may need assistance with self-care

*Level III:* Partial disability characterized by severe limitation in one or more of the major life activities; usually unable to attend school or work regularly (considered occupationally disabled); often requires assistance with self-care

*Level IV:* Total disability characterized by complete, or almost complete, dependency on others for activities of daily living, self-care, and economic support; usually unable to work or attend regular school

 **BOX 18-5**

*Variables Affecting Adaptation to a Disability*

Societal attitudes
Attitudes of health care professionals
Family variables
The stage of grief and mourning
Age at which the disabling condition occurred
Age-appropriateness of the disability
Rapidity of onset of the disability
Level of disability caused by the disabling condition
Visibility of the disability
Value of the disabled area
Attitudes regarding self
Attitudes of significant others
Community resources available and used
Coping mechanisms used
Prognosis and/or expected duration of the disability

## Societal Attitudes

As previously mentioned, societal attitudes play a major role in individual and family adaptation to disabling conditions. In fact, the debilitating aspects of a disability result not so much from the condition itself but from the manner in which others define and respond to it. Societal attitudes are some of the most difficult barriers to overcome and can be more handicapping to the individual than the disability itself (Moore, Feist-Price, 1999; President's Committee on Employment of People with Disabilities [PCEPD], 1999). "Whether born from ignorance, fear, misunderstanding or hate, these attitudes keep people from appreciating—and experiencing—the full potential a person with a disability can achieve" (PCEPD, 1999).

Societal attitudes have been described as "invisible barriers" (Kendrick, 1983, p. 17). The impact of these barriers is seen in the quote from Deborah Kendrick, a mother who is blind:

The difficulty is neither in being blind nor in being a mother. It is in the attitudes of others, the invisible barriers which can separate me from other mothers and my children from their children (Kendrick, 1983, p. 18).

Lack of knowledge and misconceptions about disabling conditions contribute to such attitudinal barriers (PCEPD, 1999). Persons who are disabled are often stereotyped as helpless, incompetent, suffering, and dependent (Gatens-Robinson, Rubin, 1995; Moore, Feist-Price, 1999). They may be held at least partially responsible for their disability.

In her classic work on disability, Safilios-Rothschild (1982), identified a number of societal variables that affect attitudes toward people who are disabled. These variables are presented in Box 18-6. Different societies view disabling conditions differently, as shown in the example of Donald Sims (Figure 18-4), who has impaired functioning of his lower extremities following a motorcycle accident. He found that when he visited the Choco Indians in Panama his strengths were respected and his differences accepted. The attitudes of the Choco Indians helped him to realize his potential, and Sims stated:

An unbelievable experience! They treated me as though I was no different—I was accepted as a person—a people, a culture with no concept of handicapped. I did what I could, they did their thing, and we all worked and played together. No one shied away from the chair. The Choco Indians made my Panama trip the most wonderful experience since my accident. They helped reinstate my faith in people, life itself, and a positive attitude toward all things.

Societal attitudes can increase the social isolation of people who are disabled. In breaking down these attitudes and barriers, "The best remedy is familiarity, getting people with and without disabilities to mingle as coworkers,

**BOX 18-6**

*Variables Affecting Societal Attitudes Toward People Who Are Disabled*

### Beliefs Regarding the Value of Physical and Mental Integrity

The value a society places on physical and mental integrity greatly affects societal acceptance of people who are disabled and the scope of services offered to them. If a society highly values physical and mental integrity and "devalues" people who are disabled, they may experience prejudice, discrimination, and be isolated from the mainstream of society in placements such as institutions for the mentally ill and mentally retarded and other long-term care facilities.

### Beliefs in Relation to Illness

In most societies, people who are acutely ill are usually allowed to be "sick" for the duration of their illness. However, once the condition becomes chronic, the person may be expected to "adjust" and may even be expected to perform "normally" in relation to societal roles and expectations, even when achieving such behavior may be difficult.

### Beliefs Regarding Condition Occurrence

If it is believed that the individual had a high degree of responsibility in the occurrence of the condition, less aid and assistance may be given. Obesity, alcoholism, mental illness, AIDS, domestic violence, and drug abuse are examples of this.

### The Role of the Government in Alleviating Social Problems

If a society does not believe that the government should assume an active role in alleviating social problems, there may be little public assistance or social support for people who are disabled. Also the government may assume a treatment or assistance role rather than a preventive one.

### Beliefs Regarding the Origins of Poverty

Many people who have disabling conditions live in poverty. If a society believes that poverty is generally a matter of self-will, there may be less willingness to assist people who are disabled.

### The Rate of Unemployment and Economic Development

When unemployment is high and/or the economy is unstable, people who are disabled may be at a disadvantage in hiring and employment practices, and there also may be less inclination to financially subsidize those who are disabled.

Modified from Safilios-Rothschild C: *The sociology and social psychology of disability rehabilitation,* New York, 1982, University Press of America, p. 4.

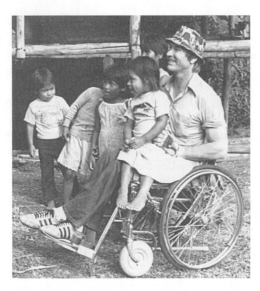

**FIGURE 18-4** Societal attitudes influence how individuals, families, and groups perceive differences among individuals in a society and can facilitate or inhibit individual growth and development. (Courtesy Donald Sims and photographer H. Morgan Smith, Explorations, Brigade Quartermasters. Morgan Smith is an honorary member of the Choco Indian tribe and is an anthropologist and naturalist who has conducted numerous archeological excavations.)

associates and social acquaintances. In time most of the attitudes will give way to comfort, respect and friendship" (PCEPD, 1999).

Language used to describe people who are disabled should emphasize abilities and competencies and not foster dependency (Richardson, 1997). Negative descriptors and language can lead to learned helplessness and social devaluation. **Learned helplessness** is largely a societal phenomena. It occurs when people with disabilities are socialized by their environment to assume a dependent role. Nurses want to encourage independence and build on the competencies of people who are disabled.

The nurse needs to evaluate her or his attitudes toward people with disabilities and work to promote positive, facilitative societal attitudes toward people who are disabled. The nurse can be a role model of interaction and caring for people who are disabled.

### Attitudes of Health Care Professionals

The attitudes of health professionals greatly influence a person's response to treatment and adaptation to the disability (Oermann, Lindgren, 1995, p. 8). Too often health care professionals look on people who are disabled in terms of their limitations instead of their strengths and promote dependence rather than independence. It is not uncommon for people who are disabled to report that health care professionals are not knowledgeable about the special needs imposed by their disability and the resources that they need.

They report that health care professionals sometimes seem insensitive and disinterested in them.

Health care professionals need to apply the "people first" philosophy discussed earlier in this chapter. The person's dignity and privacy should be maintained. Special comfort measures may need to be taken when doing exams and procedures with people who experience disabling conditions and extra time may be needed when doing health histories and physical exams. Nurses need to assess and overcome their own attitudinal barriers toward disabling conditions and develop facilitative attitudes toward clients regardless of the level of disability and potential for rehabilitation (Oermann, Lindgren, 1995, p. 8).

### Family Variables

When persons become disabled, they and their families experience stress. The protracted stress of providing care for family members with disabling conditions can cause families to dissolve or develop psychosocial issues such as emotional difficulties, substance abuse, frustration, and isolation (Breese, Mikrut, 1995, p. 39). Families of persons who are disabled may be treated as if they were different from other families or somehow to blame for the disability. This can heighten stress and make it more difficult for families to adjust.

Each family adapts and copes differently. As discussed in Chapter 8, some families are more vulnerable to stress than others, and disabling conditions can produce stress for the entire family. The availability of appropriate community resources can assist the family in adapting to the disability and prevent family burnout. Family adaptation is a significant factor in client progress and outcomes (Canam, Acorn, 1999; Thomas, Ellison, Howell, et al., 1992; Weeks, 1995).

Disabling conditions often require that a family reallocate goals and priorities, division of labor, use of time, family roles, financial resources, and caregiving—sometimes on a long-term basis. This frequently happens in families with a member who is severely disabled. Take, for example, this case scenario of parents of a child who is severely mentally disabled.

**CASE** *Scenario* With the help of community supports such as school programs and community health nursing services, Mr. and Mrs. Zelinski had been able to care at home for Joshua, their 19-year-old son who has been severely mentally retarded since birth. Mrs. Zelinski gave up her job when Joshua was born so that she would be available to take care of him. Joshua's medical care frequently strained family finances. Respite care was not readily available in their community, and the Zelinskis rarely traveled or did things together without Joshua. Joshua has reached the age of adulthood and is unable to live independently. Except for a state institution, there are no other local residential placements for him, and the Zelinskis had mutually decided that institutional placement was not an acceptable option for them. When other parents were launching their adult children, Mr. and Mrs. Zelinski were reassessing family goals, roles, finances, and resources and prepared to continue to care for their adult child at home.

Situations like this are not uncommon, and lack of appropriate community resources often creates stress. Frequently, the financial demands of the condition place economic hardships and stress on the family. While caring for a disabled family member, families are expected to carry out other day-to-day activities and responsibilities, such as school, work, and household maintenance. The stress of these multiple roles and activities can be overwhelming and result in caregiver burnout.

The emotional, physical, and financial toll of caring for a family member who is disabled can be immense. If the stress of caregiving becomes too great, a decision may be made to place the family member who is disabled outside the home. Families are likely to make placements outside the home when the person is severely disabled; the family cannot provide adequate care and resources; there is a high level of family conflict and discord, such as marital dissatisfaction; and community resources are insufficient. The recent story of a family that abandoned their 10-year-old, respirator-dependent son at a local hospital because they could no longer physically care for him is an illustration of what can happen when a family reaches the "breaking point" (El Nasser, 1999).

Eliopoulos (1997) suggests the use of *chronic care coaches* to ease caregiver stress and provide support and guidance to the person who is disabled. Virtually anyone can serve as a coach, and local support groups and other community agencies can be a source of recruitment (Eliopoulos, 1997). Coaches need to be readily available, knowledgeable about the condition, and offer optimism and encouragement.

Nursing interventions focus on minimizing family stress and promoting adaptation. The nurse serves as a case manager, coordinating activities, maintaining communication with the client and family, and linking clients to community resources. Supportive nursing interventions can help alleviate some of the stress the family is experiencing. Respite care, discussed later in this chapter, often helps alleviate family stress.

## Stage of Grief and Mourning

The stage of **grief and mourning** the individual and family have reached in relation to the condition is important. The person and family have suffered a loss. This loss may take many forms, such as loss of independence, control over life, privacy, body image, body functioning, social status, financial stability, employment, material possessions, and predetermined self-fulfillment. Losses in terms of changes in personal relationships and roles also may occur. The process may be compounded by the fact that there may be no immediate end in sight, and the individual is grieving personally while experiencing the effects of significant others

**BOX 18-7**

*Grief and Mourning Process
with Disabling Conditions*

- *Denial.* The individual/family is not prepared to accept the reality and ramifications of the disability and deny that it is occurring.
- *Awareness.* The individual/family realizes that the disability is real; the loss becomes real; and feelings of hostility, bitterness, and anger can arise in response to it.
- *Mourning.* The individual/family actively grieves for the loss that has occurred.
- *Depression.* The individual/family realizes the permanency, long-term nature, or other ramifications of the condition and experiences feelings of rejection, helplessness, altered self-esteem, and despair. This is often a very encompassing and time-consuming stage.
- *Adaptation.* The individual/family becomes capable of coping with the disability. Although periods of depression may occur periodically, the goal of this stage is equilibrium and rehabilitation.

grieving as well. Unresolved grief can seriously alter and affect interpersonal relationships and family functioning. Until grieving has been successfully accomplished, treatment, rehabilitation, and adaptation cannot be fully successful.

Community health nurses play a major role in helping families experience a healthy grieving process. Being able to accept the fact that *grief is normal* helps the nurse assist families in working through the process in a constructive manner.

The grief and mourning process in relation to a disabling condition closely resembles the stages discussed by Kubler-Ross (1969), in her classic studies on death and dying. Box 18-7 outlines the grief and mourning process that a person and family experience while adapting to a disabling condition. A phenomenon associated with the grief and mourning process is that of chronic sorrow.

CHRONIC SORROW. Chronic sorrow is a term used to describe the long-term periodic sadness and depression the client and family experience in relation to chronic illness (Lindgren, Burke, Hainsworth, Eakes, 1992, p. 27). This long-term sadness has been described as "recurring waves of grief" experienced by individuals and caregivers whose anticipated life course has been disrupted (Eakes, Burke, Hainsworth, 1998, p. 179). It is cyclical and potentially progressive in nature (Eakes, Burke, Hainsworth, 1998; North American Nursing Diagnosis Association [NANDA], 2001). It is a form of unresolved grieving and continues as long as the disparity created by the loss remains (Eakes, Burke, Hainsworth, 1998).

Chronic sorrow is commonly experienced by people who have encountered significant loss or experience ongoing loss (Eakes, Burke, Hainsworth, 1998). The critical attributes of chronic sorrow are given in Box 18-8. Although it is

**BOX 18-8**

*Critical Attributes of Chronic Sorrow*

> There is a perception of sorrow or sadness over time in a situation that has no predictable end.
> The sadness or sorrow is cyclic or recurrent.
> The sorrow or sadness is triggered either internally or externally and brings to mind the person's losses, disappointment, or fears.
> The sadness or sorrow is progressive and can intensify even years after the initial sense of disappointment, loss, or fear.

From Lindgren CL, Burke ML, Hainsworth MA, Eakes GG: Chronic sorrow: a lifespan concept, *Schol Inq Nurs Pract* 6(1):31, 1992. Used by permission of Springer Publishing Co., Inc., NY, 10013.

natural for chronic sorrow to occur, the nurse should work with the client and family to help achieve grief resolution and promote successful coping and adaptation.

## Age and Age-Appropriateness of the Condition

The *age* at which a disabling condition occurs and the *age-appropriateness* of the condition are also critical to adaptation. Disabling conditions that occur after the development of personal self-image frequently cause more difficulty with coping and adaptation. A child born without an arm will have a different adjustment process than the child who loses an arm at age 5 or the adult who loses an arm at age 50. The internalized body image of the adult makes it difficult to accept, much less incorporate, drastic alterations of body structure. An "age-appropriate" disability is often more easily accepted. For example, an elderly person with a hearing loss or arthritis may be more readily integrated and accepted, and more societal resources may be available for this person than for a preschooler with the same condition. However, an adult who is mentally retarded may have a more difficult time being mainstreamed than a child with the same condition.

## Condition Onset

The *rapidity of a condition's onset* is critical to adjustment. If a condition develops gradually, as does rheumatoid arthritis, the adjustment time is lengthened and there is an opportunity to develop skills, resources, support systems, and coping mechanisms. If the occurrence is sudden, as with traumatic injury (e.g., spinal cord injury), there is little or no adjustment time. Sudden change that affects personal functioning and self-image, as well as the image held by others, is difficult to incorporate into one's body image.

## Level of Disability

The level of disability associated with a condition has already been discussed in this chapter. Generally, the greater the *level of disability*, the more difficult it is to adjust to the condition. An individual with a paralyzed hand will likely have less difficulty in adjustment than a paraplegic or a person who is severely mentally retarded. The level of disability is a major determinant of the functional capacity of the individual and the response of society to the disability.

## Condition Visibility

The *visibility* of the condition affects the adjustment made to it. People generally have stronger reactions to visible conditions than to nonvisible ones. Visible conditions generally elicit more discriminating individual and societal responses than a nonvisible or slightly visible condition. For example, a person with severe diabetes with target organ damage due to the condition will likely elicit less societal discrimination than a person who is physically challenged or mentally retarded. Nurses need to remember that conditions that may have little or no outward visibility can still cause significant concern for the individual (e.g., sexual dysfunction). From another viewpoint, an "invisible" disability such as a serious heart condition may not be acknowledged by society even though the condition places severe functional limitation on the individual (e.g., the individual may be expected to perform as if no impairment existed).

## Attitudes Regarding Self/Attitudes of Significant Others

How one regards oneself and the attitudes of significant others have an important effect on an individual's psychosocial adjustment to the condition. The attitudes and expectations of family, friends, and health care professionals significantly influence the self-perceptions of people who are disabled (Oermann, Lindgren, 1995, p. 6). The nurse can assist clients in building positive attitudes by looking at their strengths and enhancing their self-esteem. Box 18-9 provides nursing activities that assist clients in enhancing their self-esteem. The nurse serves as a role model for promoting positive attitudes toward people with disabilities and disabling conditions.

## Value of the Disabled Area

The personal and social value placed on body parts or functions significantly affects the type and degree of stigma attached to the disability. The value placed on body parts and functions varies from individual to individual and between societies; however, some seem to have a higher value than others. The example of facial disfigurement helps illustrate the value placed on a specific part of the body. Although facial disfigurement usually causes few functional limitations, it is one of the most difficult disabling conditions to adjust to because of the high value placed on facial characteristics.

## Availability of Community Resources

*Community resources* play a key role in disability outcome, and adjustment is impeded if necessary resources are not

**BOX 18-9**

## NIC Nursing Intervention: Self-Esteem Enhancement

| | |
|---|---|
| **Definition**<br>Assisting a client to increase his/her personal judgment of self-worth<br><br>**Activities**<br>Monitor client's statements of self-worth<br>Determine client's locus of control<br>Determine client's confidence in own judgment<br>Encourage client to identify strengths<br>Encourage eye contact in communicating with others<br>Reinforce the personal strengths that client identifies<br>Provide experiences that increase client's autonomy, as appropriate<br>Assist client to identify positive responses from others<br>Refrain from negatively criticizing<br>Refrain from teasing<br>Convey confidence in client's ability to handle situation<br>Assist in setting realistic goals to achieve higher self-esteem<br>Assist client to accept dependence on others, as appropriate<br>Assist client to reexamine negative perceptions of self | Encourage increased responsibility for self, as appropriate<br>Assist client to identify the impact of peer group on feelings of self-worth<br>Explore previous achievements of success<br>Explore reasons for self-criticism or guilt<br>Encourage client to evaluate own behavior<br>Encourage client to accept new challenges<br>Reward or praise client's progress toward reaching goals<br>Facilitate an environment and activities that will increase self-esteem<br>Assist client to identify significance of culture, religion, race, gender, and age on self-esteem<br>Instruct parents on the importance of their interest and support in their children's development of a positive self-concept<br>Instruct parents to set clear expectations and to define limits with their children<br>Teach parents to recognize children's accomplishments<br>Monitor frequency of self-negating verbalizations<br>Monitor lack of follow-through in goal attainment<br>Monitor levels of self-esteem over time, as appropriate |

From McCloskey JC, Bulechek GM, editors: *Nursing interventions classification (NIC)*, ed 3, St Louis, 2000, Mosby, p. 580.

available and accessible. Nurses need to be familiar with community resources and know how to use the referral process (see Chapter 10).

Private, voluntary agencies (see Chapter 5) that provide direct services to people who are disabled are noted throughout this chapter. They include organizations such as the American Cancer Society, American Lung Association, and American Heart Association. A relatively new nationwide service for linking people to community services is the 211 dialing code (Deoudes, 2000). Much like the 911 emergency dialing code, in communities that have 211 dialing, information and referral services are provided that link people to basic humans needs resources. Communities across the nation are establishing 211 dialing systems. Appendix 18-1 gives a listing of numerous agencies that people who are disabled often use. Governmental agencies are discussed later in this chapter.

### Stop and Think About It

What resources are available in your community for people who are disabled? What role do you envision you might assume as a nurse when working with these resources? How could nurses enhance resource availability?

### Coping Abilities

The *coping abilities* of the individual and family are crucial, and how well the family is able to cope with the disabling condition will influence the client's recovery and adaptation (see Chapter 8). Using effective coping strategies can moderate the emotional and psychological impact of the condition and help mediate physical aspects. Effective coping helps reduce tension and maintain equilibrium, promote family growth, enhance sound decision making, maintain autonomy, avoid the use of negative self-evaluation, and control potential stressors before they become a problem (Miller, 1992, p. 21). Having a responsive health care delivery system and appropriate community resources aids the family in successful coping.

### Condition Prognosis

The *prognosis* of the condition is an important variable in adaptation. If the long-term prognosis does not show much hope of cure or recovery, it can be discouraging, even devastating, to the client and family. Conditions for which the prognosis is more encouraging make it easier for the family to cope and adapt. It is crucial for the community health nurse to identify variables that may hamper successful adaptation. Once such variables are identified, the nurse can develop interventions to counteract their effect and facilitate adaptation.

### Chronic Pain

Pain is an important variable in adapting to and coping with a disabling condition. People who are in chronic pain experience quality of life issues. Many people with disabilities experience chronic pain.

Chronic pain is pain that recurs or persists over an extended period of time and interferes with functioning (Simon, McTier, 1996, p. 20). Chronic pain affects more than 50 million Americans and is described by some health experts as the major cause of disability in the nation (Simon, McTier, 1996). It is a common element of many disabling conditions, and chronic pain syndrome is in itself a disabling condition. Chronic pain has a significant effect on individuals and their families and impedes a person's ability to work and to perform role function. Rehabilitation programs have been designed specifically to address chronic pain (Vines, Cox, Nicoll, et al., 1996, p. 25). The goal of a nurse in pain management is to im-

prove the level of functioning for those affected by pain (Association of Rehabilitation Nurses [ARN], 1994b).

People suffering from chronic pain evidence inactivity, depression, disruption of marital and family relationships, use of drugs to control the pain, disruptions in sleep patterns, and disruptions in eating (weight gain or loss) (Simon, 1996, p. 14). Research has resulted in the development of a Chronic Pain Assessment Tool for Nurses (Simon, McTier, 1996). The pain history section of the tool is given in Figure 18-5.

Simon (1996) found three common nursing diagnoses for clients with chronic pain: (1) ineffective coping related to chronic pain, (2) activity intolerance related to de-

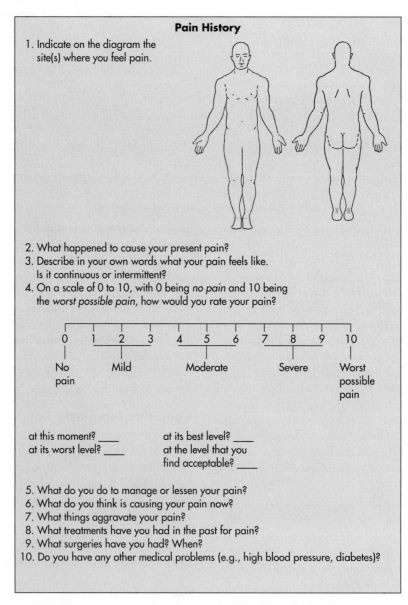

**FIGURE 18-5** Pain history section of a chronic pain assessment tool. (Reprinted from Simon JM, McTier CL: Development of a chronic pain assessment tool, *Rehabil Nurs* 21[1]:20-24, 1996, with permission of the Association of Rehabilitation Nurses, 4700 W Lake Avenue, Glenview, Ill, 60025-1485. © 1996 Association of Rehabilitation Nurses.)

creased muscle tone and strength from inactivity secondary to chronic pain, and (3) sleep pattern disturbance related to pain and distress. Nursing roles in pain management include those of educator, clinician, and case manager. Interventions should be directed at assessing and monitoring the pain, pain control and reduction, and educating the client and the family about chronic pain. This education includes information on the physiology of the affected body systems, pain cycle, exercise and body mechanics in relation to pain, the purpose and side effects of the pain medication, problem-solving skills and communication techniques, good nutrition, and sleep enhancement (Simon, 1996). Research has shown that rehabilitation programs for pain, managed and evaluated primarily by professional rehabilitation nurses, have been successful in helping clients control their pain and achieve a higher level of physical functioning and role performance (Vines, Cox, Nicoll, et al., 1996, p. 30).

## SOME AREAS OF CONCERN FOR PEOPLE WHO ARE DISABLED

Some areas of concern for people who are disabled are listed in Box 18-10 and discussed in the following sections. Many of these concerns focus on improving the quality of life and allowing the person who is disabled to lead as normal a life as possible. The degree to which these concerns are evidenced is highly individual.

### Education

Historically, people who are disabled have been at an educational disadvantage in the United States. It was not until 1975 that the federal government enacted a law mandating a free, appropriate education for all children, regardless of their disabilities (see Chapters 4 and 16). This law was the *Education for All Handicapped Children Act*, which later became the *Individuals with Disabilities Education Act (IDEA)*.

**BOX 18-10**

*Some Areas of Concern for People Who Are Disabled*

Education
Financial stability
Employment
Access to resources and services
Health care
Social, recreational, and athletic opportunities
Sexuality
Guardianship
Community residential opportunities
Attendant services
Respite care
Civil rights

Before the federal law in 1975, if a person did not fit into existing local school district programs, the school district was not responsible for the person's education, and many persons who were disabled were denied an education unless their families could afford to send them to private schools. Today, local public school districts *must* provide a free, appropriate education for all children with disabilities.

In regard to postsecondary education, the person with a disability must be considered on academic records and cannot be discriminated against because of the disability. Also, educational programs cannot limit the number of disabled students admitted and are required to accommodate the student who is disabled. The *HEATH Resource Center* in Washington, D.C., is the national clearinghouse for postsecondary education information for individuals with disabilities. This is a valuable resource because more students with disabilities are attending college than ever before. Almost 10% of entering college freshman, or 15,000 students, have a disability (Greenberg, 2000). Before the passage of the Education for All Handicapped Children Act in the 1970s this percentage was only 3% (Greenberg, 2000).

*Gallaudet University* in Washington, D.C., is funded by the federal government to provide a college education for people who are deaf, and federal funding supports the *Helen Keller National Center for Deaf-Blind Youth and Adults*. Many states operate special schools for people who are blind or deaf. The U.S. Department of Education recognizes the *Distance Education and Training Council* in Washington, D.C., and its *Directory of Accredited Institutions* as a resource for locating quality schools of home study. The *National Library Service for the Blind and Physically Handicapped* has a network of libraries throughout the United States that produce, distribute, and loan educational materials.

Education in the arts is often overlooked when planning care for people who are disabled. Some organizations that promote and enable artistic expression for people who are disabled are given in Box 18-11. Local communities often have programs in the arts available.

Other resources to facilitate the educational endeavors of people who are disabled include homebound and computerized instruction, libraries, Braille and audiobooks for the visually impaired, closed caption educational programming for people who are hard of hearing, and modified classrooms for the physically impaired.

Professional and public education about disabling conditions and disability prevention is needed. More education must be carried out by public health agencies, schools, and at home to instill in people the importance of healthful, disability preventing behaviors (Pope, Tarlov, 1991, p. 211).

**COMPUTERS AND EDUCATION.** Computers have numerous applications in the classroom, home, and community and have the potential to greatly enhance the quality of life of people who are disabled. Americans with disabilities are less than half as likely as their nondisabled counterparts to own a computer, and they are about one quarter as

### BOX 18-11
*Disability and the Arts*

Very Special Arts (VSA)
*http://www.vsarts.org*
Very Special Arts (VSA) was founded in 1974 by Jean Kennedy Smith. It is an affiliate of the John F. Kennedy Center for the Performing Arts in Washington, D.C. VSA has affiliates in 40 states and 83 countries. VSA creates and supports learning opportunities through the arts for people with disabilities and sponsors arts programs, awards, and festivals. Programs are implemented through an extensive network of state, local, and international organizations. Its *Arts for Children in Hospitals Program* links medical students with children. Its *Disability Awareness Guide* provides concise definitions of various disabilities and suggestions for productive interactions with people who are disabled. The Very Special Arts Gallery in Washington, D.C. showcases the work of artists with disabilities. It can be reached at 1-800-933-8721.

National Institute of Art and Disabilities (NIAD)
*http://www.niadart.org*
The institute is in Richmond, California. It operates programs, provides professional training and consultation, and helps establish art centers and programs for children and adults with disabilities. NIAD offers creative opportunities including print making, ceramics, textiles, decorative arts, and sculpture. Promotes exhibitions of creative art of people with disabilities. Publications include *Freedom to Create, The Creative Spirit, Art and Disabilities,* and *Disabled Artist at Work,* as well as a quarterly newsletter. It has served as a prototype for similar programs nationwide.

Kardon Institute of the Arts for People with Disabilities (KIA)
*http://www.kardoninstitute.org*
The institute is in Philadelphia, Pennsylvania. Its mission is to make the joys and benefits of participation and education in the arts accessible to persons with disabilities. Its programs include instrumental and vocal instruction and music therapy. It provides information on establishing music programs for people who are disabled and has an extensive library collection on the topic of music for the disabled, including a collection of large print and Braille music, textbooks, and supportive materials on all areas of teaching music to people who are disabled. It publishes *Guide to the Selection of Musical Instruments with Respect to Physical Ability and Disability,* the first reference book of its kind on the subject.

likely to use the internet (Kaye, 2000). Computers have the potential to greatly broaden the lives and educational opportunities of people with disabilities. For example, screen readers can provide blind people with instant access to vast quantities of online information; voice recognition can enable people with limited manual dexterity to manage finances and perform work-related tasks; and email can link people who are homebound with friends, relatives, and community resources (Kaye, 2000). People who are disabled need to be facilitated in using this valuable resource to enhance their lives. Most large computer companies offer special services and programs that help link people who are disabled with computer services and resources. Examples of these programs are Apple Computer's Disability Solutions Group and International Business Machines (IBM) Independence Series (1-800-426-4832). These companies provide services such as adaptive devices, software programs, and publications and help people use computers to enhance their quality of life.

### Financial Stability

Financial stability is a major concern for people who are disabled. Although many adults who are disabled are financially independent, some are unable to achieve this independence and must rely on assistance programs for financial support. Many families with a disabled member have financial problems as a result of the disabling condition.

Financial assistance programs for the adult who is disabled are offered through the state Department of Social Services (DSS) or the federal Social Security Administration (SSA) (see Chapter 5). Under the Social Security Administration, the person who is disabled may be eligible for *Social Security Disability Insurance* benefits or *Supplemental Security Income* (SSI). Under DSS the person may be eligible for all forms of aid such as General Assistance, Temporary Assistance to Needy Families (TANF), and Medicaid. The individual also may receive private disability insurance benefits. However, many people do not have private disability insurance coverage.

### Employment

Whatever the employment setting, the skills and talents of persons with disabilities can be used, and industries across the country employ people with disabilities. However, many adults who are disabled remain unemployed or underemployed, despite their ability to take part in meaningful work in the community. Many people who are disabled and not working believe that attitudinal barriers keep them from working (e.g., that employers are unwilling to recognize that they are capable of taking on a full-time job) (PCEPD, 1999). A majority of people with disabilities who work have encountered supervisors and co-workers who believe that a person with a disability "cannot do the job" (PCEPD, 1999).

The President's Committee on Employment of the Handicapped was established by President Harry Truman in 1947 to facilitate employment of disabled war veterans and other handicapped Americans. That committee is now the *Office of Disability Employment Policy (ODEP)* (*http://www.dol.gov/dol/odep*) and works to enhance the employment of all people with disabilities. The committee sponsors the *Job Accommodation Network (JAN)*, an information service that assists employers in accommodating the workplace for the worker who is disabled. Many states have a Governor's Committee on Employment of People with Disabilities.

The federal *Job Training Partnership Program* offers job training for people to obtain productive employment, and many people with disabilities fit the eligibility criteria for the program. *Federal Job Information Centers* have placement coordinators who provide assistance to individuals with disabilities and offer information about federal employment opportunities. Across the nation more than 2000 local branches of state Employment Service offices (see state government resources in this chapter) are mandated by law to employ a specialist trained in working with people who are disabled to assist them in finding employment. Publications such as *Job Strategies for People with Disabilities* assist people who are disabled in looking for employment.

Disabling conditions can limit a person's ability to work (Figure 18-6). Adults who are disabled are found in competitive, modified, and sheltered employment. **Competitive employment** is work with nondisabled members of the workforce on an equal basis, such as a job on the assembly line at an automotive factory. **Modified employment** is work done with nondisabled members of the workforce, but the environment has been modified to meet the needs of the workers who are disabled. **Sheltered employment** (Figure 18-7) is work that is available specifically for people who are disabled and is done under direct supervision and guidance. Private organizations such as Associations for Retarded Citizens (ARCs), Goodwill Industries, and the National Industries for the Severely Handicapped (*http://www.nish.org*) support and sponsor sheltered employment. Federal legislation provides for special preference being given in bidding on government contracts to workplaces offering sheltered employment.

Under the Americans with Disabilities Act (ADA), workplaces are required to make *reasonable accommodations* for workers who are disabled. Such accommodations are usually not expensive. Data collected by the President's Committee on Employment of People with Disabilities showed that 18% of employers reported that making such accommodations cost them nothing, 50% said the cost was $500 or less, and only 5% reported costs greater than $5000 (Reasonable accommodation, 1995, p. 6). Overall, companies have an average return of $28.69 in benefits for every dollar invested in making an accommodation (PCEPD, 1996), and the accommodations usually qualify for employer tax credits.

*Job coaches* may be provided through the employer to furnish specialized on-site training to assist an employee with a disability in learning and performing a job and adjusting to the work environment (PCEPD, 2000). *Mentors* may be used to serve as a role model, trusted counselor or teacher. Mentors provide opportunities for professional development and growth and support in career planning or devel-

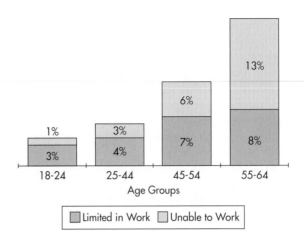

**FIGURE 18-6** Percentage of adult population unable to or limited in work, by age. (From Stucki BR: *Living in the community with a disability: demographic characteristics of the population with disabilities under age 65,* Washington, DC, 1995, American Association of Retired Persons, p. 55).

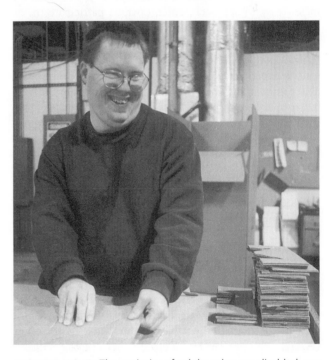

**FIGURE 18-7** The majority of adults who are disabled can achieve skills that permit them to be gainfully employed. Sheltered workshops provide job training and placement services that enhance an individual's ability to function in competitive as well as noncompetitive work environments. (Courtesy Ed Richardson.)

opment, along with information, encouragement, and advice (PCEPD, 2000).

As a result of the Americans with Disabilities Act (ADA), employers are prohibited from discriminating against any qualified individual with a disability in terms of job hiring, training, compensation, and advancement and are required to make reasonable accommodations to hire workers who are disabled. Under ADA provisions, employers cannot ask job applicants about the existence, nature, or severity of a disability; medical history; health insurance claims; or work absenteeism. Employers who discriminate against the disabled face legal action, fines, and penalties.

Persons who are disabled have proven to be loyal, trustworthy, capable, dependable employees who are willing to work, have good job performance, and reliable attendance records. Our country's work ethic makes employment a central part of life. In our society it is an expectation that people will work and be self-sufficient. Work has a great deal to do with how people identify themselves, as well as how they are identified by others. Employment offers the possibility of improving an individual's and family's financial stability, quality of life, and self-esteem.

## Access to Resources and Services

A major barrier to employment and other life activities for the person who is disabled is accessibility. Accessibility means easy to approach, enter, operate, participate in, or use safely, independently, and with dignity by a person with a disability (PCEPD, 2000).

Transportation is critical to maintaining access and personal independence. Many persons who are disabled are unable to drive, and the United States does not have an extensive public transportation system, especially in rural and suburban areas. This shortage of public transportation often prevents people who are disabled from taking part in employment and other community activities. It can prevent them from being able to do things such as grocery shopping, getting to health care appointments, and being able to participate in travel and recreation activities. Provisions of the ADA provided for increased accessibility to public transportation.

Some people who are disabled have vehicles adapted for their personal transportation use, but this is often costly. People who are disabled often have to rely heavily on friends, relatives, Dial-A-Rides, and other resources for transportation. To assist the person who is disabled in independent driving, the American Automobile Association (AAA) publishes *The Handicapped Driver's Mobility Guide*.

Accommodations such as ramps, elevators, wide aisles, and doorways assist persons who are disabled in gaining access to buildings. Although provisions of the ADA ensured physical access to buildings, in actuality this has not happened. Research that looked at mall access to people using wheelchairs found that none of the malls studied was fully compliant in any area of access (McClain, 2000). More work needs to be done to make accessibility a reality.

## *Stop and Think About It*

Think of buildings in your town, or the place where you work. What type of problems make access difficult for people who are disabled? What can the nurse do to facilitate access for people who are disabled?

## Health Care

Americans with disabilities, one sixth of the U.S. population, account for almost half of medical spending (Max, Rice, Trupin, 1996, p. 1). Adults who are unable to perform their major activity (e.g., paid work or keeping house) contact their physicians five times more each year than people who are able to perform their major activity (LaPlante, Rice, Wenger, 1995, p. 1). Attitudes of health care professionals have been discussed previously in this chapter. Access to care and health insurance as concerns of people who are disabled are discussed in the following sections.

ACCESS TO CARE. Americans with disabilities often have difficulty gaining access to health care. Transportation as an access problem has already been discussed. Transportation to health care is often difficult to arrange.

Another problem of access is having the appropriate resources available to be used. People living in rural and underserved areas may not have the health care resources they need, even if transportation was available to get to them. Health care providers may not participate in the person's health insurance program and participating providers may only be found at a great geographical distance. For example, some people in Tennessee's Medicaid waiver program, TennCare, have to travel up to 100 miles to see a specialist.

Obtaining prescriptions and health care supplies can be difficult for the person who is disabled. Examples of shop-at-home catalogs for health care supplies are Sear's *Home Health Care Catalog* (1-800-326-1750) and J.C. Penney's *For Your Special Needs: Home Health Care and Easy Dressing Fashions* catalog (1-800-222-6161). MOMS (*http://www.momsup.com*) is a catalog of aids and appliances for independent living (1-800-522-6294) and Disability Products (*http://www.disabilityproducts.com*) is another website where products can be obtained.

HEALTH INSURANCE. There is no national health insurance in the United States and millions of Americans are uninsured or underinsured (see Chapter 4). Americans with disabilities often have a difficult time obtaining private health insurance because their condition preceded their insurance application, a "preexisting" condition; they are considered high risk; or they cannot afford insurance. Some persons with disabilities are eligible for Medicaid and/or Medicare. Even when the person has health insurance, it is often inadequate to meet their special health needs (e.g., assistive devices, respite care, attendant services, physical and occupational therapy, prescriptions).

## Social, Recreational, and Athletic Opportunities

Few social, recreational, and athletic programs are available for persons who are disabled. Some adults who are disabled, especially those who are mentally retarded, find great enjoyment in participating in social and recreational activities planned especially for them (e.g., parties, camp, athletic activities). Others, such as clients with unstable diabetes, may readily integrate into existing community activities. Whatever the level of disability, people should have social and recreational opportunities available to them. A problem with many people who are disabled is that of social isolation.

Activities such as the *Special Olympics* (*http://www.specialolympics.org*) and the *Paralympics* (*http://www.paralympic.org*) provide opportunities for athletes who are disabled to participate in sporting events. The Special Olympics were founded in 1968 by Eunice Kennedy Shriver as a nonprofit program of sports training and competition for individuals with mental retardation. Today, more than 1 million athletes in nearly 150 countries and all 50 states participate. The Paralympic games had their origin after World War II. Today they draw elite athletes from all over the world and immediately follow the Olympic games.

*Disabled Sports USA* (*http://www.dsusa.org*) is an organization that works to ensure that persons of all ages with physical disabilities have access to sports, recreation, and physical education programs. With almost 100 local chapters nationwide, the organization offers year-round sports programs. Other groups such as the U.S. Electric Wheelchair Organization, the U.S. Association of Blind Athletes, and Access to Sailing all help link people who are disabled with recreational opportunities.

*The Itinerary*, a magazine for travelers with disabilities, specializes in helping people who are disabled know about "accessible" vacations. To make national parks more accessible, the National Park Service has travel guides for people who are disabled. *Mobility International USA* (*http://www.miusa.org*) and the *Society for the Advancement of Travel for the Handicapped (SATH)* (*http://www.sath.org*) are two organizations that provide information on travel for the disabled throughout the world, offer travel tips, and have listings of travel agents who are experienced in dealing with people who are disabled.

Group such as the Disability Discussion Forum (*http://www.tell-us-your-story.com*) and Encourage One Another (*http://www.encourageoneanother.com*) provide online support groups for people who are disabled. Communities across the country are making social and recreational activities more accessible to people with disabilities. Some innovative community-based programs in recent years have included the use of horses and ponies as therapeutic and recreational activities for children who are disabled (Associated Press, 2000).

## Sexuality

Sexual health is an integration of somatic, emotional, intellectual, and social aspects of sexual being, in ways that are positive and enriching and that enhance personality, communication, and love (Hoeman, 2001). **Sexuality** is an important concern for the person who is disabled.

Persons who are disabled are just as interested in romance and sex as nondisabled people (Duffy, 1996). Unfortunately, health care professionals have difficulty dealing with the sexual aspects of disability (Greco, 1996; Herson, Hart, Gordon, et al., 1999) or ignore it all together. This is unfortunate, because the sexual implications of a disability are often of great concern to the client. Adding to this, many misconceptions surround the sexuality of people who are disabled, and they are often treated as if they were asexual. Yvonne Duffy, an author who is disabled, writes:

Of all the nuances of acceptance that people with disabilities seek, the opportunity to be considered worthy of love—as spouses and lovers—has remained the most elusive. We have discovered that though we may be considered fine neighbors, co-workers or even friends, the line is often drawn when it comes to intimate relationships. (Duffy, 1996, p. R1)

Duffy goes on to state that as a teenager:

I felt uncomfortable at the few social functions to which I was invited...Occasionally, a young man approached me to inquire about the state of my health—as though having a disability meant that I was sick. Conversation seldom progressed beyond that point...Times are changing though. As an adult, I have known men who looked beyond my disability to find the real me.

Duffy's story illustrates the need to put the "people first" philosophy into practice. Health care professionals need to look closely at their own attitudes about sexuality and not let their attitudes deny, limit, or inhibit the person from sexual expression and fulfillment. Achievement of intimacy with a partner can lead to increased self-esteem and fulfillment.

The Sexuality Information and Education Council of the United States (SIECUS) advocates that persons with disabilities receive sexuality education, sexual health care, and opportunities for socializing and sexual expression, and that health care professionals work with people who are disabled and their families to help them understand and support the sexual development and expression of people who are disabled (SIECUS, 1996, p. 22). SIECUS recommends that social and health care agencies develop policies to ensure the protection of the sexual rights of people who are disabled. SIECUS regularly publishes an annotated bibliography on sexuality and disability. The SIECUS journal, *Sexuality and Disability*, offers the health care professional insightful readings.

A sexual history should be part of the nurse's assessment. When the client is asked questions concerning sexuality the nurse "leaves the door open for any questions or discussion by the client" (Greco, 1996, p. 596). The sexual implications of the client's disability should routinely be addressed. Box 18-12 gives a sexual history format that can be helpful to the nurse in obtaining assessment information from clients who are disabled. Nursing interventions include education and counseling for the client and partner and making the client aware of available resources.

Unfortunately, scarce counseling resources and the reluctance of professionals to deal with the topic of sexuality can leave the client with unanswered questions and little assistance in working out problems and concerns. Barriers cited

**BOX 18-12**

*Sexual History Form*

---

Name _____ Age ____
Marital/partnership status (includes quality, duration)

_____

Occupation _____ Highest education _____
Religion _____ Interests/hobbies _____

_____

### Medical History
Psychological/psychiatric problems_____
Behavioral/emotional problems _____
Renal insufficiency _____
Diabetes _____
Neurological conditions _____
Hereditary disorders _____
Hypertension _____
Endocrine disorders _____
Sexually transmitted diseases _____

### Current Medications
Antihypertensives _____
Antipsychotics _____
Antihistamines _____
Alcohol _____
Analgesics _____
Narcotics _____
Recreational drugs _____

### Premorbid Sexual Function
Description of sexual activities preferred _____
Frequency of sexual activity _____
Partner who generally initiates sexual activity _____
Sexual preferences of the client _____

### Specific Concerns of the Couple
Fertility _____
Birth control _____
Importance of sex in the relationship _____

Physical issues that impact sexual function _____
Transfers _____
Ability to dress/undress _____
Hemiplegia/hemiparesis _____
Paraplegia/quadriplegia _____
Range-of-motion limitations _____
Hypertonicity _____
Hypotonicity _____
Endurance _____
Balance _____
Presence of sensation versus being hypersensitive ____
Presence of pain and location _____
Presence of bowel and/or bladder incontinence _____
Presence of genitourinary or gastrointestinal collection devices and their position

Difficulty with vision, hearing, oral motor control

_____

General and genital hygiene and cleanliness _____

### Sexual Response Issues
Female
  Menstrual history _____
  Sexual interest _____
  Frequency of sexual interaction _____
  Vaginal lubrication _____
  Sensation present _____
  Orgasmic capacity _____
  Fertility _____
Male
  Sexual interest _____
  Presence of morning erections _____
  Presence of erections with manual stimulation _____
  Process for ejaculation _____
  Sensation present _____
  Type of ejaculation and volume _____
  Fertility _____

---

From Greco SB: Sexuality and education counseling. In Hoeman SP: *Rehabilitation nursing: process and application*, ed 2, St Louis, 1996, Mosby, p. 609.

by health care professionals for not providing sexuality information include too little time, lack of knowledge, perceptions as someone else's job, own attitudes and beliefs, and lack of client readiness (Herson, Hart, Gordon, Rintala, 1999). The nurse needs to understand that being disabled does not change a person's need for intimacy and incorporate the client's sexual concerns into the plan of care.

## Guardianship

Most persons who are disabled do not need guardians and are able to go through their entire lives making their own decisions. This is especially true of people who are physically disabled. However, **guardianship** is often considered for individuals who are severely disabled, especially those who are mentally ill or mentally retarded. Handling guardianship issues can be difficult for families.

Guardianship can be either plenary (complete) or partial. Partial guardianship implies that the person is able to carry out some functions independently but is not competent to carry out other functions. Competency has to do with a person's ability to make an informed decision, or with risk of harm as a result of their inability to care for themselves or manage their affairs. If no guardian is appointed, the person is responsible for making his or her own decisions, including decisions regarding health care. If a guardian is appointed, the court gives the guardian the authority to exercise certain legal rights in the person's best interest. Because guardianship involves a serious deprivation of personal liberty and dignity, the law requires that it be imposed only when other, less restrictive alternatives have been proven ineffective.

Parents are "natural" guardians of their own minor children and can make legal decisions for them. Parents are *not* natural guardians of their adult offspring, even if they are disabled, and cannot make legal decisions for them without having guardianship. Once the age of majority is reached, a person is legally responsible for himself or herself unless a legal guardian has been appointed by the court. Many parents are unaware of this fact, and anticipatory guidance about guardianship needs is helpful.

Families frequently experience a crisis when they realize that their adult offspring are not able to take care of their own decision making and parents may have to accept the reality that their offspring may never develop the skills to function independently. When this occurs, feelings of sadness and hopelessness are common. Helping families identify the strengths their adult offspring have, the potential they have for benefiting from experiences that are developmentally within their reach, and linking them with appropriate resources can reduce parents' anxiety and increase their ability to plan for the future.

In some families, siblings, relatives, or friends may be asked to assume guardianship responsibility for an adult who is disabled. In some situations this is a feasible solution and in others it is not. At times community health nurses have found that families assume that adults who are disabled are unable to care for themselves just because they have a disability. It is important to remember that not all adults who are disabled need guardians. In fact, most of them do not. The nurse can assist the family in looking at other guardianship options.

Some options that are less restrictive alternatives to guardianship include *representative or protective payee* (a person who is appointed to manage entitlement benefits, such as retirement, on behalf of the individual), *conservatorship* (a voluntary proceeding in which a person asks the Probate Court to appoint a specific individual, the conservator) to manage his or her property, and *power of attorney* (a contract between two individuals where one party gives the other the authority to make a number of decisions, such as medical, on their behalf). The National Guardianship Association provides information on guardianship (*http://www.guardianship.org*).

## Community Residential Opportunities

It is the right of people who are disabled to live their lives as normally and independently as possible. Many people who are disabled do not require any specialized form of housing and live independently in the community.

Historically, people who were disabled, especially people who were mentally impaired, were placed in state residential facilities. For example, in the 1950s hundreds of thou-

sands of people resided in psychiatric mental hospitals in the United States (Shadish, Lurigio, Lewis, 1989, p. 2). Today, many of these institutional settings have been closed or reduced in size, and the number of people with disabilities living in community settings has greatly increased. States and local communities are developing innovative ways to assist people who are disabled to live in the mainstream of community life.

### Stop and Think About It

If you had a disabling condition where would you want to live? Would you want to live in an institution? Would you want to live in a home setting adapted to your needs? What type of residential opportunities are available for people who are disabled in your community?

In 1972 the nation's first independent living center was established in Berkeley, California (Smith, Smith, Richards, et al., 1994, p. 14). The nation's independent living centers help people to live independently by providing services such as wheelchair repair, training of attendants, and referrals for employment and housing (Robert Wood Johnson Foundation, 1992, p. 76). A publication, *Independent Living*, assists people who are handicapped with independent living needs and is available through Equal Opportunity Publications, 150 Motor Parkway, Suite 400, Greenlawn, NY 11740.

Table 18-1 presents some of the options available for community living for people with disabilities. Such options are becoming more and more available in American communities. Community living arrangements should meet the needs of the individual. When selecting a residential placement, objectives for the individual should be established and the placement carefully evaluated. Nurses are involved with home visits to clients as well as helping to establish and monitor community living facilities.

ADAPTING THE LIVING ENVIRONMENT. For some persons who are disabled, especially those with mobility limitations or those who are wheelchair bound, independent living means that housing needs be accessible. Persons with disabilities who need to adapt their homes may be eligible for home improvement loans insured by the Department of Housing and Urban Development (HUD). The HUD-insured loan can be used to remove architectural barriers or hazards in the home and make home adaptations. Persons who are disabled also may be eligible for rental assistance through HUD. Box 18-13 lists some resources for adapting living environments to make them accessible.

FUNDING AND MONITORING. The funding and monitoring of residential placements will vary from state to state. People looking for specific placements can check with local offices of the state department of human or social services, departments of mental health and mental retardation, HUD, or specialty agencies dealing with the conditions involved. Some examples of such agencies are the

**TABLE 18-1**

*Residential Alternatives for Persons with Disabilities*

| RESIDENTIAL MODEL | CHARACTERISTICS |
| --- | --- |
| Public residential facilities | Institutionalized facilities with trained staff and full-time supervision for residents. Residents are segregated from the community. |
| Sheltered villages | Institutionalized facilities with trained staff and full-time supervision for residents. Privately supported, the facilities are often located in rural areas where the residents are segregated from the community. |
| Public community facilities | Institutionalized facilities with trained staff and full-time supervision for residents. (These residences also are referred to as *Intermediate Care Facilities.*) Residents are segregated from the community for some activities but integrated for other activities. |
| Public group homes | Government operated homes that are shared by groups of persons and supervised by a staff that may be part time. Residents may be segregated from the community for some activities but integrated for other activities. |
| Private group homes | Privately operated homes that otherwise have the same characteristics as *public group homes.* |
| Cooperatively owned group homes | Homes that are owned jointly by residents and for which full-time or part-time staff may be employed. Residents may be segregated from the community for some activities but integrated for other activities. |
| Foster care | Persons with disabilities live in the home and under the supervision of a caregiver. The caregiver may be paid a stipend for these services. The degree to which residents are integrated can vary according to the attitudes of caregivers. |
| Public apartments | Government operated apartments that are leased to individuals. Persons are supervised or assisted by an apartment manager who may be part time. Residents may be segregated from the community for some activities but integrated for other activities. |
| Privately apartments | Privately managed apartments that have the same characteristics as *public apartments.* |
| Cooperatively owned apartments | Cooperatively owned apartments or condominiums that are leased to individuals. Otherwise, this type of residence has the same characteristics as *public* or *private apartments.* |
| Independent living | A wide range of residential options that could include renting or purchasing a residence in ways similar to those by which residences are selected and maintained by persons without disabilities. Persons with disabilities would have unrestricted access to community activities and could request assistance from agency personnel as appropriate. |

From Giordano G, D'Alonzo BJ: The link between transition and independent living, *Am Rehab* 20(1):2-7, 1994, p. 4.

local Association for Retarded Citizens, the National Association for Multiple Sclerosis, and associations for the blind. These agencies are often aware of community placement opportunities and can refer people to appropriate resources.

ZONING AND BUILDING REGULATIONS. In many areas restrictive zoning regulations do not allow group homes for persons who are disabled. Restrictive zoning policies have led to the clustering of community residential facilities for persons who are disabled (often persons who are mentally ill or mentally retarded) in areas where zoning regulations are not restrictive; often in less desirable residential areas. Some communities have actively tried to restrict residences for the disabled.

The community health nurse needs to educate the community and its leaders regarding the residential needs of a person who is disabled. Actively participating on community advisory boards that facilitate community residential programs provides opportunities to work with community leaders, educate the public, and establish new and innovative community residential opportunities.

## Attendant Services

The person who is disabled may not be able to carry out all the activities of daily living. When this happens the person can benefit from attendant services. The attendant assists the person in such activities as maintaining personal appearance and hygiene (e.g., feeding, dressing, grooming), mobility, household maintenance, safety, companionship, and resource use.

Unfortunately, no comprehensive, uniform system for providing such services exists, and services vary greatly from state to state. Many persons who need attendant services are

**BOX 18-13**

*Some Resources for Accessible Housing*

Accessible housing is essential if persons with disabilities are to be able to live independently in the community. Builders and contractors are often unaware of modifications or regulations involving handicap accessibility, and individuals are often not aware of how to adapt housing to meet their needs. The following organizations are some resources for accessible housing:

**Center for Universal Design (CUD)**
North Carolina State University
College of Design
Campus Box 8613
Raleigh, NC, 27695-8613
*http://www.design.ncsu.edu/cud*
1-800-647-6777
The Center was established in 1989 under a National Institute on Disability and Rehabilitation Research grants. It is a leading national research, information, and technical assistance center. CUD evaluates, develops, and promotes universal design in housing, public and commercial facilities, and related products. CUD offers design solutions (including floor plan designs), training, information, referral, and technical assistance to improve the quality and availability of residential environments for people with disabilities.

**Adaptive Environments Center (AEC)**
374 Congress Street Suite 301
Boston, MA 02210
*http://www.adaptenv.org*
(617) 482-8099
AEC was founded in 1978 to address the environmental issues that confront people with disability and elders. AEC promotes accessibility as well as universal design through education programs, technical assistance, training, consulting, publications, and design advocacy. It sponsored the first biennial international conference on universal design in 1998.

**Beyond Barriers**
Access One, Inc.
25679 Gramford Avenue
Wyoming, MN 55092
*http://www.beyondbarriers.com*
1-800-561-2223
Beyond Barriers' goal is to improve the daily living conditions of persons with disabilities and the elderly who find their independence threatened by offering a full range of products designed to allow freedom and independence. It offers building and remodeling solutions to help people remain independent and active in their homes and communities.

---

unable to obtain them, often because of the limited availability and cost involved. These services are sometimes funded through Medicaid, Department of Social Services, Older Americans Act provisions, Veterans Administration, and various state and locally funded programs. If attendant services are not available, some people who are disabled may not be able to live independently, and without these services persons who are disabled may be needlessly placed in long-term care facilities such as nursing homes and institutions.

Some attendant programs involve the use of animals to help people with disabilities. *Seeing Eye Dogs* have long been a part of American communities. More recently other animals have been used. Programs such as *Helping Hands Monkeys* (*http://www.helpinghandsmonkeys.org*) and *Loving Paws Assistance Dogs* (*http://www.lovingpaws.com*) provide animals trained to assist people with disabilities in daily activities. The community health nurse can be instrumental in helping link clients with such resources and encourage communities to develop additional resources and services.

## Respite Care

Family caretakers often provide 24-hour-a-day care to disabled family members. Caretakers often experience burnout or just need time for themselves.

**Respite care** is one solution to the problem of caretaker overload and provides time away for caregivers on a short-term (e.g., a few hours away to go shopping) or long-term

(e.g., travel, health concerns) basis. It gives caregivers the opportunity to do those things they need to or want to do for themselves without having the responsibility of caregiving. Respite care can occur in settings such as the clients' homes, private homes, foster care, group homes, hospitals, and nursing homes. Providing this temporary time away for caretakers helps relieve caretaker stress and may prevent or delay institutionalization.

Many communities do not offer much in terms of respite care. When respite care is available, it is often costly. Some families and organizations have developed respite co-op groups in which they exchange periods of time in caring for their respective disabled family members. Medicaid waivers can sometimes be used for respite care reimbursement if the cost is the same or less than institutional care, realizing that it can be more economical to finance respite care services than it is to provide institutional care or long-term care. The community health nurse can be instrumental in advocating for respite care services for clients and in making this very important need known to the community.

## Civil Rights

The ADA has sometimes been referred to as the Civil Rights Act for People with Disabilities. This law and others legally guarantee the civil rights of people who are disabled. It is the responsibility of the Offices for Civil Rights in the U.S. Department of Education and the USDHHS to enforce federal laws prohibiting discrimination against persons who are disabled in federally assisted educational and health and welfare programs and to investigate discrimination complaints brought by individuals. States have *Protection and Advocacy Agencies* (see the discussion of state government resources that follows in this chapter) to help ensure that the civil rights of people who are disabled are upheld. These agencies usually have toll-free numbers and websites.

## SOME GOVERNMENTAL RESOURCES FOR PEOPLE WHO ARE DISABLED

Numerous resources for people who are disabled have already been presented in this chapter. International, federal, state, and local governments offer many services to persons who are disabled. Federal resources remain rather constant across the nation, whereas state and local resources can vary greatly. On an international level organizations such as WHO, World Institute on Disability, and Rehabilitation International address issues related to health and disability.

## FEDERAL GOVERNMENT RESOURCES

On the federal level many different agencies offer services to persons who are disabled. The U.S. Department of Education and the USDHHS are major providers of service to people who are disabled.

### U.S. Department of Education

The Department of Education is involved in information, education, and advocacy programs for people with disabilities. It also oversees compliance with federal legislation for the education of children with disabilities. It has numerous branches that provide service to people with disabilities.

OFFICE OF SPECIAL EDUCATION AND REHABILITATIVE SERVICES. The Office of Special Education and Rehabilitation Services houses the Clearinghouse on Disability Information and publishes the quarterly periodical *American Rehabilitation*. It oversees federally mandated educational programs for people with disabilities.

ERIC CLEARINGHOUSE ON DISABILITY AND GIFTED EDUCATION. The Clearinghouse on Disability Information responds to inquiries on a wide range of topics including federal programs and legislation affecting the disabled community and makes referrals to appropriate resources.

NATIONAL INSTITUTE ON DISABILITY AND REHABILITATION RESEARCH. The National Institute on Disability and Rehabilitation Research (NIDRR) contributes to the independence of people with disabilities and sponsors Rehabilitation Research and Training Centers (RRTCs), Rehabilitation Engineering Centers (RECs), research and demonstration projects, research training, and career development grants. NIDRR also gathers disability data and pub-

lishes a series, *Disability Statistics Abstract*, that highlights information on disabling conditions.

NATIONAL REHABILITATION INFORMATION CENTER. The National Rehabilitation Information Center (NARIC) (1-800-34-NARIC) describes itself as serving the nation's disabled community and providing "information for independence" (NARIC, 1996). It was established in 1977 and is funded by NIDRR to collect and disseminate disability information, including the results of federally funded research projects. NARIC publishes a directory of national disability information resources, a guide to disability and rehabilitation periodicals, resource guides, and fact sheets on rehabilitation topics. NARIC's computerized databases include REHABDATA, ABLEDATA, and ABLE INFORM. REHABDATA (1-800-346-2742) contains bibliographical information on the NARIC library; ABLEDATA (1-800-227-0216) provides information about commercial rehabilitation products; and ABLE INFORM (301-589-3563) is an electronic bulletin board of assistive technology, disability, and rehabilitation information. ABLEDATA has become one of the most important national sources of information on assistive technology and the manufacturers of products for persons with disabilities.

### U.S. Department of Health and Human Services

The USDHHS (*http://www.hhs.gov*) provides services to persons who are disabled, including grants to states for maternal and child health. The Medicaid and Medicare programs administered by the department provide funding for numerous health care services used by people with disabilities. The department's Centers for Disease Control and Prevention (CDC) works to prevent chronic disabling conditions among Americans and collects national statistics on disabling conditions. As previously mentioned, *Healthy People 2010*, a publication of the department, has national objectives relating to disabling conditions.

NATIONAL CENTER FOR CHRONIC DISEASE PREVENTION AND HEALTH PROMOTION. The National Center for Chronic Disease Prevention and Health Promotion (NCCDPHP) is part of the CDC in the USDHHS. It is a lead federal agency in chronic disease and disability prevention. The center advocates for healthier lifestyles, facilitates nationwide efforts to prevent chronic diseases, and works with communities to translate research findings into effective community health programs. It actively supports initiatives that promote good nutrition, tobacco-free lifestyles, physical activity, adolescent and school health, reproductive health, health promotion, and early disease detection. NCCDPHP programs target populations, such as older Americans and minorities, that have a disproportionate share of chronic diseases, and assists states in developing surveillance systems to monitor and track chronic diseases and related risk factors.

## National Council on Disability

The National Council on Disability is presidentially appointed and has made prevention of disability one of its highest priorities. It works closely with the Office of Disease Prevention and Health Promotion in the CDC, and its efforts include promoting the development of a national disabilities prevention plan.

## STATE GOVERNMENT RESOURCES

Numerous offices and departments on the state level offer services to people who are disabled. Programs are administered by each state and vary from one state to another. The nurse is encouraged to explore organizations that provide services in the state in which she or he is practicing.

### State Departments of Education

State departments of education are responsible for special education and related services for children in their state and have final responsibility for implementing the provisions of the Individuals with Disabilities Education Act (IDEA). They provide consultation, information services, and funding for such programs. They also answer individual questions and provide information on special education services. States often sponsor residential educational and training schools for children who are blind or deaf. Information on these schools is available through local school districts. Some states have a separate office for deaf-blind services.

### State Health Authority

State Health Authorities (SHAs) are discussed in Chapter 5. SHAs often fund and administer children's special health care services programs that target services to children with disabilities. These services are funded primarily through federal grants to states to provide health care services to children who are disabled or who have chronic health problems. Services usually provided include payment for direct care, counseling, genetic disease testing, training and education for health care professionals and caregivers, and research funding. SHAs and local health departments work collaboratively to provide these services to families.

### State Vocational Rehabilitation Agency

In each state an agency is responsible for the administration of vocational rehabilitation programs, supported employment, and independent living for people with disabilities. This vocational rehabilitation agency assists people with disabilities to achieve suitable employment, supports them in maintaining competitive employment, and assists them in living independently in the community (Office of Special Education and Rehabilitative Services, 2000). States are making efforts to enhance rehabilitation services in rural and underserved areas. Some services commonly provided by these agencies are given in Box 18-14.

**BOX 18-14**

### *State Vocational Rehabilitation Agencies: Services Frequently Offered*

- Medical, psychological, vocational, and other types of assessments to determine the functional strengths and limitations of the individual
- Counseling to assist a person in selecting suitable rehabilitation programming, including the types of services needed to achieve the person's choice of a goal
- Referral to necessary services from other agencies
- Physical and mental restoration services necessary to correct or substantially modify a physical or mental condition that is stable or slowly progressive
- Vocational and other types of training, including on-the-job training, trade schools, and training in institutions of higher education
- Interpreter and reader services
- Services to family members when necessary to achieve the rehabilitation objectives
- Rehabilitation technology services
- Placement in suitable employment
- Postemployment services necessary to maintain or regain employment
- Other services necessary to achieve rehabilitation objectives

Source: Office of Special Education and Rehabilitative Services: *Pocket guide to federal help for individuals with disabilities*, Washington, DC, 2000, Department of Education.

### State Employment Services Offices

Each state has an Employment Services office with local branches. These public employment centers assist employers in finding workers and workers in finding jobs. Helping job seekers with disabilities is a specific responsibility of the Employment Services Office.

### State Agency for People Who Are Blind or Visually Impaired

Almost half of the states have a separate agency or commission that works specifically with services to people with visual impairments (Office of Special Education and Rehabilitative Services, 2000). These agencies offer training in daily living skills, mobility training, filling out job application forms, and other rehabilitation needs. They provide funding for reader services for college students who are visually impaired.

### State Mental Retardation Agency

Such agencies plan, administer, and develop standards for mental retardation services provided in state-operated facilities and state-funded community-based programs. They provide information on programs and program eligibility. In some states these agencies are combined with the state mental health agency.

## State Mental Health Agency

These agencies often finance and administer community mental health centers and state residential facilities for people who are mentally ill and mentally retarded. They develop standards for state and local mental health programs and provide information on community and residential treatment programs and placement options. They may compile community resource lists.

## State Developmental Disabilities Council

These agencies provide services to families with members with developmental disabilities. They provide information and community resources. These councils frequently have toll free numbers where families can obtain information.

## State Protection and Advocacy Agency

Protection and advocacy agencies are responsible for pursuing legal, administrative, and other remedies to protect and guard the civil rights of persons who are developmentally disabled or mentally ill. As advocates they work to promote the quality of life for people who are disabled. They link clients to community resources; compile resource lists in areas such as housing, health, social and recreational programs, and support groups available in local communities. They are an excellent source of information and referral.

## Other

Universities in a state may have institutes that study disabling conditions (e.g., Institute for the Study of Mental Retardation and Related Disabilities) and frequently provide education and training for health, education, and social service professionals working with people who are disabled. They also may provide direct services to people with disabilities through specially designated programs and institutes. Information and listings of university-affiliated programs can be obtained by contacting the American Association of University Affiliated Programs for Persons with Developmental Disabilities at 8630 Felton Street, Suite 410, Silver Spring, MD 20910 (301-588-8252).

## LOCAL GOVERNMENT RESOURCES

Local governments, through organizations such as schools, health departments, and departments of parks and recreation, offer services to people who are disabled. These services vary greatly from one community to another. The local health department is usually a good source of information and referral to such services.

## LEGISLATION

An overview of federal legislation and voluntary efforts that facilitate service provisions for persons with disabilities is

**BOX 18-15**

### Legislation and the Person Who Is Disabled

- Social Security Act (1935)
- Developmental Disabilities Act (1971)
- Rehabilitation Act (1973)
- Developmental Disabilities and Bill of Rights Act (1975, 1984)
- Education for All Handicapped Children Act (1975)
- Mental Health Systems Act (1980)
- Civil Rights of Institutionalized Persons Act (1980)
- Protection and Advocacy for Mentally Ill Individuals Act (1986, 1988)
- Americans with Disabilities Act (1990)
- Individuals with Disabilities Education Act (1990)

presented in Appendix 18-2. Several major pieces of legislation have provided the mechanisms for meeting many needs of persons who are disabled and are given in Box 18-15. The nurse needs to be knowledgeable about legislation that affects persons who are handicapped and to advocate for necessary legislation. The nurse needs to be able to assist clients in knowing their rights under the law and how to proceed when these rights are violated. The Social Security Act, Americans with Disabilities Act, the Individuals with Disabilities Education Act, and the Rehabilitation Act, mentioned previously in Chapter 4, provide services to people who are disabled.

### Social Security Act (P.L. 74-721)

The Social Security Act of 1935 is discussed in Chapters 4 and 5. This act enabled numerous programs that serve people with disabilities. *Social Security Disability Insurance* and *Supplemental Security Income* are two programs used extensively by people who are disabled. Maternal and child health programs that provide services to children with disabilities also are provided under the act. The acts *Medicare* and *Medicaid* programs provide health care services to people who are disabled.

### Americans with Disabilities Act (P.L. 101-336)

The Americans with Disabilities Act (ADA) of 1990 is considered by many to be the most significant piece of legislation in the United States for people with disabilities (Watson, 2000). The act provides a mandate to end discrimination against individuals with disabilities. It is a comprehensive civil rights law that makes it unlawful to discriminate against a qualified individual with a disability in employment, housing, public accommodations, transportation, and telecommunication. The law empowers people who are disabled.

As a result of this legislation, all across America access to transportation, buildings, and recreational areas has been enhanced; interpreters are being provided; workplaces are accommodating people who are disabled; and people are becoming more sensitive to the needs of the disabled community and are helping make a difference in the lives of persons who are disabled. The act calls on everyone to remove barriers to access. According to Attorney General Janet Reno (1993), this law is helping break down not only physical barriers but also social barriers and has helped people with and without disabilities work together to eliminate the barriers that have kept people who are disabled from being treated equally.

## Individuals with Disabilities Education Act (P.L. 101-476)

The Education for All Handicapped Children Act became the Individuals with Disabilities Education Act (IDEA) in 1990. Consistent with the Americans with Disabilities Act, the law used the term disability rather than handicap. The law continued to mandate that local school districts must provide a free appropriate elementary and secondary education for all children with disabilities from age 6 through age 21. Final responsibility for implementing the special education and related services for 3 to 21 years old under IDEA rests with the state education agency. Funding for services to children from birth to 2 and 3 to 5 was made available to states on a state-federal sharing basis. Under the law, parents have the right to participate in and approve their child's Individualized Education Program (IEP) developed for their children. If children are placed in private schools by state or local education systems to receive an appropriate education, it must be done at no cost to the parent and services such as transportation and special aids must be provided at public expense (Office of Special Education and Rehabilitative Services, 2000, p. 8).

## Rehabilitation Act of 1973 (P.L. 93-112)

The Rehabilitation Act of 1973 replaced the Vocational Rehabilitation Act of 1920 and was a landmark piece of legislation for individuals with disabilities, helping to ensure their civil rights and provide protection and advocacy services. The purposes of the act are (1) to empower individuals with disabilities to maximize employment, economic self-sufficiency, independence, and inclusion and integration into society through research, training, demonstration projects, and the guarantee of equal opportunity; and (2) to ensure that the federal government plays a leadership role in promoting the employment of individuals with disabilities, especially individuals with severe disabilities, and in assisting states and providers of services in fulfilling the aspirations of individuals with disabilities for meaningful and gainful employment and independent living (Stafford, 1995). To qualify for programs under the act, a person must be at least 16 years old, have a physical or mental disability that constitutes an employment handicap, and be able to become employable as a result of the education, training, and rehabilitation.

---

### BOX 18-16
*Predicted Developments in Rehabilitation*

1. Community-based rehabilitation services will increase.
2. Supported employment programs will increase.
3. Individuals with disabilities will assume greater control of the programs that affect them.
4. Models of culturally sensitive rehabilitation counseling will emerge.
5. Private-sector businesses will become increasingly involved in rehabilitation.
6. Tolerance and acceptance of disabilities will expand among persons without disabilities.
7. Rehabilitation technology will have an increased impact on persons with disabilities.
8. Services for older persons with disabilities will expand.
9. Programs built on partnerships between agencies, communities, and businesses will expand.
10. Life span approaches will permeate rehabilitation.
11. Rehabilitation services will become less agency focused and more client centered.
12. Models for developing rehabilitation personnel through nontraditional programs will emerge.
13. Services for persons with severe disabilities will expand.
14. Independent living opportunities will broaden for persons with disabilities.
15. Federal and state regulations, and the implementation of those regulations, will be directed increasingly to local levels.

From Giordano G, D'Alonzo BJ: Challenge and progress in rehabilitation: a review of the past 25 years and a preview of the future, *Am Rehab* 21(3):14-21, 1995, p. 18.

## REHABILITATION

Rehabilitation is a complex, interdisciplinary process of restoring an individual to the fullest physical, emotional, social, vocational, and economic well-being possible. Rehabilitation activities are an important part of the treatment plan for many persons who are disabled. Client education is fundamental to the rehabilitation process. The process is holistic and client centered and strives to reduce the level of disability and handicap and promote client independence and empowerment (Smith, 1999a). Major goals of rehabilitation are to integrate the individual into society and provide as normal a life as possible. Rehabilitation is often a long-term process, demanding multiple resources and a high level of commitment. Some predicted developments in rehabilitation are given in Box 18-16. The National Rehabilitation Association (*http://www.nationalrehab.org*), the National Council on Disability (*http://www.ncd.gov*), and the American Association for Rehabilitation Nurses (*http://www.rehabnurse.org*) are all valuable resources on rehabilitation.

Individuals, their families, and significant others are essential members of the interdisciplinary rehabilitation team (ARN, 1994a, p. 2). Comprehensive rehabilitation programs combine medical treatment with such things as home health nursing services; social services; psychological services; and physical, occupational, and speech therapy. The use of pastors as part of the interdisciplinary rehabilitation team is successful with some clients (Easton, Andrews, 2000).

If people are to return as fully as possible to their previous level of function they must be immersed in as much of their previous lifestyle as soon as possible (Pryor, 2000). Early intervention results in successful care outcomes and the smooth transition between phases of rehabilitation and community reintegration (Breese, Mikrut, 1995). There is a direct correlation between the time the injury or illness occurred, when the rehabilitation referral was made, and the success of the rehabilitation program. The longer the time lapse between condition occurrence and rehabilitation services, the less chance that rehabilitation efforts will be optimally effective (Breese, Mikrut, 1995).

If families are supported and included during the initial phase of rehabilitation, they are often more effective in supporting the client and have better long-term adaptation to the disability (Winterhalter, 1992). Provision of early interventions, stabilization of psychosocial function, case management, and utilization of community resources (see Chapter 10) assist a family in adapting to the disability and having successful rehabilitation outcomes. Some factors related to adaptation have been previously discussed in this chapter.

The internet and its links to numerous resources is having a significant impact on the rehabilitation process (Patterson, 2000). It can provide immediate access to information and education, link clients to support groups and resources, and provide clients with career development tools (Patterson, 2000). Internet resources are presented throughout this chapter.

The rehabilitation plan of care is mutually established with the client and family and promotes active client participation. Active client participation promotes independence, compliance, and empowerment. Lack of client participation can affect the client's self-esteem and disrupt the therapeutic process. Vocational rehabilitation is an important part of the rehabilitation process.

## Vocational Rehabilitation

As previously mentioned, states have a vocational rehabilitation agency. There are also many private sector vocational rehabilitation resources. Vocational rehabilitation provides training for people to resume jobs or learn new job skills. Such services may be covered under an individual's health care insurance. A major goal of vocational rehabilitation is to have a client in an appropriate, satisfying job with a stable employer.

Vocational rehabilitation efforts involve assessment of the client's work potential; vocational education and training; obtaining the assistive devices necessary for employment; vocational counseling; and employment placement, evaluation, and follow-up. Unemployment has both emotional and financial aspects and can be devastating for individuals and their families; vocational rehabilitation can help people gain employment.

Many vocational rehabilitation services are provided under the Rehabilitation Act of 1973 discussed previously in this chapter. To apply for rehabilitation services, the person should contact the local office of the state Department of Education, Division of Vocational Services or the state Employment Services Office. Other rehabilitation programs are offered through hospitals, long-term care facilities, and outpatient settings.

## Community Rehabilitation Opportunities

Rehabilitation facilities in the United States arose out of a concern by local leaders, parents, and advocates who perceived a real need for resources and services to assist people with disabilities in their home communities (Geigel, 1995). Starting in the nineteenth century, the private sector began to develop rehabilitation facilities, workshops, work centers, and extended employment facilities (Geigel, 1995).

Today such facilities make up a national network of service providers such as local school districts, universities, Goodwill Industries, National Easter Seal Society, Jewish Vocational Services, Associations for Retarded Citizens, United Cerebral Palsy Association, and the American Rehabilitation Association. Organizations such as these provide services including sheltered workshops, employment, and training. These facilities provide many valuable services to the person who is disabled. One challenge is providing such services to the millions of Americans living in rural areas (Riemer-Reiss, 2000). People with disabilities living in rural areas commonly receive fewer resources than their urban counterparts (see Chapter 3). Telecounseling, email, and real-time video are being used in some rural areas to provide rehabilitation counseling and support (Riemer-Reiss, 2000).

New and innovative rehabilitation programs such as horseback riding and the use of animals in rehabilitation programs are emerging (All, Loving, 1999; Associated Press, 2000). More and more rehabilitation opportunities are emerging in communities.

## THE NURSE AND THE REHABILITATION PROCESS

Rehabilitation is a specialty practice within nursing, and rehabilitation nurses have experience with enabling clients and families to become experts on their condition and negotiate realistic goals (Hoeman, 2001). They are involved in assessment and innovations ranging from primary prevention through optimal health restoration (Hoeman, 1999). The rehabilitation process follows the same steps as the nursing process. It involves data gathering, formation of diagnoses and rehabilitation prognoses, goals, plans, follow-up, and evaluation. It is an interdisciplinary process that involves counseling, discharge planning, and case management (see Chapter 10).

Rehabilitation nurses must possess the special knowledge and clinical skills that help them deal with the profound impact of disability on individuals and their families, and they must realize that individuals with disabilities have intrinsic worth that transcends their disability (ARN, 1994a, p. 3). To facilitate care of clients who are disabled the rehabilitation nurse must have knowledge of growth and development, functional status, family and crisis theory, group process, role theory, adaptation and coping, learning theory, and the change process (ARN, 1994a, p. 4). Meeting the emotional needs of the patient is critical to the rehabilitation process (Lambert, 1999).

Rehabilitation nurses intervene to prevent disability, reduce the stigma of disability, restore optimal functioning, enhance quality of life, promote independence, help the individual and family adapt to an altered lifestyle, and assist people in looking beyond the disability (ARN, 1994a, p. 3). The nurse needs to maximize the wellness of clients, build on client strengths, help them compensate for negative factors, maximize the use of available energy, promote ego integrity, and inspire hope (Davidhizar, Shearer, 1997).

Nurses work to maximize the client's physical health and independence, emotional health and relationships, mobility and access, employment and leisure activities, and the ability to remain in a community environment (Smith, 1999b). Roles that the nurse uses in the rehabilitation process include technical expert and provider of care, provider of psychological support, counselor, educator, coordinator of care, team worker, client advocate, researcher, and care evaluator (Chin, Finnocchiaro, Rosebrough, 1998, pp. 10-11; Smith, 1999b).

## Evaluating the Rehabilitation Regimen

Evaluating the client's rehabilitation regimen is an important nursing role. The nurse needs to consider components of the rehabilitation plans such as resource coordination and appropriateness and client satisfaction with the plan of care. Questions that address client outcomes and satisfaction should be raised. Use of a client satisfaction survey can be helpful. It can provide data about client perceptions of care, serve as a basis for decision making about care, and help show clients and families that their opinions are valued. Sample items for such a survey are given in Figure 18-8.

Nurses are in key positions to help the client and family accept and implement the rehabilitation program. Early involvement with a skilled support person, such as a commu-

**BOX 18-17**

*Rehabilitation Nursing Practice*

Rehabilitation nurses rely on sound theoretical foundations and scientific knowledge as they work with clients and their families to:
- Set goals for maximum levels of interdependent functioning and activities of daily living
- Promote self-care, prevent complications or further disability
- Reinforce positive coping behaviors
- Ensure access with continuity of services and care
- Advocate for optimal quality of life
- Improve outcome for clients
- Contribute to reforms in the character, structure, and delivery of health care in the United States

From Hoeman SP: Conceptual bases for rehabilitation nursing. In Hoeman SP: *Rehabilitation nursing: process and application,* ed 2, St Louis, 1996, Mosby, p. 3.

**BOX 18-18**

*Nursing Diagnoses Used Most Frequently in Rehabilitation Nursing Practice*

Impaired physical mobility*
Self-care deficit*
Alteration in urinary elimination pattern*
Impaired skin integrity*
Alteration in bowel elimination pattern*
Potential for physical injury*
Knowledge deficit*
Impaired verbal communication*
Decreased activity tolerance*
Alterations in comfort
Impaired thought process
Ineffective family coping
Noncompliance
Body image disturbance
Self-esteem disturbances
Alteration in nutrition: Less than required
Health management deficit
Impaired home maintenance management
Sensory perception alterations
Uncompensated swallowing impairment

From Sawin KJ, Heard L: Nursing diagnoses used most frequently in rehabilitation nursing practice, *Rehabil Nurs* 17(5):257, 1992. Reprinted from *Rehabilitation Nursing,* vol 17, issue 5, with permission of the Association of Rehabilitation Nurses, 4700 W. Lake Avenue, Glenview, Ill, 60025-1485. © 1992 Association of Rehabilitation Nurses.
*Top 9 diagnoses.

nity health nurse, will help bridge gaps in service and help reduce frustration and lessen the likelihood of secondary disabilities occurring. Box 18-17 presents an overview of rehabilitation nursing practice. Diagnoses frequently used by rehabilitation nurses are given in the Box 18-18.

**Preadmission information**

How did you find out about the rehabilitation unit? (Check one)
- ❑ Doctor
- ❑ Nurse
- ❑ Other health person
- ❑ Friend
- ❑ Other (please name) _____

Did the nurse or doctor talk to you before you came?    ❑ Yes  ❑ No
If yes, did you get your questions answered?    ❑ Yes  ❑ No
If yes, did you understand what the unit was like?    ❑ Yes  ❑ No
What should clients know about the rehabilitation unit before coming to the unit?

| About your care | Always | Often | Sometimes | Rarely | Never | NA |
|---|---|---|---|---|---|---|
| I was included in planning my care. | ❑ | ❑ | ❑ | ❑ | ❑ | ❑ |
| The staff listened to my problems. | ❑ | ❑ | ❑ | ❑ | ❑ | ❑ |
| Questions about sex were answered. | ❑ | ❑ | ❑ | ❑ | ❑ | ❑ |
| My call light was answered quickly. | ❑ | ❑ | ❑ | ❑ | ❑ | ❑ |
| I learned about my medications. | ❑ | ❑ | ❑ | ❑ | ❑ | ❑ |
| Nurses explained things to be done to me. | ❑ | ❑ | ❑ | ❑ | ❑ | ❑ |
| Therapists explained things to be done to me. | ❑ | ❑ | ❑ | ❑ | ❑ | ❑ |
| **Family** | | | | | | |
| My family was included in planning my care. | ❑ | ❑ | ❑ | ❑ | ❑ | ❑ |
| My family was taught how to care for me. | ❑ | ❑ | ❑ | ❑ | ❑ | ❑ |
| My family had their questions answered. | ❑ | ❑ | ❑ | ❑ | ❑ | ❑ |
| My family went to family support group. | ❑ | ❑ | ❑ | ❑ | ❑ | ❑ |
| My family rated this group as helpful. | ❑ | ❑ | ❑ | ❑ | ❑ | ❑ |
| **If you had speech problems, please answer the following:** | | | | | | |
| Therapist helped me learn to talk. | ❑ | ❑ | ❑ | ❑ | ❑ | ❑ |
| My speech improved. | ❑ | ❑ | ❑ | ❑ | ❑ | ❑ |
| Staff understood my speech problem. | ❑ | ❑ | ❑ | ❑ | ❑ | ❑ |
| I learned to talk with the staff. | ❑ | ❑ | ❑ | ❑ | ❑ | ❑ |
| Family was taught to understand my speech. | ❑ | ❑ | ❑ | ❑ | ❑ | ❑ |

**Results and evaluation**

Did you have special things to learn before you came?    ❑ Yes  ❑ No
Did you learn what you wanted to learn?    ❑ Yes, definitely.  ❑ Yes, I think so.  ❑ No, I don't think so.  ❑ No, definitely not.
If needed, would you return to the unit?    ❑ Yes  ❑ Probably  ❑ No
Would you tell others to come to the unit?    ❑ Yes  ❑ Probably  ❑ No
What I liked most about the rehabilitation center:

_____
_____
_____

What I liked least about the rehabilitation center:

_____
_____
_____

**FIGURE 18-8** Sample items on a client satisfaction survey. (Reprinted from Courts NF: A patient satisfaction survey for a rehab unit, *Rehabil Nurs* 13[2]:80, 1988, with permission of the Association of Rehabilitation Nurses, 4700 W Lake Avenue, Glenview, Ill, 60025-1485. © 1988 Association of Rehabilitation Nurses.)

## THE COMMUNITY HEALTH NURSE AND THE ADULT WHO IS DISABLED

The nurse's role in working with the client who is disabled is varied and comprehensive. Nurses build on client and family strengths, establish mutually acceptable goals, and establish linkages with community resources. Nursing interventions focus on preventing disability and diminishing the severity of disabling conditions. Because of the complexities of providing therapeutic services to people who are disabled, community health nurses often use an interdisciplinary approach to providing care and may be part of a interdisciplinary team.

**BOX 18-19**

*Some Information Resources for Families*

---

Beach Center on Families and Disabilities
*http://www.lsi.ukans.edu/beach*
The center is located at the University of Kansas. For more than a decade, the Center has provided valuable services and information to families. It conducts research on families, disability, and policy and strives to individualize services to families, enhance family capabilities, provide advocacy services, and reduce family stress.

Family Village
*http://familyvillage.wisc.edu*
The Family Village is located at the University of Wisconsin. It provides informational resources on specific diagnoses, communication connections, adaptive products and technology, adaptive recreational activities, education, worship, health issues, disability-related media and literature.

Accent on Living (AOL)
*http://www.blvd.com/accent/*
AOL operates a computerized retrieval system containing information on products and devices and how-to information in areas such as eating, bathing, grooming, clothing, furniture, home management, toilet care, sexuality, mobility, and communication. It also publishes *Accent on Living,* a quarterly magazine.

4Disability
*http://www.4disability.com*
4Disability provides links to disability sites.

e-bility
*http://www.e-bility.com*
This website provides links to disability relation information, resources, services, and products

Internet Resources on Disabilities
*http://busboy.sped.ukans.edu/disabilities*
This website is maintained by the University of Kansas. It provides links to disability information and is compiled by the University's Department of Special Education.

National Council on Disability
*http://www.ncd.gov*

National Organization on Disability
*http://www.nod.org*

National Rehabilitation Information Center (NARIC)
*http://www.naric.com*

National Institute on Disability and Rehabilitation Research
*http://www.healthfinder.gov*

National Rehabilitation Association
*http://www.nationalrehab.org*

Disabled American Veterans
*http://www.dav.org*

National Industries for the Severely Handicapped (NISH)
*http://www.nish.org*

---

## Working with Clients and Their Families

Families are often the primary caregivers of family members who are disabled. It is important to identify strategies that promote family functioning, stability, growth, and coping. Improving the quality of life for people who are disabled, their families, and caregivers is an important nursing role (Canam, Acorn, 1999; Watson, 1992; Weeks, 1995; Youngblood, Hines, 1992). The nurse assists the client and family in adjusting to changes imposed by the condition and assists clients in living successfully in the community. Nurses often assume a case management role when working with families.

Family-centered nursing interventions play a key role in helping. In working with families, nurses carry out many roles, including case manager, counselor, teacher, advocate, and caregiver. In providing care, nurses must be careful to be empathetic, not sympathetic, and encourage independence. Nurses provide guidance, knowledge, and support; but it is the client and family who evoke change.

The nurse realizes that variables discussed previously in this chapter such as family coping patterns, expectations, available community resources, and economic status affect the family's ability to adapt. Often the nurse will coordinate care for the client between a number of community resources. Some information resources for families are given in Box 18-19.

Families play an important role in adapting to a disability (Pryor, 2000). Families often need assistance in planning for the long-term implications of the disability, setting realistic expectations, and using self-management techniques. Some of the long-term implications of the condition can be mitigated through the use of *anticipatory guidance*. Anticipatory guidance "anticipates" a situation before it occurs and provides the client with the skills necessary to successfully manage it. The teaching tips in Box 18-20 list some perceived needs that could be used as anticipatory guidance with families.

Allowing for meaningful expression of feelings that can range from despair and hopelessness to unrealistic optimism is a significant contribution of the community health nurse. Nurses need to assess their personal feelings, which can

Teaching TIPS BOX 18-20

## Educational Needs of Prospective Family Caregivers*

| RANK | ITEM (LEARNING TO . . .) | MEAN SCORE |
|---|---|---|
| 1 | Normalize the daily routine of a disabled adult within the bounds of his or her disabilities. | 4.86 |
| 2 | Ensure that assistance is available when a disabled adult needs help. | 4.83 |
| 3 | Evaluate the strengths and capabilities of a disabled adult. | 4.81 |
| 4 | Supervise or carry out prescribed treatments and other recommendations for maintaining a disabled adult's well-being. | 4.80 |
| 5 | Anticipate the needs of a disabled adult for future assistance and services. | 4.77 |
| 6 | Evaluate options for treatment and services for a disabled adult. | 4.71 |
| 7 | Monitor the course of the disease (or condition) and evaluate the significance of changes in a disabled adult. | 4.67 |
| 7 | Communicate adequately with a disabled adult. | 4.67 |
| 7 | Maintain or gain up-to-date knowledge of the health and human services systems and the options within these systems. | 4.67 |
| 7 | Maintain or gain up-to-date knowledge of payment mechanisms for services provided to disabled adults. | 4.67 |
| 8 | Perform basic personal care procedures for a disabled adult. | 4.65 |
| 9 | Provide structure for a disabled adult's activities. | 4.64 |
| 10 | Manage the current and future costs related to being a caregiver. | 4.63 |
| 10 | Give appropriate consideration to a disabled adult family member's opinions and preferences. | 4.63 |
| 11 | Accept emotionally the likelihood of a progressive decline in the health of a person who is significant to you. | 4.59 |
| 12 | Work through changes in the lifelong relationship between you and another person. | 4.54 |
| 13 | Avoid severe drain on your own physical strength and health. | 4.53 |
| 13 | Interact with medical and other human service providers. | 4.53 |
| 14 | Be creative in decreasing the tediousness of the daily routines of providing care to a disabled adult. | 4.52 |
| 14 | Compensate for emotional drain due to your constant responsibilities. | 4.52 |

Reprinted from Weeks SK: What are the educational needs of prospective family caregivers of newly disabled adults, *Rehabil Nurs,* 20(5):256-260, 1995, with permission of the Association of Rehabilitation Nurses, 4700 W Lake Avenue, Glenview, Ill, 60025-1485. © 1995 Association of Rehabilitation Nurses.

*Scores ranged from 1 (no importance) to 5 (high importance).

inhibit or enhance their ability to function effectively with persons who are disabled. Numerous studies have shown that health care providers have many inaccurate perceptions and negative attitudes about persons who are disabled (Lindgren, Oermann, 1993, p. 121). Lindgren and Oermann conducted a study to examine the attitudes of nursing students toward the people who are disabled to determine the effect of an educational program on these attitudes. Study results showed that students had significantly higher scores and more positive attitudes following the education program.

Nursing interventions should include assessing the entire family as a unit (see Chapters 7 and 9). The family assessment process includes examining family dynamics and characteristics and perceptions of roles, disability, health care, coping skills, and support systems (Youngblood, Hines, 1992). Box 18-21 presents some questions that help the nurse assess the family's perceptions of the disability. Nurses focus on prevention strategies for people who already have potentially disabling conditions to limit condition occurrence, impairment, and functional limitation. They promote self-care, self-management, and self-

advocacy; provide health education interventions; link clients with community resources; and take part in client advocacy.

### Promoting Self-Care, Self-Management, and Self-Advocacy

Nursing interventions should focus on self-care, self-management, and self-advocacy. Self-care interventions help keep the person independent. Self-management techniques are directed toward helping clients make informed decisions. Self-advocacy interventions help the person to be in control of the situation and be able to act effectively on his or her own behalf. Some self-advocacy behaviors are given in Box 18-22. Nurses who promote self-advocacy work in partnership with clients, assisting them in obtaining the knowledge needed to make informed decisions and in learning negotiation skills.

### Health Education Interventions

Health education historically has been a community health nursing role (see Chapter 12). Nursing interventions include teaching clients about their conditions, community

**BOX 18-21**

*Assessment of Family's Perception of Disability*

I. Family Characteristics
- What are the biological characteristics of each family member?
- What is the family's cultural/ethnic background?
- What are the socioeconomic resources available to family members?
- What are the personality characteristics of each family member?

II. The Family's Perception of Rules and Roles
- What are the rules that govern family interactions?
- How do family members interact with each other?
- What is the structure of the family unit?
- How are rules and roles assigned?
- What events cause rules and/or roles to change?

III. The Family's Perception of the Disability
- What meaning does the disability have for each family member?
- What responsibility does each member have for the management of the disability?
- How are decisions made about the management of the disability?
- How are family interactions affected by the disability?

IV. The Family's Perception of Health Care
- What experiences have family members had with health care systems?
- What experiences with health care systems have resulted from the disability?
- What expectations do family members have in regard to the management of the disability?
- How do family members expect to interact with health care professionals?

V. The Family's Perception of Coping Skills and Support Systems
- How have family members reacted to crisis in the past?
- What information does the family need about the disability?
- What resources are available to family members?
- What support systems are available to family members?

From Youngblood NM, Hines J: The influence of the family's perception of disability on rehabilitation outcomes, *Rehabil Nurs* 17(6):325, 1992. Reprinted from *Rehabilitation Nursing*, vol 17, issue 6, with permission of the Association of Rehabilitation Nurses, 4700 W Lake Avenue, Glenview, Ill, 60025-1485. © 1992 Association of Rehabilitation Nurses.

**BOX 18-22**

*Self-Advocacy*

Self-advocacy enables persons who are disabled and their families to:
- Control the type and source of treatment received
- Be free to refuse treatment or services
- Have access to all relevant information about their own treatment
- Comprehend the process of appealing any decision that affects them
- Make informed choices
- Rely on service providers to be catalysts and resources rather than decision makers
- Take reasonable risks and have the right to fail but to take responsibility for change
- Acquire skills that will maximize independence
- Engage in productive activity commensurate with their needs, abilities, and interests

Modified from Breese P, Mikrut S: Survivor training and empowerment program (S.T.E.P.), *Am Rehab* 21(3):38-42, 1995, pp. 41-42.

accepting people who are disabled. For example, in the school setting, programs that discuss disabilities, such as New Kids on the Block, can be an effective way to help children learn about disabling conditions. New Kids on the Block is a national program that assists children in developing positive attitudes toward people with disabilities. School nurses can help children understand disabling conditions and why these conditions exist, and assist children in accepting each others' differences. Local health departments and community agencies have numerous health education materials available to assist the nurse in working with families and the community.

GROUP LEARNING. Nursing interventions that involve group learning for adults with disabilities have historically been a part of community health nursing activities. Nurses have historically and successfully been involved in classes regarding conditions such as arthritis, diabetes, hypertension, stroke, myocardial infarction, and mental retardation. It appears that the commonality of emotional and physical problems shared by clients in groups is conducive to learning (Payne, 1995, p. 268). Nursing research on the use of groups with adults who are disabled has shown that group members received the following benefits from others in the group: learning from each other, reduced feelings of isolation, and enjoyment of hearing other's experiences, goals, and problems (Payne, 1993). Other studies have shown that group sessions have been helpful in treating the social isolation and loneliness often experienced by people with disabilities (Acorn, Bramptom, 1992, p. 22). Clients often hear of resources from other people experiencing the same condition, such as meetings with self-help groups.

resources, self-management, self-care, and self-advocacy. Community health nurses also "educate" communities about people who are disabled and disabling conditions. Nurses may promote community awareness by focusing on primary prevention of disabling conditions.

Health education activities in schools and workplaces can assist people in understanding disabling conditions and

## Community Resource Utilization

Assisting clients in using community resources is an important role for the nurse. Numerous resources are discussed in this chapter. Clients are often not aware of the resources available to them or how to work with these resources. The nurse links clients to appropriate community resources through the referral process (see Chapter 10). Searching out resources can be a trying experience for clients and their families. The nurse assists the client in learning how to find and utilize community resources.

The local telephone directory is a useful source of information. Some telephone directories include specific sections on community resources. Many agencies are located under the government phone listings or under specific headings in the yellow pages such as hospitals, hospital equipment, rehabilitation, and mental health. Local health departments and departments of human or social services, federal Social Security Administration offices, state developmental disability councils, United Way, and public libraries are all sources of information. Shop-at-home catalogs, previously mentioned under Health Care in this chapter, have many useful items.

Other helpful publications are *Health Information Resources in the Federal Government*, published by the Office of Disease Prevention and Health Promotion (ODPHP) (*http://www.odphp.osophs.dhhs.gov*), as well as directories of national disability organizations published by NIDRR. These publications provide listings of many resources that can be of assistance to the person who is disabled.

Box 18-23 tells a story of survivors of traumatic brain injury (TBI) and how resource utilization affected adaptation. Nationally, almost 2 million Americans experience TBI each year, and many of these cases result in a disabling condition (Forkosch, Kaye, LaPlante, 1996, p. 1). A large number of TBIs involve motor vehicle and household accidents. Health education by nurses in relation to safety, including discussions on the use of seatbelts and household safety, is a significant preventive intervention.

SELF-HELP GROUPS. Self-help groups are lay groups in which people who share some problem in their lives come together regularly to express empathy and support one another (Hildingh, Fridlund, Segesten, 2000). These groups deal with a variety of problems, have been found to be therapeutic to clients, and are an excellent way to bring

**BOX 18-23**

*A Story of Survival and Resource Management*

Survivors of traumatic brain injury (TBI) and their families face an extremely complex and potentially confusing array of services, medical professionals, and human service delivery systems. The course of rehabilitation is extensive, sometimes encompassing many years, numerous medical disciplines, service delivery systems, and bureaucratic entities. The process of rehabilitation and community reintegration following brain injury often requires years of effort and major medical and rehabilitative expenses. Survivors of TBI emerge from the medical milieu concerned about the future but unaware and uninformed of the bureaucratic and medicolegal challenges that lie ahead.

Most of the survivors of TBI receive time-limited case management services through the insurance carrier responsible for covering the accident or through a facility-based case manager who acts as an internal coordinator of the rehabilitation team. However, once the injured person leaves the facility and insurance monies are depleted, case management (service coordination) either stops or is abruptly transferred to the family. Therefore, upon transfer to the home or community, families, by default, begin to face the reality of providing long-term support and service coordination with limited financial and emotional resources.

Survivors, through extensive hospitalizations and indoctrination into the role of the client, frequently learn to passively accept medical treatment and rehabilitation options available to them. After discharge from the medical setting, they are thrust into the role of fending for themselves with few supports and are often unable to obtain information on existing service or programs that address their unique needs.

Unfortunately, little preparation is given to people with brain injury and their families to adequately function in their new role as "service coordinator." Forced to fill the role of self-advocate or service coordinator, survivors and their families learn about available services and procurement of those services in a lengthy piecemeal process that may never reveal the full spectrum of assistance available. The process is a time-consuming, frustrating, and potentially overwhelming endeavor for a family already taxed by the advent of a traumatic event.

Human service delivery systems and state social service systems, which typically assume responsibility for the provision of long-term support and case management, are unable to keep pace with the ever-increasing demand for service to a population of Americans who live longer and have more severely disabling conditions. Case management—or service coordination—specifically for people with brain injury has not been developed in most states and is not readily available to these individuals who have difficulty accessing other social service systems. As a result, many survivors of brain injury "fall through the bureaucratic cracks," are unable to access services available to people with other disabilities, and become exhausted by running the gauntlet of social services before they realize any success for their efforts.

Modified from Breese P, Mikrut S: Survivor training and empowerment program (S.T.E.P.), *Am Rehab* 21(3):38-39, 1995.

people together with similar health concerns (Kessenich, Guyatt, Patton, et al., 2000). These groups are supplementary sources of support outside the clients' existing social network and are important to consider when planning nursing care (Hildingh, Fridlund, Segesten, 2000). Nurses should be knowledgeable of such groups in the community and refer clients to them as appropriate.

## Client Advocacy

The person who is disabled is vulnerable and at risk for having unmet health care needs. The nurse uses advocacy skills to facilitate the development of relevant public policies and community services, decrease societal barriers for people who are disabled, and facilitate more positive societal attitudes. Nurses frequently are involved in advocacy for clients who are disabled; however, many health professionals hesitate to put themselves in client advocacy positions for reasons including the following:

- *Unfamiliar role.* Professionals have generally not been trained to be advocates and often do not have the skills to undertake such a role. The advocate may find advocacy difficult, awkward, and uncomfortable.
- *Fear of reprisal.* Often, the greater the impact of the advocacy action, the greater the risk of reprisal. The advocate must be aware of the possibility of reprisal and must evaluate the possible outcomes of his or her behavior.
- *Role conflict.* It is difficult to take stands contrary to the stand of other professionals in the field or contrary to the organization for which one works, and the advocate may be pressured to "conform." The advocacy role may be in conflict with the professional role or personal beliefs.
- *Apathy.* It is easier not to be involved, especially when one is not personally or directly affected.
- *Lack of support.* If one lacks the support of others, the advocacy stand becomes more difficult and sometimes risky (e.g., job security).
- *Change implications.* Advocacy often means change, and change often means stress.

Concerns such as not enough time or money, no one to help, not wanting to get involved on an emotional level, and the system not being ready for change all are common reasons for not assuming an advocacy role. It is easy to feel empathy with these concerns, and most people have probably voiced them at one time or another. Taking an advocacy stand requires time, a commitment to client rights, and the belief that clients have a right to essential health care services. The impact that a nurse can have on the system as an advocate should not be underestimated. An example of this is the case of a nurse working with a local association of parents of disabled children.

**CASE Scenario** The parents in a local association for disabled citizens were increasingly aware of instances of abuse of their children in the state institu-

tional setting in which they resided. The parents had talked with the institution administration and believed that they were not receiving adequate information; some of the parents felt intimidated. The parents were becoming increasingly concerned about the implications of their actions on their children. If they continued to press for information, they were worried about reprisals. If they did not press for information, they were worried that the situation would get worse. A nurse who was a member of the association was able to act as an advocate and take action.

The nurse met with the parents and the institution administration. After assessing and concluding that there was a problem and that the administration was resistant to change, the nurse examined the laws of the state regarding child abuse. One section of the law clearly stated that an institution must be independently investigated when there were suspected cases of child abuse or neglect. The nurse knew that state institutions were not adhering to that section of the law and were doing their own investigations. By obtaining legal counsel, working with the parent group, and using the established grievance procedure for state mental health clients, the community health nurse was able to help effect change in the system. The state now has impartial investigations of all cases of child abuse in state institutions and residential facilities, and parents or guardians have access to the results.

The advocacy efforts of this community health nurse had many positive effects. Reporting procedures for institutional cases of suspected abuse and neglect were clearly written and implemented in that state. The state legislature appropriated money to be used in further protection and advocacy services for people who are developmentally disabled. In addition, the general public became increasingly aware of the needs of people who are mentally disabled and some of the conditions under which they live.

Nurses are in a position to correct public misconceptions about people who are disabled. They can work to gain greater acceptance of individuals who are disabled in whatever setting they reside. The nurse can be a role model and be instrumental in promoting a positive attitude toward people who are considered disabled by the general public.

## NURSING ORGANIZATIONS AND DISABILITY

A number of specialty nursing organizations focus on disabling conditions (Box 18-24). The Association of Rehabilitation Nurses (ARN) is a professional organization for rehabilitation nurses and an excellent resource on rehabilitation nursing practice. ARN sponsors research and educational opportunities in rehabilitation nursing. It offers numerous publications, including *Standards and Scope of Rehabilitation Nursing Practice* (ARN, 1994a) (Box 18-25),

### BOX 18-24
*Nursing Organizations and Disability*

Association of Rehabilitation Nurses
*http://www.rehabnurse.org*
American Nephrology Nurses' Association
*http://anna.inurse.com*
American Association of Neuroscience Nurses
*http://aann.org*
American Psychiatric Nurses Association
*http://www.apna.org*
American Association of Nurses in AIDS Care
*http://www.anacnet.org*
Wound, Ostomy, Continence Nurses
*http://www.wocn.org*
American Society of Plastic and Reconstructive Surgery Nurses
*http://asprsn.inurse.com*
National Association of Orthopaedic Nurses
*http://naon.inurse.com*
Oncology Nursing Society
*http://www.ons.org*
Association of Pediatric Oncology Nursing
*http://www.apon.org*

*Scope and Standards of Advanced Clinical Practice in Rehabilitation Nursing* (ARN, 1996), and the journal *Rehabilitation Nursing*, and briefly published the journal *Rehabilitation Nursing Research*. ARN promotes rehabilitation nursing research and research-based rehabilitation nursing practice. It has offered certification in rehabilitation nursing since 1984 and advanced practice nursing certification since 1997.

## SUMMARY

The number of individuals in society who are characterized as disabled can be expected to increase as will demand for services to these individuals. Adults who are disabled are confronted with adapting to their disability amidst societal, family, and individual variables that influence adaptation and personal growth and development. Most disabling conditions are long term and require ongoing use of community resources. The need for case management interventions is great, as is the need for greater availability of services for people who are disabled.

Community health nurses are in a unique position to assist clients who are disabled in obtaining services that will enhance adaptation and promote growth. They assist

### BOX 18-25
*Standards of Rehabilitation Nursing Practice*

The goal of rehabilitation nursing is to assist the individual who has a disability and/or chronic illness in restoring, maintaining, and promoting his or her maximal health. This includes preventing chronic illness and disability. The rehabilitation nurse is skilled at treating alterations in functional ability and lifestyle that result from physical disability and chronic illness.

*Standards of Care*
*Standard I. Assessment*
   The rehabilitation nurse collects client health data.
*Standard II. Nursing Diagnosis*
   The rehabilitation nurse analyzes the assessment when determining diagnoses.
*Standard III. Outcome Identification*
   The rehabilitation nurse identifies expected outcomes individualized to the client.
*Standard IV. Planning*
   The rehabilitation nurse develops a plan of care that prescribes interventions to attain expected outcomes.
*Standard V. Intervention*
   The rehabilitation nurse implements the interventions identified in the plan of care.
*Standard VI. Evaluation*
   The rehabilitation nurse evaluates the client's progress toward attainment of outcome.

*Standards of Professional Performance*
*Standard I. Quality of Care*
   The rehabilitation nurse systematically evaluates the quality and effectiveness of rehabilitation nursing practice.
*Standard II. Performance Appraisal*
   The rehabilitation nurse evaluates his or her own nursing practice in relation to professional practice standards and relevant statutes and regulations.
*Standard III. Education*
   The rehabilitation nurse acquires and maintains current knowledge in nursing practice.
*Standard IV. Collegiality*
   The rehabilitation nurse contributes to the professional development of peers, colleagues, and others.
*Standard V. Ethics*
   The rehabilitation nurse's decisions and actions on behalf of clients are determined in an ethical manner.
*Standard VI. Collaboration*
   The rehabilitation nurse collaborates with the client, significant others, and health care providers in providing client care.
*Standard VII. Research*
   The rehabilitation nurse uses research findings in practice.
*Standard VIII. Resource Utilization*
   The rehabilitation nurse considers factors related to safety, effectiveness, and cost in planning and delivering client care.

Reprinted with permission from Association of Rehabilitation Nurses: *Standards and scope of rehabilitation nursing practice*, ed 3, Glenview, Ill, 1994a, ARN. © 1994 Association of Rehabilitation Nurses, 4700 W Lake Avenue, Glenview, Ill, 60025-1485.

clients with rehabilitation and work cooperatively with the clients and their families to establish plans of care. A sensitivity to the needs of this population group and an awareness that there are individual differences among clients who are disabled are both essential for the community health nurse to function effectively with clients who have special needs.

Increasingly, health care professionals are becoming actively involved in advocacy for this population group. Advocacy has been critical in the procurement of many essential services for these clients. While legislation in the last decade has reflected a more positive attitude toward people who are disabled, numerous needs remain unmet. Professionals must continue to facilitate public awareness about disabling conditions and the needs of people who are experiencing them. Americans who are disabled have the same human and civil rights as everyone else and deserve their share of the country's health resources.

## CRITICAL THINKING
### *exercise*

In this chapter the effect of societal values on adaptation to a disability is discussed. What are some of the values the American society holds that affect adaptation to a disability and the quality of life for people who are disabled? As a nurse, what are some things that you could do to facilitate positive attitudes toward persons who are disabled? What are your own attitudes about persons who are disabled, and how do you think these attitudes will affect your nursing practice?

## REFERENCES

Acorn S, Bramptom E: Patients, loneliness: a challenge for rehabilitation nurses, *Rehabil Nurs* 17(1):22-25, 1992.

All AC, Loving GL, Crane LL: Animals, horseback riding and implications for rehabilitation therapy, *J Rehabil* 65:49-57, 1999.

Associated Press: Horses are therapists in program for disabled children, *Knoxville News-Sentinel*, January 17, 2000, A2.

Association of Rehabilitation Nurses (ARN): *Standards and scope of rehabilitation nursing practice*, ed 3, Skokie, Ill, 1994a, ARN.

Association of Rehabilitation Nurses (ARN): *The pain management rehabilitation nurse: role description*, Skokie, Ill, 1994b, ARN.

Association of Rehabilitation Nurses (ARN): *Scope and standards of advanced clinical practice in rehabilitation nursing*, Skokie, Ill, 1996, ARN.

Breese P, Mikrut S: Survivor training and empowerment program (S.T.E.P.), *Am Rehab* 21(3):38-42, 1995.

Buscaglia LF, editor: *The disabled and their parents: a counseling challenge*, ed 2, Thorofare, NJ, 1983, Slack.

Canam C, Acorn S: Quality of life for family caregivers of people with chronic health problems, *Rehabil Nurs* 24(5):192-196, 1999.

Centers for Disease Control and Prevention (CDC): *Chronic diseases and their risk factors. The nation's leading causes of death*, Atlanta, 1999, CDC.

Chin PA, Finnocchiaro D, Rosebrough A: *Rehabilitation nursing practice*, New York, 1998, McGraw-Hill.

Courts NF: A patient satisfaction survey for a rehab unit, *Rehabil Nurs* 13(2):79-81, 1988.

Davidhizar R, Shearer R: Helping the client with chronic disability achieve high-level wellness, *Rehabil Nurs* 22(3):131-135, 1997.

Deoudes G: In the spotlight: United Way and dial 211: improving access to human services for younger and older Americans, *Together* 5(3):3, 2000.

Duffy Y: Disability shouldn't be a bar to romance, *The Atlanta Journal Constitution*, August 11, 1996, p. R1.

Eakes GG, Burke ML, Hainsworth MA: Middle-range theory of chronic sorrow, *Image* 30:179-183, 1998.

Easton KL, Andrews, JC: The roles of the pastor in the interdisciplinary rehabilitation team, *Rehabil Nurs* 25:10-12, 2000.

Eliopoulos C: Chronic care coaches: helping people to help people, *Home Healthc Nurse* 15(3):185-188, 1997.

El Nasser H: Parents of disabled kids relate to 'breaking point,' *USA Today*, Dec 30, 1999, p. A4.

Finkelstein V, French S: Towards a psychology of disability. In Swain J, Finkelstein V, French S, Oliver M, editors: *Disabling barriers—enabling environments*, London, 1993, Sage, pp. 26-33.

Forkosch JA, Kaye S, LaPlante MP: The incidence of traumatic brain injury in the United States, *Disabil Stat Abstract*, Number 14, Washington, DC, 1996, National Institute on Disability and Rehabilitation Research.

Gatens-Robinson E, Rubin SE: Societal values and ethical commitments that influence rehabilitation service delivery behavior. In SE Rubin, RT Roessler, editors: *Foundations of the vocational rehabilitation process*, ed 4, Austin, Tx, 1995, Pro-ed, pp. 157-174.

Geigel W: Rehabilitation facilities: a perspective, *Am Rehab* 21(3):28-30, 1995.

Giordano G, D'Alonzo BJ: The link between transition and independent living, *Am Rehab* 20(1):2-7, 1994.

Giordano G, D'Alonzo BJ: Challenge and progress in rehabilitation: a review of the past 25 years and a preview of the future, *Am Rehab* 21(3):14-21, 1995.

Greco SB: Sexuality and education counseling. In Hoeman SP: *Rehabilitation nursing: process and application*, ed 2, St Louis, 1996, Mosby, pp. 594-627.

Greenberg B: More learning-disabled students at college, *Knoxville News Sentinel*, February 10, 2000, p. A1.

Herson L, Hart KA, Gordon MJ, et al.: Identifying and overcoming barriers to providing sexuality information in the clinical setting, *Rehabil Nurs* 24:148-151, 1999.

Hildingh C, Fridlund B, Segesten K: Self-help groups as a support strategy in nursing: a case study, *Rehabil Nurs* 25:100-104, 2000.

Hoeman SP: Conceptual bases for rehabilitation nursing. In Hoeman SP: *Rehabilitation nursing: process and application*, ed 2, St Louis, 1996, Mosby, pp. 3-20.

Hoeman SP: Foreword. Rehabilitation—A vital nursing function. In Pryor J, editor: *Professional Development Series No. 11*, Australia, 1999, Royal College of Nursing.

Hoeman SP: *Rehabilitation nursing: process and application*, ed 3, St Louis, 2001, Mosby.

Kaye S: Disability and the digital divide, *Disability Stat Abstract*, 22(July):1-4, 2000.

Kendrick D: Invisible barriers: how you can make parenting easier, *Disabled USA* 1:17-19, 1983.

Kessenich C, Guyatt GH, Patton CL, et al: Support groups intervention for women with osteoporosis, *Rehabil Nurs* 25:88-92, 2000.

Kubler-Ross E: *On death and dying*, New York, 1969, MacMillan.

Lafata JE, Koch GG, Weissert WG: Estimating activity limitation in the noninstitutionalized population: a method for small areas, *Am J Public Health* 84(11):1813-1817, 1994.

Lambert J: Meeting the emotional needs of a patient, *Rehabil Nurs* 24:141-142, 1999.

LaPlante MP, Rice DP, Wenger BL: Medical care use, health insurance and disability in the United States, *Disabil Stat Abstract*, Number 8, Washington, DC, 1995, National Institute on Disability and Rehabilitation Research.

Lindgren CL, Burke ML, Hainsworth MA, et al.: Chronic sorrow: a lifespan concept, *Schol Inq Nurs Pract* 6(1):27-40, 1992.

Lindgren CL, Oermann MH: Effects of an educational intervention on students' attitudes toward the disabled, *J Nurs Educ* 32(3):121-126, 1993.

Marks JS: Looking back offers perspectives for meeting challenges that lie ahead, *Chronic Diseases Notes and Reports* 11:2-9, 1998, Centers for Disease Control and Prevention.

Martin N, Holt NB, Hicks D: *Comprehensive rehabilitation nursing*, New York, 1981, McGraw-Hill.

Max W, Rice DP, Trupin L: Medical expenditures for people with disabilities, *Disabil Stat Abstract*, Number 12, Washington, DC, 1996, National Institute for Disability and Rehabilitation Research.

McClain L: Shopping center wheelchair accessibility: ongoing advocacy to implement the Americans with Disabilities Act of 1990, *Public Health Nurs* 17:178-186, 2000.

McCloskey JC, Bulechek GM, editors: *Nursing interventions classification (NIC)*, ed 2, St Louis, 1996, Mosby.

Miller JF: *Coping with chronic illness: overcoming powerlessness*, ed 2, Philadelphia, 1992, FA Davis.

Moore CL, Feist-Price S: Societal attitudes and the civil rights of persons with disabilities, *J Applied Rehab Counsel* 30(2):19-24, 1999.

Mumma CM: *Rehabilitation nursing: concepts and practice—a core curriculum*, ed 2, Evanston, Ill, 1987, Rehabilitation Nursing Foundation.

National Center for Chronic Disease Prevention and Health Promotion (NCCDPHP): *CDC/NCCDPHP: turning research findings into effective community programs*, Atlanta, 1996, Centers for Disease Control and Prevention.

National Rehabilitation Information Center (NARIC): *Factsheet on the National Rehabilitation Information Center, information for independence*, Silver Spring, Md, 1996, NARIC.

North American Nursing Diagnosis Association (NANDA): *Nursing diagnosis definitions and classifications—2001-2002*, Philadelphia, 2001, NANDA.

Oermann MH, Lindgren CL: An educational program's effects on students' attitudes toward people with disabilities: a 1-year follow-up, *Rehabil Nurs* 20(1):6-10, 1995.

Office of Special Education and Rehabilitative Services: *Pocket guide to federal help for individuals with disabilities*, Washington, DC, 2000, US Department of Education.

Patrick DL: Toward an epidemiology of disablement, *Am J Public Health* 84(11):1723-1724, 1994.

Patterson JB: Using the internet to facilitate the rehabilitation process, *J Rehabil* 96:4-10, 2000.

Payne JA: The contribution of group learning to the rehabilitation of spinal cord injured adults, *Rehabil Nurs* 18(7):375-379, 1993.

Payne JA: Group learning for adults with disabilities or chronic disease, *Rehabil Nurs* 20(5):268-272, 1995.

Pope AM, Tarlov AR, editors: *Disability in America: toward a national agenda for prevention*, Washington, DC, 1991, National Academy Press.

President's Committee on Employment of People with Disabilities (PCEPD): *Ability for hire: educational kit 1996*, Washington, DC, 1996, PCEPD.

President's Committee on Employment of People with Disabilities (PCEPD): *Think ability: educational kit 1999*, Washington, DC, 1999, PCEPD.

President's Committee on Employment of People with Disabilities (PCEPD): *Ability you can bank on: educational kit 2000*, Washington, DC, 2000, PCEPD.

Pryor J: Creating a rehabilitative milieu, *Rehabil Nurs* 25:141-144, 2000.

Reasonable accommodation: what consumers and employers want to know, *NARIC Q* 4(4):2, 6, 1995.

Reno J: Disability law will be enforced, *USA Today*, Monday, July 26, 1993, p. A9

Richardson M: Addressing barriers: disabled rights and the implications for nursing of the social construct of disability, *J Adv Nurs* 25:1269-1275, 1997.

Riemer-Reiss M: Vocational rehabilitation counseling at a distance: challenges, strategies and ethics to consider, *J Rehab* 66:11-17, 2000.

Robert Wood Johnson Foundation: *Challenges in health care*, New York, 1992, The Foundation.

Safilios-Rothschild C: *The sociology and social psychology of disability rehabilitation*, New York, 1982, University Press of America.

Sawin KJ, Heard L: Nursing diagnoses used most frequently in rehabilitation nursing practice, *Rehabil Nurs* 17(5):256-262, 1992.

Sexuality Information and Education Council of the United States (SIECUS): SIECUS position statements on human sexuality, sexual health and sexuality education and information 1995-96, *SIECUS Report* 24(3):21-23, 1996.

Shadish WR, Lurigio AJ, Lewis DA: After institutionalization: the present and future of mental health long-term care policy, *J Soc Issues* 45(3):1-15, 1989.

Simon JM: Chronic pain syndrome: nursing assessment and intervention, *Rehabil Nurs* 21(1):13-19, 1996.

Simon JM, McTier CL: Development of a chronic pain assessment tool, *Rehabil Nurs* 21(1):20-24, 1996.

Smith LW, Smith QW, Richards L, et al.: Independent living centers: moving into the 21st century, *Am Rehab* 20(1):14-22, 1994.

Smith M: The nature of rehabilitation. In Smith M: *Rehabilitation in adult nursing practice*, Edinburgh, 1999a, Churchill Livingston.

Smith M: Nursing and rehabilitation. In Smith M: *Rehabilitation in adult nursing practice*, Edinburgh, 1999b, Churchill Livingston.

Stafford BJ: A legislative perspective on the Rehabilitation Act, *Am Rehabil* 21(3):37-41, 1995.

Stryker R: *Rehabilitation aspects of acute and chronic nursing care*, Philadelphia, 1977, WB Saunders.

Stucki BR: *Living in the community with a disability: demographic characteristics of the population with disabilities under age 65*, Washington, DC, 1995, American Association of Retired Persons.

Sussman MB, editor: *Sociology and rehabilitation*, Washington, DC, 1966, American Sociological Association.

Thomas VM, Ellison K, Howell EV, et al.: Caring for the person receiving ventilatory support at home: caregiver's needs and involvements, *Heart & Lung* 21:180-186, 1992.

Thorne S, Paterson B: Shifting images of chronic illness, *Image* 30:173-178, 1998.

Trupin L, Rice DP: Health status, medical care use, and number of disabling conditions in the United States, *Disabil Stat Abstract*, Number 9, Washington, DC, 1995, National Institute on Disability and Rehabilitation Research.

US Department of Commerce: *Statistical abstract of the United States: 1995*, ed 115, Washington, DC, 1995, US Government Printing Office.

US Department of Commerce: *Statistical abstract of the United States: 1999*, ed 119, Washington, DC, 1999, US Government Printing Office.

US Department of Health and Human Services (USDHHS): *Healthy People 2010, conference edition*, Washington, DC, 2000, US Government Printing Office.

Vines SW, Cox A, Nicoll L, et al.: Effects of a multimodal pain rehabilitation program: pilot study, *Rehabil Nurs* 21(1):25-30, 1996.

Watson PG: Family issues in rehabilitation, *Holistic Nurs Pract* 6(2):51-59, 1992.

Watson PG: The Americans with Disabilities Act: more rights for people with disabilities, *Rehabil Nurs* 25(4):145-149, 2000 [Reprint of article from *Rehabil Nurs* 15(6), 1990].

Weeks SK: What are the educational needs of prospective family care-givers of newly disabled adults? *Rehabil Nurs* 20(5):256-260, 272, 1995.

Winterhalter JG: Group support for families during the acute phase of rehabilitation, *Holistic Nurs Pract* 6(2):23-31, 1992.

World Health Organization (WHO), Expert Committee on Disability Prevention and Rehabilitation: *Disability prevention and rehabilitation*, Technical Report Series 668, Geneva, 1981, WHO.

Youngblood NM, Hines J: The influence of the family's perception of disability on rehabilitation outcomes, *Rehabil Nurs* 17(6):323-326, 1992.

## SELECTED BIBLIOGRAPHY

Biordi B, Oermann MH: The effect of prior experience in a rehabilitation setting on students' attitudes toward the disabled, *Rehabil Nurs* 18(2):95-98, 1993.

Burks KJ: A nursing practice model for chronic illness, *Rehabil Nurs* 24(5):197-200, 1999.

Drayton-Hargrove S: Assessing abuse of disabled older adults: a family systems approach, *Rehabil Nurs* 25:136-140, 2000.

Favazza PC, Odom SL: Promoting positive attitudes of kindergarten-age children toward people with disabilities, *Exceptional Children* 63:405-418, 1997.

Fredereicks DW, Williams WL: New definition of mental retardation for the American Association of Mental Retardation, *Image* 30:53-56, 1998.

Garske GG, Williams BT, Schiro-Griest C: The financial costs of severe mental illness, *J Rehabil* 65:39-44, 1999.

Gibbons KB: A model for professional rehabilitation nursing practice, *Rehabil Nurs* 20(1):23-28, 1995.

Harley DA, Hall M, Savage TA: Working with gay and lesbian consumers with disabilities: helping practitioners understand another frontier of diversity, *J Applied Rehab Counseling* 31(1):4-11, 2000.

Lustig DC: Families with an adult with mental retardation: predictors of family adjustment, *J Applied Rehab Counseling* 30:11-17, 1999.

Makas E: Positive attitudes toward disabled people: disabled and nondisabled persons' perspectives, *J Soc Issues* 44(1):49-61, 1988.

O'Neill DP, Kenny EK: Spirituality and chronic illness, *Image* 30:275-280, 1998.

Sanchez J, Byfield G, Brown TT, et al.: Perceived accessibility versus actual physical accessibility of healthcare facilities, *Rehabil Nurs* 25:6-9, 2000.

Weeks SK: Colors, symbols, and other communication ideas, *Rehabil Nurs* 24:190-191, 1999.

# Information Resources

HIV/AIDS Hotline
1-800-342-2437

Alcohol and Drug Helpline
1-800-821-4357

Alzheimer's Association
1-800-272-3900

Arthritis Foundation Information Line
1-800-283-7800

Asthma Information Line
1-800-822-2762

National Arthritis and Musculoskeletal and Skin Diseases
   Clearinghouse
1-877-22-NIAMS

American Council of the Blind
1-800-424-8666

Guide Dogs for the Blind
1-800-295-4050

Brain Tumor Society
1-800-770-TBTS

National Cancer Institute Information Service
1-800-422-6237

Christopher Reeve Paralysis Association
1-800-225-0292

Chron's and Colitis Foundation of America
1-800-932-2423

Cystic Fibrosis Foundation
1-800-344-4823

National Association for Continence
1-800-252-3337

Cancer Information Service
1-800-4-CANCER

American Cancer Society
1-800-227-2345

American Diabetes Association
1-800-232-3472

American Heart Association
1-800-242-8721

American Lung Association
1-800-586-4872

Asthma Information Line
1-800-822-2762

National Institute on Deafness and Other Communication
   Disorders Information Clearinghouse
1-800-241-1044

Epilepsy Foundation of America
1-800-332-1000

Hepatitis Foundation International
1-800-891-0179

The ARC (Association for Retarded Citizens)
1-800-433-5255

Multiple Sclerosis Foundation
1-800-441-7055

Muscular Dystrophy Association
1-800-572-1717

National Alliance for the Mentally Ill
1-800-950-6264

National Foundation for Depressive Illness
1-800-248-4344

National Institute of Mental Health Information Hotline
1-800-647-2642

National Mental Health Association
1-800-969-6642

American Liver Foundation
1-800-223-0179

National Stroke Association
1-800-787-6537

---

*Note, phone numbers frequently change. If one of these numbers is not correct please contact 1-800-555-1212 for 800 number information. Also, search online for other resources at sites such as *http://www.healthfinder.gov* or contact the Office of Disease Prevention and Health Promotion in the U.S. Department of Health and Human Services to obtain a copy of the publication *Toll-Free Numbers for Health Information.*

# Information Resources (cont'd)

National Institute for Neurological Disorders and Stroke
1-800-352-9424

Paralyzed Veterans of America
1-800-424-8200

American Parkinson's Disease Association
1-800-223-2732

Osteoporosis and Related Bone Diseases National Resource Center
1-800-624-BONE

United Ostomy Association
1-800-826-0826

National Psoriasis Foundation
1-800-723-9166

National STD Hotline
1-800-227-8922

Sickle Cell Disease Association
1-800-421-8453

Thyroid Foundation of America
1-800-832-8321

American Foundation of Urologic Disease
1-800-242-2383

National Fragile X/Foundation
1-800-336-4363

National Health Information Center
1-800-336-4797

National Women's Health Information Center
1-800-994-9662

National Center for Chronic Disease Prevention and Health Promotion (CDC)
1-877-CDC-DIAB

National Hospice Organization
1-800-658-8898

National Institute for Rehabilitation Engineering
1-800-736-2216

National Rehabilitation Information Center
1-800-346-2742

National Organization for Rare Disorders
1-800-999-6673

IBM Independence Series
1-800-426-4832

# Legislation and Voluntary Efforts for the Disabled: United States

1798 U.S. Congress establishes a marine hospital to provide for disabled seamen (England had established such a facility in 1588).

1902 Goodwill Industries is originated by a minister, Dr. Edgar Helms, to provide employment opportunities for people who are disabled.

1918 Federal Board of Vocational Rehabilitation established to provide vocational rehabilitation services to the disabled veterans of World War I.

   Massachusetts becomes the first state to establish public provisions to aid in the vocational rehabilitation of disabled citizens.

1920 The first Vocational Rehabilitation Act (Public Law 565) is passed. Services under the act were primarily for physically disabled military personnel. This act was administered by the Vocational Rehabilitation Administration.

1935 Social Security Act (Public Law 74-721) is passed, resulting in increased federal appropriations to states for vocational rehabilitation with direct relief provided for the disabled. Amendments to this act have provided programs for people who are disabled including Supplemental Security Income, Social Security Disability Insurance, Medicare, and Medicaid.

1943 Amendments to the Vocational Rehabilitation Act broadened vocational rehabilitation services to facilitate competitive employment and included medical services. Coverage was expanded to people who were blind, mentally ill, or mentally retarded.

   Baruch Committee on Physical Medicine is established by the son of Dr. Simon Baruch, a confederate army surgeon and pioneer in the field of physical medicine. The committee supports research and scholarship in physical medicine.

1944 The Public Health Act of 1944 (Public Law 78-410) provides for professional education, training, and research for publich health professionals.

1945 Joseph Bulova School of Watchmaking establishes a training program in watchmaking for people who are disabled. Forerunner of many companies offering employment and training opportunities to the disabled.

1946 National Mental Health Act (Public Law 79-487) authorizes extensive federal support for mental health research, diagnosis, prevention, and treatment, establishing the National Institute of Mental Health and state grant-in-aid programs for mental health under the U.S. Public Health Service.

1947 The Department of Rehabilitation and Physical Medicine is started at New York University College of Medicine at Bellevue Hospital under the direction of Dr. Howard Rusk. This department served as a model for the development of rehabilitation centers all over the world and received grant funding from the Baruch Committee.

1953 Establishment of the Department of Health, Education, and Welfare with the Office of Vocational Rehabilitation as a part.

1954 Vocational Rehabilitation Act amendments expanded to include training and education programs for professional rehabilitation personnel.

1956 Amendments to the Social Security Act give benefits to workers and their families during periods of extended disability.

   The Mental Health Study Act (Public Law 84-812) authorizes grants to facilitate a program of research into resources and methods of care for the mentally ill. The act authorized grants for participation in a national study and reevaluation of the human and economic problems of mental illness.

1963 Mental Retardation Facilities and Community Mental Health Centers Construction Act of 1963 (Public Law 88-164) provides funding for construction of research centers and facilities for people who are mentally retarded. Provides funding for construction of community mental health centers.

1965 Amendments to the Vocational Rehabilitation Act provided for increased flexibility in financing state rehabilitation programs and assisted in the expansion and improvement of rehabilitation services. The word *handicapped* was substituted for *physical disability*. The Federal Board of Vocational Education is established. The amendments expanded services to include social rehabilitation as well as vocational and medical services.

   Social Security Act Amendments created Medicaid and Medicare. Both programs provide essential health and health-related services for individuals who are disabled (see Chapter 5).

   The Mental Retardation Facilities and Community Mental Health Centers Construction Act Amendments of 1965 (Public Law 89-105) authorize assistance in meeting the initial cost of professional and technical personnel for comprehensive community mental health centers.

1968 Architectural Barriers Act (Public Law 90-480) is passed. The act mandated that almost any public building constructed or leased by federal funds must be accessible to the physically disabled and that all construction after 1968 using federal funds ensure building accessibility

# Legislation and Voluntary Efforts for the Disabled: United States (cont'd)

to disabled persons with no exceptions allowed. The act affected many educational settings and was enforced by the Architectural Barriers Compliance Board. However, the mandates of this law were ignored, and in 1978 Congress created a compliance board to enforce the law (Goldman, 1984).

1971 Developmental Disabilities Act (Public Law 91-517) is passed. The act states that each state would receive federal funds to establish and maintain services that are required by developmentally disabled children and adults. These services include diagnosis, evaluation, treatment, personal care, special living arrangements, training, education, sheltered employment, recreation, counseling, protective and sociolegal services, information services, transportation services, and follow-up services.

Urban Mass Transportation Act (Public Law 91-453) is passed. The act states that special efforts would be made in federally funded mass transportation to include usage by persons who are disabled.

1972 Social Security Act Amendments established intermediate care facilities for people with mental retardation.

1973 Rehabilitation Act of 1973 (Public Law 91-453) is a landmark piece of legislation that *replaced the 1920 act*. It authorized vocational rehabilitation services: emphasized services to those with severe disabilities, expanded the federal role in service and training programs, defined services necessary for rehabilitative programs, established the National Architectural and Transportation Barriers Board, and began affirmative action programs to facilitate employment of people who were disabled.

Social Security Act of 1935 amendments eliminate previous categories of Aid to the Blind, Aid to the Aged (Old Age Assistance), and Aid to the Disabled under which direct financial assistance was given to people who were disabled. Supplemental Security Income is established as of January 1, 1974, under which the aged, blind, and disabled could qualify.

1974 Rehabilitation Act Amendments of 1974 (Public Law 93-576) authorized the White House Conference on the Disabled.

Numerous pieces of transportation legislation included the following:

1. Amtrak Improvement Act (Public Law 93-140) stated that the Amtrak corporation must ensure that the disabled would not be denied transporta-

tion because of the disability. Provisions did not apply to commuter and short-haul service.

2. Federal Aid Highway Act (Public Law 93-87) stated that funding could not be approved for any state or federal highway not granting reasonable access for the movement of the physically disabled across curbs.

3. National Mass Transportation Act (Public Law 93-503) stated that mass transit funds could not be approved unless the rates charged persons who are disabled were reduced rates from regular fare.

4. Federal Bus Act (Public Law 93-37) stated that all federally funded projects to improve bus transportation must include plans to facilitate usage by people who are disabled.

1975 Developmental Disabilities Assistance and Bill of Rights Act (Public Law 94-103) created a system of protection and advocacy on the state level to protect the rights of the developmentally disabled and to pursue legal and other actions as necessary to eliminate the problems facing citizens with mental retardation, epilepsy, autism, and cerebral palsy.

Education for All Handicapped Children Act (Public Law 94-142) passes. Enabled by September 1, 1980, a free, appropriate public education to all persons aged 3 to 21 years old regardless of the disabling condition.

1977 Reorganization of the Department of Health, Education, and Welfare with creation of the Office of Human Development. The Administration for Handicapped Individuals (AHI) is in the Office of Human Development and oversees (1) Rehabilitation Services Administration, (2) President's Committee on Mental Retardation, (3) Architectural and Transportation Barriers Compliance Board, (4) White House Conference on Handicapped Individuals, (5) Developmental Disabilities Office, and (6) Office of Handicapped Individuals.

Federal law provided special rates (reduced) on a space-available basis to persons with severely visual physically or mentally disabled people, as well as any attendant required by such persons.

1978 Rehabilitation Act Amendments establish the Council on the Handicapped to function as a steering committee to make recommendations to the President concerning the needs of disabled individuals and establish the National Center for Rehabilitation Research.

1980 Mental Health Systems Act (Public Law 96-398) gives the states more authority to plan community mental health centers, to increase the quality of mental health

# Legislation and Voluntary Efforts for the Disabled: United States (cont'd)

services, and to reach more people. Includes advocacy provisions and a Bill of Rights of Mental Health.

Civil Rights of Institutionalized Persons Act (Public Law 96-247) authorizes actions for redress in cases involving deprivations of rights of institutionalized persons that were secured or protected by the Constitution of the United States. The act states that when an action has been commenced in any court of the United States seeking relief from conditions that deprive persons residing in such institutions of any rights, privileges, or immunities secured or protected by the Constitution or laws of the United States that causes them to suffer grievous harm, the Attorney General of the United States may intervene.

1982 Social Security Act Amendments allow children who are disabled to live at home, rather than requiring institutionalization, in order to receive services. Telecommunications for the Disabled Act (Public Law 97-140) amends the Communication Act of 1934 to provide persons with impaired hearing with reasonable access to telephone service.

1984 Rehabilitation Amendments (Public Law 98-221) modifies the definition of severely disabled and places the age limit for disability benefits at 16 years. Made the National Council on the Handicapped an agency independent from the Department of Education.

Developmental Disabilities Assistance and Bill of Rights Act (Public Law 98-527) formally establishes a Bill of Rights for the developmentally disabled.

1986 Protection and Advocacy for Mentally Ill Individuals Act of 1986 (Public Law 99-319) establishes protection and advocacy services for individuals who are mentally ill. Restated the Bill of Rights for mental health patients. Promotes the establishment of family support groups for the families of people with Alzheimer's disease.

Education of the Deaf Act (Public Law 99-371) consolidates several free-standing statutes relating to federally supported educational institutions for the deaf into one effective piece of legislation.

Rehabilitation Amendments (Public Law 99-506) emphasize the rehabilitation needs of disabled Native Americans, provide funding for disability technology, and expand the influence of the National Council on the Handicapped.

Employment Opportunities for Disabled Americans Act (Public Law 99-643) amends the Social Security Act to improve employment opportunities for disabled Americans.

Air Carrier Access Act of 1986 greatly improves access to air transportation for people who are disabled.

1988 Numerous pieces of technology-related legislation including:

1. Hearing Aid Compatibility Act of 1988 (Public Law 100-394) requires telephones manufactured or imported into the United States after August 16, 1989, be hearing aid–compatible.
2. Technology-Related Assistance for Individuals with Disabilities Act of 1988 (Public Law 100-407) establishes a competitive grant program to enable participating states to develop and implement programs to promote technology-related assistance to individuals with disabilities.
3. Telecommunications Accessibility Act (Public Law 100-542) ensures that the federal telecommunication system is fully accessible to hearing-impaired persons who use telecommunications.

Protection and Advocacy for Mentally Ill Individuals Amendments Act of 1988 (Public Law 100-509) amends the 1986 act to reauthorize the act and to establish a governing authority for protection and advocacy in each state. Fair Housing legislation clarifies the rights of people who are disabled in housing

1990 The Americans with Disabilities Act (Public Law 101-336), called a civil rights act for people with disabilities, was passed. It was a landmark piece of legislation designed to provide a clear and comprehensive mandate to end discrimination against individuals with disabilities and addressed issues such as housing, employment, public transportation, and communication services.

The 1975 Education for All Handicapped Children Act was renamed the Individuals with Disabilities Education Act (IDEA), (Public Law 101-476). Consistent with the Americans with Disabilities Act, Public Law 101-476 changed terminology (handicapped to disability) to reflect a more positive focus on individuals who have functional limitations.

# 19

# The Well Elderly: Needs and Services

*Sandra L. McGuire*

## OBJECTIVES

*Upon completion of this chapter, the reader should be able to:*

1. Construct a personal philosophy of aging.
2. Discuss societal values and attitudes in relation to aging.
3. Discuss cultural diversity and aging in the United States
4. Discuss the *Healthy People 2010* initiative in relation to aging.
5. State major causes of mortality and morbidity for the elderly.

6. Describe health promotion and wellness activities for the elderly.
7. Describe barriers to health care for the elderly.
8. Identify significant legislation in relation to older Americans.
9. Identify resources and services for the elderly.
10. Conceptualize the community health nurse's role in promoting healthy aging.

## KEY TERMS

Administration on Aging (AoA)
African-American elders
Ageism
American Association of Retired Persons (AARP)
Area agencies on aging
Asian American and Pacific Islander (AAPI) elders
Cultural competency
Depression
Developmental tasks
Elder abuse
Elder morbidity

Elder mortality
Elder neglect
Hartford Institute for Geriatric Nursing
Hispanic American elders
Life course planning
National Conference of Gerontological Nurse Practitioners (NCGNP)
National Council on the Aging (NCOA)
National Gerontological Nursing Association (NGNA)
National Institute on Aging

Native American elders
Nutrition Screening Initiative
Older Americans Act (OAA)
*Scope and Standards of Gerontological Nursing Practice*
Senior center
Sexuality
Social Security Administration (SSA)
State units on aging
Suicide
White House Conferences on Aging (WHCoA)

*In the new century...the future is aging.*

ADMINISTRATION ON AGING

*There's no shame in growing old—we're all doing it. Age is, after all, the one thing we all share.*

MAGGIE KUHN

Meet Art Johnson, a retired school principal from Waterford, Michigan. At 80 years of age he taught adult education at a local high school, golfed competitively, continued postgraduate education, and

helped with coaching Little League baseball. He was known and loved in his community.

Meet Hattie Harris of Rochester, New York, where the city declared a "Hattie Harris Day." At 91 years of age she was described as the "elder statesman of the Republican Party" and the "Mayor of Strathallan Park." In those positions she advised political candidates, set up neighborhood political rallies, and worked for the betterment of her community.

Meet Herbert Kirk of Bozeman, Montana. At 97 years of age he received his bachelor's degree from Montana State University. At the graduation ceremony Mr. Kirk received

## BOX 19-1

### *Go for It—Healthy, Active Aging*

John Glenn became an astronaut again at the age of 77.

Mary Baker Eddy directed the Christian Science Church at 89.

Harold and Bertha Soderquist joined the Peace Corps and learned a foreign language when he was 80 and she was 76.

Thomas Edison, the inventor of the electric light bulb, filed for his 1033rd patent at the age of 81.

Albert Schweitzer was in charge of an African hospital at 89 and helped build a half-mile road near the hospital at 87.

George Bernard Shaw was writing at 91.

Ronald Reagan served as President of the United States in his 70s.

Maggie Kuhn headed the Gray Panthers at 88.

Anna Mary Moses, better known as Grandma Moses, illustrated an edition of *'Twas the Night Before Christmas* when she was 100.

Frank Lloyd Wright began his most creative and prolific work at the age of 69 and was active until his death at 91.

Elizabeth Eichelbaum graduated with a doctorate in education from the University of Tennessee in 2000 at age 90. Dr. Eichelbaum earned her GED at age 65, her bachelor's degree at age 69, and her master's degree at age 81.

Dr. Leila Denmark, a pediatrician, was still seeing children every day at her office in Alpharetta, Georgia, at the age of 101.

a standing ovation from the thousands of people gathered at the university field house. Part of the ceremony included the reading of a congratulatory letter sent by President Bill Clinton. The year before he had won two gold medals in the International Track Athletic Congress in Finland.

Individuals like Art Johnson, Hattie Harris, and Herbert Kirk can be found in every American community. They are examples of older Americans who have lived life to its fullest and best. They are elder role models and show us what successful aging can be.

## AGING DEFINED

Aging and "old age" are relatively contemporary phenomena. During the Stone Age the average life span was 15 years. By the late 1700s people lived into their 30s, and the life expectancy for Americans at the beginning of the twentieth century, in 1900, was less than 50 years.

Everyone is aging, and people are living longer than ever before. Aging is a natural and lifelong process of growing and developing. Aging is a universal phenomenon as well as an individual process that incorporates personal life experi-

ences. In the United States a chronological marker, the age of 65, is often used to denote the advent of *old age*.

The designation of old age in the United States was legislatively determined by the Social Security Act of 1935, which set eligibility for federal old age retirement benefits at age 65. Interestingly, in 1935 many Americans did not live to reach age 65. Today almost 2 million Americans celebrate their sixty-fifth birthday each year—almost 5500 each day (American Association of Retired Persons [AARP], Administration on Aging [AoA], 2001). With this "graying of America" old age is being redefined both socially and politically.

Nurses are providing care to more older people than ever before and can expect to spend a large part of their professional career providing care for the elderly. Nurses can facilitate healthy aging. Box 19-1 highlights a number of active older people.

## SOME PERSPECTIVES ON AGING

The older population is growing throughout the world. Worldwide, the number of persons aged 60 and over is estimated to be 600 million, and by the year 2050 it is projected to be 2 billion, at which time the population of older persons will be larger than the population of children under the age of 14 for the first time in human history (AoA, 2000a).

Globally, we are witnessing one of society's greatest achievements—an extension of human longevity more dramatic than in the preceding 4,500 years. Advancements in medicine, public health, and technology will make it even more commonplace for people to live 80, 90, or 100 more years (AoA, 2000b).

Older people are the gatekeepers of a nation's history, values, culture, and traditions. They are "those who have gone before" and made today's accomplishments and lifestyles possible. Throughout history, aging persons have been portrayed in literature and art as wise individuals, strong in character, and leaders of people. However, cultures vary in how older people are perceived and cared for. In some cultures elderly people are given elevated status and treated with great respect. In other cultures elders face social isolation and are devalued. Attitudes about aging in the United States are largely negative and ageist.

### American Attitudes Toward Aging

America is often described as an ageist society. Dr. Robert Butler, a renowned gerontologist, coined the term **ageism** in 1968 and defined it as a process of systematic stereotyping of, and discrimination against, people because they are old. The *Gray Panthers* (Figure 19-1), an intergenerational, advocacy organization that supports the rights of older people, view ageism as the use of age to define capability and role.

Biases against aging are so deeply ingrained in our society that they unintentionally surface in everyday life—in

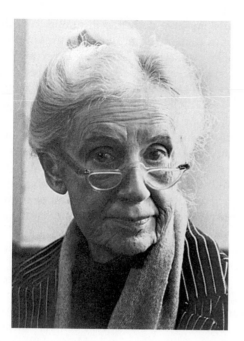

**FIGURE 19-1** Maggie Kuhn, founder of the Gray Panthers. (Courtesy Julie Jensen.)

writing, films, and even conversation—denying older persons their individuality and the opportunity to maximize their potential (AARP, 1984). Descriptors such as *vigorous, active, attractive,* and *independent* are often used to describe a person of 20, 30, or 40, but rarely one of 70, 80, or 90.

In general, Americans are not educationally, socially, or emotionally prepared for old age (McGuire, Gerber, 1996), and many myths and misconceptions about aging exist in our society (Box 19-2). People need to explore their "elder within" (Dychtwald, 1990), the older person they will be someday, and plan for old age. People need to become knowledgeable about the aging process; develop realistic, positive attitudes toward aging; and realize that older people are valuable and contributing members of society.

Organizations discussed later in this chapter such as the Administration on Aging, National Institute on Aging, American Association for Retired Persons, and National Council on Aging all work to eliminate ageism. We all need to work to eliminate such discrimination. The costs of ageism are great; as with other forms of prejudice, it is dehumanizing and inhibits people from maximizing their potential. Nurses need to evaluate their attitudes about age and aging and how these attitudes affect nursing care.

### Stop and Think About It

What are your attitudes toward age? Are you looking forward to growing older? Have you explored your "elder within," who you plan to be, and what you plan to do as an older person? How could you promote positive attitudes about aging and healthy aging with clients?

---

 **BOX 19-2**

*Myths About Aging*

*All Older People Are Alike*
Fact: Older people are uniquely individual.

*Most Older People Live in Institutional Settings*
Fact: Only 4% of older people are in institutional settings.

*The Majority of Older People Are Lonely and Isolated from Their Families*
Fact: The majority of older people live in a family setting. Many older people live near their children and have regular contact with friends and family.

*Older People Cannot Learn*
Fact: Older people are capable of learning and enjoy learning. The senior "Elderhostel" program is a good example of this.

*The Majority of Older People View Themselves as Being in Poor Health*
Fact: The majority (73%) of older people report their health as being good, very good, or excellent.

*Older People Cannot Work*
Fact: Approximately 4 million older Americans are in the labor force.

*The Majority of Older People Have Incomes Below the Poverty Level*
Fact: Only 16% of older Americans are classified as poor or near-poor.

*Most Older People Have No Interest in Sexual Activity*
Fact: The need for sexual activity does not stop with old age.

*Old Age Begins at 65*
Fact: In this country 65 was legislated as the age for Social Security retirement benefits; but when "old age" begins is very individual.

Excerpts from Harris DK: *Sociology of aging,* ed 2, New York, 1990, Harper & Row, p. 5; American Association of Retired Persons (AARP), Administration on Aging (AoA): *A profile of older Americans 2000,* Washington, DC, 2001, AARP, AoA.

## AGING AND CULTURAL DIVERSITY: UNITED STATES

By the year 2030 the U.S. minority older population will triple in number and 25% of the elderly population will belong to a minority racial or ethnic group (Administration on Aging [AoA], 2001a) up from just over 16% in 1999 (AARP, AoA, 2001). In some states, such as California, the percentage will be even higher. Figure 19-2 illustrates the increase that is projected to occur among our nation's leading minority population groups within the next few decades. As the figure indicates, while all ethnic and minority groups are expected to grow, Hispanic American and Asian American populations will dramatically increase.

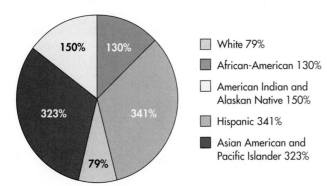

FIGURE 19-2 Census Bureau estimates of population increase. The United States is a nation with a rich mix of persons with diverse racial, ethnic, and cultural backgrounds. As evidenced by the chart above, this mix is becoming even more dynamic. The minority older population will triple by 2030. By then, about one quarter of the elderly population will belong to a minority racial or ethnic group. (From Administration on Aging [AoA]: *Fact sheet: cultural competency*, Washington, DC, 2001a, AoA, p. 1.)

**BOX 19-3**

*Characteristics of Culturally Competent Service Delivery to Elders*

Culturally competent service delivery entails:
- *Cultural appropriateness*—being sensitive to the cultural norms, values, and beliefs of the particular individual, the situation, and the environment as they pertain to the needs of the ethnic elders and the types of services to be utilized
- *Cultural access*—providing information and services in languages or through media that facilitates delivery to minority elders
- *Cultural acceptability*—encouraging ethnic elders to actively seek services.

It is necessary to understand and adopt cultural concepts and to address structural and cultural barriers in designing culturally competent services; therefore, service providers must appreciate not only how groups differ, but also how they are alike.

From Administration on Aging (AoA): *Fact sheet: cultural competency*, Washington, DC, 2001a, AoA, p. 3.

Presently, immense disparities in health, longevity, and economics exist among ethnic groups in the United States. For example, white women have a life expectancy at birth of 80 years, whereas African-American females have a life expectancy of 74 years (U.S. Department of Health and Human Services [USDHHS], 1996b). Economically, 8% of elderly whites are poor, compared with almost 23% of elderly African Americans and 20% of elderly Hispanics (AARP, AoA, 2001). The highest poverty rates are experienced by elderly Hispanic women who live alone (AARP, AoA, 2001). The AoA is committed to eliminating health disparities that adversely affect America's minority racial and ethnic groups (AoA, 2000c), and *Healthy People 2010* has as a goal to eliminate such disparities.

Health disparities for racial and ethnic minorities often involve problems of access, and practitioners and service systems need to become more responsive to these needs (AoA, 2001a). Barriers to access to care for minority populations include language barriers, lack of appropriate information, distrust of the mainstream delivery systems, and low-income and education levels (AoA, 2001a). Understanding different cultural values and attitudes in relation to aging and health is essential for community health nurses to develop strategies that enhance the quality of life for the aged and promotes cultural competency.

According to the Administration on Aging, **cultural competency** is:

A set of behaviors and attitudes integrated into the practices and policies of agencies or professional service providers that enables them to understand and work effectively in cross-cultural situations. When professionals are culturally competent they establish positive, helping relationships that engage the client and improve the quality of services provided (AoA, 2001a, p. 2).

The nurse needs to be culturally sensitive and culturally competent. The cultural assessment guide found in Appendix 7-1 assists the community health nurse in obtaining cultural data. Characteristics of culturally competent service delivery for ethnic elders are given in Box 19-3. Some health information on our nation's leading ethnic and minority groups follows.

### African-American Elders

The number of **African-American elders** is expected to increase 130% between 1990 and 2030 (AoA, 2001a). Currently, African-American life expectancy is 70.2 years as compared to 76.5 years for all population groups, and African-American men have a life expectancy of only 66.1 years (AoA, 2001b).

More than 25% of African-American elders have incomes that fall below the poverty line, and 68% are poor (AoA, 2001b). The leading disease-related causes of death among African Americans are the same as those found among whites, specifically heart disease, cancer, HIV infection, cerebrovascular disease, and diabetes (Miller,

2000). However, these diseases are more likely to cause disability and death in the African-American population (Miller, 2000). Only 14% of African-American elders receive annual vaccinations (e.g., influenza), placing them at increased risk of immunizable communicable disease (AoA, 2001b).

African American elders often seek medical care at later stages in the disease process, and this makes treatment outcomes less favorable (Miller, 2000; National Institutes of Health [NIH], 1998). There is also a tendency in this population group to use emergency services as opposed to primary care office visits, and this means that they are less likely to have a regular source of care, receive health education, or take part in preventive care (Franke, Ohene-Frempong, 1999; Miller, 2000). Nearly 25% of African-American elders rely solely on Medicare for health insurance coverage in comparison to about 10% of the general population (Kaiser Family Foundation, 1999; Miller, 2000). Inadequate health insurance coverage greatly limits access to resources and services and results in more negative health outcomes (Cornelius, 2000; Miller, 2000). Historically, African-American households have been actively involved in caregiving for family elders.

## Hispanic American Elders

The Hispanic population is the most rapidly growing ethnic group and will soon be the largest minority group in the United States. The number of **Hispanic American elders** is expected to increase almost 350% by the year 2030 (AoA, 2001a). Among Hispanic elders in the United States almost 50% are of Mexican descent, 15% are of Cuban descent, and 12% are of Puerto Rican descent (AoA, 2001c). The leading disease-related causes of death for Hispanic Americans include heart disease, cancer, HIV infection, cerebrovascular diseases, pneumonia, influenza, and diabetes. Only 15% of Hispanic American elders receive recommended annual vaccinations (AoA, 2001c).

Hispanic elders tend to live in community settings rather than institutional ones and tend to have greater familial support than other groups (Miller, 2000). More than 52% of Hispanic American elders receive care from adult children (AoA, 2001d). Almost 30% of Hispanic American households provide informal caregiving to a friend or relative, and more than 50% of these caregivers also have a child under the age of 18 living at home (AoA, 2001c).

Almost 25% of Hispanic elders live below the poverty level—more than double the rate of older white, non-Hispanic adults (AoA, 2001d). Hispanic elders are almost twice as likely to have one or more limitations in activities of daily living than other groups of elderly (Miller, 2000). Barriers to obtaining health care include no insurance, inadequate insurance, and language barriers (Guendelman, Wagner, 2000; Miller, 2000).

## Native American Elders

The number of **Native American elders** (e.g., American Indians, Alaska Natives and Native Hawaiians) is expected to increase 150% by the year 2030 (AoA, 2001c). This group of elders often does not seek medical care and reports a lack of trust in the medical system (Miller, 2000). Many American Indians and Alaskan Natives live on reservations where limited medical services exist (Miller, 2000). The *Indian Health Service (IHS)* (see Chapter 5) was established to provide health services to this population group, but it is not able to adequately cover the vast geographical areas where most reservations are located (Jones-Saumty, 1999; Miller, 2000). Of the nearly 300 reservations in the United States, only 15 provide long-term care facilities for the elderly (Miller, 2000).

Diabetes is a serious health concern among Native American elders, and they die of diabetes at three times the rate of whites (Miller, 2000; Ross, 2000). In addition to diabetes, leading causes of death among this population are heart disease, cancers, and cerebrovascular diseases. There is a high incidence of alcoholism and alcohol abuse among this ethnic group (Miller, 2000).

Native Americans receive grants from the AoA to implement congregate and home-delivered meals, transportation, and in-home supportive services (AoA, 2000d). Two resource centers for Native American elders have been established. The *Native Elder Health Care Resource Center* at the University of Colorado (*http://www.uchsc.edu/sm/nehcrc*) is developing a series of educational modules addressing some of the most prevalent and disabling illnesses affecting Native American elders, including diabetes mellitus, cancer, oral health, depression, and alcohol abuse and dependence (AoA, 2001e). The *National Resource Center on Native American Aging* at the University of North Dakota (*http://www.und.nodak.edu/dept/nrcnaa*) assists in developing community-based solutions to improve the quality of life and the delivery of care to Native American elders, including an elderly needs-assessment tool to assist tribes in planning for elder care services.

## Asian American and Pacific Islander Elders

Asian American and Pacific Islander (AAPI) elders comprise more than 30 ethnic groups, and each has a unique culture, tradition, language, and religion. The number of AAPI American elders is expected to increase by almost 325% by the year 2030 (AoA, 2001a). The largest groups of Asian Americans are those of Chinese, Japanese, Filipino, Asian Indians, and Korean descent. Pacific Islander elders include people of Micronesian, Polynesian, and Melanesian descent. The AAPI elders have high rates of chronic diseases and illnesses, and 12% live below the poverty line (as compared with 5% of the older non-Hispanic population) (AoA, 2001f).

The leading causes of death for AAPIs are heart disease, cancers, and cerebrovascular diseases (National Center for

Health Statistics [NCHS], 1996). AAPI elders have the lowest rate of physician visits when compared with other ethnic minority groups, and many do not have health insurance (Miller, 2000). The inability to speak English has been cited as a considerable barrier to seeking health care with this group (Miller, 2000).

No matter what racial or ethnic group a person belongs to, developmental tasks of aging need to be accomplished. How these tasks are achieved varies across ethnic groups. Developmental tasks have been integrated throughout this text, and developmental tasks of aging are discussed here.

## DEVELOPMENTAL TASKS OF AGING

Aging is a stage of human development with specific *developmental tasks*. Accomplishing these tasks assists the individual in self-fulfillment and personal growth (Figure 19-3). **Developmental tasks** for the elderly include maintaining appropriate and satisfying living arrangements, adjusting to retirement, safeguarding physical and mental health, continuing a social network of friends and family, and maintaining an active role in the community. Achieving developmental tasks often involves role reorientation, reversal of caregiver roles, adjustment to retirement, and adapting to changes in health status.

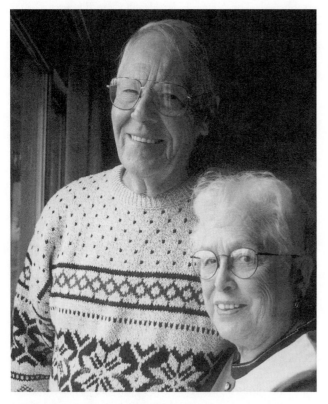

**FIGURE 19-3** Don and Mary Lue Johnson of Maryville, Tennessee, exemplify successful aging. They have been married more than 50 years and remain active in their community. (Courtesy Ed Richardson.)

According to Erikson (1982), older persons are faced with resolving the psychological conflict of *integrity versus despair*. The successful accomplishment of integrity occurs when individuals review their lives, accept what they have done, and feel satisfied with what they have accomplished. If this does not occur, the older person may experience despair and depression and may become dissatisfied with life.

The end result of the aging process is death, and nurses, the aged, and their families must come to terms with helping the client and family work through this final stage of human growth and development. Nurses should evaluate their own feelings and thoughts about death and dying to enhance client care.

## *HEALTHY PEOPLE 2010* AND AGING

*Healthy People 2010* has a national health goal to increase quality and years of healthy life (USDHHS, 2000, p. 2). The document does not separate out objectives based on age. National health objectives that relate to elder health are integrated throughout the document. Many objectives address multiple age groups and only a few objectives incorporate the words *older adults* or *elderly*. Examples of *Healthy People 2010* objectives that have importance to elder health are given in Box 19-4. The nurse should be familiar with these objectives, understand their impact on nursing care, and be at the forefront of their accomplishment.

*Healthy People 2010* focuses on primary prevention and health promotion. An important aspect of health promotion for older people is to maintain health and functional independence (USDHHS, 2000). A significant number of the health problems evidenced with aging are either preventable or can be controlled by preventive activities, and strong social support is important in promoting the health of older adults (USDHHS, 2000).

Many older Americans are not adequately participating in preventive health activities. Although vaccine coverage has increased in recent years among the elderly, it is still far from the goals set for achievement in *Healthy People 2010*. Only 29% of elders receive pneumococcal vaccine, and about 55% receive influenza vaccine (USDHHS, 1999) (Figure 19-4). When all forms of exercise are added together, two thirds of the elderly do not achieve recommended exercise levels (USDHHS, 1999), and many elders do not have adequate nutritional intake or regular physical examinations and screenings. Engaging in preventive activities can improve health and reduce the likelihood of disability, and nurses need to encourage elderly clients to take part in these activities.

Across the nation agencies are working to meet *Healthy People 2010* national health objectives and promote healthy aging. In the public sector the Administration on Aging (AoA) and the National Institute on

**BOX 19-4**

**Focus Areas and Objectives Targeting Older Adults**

## Access to Quality Health Care Services

- Increase the proportion of persons who have a specific source of ongoing care
- Reduce hospitalization rates for three ambulatory-care-sensitive conditions—pediatric asthma, uncontrolled diabetes, and immunization preventable pneumonia and influenza in *older adults*

## Arthritis, Osteoporosis, and Chronic Back Conditions

- Reduce the overall number of cases of osteoporosis
- Reduce the proportion of adults who are hospitalized for vertebral fractures associated with osteoporosis

## Cancer

- Increase the proportion of adults who receive a colorectal cancer screening examination

## Chronic Kidney Disease

- Reduce the rate of new cases of end-stage renal disease
- Increase the proportion of dialysis clients registered on the waiting list for transplantation
- Reduce kidney failure due to diabetes

## Diabetes

- Prevent diabetes
- Reduce the overall rate of diabetes that is clinically diagnosed
- Reduce diabetes death rate
- Reduce diabetes-related deaths among persons with diabetes
- Reduce deaths from cardiovascular disease in persons with diabetes
- Reduce the rate of lower extremity amputations in persons with diabetes
- Increase the proportion of adults with diabetes who have a glycosylated hemoglobin measurement at least once a year
- Increase the proportion of adults with diabetes who have an annual dilated eye examination
- Increase the proportion of adults with diabetes who have at least an annual foot examination
- Increase the proportion of persons with diabetes who have at least an annual dental examination
- Increase the proportion of adults with diabetes who perform self-glucose blood glucose monitoring at least once daily

## Disability and Secondary Conditions

- Reduce the proportion of adults with disabilities who report feelings such as sadness, unhappiness, or depression that prevent them from being active
- Increase the proportion of adults with disabilities who participated in social activities
- Increase the proportion of adults with disabilities reporting sufficient emotional support
- Reduce the number of people with disabilities in congregate care facilities, consistent with permanency planning principles
- Eliminate disparities in employment rates between working-aged adults with and without disabilities

## Educational and Community Based Programs

- Increase the proportion of *older adults* who have participated during the preceding year in at least one organized health promotion activity

## Food Safety

- Reduce infections caused by key foodborne pathogens

## Health Communication

- Increase the proportion of households with access to the internet at home

## Heart Disease and Stroke

- Reduce hospitalizations of *older adults* with heart failures as the principal diagnosis

## Immunization and Infectious Diseases

- Reduce invasive pneumococcal infections
- Increase the proportion of adults who are vaccinated annually against influenza and ever vaccinated against pneumococcal disease

## Injury and Violence Prevention

- Reduce hospitalization for nonfatal head injuries
- Reduce deaths caused by motor vehicle crashes
- Reduce pedestrian deaths on public roads
- Reduce residential fire deaths
- Reduce deaths from falls
- Reduce hip fractures among *older adults*

## Medical Product Safety

- Increase the proportion of primary care providers, pharmacists, and other health care professionals who routinely

From US Department of Health and Human Service (USDHHS): *Healthy People 2010, conference edition,* Washington, DC, 2000, US Government Printing Office.

*Continued*

Aging (NIA) have provided significant leadership in this endeavor. In the private sector, organizations such as the American Association of Retired Persons (AARP), the National Council on the Aging (NCOA), the American Nurses Association (ANA), the National Gerontological Nursing Association (NGNA), and the Hartford Institute for Geriatric Nursing have provided leadership in promoting healthy aging. These agencies work to improve the quality of life and reduce morbidity and mortality among American elders.

**BOX 19-4**

*Focus Areas and Objectives Targeting Older Adults—cont'd*

review with their clients *aged 65 years and older* and clients with chronic illnesses or disabilities all new prescribed and over-the-counter medicines

### Mental Health and Mental Disorders

- Increase the number of states, territories, and the District of Columbia with an operational mental health plan that addresses mental health crisis interventions, ongoing screening, and treatment services for *elderly persons*

### Nutrition and Overweight

- Increase the proportion of adults who are at a healthy weight
- Reduce the proportion of adults who are obese
- Increase the proportion of persons aged 2 years and older who consume at least two daily servings of fruit
- Increase the proportion of persons aged 2 years and older who consume at least three daily servings of vegetables, with at least one third being dark green or deep yellow vegetables
- Increase the proportion of persons aged 2 years and older who consume at least six daily servings of grain products, with at least three being whole grains
- Increase the proportion of persons aged 2 years and older who consume less than 10% of calories from saturated fat
- Increase the proportion of persons aged 2 years and older who consume no more than 30% of calories from fat
- Increase the proportion of persons aged 2 years and older who meet dietary requirements for calcium
- Increase the proportion of physician office visits made by clients with a diagnosis of cardiovascular disease, diabetes, or hyperlipidemia that include counseling or education related to diet and nutrition

### Oral Health

- Reduce the proportion of *elderly persons* who have had all their natural teeth extracted
- Increase the proportion of children and adults who use the oral health care system each year

### Physical Activity and Fitness

- Reduce the proportion of adults who engage in no leisure-time physical activity
- Increase the proportion of adults who engage regularly, preferably daily, in moderate physical activity for at least 30 minutes per day

- Increase the proportion of adults who engage in vigorous physical activity that promotes the development and maintenance of cardiorespiratory fitness 3 or more days per week for 20 or more minutes per occasion
- Increase the proportion of adults who perform physical activities that enhance and maintain muscular strength and endurance
- Increase the proportion of adults who perform physical activities that enhance and maintain flexibility

### Respiratory Diseases

- Reduce asthma deaths
- Reduce hospitalizations for asthma
- Reduce hospital emergency department visits for asthma
- Reduce the proportion of adults whose activity is limited due to chronic lung and breathing problems
- Reduce deaths from chronic obstructive pulmonary disease (COPD) among adults

### Substance Abuse

- Reduce cirrhosis deaths
- Reduce the proportion of adults who exceed guidelines for low-risk drinking

### Tobacco Use

- Reduce the proportion of nonsmokers exposed to environmental tobacco smoke

### Vision and Hearing

- Increase the proportion of persons who have a dilated eye examination at appropriate intervals
- Reduce visual impairment due to diabetic retinopathy
- Reduce visual impairment due to glaucoma
- Reduce visual impairment due to cataract
- Increase access by persons who have hearing impairment to hearing rehabilitation services and adaptive devices, including hearing aids, cochlear implants, or tactile or assistive augmentative devices
- Increase the proportion of persons who have had a hearing exam on schedule
- Increase the number of person who are referred by their primary care physician for hearing evaluation and treatment

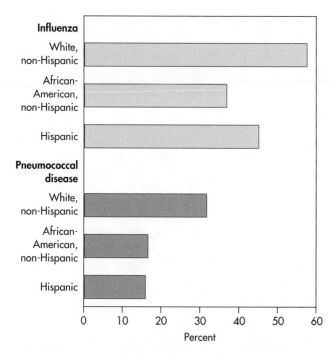

**FIGURE 19-4** Percentage of elders vaccinated against influenza and pneumococcal disease: United States. (From US Department of Health and Human Services (USDHHS): *Health and aging chartbook. Health, United States 1999*, Hyattsville, Md, 1999, National Center for Health Statistics, p. 69)

## ELDER MORBIDITY AND MORTALITY

The leading causes of **elder mortality** are heart disease, cancer, stroke, chronic obstructive pulmonary disease, pneumonia, and influenza (USDHHS, 1999, 2000). Other leading causes of death include diabetes, unintentional injuries, nephritis, Alzheimer's disease, and septicemia. The biggest decreases in mortality have been in heart disease and stroke; however, death rates for the elderly from influenza and pneumonia have increased (USDHHS, 1999, p. 18). These rising pneumonia and influenza death rates are preventable because immunizations are available for these conditions. The National Institute on Aging (NIA) has an AgePage, *Shots for Safety*, that can be ordered by dialing NIA's toll-free number (1-800-222-2225) or by downloading from the internet (*http://www.nih.gov/nia/health/agepages/shots.htm*). Nurses can use this publication to help explain the importance of adult immunizations to elders.

In relation to **elder morbidity,** the most frequently occurring chronic problems among noninstitutionalized elderly persons include arthritis (49%), hypertension (36%), hearing impairments (30%), heart disease (27%), orthopedic impairments (18%), cataracts (17%), sinusitis (12%), and diabetes (10%) (AARP, AoA, 2001). Arthritis is not only the most frequently reported chronic condition but also the leading cause of disability among the elderly

(USDHHS, 1999, p. 48). Other chronic conditions include depression, osteoporosis, incontinence, digestive disorders, constipation, chronic pain, sleep disturbance, and Alzheimer's disease. Principal reasons for office visits to primary care providers and common diagnoses in older clients are given in Table 19-1.

Chronic conditions can have a great impact on quality of life and a person's ability to carry out activities of daily living (ADLs). As discussed in Chapter 18, the incidence of chronic conditions increases with age, and these conditions can significantly affect physical functioning and ADLs. Elderly persons most affected by health limitations are women, the poor, and minorities. However, income has a greater effect than race and gender on activity limitation. Improving functional independence in late life and limiting the effects of chronic conditions are important parts of health promotion for older adults.

### Health Care Expenditures

Although the 65 and older age group represents 12% of the U.S. population, it accounts for 36% of total personal health care expenditures. Older Americans spend an average of $3000 per year in out-of-pocket health care expenditures, a 33% increase since 1990 (AARP, AoA, 2001). In contrast, people under age 65 spend about 50% of that (AARP, AoA, 2001). Medicare provides health care insurance for 96% of older Americans, but Medicare has many coverage gaps, including not paying for prescription drugs, and most elders supplement their Medicare with additional health insurance (USDHHS, 1999, p. 72). About 12% of elders receive Medicaid (AARP, 1996). Health insurance is costly and more than 50% of out-of-pocket expenditures for the elderly are for health insurance (52%) (AARP, AoA, 2001). An additional 22% of out-of-pocket expenses are for medications and 20% for medical care services (e.g., physician visits) (AARP, AoA, 2001).

## DEMOGRAPHICS AND AGING: UNITED STATES

In colonial times half of the U.S. population was under age 16, and only a few people lived to the age of 65 (AoA, 2000e). In 1900 the life expectancy in America was 47 years old, today life expectancy is more than 77 years, and most newborns can expect to live into their 80s. Since 1900 there has been over a tenfold increase in older people (from 3 million to more than 34 million), and the percentage of the population age 65 and older has risen from 4% to almost 13%. Figure 19-5 illustrates how this aging of America is expected to continue. Analysis of this figure shows that by the year 2030 there are projected to be as many people over age 65 as there will be under the age of 20. Box 19-5 gives some descriptive information on aging and the elderly in the United States.

**TABLE 19-1**

*Primary Care Office Visits Among Older Clients*

| | AGE (YEARS) | |
| --- | --- | --- |
| | **65-74** | **75 AND OLDER** |
| ***Ten Principal Reasons for Visit*** | | |
| | 1. Postoperative visit | 1. General medical examination |
| | 2. General medical examination | 2. Vision dysfunction |
| | 3. Vision dysfunction | 3. Postoperative visit |
| | 4. Glaucoma | 4. Glaucoma |
| | 5. Cough | 5. Blood pressure check |
| | 6. Diabetes mellitus | 6. Cough |
| | 7. Back symptoms | 7. Cataract |
| | 8. Hypertension | 8. Vertigo or dizziness |
| | 9. Blood pressure check | 9. Hypertension |
| | 10. Skin lesion | 10. Back symptoms |
| ***Ten Most Common Diagnoses*** | | |
| | 1. Essential hypertension | 1. Essential hypertension |
| | 2. Diabetes mellitus | 2. Glaucoma |
| | 3. Glaucoma | 3. Cataract |
| | 4. Cataract | 4. Diabetes mellitus |
| | 5. Chronic ischemic heart disease | 5. Chronic ischemic heart disease |
| | 6. Osteoarthritis | 6. Osteoarthritis |
| | 7. Dermatoses | 7. Cardiac dysrhythmias |
| | 8. Cardiac dysrhythmias | 8. Organ or tissue replacement |
| | 9. Lipid disorders | 9. Dermatoses |
| | 10. Bronchitis | 10. Heart failure |

From US Department of Health and Human Services, (USDHHS), Public Health Service: National ambulatory medical care survey: 1991 summary, *Vital Health Statistics,* Series 13, No. 116, May 1994. In Ham RJ, Sloane PD: *Primary care geriatrics: a case-based approach,* ed 3, St Louis, 1997, Mosby, p. 5.

**BOX 19-5**

*Aging in the United States*

A child born today can expect to live to be almost 77 years of age, compared with age 47 for a child born in 1900.

Since 1900 the percentage of Americans 65+ has tripled. (Among American elderly, 18 million are age 65 to 74, 12 million are age 75 to 84, and 4 million are 85+.)

By 2030 there will be about 70 million older persons, 20% of the U.S. population, that will be age 65+. This is more than twice the number in 1999.

Elders age 85+ are the most rapidly growing segment of our population.

More than half of the elderly live in the nine states of California, Florida, New York, Texas, Pennsylvania, Ohio, Illinois, Michigan, and New Jersey. Each of these states has more than 1 million elderly residents, and California has the largest number (over 3.6 million) while Florida has the largest proportion (18.1%).

The states and jurisdictions with the highest poverty rates for elders are Mississippi (19.1%), Louisiana (17.1%), District of Columbia (16.5%), Arkansas (15.8%), West Virginia (15.1%), New Mexico (14.8%), Texas (14.4%), Alabama (13.3%), New York (13.2%), and North Carolina (12.7%).

Elderly women outnumber elderly men three to two.

Only 4% of American elderly reside in institutional settings such as nursing homes. However, this percentage increases dramatically with age, rising from 1.1% for persons aged 65 to 74 to 19% for persons 85+.

The majority of noninstitutionalized elderly (67%) live in a family setting, and about 31% live alone.

Data from American Association of Retired Persons (AARP), Administration on Aging (AoA): *A profile of older Americans 2000,* Washington, DC, 2001, AARP/AoA.

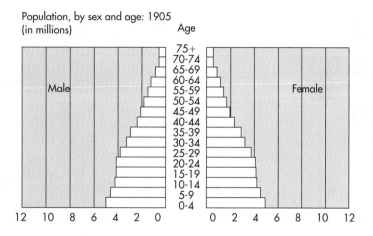

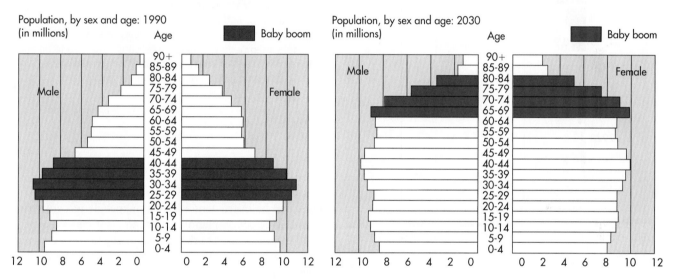

**FIGURE 19-5** Population characteristics by age and sex, United States 1905, 1990, and 2030. (From US Bureau of the Census: *Sixty-five plus in America*, Washington, DC, 1992, US Government Printing Office, pp. 1-2, 2-4, 2-9.)

Americans age 85 and older, the "oldest old," are the most rapidly growing age group in the United States. Figure 19-6 displays the growth of this age group in the United States from 1900 to 2050. The number of centenarians, people at least 100 years old, has doubled in the last 10 years (AoA, 2000d), and it is predicted that there will be more than 1 million centenarians within the next 40 years (U.S. Bureau of the Census, 1992, p. 1). Although the more than 4 million Americans over age 85 constitute less than 2% of the total population, the rapid growth of this segment of the population has significant implications for nursing and health care.

## Employment and Retirement

Almost 4 million older Americans are employed, and about half work part-time (AARP, AoA, 2001). Many older workers are poor (incomes below the poverty level) and near poor (incomes less than 125% of poverty) (AoA, 2000e). In the future, it is predicted that more seniors will remain in or reenter the work force. Many people retire only to start second careers, volunteer in their communities, or start businesses of their own.

Numerous resources exist to assist older people who want to work. The Department of Labor has the *Division of Older Worker Programs*, the American Association of Retired Persons (AARP) offers the *Senior Community Service Employment Program* and the National Council on the Aging (NCOA) sponsors the *National Association of Older Worker Employment Services* (NAOWES).

Many older people work as volunteers in their communities. Programs such as the *Retired Senior Volunteer Program* (RSVP) and the *Service Corps of Retired Executives* (SCORE) are active in many communities. Information on such programs can be obtained through local *Area Agencies on Aging*. Many seniors volunteer to work through their

Population 85 years and over:
1900 to 2050 (in millions)

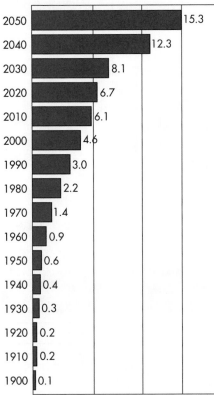

| Year | Value |
|------|-------|
| 2050 | 15.3 |
| 2040 | 12.3 |
| 2030 | 8.1 |
| 2020 | 6.7 |
| 2010 | 6.1 |
| 2000 | 4.6 |
| 1990 | 3.0 |
| 1980 | 2.2 |
| 1970 | 1.4 |
| 1960 | 0.9 |
| 1950 | 0.6 |
| 1940 | 0.4 |
| 1930 | 0.3 |
| 1920 | 0.2 |
| 1910 | 0.2 |
| 1900 | 0.1 |

**FIGURE 19-6** U.S. population 85 years and over: 1900 to 2050. (From US Bureau of the Census: *Sixty-five plus in America*, Washington, DC, 1992, US Government Printing Office, pp. 2-10).

 **BOX 19-6**

*Life Course Planning*

A life course planning approach maximizes access to information and realistic options so people can do the following:

- Maintain the best possible health status and address long-term care needs that they or family members might have
- Establish long-term economic security and contribute to pension, savings, investments, and public benefits
- Secure living arrangements that accommodate any special needs
- Engage in productive, satisfying activities including volunteer work, employment, and community participation, which are expressions of active aging
- Be an informed consumer

Through life course planning, everyone—from secure, middle-aged people to older Americans who tend to be at greatest risk—can make responsible, informed personal choices in anticipation of their later years.

Source: Administration on Aging (AoA): *Life course planning*, Washington, DC, 2000b, The Administration.

churches, local schools, community groups (e.g., Habitat for Humanity) and on an individual basis.

*Retirement* is a contemporary phenomenon. Before the passage of the retirement provisions of the Social Security Act of 1935 (see Chapter 4), few Americans could afford to retire. With the advent of retirement insurance, people were able to retire from work and enjoy life's later years. In order to achieve and maintain quality of life in their older years, people must anticipate their needs and engage in comprehensive **life course planning** (AoA, 2000b) (Box 19-6).

The AoA offers pension counseling projects and sponsors the *Pension Rights Center* (AoA, 2000f). Numerous private organizations such as businesses, NCOA, and AARP have information and programs available that assist in life course planning. Life course planning is more than just financial planning. It includes planning for the entire retirement experience. Retirement is a time for role restructuring and major decisions such as choosing where one will live; deciding on a new or part-time career; determining educational, recreational, and leisure pursuits; addressing relationships with friends and family; and reassessing finances. For many, retirement is when they finally have significant

amounts of time for leisure and recreational pursuits. The nurse can be instrumental in helping people recognize the need for life course planning and can assist persons in seeing the options open to them, make them aware of community resources, and offer support and guidance during this stage of transition.

## Income

After retirement, many Americans live on a relatively *fixed income*. The median income of older persons is just over $19,000 a year for men and almost $11,000 for women (AARP, AoA, 2001). More than 3 million older Americans live in poverty, and another 2 million are classified as "near-poor" (having incomes between the poverty level and 125% of this level) (AARP, AoA, 2001). Older women, minorities, and the "oldest old" are more likely to live in poverty.

Ninety percent of older Americans receive Social Security, making it the major source of income for older Americans (AARP, AoA, 2001). Income from assets is reported by 62% of older Americans, income from private pensions by 44%, and income from earnings by 21% (AARP, AoA, 2001). Only 8% of the elderly receive public assistance and only 6% receive food stamps (AARP, 1996). Adequate income and assets are critically important to enable well-being in all dimensions of life in later years, and it is estimated that retirees will need at least 70% of their preretirement income to maintain their standard of living after they stop working (AoA, 2000b). People need to start planning for the financial aspects of their old age long before old age begins.

## Housing

Safe, appropriate housing is a major concern for the elderly. Many elders continue to live independently in their own homes. Of the almost 21 million households headed by older Americans, almost 80% were owners and approximately 20% were renters (AARP, AoA, 2001). Of the 5 million households that include a senior citizen with a disability, more than 2 million expressed the need for home modifications in order to be able to stay in the home environment (AoA, 2000g).

Many communities offer publicly subsidized "senior housing" units to the elderly that are rented on a sliding scale basis. However, such units often have waiting lists. Other housing opportunities range from single family dwellings, apartment or condominium living, congregated living, shared group homes, board and care homes, and living with family to assisted living and long-term care. Senior continuing care housing communities are being developed across the country. In such communities housing options range from independent living to nursing home placements. Such housing communities are often in the private, for-profit sector, and many are priced out of the reach of the low- to middle-income seniors.

The NCOAs *National Institute on Senior Housing* has a goal to help older Americans remain in their homes as long as possible and to have affordable, safe, and appropriate housing available for senior citizens (NCOA, 2000). The AARP has information on housing options to older persons, provides information on the *Elder Cottage Housing Opportunity* (ECHO) where elders live in a separate unit in the yard of their child's home, and has information on home modifications to help people age in place. Innovative housing ideas for the elderly are being developed, including home sharing, ECHO, home equity conversion, group homes, "granny flats," and home renovations that suit the individual's changing needs. Groups such as the *Center for Universal Design* (see Chapter 18) have innovative floor plans, interior designs, and home modifications that aid the elderly person in independent living.

Deciding whether to live in their own homes or apartments, live with relatives, or live in a long-term care facility is just one of the many issues the elderly confront. Appropriate housing helps promote self-esteem, provides comfort, encourages socialization, and prevents or delays the costly alternative of institutionalization. Trying to decide where to live is an important decision. Box 19-7 looks at some questions to answer when choosing the most appropriate housing option.

## Education

The educational level of the older population is increasing. In the last 30 years the percentage of elders who had completed high school in the United States rose from 28% to 68%, and about 15% of these had a bachelor's degree or higher (AARP, AoA, 2001). The percentage of elders who have completed high school varies considerably by race and

### BOX 19-7

*Questions to Answer in Choosing the Most Appropriate Housing Option*

- Does this arrangement provide a supportive environment for retaining maximum independence?
- Is it easy to move about in the home environment or can home modifications enhance continued mobility?
- Is this a comfortable and safe place to live?
- Is the cost affordable?
- Is there access to in-home and community services when and if needed?
- Is the location convenient and accessible to transportation, shopping, and health services?
- Are opportunities for socializing and participation in daily life adequate, including family, friends, church, and community activities?

Source: Administration on Aging (AoA): *Housing options for older Americans*, Washington, DC, 2000g, The Administration.

ethnic origin. Among older persons, 73% of whites, 68% of Asians and Pacific Islanders, 45% of African Americans, and 32% of Hispanics have completed high school (AARP, AoA, 2001). It is becoming increasingly common for older people to return to school or have advanced degrees. Programs such as *Elderhostel* (*http://www.elderhostel.org*) enable elders to continue their education throughout life. Better-educated consumers are scrutinizing their health care more and demanding higher quality and more appropriate health care.

## NORMAL BODY CHANGES OF AGING

Aging is a natural and lifelong process. As we age, physical, psychosocial, and emotional changes occur. The physical, mental, and psychological changes associated with aging occur very gradually and are highly individual (e.g., less than 1% of the physical function an individual has at age 30 is lost each succeeding year). Listed in Table 19-2 are some physical changes that occur with aging and their implications for care. These changes must be taken into account if the client's potential for health and wellness is to be maximized. For instance, smooth muscle weakness and muscle atrophy often lead to constipation with older people. However, diet and exercise can help overcome this problem.

Numerous books have been written for elders who wish to remain healthy and enjoy old age. The noted psychologist B.F. Skinner has written (with M.E. Vaughn) *Enjoy Old Age: A Program of Self-Management* (1983) out of his own life experience; Maggie Kuhn has written *Maggie Kuhn on Aging* (1977); Alex Comfort has written *Say Yes to Old Age: Developing a Positive Attitude Toward Aging* (1990); and Lydia Bronte has written *The Longevity Factor: The New Reality of Long Careers and How It Can Lead to Richer Lives* (1993). A common theme in all of these books is that aging is individual, and old age is a time of continued growth,

**TABLE 19-2**

*Physical Changes with Age*

| CHANGE | IMPLICATIONS |
| --- | --- |
| *Skeletal System* | |
| 1. Compression of vertebral disks | 1. Postural changes and decreased stature (average loss of 1-2 inches) |
| 2. Muscle atrophy | 2. Diminished strength and balance |
| 3. Decalcification of bones | 3. Osteoporosis, increased risk of fractures |
| 4. Ossification of joint cartilage | 4. Joint pain and stiffness |
| *Gastrointestinal System* | |
| 1. Diminished production of hydrochloric acid | 1. Impaired digestion and absorption |
| 2. Decreased salivary gland secretion | 2. Impaired digestion |
| 3. Delayed emptying of the stomach and esophagus | 3. Feeling of "fullness," gastric reflux |
| 4. Decreased peristalsis | 4. Slowed digestion and absorption; bloating |
| 5. Taste buds atrophy | 5. Taste sensation decreases |
| 6. Diminished anal sphincter control | 6. Fecal incontinence |
| *Respiratory System* | |
| 1. Increase in residual lung volume and decrease in vital capacity | 1. Impaired ventilation and reduced ability to cough or breathe deeply |
| 2. Loss of elasticity of lung tissue and decrease in muscle structure | 2. Difficulty breathing; increased episodes of shortness of breath and dyspnea on exertion |
| 3. Decrease in oxygen exchange between the alveoli and capillaries | 3. Less oxygen available; dyspnea on exertion |
| *Neurological System* | |
| 1. Decrease in size and weight of brain and in number of neurons | 1. Slower nerve transmission; thought and memory changes |
| 2. Spinal cord synapse degeneration | 2. Diminished coordination |
| 3. Optic and auditory nerve degeneration | 3. Diminished vision and hearing |
| *Genitourinary System* | |
| 1. Bladder: loss of muscle tone | 1. Incomplete bladder emptying that can result in urinary retention and cystitis |
| 2. Pelvic muscle and sphincter relaxation | 2. Urinary incontinence |
| 3. Kidney: reduced blood flow and filtration; interstitial fibrosis | 3. Fluid and electrolyte imbalance |
| 4. Atrophy of ovarian, uterine, vaginal tissues; thinning of vaginal walls | 4. Decreased vaginal lubrication; decreased vaginal elasticity; loss of fertility; stress incontinence; dyspareunia |
| 5. Diminished spermatogenesis; atrophy of testes, enlargement of prostrate | 5. Increased time for erection; reduced volume of seminal fluid; reduced force of ejaculation; frequency of urination |

development, and fulfillment. Americans are fortunate to live in a country where they are able to grow old. They need to take advantage of, and look forward to, this opportunity for a long and active life.

## HEALTH PROMOTION AND THE ELDERLY

The NCOA sponsors the *Health Promotion Institute*, which works to promote the ongoing development of preventive services that will enhance awareness among older Ameri-

cans of the importance of health promotion activities. AARP sponsors the *National Eldercare Institute on Health Promotion*, which works to promote wellness among older Americans and to stimulate development of health promotion programs. *Healthy People 2010* has an objective to increase to 90% the proportion of older adults who have participated in at least one organized health promotion activity each year (USDHHS, 2000). The NIA encourages health promotion activities for elders and publishes a series of *AgePages* on various health education topics.

**TABLE 19-2**

*Physical Changes with Age—cont'd*

| CHANGE | IMPLICATIONS |
|---|---|
| *Nutrition and Metabolism* | |
| 1. Vitamin and mineral deficiencies | 1. Capillary fragility and bruising; anemia; malnutrition; bone demineralization; inflammation of mucous membranes |
| 2. Altered digestive processes | 2. Impaired taste, digestion, and absorption of food |
| 3. Dentition: lost teeth, ill-fitting dentures | 3. Impaired appetite; malnutrition; dehydration |
| 4. Inadequate fluid intake | 4. Dehydration; fluid and electrolyte imbalance |
| *Cardiovascular System* | |
| 1. Thickening and fibrosis of blood vessels | 1. Atherosclerotic changes; increased risk for hypertension, heart ischemia, stroke, and myocardial infarction |
| 2. Enlargement of left ventricle | 2. Increased risk of congestive heart failure and impaired tissue perfusion; edema |
| 3. Enlargement of right ventricle | 3. Reduced oxygenation of blood; pulmonary hypertension |
| 4. Impaired peripheral vascular circulation | 4. Decreased tissue nourishment; edema |
| 5. Diminished cardiac output | 5. Decreased blood flow and tissue oxygenation |
| 6. Calcification of cardiac valves | 6. Heart murmurs and disorders |
| 7. Changes in atrioventricular and sinoatrial nodes | 7. Conduction abnormalities |
| *Skin and Cutaneous Tissue* | |
| 1. Atrophy of sweat glands and sebaceous glands produce less sebum | 1. Decreased perspiration; increased susceptibility to trauma, abrasions, bedsores; skin becomes drier; impaired heat dissipation |
| 2. Deposits of melanin | 2. "Age spots" occur |
| 3. Thickening of finger and toenails | 3. Splintering of nails; difficulty in cutting nails; increased risk of infection |
| 4. Loss of subcutaneous fat and water in the epidermis | 4. Wrinkling of skin; decreased turgor; slower wound healing |
| 5. Thinning of skin | 5. Increased risk of tearing, abrasions |
| *Immune System* | |
| 1. Decreased ability to make antibodies and mount an immune response | 1. Increased risk of infection |
| *Sensory* | |
| 1. Lens of eye becomes more opaque and rigid; lens yellows | 1. Decreased ability to focus on near objects (presbyopia); increased sensitivity to glare; increased difficulty with color discrimination; peripheral vision decreases |
| 2. Size of pupil decreases | 2. Need brighter light to see, decreased night vision |
| 3. Odor identification declines | 3. Decreased appetite |
| 4. Taste buds decrease in number | 4. Decreased sense of taste and diminished appetite |
| 5. Cochlear damage | 5. Sensory hearing loss |

These AgePages can be ordered through NIA's toll free number (1-800-222-2225) or downloaded from the internet (*http://www.nia.nih.gov*).

It once seemed that health problems were inevitable in old age; however, there is conclusive evidence that many diseases can be controlled or prevented through a healthy lifestyle (AoA, 2000h). Changes in lifestyle can preserve function, delay or prevent the onset of disease and disability, and improve quality of life. Some healthy lifestyle activities are given in Box 19-8.

A medical model that focuses on disease pathology has historically dominated the provision of health care in the United States, and older people grew up with a health care system that did not focus on preventive health. Studies have shown that older people go to the doctor primarily when something is wrong, have trouble with the idea of having tests done when they have no symptoms, and do not know when to request tests or what to expect from them (AARP, 1991, p. 15). The nurse needs to work with older clients to help them see the benefit of health promotion activities.

Fortunately, most older people generally view their health positively. More than 70% of older people living in the community describe their health as excellent, very good, or good (AARP, AoA, 2001). There was little difference between the sexes on their rating of health; however, older African Americans (42%) and older Hispanic Americans (35%) were much more likely to relate their health as fair or poor than older whites (26%) (AARP, AoA, 2001). Health promotion activities can make elders healthier and change or eliminate risk factors such as lack of exercise, cigarette smoking, excessive alcohol intake, and high-cholesterol diets. Health promotion activities such as regular physical examinations, exercise, safety, and good nutrition play a significant role in promoting healthy aging.

### BOX 19-8

### *Longevity and the Power of A Healthy Lifestyle*

Virtually all older people can reap health benefits if they:
- Improve their diet and nutrition
- Maintain an appropriate weight
- Stop smoking
- Stick with regular physical activity and exercise
- Get regular health checkups
- Keep physically and mentally active and socially engaged

Source: Administration on Aging (AoA): *Longevity and the power of a healthy lifestyle*, Washington, DC, 2000h, The Administration.

## Physical Examinations

The report of the U.S. Public Health Service (2000), *Put Prevention Into Practice*, outlined a preventive care timeline for periodic health examination of adults. Physical examinations can help detect conditions early and prevent complications. For example, a sigmoidoscopy can detect polyps that 10 years later might have become cancer of the colon, and early detection of diabetes can help keep the disease and its related conditions under control. Physical examinations are a perfect time to discuss personal health habits regarding sleep, nutrition, exercise, alcohol, and smoking. They are also a time when the elder can share health concerns with the provider and work in partnership to develop a plan of care. A schedule of when periodic health examinations are recommended is given in Figure 19-7. An NIA publication, *Talking to Your Doctor*, assists older people in preparing for physical examinations and other health care visits and can be ordered through NIA's toll free number (1-800-222-2225).

## Exercise

Exercise can help older people feel better and enjoy life more, even those who think that they are too old or out of shape (NIA, 1998). The effects of exercise can assist in slowing the physiological aging process, allow more independence and freedom, reduce risk factors for chronic disease, and optimize physical and mental health (Perkins, 2000).

Increased levels of physical activity are associated with reduced incidence of coronary artery disease, hypertension,

| Periodic health examination protocol | | | | | | |
|---|---|---|---|---|---|---|
| Age | 20 | 30 | 40 | 50 | 60 | 70+ |
| Physical examination and health risk assessment | | Every 5 years | 3 years | Every 2 years | | Yearly |
| Blood pressure | Yearly | | | | | |
| Cholesterol | Every 5 years | | | | | |
| Breast and pelvic examination | | Every 3 years | Yearly | | | |
| Pap smear | Yearly | | | | | |
| Mammography | | Baseline at 35 | 2 years | Yearly | | |
| Stool for blood | | | 3 years | Yearly | | |
| Proctosigmoidoscopy | | | | Every 3 years (after 2 yearly negatives) | | |
| Immunizations | Tetanus/diphtheria—every 10 years Influenza—yearly after age 65 Pneumovax—at age 65 and then every 5 years | | | | | |

**FIGURE 19-7** Periodic health examinations. (From Annual checkups—who needs them, *Aging* 365:2, 1993.)

obesity, stroke, and osteoporosis (Ham, Sloane, 2001). Clinical evidence indicates that conditions such as osteoporosis, arterial and venous insufficiency, gastrointestinal stasis, and musculoskeletal stiffness actually have more adverse symptoms in inactive elders (Ham, Sloane, 2001). Exercise has the potential to improve sleep, digestion, cardiovascular status, mobility, strength and balance, mood, and bone density and increase life span. Exercise can prevent and improve some disabilities and diseases in older people (NIA, 1998).

Unfortunately, only one third of older Americans exercise regularly (USDHHS, 1999). In addition 50% of people over age 65 do not participate in any leisure activity (Perkins, 2000). Research by O'Neill and Reid (1991) found that 87% the elderly perceived at least one major barrier that prevented their involvement in physical activity, such as an existing health problem or lack of knowledge about exercise resources and regimens (Figure 19-8).

*Healthy People 2010* has objectives to increase the proportion of elderly people who engage in moderate physical activity for 30 minutes each day, take part in leisure-time physical activity, participate in physical activities that enhance and maintain muscular strength and endurance, and participate in physical activities that enhance and maintain flexibility (USDHHS, 2000). The NIA encourages elders to make physical activity a part of their everyday life and publishes an AgePage, *Exercise: Feeling Fit for Life* (NIA, 1998). The NIA and organizations such as the Arthritis Foundation have exercise videos available specifically for elders.

According to Ham and Sloane (1997), "The right amount of exercise in old age is 'more exercise than yesterday.' For the sedentary older person the recommendation should be for slow reacquisition of regular, low-impact, unstressed but progressively increasing exercise" (p. 105). Research by Schaller

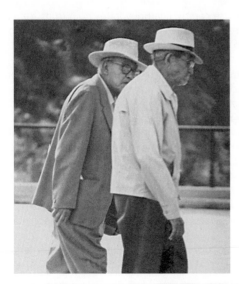

**FIGURE 19-8** Nurses should stress the benefit of exercise to health. Exercising with a friend battles loneliness. (Courtesy Ken Yamaguchi. In Castillo HM: *The nurse assistant in long-term care: a rehabilitative approach*, St Louis, 1992, Mosby.)

(1996) indicated that Tai Chi was a safe and enjoyable form of exercise in older adults. In general, swimming, walking, and bicycling are all excellent exercises for the elderly (Ham, Sloane, 2001).

Many communities have YMCAs, YWCAs, and senior and fitness centers that offer senior exercise programs. The National Senior Games Association (*http://www.nsga.com*) is a sponsor of *Senior Olympics* where elite senior athletes compete in athletic activities. Communities across the country have elders who participate in Senior Olympics. Many senior Olympians go on to compete in state and national competitions. As with everyone else, older people with existing diseases and conditions should consult their primary care provider before beginning an exercise program.

## Stop and Think About It

Does your local community have Senior Olympic games? What agency in the community sponsors these games? Have you ever attended Senior Olympics? How could nurses be active in supporting exercise, athletic, and recreational activities with seniors?

## Safety

Safety is a concern for all age groups. Factors that contribute to accidents and injuries in elders include muscle weakness, demineralization of bone, slowed reaction time, unsteady gait, changes in hearing and vision, changes in short-term memory, and polypharmacy. A particularly high risk to safety occurs when a person is functionally impaired, as with Alzheimer's disease (Eliopoulos, 2001).

Postural hypotension is frequently associated with falling in the elderly. Falls are a leading cause of accidental injury and death with elders. *Healthy People 2010* has an objective to reduce the incidence of hip fractures in older adults and numerous objectives that address the need to reduce accidental injuries in older adults from falls, motor vehicle accidents, pedestrian accidents, and fires (USDHHS, 2000).

One third of community-dwelling elders experience at least one episode of falling each year, and the incidence is greatly increased in nursing home residents (Farmer, 2000). About 50% of people over 80 experience at least one fall each year (Ham, Sloane, 2001). Many hospital and nursing home admissions are the result of falls. About 50% of elders discharged from the hospital after a fall experience decreased independence (Leccese, 1999).

Fear of falls and their resultant injuries limits the activities of many older people. In assessing the individual's fall risk, the nurse needs to consider factors such as a history of falls, confusion, impaired judgement, sensory deficits, ambulation capabilities, medications, postural hypotension, diseases that affect perfusion and oxygenation, and environmental risk factors such as poor lighting, highly polished floors, and throw rugs (Farmer, 2000). Most falls are preventable.

Many accidents occur in the home and could be prevented if people followed simple safety rules. The home should be assessed for safety hazards and made as safe as possible. Stairs and bathrooms are the most dangerous locations for falls. Stairs should be adequately lighted, free of clutter, and equipped with handrails and nonskid surfaces. It may be helpful to outline the edge of each step with a luminescent or contrast tape or color and to paint top and bottom steps in colors that make them easily noticed. Bathrooms should have handrails, nonslip adhesive surfaces in tubs and showers, and nonslip flooring.

Other safety precautions around the home include having enough light; having light switches within easy reach; using a light when getting up at night; using nonskid soles on shoes; eliminating throw rugs, casters on chairs, and extension cords; avoiding sedation; and placing distinct labels on medications and toxic substances. Smoking in bed should be eliminated. To avoid accidental scaldings and burns, lowering hot water heater temperatures and labeling hot and cold water faucets is helpful. Only safe home heating methods should be used to minimize the chance of smoke and fires. Carbon monoxide and smoke detectors should be a part of every elder's home.

Having a telephone or emergency responder system in the home is an important safety measure. The telephone and emergency numbers should be in a convenient, accessible location—often at the bedside. Telephone services such as "Friendly Caller" programs help give the elderly person contact with the outside world, reduce social isolation, and promote safety.

Crime and the elderly is another safety concern. Contrary to popular belief, the elderly have the lowest victimization rates of any age group in our society except for "personal larceny with contact" (i.e., purse snatching and pickpocketing) (Harris, 1990, p. 400). Common crimes against the elderly include purse snatchings, fraud, theft, vandalism, and harassment. Consumer fraud, confidence games, and medical quackery are major forms of crime against the elderly (Harris, 1990, p. 406). Telemarketing fraud is a concern and elders should exhibit caution in negotiating telemarketing contracts. Research shows that the elderly rank fear of crime as a major concern (Harris, 1990, p. 401) and that this fear may add to their social isolation.

The nurse can be of assistance in making seniors aware of the health risks of accidents and in helping to prevent them. The nurse also can help older adults understand that safety is an area over which they have control and that safety precautions can help promote health and maintain quality of life. Primary prevention measures can greatly decrease accidental injury and illness in the elderly.

## Nutrition

The Surgeon General's *Report on Nutrition on Health* noted that two thirds of all deaths are due to diseases associated with poor diets and dietary habits and what we eat affects our health, quality of life, and longevity (AoA, 2000i). Good nutrition is essential to maintaining cognitive and physical functioning and plays an essential role in the control and management of many chronic diseases.

Older adults are at risk of dehydration and nutrition problems (Orr, 2000). Researchers have estimated that up to 50% of those age 65 and older have poor nutrition or are malnourished (Greely, 1991). Undernutrition is a common problem among elders, and more than 50% of elderly persons who are hospitalized or experiencing a disease have protein-energy malnutrition (Lesourd, 1999; Turner, Fitch-Hilgenberg, DiBrezzo, et al., 2000).

Poor nutrition among older people occurs as a result of a number of problems such as tooth loss and gum disease, ill-fitting dentures, illness, lack of proper hydration, poverty, medication side effects, social isolation, and mobility limitations. Normal age-related changes that affect nutrition include a decrease in thirst response, muscle mass, and metabolic rate; delayed gastric motility; and diminished taste sensation. Some suggestions for a longer, healthier life through good nutrition, along with select dietary recommendations for the elderly, are given in Box 19-9.

Many programs help improve senior nutrition. Qualifying seniors are eligible for food stamps. The AoA's *Elderly Nutrition Program* helps older Americans build a foundation for health through improved diets, increased physical activity, and improved lifestyle choices (AoA, 2000i). The Older

**BOX 19-9**
### Nutrition for the Elderly

*Teaching TIPS*

**Some Suggestions for Elders: A Healthier Life through Good Nutrition**

- Establish and maintain good eating patterns and eat a variety of foods.
- Reduce caloric intake by 5% per decade for individuals 51 years of age or older.
- Increase complex carbohydrates from fruits, vegetables, cereals, and whole wheat breads. (At least 55% of daily caloric intake should be from carbohydrates.)
- Limit fats to 30% or less of daily calories.
- About 15% of daily food intake should be from protein.
- Calcium, vitamin D, and vitamin $B_{12}$ have decreased absorption with age and need to be supplemented. (Calcium and vitamin D are important to healthy bones.)
- Unless a medical condition dictates otherwise, drink at least 8 glasses of water a day (a minimum of 1500 ml).
- Reduce salt intake.
- Eat 4 or 5 small meals a day rather than 3 large meals.
- Maintain good dental health.
- To keep your appetite hearty and your muscles healthy, mix aerobic exercises (walking or swimming) with activities that strengthen muscle.
- Stay socially active and mentally alert. Both tend to increase appetite.

Sources: Eliopoulos C: *Gerontological nursing,* ed 5, Philadelphia, 2001, JB Lippincott; Hogstel MO: *Gerontology. Nursing care of the older adult,* Albany, NY, 2001, Delmar; Rosenburg IH: *As you age: 10 keys to a longer, healthier, more vital life, Worldview* 5(2):2-3, 1993.

Americans Act provides for congregate and home-delivered meals. The U.S. Department of Agriculture has a new program for low-income seniors, the *Seniors Farmers' Market Nutrition Pilot Program*, that offers coupons to low-income seniors that can be exchanged for foods at farmers' markets, roadside stands, and community supported agricultural programs. Local nutritional services to the elderly are often coordinated through senior centers and Area Offices on Aging. *Healthy People 2010* has objectives to increase the proportion of older adults who are at a healthy weight, reduce the proportion of elder obesity, improve the nutritional status of older adults, and increase the incidence of older adults receiving nutrition counseling or education (USDHHS, 2000).

GETTING SENIORS TO EAT WELL. The community health nurse plays an important role in senior nutrition counseling and education and in referring seniors to nutrition resources. Getting seniors to eat well is a complex challenge. Problems such as ill-fitting dentures, loss of teeth, and periodontal disease make chewing painful and can make it difficult to maintain good nutrition. Physical changes of aging that can affect nutrition have been mentioned previously. In addition, certain medications can depress appetite or taste sensations. The frail elderly may actually lack the dexterity and energy to feed themselves.

Older people living alone are especially vulnerable to the problems of inadequate nutrition, often losing interest in meal planning and preparation. Alternating meal preparation with someone else and "Meal Clubs," in which meal preparation responsibilities are shared, can help curb food costs, offer variety to meals, and provide companionship. Cooking in larger quantities and freezing foods may be a helpful idea. Many local restaurants offer senior discounts, and local churches frequently sponsor meals for seniors.

Serving foods in an attractive, pleasant manner often enhances appetite. Fixing foods with different textures and aromas and using flavor boosters such as commercially prepared flavor enhancers and spices can enhance appetite. Switching around from food to food during meals may help prevent sensory adaptation and increase appetite. Also, eating each food separately, rather than mixing them, helps increase the ability to taste the food. Good oral hygiene should be encouraged and helps promote appetite.

Economics enters into senior nutrition. Food prices keep increasing and senior income generally remains relatively constant. The nurse can counsel the elderly on low-cost food buying and preparation such as using dried legumes, beans, whole cereal grains, dried fortified milk, and less expensive cuts of meat to save on cost.

Physical barriers to proper nutrition need to be considered. Physical disabilities such as orthopedic problems and poor vision can inhibit the ability to shop. Shopping assistance may be available through local homemaker services, senior centers, or friends and family. Many grocery stores are now providing electric shopping carts that could be useful to the older shopper. Lack of transportation to cost-efficient grocery stores, restaurants, and food programs can pose a nutrition problem.

NUTRITION SCREENING. It is essential for the nurse to do an in-depth assessment of hydration and nutritional status with the elderly client (Zembrzuski, 2000). Adequate hydration is important and fluids are necessary to maintain kidney function, aid in food and medication absorption, decrease medication side effects, aid in expectoration, soften stools, and prevent dehydration. The **Nutrition Screening Initiative** (2000) is a national program sponsored by the American Academy of Family Physicians, the American Dietetic Association, and the NCOA. It is committed to the identification of nutritional problems in older persons, improved elder nutrition, and improved delivery of nutrition services to the elderly. The Initiative has developed a checklist that can be helpful to the nurse when initiating discussion about diet and nutrition (Appendix 19-1).

The nurse should implement a nutritional assessment such as a 3-day diet recall to assist in evaluating a client's nutritional status and needs. Diet recall can lead to discussions of food preparation and preferences, buying habits, and eating problems, and can be an excellent teaching tool. Older persons have developed a lifetime of food practices, and the nurse needs to remember that nutritional habits are not easy to change. Also, cultural, ethnic, and religious beliefs, as well as income, strongly influence nutritional practices. The nurse can help link clients to community nutrition resources and services. When the nutrition problems of the client are beyond the scope of the nurse, a nutritionist or physician should be contacted. Many local health departments have nutritionists on the staff; nutritionists also are available through local hospitals and county extension services. A modified food pyramid guide for seniors is given in Table 19-3.

**TABLE 19-3**

*Modified Food Guide Pyramid for Older Adults Compared with Original Food Guide Pyramid*

| ITEM | MODIFIED FOOD GUIDE PYRAMID |
|---|---|
| Supplements | Calcium, vitamin D, and $B_{12}$ |
| Fats, oils, and sweets | Use sparingly |
| Milk, yogurt, and cheese group | 3 servings |
| Meat, poultry, fish, dry beans, eggs, and nut group | ≥2 servings |
| Vegetable group | ≥3 servings |
| Fruit group | ≥2 servings |
| Bread, cereal, rice, and pasta group | ≥6 servings |
| Water | ≥8 servings |

Adapted from Russell RM, Rasmussen H, Lichtenstein AH: Modified food guide pyramid for people over seventy years of age, *J Nutrition* 129:751-753, 1999.

## SELECTED HEALTH CONCERNS AMONG THE ELDERLY

Common causes of morbidity and mortality have already been presented in this chapter. Some selected health concerns are discussed in the following sections.

### Inadequate Health Insurance

Most older Americans receive health insurance through the federal health insurance program of Medicare. This program is discussed in Chapter 5, where it was noted that Medicare has many gaps in service provision. A major gap in Medicare coverage is the program's lack of prescription drug coverage for the elderly. Medicare also has restrictions on long-term care, home health care, and preventive health services. Many elders purchase Medigap insurance to supplement their Medicare coverage.

### Medications

It has already been noted that Medicare does *not* pay for the cost of prescription drugs. Some older Americans do not take their prescribed medications properly because they cannot afford to buy them. They often omit medications or take less than the prescribed dosage to decrease cost. Federal legislation has been proposed to cover the cost of prescription medications for the elderly, but none has been enacted. Some states are looking at their own solutions to this problem. For example, Tennessee is presently considering the *Senior Citizen Prescription Drug Discount Program Act* to help seniors who lack prescription drug coverage to get discounted drug prices (Ferrar, 2001).

Older people frequently have chronic disease conditions that require long-term and/or multiple-drug therapy. Taking several drugs concurrently, *polypharmacy,* and having more than one chronic condition markedly increases the risk of drug reactions. The elderly account for approximately one third of all prescription drug use in the United States (Beers, Berkow, 2000). Women use more medications than men, and frail elders use the most drugs. Taking all medications into consideration, elders take an average of seven medications daily (Beers, Berkow, 2000). Research has repeatedly cited overuse of medications in elders as a major health concern (Johnson, 2000). However, discontinuing medications also can pose problems. Research has shown adverse drug withdrawal events in older clients who had certain medications discontinued (Johnson, 2000).

Many elders make errors in their medication regimens, are confused about their medication regimens, and tend to self-medicate. The elderly are at higher risk of nonadherence to their drug regimen than any other age group (Yee, Weaver, 2000). A number of all hospital and nursing home admissions of older Americans result from taking prescriptions incorrectly. Millions of older Americans are prescribed potentially inappropriate medications each year by their health care providers (Johnson, 2000).

Elders suffer side effects from medications 2 to 3 times more frequently than do younger clients (White, 1995, p. 545). Many drugs induce impairments in elders' mobility and can be a risk factor for falls and other injuries. The physiological changes that come with aging alter how older adults distribute, metabolize, and excrete drugs; make them susceptible to adverse drug effects; and can cause increased plasma levels of drugs. Numerous medications can cause changes in behavior and mental status with elders. *Healthy People 2010* has an age-related objective to increase the number of primary health care providers who routinely review with their clients age 65 and older any new medication prescribed (USDHHS, 2000).

The nurse needs to carefully monitor the medications of elderly clients, assess if they are taking their medications as prescribed, and help make sure that elders understand their medication regimens and what their medications are for. The nurse is in an excellent position to help clients avoid medication errors and adhere to medication regimens. Nurses need to elicit a medication history from each client. Clients should be encouraged to keep an up-to-date list of medications with drug name, dosage, times of administration and reason for taking the drug. Such information needs to be regularly reviewed with clients on office visits, in the clinic setting, and on home visits. Appendix 19-2 provides a guide to use when doing a medication assessment with elderly persons.

ELDER ABUSE AND NEGLECT. It has been estimated that over 3% of the elder population, more than 1 million older Americans, are abused and neglected each year (Beers, Berkow, 2000, p. 150). The number of reports of elder abuse is increasing (AoA, 2000j; Drayton-Hargrove, 2000).

Mistreated elders are often frail, disabled, dependent, over age 70, and women. Persons aged 80 years and older suffer abuse and neglect two to three times the proportion of the older population (AoA, 2000j). Typically family members, not strangers, are the perpetrators of this abuse and two thirds of perpetrators are adult children or spouses (AoA, 2000j). A major problem with elder abuse and neglect is the "invisibility" of the problem (Molony, Waszynski, Lyder, 1999, p. 531).

**Elder abuse** may be *physical* (e.g., slapping, bruising, sexually molesting, pushing, restraining), *psychological* (e.g., threats, intimidation, humiliating), *financial/material* (e.g., misuse or misappropriation of funds or property), or involve *violation of rights* (e.g., forced institutionalization).

**Elder neglect** includes passive, active, or self-neglect. It typically involves withholding necessities of life such as food, proper clothing, medications, and comfort measures. *Passive neglect* is the unintentional failure to fulfill a caretaking obligation as a result of things such as ignorance or lack of ability. *Active neglect* is an intentional failure to fulfill a caretaking obligation. *Self-neglect* is a common form of neglect. Lack of knowledge regarding the elder's health needs can lead to neglect. *Abandonment* is a form of neglect. Some have adopted the term "granny dumping" to describe abandonment.

Elder abuse and neglect is frequently not reported to authorities. Without intervention it is unlikely that the abuse will go away, and it often tends to intensify over time (Lynch, 1997). As with other forms of family violence, when it is reported, authorities may hesitate to become involved.

SIGNS AND SYMPTOMS. Detecting elder abuse and neglect is not always easy. Signs and symptoms of elder abuse include bruises, lacerations, pressure sores, fractures; malnutrition; conflicting explanations about the elder's condition; a caregiver describing an elder as "clumsy" or "accident-prone"; sudden changes in the elder's physical or mental state; unusual fears exhibited by the elder; abnormal caregiver behavior; social isolation of the elder by a caregiver; and indifference or hostility displayed by the caregiver in response to questions. A recent, unexpected change in the financial status of the caregiver can be a sign of financial abuse.

Risk factors play a part in elder abuse, including social isolation of the victim, substance abuse or psychological disorder of the abuser, history of family violence, crowded or inadequate family living conditions, marital problems in the caregiving family, insufficient income, increasing dependency needs of the elderly, and pathological parent-child relationships (e.g., children who were mistreated by parents now mistreating parents) (Beers, Berkow, 2000, p. 151; Molony, Waszynski, Lyder, 1999, p. 531). Nursing research has identified elder abuse risk factors that include functional disability, confusion, minority status, and poor social networks (Campbell, Harris, Lee, 1995).

LEGISLATION AND REPORTING. Each state has elder abuse reporting and adult protective services legislation. Laws and definitions of terms vary greatly from one state to another, but all states have reporting systems. Generally state *Adult Protective Service* (APS) agencies receive and investigate reports of suspected abuse and neglect. Nurses are routinely identified under state protective service laws as mandatory reporters of suspected abuse or neglect.

DOCUMENTATION. According to Miller (1995, p. 541), in assessing cases of suspected abuse or neglect, the health professional should document (1) background data (e.g., client's name, address, phone number, caregiver name, documentation of previous maltreatment), (2) signs of maltreatment or self-neglect (e.g., bruises, burns, broken bones), (3) severity of signs, (4) indicators of maltreatment intentionality (e.g., caregiver will not allow nurse to be alone with client), (5) symptoms of acute or chronic illness (e.g., incontinence), (6) functional incapacity (e.g., an inability to dress or toilet without assistance), (7) aggravating social condi-

tions (e.g., client lives alone and is isolated), (8) source of information (e.g., agency referral), and (9) recommendations (e.g., opening the case for home health care services). A well-documented history of injury and illness is important. The nurse is mandated by most state law to report suspected cases of elder abuse or neglect.

PREVENTION AND INTERVENTION. Nursing research on elder abuse has resulted in the development of assessment tools for elder abuse, prevention strategies, and nursing interventions (Campbell, Harris, Lee, 1995). Primary prevention is the key to resolving the serious problem of elder abuse. Primary prevention activities include encouraging people to plan for future care needs while they are healthy and capable of making such decisions, providing adequate community resources to prevent caregiver burnout (e.g., respite care, financial aid, counseling), fostering personal self-esteem, and promoting positive attitudes about aging. Secondary prevention efforts focus on early casefinding and treatment (e.g., crisis intervention, Neighborhood Watches, and "buddy" systems). Tertiary prevention interventions involve family and caregiver rehabilitation activities in relation to counseling and care management, and in some cases, the removal of the elderly person from the setting. However, community placement options for such elders are limited and elders may prefer to remain in the abusive situation rather than be placed outside the home.

Interventions can be complicated, and an abused elder may be loyal or fearful of the abuser, ashamed to acknowledge the abuse, or unaware of the services available to them (Lynch, 1997, p. 27). If the nurse suspects abuse, she or he should try to interview the client privately, avoid asking leading questions, and keep questions simple and direct (Lynch, 1997, pp. 27-28).

The AoA funds the *National Center on Elder Abuse* (*http://www.elderabusecenter.org*). The center provides information, training, and research on elder abuse and is engaged in activities to prevent abuse and neglect from occurring. Its website includes a state-by-state listing of toll-free telephone numbers to report suspected elder abuse and neglect.

## Depression

Mental health is an important aspect of healthy aging. The United States has failed to ensure older persons' access to community mental health services, and many older persons have unmet mental health needs (USDHHS, 2000).

**Depression** is not a normal part of growing old, but it is a common problem for the elderly (Beers, Berkow, 2000, p. 310; Kurlowicz, 1999; NIA, 1996; USDHHS, 2000). It is estimated that depression affects more than 5 million elders in the United States (Kurlowicz, 1999). The prevalence of depression with elders tends to vary by setting, with major

### BOX 19-10

## Symptoms and Signs of Depression in Late Life

| SYMPTOMS | OBSERVABLE SIGNS |
|---|---|
| **Emotional** | **Appearance** |
| Dejected mood or sadness | Stooped posture |
| Decreased life satisfaction | Sad face |
| Loss of interest | Uncooperativeness |
| Impulse to cry | Social withdrawal |
| Irritability | Hostility |
| Emptiness | Suspiciousness |
| Fearfulness and anxiety | Confusion and clouding of |
| Negative feelings toward self | consciousness |
| Worry | Diurnal variations of mood |
| Helplessness | Drooling (in severe cases) |
| Hopelessness | Unkempt appearance (in |
| Sense of failure | severe cases) |
| Loneliness | Occasional ulcerations of |
| Uselessness | skin secondary to picking |
| | Crying or whining |
| **Cognitive** | Occasional ulcerations of |
| Low self-esteem | cornea secondary to |
| Pessimism | decreased blinking |
| Self-blame and criticism | Weight loss |
| Rumination about problems | Bowel impaction |
| Suicidal thoughts | |
| Delusions: | **Psychomotor** |
| Of uselessness | **Retardation** |
| Of unforgivable behavior | Slowed speech |
| Nihilistic | Slowed movements |
| Somatic | Gestures minimized |
| Hallucinations: | Shuffling slow gait |
| Auditory | Mutism (in severe cases) |
| Visual | Cessation of mastication |
| Kinesthetic | and swallowing (in severe |
| Doubt of values and beliefs | cases) |
| Difficulty concentrating | Decreased or inhibited |
| Poor memory | blinking (in severe cases) |
| | |
| **Physical** | **Psychomotor Agitation** |
| Loss of appetite | Continued motor activity |
| Fatigability | Wringing of hands |
| Sleep disturbance: | Picking at skin |
| Initial insomnia | Pacing |
| Terminal insomnia | Restless sleep |
| Frequent awakenings | Grasping others |
| Constipation | |
| Loss of libido | **Bizarre or** |
| Pain | **Inappropriate Behavior** |
| Restlessness | Suicidal gestures or |
| | attempts |
| **Volitional** | Negativism, such as refusal |
| Loss of motivation | to eat or drink and stiff- |
| or "paralysis of will" | ness of the body |
| Suicidal impulses | Outbursts of aggression |
| Desire to withdraw socially | Falling backward |

From Blazer DG: *Depression in late life,* ed 2, St Louis, 1993, Mosby, p. 30.

depression affecting up to 15% of elderly living in the community, and about 30% of the institutionalized elderly (Beers, Berkow, 2000, p. 13).

Most of our knowledge about the etiology and treatment of depression has come from studies conducted on clients experiencing major depression under the care of psychiatrists and/or residing in hospital and nursing home settings (Baldwin, 1995; Caine, Lyness, King, 1993). Little research has been done on people under the care of their primary care provider and/or residing in community settings. Ham and Sloane (1997) state that "depression should be regarded as a communicable disease...if the depression has become persistent and unaddressed, the spouse or other family members may have become depressed themselves or begun to feel hopeless about the situation" (p. 262).

Depression can be difficult to recognize in the elderly. The elderly frequently describe physical rather than emotional manifestations of illness, and as a result, depression often goes undetected by families and health professionals (USDHHS, 1991, p. 26). Confusion or attention problems caused by depression can sometimes look like Alzheimer's disease or other brain disorders. Signs and symptoms of depression in the elderly often do not follow the patterns seen in younger individuals. Depression may occur for no obvious or clear reason.

Depression can result from things such as disability, declining health, physical illness, medications, financial problems, and loneliness. Depression in older people is often related to experiencing losses such as retirement, disability, or death of a spouse or loved one, and an accumulation of such losses can result in major depression. "An important component of depression among older adults may be a perceived lack of control over their lives or their current situation" (Staab, Hodges, 1996, p. 354).

Classic symptoms of depression in elders include anxiety; tiredness and lack of energy; loss of interest in everyday activities; feeling worthless, hopeless, irritable, and/or fearful; overwhelming sadness or grief; sleeping and eating disturbances (including significant weight loss or gain); difficulty concentrating or thinking; recurring thoughts of death or suicide; and aches and pains that do not go away (NIA, 1996). Some of the first symptoms noted are often decreased concentration, mobility, and zest for life, followed by signs of sleep and appetite disturbance, inattention to grooming and daily living tasks, and feelings of hopelessness and isolation (Huysman, 1996). Signs and symptoms of depression and drugs that can cause symptoms of depression are given in Boxes 19-10 and 19-11.

**DEPRESSION: A TREATABLE CONDITION.** Depression is the most treatable of all mental illnesses (NIA, 1996). Elders need to be routinely screened for depression by families, friends, and health care workers. The *Geriatric Depression Scale* (Yesage, Brink, Rose, 1983) has been tested and used extensively with the elder population to screen for depression (Beers, Berkow, 2000; Kurlowicz, 1999). The *Mini-*

**BOX 19-11**

## Drugs That Can Cause Symptoms of Depression

| | | |
|---|---|---|
| **Antihypertensives**<br>Reserpine<br>Methyldopa<br>Propranolol<br>Clonidine<br>Hydralazine<br>Guanethidine<br><br>**Analgesics**<br>**NARCOTIC**<br>　Morphine<br>　Codeine<br>　Meperidine<br>　Pentazocine<br>　Propoxyphene<br><br>**NONNARCOTIC**<br>　Indomethacin | **Antiparkinsonism Drugs**<br>Levodopa<br><br>**Antimicrobials**<br>Sulfonamides<br>Isoniazid<br><br>**Cardiovascular Preparations**<br>Digitalis<br>Diuretics<br>Lidocaine<br><br>**Hypoglycemic Agents**<br>**Psychotropic Agents**<br>**SEDATIVES**<br>　Barbiturates<br>　Benzodiazepines<br>　Meprobamate | **ANTIPSYCHOTICS**<br>　Chlorpromazine<br>　Haloperidol<br>　Thiothixene<br><br>**HYPNOTICS**<br>　Chloral hydrate<br>　Flurazepam<br><br>**Steroids**<br>Corticosteroids<br>Estrogens<br><br>**Other**<br>Cimetidine<br>Cancer chemotherapeutic agents<br>Alcohol |

Source: Kane RL, Ouslander JG, Abrass IB, editors: *Essentials of clinical geriatrics,* New York, 1994, McGraw-Hill; Levenson AJ, Hall RCW, editors: *Neuropsychiatric manifestations of physical disorders in the elderly,* New York, 1981, Raven Press. In Ham RJ, Sloane PD: *Primary care geriatrics: a case-based approach,* ed 3, St Louis, 1997, Mosby, p. 264.

*Mental State Exam* (Folstein, Folstein, McHugh, 1975) is a frequently used mental health and cognition tool that is not specifically for depression, but aids in assessing the mental status of an elder (Beers, Berkow, 2000; Kurlowicz, Wallace, 1999).

Most people who are depressed can be treated successfully on an outpatient basis, and depression in older people typically responds to treatment (NIA, 1996). Many therapies are used to treat depression. Antidepressant drugs can improve mood, sleep, appetite, and concentration; however, it may take 6 to 12 weeks before there are real signs of progress (NIA, 1996).

Hospitalization may be effective in stabilizing depression among the elderly and provides an opportunity to monitor for suicidal tendencies (Huysman, 1996). Exercise and social interactions can be important interventions in affecting mood and relieving depression. Some researchers recommend walking to alleviate depression (McAuliffe, 1994). Unresolved depression can result in serious physical and psychological consequences. A fatal outcome of depression is suicide.

SUICIDE AND DEPRESSION. Depression is one of the most common risk factors for suicide (Beers, Berkow, 2000, p. 310; U.S. Preventive Services Task Force, 1996, p. 541). The highest rates of suicide in the United States occur in people older than 70 years (Beers, Berkow, 2000, p. 310; USDHHS, 2000) and men age 65 and older have the highest rate of suicide in the United States (U.S. Preventive Services Task Force, 1996, p. 547). *Healthy People 2010* ad-

dresses the need to reduce the incidence of suicide in the elderly (USDHHS, 2000).

Important high-risk indicators for suicide include social isolation and loneliness, bereavement, low self-esteem, pain and illness, history of drug or alcohol abuse, history of prior suicide attempts, and a sense of hopelessness. The elderly are less likely than younger people to seek help to prevent suicide and the elderly often succeed at suicide attempts (Beers, Berkow, 2000). Few suicide prevention and intervention programs specifically target older persons, and few professionals are specifically trained in elder suicide prevention and counseling (AARP, 1989).

Health professionals "need to consider how current approaches to suicide prevention can better reflect the special circumstances of older persons" (Meehan, Saltzman, Sattin, 1991, p. 1200). As many as 70% of elderly persons who committed suicide visited their primary care provider within the previous 4 weeks (Beers, Berkow, 2000, p. 311). This gives practitioners a "window of opportunity" to assess, diagnose, and intervene (U.S. Preventive Services Task Force, 1996, p. 548). Another window of opportunity that is frequently overlooked is the "window" through which health care providers can look at "chronic suicide" activities evidenced by elders. Butler (1992) states that chronic suicide involves activities such as refusal to take medication, refusal to eat, and not following elementary safety procedures (e.g., walking out in traffic, falling down stairs). Such activities can result in death by "chronic suicide" (Butler, 1992).

Nurses and other health professionals need to take the suicidal thoughts of elders seriously. If older persons say they are going to kill themselves, they usually mean it and are successful in carrying out the task (Butler, 1992). AARP has published *Elder Suicide: A National Survey of Prevention and Intervention Programs* to increase understanding among the general public about this problem. Nurses need to recognize the clinical symptoms and risk factors for depression, work to prevent depression, and facilitate early diagnosis and treatment.

## Sexuality

"**Sexuality** includes love, warmth, caring, and sharing between people and the identification with a sexual role" (Eliopoulos, 2001, p. 162). Most older people want and are able to enjoy an active, fulfilling sex life (NIA, 1994). Sexual desire persists throughout the life span (Wallace, 2000a, p. 217; Wallace, 2000b) and regular sexual activity helps maintain sexual ability. Sexuality is an important component of the lives of elders, which is often overlooked by health care professionals. The expression of sexuality for elders results in a higher quality of life (Wallace, 2000a). Research by Johnson (1996) found elders to be interested and satisfied with a variety of sexual activities even in the presence of a number of health concerns. The unavailability of a partner, ageism, changes in body image, physical conditions, medications, and cognitive impairments are some of the factors that affect sexual function in later life (Eliopoulos, 2001, pp. 167-169).

Older adults have the need to touch and be touched. This need often goes unmet, especially in elders who have lost a spouse and live alone. When human beings are deprived of touch, the experience can lead to depression, feelings of isolation, and mental health problems. Touch is a way older adults may fulfill their sexuality with each other (Wallace, 2000a, p. 218).

Although sexual desire continues throughout life, physical changes of aging and medical conditions can alter sexual ability and response. Physical changes that come with aging include thinning of the vaginal walls, increasing vaginal dryness, and atrophy of the testes. As a result of physical changes, sexual experiences may differ from those of earlier years but can still be fulfilling and pleasurable. Some questions that the nurse can ask in obtaining a sexual health history from the older adult are given in Box 19-12. Alcohol is a factor that can affect sexual ability. Too much alcohol can reduce potency in men and delay orgasm in women. Certain medications such as antidepressants, tranquilizers, and certain antihypertensive medications can cause impotence.

The nurse can foster sexuality and intimacy with elders, help answer their questions, and assist them in feeling comfortable with fulfilling their sexuality. Nurses can assess normal changes of aging, as well as those caused by medications

**BOX 19-12**

### *Sexual Health History*

Please put a check in the box next to any question you are unsure of how to answer, or that you would like to discuss further with your nurse or physician.

- ❑ 1. Are you currently sexually active?
- ❑ 2. Are you currently active with more than one partner?
- ❑ 3. What kinds of protection do you and your partner use during sexual activity?
- ❑ 4. How has your illness and/or medications affected your sexual activity?
- ❑ 5. Do you have questions or concerns about your sexual activity?
- ❑ 6. Have you ever had a sexually transmitted disease, or knowingly been exposed to somebody with a sexually transmitted disease?
- ❑ 7. Have you ever had, or do you now have, discharge, rashes, or sores in the genital area?
- ❑ 8. Is there anything you would like to discuss concerning sexual issues?

From Letvak S, Schoder D: Sexually transmitted diseases in the elderly: what you need to know, *Geriatr Nurs* 17(4):159, 1996.

and medical conditions, and intervene to prevent or correct sexual problems (Wallace, 2000a, p. 217). The nurse can help educate clients about the normal sexual changes associated with aging and refer clients to additional resources as necessary.

GAY AND LESBIAN AGING. It is estimated that as many as 3.5 million Americans over the age of 60 are lesbian, gay, bisexual, or transgender (LGBT), and these numbers are expected to increase (AoA, 2001g). Older persons who are gay or lesbian are more likely to live alone than other elders, which puts them at higher risk for poor nutrition, depression, and long-term care placement (AoA, 2001g).

Older LGBT persons express concerns about access to high-quality health care, and some are reluctant to reveal their sexual orientation to health care providers because of fear of discrimination and confidentiality not being maintained (AoA, 2001g). Many insurance programs do not recognize same-sex partners for receiving family insurance coverage benefits. Unmarried partners currently are not eligible for spousal or survivor's benefits through federal programs such as Social Security and most private pension plans. Property inheritance by an unmarried partner requires careful estate planning. The disability or death of a partner often adversely affects the financial security of the surviving partner.

There is little research on this population group, and information on their health care needs is scarce. Existing research suggests that older LGBT adults are satisfied with their lives (AoA, 2001g). This research also notes that they face discrimination based on both age and sexual orientation and may not feel comfortable participating in organizations and activities that typically serve older people. Existing studies report that LGBT elders report high levels of satisfaction with their social support networks (AoA, 2001g).

In the past, LGBT partners have not received the community support and assistance that other family caregivers do. For example, a seriously ill lesbian may find that her partner is excluded from making health care and end-of-life decisions. The AoA's *National Family Caregiver Support Program* signed into law in November of 2000 provides assistance to anyone caring for a frail elder, including unrelated individuals. Such legislation is helping protect the rights of LBGT elders. The AoA is working to expand knowledge about health risks that disproportionately affect LGBT Americans.

Some research has indicated that lesbians are more likely than heterosexual women to smoke, be overweight, and abuse alcohol (AoA, 2001g). A major health concern for gay men is human immunodeficiency virus/acquired immunodeficiency syndrome (HIV/AIDS), although this is not the only population group at high risk. It is expected that the number of elders with HIV will increase in the future as drugs, possible vaccines, and technology increase the life span of those with the condition.

## BARRIERS TO HEALTH CARE

Societal attitudes about age and aging are barriers to all care, including health care. These attitudes often inhibit healthy aging, affect resource availability, and have an impact on the care that is given. Other major barriers to health care for the elderly include the *cost* of health services and ability to *access* health services. Health care services are generally costly and may not be covered under private insurance, Medicare, or Medicaid (see Chapter 5). If services are too expensive, the elderly may not use them. The prices of food, medicine, doctors' visits, and gas continually rise, yet many older persons live on a fixed income, making it difficult to afford the health care services they need.

A major access barrier is that of transportation. There is little public transportation in the United States, so the elderly frequently have to rely on friends and family, taxis, Dial-a-Ride, and church or volunteer groups for transportation services. As a result of the Americans with Disabilities Act of 1990, buildings are now becoming more accessible for people who need to use wheelchairs, walkers, and other mobility appliances, but "accessibility" remains a problem. Seniors living in rural areas are especially affected by the problems of transportation and access to service.

## RURAL ELDERLY

Health concerns of people in rural communities is discussed in Chapter 3. In the United States almost one out of four older Americans lives in a rural setting (AARP, AoA, 2001). In many cases the elderly in these rural towns are the "oldest-old," those 85 and older. The rural elderly have a greater incidence of chronic health problems than elderly living in metropolitan areas (Growing old, 1993). Minority rural elders have poorer health than other rural elders. The health promotion needs of the rural elderly are extensive.

The elderly in rural America are often isolated from access to health care services and have inadequate health care. Rural hospitals continue to close at an alarming rate. Many rural areas have a shortage of health care professionals. Studies have shown that rural areas have almost 44% fewer physicians than metropolitan areas (Where doctors are few and far between, 1993).

Numerous organizations are working to address the health care needs of the nation's rural elders. NCOA's *National Center on Rural Aging* (NCRA) works to increase service provision to the rural elderly. The *National Resource Center for Rural Elderly* (University of Missouri, Kansas City, Missouri) focuses on service provision, housing, and health care for the elderly and serves as an information clearinghouse. Elders who are members of AARP can obtain prescribed medications at a reduced cost by mail if there is no drugstore in their community. Community health nurses need to help link rural elders to such organizations and services and advocate for further services.

## SIGNIFICANT LEGISLATION

Two extremely significant pieces of legislation for the elderly are the Social Security Act of 1935 and the Older Americans Act of 1965. Other pieces of legislation also have affected senior health and quality of life.

### Older Americans Act

The **Older Americans Act** (OAA) evolved over a period that spanned 15 years and 4 presidential administrations (Wallace, McGuire, Lee, et al., 1999). Under President Lyndon B. Johnson, Congress passed the act in 1965. It was the first legislation in the United States with the mission of organizing and delivering services to senior citizens and remains the only piece of legislation focusing on the needs of this population group.

The act authorized the Administration on Aging within the Department of Health and Human Services; authorized grants to states for community planning and services programs, and funded research and training in gerontology. It proposed broad, comprehensive goals to improve the quality of life for older Americans. These goals are displayed in Box 19-13.

### BOX 19-13
*Goals of the Older Americans Act*

The Older Americans Act was designed to help elders achieve the following goals:
- An adequate retirement income
- The best possible physical and mental health available
- Suitable, affordable housing
- Necessary restorative services
- Employment without age discrimination
- Retirement in health, honor, and dignity
- Meaningful activity within the widest range of civic, cultural, and recreational opportunities
- Provision of efficient and coordinated community services
- Benefits from research knowledge that can sustain and improve health and quality of life
- Freedom, independence, and the free exercise of individual initiative in planning and managing their own lives

### BOX 19-14
*Some Services and Programs Under the Older Americans Act*

- Senior centers
- National Family Caregiver Support Program
- Retired Senior Volunteer Program (RSVP)
- Foster grandparents
- Nutrition Services Incentive Program
- Congregate meals
- Home-delivered meals
- Home care services
- Health education
- Elder Abuse Prevention Program
- Ombudsman Program
- Caregiver support services
- Legal assistance programs
- Senior information and referral services

Over the years the act has been amended to include the establishment of Area Agencies on Aging, multipurpose senior centers (discussed later in this chapter), senior nutrition programs, senior employment and volunteer programs, health promotion and disease prevention activities, and in-home services for elders. Examples of services and programs provided for under the act are given in Box 19-14. The act remains a major piece of legislation relating to services for older Americans. It was reauthorized by President Bill Clinton in 2000 (P.L. 106-501). The reauthorization extends the Act's programs through fiscal year 2005. The reauthorized act contains an important new program, the *National Family Caregiver Support Program*, which helps families caring for frail elder members. The reauthorized act also made provisions for services for grandparents who are caregivers of grandchildren and other older individuals who are relative caregivers of children under the age of 18. Also, new provisions require that state plans show efforts to coordinate services with agencies and organizations that provide multigenerational activities and programs. Appendix 19-3 presents some amendments to the act.

### Social Security Act

The Social Security Act of 1935 is discussed in Chapters 4 and 5. This act mandates many programs that serve elderly people including Old Age, Survivors and Disability Insurance (OASDI), Supplemental Security Income (SSI), and the health programs of Medicare and Medicaid. Information on these programs is readily available at local branches of the federal Social Security Administration and at the administration's website (*http://www.ssa.gov*).

### Other Legislation

Several other pieces of legislation have helped improve the quality of life for the elderly. Examples of this legislation include the *Age Discrimination in Employment Act of*

1967, which prevented age discrimination in employment and protected workers from forced retirement; the *Rehabilitation Act of 1973*, which provided for rehabilitation services to Americans; the *Research on Aging Act of 1974*, which created the National Institute of Aging in the National Institutes of Health; and the *Americans with Disabilities Act of 1990*, which assured the rights of Americans with disabilities. These pieces of legislation have helped provide important resources and services to older Americans.

## SOME GOVERNMENT RESOURCES FOR ELDERS

Many resources for older Americans are available in both the public and private sectors. Public-sector resources are supported by tax dollars and exist on federal, state, and local levels. Numerous agencies exist within federal, state, and local government to provide services to elders. The U.S. Department of Health and Human Services (USDHHS) and the Social Security Administration are major federal agencies involved in providing services to older people. Within the USDHHS agencies that provide extensive services to elders are the Administration on Aging and the National Institute on Aging.

### Social Security Administration

In 1936 the Social Security Administration (SSA) (*http://www.ssa.gov*) started operations in a converted Coca-Cola bottling factory on the harbor in downtown Baltimore, Maryland (Social Security Administration, 2001). Today it is a freestanding agency of the federal government with its own headquarters in the Baltimore suburbs. The administration is discussed in Chapter 5. Its website has extensive information including how to apply

**National Aging Services Network**

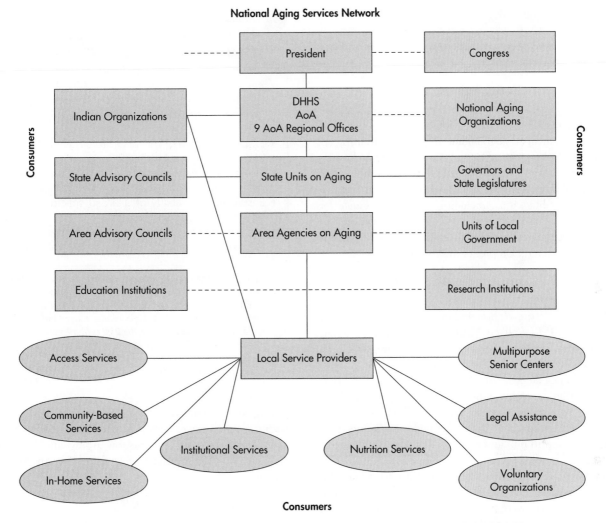

**FIGURE 19-9** National Aging Services Network. (From Administration on Aging [AoA]: *National Aging Services Network Organizational Chart.* Retrieved from the internet March 2001. *http://www.aoa.dhhs.gov/aoa/pages/orgchart-med2.gif*)

for benefits, policy papers, social security statistics, and information on publications.

The SSA administers the Social Security Act programs of Old Age, Survivors and Disability Insurance ("Social Security") and Supplemental Security Income (SSI) that are used extensively by senior citizens. SSA branch offices are located in communities across the country and are found in the local telephone directory under federal government listings.

## Administration on Aging

Amendments to the Older Americans Act created the **Administration on Aging (AoA)** (*http://www.aoa.gov*). The AoA provides leadership in the federal government for the provision of supportive home and community-based services, promotes activities to meet the needs of older adults and their caregivers, and assists in protecting the rights of vulnerable and at-risk elders (AoA, 2000k). The adminis-

tration leads a national aging network of 57 State Units on Aging and 655 Area Agencies on Aging (Figure 19-9).

Its *National Aging Information Center* (NAIC) offers information, searchable databases, publications, and statistical resources on aging. The *Eldercare Locator* (1-800-677-1116) is an AoA service that helps link people in every community in the country with community resources for elders. The Eldercare Locator has information on home and community-based care services (e.g., meal delivery, transportation and chore services), housing options, community senior centers, adult day care and respite care, financial and legal services, and specialized services for older individuals with conditions such as Alzheimer's disease. The AoA's *Long Term Care Ombudsman Program* is an elder rights protection service that investigates and resolves complaints about nursing homes, board and care homes, and adult care homes. The administration publishes *Aging* magazine and each year during the month of May sponsors *Older Ameri-*

cans Month. During Older Americans Month communities across the country honor older Americans with activities and events. The AoA offers numerous publications and fact sheets on aging-related topics.

## National Institute on Aging

The National Institute on Aging (1-800-222-2225) (*http://www.nia.nih.gov*) was established to conduct and support biomedical and behavioral research and training related to the aging process. Its purpose is to increase knowledge about aging and the associated physical, psychological, and social factors resulting from advanced age. It has numerous free publications, including *A Resource Guide for Older Americans* and *AgePages*. AgePages are usually one- to two-page documents that present easily understandable information on different topics of interest to elders.

## White House Conferences on Aging

Forerunners to the White House Conferences on Aging (WHCoA) were the National Conferences on Aging held in 1950 and 1952 (Wallace, McGuire, Lee, Sauter, 1999). In 1961 the first White House Conference on Aging was held. At this conference it was recommended that a federal coordinating agency be established in the field of aging and that federal legislation on aging needed to be enacted (Wallace, McGuire, Lee, Sauter, 1999). The 1961 WHCoA conference document, *Education and Aging*, endorsed the need for aging education in public schools, higher education institutions, and libraries (McGuire, 1987; USDHEW, 1961). The 1961 conference was a major impetus to the passage of the Older Americans Act in 1965 and the formation of the AoA. Conferences were planned to be held every 10 years, with the next conference scheduled for 1971.

In 1971 the second WHCoA was held, and the conference document, *Toward a National Policy on Aging*, focused on the need to develop national policy on aging and reinforced the need for aging education throughout life (USDHEW, 1971). A third WHCoA conference was held in 1981 and the fourth, the last of the twentieth century, was held in 1995. Many in the field of aging viewed the prolonged gap between the 1981 and 1995 conferences to indicate a lack of interest on the federal level in maintaining and expanding services to elders. Resolutions that came from the 1995 conference are given in Box 19-15. A fifth WHCoA is scheduled to be held by December 31, 2005. These conferences help increase public awareness of the needs and concerns of older Americans and lay the groundwork for providing essential resources and services.

## Action

This agency is an independent federal organization that administers volunteer programs. Its purpose is to mobilize Americans for voluntary service throughout the United States through programs that help meet basic human needs and support self-help efforts of low-income families and im-

## BOX 19-15

### *Resolutions of the White House Conference on Aging 1995*

- Keep Social Security sound now and for the future
- Preserve the integrity of the Older Americans Act
- Preserve the nature of Medicaid
- Reauthorize the Older Americans Act
- Ensure the future of the Medicare program
- Increase funding for Alzheimer's research
- Preserve advocacy functions under the Older Americans Act
- Ensure the availability of a broad spectrum of elder services
- Finance and provide long-term care services
- Acknowledge the contributions of older volunteers

Sources: US Department of Health and Human Services (USDHHS): *1995 White House Conference on Aging: adopted resolutions,* Washington, DC, 1996a, US Government Printing Office; US Department of Health and Human Services (USDHHS): *1995 White House Conference on Aging. The road to an aging policy for the 21st century: executive summary,* Washington, DC, 1996b, US Government Printing Office; Wallace D, McGuire SL, Lee HT, et al.: Older Americans Act: implications for nursing, *Nurs Outlook* 47:181-185, 1999.

poverished communities. ACTION sponsors *Foster Grandparents, Retired Senior Volunteers Program (RSVP),* and *Senior Companions.* State Units on Aging and local Area Agencies on Aging often have information on ACTION programs.

## Other Federal Agencies

Numerous other federal agencies provide assistance to the elderly. The *Department of Agriculture* offers many food and nutrition programs. The *Department of Housing and Urban Development* subsidizes low-cost public housing for the elderly. The *Department of the Treasury* offers assistance with income tax problems and filing taxes through the Internal Revenue Service. The *Department of Labor* enforces the Age Discrimination in Employment Act. The *Department of the Interior* issues Gold Age Passports (free) and Golden Eagle Passports (low-cost) to seniors for the federal park system. The *Department of Transportation* underwrites funding to assist in providing mass transportation that services the elderly. The *Department of Defense* offers programs for retired veterans, often through Veterans Administration hospitals.

## State and Local Agencies on Aging

The Older Americans Act of 1965 provides funding to states to establish State Units on Aging and local Area Agencies on Aging. These agencies plan and coordinate programs for older Americans (see Appendix 19-3). Area Agencies on Aging are active in service provision to local communities. Figure 19-9 illustrates how these agencies fit into the national aging network.

**BOX 19-16**

*Senior Centers*

Senior centers receive funding through the Older Americans Act and are located in communities across the country. They play a vital role in service provision to older Americans and their families. These centers provide services that help older Americans remain independent and active in their communities. Some of the services provided at senior centers include the following:

- Meal and nutrition programs
- Information and assistance
- Health, fitness, and wellness programs
- Recreational opportunities
- Transportation services
- Arts programs
- Volunteer opportunities
- Educational opportunities
- Employment assistance
- Intergenerational programs
- Social opportunities

Source: Administration on Aging (AoA): *Fact sheet. Senior centers*, Washington, DC, 2001h, The Administration.

## Senior Centers

The first **senior center** was the William Hodson Senior Center established by the New York City Department of Welfare in 1943 (The first half-century, 1993). Today, the nation has more than 12,000 senior centers that serve millions of older Americans each year. The Older Americans Act helps provide funding for the centers. Senior centers routinely provide social, recreational, educational, and nutritional services. Some centers offer health care screening. Senior centers are a hub of activity for elders in the community and provide valuable services. Information about these centers can often be found under local government listings in the phone book. Some services provided through senior centers are given in Box 19-16.

## SOME PRIVATE RESOURCES FOR ELDERS

Private/voluntary resources for elders are numerous and vary from community to community. On a national level two private, voluntary agencies that work actively for the elderly are the **National Council on the Aging (NCOA)** and the **American Association for Retired Persons (AARP).** These two groups, along with groups such as Generations United (*http://www.gu.org*), the National Academy for Teaching and Learning About Aging (*http://www.unt.edu/natla*), Generations Together (*http://www.gt.pitt.edu*), and the Gray Panthers (*http://www.graypanthers.org*) provide many valuable resources and services to elders, their families, and the community. Nursing organizations are discussed later in the chapter.

Local communities have numerous resources targeted at service provision to elders. Each year in May communities across the nation highlight activities for seniors as a part of *Older Americans Month.* Community resources include church-sponsored activities, adult day care programs, care management agencies, family service agencies, geriatric counselors, health care professionals, and caregiver support groups. The nurse needs to be aware of resources and services for the elderly in the community and be an advocate for service provision.

### Stop and Think About It

What are some of the resources and services for elders in your community? What are the services offered by your local Senior Center? What does your community do to celebrate Older Americans Month? How could nurses be involved in expanding the scope of services available to seniors in local communities?

### National Council on the Aging (NCOA)

Established in 1950, the NCOA (*http://www.ncoa.org*) is a private, nonprofit organization that serves as a national resource for information and consultation and sponsors publications, special programs, advocacy activities, research, and training to meet older persons' needs and improve their lives. NCOA forms cooperative relationships with government and private agencies to educate the public and professionals about the aged and to provide services to the aged.

In 1987 NCOA and the Child Welfare League of America cofounded *Generations United*, a coalition of more than 100 national organizations dedicated to linking the needs and resources of generations. Generations United focuses on themes and programs that help bring young and old together. Such affiliations have been successful in developing programs such as the Senior Center/Latchkey program that links seniors with young children who are home alone after school.

### American Association of Retired Persons (AARP)

The AARP (*http://www.aarp.org*) was established in 1958 by Dr. Ethel Percy Andrus, founder of the National Retired Teachers Association. AARP today has over 30 million members across the United States in almost 4000 local chapters and is the largest nonprofit, nonpartisan membership organization in the world. The purposes of AARP are to enhance the quality of life for older persons; promote independence, dignity, and purpose for older persons; provide leadership in determining the role of older persons in society; and improve the image of aging. Membership in the group is limited to those age 50 years and older.

AARP publishes a bimonthly magazine, *Modern Maturity*, that offers retirement advice, travel ideas, and health tips, and also publishes the monthly *AARP News Bulletin*. It sponsors a tax assistance program to help older taxpayers, provides leadership in legislative issues, and is an advocate for the elderly.

## INTERNET RESOURCES

Internet resources are mentioned separately to make note of the abundance of resource information available for elders at these sites. The nurse can be helpful in assisting elders select sites for health information and in evaluating the quality of the information available.

To help seniors become more proficient at using computer resources, the federal government has provided funding for computer classes to be taught at low or no-cost to seniors at senior centers around the country. Many universities and junior colleges offer courses at low or no-cost to seniors, and many seniors are using this opportunity to learn about computers. Local communities are using volunteers to help link homebound elders with computer resources. Internet resources help link seniors to many valuable resources and services. Various websites have been listed throughout this chapter.

## THE NURSING ROLE

Community health nurses have unique opportunities to facilitate healthy aging. For example, they can implement aging education programs in schools, teach elderly clients about available resources in the community, work with area agencies on aging to enhance service provision to the elderly (e.g., senior centers, local offices on aging, senior apartments), provide direct nursing care, and develop creative learning opportunities and programs. Innovative nurses have developed nurse-run clinics for senior citizens that provide essential health services; developed and implemented aging education programs; and participated in community planning activities for the elderly. Nurse-managed centers for older adults can provide quality, comprehensive care and can be a vital part of the plan to help meet the health needs of the rapidly expanding elderly population.

As early as 1925 an editorial in the *American Journal of Nursing* alerted nurses to the increasing need to prepare for care of the elderly (Editorial, 1925). This editorial was well ahead of its time, and the number of elders has continued to rise. The role of the nurse in working with the elderly client has been discussed throughout this chapter in reference to healthy aging, health promotion, and concerns of the elderly.

Gerontological nursing involves assessing the health and functional status of elders; planning, providing, and coordinating appropriate nursing and health care services; and evaluating the effectiveness of care (ANA, 1995, p. 7). The nurse works to maximize the elder's functional ability in ADLs, strives to identify and build on elder strengths, and assists the client in maintaining independence (ANA, 1995, p. 7). The nurse often assumes the role of advocate for the elderly client and helps link the client to community resources.

Graduates of nursing programs are entering practice where the majority of clients are over age 65 and many are the oldest old. No matter what the setting, nurses will find themselves working with elders. Even in pediatrician offices the nurse can find him or herself working with grandparents or seniors who are providing care to children. Nurses need to evaluate their own attitudes about aging, understand the aging process, be familiar with public policy and economics on aging, and encourage elders to take part in health promotion activities. Nurses need to be knowledgeable of community resources and help link elders to them.

The ANA established certification of gerontological nurses in 1973, and the ANA's Council on Gerontological Nursing has been involved in many important gerontological nursing initiatives. The National League for Nursing is committed to the improvement of education and practice in gerontological nursing. Unfortunately, education in gerontology is frequently lacking in the educational programs of nurses and other health care professionals. Recently, the Hartford Institute for Geriatric Nursing, discussed later in this chapter, is championing the quest to integrate gerontological nursing content into nursing education.

No health profession has claimed service to the elderly as its unique task, leaving open a window of opportunity for nurses to step forward and assume primary responsibility for providing comprehensive health care to the elderly. Nurses need to remain integrally involved in the provision of quality care to elders.

### Standards of Practice

The ANA's (1995) *Scope and Standards of Gerontological Nursing Practice* are presented in Box 19-17. These standards address the application of the nursing process to gerontological nursing, interdisciplinary collaboration, the integration of theory and research in practice, and professional performance. The standards guide gerontological nursing practice.

### Levels of Prevention

Getting older people to take part in health promotion activities can be a challenging but rewarding experience. The nurse can help the elderly client to see that "an ounce of prevention is worth a pound of cure." Nurses can assist people in taking responsibility for maintaining their health and promoting healthy aging.

When implementing health promotion and wellness activities for the elderly client, community health nurses emphasize *primary prevention interventions*. Such activities have the potential to facilitate wellness, reduce premature death and disability, maintain health and functional independence of older adults, and improve the overall quality of life.

Primary prevention is integrally linked with health promotion and wellness. A goal of primary prevention activities is to help the elderly maintain physical functioning and independence as long as possible (USDHHS, 1991; USDHHS, 2000). Wellness programs for seniors are often located in local senior centers, churches, and fitness organizations.

**BOX 19-17**

*Scope and Standards of Gerontological Nursing Practice*

## Standards of Clinical Gerontological Nursing Care

### STANDARD I. ASSESSMENT

**The gerontological nurse collects patient health data.**
Information obtained from older adults, families, significant others, and the interdisciplinary team and nursing knowledge is used to develop the comprehensive plan of care. These assessments must always be culturally and ethnically appropriate.

### STANDARD II. DIAGNOSIS

**The gerontological nurse analyzes the assessment data in determining diagnoses.**
The gerontological nurse, either independently or in collaboration with interdisciplinary care providers, evaluates health assessment data to develop comprehensive diagnoses that guide interventions.

### STANDARD III. OUTCOME IDENTIFICATION

**The gerontological nurse identifies expected outcomes individualized to the older adult.**
The ultimate goals of providing gerontological nursing care are to influence health outcomes and improve or maintain the health status of the older adult. Outcomes often focus on maximizing the state of well-being, functional status, and quality of life.

### STANDARD IV. PLANNING

**The gerontological nurse develops a plan of care that prescribes interventions to attain expected outcomes.**
A plan of care is used to structure and guide therapeutic interventions and achieve expected outcomes. It is developed in conjunction with the older adult, significant others, and interdisciplinary team members.

### STANDARD V. IMPLEMENTATION

**The gerontological nurse implements the interventions identified in the plan of care.**
The gerontological nurse uses a wide range of culturally competent interventions including health promotion, health maintenance, prevention of illness, health restoration, rehabilitation, and palliation. The gerontological nurse implements the plan of care in collaboration with the older adult and others.

### STANDARD VI. EVALUATION

**The gerontological nurse evaluates the older adult's progress toward attainment of expected outcomes.**
Nursing practice is dynamic and evolving. The gerontological nurse continually evaluates the older adult's responses to treatment and interventions. Collection of new data, revision of the database, alteration of diagnoses, and modification of the plan of care are essential.

## Standards of Professional Gerontological Nursing Performance

### STANDARD I. QUALITY OF CARE

**The gerontological nurse systematically evaluates the quality of care and effectiveness of nursing practice.**
The dynamic nature and growing body of gerontological knowledge and research provide both the impetus and the means for gerontological nurses to improve the quality of patient care.

### STANDARD II. PERFORMANCE APPRAISAL

**The gerontological nurse evaluates his or her own nursing practice in relation to professional practice standards and relevant statutes and regulations.**
The gerontological nurse is accountable to the public for providing competent clinical care and has an inherent responsibility to practice according to standards established by the professional and regulatory bodies.

### STANDARD III. EDUCATION

**The gerontological nurse acquires and maintains current knowledge applicable to nursing practice.**
Scientific, cultural, societal, and political changes require a continuing commitment from the gerontological nurse to pursue knowledge to maintain competency, enhance nursing expertise, and advance the profession. Formal education, continuing education, certification, and experiential learning are some of the means for professional growth.

### STANDARD IV. COLLEGIALITY

**The gerontological nurse contributes to the professional development of peers, colleagues, and others.**
The gerontological nurse is responsible for sharing knowledge, research, and clinical information with colleagues and others through formal and informal teaching methods and collaborative educational programs.

### STANDARD V. ETHICS

**The gerontological nurse's decisions and actions on behalf of older adults are determined in an ethical manner.**
The gerontological nurse is responsible for providing nursing services and health care that are responsive to the public's trust and the older adult's rights. Formal and informal care providers must also be prepared to provide the care needed and desired by the older adult and to render services in an appropriate setting.

From American Nurses Association: *Scope and standards of gerontological nursing practice,* ed 2, Washington, DC, 2001, American Nurses Publishing.

*Continued*

**BOX 19-17**

*Scope and Standards of Gerontological Nursing Practice—cont'd*

**STANDARD VI. COLLABORATION**

**The gerontological nurse collaborates with the older adult, the older adult's caregivers, and all members of the interdisciplinary team to provide comprehensive care.**

The complex nature of comprehensive care for older adults and their caregivers requires expertise from all members of the interdisciplinary team. Collaboration between health care consumers and providers is optimal for planning, implementing, and evaluating care. Communication among members of the interdisciplinary team provides a forum to evaluate the effectiveness of the plan of care and to utilize appropriate resources to achieve identified goals.

**STANDARD VII. RESEARCH**

**The gerontological nurse interprets, applies, and evaluates research findings to inform and improve gerontological nursing practice.**

Gerontological nurses are responsible for improving current nursing practice and future health care for older adults by participating in the generation, testing, utilization, and evaluation of research findings. At the basic level of practice, the gerontological nurse participates in research studies, identifies clinical problems, and interprets and utilizes research findings to improve clinical care to older adults. At the advanced practice level, the gerontological nurse may be a full research participant in the generation, testing, utilization, critical evaluation, and dissemination of knowledge related to gerontological health care research.

**STANDARD VIII. RESOURCE UTILIZATION**

**The gerontological nurse considers factors related to safety, effectiveness, and cost in planning and delivering patient care.**

The older adult is entitled to health care that is safe, ethical, effective, acceptable, and affordable. Treatment decisions consider quality of care and appropriate utilization of resources.

From American Nurses Association: *Scope and standards of gerontological nursing practice,* ed 2, Washington, DC, 2001, American Nurses Publishing.

Examples of primary prevention interventions include health education measures in relation to the normal changes of aging; need for preventive medical care (e.g. regular physical examinations, receiving immunizations for pneumonia and influenza); proper exercise, nutrition, and oral health; safety measures; and health assessment. These activities also include anticipatory guidance that can help prepare the individual and family for significant life changes such as retirement. Predisposition to conditions such as coronary artery disease can be altered with a preventive program of exercise, good nutrition, avoidance of smoking, and protection from stress.

*Secondary prevention* activities involve early diagnosis and treatment, including encouraging and facilitating regular medical and dental care and periodic screening for conditions (e.g., hypertension and diabetes); encouraging adherence to medical treatment regimens; carrying out self-monitoring activities such as breast and testicular self-examinations; and assessing for the warning signs of cancer. *Tertiary prevention* involves rehabilitative and restorative activities and includes physical, occupational, recreational, and speech therapy and adjusting to activities of daily living in relation to changing levels of functioning.

## Nursing Organizations

The American Nurses Association (ANA) (*http://www.ana.org*), National League for Nursing (NLN) (*http://www.nln.org*), National Gerontological Nursing Association (NGNA) (*http://www.ngna.org*), and the **National Conference of Gerontological Nurse Practitioners (NCGNP)** (*http://www.ncgnp.org*) have all contributed to advancing the practice of geriatric nursing. As previously mentioned the ANA publishes standards of gerontological nursing practice. ANA offers certification in gerontological nursing through it its American Nurses Credentialing Center (ANCC). The NGNA is the specialty organization for nurses in the field of geriatrics, and the NCGNP is the specialty organization for gerontological nurse practitioners.

A relatively new group, the **Hartford Institute for Geriatric Nursing** (*http://www.hartfordign.org*) was founded at New York University in 1996 to create a major national movement to improve health care for older adults by helping to train nurses in the care of older adults. The Institute was funded with a grant from the Hartford Foundation and offers a wide range of activities and publications in education, practice, research, public policy, and consumer education. The Institute publishes a *Best Practice Curriculum Guide* to be used to integrate geriatric nursing concepts into undergraduate nursing content and the *Try This* series in which topics of interest in geriatrics are presented in a user-friendly clinically based format. A visit to the Institute's website provides an abundance of information on gerontological nursing.

## Advanced Practice Nursing Roles

The advanced practice gerontological nurse holds a master's degree in nursing, with a concentration in gerontological nursing and a mandatory number of hours in advanced clinical placement. Advanced practice nurses can be gerontological nurse practitioners (GNP) or clinical nurses specialists (CNS). Certification is available to these nurses through the ANCC.

A GNP is an expert in providing primary health care to older adults in a variety of settings. Practicing independently and collaboratively with other health care professionals, the GNP works to maximize the person's functional abilities; promotes, maintains, and restores health; and prevents or minimizes disabilities (ANCC, 2000a). GNPs take part in advanced practice, case management, education, consultation, research, administration, and advocacy for older adults (ANCC, 2000a).

Clinical nurse specialists in gerontology are experts in providing, directing, and influencing the care of older adults and their families and significant others in a variety of settings and demonstrate an in-depth understanding of the dynamics of aging, as well as the interventions necessary for health promotion and management of health status alterations (ANCC, 2000b).

Such programs are scattered throughout the nation, and nurses graduating from such programs fall under each state's nurse practice acts for their scope of practice. There is presently a shortage of advanced practice gerontological nurses, and it is hoped more nurses will pursue these advanced practice roles.

## SUMMARY

Aging is a universal phenomena—everyone is aging. The expected growth of the population over 65 signals an expanding nursing role and opportunity to work with older people. Most nurses will spend a large part of their professional practice providing care for elders. Nurses need to be educated to provide such care. Challenging and enriching opportunities exist for nurses in the area of geriatrics.

Nurses need to promote positive attitudes about aging, be educated about aging, and be familiar with the aging process. Nursing efforts need to focus on health promotion and disease prevention and facilitate wellness and healthy aging. Unfortunately, our society's ageist attitudes often become self-fulfilling prophecies in old age and inhibit healthy aging. Nurses need to be aware of their own attitudes about aging and how these attitudes affect nursing care and caring.

*Healthy People 2010* has addressed health needs of the elderly and established numerous national health objectives related to elder health. Nurses frequently need to be aware of national elder health objectives and initiatives, the physiological changes of aging, public and social policy on aging, and community resources and services. Nurses are advocates for elder health and work to minimize barriers to care such as societal attitudes, inadequate resources and services, and problems of accessibility.

Nursing has the opportunity to be the leader in the delivery of health care services to the elderly. Planning and implementing policy for the elderly client is a significant challenge for community health nurses. It is important to remember that the elderly person is a unique individual with unique health care needs.

## CRITICAL THINKING
*exercise*

After reading this chapter you are aware of the *Healthy People 2010* national health objectives for older people and numerous needs, resources, and services in relation to the elderly client. What do you see as the greatest major health care concern for today's older Americans? What can nurses in your community do to help meet this health care need?

## REFERENCES

Administration on Aging (AoA): *AoA's response to global aging*, Washington, DC, 2000a, AoA.

Administration on Aging (AoA): *Life course planning*, Washington, DC, 2000b, AoA.

Administration on Aging (AoA): *A diverse aging population: working towards a healthier, longer life*, Washington, DC, 2000c, AoA.

Administration on Aging (AoA): *The growth of America's older population*, Washington, DC, 2000d, AoA.

Administration on Aging (AoA): *Employment and the older worker*, Washington, DC, 2000e, AoA.

Administration on Aging (AoA): *Pension and benefits counseling*, Washington, DC, 2000f, AoA.

Administration on Aging (AoA): *Housing options for older Americans*, Washington, DC, 2000g, AoA.

Administration on Aging (AoA): *Longevity and the power of a healthy lifestyle*, Washington, DC, 2000h, AoA.

Administration on Aging (AoA): *Good nutrition! Essential for health!* Washington, DC, 2000i, AoA.

Administration on Aging (AoA): *Elder abuse prevention*, Washington, DC, 2000j, AoA.

Administration on Aging (AoA): *AoA on Aging*, Washington, DC, 2000k, AoA.

Administration on Aging (AoA): *Fact sheet: cultural competency*, Washington, DC, 2001a, AoA.

Administration on Aging (AoA): *Fact sheet: serving our African American elders*, Washington, DC, 2001b, AoA.

Administration on Aging (AoA): *Fact sheet: serving our Hispanic American elders*, Washington, DC, 2001c, AoA.

Administration on Aging (AoA): *Fact sheet: caregiver diversity*, Washington, DC, 2001d, AoA.

Administration on Aging (AoA): *Fact sheet: American Indian, Alaska native and native Hawaiian program*, Washington, DC, 2001e, AoA.

Administration on Aging (AoA): *Fact sheet: serving our Asian American and Pacific Islander elders*, Washington, DC, 2001f, AoA.

Administration on Aging (AoA): *Lesbian, gay, bisexual, and transgender older persons*, Washington, DC, 2001g, AoA.

Administration on Aging (AoA): *Fact sheet: senior centers*, Washington, DC, 2001h, AoA.

Administration on Aging (AoA): *National aging services network organizational chart*. Retrieved from the internet March 2001. *http://www.aoa.dhhs.gov/aoa/pages/orgchart-med2.gif*

American Association of Retired Persons (AARP): *Truth about aging: guidelines for accurate communications*, Washington, DC, 1984, AARP.

American Association of Retired Persons (AARP): *Elder suicide: a national survey of prevention and intervention programs*, Washington, DC, 1989, AARP.

American Association of Retired Persons (AARP): *Healthy older adults*, Washington, DC, 1991, AARP.

American Association of Retired Persons (AARP): *A profile of older Americans 1995*, Washington, DC, 1996, AARP.

American Association of Retired Persons (AARP), Administration on Aging (AoA): *A profile of older Americans 2000*, Washington, DC, 2001, AARP/AoA.

American Nurses Association (ANA): *Scope and standards of gerontological nursing practice*, Washington, DC, 1995, ANA.

American Nurses Credentialing Center (ANCC): *Computer-based testing for ANCC board certification. Nurse practitioners and informatics nurse*, Washington, DC, 2000a, ANCC.

American Nurses Credentialing Center (ANCC): *ANCC board certification. Clinical nurse specialist, nursing administration, generalist, and modular exams*, Washington, DC, 2000b, ANCC.

Annual checkups—who needs them, *Aging* 365:2-3, 1993.

Baldwin RC: Antidepressants in geriatric depression: what difference have they made? *Int Psychogeriatrics* 7(Suppl):55-68, 1995.

Beers, MH, Berkow MD: *The Merck manual of geriatrics*, ed 3, Whitehouse Station, NJ, 2000, Merck Research Laboratories.

Blazer DG: *Depression in late life*, ed 2, St Louis, 1993, Mosby.

Bronte L: *The longevity factor: the new reality of long careers and how it can lead to richer lives*, New York, 1993, Harper Collins.

Butler R: *Treatment of the aged*, Network for Continuing Medical Education, Continuing Medical Education Series, Video #629, 1992.

Caine ED, Lyness MM, King DA: Reconsidering depression in the elderly, *Am J Geriatric Psychiatry* 1:4-20, 1993.

Campbell JC, Harris MJ, Lee RK: Violence research: an overview, *Scholar Inq Nurs Pract* 9(2):105-126, 1995.

Castillo HM: *The nurse assistant in long-term care: a rehabilitative approach*, St Louis, 1992, Mosby.

Comfort A: *Say yes to old age: developing a positive attitude toward aging*, New York, 1990, Crown.

Cornelius LJ: Limited choices for medical care among minority populations. In Hogue CJR, Hargraves MA, Collins KS, editors: *Minority health in America: findings and policy implications from the Commonwealth Fund Minority Health Survey*, Baltimore, 2000, Johns Hopkins University Press.

Drayton-Hargrove S: Assessing abuse of disabled older adults: a family systems approach, *Rehabil Nurs* 25(4):136-140, 2000.

Dychtwald K: *AgeWave*, New York, 1990, Bantam Books.

Editorial, *Am J Nurs* 25(5):394, 1925.

Eliopoulos C: *Gerontological nursing*, ed 5, Philadelphia, 2001, Lippincott.

Erikson EH: *The life cycle completed: a review*, New York, 1982, Norton.

Farmer BC: *Try this: best practices in nursing care to older adults, Fall risk assessment*, 2(1), New York, May 2000, Hartford Institute for Geriatric Nursing.

Ferrar R: Bill aims to lower seniors' drug cost, *Knoxville-News Sentinel*, March 9, 2001, A1, A3.

The first half-century of senior centers charts the way for decades to come, *Perspect Aging* 22(2):2-6, 1993.

Folstein ME, Folstein SE, McHugh PR: Mini-mental state: a practical method for grading the cognitive state of patients for the clinician, *J Psych Research* 12:189-198, 1975.

Franke N, Ohene-Frempong J: Health care for African-Americans: availability, accessibility, and usability. In Ma GX, Henderson G, editors: *Rethinking ethnicity and health care: a sociocultural perspective*, Springfield, Ill, 1999, Charles C. Thomas.

Greely A: *Nutrition and the elderly*, Pub No (FDA) 91-2243, Washington, DC, 1991, US Department of Health and Human Services.

Growing old in rural America: new approach needed in rural health care, *Aging* 365:18-25, 1993.

Guendelman S, Wagner T: Hispanics' experience with the health care system: access, utilization and satisfaction. In Hogue CJR, Hargraves MA, Collins KS, editors: *Minority health in America: findings and policy implications from the Commonwealth Fund Minority Health Survey*, Baltimore, 2000, The John Hopkins University Press.

Ham RJ, Sloane PD: *Primary care geriatrics: a case-based approach*, ed 3, St Louis, 1997, Mosby.

Ham RJ, Sloane PD: *Primary care geriatrics: a case-based approach*, ed 4, St Louis, 2001, Mosby.

Harris DK: *Sociology of aging*, ed 2, New York, 1990, Harper & Row.

Hogstel MO: *Gerontology. Nursing care of the older adult*, Albany, NY, 2001, Delmar.

Huysman AM: Depression in older people and its implications in health care, *Topics in Geriatric Rehab* 11(4):16-24, 1996.

Johnson BK: Older adults and sexuality: a multidimensional perspective, *J Gerontol Nurs* 22(2):6-15, 1996.

Johnson JF: Pharmacologic management, In Lueckenotte AG: *Gerontologic nursing*, ed 2, St Louis, 2000, Mosby.

Jones-Saumty DJ: Contemporary healthcare issues of Native Americans and Alaska Natives. In Ma GX, Henderson G, editors: *Rethinking ethnicity and health care: a sociocultural perspective*, Springfield, Ill, 1999, Charles C. Thomas.

Kaiser Family Foundation: *Key facts: race, ethnicity and medical care* (Report #1523), Menlo Park, Calif, 1999, The Foundation.

Kane RL, Ouslander JG, Abrass IB, editors: *Essentials of clinical geriatrics*, New York, 1994, McGraw-Hill.

Kuhn ME: *Maggie Kuhn on aging*, Philadelphia, 1977, Westminister.

Kurlowicz L: The geriatric depression scale, *Try this: best practices in nursing care to older adults* 1(4), New York, May 1999, Hartford Institute for Geriatric Nursing.

Kurlowicz L, Wallace M: The Mini Mental State Examination (MMSE), *Try this: best practices in nursing care to older adults* 1(3), New York, January 1999, Hartford Institute for Geriatric Nursing.

Leccese C: Reducing falls in the elderly. Practical solutions, *ADVANCE Nurs Practitioners* August:59-62, 1999.

Lesourd B: Immune response during disease and recovery in the elderly, *Proc Nutr Soc* 58:85-98, 1999.

Letvak S, Schoder D: Sexually transmitted diseases in the elderly: what you need to know, *Geriatr Nurs* 17(4):156-160, 1996.

Levenson AJ, Hall RCW, editors: *Neuropsychiatric manifestations of physical disorders in the elderly*, New York, 1981, Raven Press.

Lynch SH: Elder abuse: what to look for, how to intervene, *Am J Nurs* 97:27-32, 1997.

McAuliffe K: Out of the blues, *Walking*, March/April:42-44, 46-47, 1994.

McGuire SL: Aging education in schools, *J Sch Health* 57(5):174-176, 1987.

McGuire SL, Gerber DE: Prevention starts early: aging education for children. In Edwards RB, Bittar EE, editors: *Advances in bioethics: violence, neglect and the elderly*, Greenwich, Conn, 1996, JAI Press.

Meehan P, Saltzman L, Sattin R: Suicides among older United States residents: epidemiologic characteristics and trends, *Am J Public Health* 81(9):1198-1200, 1991.

Miller CA: *Nursing care of older adults: theory and practice*, ed 2, Philadelphia, 1995, Lippincott.

Miller KH: A changing landscape: health issues among minority elders in the United States, *Health Ed Monograph Series* 18(2):33-37, 2000.

Molony SL, Waszynski CM, Lyder CH: *Gerontological nursing: an advanced practice approach*, Stamford, Conn, 1999, Appleton & Lange.

National Center for Health Statistics (NCHS): *National health interview survey*, Washington, DC, 1996, USPHS.

National Council on the Aging (NCOA): *NISH. The National Institute on Senior Housing*, Washington, DC, 2000, NCOA.

The National Institute of Senior Centers and the Senior Center Field: a chronology, *Perspect Aging* 22(2):10-11, 1993.

National Institute on Aging (NIA): *Sexuality in later life*, AgePage, Washington, DC, 1994, NIA.

National Institute on Aging (NIA): *Depression: a serious but treatable illness*, AgePage, Washington, DC, 1996, NIA.

National Institute on Aging (NIA): *Exercise: feeling fit for life*, AgePage, Washington, DC, 1998, NIA.

National Institutes of Health (NIH), Office of Research on Women's Health: *Women of color health data book*, NIH Pub No 98-4247, Washington, DC, 1998, US Government Printing Office.

Nutrition Screening Initiative: *Nutrition screening checklist*, Washington, DC, 2000, A cooperative effort of the American Dietetic Association, the American Academy of Family Physicians, and the National Council on the Aging.

O'Neill K, Reid G: Perceived barriers to physical activity by older adults, *Can J Public Health* 82(6):392-396, 1991.

Orr ME: Nutrition. In Lueckenotte AG: *Gerontologic nursing*, ed 2, St Louis, 2000, Mosby.

Perkins S: Physical activity and the healthy older adult, *Health Ed Monograph Series* 18(2):38-43, 2000.

Rosenburg IH: As you age: 10 keys to a longer, healthier, more vital life, *Worldview* 5(2):2-3, 1993.

Ross H: Growing older: health issues for minorities, *Closing the Gap*, Washington, DC, May 2000, USDHHS.

Russell RM, Rasmussen J, Lichtenstein AH: Modified food guide pyramid for people over seventy years of age, *J Nutrition* 129:751-753, 1999.

Schaller KJ: Tai Chi Chih: an exercise option for older adults, *J Gerontol Nurs* 22(10):12-17, 1996.

Skinner BF, Vaughn ME: *Enjoy old age: a program of self-management*, New York, 1983, Norton.

Social Security Administration: Operations in the Candler Building 1936-1960. Retrieved from the internet on March 8, 2001. *http://www.ssa.gov/history/candlerops.html*

Staab AS, Hodges LC: *Essentials of gerontological nursing: adaptation to the aging process*, Philadelphia, 1996, Lippincott.

Turner LW, Fitch-Hilgenberg M, DiBrezzo R, et al.: Enhancing the quality of the later years: nutrition and aging, *Health Ed Monograph Series* 18(2):44-50, 2000.

US Bureau of the Census: *Sixty-five plus in America*, Washington, DC, 1992, US Government Printing Office.

US Department of Health and Human Services (USDHHS): *Healthy People 2000, full report, with commentary*, Washington, DC, 1991, US Government Printing Office.

US Department of Health and Human Services (USDHHS), Public Health Service: National ambulatory medical care surgery: 1991 summary, *Vital Health Statistics*, Series 13, No. 116, May 1994.

US Department of Health and Human Services (USDHHS): *1995 White House Conference on Aging: adopted resolutions*, Washington, DC, 1996a, US Government Printing Office.

US Department of Health and Human Services (USDHHS): *1995 White House Conference on Aging. The road to an aging policy for the 21st century: executive summary*, Washington, DC, 1996b, US Government Printing Office.

US Department of Health and Human Services (USDHHS): *Health and aging chartbook. Health, United States 1999*, Hyattsville, Md, 1999, National Center for Health Statistics.

US Department of Health and Human Services (USDHHS): *Healthy People 2010, conference edition*, Washington, DC, 2000, US Government Printing Office.

US Department of Health, Education and Welfare (USDHEW): *1961 White House Conference on Aging: education and aging*, Washington, DC, 1961, US Government Printing Office.

US Department of Health, Education and Welfare (USDHEW): *1971 White House Conference on Aging: toward a national policy on aging*, Washington, DC, 1971, US Government Printing Office.

US Preventive Services Task Force: *Guide to clinical preventive services: report of the U.S. Preventive Services Task Force*, ed 2, Baltimore, 1996, Williams & Wilkins.

US Public Health Service (USPHS): *Put prevention into practice*, Waldorf, Md, 2000, American Nurses Publishing.

Wallace D, McGuire SL, Lee HT, et al.: Older Americans Act: implications for nursing, *Nurs Outlook* 47:181-185, 1999.

Wallace M: Intimacy and sexuality. In Lueckenotte AG, editor: *Gerontologic nursing*, ed 2, St Louis, 2000a, Mosby.

Wallace M: Sexuality. *Try this: best practices in nursing care of older adults* 2(3), New York, November 2000b, Hartford Institute of Geriatric Nursing.

Where doctors are few and far between, *Aging* 365:12-17, 1993.

White P: Pearls for practice: polypharmacy and the older adult, *J Am Acad Nurse Pract* 7(11):545-548, 1995.

Yee BWK, Weaver GD: Medication issues and aging, *Health Ed Monograph Series* 18(2):51-57, 2000.

Yesage JA, Brink TL, Rose TL, et al.: Development and validation of a geriatric depression screening scale: a preliminary report, *J Psych Research* 17:37-49, 1983.

Zembrzuski C: *Try this: best practices in nursing care to older adults. Nutrition and hydration*, 2(2), New York, September 2000, The Hartford Institute for Geriatric Nursing.

## SELECTED BIBLIOGRAPHY

Ayello EA: Predicting pressure ulcer sore risk, *Try this: best practices in nursing care to older adults* 1(5):1-2, 1999.

Burgratt V: The older woman: ethnicity and health, *Geriatr Nurs* 21:183-186, 2000.

Flahaerty E: Assessing pain in older adults. *Try this: best practices in nursing care to older adults* 1(6):1-2, May, 2000.

Hofland SL, Powers J: Sexual dysfunction in the menopausal woman: hormonal causes and management issues, *Geriatr Nurs* 17(4):161-165, 1996.

Hungelmann J, Kenkel-Rossi E, Klasser L, et al.: Focus on spiritual well-being: harmonious interconnectedness of mind-body-spirit—use of the JAREL spiritual well-being scale, *Geriatr Nurs* 17(6):262-265, 1996.

Jurkowski ET, Tracy MB: Social policy and the aged: implications for health planning, health education, and health promotion, *Health Ed Monograph Series* 18(2):20-26, 2000.

Marchi-Jones S, Murphy JF, Rosseau P: Caring for the caregivers, *J Gerontol Nurs* 22(8):7-13, 1996.

McGuire SL: Promoting positive attitudes toward aging: literature for young children, *Childhood Education* 69(4):204-210, 1993.

McGuire SL: Promoting positive attitudes through aging education: a study with preschool children, *Gerontol Geriatrics Ed* 13(4):3-12, 1993.

Phillips LR: Domestic violence and aging women, *Geriatr Nurs* 21:188-193, 2000.

Smyth C: The Pittsburgh Sleep Quality Index, *Try this: best practices in nursing care to older adults* 1(6):1-2, 1999.

# Nutrition Screening Checklist

The warning signs of poor nutritional health are often overlooked. Use this checklist to find out if you or someone you know is at nutritional risk.

Read the statements below. Circle the number in the yes column for those that apply to you or someone you know. For each yes answer, score the number in the box. Total your nutritional score.

## Determine Your Nutritional Health

| | Yes |
|---|---|
| I have an illness or condition that made me change the kind and/or amount of food I eat. | 2 |
| I eat fewer than 2 meals per day. | 3 |
| I eat few fruits or vegetables, or milk products. | 2 |
| I have 3 or more drinks of beer, liquor, or wine almost every day. | 2 |
| I have tooth or mouth problems that make it hard for me to eat. | 2 |
| I don't always have enough money to buy the food I need. | 4 |
| I eat alone most of the time. | 1 |
| I take 3 or more different prescribed or over-the-counter drugs a day. | 1 |
| Without wanting to, I have lost or gained 10 pounds in the last 6 months. | 2 |
| I am not always physically able to shop, cook, and/or feed myself. | 2 |
| | Total |

## Total your nutritional score. If it's —

**0-2**  **Good!** Recheck your nutritional score in 6 months.

**3-5**  **You are at moderate nutritional risk.** See what can be done to improve your eating habits and lifestyle. Your office on aging, senior nutrition program, senior citizens center, or health department can help. Recheck your nutritional score in 3 months.

**6 or more**  **You are at high nutritional risk.** Bring this checklist the next time you see your doctor, dietitian, or other qualified health or social service professional. Talk with them about any problems you may have. Ask for help to improve your nutritional health.

These materials are developed and distributed by the Nutrition Screening Initiative, a project of:

American Academy of Family Physicians

The American Dietetic Association

National Council on the Aging, Inc.

Remember that warning signs suggest risk but do not represent diagnosis of any condition.

From Nutrition Screening Initiative: *Nutrition screening checklist,* Washington, DC, 2000, a cooperative effort of the American Dietetic Association, the American Academy of Family Physicians, and the National Council on the Aging. Used with permission.

# Nutrition Screening Checklist (cont'd)

**The Nutrition Checklist is based on the Warning Signs described below.
Use the word DETERMINE to remind you of the Warning Signs.**

## Disease

Any disease, illness, or chronic condition that causes you to change the way you eat, or makes it hard for you to eat, puts your nutritional health at risk. Four of five adults have chronic diseases that are affected by diet. Confusion or memory loss that keeps getting worse is estimated to affect one of five or more of older adults. This can make it hard to remember what, when, or if you've eaten. Feeling sad or depressed, which happens to about one in eight older adults, can cause big changes in appetite, digestion, energy level, weight, and well-being.

## Eating Poorly

Eating too little and eating too much both lead to poor health. Eating the same foods day after day or not eating fruit, vegetables, and milk products daily also will cause poor nutritional health. One in five adults skip meals daily. Only 13% of adults eat the minimum amount of fruit and vegetables needed. One in four older adults drink too much alcohol. Many health problems become worse if you drink more than one or two alcoholic beverages per day.

## Tooth Loss/Mouth Pain

A healthy mouth, teeth, and gums are needed to eat. Missing, loose, or rotten teeth or dentures that don't fit well or cause mouth sores make it hard to eat.

## Economic Hardship

As many as 40% of older Americans have incomes of less than $6000 per year. Having less—or choosing to spend less—than $25 to 30 per week for food makes it very hard to get the foods you need to stay healthy.

## Reduced Social Contact

One third of all older people live alone. Being with people daily has a positive effect on morale, well-being, and eating.

## Multiple Medicines

Many older Americans must take medicines for health problems. Almost half of older Americans take multiple medicines daily. Growing old may change the way we respond to drugs. The more medicines you take, the greater the chance for side effects such as increased or decreased appetite, change in taste, constipation, weakness, drowsiness, diarrhea, nausea, and others. Vitamins or minerals when taken in large doses act like drugs and can cause harm. Alert your doctor to everything you take.

## Involuntary Weight Loss/Gain

Losing or gaining a lot of weight when you are not trying to do so is an important warning sign that must not be ignored. Being overweight or underweight also increases your chance of poor health.

## Needs Assistance in Self-Care

Although most older people are able to eat, one of every five have trouble walking, and with shopping, buying, and cooking food, especially as they get older.

## Elder Years Above Age 80

Most older people lead full and productive lives. But as age increases, risk of frailty and health problems increase. Checking your nutritional health regularly makes good sense.

**The Nutrition Screening Initiative, 1010 Wisconsin, NW, Suite 800, Washington, DC 20007.**

The Nutrition Screening Initiative is funded in part by a grant from Ross Laboratories, a division of Abbott Laboratories.

# Seniors Substance Abuse Project

ASSESSMENT FORM

Name _____ ID# _____

Occupation _____

Language in the home _____

Current living arrangements _____

_____

Number of children _____

Significant others _____

_____

---

### RELEASE OF INFORMATION

I, _____, agree to participate in a Seniors Substance Abuse Project conducted by the Kent County Health Department. I authorize Donna Spruit, R.N., from the Kent County Health Department to release information regarding my medication and health status to _____

_____
(doctor or agency).

I also authorize _____ (doctor or agency) to give information regarding my medication and health status to Donna Spruit, R.N.

Recipients of substance abuse services have rights protected by State and Federal Law and promulgated rules. For information, contact Seniors Project Supervisor, Kent County Health Dept., 700 Fuller NE, Grand Rapids, MI, 49503, 616-336-3040, or the Office of Substance Abuse Services, Recipient Rights Coordinator, P.O. Box 30035, 3500 North Logan, Lansing, MI 48909.

Client's signature _____

Date _____

Witness _____

Relationship to Client _____

---

Interviewer's name _____ Date _____

Site of interview _____

# Seniors Substance Abuse Project (cont'd)

Seniors Project Questionnaire

ID# _____

Date _____

## KNOWLEDGE OF MEDICATIONS

List each medication (including over-the-counter and home remedies) the client is taking in the left-hand column. In the center column, write down what the client says is the reason [for] taking this drug. Include how much and how often he [or she] claims to take each in the right column. Use the client's words if possible. It is important that the *client's perceptions* be recorded, not the interviewer's.

| Name of Drug | Reason for Taking | Amount and Frequency (with Meals/without Meals) |
|---|---|---|
|  |  |  |
|  |  |  |
|  |  |  |
|  |  |  |
|  |  |  |
|  |  |  |
|  |  |  |
|  |  |  |
|  |  |  |
|  |  |  |
|  |  |  |
|  |  |  |
|  |  |  |
|  |  |  |
|  |  |  |
|  |  |  |
|  |  |  |
|  |  |  |

*Continued*

# Seniors Substance Abuse Project (cont'd)

## SENIOR SUBSTANCE ABUSE QUESTIONNAIRE MEDICATION USE/MISUSE

*Risk Factor Analysis*　　　　　　Date: _____　ID# _____

Evaluate the status of risk factor and circle the number on the left that best describes the client's risk. 0 for not-at-all to 5 for very much a problem. On the right of each risk factor write in any comments that may help clarify the specific situation; for example, "diet implications"—*special weight reduction 1500 cal. diet, lo Na lo chol.*; "side effects"—*C/O dry mouth, excessive tiredness*; "sensory deprivation"—*poor vision, cataracts both eyes.*

0  1  2  3  4  5　Cost _____

0  1  2  3  4  5　Confusion _____

0  1  2  3  4  5　Diet implications _____

0  1  2  3  4  5　Difficulty opening safety closures _____

0  1  2  3  4  5　Depression _____

0  1  2  3  4  5　Drug intolerance _____

0  1  2  3  4  5　Forgets to take medication _____

0  1  2  3  4  5　Fear of taking medication _____

0  1  2  3  4  5　Inappropriate storage:

　　　　　　　　　____ temperature, humidity _____

　　　　　　　　　____ removal from original container _____

　　　　　　　　　____ medication stored at bedside _____

0  1  2  3  4  5　Language barrier _____

0  1  2  3  4  5　Lack of knowledge regarding meds _____

0  1  2  3  4  5　Living alone _____

0  1  2  3  4  5　Multiple prescriptions _____

0  1  2  3  4  5　Multiple pharmacies _____

0  1  2  3  4  5　Multiple physicians _____

0  1  2  3  4  5　Physician hopping _____

0  1  2  3  4  5　Outdated medications _____

0  1  2  3  4  5　Over-the-counter use _____

0  1  2  3  4  5　Reading disability _____

0  1  2  3  4  5　Sensory deprivation _____

0  1  2  3  4  5　Side effects _____

0  1  2  3  4  5　Stopping medication _____

0  1  2  3  4  5　Stretching medication _____

0  1  2  3  4  5　Sharing medication _____

0  1  2  3  4  5　Not following prescribed regimen _____

0  1  2  3  4  5　Transportation difficulty _____

0  1  2  3  4  5　Use of household remedies (e.g., baking soda) _____

0  1  2  3  4  5　Mood-altering drugs _____

0  1  2  3  4  5　Use of alcohol _____

0  1  2  3  4  5　Other (list):

0  1  2  3  4  5　_____

0  1  2  3  4  5　_____

0  1  2  3  4  5　_____

0  1  2  3  4  5　_____

Total Risk Factor Score _____

*Interviewer's Signature* _____

# Seniors Substance Abuse Project (cont'd)

## SENIORS SUBSTANCE ABUSE QUESTIONNAIRE GUIDE
## RISK FACTOR ANALYSIS

Review each risk factor with the client and determine applicability. Rate the risk factor from 0 (not applicable, no risk) to 5 (high risk), and circle the appropriate number. This analysis requires your professional judgment and is based on your assessment of the client and his or her personal situation.

### Cost

Clients may consider some of their medications to be very costly. If their income level is low and/or fixed, they may not be able to afford these medications. Determine their priority for expenses—medications may not be high priority, and therefore, the risk of omission is increased.

### Confusion

Rate this according to how well oriented the client seems to be. Does he or she relate appropriately to time and place, etc.?

### Diet Implications

Is the client on a special diet such as low sodium, low cholesterol, weight reduction, diabetic? Some medications contain sodium (e.g., Mylanta, Maalox). Some medications are to be taken on an empty stomach, while others are to be taken with meals. Milk is to be avoided with certain drugs. It is important to determine whether the client adheres to these recommendations.

### Difficulty Opening Safety Closures

Clients with arthritis may have increased difficulty opening safety caps. They may omit a dose just because of the hassle or worse yet, they may transfer drugs to an unmarked container (see inappropriate storage). Determine how likely this risk is. Client may be unaware that easy-open caps are available from the pharmacy.

### Depression

Is the client now depressed or does he or she have a history of depression? Because of the many losses suffered by the elderly, some degree of depression is fairly common. Depression may influence adherence to a medical regimen. Likewise, depression may be a side effect of some drugs.

### Drug Intolerance or Allergy

History of intolerance or allergy would have implications for current drug use. It would be important that this information be readily available in case of emergency. Rate this risk according to the severity and likelihood of recurrence.

### Forgets to Take Medication

Does the client state that he or she sometimes forgets to take medication? Determine how likely this is. This risk may go hand-in-hand with confusion, or it may stand alone. Not all persons who forget to take medication are confused. They may be overwhelmed by the number of medications they are to take or they may be distracted by other activities. Listen for key phrases like, "Don't know if I remembered." Client may be threatened or embarrassed to admit forgetfulness. Good, nonthreatening interviewing is helpful here.

### Fear of Taking Medication

Some clients are reluctant to take drugs, even those that are prescribed. Determine if the client has any such reluctance. Some clients may be very open and verbal about this fear. Rate this risk according to how likely it is that the client would not take needed medication.

### Inappropriate Storage

TEMPERATURE, HUMIDITY. Medications are subject to deterioration in certain temperature extremes and high humidity. Storage in the bathroom is undesirable. Storage in the refrigerator is required for certain drugs and contraindicated for others. Check labels or check with pharmacist if necessary.

REMOVAL FROM ORIGINAL CONTAINERS. Many clients are tempted to put all pills together in one container, especially when they travel. This is a very unsafe practice. All medications should remain in the original containers until needed. It is considered safe to place medications in special dispensers. These are best when divided by time of day they are to be taken. This helps the problem of forgetfulness. However, a list of what each drug is should be available nearby for emergency information, especially if traveling.

MEDICATION STORED AT BEDSIDE. Although this may seem like a very convenient storage site, it runs the risk of error if the client should happen to take medications when not fully awake. Also, too easy access may make overusing certain medications more likely, such as pain medication or mood-altering drugs. Having to go to the storage site allows a more purposeful effort and hopefully a more accurate dosage.

# Seniors Substance Abuse Project (cont'd)

## SENIORS SUBSTANCE ABUSE QUESTIONNAIRE GUIDE
## RISK FACTOR ANALYSIS

LANGUAGE BARRIER. Labels and directions written in a language not understood by a client could lead to misuse. Also, if the client does not understand verbal instructions given by the doctor or pharmacist, there is increased potential for misuse.

LACK OF KNOWLEDGE REGARDING MEDICATIONS. See first part of questionnaire, "Knowledge of Medications." How well does the client understand what the medications he or she is taking are for, how to take them, how much to take, and how often?

LIVING ALONE. This may or may not be a risk factor, depending on how well the client has adapted to living alone. Living alone can be a problem if there is no support system to encourage the client to take good care of himself or herself. Motivation to comply with a medical regimen will be affected in some cases.

### Multiple Prescriptions

The more medications the clients are taking, the more likely they are to have a problem with adverse drug interactions, side effects, inclusion about dosage and schedule, etc.

### Multiple Pharmacies

Going to more than one pharmacy to have prescriptions filled is undesirable. The pharmacist may be unaware of other drugs the client is taking and the pharmacist will be hampered in his or her ability to do a drug profile and advise the client on possible incompatibility of certain drugs.

### Multiple Physicians

Because the elderly tend to have a number of chronic illnesses, they frequently find themselves being treated by a number of specialists (e.g., internist, rheumatologist, cardiac specialist, gastroenterologist). This is sometimes unavoidable, and it is important that each physician be aware of what drugs the other has prescribed. The client has responsibility for conveying that information.

### Physician Hopping

This is different from "multiple physicians." Here clients go from one doctor to another within a short span of time because they are not satisfied with their care. This can be a dangerous and fruitless practice and frequently results in multiple prescriptions for similar drugs (e.g., mood-altering drugs, antibiotics, pain medication). The client rarely informs the new doctor of his recent previous visits to other doctors. There are clients who have gotten three prescriptions for the same drug from three different doctors and ended up taking all three, and therefore, three times the desired dosage.

### Outdated Medication

All drugs should be discarded once they are outdated. *Saving drugs* is a potentially dangerous practice because they can change in composition and may be harmful if used. Also their presence in the medicine chest could result in someone accidentally taking the old drug instead of the desired one. The risk factor can be most accurately evaluated by a home visit where the medicine chest can be viewed or by asking the client to bring all drugs to the next visit.

### Over-the-Counter Use

Clients who regularly use over-the-counter drugs run the risk of drug interactions, especially if they are taking other prescription medication. Sometimes clients do not count over-the-counter drugs as "real" drugs. They do not realize that these drugs also have side effects and contraindications. The more over-the-counter drugs used by the client and the greater the frequency, the higher the risk rating they would receive from this risk factor.

### Reading Disability (Comprehension)

This is not to be confused with the "language barrier" problem. What is considered here are perceptual difficulties that could be the result of a stroke (aphasia) or possibly a lifelong condition. If a client is unable to read and understand the information on the label, it would signal a risk of misuse.

### Sensory Deprivation

Sensory deprivation includes visual, auditory, or other sensory-related problems that may influence the client's ability to follow directions or correctly self-administer medications, such as reduced vision or blindness, loss of feeling in fingertips, deafness.

### Side Effects

Undesirable effects caused by the drug may influence a client to avoid taking a needed drug (e.g., disagreeable

# Seniors Substance Abuse Project (cont'd)

## SENIORS SUBSTANCE ABUSE QUESTIONNAIRE GUIDE
## RISK FACTOR ANALYSIS

taste, dry mouth, dizziness, nausea, drowsiness, lingering bad taste in mouth, impotence).

### Stopping Medication

When the client stops taking a prescribed drug before the desired therapeutic results are obtained, this is a medication misuse. This risk factor could occur as a result of unpleasant side effects, cost, emotional reasons, denial of illness, symptoms reduction (e.g., blood pressure medication, antibiotics), or embarrassment.

### Stretching Medication

The client tries to make the medication last longer by skipping doses or taking less than the prescribed dose. This is usually done for financial reasons or because the client desires to minimize the amount of drugs he or she is taking.

### Sharing Medication

Usually a misplaced friendship gesture. The friend tells the client that this drug worked for him, "why doesn't he or she take one." A very dangerous practice.

### Not Following Prescribed Regimen

This may or may not be a *deliberate* act on the part of the client. It could be the result of "confusion," "forgetfulness," or "stretching medication." Adjusting dosage schedules ad lib can be potentially hazardous, depending on the drug and its intended action.

### Transportation Difficulty

This may not be a problem unless it results in not getting a prescripton filled or related effect such as not making a follow-up visit to the doctor, which might be a necessary component in monitoring a drug's effectiveness.

### Use of Household Remedies

The use of such items as baking soda for upset stomach could be a problem if the client were on a low-sodium diet and/or hypertensive, because baking soda is high in sodium.

The household remedy would need to be evaluated as to the contents, amount taken, and frequency.

### Mood-Altering Drugs

This category of drug runs a risk of its own because of the nature of the drug and the condition it is intended to alleviate. These drugs may be habit forming. A depressed client may overdose himself.

### Use of Alcohol

Some drugs interact or are increased by the use of alcohol. It would be important to determine how much and how often the client used alcohol. A history of alcohol abuse would be significant.

Asking the following questions developed by John A. Ewing, Director for the Center for Alcohol Studies at the University of North Carolina, may be helpful:
1. Have you felt the need to cut down your drinking?
2. Have you ever felt annoyed by criticism of your drinking?
3. Have you had guilty feelings about drinking?
4. Do you ever take a morning eye-opener?

If two or three questions receive a positive response, the likelihood that the person is an alcoholic is high.

Add up the total risk factor score and place in the designated space. By looking over the form, you can determine which risk factors you can help eliminate or reduce through intervention. Write up a plan with the client. After 6 to 8 weeks, readminister the tool and determine if the total risk factor score has been lowered.

Reproduced by permission of and modified from the Nursing Division, Kent County Health Department, Grand Rapids, MI; Wanda Bierman, RN, MS, Family Health Services Supervisor and Donna Spruit, RN, Geriatric Services, Principal Developers.

# The Older Americans Act of 1965: Significant Amendments and Changes

1967 *Older Americans Act; Amendments of 1967 (Public Law 90-42)*—Authorized studies to look at the availability and adequacy of training resources in gerontology and to evaluate present and future trends and needs for such personnel and programs. Resulted in increased funding and training in the field of gerontology. Placed new emphasis on providing services to seniors.

1969 *Older Americans Act; Amendments of 1969 (Public Law 91-69)*—Mandated increased state planning for act programs through state agencies on aging. Increased the emphasis on coordination with local programs and program evaluation. Authorized grants to states and communities for model projects on services to the elderly. Established the *National Older Americans Volunteer Program (NOAVP)*. NOAVP's main purpose was to help retired persons avail themselves of opportunities for voluntary service in their communities and helped to subsidize this through provision of transportation, meals, and other necessary services needed for them to participate. Major components of NOAVP were (1) *Retired Senior Volunteer Program (RSVP)* and (2) *Foster Grandparents*.

1972 *Older Americans Act; Amendments of 1972 (Public Law 92-258)*—Amended the act to provide grants to states for the establishment, maintenance, operation, and expansion of low-cost meal projects, nutrition training, and education, as well as opportunity for social contacts for the elderly. Established the *Nutrition Program for the Elderly* and brought the nutrition of the elderly into the national limelight. From this legislation sprang many senior nutrition services.

1973 *Older Americans Act; Comprehensive Amendments of 1973 (Public Law 93-29)*—Established the *Federal Council on Aging* and the *National Information and Resources Clearinghouse for the Aging*. Required that a sole state agency administer the provisions of the act in conjunction with local agencies on aging. Established *Multipurpose Senior Centers* and *Older Readers Services*. These multipurpose centers combined social, recreational, health, and nutrition aspects for seniors into one accessible program. These centers also placed a new and increasing emphasis on the social needs of seniors and attempted to decrease social isolation for seniors through a community-based program.

1974 *Older Americans Act; Amendments of 1974 (Public Law 93-351)*—Provided for increased funding for transportation for the elderly, especially transportation services that facilitated the elderly in using the nutrition programs and multipurpose centers already designated under the act.

The transportation needs of the elderly living in rural areas were explored. This same year a separate presidential proclamation declared May to be Older Americans Month, and this tradition has been carried on by a presidential proclamation each year since.

1975 *Older Americans Act; Amendments of 1975 (Public Law 94-135)*—Established social services programs especially for seniors. A significant part of these amendments involved two separate acts: *Age Discrimination Act of 1975 and Older Americans Community Service Employment Act of 1975*. Both of these acts carry the same public law number as the amendments and are incorporated into the amendments. The Age Discrimination Act prohibited discrimination on the basis of age, largely in relation to employment. The Community Service Employment Act section of the amendments provided for community service employment for seniors where they were eligible to receive a wage. Most employment programs under the act, before this time, had involved voluntary employment for seniors. These amendments also attempted to attract more qualified people into the field of gerontology through increased funding for training.

1978 *Comprehensive Older Americans Act; Amendments of 1978 (Public Law 95-478)*—The Amendments of 1978 were extensive and provided for improved and increased programs for older Americans. These amendments called for a great reduction in the paperwork necessary to run the program; increased planning, coordination, evaluation, and administration efforts; and facilitated the quality of programs. They also established the Advisory Council on Aging; provided for area agencies on aging to contract for legal services and to carry out demonstration projects on the legal services necessary for older Americans; provided for exploring alternative work modes for older Americans such as the Senior Environmental Protection Corps with the Environmental Protection Agency (EPA); provided for grants to Indian tribes for older American services to tribes members; set up a White House Conference on Aging for 1981 (there had previously been such conferences in 1961 and 1971); provided for a study of racial and ethnic discrimination in programs for older Americans; and outlined the programs of (1) *Congregate Nutrition Services* and (2) *Home Delivered Nutrition Services for the Elderly*. In addition, these amendments mandated development and implementation of national labor policy for the field of aging; discussed the concept of "preretirement" education and planning services; authorized special projects on long-

# The Older Americans Act of 1965:
## Significant Amendments and Changes (cont'd)

term care and alternatives to institutionalization such as adult day care, supervised living in public or non-profit housing, family respite, preventive health services, home health and homemaker services, home maintenance programs, and geriatric health maintenance organizations; and authorized demonstration projects for community model programs to improve and expand social services and nutrition services, and to promote the well-being of older Americans. High priority for placement of these demonstration projects was given to rural areas and rural agencies on aging.

1981 *Older Americans Act; Amendments of 1981 (Public Law 97-115)*—Emphasized the provision of nutritional programs in congregate settings and facilitated access to such programs. These amendments also encouraged the formation of university-affiliated and other multidisciplinary centers on aging as well as long-term care projects and brought migrant and seasonal farm workers and organizations more in line with the provisions of the act.

1984 *Older Americans Act; Amendments of 1984 (Public Law 98-459)*—Often referred to as the Older Americans Personal Health Education and Training Act. Provided for a comprehensive array of community-based, long-term care services to appropriately sustain older people in their communities and homes. Authorized the designing of a uniform, standardized program of health education and training for older Americans with direct involvement of graduate educational institutions of public health in the design of such a program and direct involvement of graduate education institutions of public health, medical sciences, psychology, pharmacology, nursing, social work, health education, nutrition, and gerontology in the implementation of such a program. Planned for such education and training programs to be carried out in multipurpose senior centers as already provided for under the act.

1986 *Older Americans Act; Amendments of 1986 (Public Law 99-269)*—Amended the Older Americans Act to increase the federal contribution to senior nutrition programs covered under the act to about 57 cents per meal. Mandated that the Secretary of Agriculture and the Secretary of Health and Human Services jointly disseminate to state agencies, area agencies on aging, and providers of nutrition services covered under the act information concerning the existence of all federal commodity processing programs in which they would be eligible to participate, and the procedures necessary to participate in such programs.

1987 *Older Americans Act; Amendments of 1987 (Public Law 100-175)*—Often referred to as the Health Care Services in the Home Act of 1987. Established grants to states for in-home health care services for the frail elderly, for periodic preventive health services to be provided at senior centers or appropriate alternative sites, and to implement programs with respect to the prevention of abuse, neglect, and exploitation of the elderly. Authorized a *1991 White House Conference on Aging,* and reauthorized the Act through fiscal year 1991. Required a direct reporting relationship between the Commissioner on Aging and the Secretary of Health and Human Services; added an outreach program on Supplemental Security Income, food stamps, and Medicaid benefits; increased funds for administration of area agencies on aging and community service employment projects; added a Demonstration Project Authority in areas of health education and promotion, volunteerism, and consumer protection from home care services; and added a program for grants to assist older Hawaiian natives.

1992 *Older Americans Act; Amendments of 1992 (Public Law 102-375)*—A four-year reauthorization of the Older Americans Act that established a study committee to look at the quality of home care services for older adults; established funding for in-school intergenerational activities where older adults could serve as tutors, teacher aides, living historians, speakers, playground supervisors, lunchroom assistants, and other roles; directed more services to minorities and rural elderly; placed increased emphasis on health promotion for the elderly; increased funding for senior nutrition programs and added supportive services for family caregivers of the frail elderly; and authorized a White House Conference on Aging before December 31, 1994.

2000 *Older Americans Act: Amendments of 2000 (Public Law 106-501)*—Reauthorized the act through 2005. Created the *National Family Caregiver Support Program*, which will help families caring for frail elder members. Made provisions for grandparents who are caregivers of grandchildren and other older individuals who are relative caregivers of children under the age of 18. New provisions require that states show efforts to coordinate services with agencies and organizations that provide multigenerational activities and programs.

# School Health Nursing

*Mary Anne Modrcin-Talbott*

---

## OBJECTIVES

*Upon completion of this chapter, the reader should be able to:*

1. Discuss the history of school nursing in the United States.
2. Discuss the components of a comprehensive school health program.
3. Describe the roles of the school nurse.
4. Discuss patterns of school nursing practice.
5. Be familiar with standards of practice for school nursing.

---

## KEY TERMS

Comprehensive school health program (CSHP)
Generalized nursing services
Healthy school environment
National Association of School Nurses (NASN)

Lina Rogers
Roles of the school nurse
School health clinics
School health education
School health services
School nurse practitioner

School nursing
*Scope and Standards of Professional School Nursing Practice*
Specialized nursing services

---

As early as 1850, educators and health professionals recognized that the school was an important focal point for health promotion activities. At that time Lemuel Shattuck published the *Shattuck Report* and wrote the following:

Every child should be taught, early in life, that, to preserve his own life and his own health and the lives and health of others, is one of his most important and constantly abiding duties. Some measure is needed which shall compel children to make a sanitary examination of themselves and their associates, and thus elicit a practical application of the lessons of sanitary science in the everyday duties of life. The recommendation now under consideration is designed to furnish this measure. It is to be carried into operation in the use of a blank schedule, which is to be printed on a letter sheet, in the form prescribed in the appendix, and furnished to the teacher of each school. He is to appoint a sanitary committee of the scholars, at the commencement of school, and, on the first day of each month, to fill it out under his superintendence.... Such a measure is simple, would take a few minutes each day, and cannot operate otherwise than usefully upon the children, in forming habits of exact observation, and in making a personal application of the laws of health and life to themselves. This is education of an eminently practical character, and of the highest importance. (Shattuck, 1850, pp. 178-179)

Shattuck was advanced in his thinking about school health. He recognized that health education was an appropriate function of the school and that this function can best be coordinated by a "sanitary committee," or health council. His writings emphasized the responsibility that all citizens have for preserving life and promoting health. Today's comprehensive school health programming incorporates Shattuck's ideas.

## HISTORY OF SCHOOL NURSING IN THE UNITED STATES

The roots of **school nursing** in the United States can be traced to late nineteenth century London when the unhealthy conditions of school children resulted in the Metropolitan Association of Nursing providing the services of one of its nurses to work in the schools (Hawkins, Hayes, Corliss, 1994). This experiment was successful, and more nurses were assigned to do school nursing. The experiment was reported in the *American Journal of Nursing* in 1901 and caught the eye of Lillian Wald (Hawkins, Hayes, Corliss, 1994; Morten, 1901; Struthers, 1917).

School nursing originated in the United States in 1902 when Lillian Wald (see Chapter 1) placed a Henry Street

Settlement nurse in the New York City schools. Medical inspection of schools in New York City had been in place since 1897 but only to exclude children from school because of communicable disease (Hawkins, Hayes, Corliss, 1994). No effort was made to treat sick children, provide health education, or make referrals (Rogers, 1905).

By 1902 health conditions of school children in New York City were appalling, and it was not uncommon for a significant number of school children to be absent each day. Thousands of students were sent home from school with diseases such as pediculosis, inflamed eyes, ringworm, scabies, and impetigo. Wald proposed to New York school officials that with a nurse in the schools, children would be healthier and fewer children would be absent. Wald loaned a Henry Street Settlement nurse, **Lina Rogers,** to the New York City Health Department to do school nursing. Miss Rogers was at school in the mornings, and in the afternoons she made visits to the homes of sick children (Dock, 1902; Hawkins, Hayes, Corliss, 1994; Struthers, 1917). A 1-month trial with Miss Rogers was so successful that the New York City Health Department appointed twelve other nurses to do school nursing (Brainard, 1922, p. 269). Miss Rogers is considered the first school nurse in the United States and wrote the first book on school nursing under her married name of Lina Rogers Struthers.

By 1909 many visiting nurse associations were providing school nursing services. In 1913 a *School Nursing Committee* was founded by the National Organization for Public Health Nursing (NOPHN), and Lina Rogers Struthers was its chairperson. By 1920 the American Red Cross was providing school nursing services to rural America, and school nurses also were being employed across the country as employees of schools, local health departments, and visiting nurse associations.

As communicable diseases came more under control in the schools, school nurses expanded their activities to include health education, counseling, and screening. During this time school nursing began to develop two primary paths of employment: being employed through health departments or being employed by schools. In 1926 the NOPHN published on the scope and functions of school nursing for the first time.

In 1937 school nurses became part of the new section of *School Health and Physical Education* of the National Education Association. This section later became the **National Association of School Nurses (NASN).** The NASN (*http://www.nasn.org*) remains a professional organization for school nurses and writes standards of school nursing practice.

By 1940, almost 3500 nurses were employed by schools in the United States (Cromwell, 1946; Hawkins, Hayes, Corliss, 1994). The first edition of *The Nurse in the School* was published by the Joint Committee of the National Education Association and the American Medical Association in 1941.

In 1969 the first **school nurse practitioner** program was developed at the University of Colorado by Loretta Ford, RN, and Dr. Henry Silvers. This pilot program in the Denver public schools laid the foundation for primary health care in schools by nurses. In 1980 the Robert Wood Johnson Foundation *National School Health Services Program* demonstrated the effectiveness of school nurse practitioners in the elementary setting. Today, both advanced practice nursing and certification is available in school nursing. School nurse practitioner education is available at many nursing schools throughout the country.

In 1983 the *Scope and Standards for School Nursing Practice* were published for the first time by the American Nurses Association (ANA). These standards are now published jointly by the NASN and ANA. In addition, the *National Nurse's Coalition for School Health* was formed in 1994 to promote school health. This coalition included representatives from the National Association of School Nurses, National State School Nurses Consultants Association, American School Health Association, American Nurses' Association, and the American Public Health Association. Today school nurses remain a vital component of a comprehensive school health program.

## COMPREHENSIVE SCHOOL HEALTH PROGRAM: MODELS OF SCHOOL HEALTH

The Institute of Medicine's *Committee on Comprehensive School Health Programs* adopted an interim statement that provides a definition of a **comprehensive school health program (CSHP).** This definition is given below (Allensworth, Wyche, Lawson, et al., 1995):

A comprehensive school health program is an integrated set of planned, sequential, school-affiliated strategies, activities, and services designed to promote the optimal physical, emotional, social, and educational development of students. The program involves and is supportive of families and is determined by the local community, based on community needs, resources, standards, and requirements. It is coordinated by a multidisciplinary team and accountable to the community for program quality and effectiveness (p. 2).

Currently, no one single model is used to guide health programming in the school setting. Recently Resnicow and Allensworth (1996) proposed a coordinated eight-component model (Figure 20-1) that was a refinement of the CSHP model developed by Allensworth and Kolbe (1987) in the late 1980s. Resnicow's and Allensworth's model "extended the classic triad of health services, health education, and healthful environment to include physical education, counseling, psychology, and social services, food service, staff wellness, and family/community involvement" (Resnicow, Allensworth, 1996, p. 59).

Resnicow and Allenworth believed that in the classic school health model, healthy environment, staff wellness,

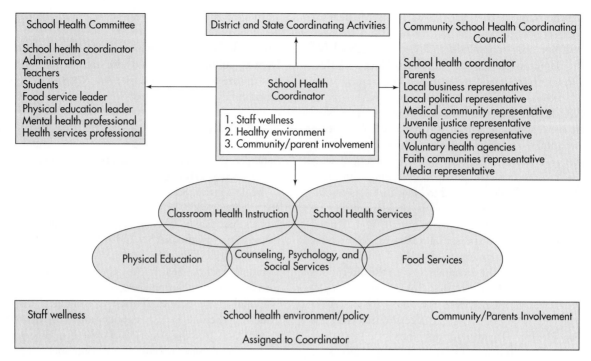

**FIGURE 20-1** The comprehensive school health program revisited. (From Resnicow K, Allensworth D: Conducting a comprehensive school health program, *J Sch Health* 66:59-63, 1996, p. 61).

and community activities often were neglected because no one had the designated responsibility for addressing them, so they refined the CSHP model by including a school health coordinator. The coordinator plays a central role in the integration, coordination, and management of school health programming. Because the school often assumes a central role in promoting community action for health, the coordinator would intervene with staff, parents, students, and the community to promote school- and community-based health programming. Such links to the community are extremely important because they help school health service providers and meet community health needs and facilitate use of community resources.

When communities develop school health programs, they often focus on the most pressing health issues of the students in their communities, such as sexual activity, substance abuse, violence, cardiovascular health risks, and poor nutrition (U.S. Department of Health and Human Services [USDHHS], 2000). Results from a recent nationwide survey of a systematic random sample of school districts reflect that although student health problems vary remarkably by grade level (Table 20-1), high-risk social behavior is the single most significant health concern at every level (Fryer, Igoe, 1996). Data suggest a relationship between economic investment in children (e.g., health insurance and mandated school health programs) and children's well-being" (Baker, 1994, p. 182).

Other comprehensive models for school health programming have been proposed. The Centers for Disease Control

and Prevention's Division of Adolescent and School Health (USDHHS, 1993) identified eight components in a CSHP (Box 20-1). There is a general consensus that a successful school health program uses an interagency, interdisciplinary approach to service delivery. However, "there is no special definition of school health to which all the various professions and organizations involved in this field subscribe... There is general consensus that school health programs are composed of three major functional areas: health services, health education, and environmental health" (Igoe, Parcel, 1992, p. 307). No one professional discipline alone can plan and implement these three components of a total school health program. Effective teamwork is critical for a successful school health program.

## Health Services

School health services are designed to protect and promote the health of all students and all school personnel. Approximately one third of school-age children in the United States have no regular form of health care (Passarelli, 1994), and many children are uninsured or underinsured. School-based health care services can play a vital role in filling this gap and in promoting children's health.

Health service programming includes such things as (1) periodic screenings for hearing and vision disorders and scoliosis, (2) emergency care, (3) development and implementation of a care management plan for children with disabilities, and (4) the linking of children and families to community resources. The type of health services needed in

**TABLE 20-1**

*Single Most Significant Health Problem Reported by Districts by Grade Level (%)*

| PROBLEM | ELEMENTARY SCHOOL | MIDDLE SCHOOL | HIGH SCHOOL |
|---|---|---|---|
| Accident/injury prevention | 6.4 | 3.1 | 0.8 |
| Chronic health problem | 11.2 | 5.2 | 2.9 |
| Communicable disease | 5.6 | 1.9 | 1.0 |
| Dental problems | 1.2 | 0.6 | 0.0 |
| Drug/substance abuse | 0.6 | 2.7 | 6.8 |
| Environmental concerns | 0.6 | 0.0 | 0.0 |
| High-risk social behaviors | 18.9 | 33.8 | 45.6 |
| Inadequate immunizations | 1.9 | 0.6 | 0.2 |
| Infectious disease | 3.3 | 0.8 | 1.0 |
| Lack of access to health care | 9.5 | 4.1 | 2.9 |
| Mental illness/ emotional problems | 4.8 | 6.4 | 5.0 |
| Poor school attendance | 2.3 | 2.3 | 2.9 |
| Poverty | 5.8 | 2.1 | 2.1 |
| Self-esteem problems | 8.7 | 19.9 | 7.7 |
| Special health needs | 9.1 | 2.9 | 1.9 |
| Suicide | 0.6 | 1.0 | 0.2 |
| Teen pregnancy | 0.0 | 1.7 | 6.6 |
| Unhealthy lifestyle habits | 6.4 | 8.1 | 8.5 |
| Violence | 0.0 | 1.2 | 2.3 |
| Vision problems | 0.6 | 0.2 | 0.4 |

From Fryer G, Igoe J: Functions of school nurses and health assistants in U.S. school health programs, *J Sch Health* 66:55-58, 1996.

a school setting varies, based on community strengths and needs and the population characteristics. Before developing a school health program, health professionals, school personnel, and community citizens need to work in partnership to assess community health needs (see Chapter 14).

School health services should not duplicate services already available in the community. Rather, they should augment community resources to enhance health care service delivery in the community. For example, if a community lacks accessible health services for children and youth, the school may provide primary health care services through a school-based clinic.

SCHOOL HEALTH CLINICS. School health clinics or centers have been in operation for over 25 years (Friedrich, 1999). These clinics that began operation in the early 1970s were designed to provide quality health care for all school-age children. Although school-based clinics gained momentum slowly, it was found that with community support and involvement, these health clinics became increasingly

 **BOX 20-1**

*Key Components of a Comprehensive School Health Program*

Addressing the full range of health needs of school-aged children calls for a broad and comprehensive approach. A comprehensive school health program includes eight key components:

- **Health education,** providing planned, sequential instructional programs for prekindergarten through twelfth-grade students. Health education programs are designed to impact positively the knowledge, attitudes, beliefs, and behaviors of the intervention group.
- **Clinical services,** offering first aid and other clinical services to students and sometimes their families, through school-based or school-linked programs. Screening, diagnosis, and treatment are frequently performed as well as case management for children with special health care needs.
- **Counseling and mental health services,** providing vocational guidance and psychological assessments. Consultations and interventions are also conducted. Issues involving self-esteem, self-control, and peer pressure are addressed with students.
- **School environment,** ensuring a safe and secure setting for learning. Aspects of a healthy environment include prevention of lead poisoning; removal of asbestos; the regulation of noise, heating, and lighting; as well as fostering secure, nonthreatening relationships among students and faculty.
- **School food programs,** providing school food services offering healthy choices, as well as education on healthy eating habits and food preparation.
- **Physical education and physical fitness,** providing age-appropriate activities for students to improve their health status, reduce stress, and increase social development.
- **Faculty and staff health promotion,** placing schools in the role of the worksite and offering a range of health promotion and disease prevention services to school faculty and staff. Adult participation in health promotion activities may also serve to model healthful behavior to students.
- **Community coordination,** increasing the school's constituency of supporters and building coalitions within the community.

From Office of Disease Prevention and Health Promotion: *School health: findings from evaluated programs,* Washington, DC, 1993, US Government Printing Office, pp. 1-1 - 1-2.

accepted and were a valuable asset to the physical and mental well-being of children. By the 1990s, school-based health centers caught on and currently over 1157 school-based clinics operate in elementary, middle, and high schools in the United States (Friedrich, 1999), and this number is growing.

Typically, funding for these centers comes from local, state, federal, and private grants. Local funding may be available through the school board, local health department, and other community organizations such as hospitals. Because these monies can be uncertain and variable from year-to-year, school-based health clinics are considering and seeking reimbursement from third-party payers and negotiating contracts with managed care organizations (Friedrich, 1999). Some schools of nursing are developing nursing practice or research centers in the school environment. These centers provide practice and/or research opportunities for nursing students and faculty and nursing services for the school community. The services provided in school-based clinics vary tremendously, from being managed by American Red Cross volunteers to primary health care centers staffed by RNs and advanced practice nurses.

Certain basic health services should be provided in all school systems. Communities need to develop strategies to achieve the following objectives:

- Appraise the health status of students and school personnel on a continual basis
- Counsel students, parents, teachers, and others regarding appraisal findings
- Encourage health care to correct remedial defects
- Provide emergency care for injury or sudden illness
- Prevent and control infectious diseases
- Identify children with disabling conditions and to arrange for educational programming that will enhance the maximum potential of these children
- Maintain a record-keeping system that complies with state laws (e.g., documentation of immunization status) and that documents the health needs of special children

The school nurse is in an excellent position to promote and coordinate school health services and assist in accomplishing these objectives. Health education activities are an important activity for the school nurse.

### Stop and Think About It

In your community are there any school-based nursing clinics at this time? If so, describe them. If not, why type of school-based services would be most appropriate?

## Health Education

*Health education* is a process that helps people make sound decisions about personal health practices and about individual, family, and community well-being. Knowledge alone does not foster appropriate health habits. To facilitate effective decision making in health matters, the school system should provide every child with the opportunity to acquire *knowledge* essential for understanding healthy functioning, develop *attitudes* and *habits* that promote healthy lifestyle behaviors, and practice health *skills* conducive to effective living (Stone, Perry, Luepker, 1989). To achieve these goals, the child, the family, and the community must be involved in the educational process. The nursing process is a useful tool when determining the health education needs of children and their families.

**School health education** is a *planned* series of *integrated* health educational activities based on input received from students, parents, community citizens, health care professionals, and educators. Health education activities in the school should be aimed at promoting both physiological and psychosocial functioning. The need for mental health education and services is imperative and cannot be overemphasized; almost half of the visits to the clinic are related to mental health concerns (Bradley, 1998; Friedrich, 1999). Students must be helped to understand normal growth and development and facilitated in discussing their needs in relation to the maturational process. The emphasis in a sound health education curriculum is on developing healthy lifestyle patterns. "Rigorous studies show that comprehensive health education in schools is effective in reducing the prevalence of health risk behaviors among youth" (Centers for Disease Control and Prevention [CDC], 1995, p. 3).

Curriculum planning for health instruction is the responsibility of all professionals in the school system. In addition to planning and providing health promotion programs for students, it is essential that health promotion programs be designed to meet the needs of faculty, staff, and parents (NASN, 1999). The school nurse is often asked to assume a major role in organizing health education activities. Although a school nurse is in a favorable position for understanding the essential concepts of health and illness and coordinating activities between the school and the community, it is crucial to remember that the nurse alone cannot implement a sound health education program. Without administrative support and active involvement of families, school administration, and teachers, it would be impossible to achieve appropriate selection, sequencing, and implementation of health content.

## Healthy School Environment

**A healthy school environment** is one that promotes optimum psychosocial and physical growth and development among school-age children and school personnel. It provides an atmosphere that fosters sound mental health and favorable social conditions. It is organized in a way that reduces unhealthy stress and eliminates safety hazards for all students and school personnel. A major concern in the current school environment is the potential for violence.

Environmental factors that affect the health and wellbeing of children in the school setting are numerous. Psychosocial and physical aspects of the environment need to be monitored to ensure an optimal setting for student learning. A healthful school environment has the following features (Comer, 1992; Igoe, 1992; Nader, 1992):

- An architectural design that takes into consideration the developmental characteristics of the population being served, the needs of disabled students and staff, and the needs of the instructional program

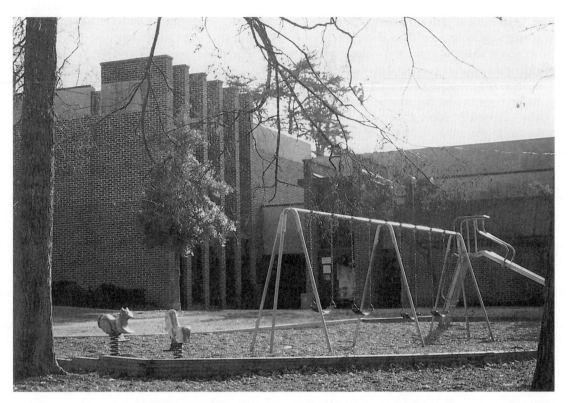

**FIGURE 20-2** School environment. (Courtesy Ed Richardson.)

- A comfortable environment that has adequate seating, lighting, heating, ventilation, toilet facilities, and drinking fountains
- An organized safety program, including procedures for emergency care
- An established procedure to ensure safe, sanitary conditions free from environmental hazards
- A recreational program that allows all students to participate
- A planned schedule of school activities that takes into account the physical and psychosocial needs of children at varying grade levels
- An organized school lunch program that provides nutritious foods, adequate time for good personal hygiene, and sufficient facilities for comfortable eating
- An established program that provides psychosocial counseling and consultation services for staff and students

A healthy school environment is conducive to promoting children's health. As part of the school health team, the nurse needs to facilitate a healthy school environment. Figure 20-2 illustrates aspects of the school environment.

## *HEALTHY PEOPLE 2010* AND SCHOOL HEALTH

The Healthy People Initiative highlights the need to focus attention on school-age children. Although no specific focus area in *Healthy People 2010* is devoted to children or

school health, objectives throughout the document address children's health and all of the document's focus areas have implications for children's health. Objectives that specifically address children's health can be retrieved from the document by using the Healthy People website (*http://www.health.gov/healthypeople*) and doing a search for "children."

The document suggests using the school as a setting for health education and health promotion. An objective in the document addresses the need to provide comprehensive school health education to prevent health problems involving unintentional injury, violence, suicide, tobacco use and addiction, alcohol or other drug use, unintended pregnancy, human immunodeficiency virus/acquired immunodeficiency syndrome (HIV/AIDS) and sexually transmitted diseases (STDs), unhealthy dietary patterns, inadequate physical activity, and environmental health (USDHHS, 2000). The document also recommends improved nurse-to-student ratios in our nation's schools (USDHHS, 2000).

National health objectives provide a framework for developing a sound health services and health education program in the school setting. They help schools develop curriculum offerings that target critical health issues such as substance abuse, violence, and sexuality concerns. They also provide support for developing a planned, sequential preschool-to-twelfth-grade comprehensive health curriculum.

The document's *Leading Health Indicators* (LHIs) (see Chapter 4) reflect major public health concerns in the

United States. LHIs such as physical activity, overweight and obesity, tobacco use, substance abuse, responsible sexual behavior, mental health, and injury and violence are excellent topics for health education in the school setting. For example, in relation to physical activity only two thirds of adolescents are engaged in the recommended amount of physical activity (USDHHS, 2000, p. 26). *Healthy People 2010* has a goal to increase the proportion of adolescents who engage in vigorous physical activity that promotes cardiorespiratory fitness 3 or more days per week for 20 or more minutes per occasion. Regular physical activity is associated with lower morbidity and mortality rates (USDHHS, 2000, p. 27), and health education programs and activities should address physical activity and provide opportunities for physical activity in the school setting.

More than 10% of children and adolescents aged 6 to 19 are overweight or obese (USDHHS, 2000, p. 28). *Healthy People 2010* has an objective to reduce the proportion of children and adolescents who are overweight or obese. Health education programs by the school nurse on nutrition and exercise can help address this issue and serve as a primary prevention tool for conditions such as high blood pressure, high cholesterol, type 2 diabetes, heart disease and stroke, gallbladder disease, arthritis, and certain cancers.

The school nurse also can help implement interventions that address the *Healthy People 2010* objective to reduce cigarette smoking by adolescents. Overall, the percentage of adolescents in grades 9 through 12 who smoked increased throughout the 1990s, and every day an estimated 3000 young persons start smoking (USDHHS, 2000, p. 31). Almost 50% of all adolescents who continue smoking regularly will eventually die from a smoking-related illness (USDHHS, 2000). School health programs and activities can encourage children to not start smoking and offer smoking cessation programs.

Other *Healthy People 2010* objectives that the nurse should routinely address in the school setting include increasing the proportion of adolescents not using alcohol or any illicit drugs and increasing the proportion of adolescents who abstain from sexual intercourse or use condoms if currently sexually active. Some schools are actually distributing condoms, and many are engaged in sex education and birth control education. These activities vary from state to state, based on laws that influence what can be addressed in the school environment.

As previously noted, many complaints that the school nurse addresses have to do with mental health. *Healthy People 2010* has a focus area on mental health that can help guide the nurse in relation to prevention and treatment activities. Of particular interest in this area is depression, anger, and self-esteem (Modrcin-McCarthy, Dalton, 1996; Modrcin-Talbott, Pullen, Barnes, et al., 1998; Modrcin-Talbott, Pullen, Zandstra, et al., 1998; Pullen, Modrcin-Talbott, Graf, 2000). School nurses can actively address mental health issues in the school setting. Unfortunately, we have not met national objectives in the area of depression and are actually regressing in the area. Our youth are experiencing a higher incidence of depression than ever before.

The objectives in *Healthy People 2010* help guide the nurse in school health programming by helping the nurse identify the significant health issues and health outcomes to reach in relation to these issues. Legislation and health issues also shape CSHPs.

## LEGISLATIVE AND LEGAL ISSUES

Federal and state legislation significantly influence nursing practice in the school setting. To function effectively in the schools, the nurse must be familiar with the legal issues involved in delivering care to children and knowledgeable about legislative programs that finance health care services for our youth. Chapters 5 and 16 discuss the major federal assistance programs that support the delivery of services to children, including Medicaid; Temporary Assistance to Needy Families (TANF); the Children with Special Health Care Needs Title V Program; Supplemental Security Income (SSI); Women, Infants, and Children (WIC); and the Food Stamp Program. Legislation related to school nutrition programs (e.g., National School Lunch Program and School Breakfast Program) also is designed to safeguard the health and well-being of American children. These programs provide nutritionally adequate food and encourage the development of healthy lifestyle behaviors through education. For many children in the United States, the school nutrition programs provide their major source of food.

From a state perspective, laws that govern school health vary significantly. It is important for all school nurses to understand their state laws because these laws provide the legal basis for the scope of nursing practice, malpractice, the reporting of abuse and neglect, and health service delivery. All school personnel are required to report suspected abuse and neglect.

State mandated school health requirements cover programs like health screening for scoliosis, hearing and vision, immunizations, disaster management, and food handling and preparation. As discussed in Chapters 4 and 16, both state and federal laws mandate special education programming for children with disabilities. School nurses actively participate in the educational planning for children with special needs.

School nurses also actively participate in implementing the provisions of the Occupational Safety and Health Act (OSHA). In many school districts, the nurse assumes major responsibility for staff in-service on OSHA's bloodborne pathogens standards. Chapter 17 discusses the mandates of OSHA.

One of the nation's strongest privacy protection laws, the *Family Educational Rights and Privacy Act (FERPA)* mandates safeguarding of student records (Policy Studies Associates, 1997). FERPA "defines education records as *all* records that schools or education agencies maintain about students. It guarantees parents' review and appeal of the records about their child, and restricts release of students' records" (Policy Studies Associates, 1997, p. 139). Schools that do not comply with FERPA regulations will lose their federal education funds.

All nurses working with children also must address *informed consent* issues. Informed parental consent is generally required for children to receive health care services, including immunizations, medical treatment by a physician, and special psychological testing for learning difficulties. An exception to this requirement occurs when children need emergency care and a parent is not readily available to give consent or refuses to give consent (Wong, 2000). However, because it is very difficult to establish what constitutes an emergency, every school needs well-developed policies that address emergency situations.

Laws that allow minors to seek treatment without parental consent usually deal with human sexuality problems, drug abuse, and mental health services. In almost all states, minors can seek and receive medical treatment for STDs without parental knowledge or consent. In some states physicians can diagnose pregnancy and provide prenatal care, contraceptive services, and drug abuse and other mental health assistance without parent consent. Although emancipated minors can give informed consent for certain types of health care, it is important for school nurses to recognize there are significant variations in state laws regarding this issue.

State and federal legislation is written to promote and protect the health of children. Knowledge of federal and state laws may assist school nurses to speak out on behalf of children when required services are not provided or when a child's rights are being violated. Advocating for strong health policy is a significant nursing intervention.

## THE ROLE OF THE COMMUNITY HEALTH NURSE IN THE SCHOOL HEALTH PROGRAM

The role of nursing in the school health program has been evolving since the beginning of the century when Lillian Wald placed Lina Rogers in the New York City schools. Control of communicable disease is no longer the primary emphasis of nursing service in the school setting. It is now recognized that the school nurse has a significant contribution to make in all aspects of the CSHP. School nurses are currently providing a complex array of school health services, such as case management for chronic health problems, primary health care services, and family counseling.

However, the general public and other health professionals are often unaware of what the school nurse does or does not do (Bradley, 1998). The challenging nature of the role of the nurse in the school setting was illustrated by Burton (1992) as she provided an accounting of the "A Day in the Life of a School Nurse" (see *A View from the Field*). It is becoming increasingly apparent to the nursing professional that the scope of school nursing practice will expand in the future as a growing number of communities use school-based health clinics to provide primary care services to children.

### The Essence and Standards of School Nursing

"School nursing is a specialized practice of professional nursing that advances the well-being, academic success, and lifelong achievement of students" (NASN/ANA, 2001, p. 1). School nursing services are provided in a variety of educational settings, such as day care centers and public schools, as well as numerous other settings including juvenile justice facilities, field trips, and sporting occasions.

NASN and ANA have provided standards for practice to guide nurses' efforts in the school setting. Criteria to measure the achievement of these standards can be found in the document *Scope and Standards of Professional School Nursing Practice* (NASN/ANA, 2001). Standards of practice guide a profession. "Standards are authoritative statements by which the nursing profession describes responsibilities for which its practitioners are accountable" (ANA, 1998, p. 1). For example, in the NASN/ANA standards, one identified outcome is that "interventions reflect current standards of school nursing practice" (NASN/ANA, 2001, p. 1). Standards and criteria are used to guide quality measurement. Nurses need to be familiar with these standards.

### Patterns for Providing School Nursing Services

Two administrative patterns are commonly used to provide nursing services in the school setting: specialized nursing services and generalized nursing services. **Specialized nursing services** are those provided by nurses who are employed to provide services to schools. These nurses are often employed by local boards of education and are accountable to school administrators. Some health departments have school-health units within the health department to provide specialized nursing services. These services are often provided on a contractual basis to the schools.

**Generalized nursing services** are those provided by nurses that serve the school on a part-time basis, as part of a generalized community health nursing program. They often work with all at-risk populations in their assigned area and are often employed by local health departments.

There is controversy about which pattern for delivering school nursing services is most appropriate. Clinical experience has shown that a variety of service delivery patterns can be used effectively to promote the health of the school community. Regardless of the administrative pattern used for delivering nursing services in the school setting, the nurse should establish strategies for ensuring that he or she is a sanctioned member of the school health team.

The activities of generalized and specialized school nurses vary among school systems. Some educational systems use

A view
from the field

## A DAY IN THE LIFE OF A SCHOOL NURSE

If you had told me 10 years ago that I would be working for a public school system, I would have said you were crazy! But here I am, in 1992, working in a field that I believe is truly on the "cutting edge" of health care—school nursing.

When I took this job, I really had no idea what I was getting into. In fact, my husband encouraged me to take this position because he thought that it would be a "fluff" position—supervising nurses as they handed out bandages—and that the vacation time looked good.

For the past five years, I have held the position of nursing supervisor for the Lawrence Public Schools in Lawrence, Mass.

Lawrence is a poor city of 63,000 people, known for its negative health status indicators and largely minority population. The public school population of 11,000 students is 77 percent minority, mostly Hispanic newcomers. Lawrence has the highest teen pregnancy rate and one of the worst drug abuse problems in Massachusetts. Those problems, combined with a 44 percent high school drop-out rate and the lowest basic skills scores in the state, make our youth some of the neediest in the country.

A solid grasp of the nursing process has been the cornerstone of my practice. In the first months of employment as the nursing supervisor for the school district, I undertook a complete needs assessment that included interviews with principals, nursing staff, and the community as a whole. I then invited these people to work with me on the Lawrence School Health Advisory Council. When the assessment was completed, I developed a plan for comprehensive health education and school health services, including school-based health centers at the high school, and at the elementary/middle level, developed and implemented a comprehensive health education program in grades K-12, integrated AIDS education into the health education program, and developed a comprehensive substance abuse program. I am proud to say that even with severe budget cuts, five years later, we are right on target.

What I have discovered is that school nursing is truly an opportunity to practice primary prevention at its best. It is exciting, challenging, and fun! Every day is different, so it is difficult to choose one day to describe my life.

This day begins at 7:30 AM. I need to deliver syringes and sharps containers to a middle school and make sure everything is in order for the school nurse to immunize sixth-grade students with the second dose of measles, mumps, rubella (MMR) vaccine. I have arranged for two other school nurses to help. There are about 100 students who need to be immunized today.

The next stop is an 8 AM meeting with my boss, the assistant superintendent of schools. I am meeting with him to bring him up to date on the Drug Free Schools Project. We have been fortunate this year to have received over $1 million in grants to develop and implement a comprehensive substance abuse prevention program in the schools. The project includes curriculum development, setting up student assistance teams, peer leadership, children of alcoholics support groups, parent education groups, teacher and administrator training, and policy development. Since I am the "health person" in the school district, anything to do with health, AIDS, drugs, sex, teen pregnancy, or violence gets directed to me. This is primary prevention!

It is now 9 AM. On the way to my office I stop at the community health center to meet with staff who serve the teen health center at the high school. I need to bring them up to date on Medicaid billing issues and new forms that were presented at a meeting with the state health department last week.

I arrive at my office that is located in a K-8 elementary school around 10 AM. There is a stack of messages waiting for me that need to be returned. I answer these calls. One of the calls is to a parent who needs bus transportation for her child who just had surgery. I need to approve all medical transportation. Another call is from the superintendent's office. "Send over copies of our AIDS curriculum...another school district is interested in what

Modified from Burton PT: A day in the life of a nurse: school nursing on cutting edge of prevention, *Am Nurse* 24:23, 1992, September.

the nurse in limited ways. Others use the nurse in a comprehensive manner, such as described in this chapter.

### Roles of the Nurse on the School Health Team

Roles of the school nurse vary and include carrying out a complex array of activities to promote health and prevent disease within a school community. Rustia's school health

promotion model (Figure 20-3) clearly illustrates the range of interventions used by nurses to promote healthy living and to improve quality of life. It also reflects the comprehensive nature of school nursing and can be used by the school nurse as a framework for articulating roles and functions. A school nurse who is able to clearly articulate his or her role and functions, and who demonstrates clinical ex-

*A view
from the field*

we are doing." They need the information yesterday! Another call is from a principal—she needs a nurse in the building every day for a child with a G-tube. Still another call is from one of the school nurses—there are 15 cases of chicken pox in her school today!

It is now 10:30 AM, and I need to prepare for a School Health Advisory Council meeting scheduled for this afternoon.

At noon, I attend a meeting of the Lawrence Violence Prevention Coalition. This community coalition was formed to develop a community response to increasing violence in the city. The question here, as in most community groups, is "What are the schools doing, and why are they not doing more?"

At 2 PM, the School Health Advisory Council meets. This council is made up of students, parents, teachers, school administrators, school nurses, as well as health and human services professionals from the community. This group of people provides me with the guidance and support I need to do my job. Because several parents on the council are more comfortable speaking Spanish, I meet with them 30 minutes before the meeting to provide them with an orientation to the agenda so that they will feel more comfortable and be able to provide input during the meeting.

At this council meeting, I present our health services budget as well as a review of the health services staffing pattern and health status of our kids. Today, I do not have good news to report. I have been instructed to present a level-funded budget to the school committee, but this actually means a budget cut. A nurse who left the system five months ago will probably not be replaced.

We have 1218 children with some type of health problem, an increase of more than 200 since last year. This includes 428 children with asthma, an increase of 125 students since last year. We also have a significant increase in the number of students with active seizure disorders, kidney disease, heart disease, and leukemia. The need for direct nursing services has increased with twice the number of children requiring medication in school this year.

Also with the mandates of Special Education, more children with complex needs are being brought into the system. The needs of these children range from intermittent catheterization and G-tube feedings to case management and clinical services. The council discusses my report in detail. They are concerned about decreases in staff with the increased need for services. Council members, including parents, offer to speak at upcoming school committee meetings in support of the health program.

It has been a busy day, but a good one. I believe that, at least for this day, I have shown how effective school nurses can be and what a vital role nurses play in bridging the gap between the health care and education communities. With the severe fiscal constraints faced by school districts, difficult decisions are made everyday. The purpose of the school system is to educate children. However, the basic health and safety needs of children must be met in order for them to learn. Because attitudes and health behaviors that school-age children develop will be carried into adulthood, the schools need to accept responsibility for educating the whole child.

School nurses play a vital role in helping the school meet this responsibility. They are truly on the cutting edge of health promotion and health services. They practice primary prevention at its best!

As a final note, I add that my husband now says I am the only person he knows who can take a perfectly simple job and make it complicated.

*Peg Trainor Burton is the nursing supervisor for the Lawrence Public Schools in Lawrence, Mass. A diploma graduate of St. Mary's School of Nursing in Clarksburg, W. Va., Burton earned a BSN at Duquesne University, Pittsburgh, and a master's degree at Boston University School of Nursing, where she specialized in community health nursing. She holds current certification as a family nurse practitioner. Burton is a member of ANA, the National Association of School Nurses, the American School Health Association, and the American Public Health Association.*

pertise to all members of the school health team, is more likely to be used appropriately than one who has trouble defining what it is a school nurse has to offer.

ADVOCATE. Many disadvantaged families have inadequate resources to obtain essential health care services for their children. The school nurse becomes an advocate for these families to help them obtain the health care they

need. This can involve linking families to resources or reaching out to families to assist them in understanding their child's health care needs. The nurse also may work with other health service providers to improve a child's access to specialized equipment or services, which in turn, may allow the child to attend school instead of being home schooled. It is not uncommon for the school nurse to

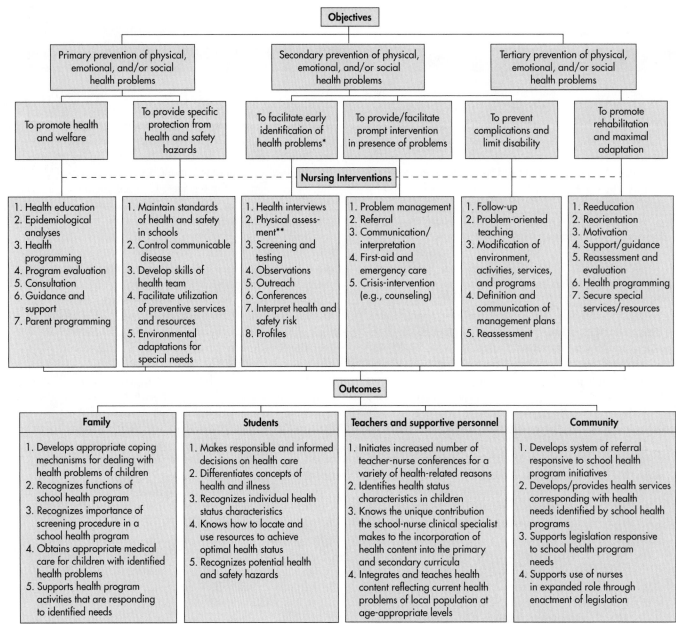

**Objectives**

**Primary prevention of physical, emotional, and/or social health problems**

**Secondary prevention of physical, emotional, and/or social health problems**

**Tertiary prevention of physical, emotional, and/or social health problems**

| To promote health and welfare | To provide specific protection from health and safety hazards | To facilitate early identification of health problems* | To provide/facilitate prompt intervention in presence of problems | To prevent complications and limit disability | To promote rehabilitation and maximal adaptation |

**Nursing Interventions**

| 1. Health education<br>2. Epidemiological analyses<br>3. Health programming<br>4. Program evaluation<br>5. Consultation<br>6. Guidance and support<br>7. Parent programming | 1. Maintain standards of health and safety in schools<br>2. Control communicable disease<br>3. Develop skills of health team<br>4. Facilitate utilization of preventive services and resources<br>5. Environmental adaptations for special needs | 1. Health interviews<br>2. Physical assessment**<br>3. Screening and testing<br>4. Observations<br>5. Outreach<br>6. Conferences<br>7. Interpret health and safety risk<br>8. Profiles | 1. Problem management<br>2. Referral<br>3. Communication/ interpretation<br>4. First-aid and emergency care<br>5. Crisis-intervention (e.g., counseling) | 1. Follow-up<br>2. Problem-oriented teaching<br>3. Modification of environment, activities, services, and programs<br>4. Definition and communication of management plans<br>5. Reassessment | 1. Reeducation<br>2. Reorientation<br>3. Motivation<br>4. Support/guidance<br>5. Reassessment and evaluation<br>6. Health programming<br>7. Secure special services/resources |

**Outcomes**

| **Family** | **Students** | **Teachers and supportive personnel** | **Community** |
| --- | --- | --- | --- |
| 1. Develops appropriate coping mechanisms for dealing with health problems of children<br>2. Recognizes functions of school health program<br>3. Recognizes importance of screening procedure in a school health program<br>4. Obtains appropriate medical care for children with identified health problems<br>5. Supports health program activities that are responding to identified needs | 1. Makes responsible and informed decisions on health care<br>2. Differentiates concepts of health and illness<br>3. Recognizes individual health status characteristics<br>4. Knows how to locate and use resources to achieve optimal health status<br>5. Recognizes potential health and safety hazards | 1. Initiates increased number of teacher-nurse conferences for a variety of health-related reasons<br>2. Identifies health status characteristics in children<br>3. Knows the unique contribution the school-nurse clinical specialist makes to the incorporation of health content into the primary and secondary curricula<br>4. Integrates and teaches health content reflecting current health problems of local population at age-appropriate levels | 1. Develops system of referral responsive to school health program initiatives<br>2. Develops/provides health services corresponding with health needs identified by school health programs<br>3. Supports legislation responsive to school health program needs<br>4. Supports use of nurses in expanded role through enactment of legislation |

*Health problem refers to physical, emotional, and/or social.

**Physical assessment includes thorough systems review as well as emotional, social, and developmental assessments when appropriate.

**FIGURE 20-3** Rustia's school health promotion model: delineation of nursing interventions and client outcomes. (From Rustia J: Rustia's school health promotion model, *J Sch Health* 52[2]:109, 1982).

identify environmental conditions that are unsafe, gaps in health education programming, or deficiencies in the delivery of personal health services. A concerned school nurse does not ignore these situations and advocates for health in the school setting.

As noted in *Healthy People 2010* there are many gaps in health care services to adolescents, and the school nurses frequently advocate for school and community-based adolescent health care services and funding for such services.

Health care services to adolescents often differ significantly from services needed by younger school-age children.

**CASEFINDER.** Casefinding is essential if these goals are to be accomplished. All personnel in the school system have a responsibility to identify as early as possible children at risk for physical, behavioral, social, or academic problems.

School nurses use various methods to identify at-risk children. School nurses can casefind through observation. Nurses observe children performing their daily school activities and interacting with peers and adults. For example, a school nurse may casefind for orthopedic problems by observing children walking down the hall between classes or during recess while playing. Eating lunch in the school cafeteria has helped other school nurses collect assessment data on children with poor dietary habits. Walking out on the playground during recess frequently assists school nurses in determining which children are having difficulty relating to their peers.

Teachers have frequent opportunities to observe the health status of students and play an important role in a health appraisal program. School nurses meet regularly with teachers to encourage them to regularly observe the health status of all students. For example, one teacher assisted the school nurse in identifying a child with an undiagnosed congenital heart defect. The teacher became concerned because a student in her class always "looked pale, tired easily, and had difficulty doing strenuous activity." The teacher shared her concerns with the school nurse, who helped link the family to a local pediatrician. Medical follow-up revealed that the child had a heart problem.

Screening programs are important casefinding tools. Screening programs such as height and weight measurements, hearing and vision tests, dental examinations, and immunization checks traditionally have been conducted in the school setting. In school-based clinics that provide primary health care services, comprehensive screening is done to identify children at risk for various health concerns such as scoliosis, urinary tract infections, anemia, STDs, teenage pregnancy, depression, and other mental health concerns.

School nurses find that by reviewing medical records, school health records, and absenteeism reports, they can frequently identify children who need follow-up. For example, one school nurse noted on school health records that at a routine blood pressure screening, a child's blood pressure had been elevated. The nurse did a repeat blood pressure measurement on the child and found that it was still elevated. She followed up by talking with the child's parents, found that there was a strong family history of hypertension, and assisted the family in locating a pediatrician for further follow-up.

Review of absenteeism records can help school nurses identify children at risk for future illnesses and absenteeism, and often, families that need nursing interventions. It is not unusual for families that are ineffectively dealing with stress to neglect family roles and responsibilities, such as ensuring regular school attendance by school-age children. Assisting these families to find coping strategies and problem-solving techniques that remove or diminish current stressors is pivotal in meeting the needs of their children.

**CASE MANAGER.** Case management is a model of practice that focuses on need assessment and planning a continuum of care for students and families (NASN, 1995). The nurse case manager traditionally ensures the provision for and evaluation of comprehensive school-based health

services and other related services for children. This role is an essential part of the school nurse's job because of the varied and continued contact and function he or she has in the community, school, and with children and families.

NASN believes that school nurses should have the expertise to be a successful case manager. This includes, but is not limited to, having the following knowledge and skills: knowledge about existing services for school-age children and their families; ability to develop a collaborated care plan based on professional standards of care; skills in continually coordinating all services for children and families, which includes understanding, selection, and obtainment of health-related services; and knowledge of evaluation procedures (NASN, 1995).

The school nurse as case manager could be instrumental in many situations where children need ongoing services for identified health concerns. This could be a child with a hard-to-manage seizure disorder or a child newly diagnosed with leukemia. Other children may be struggling with an attention deficit disorder or depression that requires coordination and collaboration with mental health services.

With the recent attention on school violence and the increasing number of school shootings that have both shocked and shattered school systems, families, and communities, it is imperative that the school nurse as a case manager takes school safety into consideration. This would include using the nursing process to identify and evaluate students who are angry; depressed; have a history of violent behavior, mental illness and/or drug use; have adjustment problems and/or low self-esteem; and demonstrate other at-risk behaviors.

### Stop and Think About It

What is your community doing to protect students and families from violence in elementary, middle, and high schools? What is the role of the nurse in these schools to assist in this endeavor?

The school nurse case manager could share knowledge about services available for students at-risk with the students and their families. Additionally, nurse case managers could assist in the selection of appropriate services for children and their families, collaborate with other related health team members to provide effective interventions, coordinate continuity of all services, and evaluate outcomes according to previously determined measurable criteria. Grabeel and Zaiger (1998) suggest that standards of school nursing practice aid in managing school health services systems effectively.

**COMMUNITY LIAISON.** School nurses must engage in community liaison activities to meet the needs of all school-age children. No school system has adequate resources to handle all the health problems experienced by the children it serves. Cooperative planning and collaboration between the educational system and other community agencies that provide services for children can serve to enhance the effectiveness of the school's health program.

Community involvement is essential during all stages of the health-planning process. Health programs that are conducted to fulfill health needs as identified by the community are far more successful than programs that ignore community priorities. Perceptions of health problems and community needs vary among communities. It is important for community health nurses working in the school setting to work in partnership with the community in addressing health needs.

Coordinating community activities can be rewarding. For example, working with others in parent-teacher organizations or community agencies can help the school nurse make the school health program more socially and culturally relevant. Community coordinating activities also expose school nurses to different viewpoints, which help nurses expand their range of solutions for addressing health needs. Such activities enhance creative thinking through stimulation by others, facilitate continuity of care, and increase community participation in health programming. Community interest groups are more motivated to implement a health program if they have participated in designing that health program.

CONSULTANT. Nurses bring to the school setting a unique set of skills that allow them to become valuable, contributing members of the school health team. Nurses have been prepared to assess comprehensively all the variables that influence a child's health status. Their understanding of normal growth and development, as well as disease processes, provides them with the knowledge needed for identifying both physical and psychosocial health problems and for determining how to handle health concerns. School personnel frequently ask school nurses questions about disease conditions such as diabetes, epilepsy, hepatitis, or scabies. They may question whether a child is ill, when to send a child home when he or she is not feeling well, or whether a child with a chronic condition should be allowed to participate in recreational activities.

School personnel often have questions and concerns about how to manage children with chronic health conditions and infectious conditions in the school setting. It is not uncommon for the school nurse to encounter fear and misconceptions about such conditions. Personnel often do not understand the etiology of communicable diseases or how to prevent the spread of these diseases. Illustrative of this, is a teacher who became so upset after she heard that one of her students had hepatitis that she moved the child's desk into the hall. The teacher was sure that everyone in the classroom would become ill because all she knew about this condition was that it was contagious. Once the nurse explained the etiology, mode of transmission, and disease process, the child was allowed to rejoin the classroom and the teacher expressed that he felt more comfortable in dealing with the condition. Appendix 11-3 summarizes some of the common communicable diseases encountered by community health nurses in the school settings.

The nurse is often used as a consultant by school personnel in dealing with health care issues involving the family. Family problems can affect a child's functioning in school and often these problems need to be addressed. Problem behavior such as poor school attendance, aggression, use of drugs, or withdrawal from school activities often signals that a child's family is having difficulty. The adolescent depicted in the following case scenario illustrates this point. The child in this case scenario had a consistently high absenteeism record until the school nurse provided family-centered nursing intervention.

**CASE Scenario** Ashley Babcock was a 14-year-old junior high school student who was missing an average of 2 days of school per week when the school social worker referred her to the school's nurse. Ashley had a functional heart murmur and her mother frequently encouraged her to stay home fearing her daughter might have a heart attack. The school social worker felt that Ashley's mother needed help with understanding how her fears were affecting Ashley's perceptions of her health as well as her school attendance and performance. Mrs. Babcock was very receptive to the nurse's visit and related to the nurse that she wasn't sure how to "care for Ashley properly" and that she has had increased fears for Ashley's health since her husband died from a heart attack a year ago. The nurse talked to Mrs. Babcock about her fears and Ashley's heart condition and encouraged her to speak to Ashley's cardiologist about her plan of care. The nurse also encouraged Mrs. Babcock to call her at school if she had additional questions. During the next few weeks the nurse contacted Mrs. Babcock weekly by phone and helped link Mrs. Babcock to resources in the community. Mrs. Babcock worked with a mental health counselor who helped her deal with her grief and her fears about Ashley's condition. She contacted Ashley's cardiologist and was much less fearful about Ashley's condition. The cardiologist had assured her that regular school activity was not a strain on Ashley's heart. Ashley's attendance record improved dramatically after her mother received the help she needed.

Extensive knowledge of community resources and the referral process is a unique skill the school nurse has to contribute in the school setting. Many families within school systems do not have a regular source of primary care and are not aware of available community health resources. The nurse can help link families to resources. An additional example of helping link families to resources follows:

**CASE Scenario** A student community health nurse came back to the health department following her visit to an inner-city junior high school. She was disturbed by the number of children who had obvious dental caries and questioned why their parents did not "care enough about them to obtain dental care." A staff nurse suggested to her that limited financial resources might be preventing many of these families from obtaining the care that was needed and suggested that they explore the situation further. When the student contacted the parents of these children, she found that financial difficulties as well as access to services were major problems. Most of the families could not afford dental care. One family was able to afford dental services but could not find a dentist who was willing to care for their daughter who was mentally retarded. The student made the families aware of the dental clinic at the health department and helped link them with possible resources in the community, including a sliding scale dental clinic through the university. Two families immediately made appointments at the health department clinic. The student was able to find a local dentist who was willing to provide care to children who were mentally retarded. Both the families and school personnel were appreciative of these referrals.

EPIDEMIOLOGIST. Nurses must become epidemiologists (see Chapter 11). They need to identify *aggregates at risk* to plan effective school health programs. In this way health services in a school setting can be designed to meet the needs of the total school population. An epidemiological approach to school health is a prevention-oriented approach.

School nurses use the epidemiological process to identify factors that influence the health status of school-age populations. The characteristics of populations are studied to determine the most appropriate intervention strategies to meet their needs. How this is done is illustrated in the following situation.

**CASE Scenario** One school nurse used health record information, data obtained during home visits, contact with students in the health clinic, and census tract information to substantiate the need for a breakfast program in the school system. The combined information from all of these data sources revealed that the children in this school had significant nutritional deficiencies, and many were not eating breakfast before coming to school (e.g., there was a high prevalence of nutritional anemia among the children). These data showed that a large percentage of the children came from impoverished families that had difficulty meeting the families' basic needs. When the school nurse shared these facts with the school administrator, she helped the nurse apply for federal funds that would support a breakfast program.

In this situation the nurse used a prevention-oriented approach to prevent nutritional problems. Prevention improves quality of life and is far less costly than curative care.

Accurate and complete record keeping is essential for epidemiological studies. A record system must be designed to allow for complete, accurate, and efficient recording of data. Each child should have an up-to-date, cumulative school health record, and records of children with special health problems should be tagged. A tagging system allows for quick analysis of the needs of the population as a whole. For example, if a number of children in a school have specific health problems (e.g., obesity, lack of exercise), health education, changes in the health curriculum, or counseling may be warranted. *Nurses need to record what they have accomplished so that nursing outcomes can be documented, measured, and recognized.*

Evaluation is part of the epidemiological process and it is imperative for community health nurses in the school setting to evaluate the results of their interventions. When nurses work with aggregates, the epidemiological process is the tool that most appropriately helps them examine the results of their group intervention strategies.

HEALTH COUNSELOR. Children and youth are currently facing difficult and complex health problems and concerns. They are exposed much earlier than their previous counterparts to issues such as sexuality concerns, varying lifestyles, pressures from peers to use alcohol and drugs, decisions regarding future career planning in a highly unstable employment environment, and family disruption and disorganization. Often they have knowledge about these issues but lack experience in dealing with them. They have a need to discuss their feelings and emotions with a nonthreatening adult, and this is often the school nurse.

The school nurse does not evaluate a student's academic performance, which helps students view her or him as less threatening. The school nurse is frequently the first member of the school health team to identify a student's need for counseling, and in many cases is the person that the student approaches about the need for such services. The nurse helps link the student to appropriate community resources.

The nurse in the school uses the family-centered nursing process to determine appropriate management goals and intervention strategies. When the child visits the health center, the nurse assesses the situation to identify actual as well as potential needs. If the nurse has insufficient data, problems can easily be missed and health care needs go unmet. The case scenario that follows illustrates the need to collect adequate data to diagnose a child's actual health problems and to plan a variety of intervention strategies to resolve these problems.

**CASE Scenario** Lindsey Smith, a first-grader, was lying on the cot in the health clinic when the community health nurse arrived for her weekly visit. The school secretary reported that Lindsey had just come to the office crying because she had a stomachache. Sobbing, Lindsey shared with the nurse that, "My stomach hurts." As the nurse examined the child she noticed that Lindsey stopped crying with a little attention. When asked if her parents knew she did not feel well this morning, her answer was, "My mother doesn't love me anymore. She went away." The nurse encouraged Lindsey to verbalize her feelings of rejection and let her know that she understood how much it hurts to lose someone you love. Although a hug provided the support Lindsey needed to return to class, the nurse realized that Lindsey needed other types of assistance to cope with her situation. With Lindsey's teachers, the nurse discussed the situation and possible interventions to reduce stress. The nurse also contacted Lindsey's father. He was very angry that his wife had left and found it extremely difficult to talk to his children about what was happening. He was concerned about how his separation was affecting his children and agreed to seek family counseling at a local mental health clinic. Lindsey's mother never returned home to her family. However, Lindsey's father, learned how to cope with the family situation and his anger. This, coupled with support from an empathic teacher, helped Lindsey function more effectively in the school setting.

Younger school children often verbalize their feelings more readily than older children. Because one of the developmental tasks of adolescence is to achieve emotional independence from parents and other adults, students at the junior or senior high level may test the school nurse before they share their real concerns. One such case is described here:

**CASE** *Scenario* Noel, a 14-year-old junior high student, wandered into the health clinic during class breaks 3 weeks in a row with minor physical complaints. Finally he asked the nurse if he could talk with her alone. He wanted to know "how a person could tell if he had a STD." Further discussion revealed that Noel was having nocturnal emissions and thought he had gonorrhea because he had learned in a health class that a purulent discharge occurred with this disease. Noel had never heard about nocturnal emissions and was fearful that he had gonorrhea. He was greatly relieved when he found out that what he was experiencing was normal. The nurse encouraged him to return to the clinic if he had other questions and suggested that his father might be able to talk with him about other developmental changes that occur during adolescence. The need to discuss normal developmental changes, as well as to review how STDs are transmitted, was also shared with the teacher responsible for the eighth-grade health class.

Health counseling opportunities such as the ones described above are numerous and present in all school settings. Nurses who are attuned to the developmental needs and the social characteristics of the population they are serving will not be "Band-Aid pushers." Rather, they will take time to find out from other school personnel which students have health problems and will be alert for students who need health counseling.

HEALTH EDUCATOR. Health education has been discussed as an integral part of an CSHP. Health education is an integral part of the school nursing role. Through health education activities, school nurses help prepare children and their families, school personnel, and the community to make sound health decisions.

NASN views health education as an important function for nurses in the school setting. The organization believes that the school nurse should be involved in a broad range of health education activities. Box 20-2 provides Teaching Tips that reflect this belief and provides examples of health education activities carried out by nurses in the school setting. Health education promotes the well-being of students, families, and the school community. Schools are not only places for health education but also places where our nation's children and young adults spend a major portion of their lives.

HOME VISITOR. Parents are vital members of the school health team. They are responsible for the health care of their children, and they greatly influence their children's health practices. Contact with parents in the home environment is an effective way of increasing their understanding and involvement with their child's health problems. Home visits help demonstrate that the school nurse cares about families and wants to include parents in their child's plan of care.

At times home visiting is the only way to obtain a comprehensive picture of a child's health status. This is particularly true if the nurse perceives that family dynamics are adversely affecting a child's level of functioning. Assessment of parent-child relationships is best obtained in the family's natural setting. Observations of how the child is physically handled, of environmental conditions, and of interactions between children, parents, and siblings are more easily assessed in the home environment. These observations provide a different type of data than a conference with a parent in the health clinic.

The school nurse cannot possibly visit at home every child served in the school system. Children who manifest needs or difficulties such as the following should receive priority for home visits:
- History of many absences as a result of illness
- Behavioral problems that interfere with academic functioning or that adversely affect social relationships with peers
- Adjustment difficulties related to a chronic condition such as diabetes, epilepsy, heart defects, or obesity
- Suspected child abuse or neglect
- Special programming needs in relation to a developmental disability
- Lack of medical follow-up on an identified health problem
- Pregnancy
- Frequent exposure to infectious diseases

Home visiting can be rewarding and extremely beneficial. It frequently is the key that opens the door to a happier

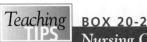

## BOX 20-2
### Nursing Opportunities for Health Education in the School Setting

### Advocate

School nurses act as advocates for sound health education practices within the school and the larger community. They work with school personnel to ensure that certified health education teachers are employed by the school district. They also lobby for a planned, comprehensive, sequential pre-K to 12 curriculum, based on students' needs and current and emerging societal and health trends. Additionally, they lobby in the community to promote community action for health. This action might include health education activities that promote healthy lifestyles or contact with governmental officials to encourage increased funding for school health education.

### Classroom Instruction

School nurses provide formal health instruction within the classroom on a variety of subjects such as health careers, substance abuse, violence prevention, consumer self-help, and sexuality. They also may provide formal health instruction for parents and other community residents within classes open to the community. Some school districts, for example, offer health career and consumer self-help classes after school hours to community residents. Additionally, the school nurse is involved in providing formal instruction to employees, especially in relation to universal precautions for bloodborne pathogens. Generally, the school nurse does not assume total responsibility for teaching a health class unless she or he was specifically hired for that purpose. Usually the nurse guest lectures or assumes responsibility for a health unit within a class.

### Client Teaching

Nurses in the school setting work with several client groups, including students, teachers, parents, and communities. In relation to these client groups, they have numerous health instruction opportunities. The school nurse, for example, would help a 14-year-old junior high student to understand body changes during adolescence after frequent visits to the health clinic with menstrual cramps. Or she or he would talk with individual teachers about the need for medical follow-up after a health screening for hypertension. Additionally, the school nurse would talk with parents about the neurological signs and symptoms of brain concussion if their child was hit on the head by a swing in the playground. On a broader level, the school nurse might provide health instruction for a group of community residents who expressed an interest in learning about resources to assist with the care of elderly parents.

### Curriculum Planning

School nurses actively participate in planning and evaluating a school health curriculum that addresses major community needs. They also assist school personnel to select age-appropriate, culturally relevant instructional materials that are scientifically sound. Frequently they develop an instructional resource file to help teachers address common health issues in the classroom.

### Resource Person

School nurses frequently consult with teachers, parents, and school administrators about concerns they may have about their own health status or the health status of one of the children in the school. They also consult with teachers who request assistance with developing a health education class. Additionally, they provide inservice programming for all staff regarding student health concerns, or for parents who are interested in gaining knowledge about what their children are learning in school.

### Role Modeling

School nurses can educate students, staff, and parents by role modeling positive health behaviors. They might reinforce nutritional instruction by the foods they select for lunch. Or they might promote healthy relationship building by the way they interact with others. They may also role model effective infectious disease control measures. It is important for the school nurse to recognize that their health actions can significantly influence the health actions of others.

Modified from Bradley BJ: The school nurse as health educator, *J Sch Health* 67:3-8, 1997; Proctor ST, Lordi SL, Zaiger DS: *School nursing practice: roles and standards,* Scarborough, Me, 1993, National Association of School Nurses, Inc.

---

life for many children. The following case scenario describes how a home visit helped one 8-year-old child positively increase her interactions with peers:

**CASE Scenario** Tammie Baxter was referred to the school nurse because she had a pronounced body odor. Her peers shunned her, and she appeared to be a lonely child. Tammie's teacher had many questions about her home environment and the health status of her parents. She had heard that Tammie's father was ill as a result of complications of diabetes. A very receptive mother answered the door when the school nurse made her first home visit. The nurse discovered that a family of seven was living in a five-room home that was composed of a living room, a kitchen, two bedrooms, and a bath. All five Baxter children, ages 8, 6, 4, 2, and 1, were sleeping on mattresses on the floor in one bedroom. Tammie smelled like urine, not because she was ill, but because two of her siblings had enuresis. She had limited clothes because the family was having severe financial problems. Tammie's difficulties with personal hygiene were resolved quickly once her mother discovered how the other children were treating her. A referral was made to a community clothes closet so that Tammie could be dressed like her peers. Tammie's teacher was amazed at how quickly her personal hygiene changed after this referral. A little extra attention from the teacher also helped alter Tammie's relationships with her classmates.

A long-term helping relationship between the Baxter family and the school nurse evolved from this one simple teacher referral.

TEAM MEMBER. No one discipline can meet the needs of all the school-age children. Team cooperation and collaboration are essential for children to receive the health services they deserve. The school nurse who has a "me" philosophy rather than a "we" philosophy will quickly become frustrated and will find that it is impossible to achieve school health goals.

Successful school nurses function within the framework of the total school health program, working cooperatively with other school personnel. Understanding the roles of each member of the school team can facilitate planning and implementation of nursing services. The role definitions presented in Table 20-2 are guidelines. When entering a new school system, every nurse should spend time identifying specified role responsibilities for each discipline in his or her school district. For an interdisciplinary team to function effectively, all team members must define how they can integrate their specific skills into an effective group effort that emphasizes a common endeavor. No team effort will be successful unless the central figures on the team are the child and involved family.

RESEARCHER. The majority of research about the effectiveness of health care is focused on medical care rather than nursing care. At this time, "there is minimal research-based information about school nursing services to provide the underpinnings for statements that will survive scrutiny" (Bradley, 1998, p. 53).

To improve services provided to elementary, middle, and high school students, it is imperative to conduct nursing research about school health services, a recognized specialty practice in nursing. Therefore it is critical that nurses who work in school settings have the necessary skills to assist in or conduct nursing research. Because of the collaborative nature of health services provided in school-based clinics, the research team may be composed of individuals from many disciplines.

There are several barriers to conducting school nursing research. These include, but are not limited to, the special challenges of using minors and protecting them from injury during research endeavors, the need to protect confidentiality of students, and the lack of consistent nomenclature in school nursing. The call for parental/guardian and school administrative approval; the desire to have faculty and staff support and involvement; the ownership of data and study results; and the economic, time, and feasibility constraints

of the research also present challenges to a school research team (Bradley, 1998).

These challenges should not discourage the school nurse from participating in school health research. Information gleaned from research studies may provide the school nurse with critical information in meeting student needs and improving both school nursing and related health care services. In addition, nursing interventions can be evaluated for both appropriateness and cost effectiveness through research. Identifying health outcomes can provide data that support the value of school nursing services.

## PRACTICAL TIPS FOR ROLE IMPLEMENTATION

Implementing multiple and varied roles is a formidable task. It is important for school nurses to avoid panic or withdrawal when they do not initially accomplish their goals. It takes time to develop a meaningful role in any setting. Provided below are some suggestions for facilitating role implementation in the school setting.

### Define Your Philosophy of Nursing Practice

If school nurses cannot articulate the role of the nurse in the school health program, they cannot expect other members of the health care team to use them as they would like to be used. Reviewing the literature devoted to school nursing and the school health policies developed by your agency will provide you with information needed to formulate a philosophy of practice with which you can feel comfortable.

### Study Your Community

Understanding the needs of the population you are serving is essential. Children, families, and school personnel will respond more quickly to your suggestions if you demonstrate a sensitivity to their concerns and if you support your comments with data. Review the students' health records to identify their pressing health problems. Analyze census tract data to determine the characteristics of the families in the school district. Talk with students and teachers as you walk around the school building. Avoid sitting in the health clinic. Leave the school setting and drive through the area in which your school is located. Do a community analysis (see Chapters 3 and 14).

### Contact Key People

A school nurse who takes the initiative to contact school personnel and community groups responsible for the implementation of the school health program is more likely to become involved quickly than one who functions in isolation. Meet with the school principal before school starts. Explain your role and determine a time when you can orient teachers to the nursing services you have to offer. Find out the name of the president of the parent teacher organization (PTA) and the student health council. A telephone

**TABLE 20-2**

*Role Descriptions for Selected Members of the School Health Team*

| DISCIPLINE | ROLE DESCRIPTION |
|---|---|
| Principals | School administrators who are responsible for planning and providing direction for all activities carried out to meet the goals of the school, including nursing services. |
| Teachers | Staff members who are responsible for the educational aspects of the school program. Teachers enhance the total school health program by conducting health education activities in the classroom and by identifying children who have physical and emotional health problems that impede learning. |
| Teacher consultants | Pupil personnel specialists* who have advanced training for handling educational programming for children with special learning needs such as reading problems, mental disabilities, and emotional disturbances. |
| Teachers, homebound | Pupil personnel teachers, specially trained to deal with physical disabilities and the educational implications of these conditions. These persons work in the home with children who have been certified by a physician as being unable to attend school. These individuals provide both educational instruction and counseling services for homebound students. |
| School social workers | Pupil personnel specialists who provide direct counseling services for a child and family, if the child is demonstrating adjustment difficulties in the school setting. School social workers apply the principles and methods of social casework to help students to enhance their social and emotional adjustment and to adapt to change. The primary purpose of their intervention is to reduce impediments to learning. These individuals are often used as resource persons by all other members of the school health team. |
| Screening technicians | Pupil personnel staff trained to identify particular health problems, usually vision and hearing difficulties, through the use of screening tests. |
| Volunteers | Lay staff who receive in-service education to carry out defined tasks for other staff members. Responsibilities should relate to the in-service training they have received. Careful selection, training, and supervision by professional staff is a must if these individuals are to be used successfully in the school setting. |
| Therapists, physical | Pupil personnel specialists who treat muscular disabilities of children on a prescriptive order from the child's physician. Their services are designed to enable students to improve their physical health status so that their physical health problems do not impede learning. |
| Therapists, speech | Pupil personnel specialists who work with children who have difficulty producing and combining certain sounds in words, who are unable to speak with reasonable fluency, who speak with an abnormally pitched voice, or who have physical anomalies such as cerebral palsy. Speech therapists help children to develop normal speech patterns that help them to more effectively develop social relationships and to advance academically. |
| School psychologists | Pupil personnel specialists whose major responsibility is to determine the reasons for a child's inability to learn. These specialists are often known as the school diagnosticians because the primary purpose of their service is to identify or diagnose causes of learning problems. These individuals use psychological tests, such as IQ and personality tests, during the psychological assessment. Parental permission must be obtained before a child can be tested by these specialists. The amount of direct counseling a psychologist does with a child varies from one school to another. Usually, however, this person functions as a consultant to other school personnel. Psychologists in other settings are often more involved in direct counseling services. |

Modified from Jackson County Intermediate School District: *Special education services available to Jackson County,* Jackson, Miss, undated, The School District.
*Pupil personnel division—a special service division of a local board of education. Pupil personnel specialists in this division are accountable to the superintendent of schools.

call to these individuals may open the doors to the community and the student body.

## Demonstrate Your Skills

The best way to help others understand what it is you do is to show them what you can do. Follow up quickly on the referrals sent to you by other school personnel. Share with them the results of your interventions. A nurse who too quickly states that an activity is not the nurse's responsibility is apt to make other members of the team hesitant to use him or her. Often the nurse is requested to provide first aid or to inspect for communicable disease because individuals making these requests are afraid to handle these situations. Respond to their concerns by first caring for the children and then providing school personnel with information so that they can handle these situations in the future.

## Communicate with All Members of the School Health Team

Do not wait for others to come to you. Relate with teachers in their lounge and in their classroom. Ask questions about the students that will help you determine where your services are most needed. Share in writing or in person when you have followed up on a referral. Use the bulletin board to provide health information to students. *Talk with the school secretary.* She or he probably knows the students and their families as well as any other person in the building.

## Organize Your Activities

A school nurse who just "lets things happen" frequently does not accomplish goals. Establish a calendar of activities for the year. Be specific about the goals you want to accomplish. Know when you will orient the teachers to your services, when you will provide in-service education, when you will review student records, and when you will follow up on student health problems. The school nurse must develop a follow-up system. *A calendar is a must.* If you need to, plan your time.

## Set Priorities

Setting priorities is discussed in Chapter 24 as a nursing management function. A nurse cannot be all things to all people. Identify what needs to be done and then determine what you can handle, considering the time you have available. Request consultation from the school health team to determine priorities significant to the needs of the population being served.

## Document Your Activities

People respond favorably to concrete data. Keep a daily record of your activities. Use these records with others to substantiate what you have done, to support the need to set priorities, and to document the need for a new health program or changes in the existing health program. *Remember, changes generally do not occur when concrete data are lacking.*

## SUMMARY

Historically, community health nurses have assumed a major role in planning health services for school-age children. Currently they work with this population group in a variety of settings such as the home, the school, clinics, and residential settings for children with special needs. A family-centered, prevention-oriented, interdisciplinary approach is the most effective way to meet the needs of school-age children, regardless of the setting in which the nurse is functioning.

Community health nurses who work with school-age children encounter an array of physical, psychosocial, cultural, environmental, and developmental health problems and concerns. A well-organized, comprehensive health care program that takes into consideration the developmental needs and characteristics of children is essential if youth are to reach their maximum potential.

Because most children attend school, the school is a logical environment in which to promote the health of all children. The role of the community health nurse in the school health program has been evolving since the turn of the century. The school nurse role is an advocate, a casefinder, a case manager, a health counselor, a health educator, an epidemiologist, a consultant, a community health planner and coordinator, and a researcher. Teamwork is essential for successful implementation of these roles, and central figures on the team are the child and his or her family.

Working with elementary, middle school, and high school children and their families can be challenging and rewarding. Nurses who have a philosophy of nursing that stresses the need to help others help themselves, and focuses on the client's strengths, find school nursing particularly rewarding.

School nursing is an exciting, rewarding field of nursing practice that provides numerous opportunities for creative, independent functioning. The needs of the population being served; community resources; patterns for delivery of service; and federal, state, and local funding and regulations influence how each of these nurses functions.

## CRITICAL THINKING
*exercise*

Considering the characteristics of the students in the high school you attended and the school environment, discuss the health needs of this group of adolescents and strategies you would implement to address these needs. Additionally, identify factors in that environment that would facilitate or hinder the implementation of health education efforts, health services programming, and environmental engineering strategies.

## REFERENCES

Allensworth D, Kolbe J: The comprehensive school health program: exploring an expanded concept, *J Sch Health* 57:409-412, 1987.

Allensworth D, Wyche J, Lawson E, et al., editors: *Defining a comprehensive school health program: an interim statement*, Washington, DC, 1995, National Academy Press.

American Nurses Association (ANA): *Standards of clinical nursing practice*, ed 2, Washington, DC, 1998, American Nurses Publishing.

Baker C: School health policy issues, *Nurs Health Care* 15:178-184, 1994.

Bradley BJ: The school nurse as health educator, *J Sch Health* 67:3-8, 1997.

Bradley BJ: Establishing a research agenda for school nursing, *J Sch Health* 68:53-61, 1998.

Brainard AM: *The evolution of public health nursing*, Philadelphia, 1922, Saunders.

Burton PT: A day in the life of a nurse: school nursing on cutting edge of prevention, *Am Nurse* 24:23, 1992.

Centers for Disease Control and Prevention (CDC): *School health programs: an investment in our future: at-a-glance, 1995,* Atlanta, 1995, CDC.

Comer JP: Environmental health: the psychosocial climate. In Wallace HM, Patrick K, Parcel GS, et al., editors: *Principles and practices of student health,* vol II, Oakland, Calif, 1992, Third Party Publishing.

Cromwell GE: *The health of the school child,* Philadelphia, 1946, Saunders.

Dock LL: School nurse experiment in New York, *Am J Nurs* 3(2):108-110, 1902.

Friedrich MJ: 25 years of school-based health centers, *JAMA* 281:781-782, 1999.

Fryer G, Igoe J: Functions of school nurses and health assistants in U.S. school health programs, *J Sch Health* 66:55-58, 1996.

Grabeel J, Zaiger D: Utilizing standards of nursing practice for effective school nursing management, *J Sch Nurs* 14(2):47-48, 1998.

Hawkins JW, Hayes ER, Corliss CP: School nursing in America—1902-1994: a return to public health nursing, *Public Health Nurs* 11(6):416-425, 1994.

Igoe JB: Environmental health: the physical environment. In Wallace HM, Patrick K, Parcel GS, et al., editors: *Principles and practices of student health,* vol II, Oakland, Calif, 1992, Third Party Publishing.

Igoe J, Parcel G: Contemporary issues of school health: mechanisms for change. In Wallace HM, Patrick K, Parcel GS, et al., editors: *Principles and practices of student health,* vol II, Oakland, Calif, 1992, Third Party Publishing.

Jackson County Intermediate School District: *Special education services available to Jackson County,* Jackson, Miss, undated, The School District.

Katz J, Green E: *Managing quality: a guide to system-wide performance management in health care,* St Louis, 1997, Mosby.

Modrcin-McCarthy MA, Dalton M: Responding to Healthy People 2000: depression in our youth, common yet misunderstood, *Issues Comprehensive Pediatr Nurs* 19(4):275-290, 1996.

Modrcin-Talbott MA, Pullen L, Barnes A, et al.: Childhood anger: so common yet so misunderstood, *J Child Adolescent Psych Nurs* 11(2):69-73, 1998.

Modrcin-Talbott MA, Pullen L, Zandstra K, et al.: A study of self-esteem among well adolescents: seeking a new direction, *Issues Comprehensive Pediatr Nurs* 21(4):229-241, 1998.

Morten H: The London public-school nurse, *Am J Nurs* 1(4):274-276, 1901.

Nader PR: Comprehensive school health. In Wallace HM, Patrick K, Parcel GS, et al., editors: *Principles and practices of student health,* vol II, Oakland, Calif, 1992, Third Party Publishing.

National Association of School Nurses (NASN): *Philosophy of school health services and school nursing,* Scarborough, Me, 1988, NASN.

National Association of School Nurses (NASN): *NASN position statement. Case management,* Scarborough, Me, 1995, NASN.

National Association of School Nurses (NASN): *NASN position statement. Coordinated school health program,* Scarborough, Me, 1999, NASN.

National Association of School Nurses (NASN)/American Nurses Association (ANA): *Scope and Standards of Professional School Nursing Practice,* Washington, DC, 2001, American Nurses Publishing.

Office of Disease Prevention and Health Promotion: *School health: findings from evaluated programs,* Washington, DC, 1993, US Government Printing Office.

Passarelli C: School nursing trends for the future, *J Sch Health* 64:141-146, 1994.

Policy Studies Associates: Protecting the privacy of student education records, *J Sch Health* 67:139-140, 1997.

Proctor ST, Lordi SL, Zaiger DS: *School nursing practice: roles and standards,* Scarborough, Me, 1993, National Association of School Nurses, Inc.

Pullen L, Modrcin-Talbott MA, Graf E: Adolescent depression: important facts that matter, *J Child Adolesc Psych Nurs* 13(2), 2000.

Resnicow K, Allensworth D: Conducting a comprehensive school health program, *J Sch Health* 66:59-63, 1996.

Rogers L: The nurse in the public school, *Am J Nurs* 5(11):764-773, 1905.

Rustia J: Rustia school health promotion model, *J Sch Health* 52(2):108-115, 1982.

Shattuck L: *Report of the Sanitary Commission of Massachusetts,* New York, 1850, Dutton & Wentworth.

Stone EJ, Perry CL, Luepker RV: Synthesis of cardiovascular behavioral research for youth health promotion, *Health Educ Q* 16:155-169, 1989.

Struthers LR: *The school nurse,* New York, 1917, Putnam.

US Department of Health and Human Services (USDHHS): *School health: findings from evaluated programs,* Washington, DC, 1993, US Government Printing Office.

US Department of Health and Human Services (USDHHS): *Healthy People 2010: conference edition,* Washington, DC, 2000, US Government Printing Office.

Wong DL: *Whaley and Wong's nursing care of infants and children,* ed 6, St Louis, 2000, Mosby.

## SELECTED BIBLIOGRAPHY

Caccamo JM: Sharing the vision: healthy, achieving students. What can schools do? *J Sch Health* 70(5):216-218, 2000.

Farrior KC, Engelke MK, Collins SC, et al.: A community pediatric prevention partnership linking schools, providers, and tertiary care services, *J Sch Health* 70(3):79-83, 2000.

Juhn G, Tang J, Piessens P, et al.: Community learning: the reach for health nursing program-middle school collaboration, *J Nurs Educ* 38(5):215-221, 1999.

Kaplan DW, Brindis CD, Phibbs SL, et al.: A comparison study of an elementary school-based health center, *Arch Pediatric Adolesc Med* 153:235-243, 1999.

Koppelman J, Lear JG: The new child health insurance expansions: how will school-based health centers fit in? *J Sch Health* 68(10):441-446.

Oros MT, Perry LA, Heller BR: School-based health services: an essential component of neighborhood transformation, *Fam Comm Health* 23(2):31-35, 2000.

Parker VG, Logan BN: Students, parents, and teachers—perceptions of health needs of school-age children: implications for nurse practitioners, *Fam Comm Health* 23(2):62-71, 2000.

Perry CS, Toole KA: Impact of school nurse case management on asthma control in school-age children, *J Sch Health* 70(7):303-304, 2000.

Rienzo BA, Button JW, Wald KD: Politics and the success of school-based health centers, *J Sch Health* 70(8):331-336, 2000.

Wyatt TH, Novak JC: Collaborative partnerships: a critical element in school health programs, *Fam Comm Health* 23(2):1-11, 2000.

# 21

# Occupational Health Nursing

*Sandra L. McGuire*

## OBJECTIVES

*Upon completion of this chapter, the reader should be able to:*

1. Discuss the *Healthy People 2010* national health objectives for occupational health.
2. Summarize the purpose, intents, and mandates of the Occupational Safety and Health Act of 1970.
3. Discuss the evolution of occupational health nursing in the United States.
4. Describe recommended educational preparation and professional opportunities for the occupational health nurse.
5. Understand the objectives and scope of practice of the occupational health nurse.
6. Discuss the leading work-related diseases/injuries in the United States.
7. Discuss communicable diseases that are contemporary workplace concerns.
8. Discuss smoking and violence as occupational health concerns.
9. Understand some major health concerns of agricultural workers.

## KEY TERMS

Agricultural workers
American Association of Occupational Health Nurses (AAOHN)
Cardiovascular diseases
Dr. Alice Hamilton
Hearing loss
Migrant farm workers
Migrant health centers
Minority health
Musculoskeletal disorders

National Institute for Occupational Safety and Health (NIOSH)
Neurotoxic disorders
NIOSH Education and Research Centers
Occupational cancers
Occupational history
Occupational lung diseases
Occupational Safety and Health Act of 1970
Occupational Safety and Health Administration (OSHA)

Occupational skin disorder (OSD)
Occupational stressors
Occupational surveillance
Psychological disorders
Reproductive disorders
Scope of practice
*Standards of Occupational and Environmental Health Nursing*
Ada Mayo Stewart
Traumatic injury

*Occupational health is the application of public health principles and medical, nursing and engineering practice for the purpose of conserving, promoting and restoring the health and effectiveness of workers through their place of employment.*

MARY LOUISE BROWN, *OCCUPATIONAL HEALTH NURSING*, NEW YORK, 1956, SPRINGER, P. 1.

The first census in 1790 showed the United States to be an agricultural nation. However, this rapidly changed with the Industrial Revolution. Between 1870 and 1910 the U.S. population rose 132%, but the number of persons working in industry rose almost 400% (Morris, 1976, p. 109). Today there are more than 130 million workers in the United States (National Institute for Occupational Safety and Health [NIOSH], 2000a).

The American workforce is diverse, representing all socioeconomic levels, ethnic and racial groups, and cultural and religious backgrounds. Women comprise 46% of the labor force, 23% of the workforce are minorities, and the median age of the American worker is 37.9 years (U.S. Department of Health and Human Services [USDHHS], 1995, p. 74). Americans spend almost one third of their time at work, and work has a profound impact on a person's physical, emotional, and social well-being (NIOSH, 1995, p. 2; Sophie, 2000, p. 125).

The working population is basically a well adult population. Occupational health professionals strive to make the workplace safe and healthy and emphasize primary prevention activities such as health education, health promotion, and worker protection. This chapter addresses occupational health in the United States and the role of the occupational health nurse (OHN) in promoting worker health.

## OCCUPATIONAL HEALTH IN THE UNITED STATES

By the mid-1800s many Americans worked under unsafe or unhealthy conditions, and workers rallied for shorter work days, health and safety measures, and child labor laws. It was common to have young children employed in the workplace and almost half of all employees in New England factories were children aged 7 to 16 years. In 1836 Massachusetts became the first state to enact a child labor law. Massachusetts continued a leadership role in occupational health and in 1850 became the first state to study occupational health; in 1879, the first to pass legislation requiring factory safety inspections; and in 1886, the first to require reporting of industrial accidents.

Around the turn of the twentieth century, occupational medicine and occupational health nursing began to emerge in the United States. The Homestake Mining Company sponsored the first industrial medical department in 1887 (U.S. Department of Labor [USDL], 1977, p. 15), and about the same time some companies began hiring nurses. Public awareness of occupational health hazards was increasing, and physicians began to write about occupational disease.

The federal government issued its first major report on occupational safety and health in 1903 (USDL, 1977, pp. 15-16). About this time a pioneer in occupational medicine and occupational epidemiology, **Dr. Alice Hamilton,** began her work. In 1910 she became the chair of the Occupational Disease Commission in Illinois; it was the first such commission in the country. In 1911 she was chosen to head the newly formed *Federal Occupational Disease Commission*.

Dr. Hamilton achieved international recognition for her research and writings on occupational diseases and conditions. She is considered by many to be the founder of occupational medicine in this country (NIOSH, 2000b). Among her numerous publications are the classic *Industrial Poisons in the United States* (1925), considered to be the first occupational medicine text in the United States, and *Exploring the Dangerous Trades: The Autobiography of Alice Hamilton, M.D.* (1943). Dr. Hamilton lived a long and remarkable life. During her time the emergence of labor unions and the formation of the U.S. Department of Labor placed new emphasis on occupational health and safety. Dr. Hamilton died the year that the Occupational Safety and Health Act of 1970 was passed, at the age of 101.

*Workers' compensation legislation* was a major influence in shaping the nature of occupational health (Rosenstock,

Landrigan, 1986, p, 338). In the early 1900s work-related illness became a growing concern among workers (Bale, 1988, p. 499), and workers began to take a firm stand on the right to be compensated for job-related illness, injury, or disability. As a result state workers' compensation legislation began to emerge. The first workers' compensation acts met with much resistance from employers, and many were ruled to be unconstitutional. In 1911 New Jersey passed the first workers' compensation act to be upheld by the courts, and other states quickly followed. Workers' compensation covers the cost of medical care and rehabilitation and provides lost wages during periods of disability due to work-related diseases and injuries. It was an impetus to the development of industrial health services in the workplace (Haag, Glazner, 1992, p. 56).

In the early 1900s much was happening in occupational health. Cornell University Medical College established an occupational disease clinic in 1910, and others soon opened around the country (Felton, 1976, p. 814). The U.S. Department of Labor was elevated to a cabinet-level position in 1913. The Office of Industrial Hygiene and Sanitation in the U.S. Public Health Service and the Industrial Hygiene Section of the American Public Health Association were both established in 1914, and in 1916 the American Association of Industrial Physicians and Surgeons was organized in Detroit, Michigan (Felton, 1976, pp. 812-813).

The Social Security Act of 1935 enacted unemployment insurance and made funds available to expand industrial hygiene programs that led to the establishment of divisions of industrial hygiene in many state and local health departments (McGrath, 1945, p. 123). Selected legislation and events in occupational health in the United States since 1935 are in Box 21-1.

Unfortunately, each year millions of preventable work-related injuries and diseases still occur in the United States (U.S. Department of Labor, Bureau of Labor Statistics, 1998a). Work is an expected part of life, worker health needs to be safeguarded, and the OHN is in an excellent position to promote worker health.

## WORK AS A DEVELOPMENTAL TASK

A developmental framework is used throughout this text to address significant developmental tasks and life transitions. Work is a developmental task for the adult (Duvall, Miller, 1985; Stevenson, 1977), and is a basic part of life and social roles (Rogers, 1994a, p. 1). Our nation promotes the work ethic and expects that adults will work, be self-sufficient, and support their families. Work is a major means of establishing individual, family, and national economic security. Work is a source of productivity, social contact, personal development, and self-expression.

Duvall and Miller (1985) described the young adult as facing the work-related task of selecting and training for an

**BOX 21-1**

*Selected Legislation and Events in Occupational Health in the United States—1936 to Present*

| | |
|---|---|
| **1936** | *Walsh-Healy Act* sets occupational safety and health standards and minimum age limitations for workers employed in government contract work. |
| **1938** | *Fair Labor Standards Act* sets a minimum age for child labor: 16 years old for general work and 18 years old for hazardous work, applicable to most industrial settings. Also establishes maximum hours and minimum wages for interstate commerce workers. |
| **1939** | American Industrial Hygiene Association established. |
| **1941** | *Federal Mine Inspection Act* passes, helping to ensure greater safety in the mining industry. |
| **1946** | American Academy of Occupational Medicine established. It merges with the American Occupational Medicine Association to form the American Academy of Occupational and Environmental Medicine in 1988. |
| **1948** | All states have enacted *Workers' Compensation* acts. |
| **1952** | *Coal Mine Safety Act* is passed, ensuring greater coal mine safety. |
| **1966** | *Mine-Safety Act* is passed, requiring mandatory inspections and health and safety standards. |
| **1969** | *Coal Mine Health and Safety Act* is passed, setting mandatory health and safety standards for underground mines. |
| **1970** | *Occupational Safety and Health Act of 1970* is passed. It is the most significant piece of occupational safety and health legislation in the United States, establishing the Occupational Safety and Health Administration (OSHA) and the National Institute of Occupational Safety and Health (NIOSH). |
| **1972** | *Black Lung Benefits Act* provides benefits to black lung victims. |
| **1977** | *Federal Mine Safety and Health Act* is passed, consolidating all existing mine legislation into one act. |
| **1979** | *Healthy People* is published by the U.S. Public Health Service, establishing occupational health as a national health priority area and setting national occupational health objectives. |
| **1990** | The *Americans with Disabilities Act* is passed, safeguarding the rights of the disabled worker. |
| **1991** | *Healthy People 2000* is published by the U.S. Public Health Service, continuing occupational health as a national health priority area. |
| **1993** | *Family Leave Act* provides protection from loss of employment when time is needed by an employee to care for ill children, spouse, parent, or the employee's own illness; employees are entitled to up to 12 weeks unpaid leave during the year. |
| **2000** | *Healthy People 2010* is published by the U.S. Public Health Service and occupational health is one of the 28 national focus areas. |

occupation; the adult and middlescent as carrying out a socially adequate worker role and creating a balance between family, community, work, and leisure; and the aged adult as adjusting to retirement. The developmental tasks of the young adult involve integrating personal values with career development and socioeconomic constraints; the early-middle-years adult as developing socioeconomic consolidation and assuming responsible positions in occupational activities; the late-middle-years adult as maintaining flexible views in occupational positions, preparing for another career when feasible, and preparing for retirement; and the adult in late adulthood as pursuing a second or third career and/or adjusting to retirement. Maintaining the health of the worker is an important role of occupational health nursing.

The developmental tasks of work are carried out simultaneously with family and individual developmental tasks. If work-related developmental tasks are not achieved, sequential development can be affected and stress can occur. For example, being out of work (unemployment) can be stressful and carry with it negative experiences and societal connotations. Unemployment as a crisis for the adult is discussed in Chapter 17.

## OCCUPATIONAL HEALTH AND *HEALTHY PEOPLE 2010*

A significant event in occupational health was the development of national health occupational health objectives in 1980 as part of the Healthy People Initiative (see Chapter 4). These objectives continued in *Healthy People 2000*, are now in *Healthy People 2010*, and are given in Box 21-2. Worksite educational topics that address these objectives are given in Box 21-3.

Progress on achieving national occupational health objectives has been mixed. In the last decade, progress has been made toward reducing work-related injury and death and the incidence of hepatitis B infection among occupationally exposed workers (USDHHS, 2000, p. 20-7). The nation is moving away from target in some areas, as evidenced by the significant increase in cumulative trauma disorders and occupational skin disorders (USDHHS, 1995, p. 74). Work-related homicides and work-related stress continue to be national concerns.

National health objectives focus on protecting worker health, keeping workers healthy, and providing a safe and healthful work environment. Accomplishment of these ob-

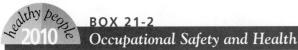

## BOX 21-2
### *Occupational Safety and Health*

Focus Area: OCCUPATIONAL SAFETY AND HEALTH
Goal: Promote the health and safety of people at work through prevention and early intervention.

*Objectives*

1. Reduce deaths from work-related injuries.
2. Reduce work-related injuries resulting in medical treatment, lost time from work, or restricted work activity.
3. Reduce the rate of injury and illness cases involving days away from work due to overexertion or repetitive motion.
4. Reduce pneumoconiosis deaths.
5. Reduce deaths from work-related homicides.
6. Reduce work-related assault.
7. Reduce the number of persons who have elevated blood lead concentrations from work exposures.
8. Reduce occupational skin diseases or disorders among full-time workers.
9. Increase the proportion of worksites employing 50 or more persons that provide programs to prevent or reduce employee stress.
10. Reduce occupational needlestick injuries among health care workers.
11. Reduce new cases of work-related, noise-induced hearing loss.

*Related Objectives from Other Focus Areas*

**IMMUNIZATION AND INFECTIOUS DISEASES**
• Reduce hepatitis B in adults and high risk populations.
• Increase hepatitis B vaccination among high risk groups.

**TOBACCO USE**
• Worksite smoking policies
• Smoke-free indoor air laws

**VISION AND HEARING**
• Occupational eye injury
• Hearing protection

From USDHHS: *Healthy People 2010, conference edition*, Washington, DC, 2000, US Government Printing Office.

---

jectives will require implementation of occupational safety and health education—not just in the workplace but in American schools and homes. "The time has come to protect one of our most valuable resources: the American worker" (NIOSH, 1995, p. 2).

## OCCUPATIONAL HEALTH LEGISLATION IN THE UNITED STATES

The United States was "backward" among industrialized nations in developing occupational safety and health programs and legislation (Cullen, 1999, p. 2). By 1884 Germany had already enacted a law that provided for a comprehensive system of occupational health, including compensation for occupational illness, injury, or disability irrespective of who was responsible for the occurrence of the condition (McCall, 1977, p. 21). In comparison, there was no established system in the United States for control of injury or disease in the workplace and no federal occupational health legislation.

For years OHNs, occupational physicians, and countless workers stressed the hazards in the American workplace and the need for occupational health legislation. In 1968 the Surgeon General, Dr. William Steward, told Congress that U.S. Public Health Service studies showed 65% of industrial workers were exposed to toxic or harmful substances or conditions in the workplace (Stellman, Daum, 1973, pp. xiii-xiv); in that same year an occupational health law was defeated by Congress.

## *Teaching* TIPS
### BOX 21-3
### *Worksite Educational Topics that Address* Healthy People *2010 Objectives*

• Violence prevention in the worksite, including how to handle disruptive employees and visitors
• Stress reduction
• Prevention of infectious diseases (e.g., hepatitis B, tuberculosis [TB], acquired immunodeficiency syndrome [AIDS]) including information on universal precautions
• Health education addressing weight loss and control, exercise activities, stress management, and smoking cessation
• Information on the use of protective equipment (e.g., safety belts, hearing protection devices, head and eye protection, protective clothing) to reduce the risk of workplace injury
• Information on worksite hazards for the pregnant woman
• Ergonomic education to prevent back injuries and cumulative trauma disorder
• Motor vehicle safety at work
• Information on community health resources

Many Americans thought that legislation in the workplace would endanger the free enterprise system. However, with the support of workers and labor unions, the Occupational Safety and Health Act of 1970 was passed. The act was passed to ensure Americans the right to "safe and healthful working conditions" (NIOSH, 1995, p. 2). It is the most significant piece of occupational safety and health legislation in the United States.

## Occupational Safety and Health Act of 1970

The Occupational Safety and Health Act of 1970 (Public Law 91-596) made a national commitment to maintaining worker health and preventing work-related disease, disability, and death. As a result of the act, and for the first time in our country's history, federal occupational safety and health standards were established. The nation had made occupational health a public concern.

INTENTS AND MANDATES OF THE ACT. The intents of this act were (1) to prevent placing toxic substances in the workplace, (2) to regulate exposure to toxic and dangerous substances already in the workplace, and (3) to com-

pensate workers for occupational illness and injury. The act resulted in the formation of federal agencies; the most well-known are the **Occupational Safety and Health Administration (OSHA)** and the **National Institute for Occupational Safety and Health (NIOSH)** (Box 21-4). The OHN works frequently with OSHA and may receive training at **NIOSH Education and Research Centers,** discussed later in this chapter.

SOME PROBLEMS WITH THE ACT. Since its inception, there have been a number of problems with the act. It has often been challenged in the courts, and funding generally has been inadequate to carry out the act's intents and mandates. Some of these problems are discussed in the following sections.

*Funding.* Funding for the act has been grossly inadequate and has affected the ability of OSHA to carry out its intents and mandates. According to the *Budget of the United States,* estimated funding is set at approximately $426 million for OSHA with an additional $68 million available in grants to states for the cost of their OSHA programs, and $220 million to NIOSH. This amounts to less than $3 per citizen per year in federal occupational safety and health spending (Office of Management and Budget, 2000).

*Coordination of services.* OSHA and NIOSH are under the jurisdiction of two different federal departments: OSHA is under the Department of Labor and NIOSH is under the Department of Health and Human Services. Their resources and services have not always been well coordinated, and interagency problems have existed. NIOSH researches occupational safety and health standards, and OSHA has the authority to set and enforce them.

*Fines and sentences.* Historically, fines and sentences set by the original provisions of the act were very low. OSHA can fine employers up to $7000 for each violation that is discovered during a workplace inspection—up to $70,000 or up to 6 months imprisonment if the violation is willful or repeated—and the failure to abate hazards can result in a $7000 per day fine (Ashford, 2000, p. 223). However, these fines and sentences are often not severe enough to act as incentives to employers to improve working conditions.

*Economic impact statements.* Economic impact statements involve a cost analysis study of a proposed OSHA standard or regulation by a company that shows what the economic impact would be on the company. If a company can show it would not be economically feasible to comply with a standard or regulation, it can appeal the proposed regulation and possibly not have to abide by it.

*Scope of the problem.* Because hundreds of thousands of workplaces are covered under the act, it can be difficult to monitor worksite problems. Added to this is the fact that there are millions of chemicals, and thousands of chemicals in the workplace are considered toxic or carcinogenic. A look later in this chapter at occupational stressors and the leading causes of work-related illness and injury illustrates the enormity of the problem.

## BOX 21-4

### *Agencies Created by the Occupational Safety and Health Act*

- *Occupational Safety and Health Administration (OSHA).* This administration sets and enforces standards for occupational safety and health. OSHA requires employers to report and keep records of work-related deaths, injuries, and illnesses and maintains a database of this information. OSHA encourages hazard reduction in the workplace and the implementation of occupational health and safety programs. States can develop their own OSHA as long as their standards meet or exceed federal standards. OSHA is part of the Department of Labor.

- *National Institute for Occupational Safety and Health (NIOSH).* This institute makes recommendations for federal occupational health standards to OSHA. It conducts research and training and provides educational opportunities for occupational health professionals at its NIOSH Education and Resource Centers. Its philosophy is reflected in the statement: "Delivering on the nation's promise: safety and health at work for all people... through research and prevention" (NIOSH, 1995, p. 3). It is part of the Department of Health and Human Services. Other agencies formed by the law were the *Occupational Safety and Health Review Commission,* a quasijudicial agency charged with ruling on contested OSHA citations that have been forwarded by the Department of Labor, and the *National Advisory Council on Occupational Safety and Health,* a consumer and professional group that makes occupational safety and health recommendations to OSHA and NIOSH. The act also mandated the formation of the *National Commission on State Workers' Compensation Laws,* but it was a temporary commission to study and make recommendations on state workers' compensation laws to the President.

*Legal challenges.* In the first year of the act alone approximately 100 bills were introduced in Congress to amend or repeal it (McNeely, 1992, p. 19). Almost every occupational health standard established by OSHA has been challenged in the courts, leading to costly and time-consuming delays in establishing standards (McNeely, 1992, p. 19). Legal arguments challenging the right of OSHA to set and enforce occupational safety and health standards continue.

*Lack of trained personnel.* There is no minimum qualification for the personnel responsible for interpreting the complex OSHA regulations and implementing compliance activities (Sattler, 1996, p. 233). There are severe shortages of industrial hygienists, OHNs, and physicians. Currently only 1500 physicians and 4000 nurses are certified in occupational health—that equates to one occupational physician and fewer than three OHNs to care for every 80,000 active workers and 20,000 retired or disabled workers (NIOSH, 1995, p. 8). OSHA can inspect only about 2% of the nation's workplaces in any given year (McNeely, 1992, p. 20). It has been noted that there are more park rangers than OSHA inspectors and that typical workplaces will see an inspector once every 77 years—about as often as we see Halley's Comet! (McNeely, 1992, p. 20). NIOSH Education and Research Centers are making strides to train and educate professionals in the field but have been unable to keep up with the demand. The American Association of Occupational Health Nurses (AAOHN) advocates the use of advanced practice nurses in occupational health settings (AAOHN, 1999a).

*Rule-making process.* NIOSH first researches standards, then OSHA establishes the proposed standard, or "rule." The OSHA rule-making process is cumbersome, time-consuming, and often slow. It includes public hearings on proposed standards (with a prehearing public comment period provided) and a posthearing public comment period before the final rule is posted.

*Dissemination of information.* Disseminating occupational health information has consistently been a problem. Once a regulation is promulgated, the only requirement of the federal government is to place the final standard in the *Federal Register*. The vast majority of employers do not have ready access to this document. Also, there is no mandate that training materials be developed to help employers implement standards (Sattler, 1996, p. 233). This means that people often have difficulty obtaining information on rules, regulations, and training materials.

### The Occupational Safety and Health Act and the OHN

The provisions of the Occupational Safety and Health Act of 1970 greatly affect occupational health nursing practice. The nurse needs to be knowledgeable of the OSHA standards and assure that the workplace is in compliance with OSHA rules and regulations. The nurse often participates in OSHA workplace visits, and assists workers in understanding their rights under the act. OHNs have indicated that an important challenge facing them in the workplace is keeping up with OSHA regulations (Rogers, Cox, 1994, p. 161). NIOSH education and training programs offer the nurse continuing education opportunities.

## OCCUPATIONAL HEALTH NURSING IN THE UNITED STATES

In her classic text *Occupational Health Nursing*, Mary Louise Brown defined occupational health nursing as, "The application of nursing and public health procedures for the purpose of conserving, promoting and restoring the health of individuals and groups through their places of employment" (Brown, 1956, p. 15). This definition is applicable to occupational health nursing practice today.

The contemporary role of the OHN emphasizes independent functioning, health promotion, prevention, investigative skills, and management of health care services (Rogers, 1994a, p. 34). The scope of practice of the OHN is broad, and the practice is a synthesis of knowledge from nursing, medicine, public health, occupational health, social/behavioral sciences, and management/administration theories and legal principles (Rogers, 1994a, p. 34). According to the American Association of Occupational Health Nurses (1999a), occupational health nursing practice is:

The specialty practice that provides for and delivers health and safety services to employees, employee populations, and community groups. The practice focuses on promotion and restoration of health, prevention of illness and injury, and protection from occupational and environmental hazards. Occupational and environmental health nurses make independent nursing judgements in providing health care services within this autonomous specialty (p. 2).

A model for contemporary occupational health nursing practice is given in Figure 21-1. The OHN has historically been a key figure in the management and delivery of occupational health services at the worksite, and the role is an autonomous one. As illustrated in Figure 21-1, the OHN's practice is affected by a variety of internal and external factors. For example, in some worksites comprehensive primary prevention and health promotion programs are emphasized, but in others emphasis is on the treatment of ill and injured workers, with little attention placed on health promotion. These differences are influenced by things such as resources allocated by the worksite for occupational health and the intrinsic values of the organization.

### The History of Occupational Health Nursing in the United States

OHNs originally were called *industrial nurses.* As the scope of practice broadened the title was changed. Box 21-5 gives

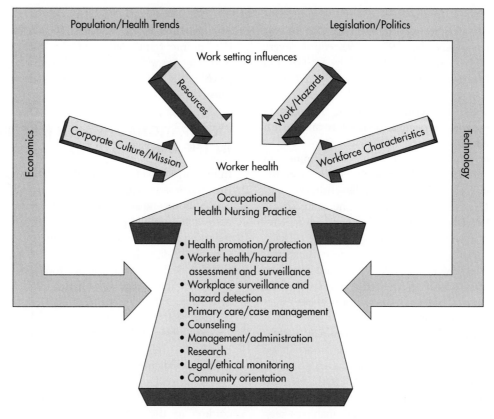

**FIGURE 21-1** Conceptual model for occupational health nursing practice. (From Rogers B: *Occupational health nursing: concepts and practice,* Philadelphia, 1994a, WB Saunders, p. 39. © Bonnie Rogers.)

a chronological overview of occupational health nursing in the United States. The evolution of occupational health nursing closely follows advances in public health and occupational health.

In 1888 Betty Moulder, a nurse, was hired by a group of Pennsylvania coal mining companies to care for the miners and their families, but little is known of her duties or accomplishments (Haag, Glazner, 1992; Parker-Conrad, 1988, p. 156). In 1895 the woman many consider the first OHN in the United States, **Ada Mayo Stewart,** was hired by the Vermont Marble Company and much has been written about her. Miss Stewart's sister, Harriet, also a nurse, worked with her during the first year of her practice (Rogers, 1994a, p. 23).

The Vermont Marble Company hired an OHN years before other companies and provided worker benefits such as housing, a library, general accident insurance, and a company store (Felton, 1988; Pinkham, 1988, p. 20). Miss Stewart was employed as a visiting nurse who gave care in the home to sick company employees and family members and went into the schools to teach health practices to the children of employees. She was an outstanding candidate for the job having studied the classics, history, mathematics, English, and Latin and graduated from Waltham Training School for Nurses where she received training in "district nursing" (see Chapter 1) (Pinkham, 1988, p. 20).

Miss Stewart often traveled through town on a bicycle and "conversed" in a form of sign language with many non–English-speaking residents (Markolf, 1945, p. 127). In addition to her other nursing responsibilities she learned about the health care customs of the native countries of the people she cared for and taught health education in the schools (Markolf, 1945, pp. 127-128), making her an early practitioner of both transcultural and school nursing. The March 1945 issue of *Public Health Nursing* celebrated the fiftieth anniversary of Miss Stewart's work. For that issue Miss Stewart, now Ada Markolf, wrote a manuscript titled "Industrial Nursing Begins in Vermont." This interesting article was written in third person, as she told the story of the "first" occupational health nursing experience in the United States (Brown, 1988, p. 434).

In the early part of the twentieth century many significant events occurred in occupational health nursing. At this time retail stores, cotton mills, and the mining industry began to have programs staffed by nurses (Felton, 1976, p. 814; Gardner, 1916, p. 301; McGrath, 1946; Waters, 1919, p. 728). *Florence S. Wright* wrote the first book on industrial nursing in 1919. In 1920 the National Organization for Public Health Nursing established an Industrial Nursing Section that defined industrial health nursing (Brown, 1988, p. 435; Pravikoff, 1992, p. 532). In 1941 *Olive Whitlock Kulp* became the first industrial nurse to

**BOX 21-5**

*An Overview of Occupational Health Nursing in the United States*

| | |
|---|---|
| **1895** | Ada Mayo Stewart (Markolf) is hired by the Vermont Marble Company. |
| **1897** | Anna B. Duncan is hired by the Benefit Association of John Wanamaker Company (New York). |
| **1913** | First registry for industrial nurses originates in Boston. |
| **1915** | Boston Industrial Nurses' Club organized. |
| **1916** | Factory Nurses' Conference organized (forerunner of the American Association of Industrial Nurses). |
| **1917** | First training course to educate occupational health nurses: *Industrial Service for Nurses*, offered at Boston College. |
| **1919** | Florence S. Wright writes *Industrial Nursing*. |
| **1920** | The National Organization for Public Health Nursing (NOPHN) establishes an Industrial Nursing section. |
| **1942** | American Association of Industrial Nurses is founded (becomes the American Association of Occupational Health Nurses in 1977). |
| **1945** | *Industrial Nursing* journal begins publication (1945-1949). |
| **1946** | Bertha McGrath writes a manual on industrial nursing, *Nursing in Industry*, in collaboration with the National Organization for Public Health Nursing. |
| **1953** | *American Association of Industrial Nurses Journal* established (becomes *Occupational Health Nursing* in 1969 and *AAOHN Journal* in 1986). |
| **1956** | Mary Louise Brown writes the classic book *Occupational Health Nursing*. |
| **1970** | *Occupational Safety and Health Act of 1970* passes, having numerous implications for occupational health nursing practice. |
| **1971** | American Board of Occupational Health Nurses (ABOHN) is formed to establish certification standards and examinations; first examination is given in 1974. |
| **1979** | *Healthy People* establishes occupational health as a national health priority area, and national health objectives are developed for occupational safety. |
| **1981** | American Association of Occupational Health Nurses (AAOHN) establishes a research committee. |
| **1982** | First research session held at the annual AAOHN Conference, and the following year the first research award is given. |
| **1989** | AAOHN established priority research areas in occupational health nursing. |
| **1991** | *Healthy People 2000* continues occupational health as a national health priority area. AAOHN revises its publication *Standards of Occupational Health Nursing Practice*. |
| **1994** | Dr. Bonnie Rogers writes *Occupational Health Nursing: Concepts and Practice*. |
| **1996** | The word environmental is added to AAOHN's mission statement and the term "occupational and environmental health nursing" begins to be used in AAOHN documents. |
| **1998** | AAOHN revises priority research areas in occupational health nursing (see Box 21-8). |
| **1999** | AAOHN writes *Standards of Occupational and Environmental Health Nursing*. |

work for the federal government (Parker-Conrad, 1988; Parrish, Allred, 1995).

In 1942 an important event occurred, the American Association of Industrial Nurses (AAIN), a forerunner of today's American Association of Occupational Health Nurses, was founded, with *Catherine Dempsey* as its first president. The new association published the journal *Industrial Nursing*. At its founding the AAIN had annual membership dues of 50¢ (Parker-Conrad, 1988, p. 158), and its membership numbered approximately 300 nurses from 16 states (Martin, 1977, p. 10). In 1958 the association began publishing the *American Journal of Industrial Nursing*. In 1956 *Mary Louise Brown* wrote the classic occupational health nursing text, *Occupational Health Nursing*.

In 1970 the Occupational Safety and Health Act provided an impetus to occupational health nursing education and practice. On January 1, 1977, the AAIN changed its name to the **American Association of Occupational Health Nurses (AAOHN)** to help reflect the broadening scope of practice. In 1983 the AAOHN established the first research award in occupational health nursing and began to

actively promote research as part of the OHN's role. In 1988 OSHA hired the first OHN consultant.

In 1990 AAOHN established research priorities and in 1998 revised them. In 1993 the Office of Occupational Health Nursing was established at OSHA. Today more than 13,000 nurses representing every state have membership in AAOHN. There are an estimated 23,000 OHNs in the United States, and many more are needed. The twenty-first century looks promising for occupational health nursing.

## Occupational Health Nursing Education and Certification

In 1945 the National Organization for Public Health Nursing and the AAIN took a position that specific courses in industrial nursing should *not* be a part of the undergraduate nursing program and recommended that *specialty education* be at the graduate level; similar to what was occurring for public health nurses (AAIN, 1976; Olson, Kochevar, 1989, p. 33). However, these organizations strongly recommended that schools of nursing integrate such content throughout the student's educational program (Markolf, 1945, p. 129).

Almost 60 years later, the integration of occupational health nursing theory and concepts into undergraduate nursing education remains limited. When occupational health nursing content is taught, it is often in community health nursing courses.

Early OHNs received most of their education on the job, and few specialized educational opportunities existed. When courses were offered, they were often short courses offered after graduation (Rogers, 1991, p. 101). One of the first such courses was offered by Boston University College of Business Administration in 1917 (Barlow, 1992, p. 464; Parker-Conrad, 1988, p. 159). It consisted of 10 lectures per week for 16 weeks, a 2-week practicum, and assistance with job placement (Parker-Conrad, 1988, p. 159). Early course content frequently focused on industrial injuries and worksite medical problems (Barlow, 1992, p. 464; Rogers, 1991, p. 101).

The USDHHS has recommended that the professional education of all primary health care providers should include instruction in occupational safety and health and content that provides an understanding of the relationship between work and health (USDHHS, 1991a, p. 297). The educational and theoretical content of occupational health nursing is grounded in public health and nursing theory, with an emphasis on community health nursing (Rogers, 1994a, p. 31). The AAOHN has published the *AAOHN Core Curriculum for Occupational Health Nursing* (Salazar, 1997) as an educational model.

The AAOHN supports the baccalaureate degree in nursing as basic preparation for entry into occupational health nursing practice (AAOHN, 1996a). However, only about 25% of OHNs are baccalaureate prepared (Rogers, Cox, 1994, p. 159). The baccalaureate degree provides an excellent framework from which to practice and to move to advanced practice roles. More baccalaureate nurses are needed in this specialty field.

Occupational health nursing education has a foundation in nursing and medical and public health sciences, with content from the occupational health sciences (e.g., toxicology, safety, industrial hygiene, and ergonomics), environmental health, epidemiology, social and behavioral sciences, legal and ethical issues, and management and administration principles (Rogers, 1998; AAOHN 1999a). Graduate education in occupational health nursing is available in several universities across the country. AAOHN recommends use of advanced practice OHNs at the worksite (AAOHN, 1999b).

### Stop and Think About It

One day you might be practicing in occupational health nursing. How has your nursing education prepared you for this role? Is there a NIOSH Education and Research Center in your area?

GRADUATE EDUCATION. The National Institute for Occupational Safety and Health Education and Research Centers (NIOSH ERCs) offer graduate and continuing education in occupational health and safety for health professionals. All ERCs have a nursing component, and some offer doctoral education in nursing. They operate under federal grants, with student stipends often available. There are 16 ERCs at major universities across the nation (Appendix 21-1); information on them can be obtained at *http://www.niosh-ERC.org*.

Many OHNs cannot take advantage of graduate education because they are not prepared at the baccalaureate level. A significant role of an OHN leader at the worksite is to help nursing staff advance their practice through education.

CERTIFICATION. Certification for OHNs has been available since 1974. It involves a combination of work experience, coursework, and written examination. Areas of certification testing often include knowledge of toxicology, treatment of chemical exposures, ergonomics, the Occupational Safety and Health Act and workers' compensation legislation, and competence in physical assessment. Beginning in 1996 a baccalaureate degree was required for OHN certification. Further information can be obtained by contacting AAOHN. Approximately 30% of OHNs are certified (Rogers, Cox, 1994, p. 159).

### Standards of Practice

Standards of practice guide the profession and are a baseline against which nursing actions can be measured. The AAOHN (discussed later in this chapter) publishes *Standards of Occupational and Environmental Health Nursing* (AAOHN, 1999a). These standards recently were revised to add environmental health and to reflect the changing and expanding scope of practice. The standards address multiple areas of responsibility including assessment, diagnosis, outcome identification, planning, implementation, evaluation, resource management, professional development, collaboration, research, and ethics.

### Objectives of Occupational Health Nursing

OHNs have standards of practice and a code of ethics on which to base their practice. They use interdisciplinary collaboration to promote worker and workplace health. Some major objectives for the OHN are to

1. Protect the worker from occupational safety and health hazards
2. Promote a safe and healthful workplace
3. Facilitate efforts of workers and workers' families to meet their health and welfare needs
4. Promote education and research in the field

The nurse works cooperatively with the worker, the worker's family, the workplace, and the community to accomplish these objectives. Fulfillment of these objectives will provide outcomes such as improvement in employee and community health status, reduction in worker morbidity and mortality, appropriate use of community resources, increased job productivity, and a safer work environment with reduced workplace hazards (AAOHN, 1999a, p. 11).

**BOX 21-6**

*Philosophy of Occupational Health Nursing Service*

The occupational health service contributes to a safe and healthful work environment through programs aimed at reducing and eliminating work-related hazards and enhancing health promotion. Occupational health services are provided to individual workers and the collective workforce within an environment that considers and meets the needs of a diverse workforce.

The occupational health nursing service is central and integral to an effective occupational health program. The occupational health nurse professional is an advocate for the worker and often manages the occupational health service. As such the occupational health nurse is concerned not only with how the worker's health is affected or influenced by the worksite and organization but also by how the worker, her or his family, the community, and the environment interact to affect worker health and productivity.

To protect worker rights, workers are given information regarding work-related hazards so that informed decisions can be made. In addition, confidentiality of health records and information is safeguarded.

The occupational health nurse professional is part of a collaborative team that has the responsibility to inform the employer of unsafe and unhealthful working conditions and practices and of the need for workplace controls. The employer has the responsibility to provide a safe and healthful work environment and to recognize and support the occupational health nurse as a professional with specialized knowledge and skills.

The occupational health nurse professional has an obligation to maintain and improve knowledge and skills relative to her or his position and to keep current with research and legislation affecting occupational health and nursing practice; the occupational health nurse professional is accountable for interventions, judgments, and decisions made according to practice standards.

The occupational health nursing service encourages a mutually supportive relationship with the community through referrals and utilization of resources and by being a productive part of the larger ecosystem that enhances the environment.

High-quality occupational health care is provided in a cost-effective manner that promotes productivity through good health.

From Rogers B: *Occupational health nursing: concepts and practice,* Philadelphia, 1994a, Saunders, p. 34. Copyright © 1994 by Bonnie Rogers.

A philosophy of occupational health nursing is given in the accompanying Box 21-6.

## Professional Organizations

The AAOHN is the specialty professional organization for OHNs. It has chapters in every state and a membership of 13,000 nurses. The association works in close cooperation with OHNs across the United States, serves as an advocate for occupational health and occupational health nursing, establishes standards of practice and a code of ethics, publishes a professional journal (*AAOHN Journal*), supports occupational health nursing research, and provides continuing education and certification in the specialty.

AAOHN actively assisted in developing the *Healthy People 2010* occupational health objectives. The association was instrumental in having OHNs placed on the staff of OSHA (Barlow, 1992, p. 465; Haag, Glazner, 1992, p. 59) and actively works to advance occupational health nursing. For further information on the association contact the AAOHN at 2920 Brandywine Rd. 5, Atlanta, GA 30341-7271 (770-455-7757).

## Scope of Practice for the OHN

The **scope of practice** of the OHN is broad, comprehensive, and dynamic. OHNs often work autonomously. Although the practice focuses heavily on primary prevention, the nurse is involved in secondary and tertiary prevention through treatment and rehabilitation of acute and chronic conditions.

**BOX 21-7**

*Staffing Recommendations for an Effective Occupational Health Nursing Program*

- One occupational health nurse for up to 300 employees in an industrial setting and up to 750 in a nonindustrial setting
- Two or more occupational health nurses for up to 600 industrial employees
- Three or more occupational health nurses for up to 1000 employees in an industrial setting
- One occupational health nurse for each additional 1000 employees in either setting
  Note: Larger and more hazardous occupational settings require more nursing personnel. Smaller organizations can implement an effective program with part-time nursing services.

From American Association of Occupational Health Nurses: *Occupational health nursing: the answer to health care cost containment,* Atlanta, 1991, AAOHN.

The scope of the practice is demanding. The number of nurses needed at a work setting is determined by factors such as the size of the workplace, type of work done, number of workers, and employee health status. Staffing recommendations for OHNs are given in Box 21-7. If these staffing recommendations are not met, it can be difficult to achieve nursing objectives.

Research has identified that management viewed occupational health nursing practice as focusing on care of illness and emergencies, counseling, follow-up on workers' compensation claims, and performing health assessments (Lusk, 1990). Activities selected by managers for greater OHN emphasis in the future were cost-containment, developing health programs, analyzing health trends, conducting research, and interdisciplinary problem solving (Lusk, 1990). The scope of practice of today's OHN has expanded and incorporates *administration and management, assessment and surveillance, direct nursing care, case management, health education, counseling, legal/ethical,* and *research* components. Roles that the nurse plays include care provider, casefinder, health educator, nurse educator, counselor, case manager, consultant and researcher. The role is increasingly expanding to incorporate more responsibilities for workplace health.

ADMINISTRATION AND MANAGEMENT. The nurse has numerous administration and management responsibilities. The operation of the occupational health service is a major part of the nurse's administrative and management function. In addition, maintenance of occupational health records, quality assurance activities, community resource utilization, and student education are all part of the nurse's administrative role.

*Managing the Occupational Health Service.* Administration and management activities include managing the occupational health service at the worksite. This involves ordering supplies, assisting in developing protocols, maintenance and revision of an occupational health nursing policy and procedure manual, strategic planning, training and supervision of auxiliary health personnel, and cooperation with federal and state occupational health regulatory bodies.

*Record keeping.* Record keeping is an important administrative function and the nurse has both legal and professional responsibilities to keep accurate, comprehensive, up-to-date written records. OSHA regulations and company policy require specific record keeping activities (AAOHN, 1996b; Maddux, 1995) and inadequate record keeping can result in OSHA citations. Records should note all employee contacts with the health service, beginning with the preemployment physical and interview, including the reason for the visit; nursing plans of care; results of screening procedures; periodic health appraisals; health risk assessments; rehabilitation activities; community referrals; and participation in worksite educational programs. *These records are confidential!*

*Quality management.* Quality management is an extremely important and ongoing occupational health nursing responsibility. Chapter 25 presents concepts of quality management such as peer review, performance management, and overall program evaluation. Figure 21-2 depicts interacting elements working together to define the scope of nursing practice and promote accountability and quality care. Standards of practice assist the OHN in providing quality nursing care and in assuring accountability for nursing functions. One measure of quality of care is employee satisfaction with the services. Research has indicated that employees are generally satisfied with occupational health nursing services (Mitchell, Leanna, Hyde, 1999; Rogers, Winslow, Higgins, 1993, p. 61).

*Community linkages.* Community resource collaboration and utilization is crucial to providing comprehensive care to workers and their families. The nurse needs to be knowledgeable about community resources, network with community agencies, and link clients to community resources (see Chapter 10). Resources of particular interest to the OHN include local health departments; local hospitals; physical and occupational therapy providers; state vocational rehabilitation agencies; state employment agencies; agencies providing counseling services for problems such as alcoholism, drug abuse, and domestic violence; voluntary organizations such as the American Heart Association,

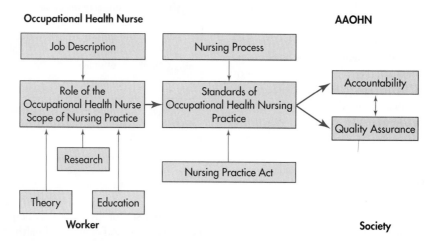

**FIGURE 21-2** Quality care in occupational health nursing. (From Randolph SA: Occupational health nursing: a commitment to excellence, *AAOHN J* 36:166, 1988.)

American Lung Association, American Diabetic Association, and American Cancer Society; and home health care agencies. The nurse may want to sponsor a health fair or other activity to help familiarize workers with the resources in their community. If the nurse finds a gap in community resource provision she or he can work in partnership with the community for resource development (e.g., adequate day care for working parents).

*Student education.* Providing supervision and training for nurses in occupational health nursing is an important role (Thomas, 1995). The nurse has historically worked with nursing students and may be involved in the educational programs of other disciplines, such as occupational safety and health, social work, vocational rehabilitation, toxicology, public health, and audiology. Historically, the OHN has mentored physicians involved in occupational medicine residency programs.

A relatively "uncharted" area for OHNs is that of educating school children about occupational safety and health. Comprehensive school health education curricula that incorporate concepts of occupational health were recommended more than 20 years ago in the document *Promoting Health, Preventing Disease: Objectives for the Nation* (USDHHS, 1980, p. 42). To date, little progress has been made in this endeavor. However, some innovative projects are beginning to emerge. An example is the hearing conservation education program offered to junior and senior high students that was developed and implemented by OHNs in collaboration with school nurses (Lukes, Johnson, 1998). The program was well received and helped educate the students about occupational and nonoccupational hearing loss and how they could conserve their hearing throughout life.

**ASSESSMENT AND SURVEILLANCE.** The OHN needs to be skilled in health history and physical assessment. An important part of the health history is the **occupational history.** Two main components of the occupational history are the employment and exposure history and the work-related health history (Rosenstock, Landrigan, 1986, p. 343).

Physical examination is an important OHN responsibility. It is the nurse who frequently does preemployment, job placement, periodic physical examinations, fitness for work, and return-to-work physicals. *Fitness for work* is the ability of the individual to perform a job based on the specific job requirements (Fielder, Caccappolo, 2000, p. 584). Such evaluations are often performed when employees are returning to work following an illness and disability.

*Screening procedures* such as audiometrics, electrocardiograms, vision screening, and pulmonary function analysis are often the responsibility of the OHN, and the nurse may order laboratory tests to provide baseline and follow-up data for diagnosis and treatment.

*Health risk appraisals* are done by the OHN to identify individual health risks, guide health counseling, and provide direction for health educational programs (Adams, Mackey,

Lindenberg, Baden, 1995). For example, in analyzing a compilation of health risk data, it was found that 70% of the workers at a plant smoked. As a result, the nurse worked with plant management and the workers, and a smoking cessation program was started at the workplace.

**Occupational surveillance** involves systematically monitoring the health status of work populations to gather data about the effects of workplace exposures and hazards to prevent worker illness or injury (AAOHN, 1996c; Merservy, Bass, Toth, 1997; Rogers, Livsey, 2000, p. 93). Surveillance is an excellent primary prevention measure. The nurse continuously surveys the work environment to identify existing and potential health hazards and to establish cause-and-effect relationships between these hazards and occupational health conditions. Surveillance activities are usually implemented in conjunction with other members of the occupational health team, including members of management, occupational safety personnel, industrial hygienists, physicians, and OSHA inspectors. These activities can result in lower workplace morbidity and mortality and fewer workers' compensation claims (Kosinski, 1999). An example of a nurse carrying out environmental surveillance is given in the following case scenario.

**CASE Scenario**    An occupational health nurse suspected that one area of the plant in which she worked had a higher-than-average noise area. After obtaining permission from the plant management to do periodic audiometric testing on the workers in this area in combination with testing on a control group, she began to collect data to confirm her hypothesis. Employees in both areas were tested every 6 months. Over time the nurse was able to show that the workers in this one area had increasingly abnormal audiograms and that the control group had consistently normal ones. The workers themselves had not noticed any change in hearing, but the audiograms told a different story. As a result of the study, corrective measures were taken. In this example, the nurse's actions assisted in facilitating the health and quality of life of the workers.

Appendix 21-2 represents an assessment guide that assists OHNs to systematically complete an environmental survey. OHNs apply the principles of epidemiology, primary prevention, and community assessment when they implement surveillance activities at the worksite (see Chapters 11 and 14).

**DIRECT NURSING CARE.** Historically, "the provision of health care for work related illness and injury has been an integral part of the nurse's work" (Rogers, 1998, p. 479). The nurse is often the primary provider of care at the worksite. Many occupational health clinics are equipped as outpatient departments, and the nurse has the resources at hand to evaluate and treat illness and injuries.

The direct nursing care functions of the OHN are diverse and demand a high level of nursing skill, flexibility, and independence. This care encompasses primary, secondary, and tertiary prevention, with nursing interventions ranging from assessment to rehabilitation. Physical assessment and screening as part of nursing care were mentioned previously. In addition, the nursing care activities include, but are not limited to, *preventive health* (e.g., giving immunizations), *acute care* (e.g., communicable disease, acute minor injury, headaches, back strain), *emergency care, treatment of nonoccupational injuries and illnesses, treatment of chronic conditions* (e.g., diabetes, hypertension, chronic obstructive pulmonary disease, arthritis), and *rehabilitation.*

*Preventive health.* Preventive health activities often involve giving immunizations, conducting health and safety education, and promoting environment conditions that are conducive to the health of workers. Health education and health promotion as primary prevention activities are discussed later in this chapter.

*Acute care.* The skills demanded for treatment of acute occupational injuries and illnesses are comprehensive, and some of these situations can be life threatening. It is estimated that more than 100,000 deaths, and an incalculable number of diseases and illnesses, occur each year as a direct result of occupational disease and illness (USDHHS, 1995). Acute care can involve treating occupational (e.g., dermatitis) as well as nonoccupational (e.g., bronchitis, flu) conditions. The nurse has standing orders and protocols that are used to treat such cases. Although nonoccupational illnesses occur outside the workplace, they have an effect on work and the work setting. The OHN initially treats these conditions and then refers the client back to his or her primary care provider and other appropriate community resources. Among the nonoccupational conditions the nurse encounters are alcoholism and drug abuse. These conditions are discussed under substance abuse later in the chapter.

*Emergency care.* Emergency care is probably the most dramatic of the OHN's direct care functions. Each year millions of traumatic injuries occur on the job; over 3 million of these are severe, and many result in permanent disabilities. Seventeen workers die on the job from work-related injuries every day in the United States (USDHHS, 2000, p. 20-10). Although fatal occupational injuries have gradually declined, injuries resulting in permanent disabilities are increasing (USDHHS, 1995). The nurse must be skilled in cardiopulmonary resuscitation, first aid, and emergency care techniques. The nurse is often the first health professional in the workplace to have contact with the ill or injured worker and has to make a decision about what immediate action to take.

*Managing chronic conditions.* Chronic conditions are occupational and nonoccupational in origin and frequently involve long-term follow-up and rehabilitation. They are discussed throughout the text and are specifically addressed in Chapter 18. Many of the leading work-related diseases and conditions discussed later in this chapter become chronic conditions. Agencies in the community (e.g., American Heart Association, American Lung Association, American Diabetes Association, Arthritis Foundation) provide excellent services. The nurse helps link workers with these resources and may provide services such as monitoring blood pressure, facilitating placement of workers in activities that do not aggravate these conditions, and assisting workers with rehabilitation activities.

*Rehabilitation.* The nurse is often involved in rehabilitation activities. These activities should begin as soon as possible and may be carried out in the workplace. Rehabilitation planning incorporates the worker and his or her family and appropriate community resources. Following rehabilitation, the nurse may be involved in assessing and facilitating the employee's ability to return to work.

CASE MANAGEMENT. Case management is discussed in Chapter 10. It is a process of coordinating a client's health care services to achieve optimal, quality care delivered in a cost-effective manner. OHNs manage complex worker health problems that are occupational or nonoccupational in nature (Rogers, 1998, p. 479). All cases can benefit from case management, although this process is more often used with complex cases. OHNs are in a unique position to implement such coordination, recommend treatment plans that ensure quality and efficacy while controlling costs, monitor care outcomes, and maintain collaborative communication and are becoming increasingly involved in case management (AAOHN, 1996d). As a case manager the OHN "establishes a provider network, recommends treatment plants that assure quality and efficacy while controlling costs, monitors outcomes and maintains a strong communication link with all parties" (AAOHN, 1998a, p.1). Case management requires a holistic approach and the nurse must look at psychological, financial, spiritual, and cultural issues in addition to the physical condition (Rogers, 1998, p. 479).

HEALTH EDUCATION AND HEALTH PROMOTION. Health education interventions are being used more and more at the workplace and often are implemented by the OHN. Employers pay a significant part of the national medical expenditures and rising health care costs are limiting company profits and necessitating cost control measures. Research has shown that worksite health education and health promotion efforts are cost effective (Breckon, Harvey, Lancaster, 1998).

Employers are realizing that it often costs less to educate workers about health care risks than to pay for illness, injury, and disability. Health education and health promotion programs help reduce workers' compensation costs, result in fewer medical benefits being used and less time lost from work, and enhance worker productivity. For example, employees who smoke cost employers 31% higher health care claim costs than those who do not smoke (Breckon, Harvey, Lancaster, 1998, p. 92). If successful smoking cessation programs can be implemented in the workplace, this cost to the employer can be greatly reduced. Other frequently used worksite health promotion programs include blood pressure control, weight control, nutrition education, and lifestyle and behavioral change. Employers are quick to use nurses in such health education programs.

The Occupational Safety and Health Act of 1970 stipulates that workers have the right to know the health hazards they are exposed to in the workplace. Educating the worker to the hazards of the workplace and actions that can be taken to minimize them is a critical step in illness and injury reduction. One problem related to this can be the difficulty of overcoming the attitudes and actions of the workers themselves. Many people who are exposed to occupational hazards deny the risks of working around such hazards and do not take steps to lessen their chances of developing health problems. It also may be difficult to get the worker to realize that a stressor exists, especially if the stressor is invisible to the human eye (e.g., gases, asbestos). People are less suspicious of, and tend to minimize the effects of, hazards they cannot see. Making the worker aware of these hazards is frequently a role of the OHN.

Another important aspect of health education and health promotion is the interpretation of health and welfare benefits to the employee. This means interpreting benefits offered through the employer, as well as providing information about available community resources and services.

Finding time at the workplace to implement health education activities can be a challenge because employers may not be willing to grant work time, and employees have little free time on the job except for lunch and coffee breaks. Contests and competitions, bulletin board postings, posters, fliers, distributing educational materials in the lunchroom or in pay envelopes, wellness articles in the company newsletter, ongoing classes, health screenings, health fairs, and short videos are examples of health education strategies used in the workplace. The nurse also can coordinate health education activities in the workplace with those going on in the community and develop university and community partnerships for health promotion (Walton, Timms, 1999, p. 449). For example, if the community is celebrating health and fitness week, or having a smoking cessation activity such as a "Smokebusters Program," the nurse can build on these activities in the workplace.

COUNSELING. Health counseling is an important occupational health nursing function that focuses on normal growth and development, family health, workplace stressors, at-risk health behaviors, and results of tests and screenings. Counseling often involves health education content. If the counseling required is beyond the scope of the nurse and the client is in agreement, a referral can be made to a counseling resource in the community.

LEGAL/ETHICAL. The importance of being knowledgeable about legislation such as the Occupational Safety and Health Act has already been mentioned. Other legislation with which the OHN will regularly work is workers' compensation, the Family and Medical Leave Act, and the Americans with Disabilities Act (Guzik, 1999). The Americans with Disabilities Act has many workplace implications such as the responsibility of the workplace to provide reasonable access and accommodations and return-to-work job accommodations (Keim, 1999; Mueller, 1999). In order to provide guidance and appropriate interventions, the nurse needs knowledge of these laws. Sometimes employees can be entitled benefits under multiple laws, and the process of determining worker benefits and responsibilities can become complicated (Guzik, 1999, p. 261).

Ethics play an important role in all occupational health nursing functions. The AAOHN (1998c) publishes a *Code of Ethics* for OHNs to assist them in dealing with ethical issues. Health professionals who work for companies face many ethical issues that test their allegiance and values (Rest, 2000, p. 283). The companies' primary purpose is to profitably provide a product or service and sometimes this can get in the way of doing what is right for the worker. Ethical issues confronting the OHN include informed consent, confidentiality of health care records, worker rights, drug testing in the workplace, right-to-know issues, and concerns related to acquired immunodeficiency syndrome (AIDS). The AAOHN code of ethics stresses the need to protect and promote the health and safety of the worker and safeguard workers' rights.

The confidential treatment of worker health information and the worker's right to privacy are professional obligations of the OHN (AAOHN, 1998d; Vaught, Paranzino, 2000). The nurse is frequently caught between management's demands to know medical information about an employee and the nurse's responsibility to protect employee privacy. Unjustified disclosure can damage the client and the nurse-client relationship, inhibit the client from freely disclosing pertinent health matters, and put the nurse at legal risk (AAOHN, 1998d).

To protect employees from unauthorized or indiscriminate access to their health information, it is recommended that written policies and procedures should guide the access, release, transmittal, and storage of health information, including computer records (AAOHN, 1998d). Educational activities should be implemented to let employees, employers, and other health care providers know about policies regarding record access. The "nurse acts as an advocate to promote client self-determination and to preserve autonomy, dignity, and rights" (AAOHN, 1998d, p. 9).

RESEARCH. "Not all nurses need to conduct research but all nurses need to use research findings in their practice" (Lusk, 1993, p. 153). Research links theory, education, and practice. Furthermore, research tests theory, builds a knowledge base in the field, and serves as the basis for practice in the profession. OHNs can play a vital role in the conduct of research to improve worker health and productivity and prevent illness and injury (Rogers, 1994b, p. 190). Nurses and nurse researchers need to work

### BOX 21-8

*American Association of Occupational Health Nurses: Research Priorities in Occupational Health Nursing*

- Effectiveness of primary health care delivery at the worksite
- Effectiveness of health promotion nursing intervention strategies
- Methods for handling complex ethical issues related to occupational health
- Strategies that minimize work-related health outcomes
- Health effects resulting from chemical exposures in the workplace
- Occupational hazards of health care workers
- Factors that influence worker rehabilitation and return to work
- Effectiveness of ergonomic strategies to reduce worker injury and illness
- Effectiveness of case management approaches in occupational illness/injury
- Evaluation of critical pathways to effectively improve worker health and safety and to enhance maximum recovery and safe return to work
- Effects of shift work on worker health and safety
- Strategies for increasing compliance with or motivating workers to use personal protective equipment

From American Association of Occupational Health Nurses (AAOHN): *AAOHN research priorities in occupational and environmental health nursing,* Atlanta, 1998b, AAOHN.

collaboratively to disseminate nursing research findings and incorporate these findings in practice.

The National Institute for Nursing Research (NINR) (see Chapter 1) has assisted nursing researchers in making significant strides in the development of knowledge for guiding nursing practice. In 1981 the AAOHN established a research committee for the purpose of promoting occupational health nursing research, and in 1983 its first research award was given. Vigorous strides have been made in occupational health nursing research over the last decade. The AAOHN encourages nursing research, and the *AAOHN Journal* regularly publishes research articles and information. In 1989 research priorities were established by AAOHN, and these priorities were revised in 1998 (AAOHN, 1998b). Box 21-8 lists these research priorities. The National Occupational Research Agenda (NORA) developed by NIOSH is given in Box 21-9 (NIOSH, 1999a). These research priorities focus on occupational health stressors and promoting worker health.

## OCCUPATIONAL STRESSORS

Although most occupational illnesses, injuries, and deaths are preventable, they are still prevalent in the workplace. Every 5 seconds a worker is injured in the United States;

### BOX 21-9

*National Occupational Research Agenda (NORA)*

The National Occupational Research Agenda (NORA) was developed by NIOSH in partnership with more than 500 organizations and individuals. It was first released in 1996 and is regularly updated. Its 3 categories and 21 research priority areas serve as a framework to guide occupational safety and health research into the twenty-first century.

*Disease and Injury*
- Allergic and irritant dermatitis
- Asthma and chronic obstructive pulmonary disease
- Fertility and pregnancy abnormalities
- Hearing loss
- Infectious diseases
- Low back disorders
- Musculoskeletal disorders of the upper extremities
- Traumatic injuries

*Work Environment and Workforce*
- Emerging technologies
- Indoor environment
- Mixed exposures
- Organization of work
- Special populations at risk

*Research Tools and Approaches*
- Cancer research methods
- Control technology and personal protective equipment
- Exposure assessment methods
- Health services research
- Intervention effectiveness research
- Risk assessment methods
- Social and economic consequences of workplace illness and injury
- Surveillance research methods

From National Institute of Occupational Safety and Health (NIOSH): *National occupational research agenda,* Pub no 99-108, Cincinnati, Ohio, 1999a, NIOSH; National Institute of Occupational Safety and Health (NIOSH): *National occupational research agenda.* Update May 2000, Cincinnati, Ohio, 2000c, NIOSH.

every 10 seconds a worker is temporarily or permanently disabled; and an estimated 11,000 workers are disabled each day as a result of work-related injuries (USDHHS, 2000, p. 20-3). Each day an average of 137 Americans die from work-related diseases, and an additional 17 die from injuries on the job (USDHHS, 2000, p. 20-3). The agricultural and mining industries have the highest rates of death from work-related injuries.

**Occupational stressors** result in occupational illness, injury, and death. These stressors can be categorized as chemical, physical, biological, ergonomic, and psychosocial (Table 21-1).

**TABLE 21-1**

*Occupational Stressors*

Occupational stressors occur in the work environment and are potentially toxic to the human system. They can cause injury, illness, and even death. Some are known to be carcinogens.

| STRESSOR | EXAMPLE | POSSIBLE EFFECTS |
|---|---|---|
| **Chemical** | Toxic chemicals include various liquids, gases, dusts, particles, fumes, mists, aerosols, and vapors | Cancer, shortness of breath, rhinitis, contact dermatitis, headaches, memory problems, allergic reactions, joint pain |
| **Physical** | Exposure to electromagnetic and ionizing radiation, noise, pressure, vibration, extreme heat and cold | Burns, hypothermia, cancer, hearing loss, Raynaud's phenomenon, cumulative trauma disorder |
| **Biological** | Infectious agents such as bacteria, viruses, mold, fungi; zoonoses; and fomites | Infectious diseases with possible sequelea |
| **Ergonomic** | Interactions between persons and their total working environment, including monotony; fatigue; boredom; stress; repetitive motion; unsafe equipment; inadequate equipment; the organization of work, tools, and equipment; and the social and behavioral elements of the workplace | Musculoskeletal disorders, accidents and injuries, emotional stress |
| **Psychosocial** | Physical and verbal aggression | Stress, emotional strain, interpersonal problems, accidents, and injuries |

## Problems with Linking Occupational Stressors to Disease

It can be difficult to link occupational stressors to work-related illnesses and conditions and more difficult to formulate cause-and-effect relationships. Factors such as long latency periods; multiple stressors; scope of the problem; and lack of comprehensive, up-to-date statistics complicate the process of linking occupational stressors to diseases and conditions.

LONG LATENCY PERIODS. A primary problem in formulating cause-and-effect relationships is that no immediate, observable effect of the occupational stressor may be apparent. Long latency periods may exist between contact with the stressor and its effects. Some occupational diseases (e.g., asbestosis) and cancers (e.g., mesothelioma) do not become evident until many years after the initial exposure to the carcinogen. Asbestosis often has a 30-year or longer latency period. In diseases and conditions with long latency periods, the worker may already have left the job where contact occurred by the time the condition is apparent, making it increasingly difficult to remember, identify, and trace the stressor.

MULTIPLE STRESSORS. The influence of multiple stressors affects establishing cause-and-effect relationships. A person may have been occupationally and environmentally exposed to many stressors; the interactions between them may greatly increase the risk of developing the condition, and their effects may not be easily separated. It can be difficult to determine which stressor caused the problem. How can the miner with emphysema prove that mine work, rather than his heavy smoking habit, was the primary factor in the causation of the disease?

SCOPE OF THE PROBLEM. The scope of the problem in relation to occupational stressors was mentioned previously in this chapter when discussing the Occupational Safety and Health Act. There are millions of chemicals in existence today, thousands of these chemicals are suspected to be toxic or carcinogens, and we have developed standards for only a few hundred. When one adds the impact of physical, biological, ergonomic, and psychosocial stressors to the chemical ones, it is easily seen that the problem is enormous.

LACK OF COMPREHENSIVE, UP-TO-DATE STATISTICS. Current, comprehensive occupational health statistics are often not readily available (USDHHS, 1995, p. 209). Health care professionals often do not elicit occupational health data as part of a health history, and many do not seriously explore the possible occupational etiology of conditions.

Birth and death certificates are commonly used in this country to obtain health statistics, but occupational information such as job and place of employment is generally missing or incomplete. In an attempt to develop preventive strategies for conditions such as low-birth-weight infants, to determine teratogens, and to decrease the incidence of infant mortality, parental employment has become a part of the standard *U.S. fetal death certificate*.

National health objectives address the need for primary care health professionals to routinely elicit occupational health data as part of a client's health history and routinely collect and analyze work-related injury and illness data. Health care professionals need to elicit information from clients about known or potential workplace stressors or exposures. Without such data it will continue to be difficult to formulate cause-and-effect relationships for work-related diseases and injuries, develop prevention plans, obtain comprehensive occupational health statistics, and treat occupational conditions.

## Hazard Communication

Under OSHA's Hazard Communication Standards, employers have a duty to inform workers of hazardous substances in the workplace. Workers have the right-to-know what they are being exposed to at the workplace. However, employers are under no obligation to inform the worker of inadequate, insufficient, or incorrect information provided by the manufacturer (Ashford, 2000, p. 225). Nurses are often involved in educating workers about hazards in the workplace.

*Stop and Think About It*

Health professionals need to routinely collect and analyze work-related health data. In what situations can you picture yourself as a nurse collecting occupational health data from a client? What type of data would it be important for you to collect?

## LEADING CAUSES OF WORK-RELATED DISEASES AND INJURIES

The NIOSH has developed a "classic" list of the 10 leading work-related diseases and injuries in the United States, which continues to guide occupational health practice (Table 21-2). Problems were placed on the list based on the frequency of their occurrence, severity of effect, and likelihood that preventive strategies could be developed and implemented (NIOSH, 1988a). Subsequently, NIOSH has de-

veloped strategies to prevent these conditions, and the Healthy People Initiative has developed national occupational safety and health objectives.

Occupational health is a focus for the nation and affects the quality of life of individuals, families, and communities (USDHHS, 2000). From a financial standpoint, it is estimated that more than $120 billion is spent annually in the United States for on-the-job-injuries (USDHHS, 2000, p. 20-3). Millions of workdays are lost each year to work-related illness and absenteeism. In addition to their potential for causing serious physical illness and injury, such conditions have an impact on the worker's psychosocial well-being. For personal, societal, and economic reasons, there is a great need to reduce the incidence of work-related disease, injury, and death.

## Occupational Lung Diseases

Occupational lung diseases encompass many disorders. Pulmonary fibrosis, often referred to as *pneumoconiosis*, is a common result of long-term worker exposure to hazardous airborne particles. *Pneumoconiosis* includes *byssinosis* (often caused by cotton dust and frequently called "brown lung"), *coal workers' pneumoconiosis* (caused by coal mine dust and often called "black lung"), *asbestosis* (caused by microscopic asbestos fibers), and *silicosis* (caused by crystalline silica dust). Asbestosis has been linked to mesothelioma, a rare and highly fatal form of lung cancer. Flock worker's lung, a chronic, fibrotic interstitial lung disease found in nylon flocking workers, recently has been described in the literature (Davidhoff, 1998; Kern, Crausman, Durand, et al., 1998). The clinical features of all pneumoconiosis are simi-

**TABLE 21-2**

*Leading Work-Related Diseases and Injuries: United States*

| CONDITION/DISORDER | EXAMPLES |
| --- | --- |
| 1. Occupational lung disorders | Asbestosis, byssinosis, silicosis, coal workers' pneumoconiosis, lung cancer, occupational asthma |
| 2. Musculoskeletal disorders | Disorders of the back, trunk, upper extremity, neck, lower extremity; traumatically induced Raynaud's phenomenon |
| 3. Occupational cancers (other than lung) | Leukemia, mesothelioma; cancers of the bladder, nose, and liver |
| 4. Work-related injury (fatal or nonfatal) | Amputations, fractures, eye loss, lacerations |
| 5. Cardiovascular disorders | Hypertension, coronary artery disease, acute myocardial infarction |
| 6. Disorders of reproduction | Infertility, spontaneous abortion, teratogenesis |
| 7. Neurotoxic disorders | Peripheral neuropathy, toxic encephalitis, psychoses, extreme personality changes |
| 8. Hearing loss | Noise-induced hearing loss |
| 9. Occupational skin disorders (OSDs) | Contact dermatitis, allergic skin reactions, burns or scaldings, chemical burns, contusions or abrasions |
| 10. Psychological disorders | Neuroses, personality disorders, alcoholism, drug dependency, stress reactions |

Modified from Centers for Disease Control (CDC): Leading work-related diseases and injuries—U.S. (occupational lung diseases), *MMWR* 32:25, January 21, 1983a; USDHHS: *Healthy people 2000: health promotion and disease prevention objectives for the nation, full report, with commentary,* Washington, DC, 1991a, US Government Printing Office.

lar and include an initial nonproductive cough that progresses to productive, progressive shortness of breath; distant breath sounds; and signs of right-sided heart failure (Christiani, Wegman, 2000, p. 492). These conditions are disabling and nonreversible. Although there is no cure for these diseases, they are preventable.

Other occupational lung diseases include farmer's lung, chronic bronchitis, emphysema, asthma, and lung cancer. Adult-onset asthma is frequently work-related, and people with preexisting asthma may have exacerbations related to work (Levy, Wegman, Halperin, 2000, p. 106). Pulmonary edema can be caused by exposure to workplace chemicals such as phosgene or oxides of nitrogen (Levy, Wegman, Halperin, 2000).

The illness, disability, and death caused by these chronic, obstructive pulmonary diseases is enormous. Early recognition of them is often difficult because of long latency periods before they are detectable. Two occupational lung diseases with exceptionally long latency periods are silicosis (latency period of approximately 15 years) and asbestosis (latency period of approximately 30 years). Once long periods of time have elapsed, it becomes increasingly difficult to link the occupational stressor to the occupational disease. Multiple causative factors, such as smoking, can contribute to the disease process and obscure the link between disease and toxic exposure at work.

Prevention strategies for occupational lung disease include stricter standards and regulations, increased disease, disability and hazard surveillance, dissemination of surveillance and prevention information, hazard removal, health education and training, and technology such as engineering designs for better ventilation and substance isolation (USDHHS, 2000, p. 20-13). Today, almost all states have exposure standards adequate to prevent these major occupational lung diseases. *Healthy People 2010* has an objective to reduce all forms of pneumoconiosis deaths among American workers (USDHHS, 2000, p. 20-12).

## Musculoskeletal Disorders

**Musculoskeletal disorders** are conditions that involve supporting structures (e.g., bones, intervertebral discs) and soft tissues of the body (including muscles, tendons, nerves) (USDHHS, 2000, p. 20-18). Such disorders often involve the large joints including the neck, shoulder, elbow, hand and wrist, back, and knee (USDHHS, 2000, p. 20-18). Examples include carpal tunnel syndrome, tension neck syndrome, and low back pain. Occupational musculoskeletal disorders account for up to $20 billion in direct costs annually in the United States (Martin, Andrew-Tuthill, 1999, p. 479; National Research Council, 1998; Ostendorf, Rogers, Bertsche, 2000, p. 17); the indirect costs such as absenteeism and decreased productivity double or triple this cost.

Factors that contribute to occupational musculoskeletal disorders are *environmental hazards*, such as equipment design; *human biological factors*, such as a person's size,

strength, or range of motion; *behavioral or lifestyle factors*, such as insufficient sleep, mental lapses, and lack of adequate fitness; and *inadequacies in health care diagnosis and treatment* (NIOSH, 1986, pp. 1-2). Many of these factors have an ergonomic component. It is often difficult to separate the occupational from nonoccupational causes of musculoskeletal disorders.

Musculoskeletal disorders are often a result of *traumatogenics*, a source of biomechanical stress stemming from job demands that exceed the worker's strength and/or endurance, such as heavy lifting or repetitive, forceful manual twisting (NIOSH, 1986, p. 1). Research suggests there is an association between musculoskeletal disorders and work-related risk factors, especially when there is a combination of such factors including repetitive lifting of heavy objects, prolonged awkward postures and vibrations, or poorly designed equipment (NIOSH, 1997a; USDHHS, 2000, p. 20-12). Although such injuries result in few work-related deaths, they account for a great deal of human suffering, cost, and loss of productivity. Musculoskeletal disorders are often the result of overexertion (e.g., back disorders) or repetitive motion.

Most back pain is at least partially related to work, but it is difficult to differentiate work-related from nonwork-related back problems (Levy, Wegman, Halperin, 2000, p. 107). Back injuries are a major component of musculoskeletal injuries, and national health objectives address the need to increase the number of worksites offering back injury prevention programs to decrease the number of back injuries. Back injuries are associated with ineffective job and equipment design, improper body mechanics, repetitive motion, and vibration injuries. Back injuries account for one third of all workers' compensation claims (Karas, Conrad, 1996, p. 189). Almost 50% of back injuries occur in the health care field (DiBenedetto, 1995, p. 134). At least 1 in 15 nurses will experience back injury serious enough to interfere with their professional career, and each year more than 40,000 nurses will report illness caused by back pain, resulting in a loss of more 764,000 workdays (DiBenedetto, 1995, p. 134).

Repetitive motion disorders also are called cumulative trauma disorders (CTD) and are an escalating workplace concern. Bernardino Ramazzini, the father of occupational medicine, first described CTD more than 200 years ago (Ostendorf, Rogers, Bertsche, 2000, p. 17). Today, industrial, agricultural, mining, and office workers all suffer from repetitive motion disorders. Common complaints with CTD are pain, restricted joint movement, numbness, and reduced manual dexterity (Ostendorf, Rogers, Bertsche, 2000, p. 18).

Each year in the United States more than 75,000 injuries or illnesses are due to repetitive motion, including typing or key entry; repetitive use of tools; and repetitive placing, grasping, or moving of objects (USDHHS, 2000, p. 20-12). Risk factors for CTD include awkward postures, force, repetitive motion, duration of activity, vibration, contact stressors, and exposure to cold (Ostendorf, Rogers, Bertsche, 2000, pp. 18-19). Repetitive motion may lead to disorders such as carpal tunnel syndrome, tendinitis, ganglionitis, and bursitis, as well as damage to muscles, tendons, ligaments, and joints. It is estimated that 40% of carpal tunnel syndrome cases involve repetitive typing (Martin, Andrew-Tuthill, 1999, p. 479; U.S. Department of Labor, Bureau of Labor Statistics, 1998b). Successful office ergonomics means properly designed work stations that include items such as adjustable office chairs, keyboard trays, and work surfaces as well as employee training and empowerment to adjust their work areas to meet their needs (Martin, Andrew-Tuthill, 1999, pp. 489-490; Ostendorf, Rogers, Bertsche, 2000, p. 19).

Strategies for reducing musculoskeletal illness and injury include having states and communities involved in prevention and control and evaluation of these disorders. This includes providing technical support and engineering technology to control ergonomic hazards, developing standardized diagnostic criteria for early detection and treatment, developing measures to prevent impairment and disability, instituting ergonomic approaches in building and equipment design to prevent musculoskeletal injury, rotation of workers to other jobs, and increasing public awareness and education through media campaigns (USDHHS, 2000, p. 20-12). Tools and products should incorporate in their design the limitations of the human body to reduce the risk of musculoskeletal disorders and improve ergonomics (Gross, Fuchs, 1990; Ostendorf, Rogers, Bertsche, 2000, p. 19).

## Occupational Cancers

Occupational cancers are cancers directly related to work-site exposure to a carcinogen. More than 200 years ago, in 1761, Dr. John Hill of London published a report on cancer of the nasal passages among tobacco snuff users, and in 1775 another London physician, Sir Percivall Pott, linked cancer of the scrotum in chimney sweeps to their occupational exposure to soot (Frumkin, Thun, 2000, p. 339). By the 1800s skin cancer was linked with occupational exposure to arsenic, tar, and paraffin oils, and bladder cancer was linked to exposure to certain workplace dyes (Frumkin, Thun, 2000). The potent hematotoxicity of benzene was described in workers in the 1800s, and a link has been made between benzene and acute myelogenous leukemia (Goldstein, Kipen, 2000, p. 615). A significant percentage of cancers are caused by work exposures (Levy, Wegman, Halperin, 2000, p. 107). Today, suspected occupational cancers and carcinogens are being investigated. Researchers are exploring the link between thyroid cancer and occupational stressors, including inonizing radiation, hydrocarbon exposure, and work in the wood processing or papermaking industries (Fincham, Ugnat, Hill, et al., 2000). Table 21-3 lists some occupationally linked cancers and carcinogens.

## TABLE 21-3

*Selected Occupational Carcinogens*

| CARCINOGEN | EXPOSURE | TARGET ORGANS/DISORDER |
|---|---|---|
| Arsenic | Insecticides | Lung, skin, hemangiosarcoma |
| Asbestos | Insulation, friction products, caulking products | Lung, mesothelioma, gastrointestional system |
| Benzene | Chemical industry | Leukemia |
| Beryllium | Aerospace, nuclear, electric and electronics industries | Lung |
| Chromium | Metal plating, pigments | Lung |
| Coal tar | Coal industry | Skin, scrotum, lung, bladder |
| Coke oven emissions | Coke oven workers | Kidney |
| Dioxin | Herbicides | Lung |
| Hardwood dust | Woodworkers | Nose |
| Ionizing radiation | Radiologists, nurses | Leukemia |
| Nickel | Nickel smelting and refining | Nose, lung |
| Radium | Radium chemists, dial painters | Nose, bone |
| Radon | Indoor environments | Lung |
| Silicia | Sandblasting, glass and porcelain manufacturing, hard rock mining | Lung |
| Solar radiation | Outdoor work | Skin, eye |
| Vinyl chloride | Vinyl chloride polymerization, Plastic industry | Liver |

Modified from Frumkin J, Thun M: Carcinogens. In Levy BS, Wegman DH, editors: *Occupational health. Recognizing and preventing work-related disease and injury*, Philadelphia, 2000, Lippincott, Williams & Wilkins, p. 340; Centers for Disease Control (CDC): Leading work-related diseases and injuries—U.S. (occupational cancers other than lung), *MMWR Morbid Mortal Wkly Rep* 33:126, March 9, 1984; Rutstein DD, Mullan RJ, Frazier TM, et al.: Sentinel health events (occupational): a basis for physician recognition and public health surveillance, *Am J Public Health* 73:1054-1062, 1984.

Numerous problems exist in linking occupational carcinogens to cancer. Many cancers have multiple etiologies, and it can be difficult to determine the workplace as the cause of exposure (e.g., lung cancer). Some cancers, such as mesothelioma, have long latency periods, making it difficult to link the cancer to an occupational exposure. Another problem in documenting occupationally induced cancers is that significant differences in the rates of cancer among small subgroups of a population may be overlooked because these rates affect the overall rate in the larger population only slightly, if at all—creating a "dilution factor" that obscures the occupational cancer. Research is looking more closely at occupational cancer links. It is important to obtain good occupational health histories from all clients with cancer (Levy, Wegman, Halperin, 2000, p. 107).

The incidence rate of cancer among certain occupational groups is significant (e.g., cancer of the bone in radium dial workers, mesothelioma in asbestosis workers). Thousands of suspected carcinogens in the workplace are not regulated. Exposure to carcinogens does not always cause cancer. The *dose, frequency of exposure*, and *duration of contact* are often the key to the toxicity of a substance. For example, many chemicals such as zinc, nickel, tin, and potassium are essential for health in small quantities but are toxic in larger quantities.

Breast cancer is a leading cause of cancer morbidity and mortality in American women. NIOSH is presently looking at the incidence of breast cancer in women exposed to the potential breast carcinogens of polychlorinate biphenyls, ethylene oxide, and serum organochlorines at their places of work (NIOSH, 1997b). Worksite screening programs for breast cancer have proved to be very successful (Caplan, Coughlin, 1998).

Nursing interventions that can assist in documenting, preventing, and treating occupationally induced cancers include cancer prevention education; cancer screening programs; risk assessment; and a comprehensive occupational history that identifies past, present, and potential exposure to occupational carcinogens by type, dose, frequency of exposure, and length of exposure, which can assist in documenting occupationally induced cancers. Early diagnosis and treatment is important, and survival rates increase significantly when cancer is discovered early.

### Traumatic Injury and Death

**Traumatic injury** includes amputations, fractures, lacerations, eye loss, acute poisonings, burns, and death. NIOSH estimates that more than 6 million injuries occur on the job each year that are serious enough to result in either lost time from work, medical treatment, or restricted work activity (USDHHS, 2000, p. 20-11). Each year up to 70,000 Americans die from work-related diseases and more than 5,000 lose their lives at the workplace (USDHHS, 2000, p. 20-5). Motor-vehicle accidents are the leading cause of death at work and workplace homicides are the second.

There are more workplace homicides than machine-related workplace deaths (USDHHS, 2000). The largest number of traumatic occupational death rates is consistently found in mining, agriculture, forestry, fishing, and construction (USDHHS, 2000, p. 20-5). Injuries among nurses and personal caregivers have increased in recent years.

The *Healthy People 2010* occupational health objectives address the need for reduction of deaths from work-related injuries, reducing work-related injuries that require medical treatment, and reducing lost time from work and restricted work activity. Progress has been made on national health objectives in relation to decreasing work-related injury death; however, nonfatal work-related injuries have increased (USDHHS, 2000, p. 20-7). Further reductions in work-related injury and death will require focused efforts to more fully identify and prioritize problems (injury surveillance). There is also a need to identify strategies to prevent occupational injuries (prevention and control), implement effective injury control measures, and monitor the results of intervention efforts (USDHHS, 2000, p. 20-10). Nurses can be part of all of these efforts as well as health education efforts that address workplace hazards and injury prevention and support enforcement of workplace safety regulations.

### Cardiovascular Disease

**Cardiovascular diseases** are the leading cause of death in the United States. Personal risk factors play an important role in developing these diseases, but factors in the workplace such as stress and exposure to cardiotoxins also contribute (Levy, Wegman, Halperin, 2000, p. 107). *Cardiotoxins* are substances toxic to the cardiovascular system such as carbon monoxide and nitrates.

The acute cardiac effect of carbon monoxide is well known. Research has linked workers exposed to carbon disulfide with cardiovascular symptoms and arteriosclerotic heart disease and associated acute episodes of anginal pain, myocardial infarction, and occupational exposure to nitroglycerine and other aliphatic nitrates can result in cardiovascular death (Theriault, Amre, 2000, p. 605). Other occupational exposures that may increase the risk of cardiovascular disease include stress, shift work, lead, cadmium, arsenic, and solvents (Theriault, Amre, 2000, pp. 610-611). Environmental smoke in the workplace needs to be considered in relation to cardiovascular disease, and many workplaces are placing restrictions on smoking or prohibiting it all together. Table 21-4 lists selected occupational hazards associated with cardiovascular disorders.

Control of cardiovascular disease is addressed in the *Healthy People 2010*. The worksite is an excellent location for teaching individuals about positive health practices and implementing preventive programs on personal risk factors such as smoking cessation, proper diet, blood pressure control, exercise, and stress reduction. An increasing number of workplaces have established health promotion and wellness programs designed to prevent premature deaths related to

**TABLE 21-4**

*Occupational Hazards Associated with Cardiovascular Disorders*

| HAZARD | CARDIOVASCULAR DISORDERS | STRENGTH OF THE SCIENTIFIC EVIDENCE |
|---|---|---|
| Carbon monoxide | Arteriosclerosis | Weak |
| Carbon disulfite | Arteriosclerosis | Strong |
| Certain aliphatic nitrates (e.g., nitroglycerin, ethylene glycol dinitrate) | Coronary spasm | Strong |
| | Arteriosclerosis | Satisfactory |
| Lead | Hypertension (renal) | Weak |
| Cadmium | Hypertension (renal) | Insufficient |
| Arsenic | Coronary heart disease | Insufficient |
| Cobalt | Cardiomyopathies | Satisfactory |
| Physical inactivity | Coronary heart disease | Strong |
| Noise | Transient high blood pressure | Strong |
| | Long-term high blood pressure | Insufficient |
| Shift work | Coronary heart disease | Weak |
| Halogenated solvents | Arrhythmia | Satisfactory |
| Chronic hand-arm vibration | Vibration white finger | Strong |
| Electromagnetic fields, radio-frequency radiation | Malfunction of electrical implants | Satisfactory |
| Work in aluminum production industry | Telangiectasis | Satisfactory |

From Theriault G, Amre D: Cardiovascular disorders. In Levy BS, Wegman DH, editors: *Occupational health. Recognizing and preventing work-related disease and injury*, Philadelphia, 2000, Lippincott, Williams & Wilkins, p. 606.

cardiovascular disease. These programs often work in partnership with community resources such as the American Heart Association.

## Reproductive Disorders

**Reproductive disorders** in the work setting occur when women or men are exposed to reproductive hazards. Reproductive hazards are substances that affect the reproductive health of women or men or their ability to have healthy children (NIOSH, 1999b). Reproductive hazards can be physical (e.g., ionizing radiation), chemical (e.g., lead, carbon disulfide, ethers, cancer drugs), biological (e.g., disease-causing agents such as bacteria and viruses) (Table 21-5),

**TABLE 21-5**

*Workplace Reproductive Hazards: Disease-Causing Agents*

| AGENT | OBSERVED EFFECTS |
|---|---|
| Cytomegalovirus (CMV) | Birth defects, low birth weight, developmental disorders |
| Hepatitis B virus | Low birth weight |
| Human immuno-deficiency virus (HIV) | Low birth weight, childhood cancer |
| Human parvovirus | Miscarriage |
| Rubella (German measles) | Birth defects, low birth weight |
| Toxoplasmosis | Miscarriage, birth defects, developmental disorders |
| Varicella-zoster virus (chickenpox) | Birth defects, low birth weight |

Source: National Institute of Occupational Safety and Health (NIOSH): *The effects of workplace hazards on female reproductive health*, Cincinnati, Ohio, 1999b, NIOSH.

and ergonomic (e.g., stress, strenuous physical labor). As many as 20 million Americans are exposed to reproductive hazards each year in the workplace (Barrett, Phillips, 1995, p. 40).

Lead is a reproductive hazard; more than 100 years ago, it was discovered to cause excess miscarriages, stillbirths, infertility, and macrocephaly in communities where lead-working was a primary occupation (NIOSH 1999a, p. 2). More recently some industrial chemicals, ionizing radiation, and specific disease-causing agents have been noted to be reproductive hazards. OSHA now has standards for the reproductive hazards of lead, dibromochloropropane, ethylene oxide, and ionizing radiation (Killien, 1999, p. 469).

Two thirds of all women in the labor force are of childbearing age, more than 1 million infants are born each year to women who worked during pregnancy, and an estimated 85% of the female work force will become pregnant at some time during their working years (Killien, 1999, p. 467). Maternal exposure to reproductive hazards can cause menstrual disorders, infertility, illness during pregnancy, miscarriage, stillbirth, chromosome or breast milk alteration, early onset of menopause, and libido suppression (Killien, 1999; LeMasters, 1992, p. 153). Fetal exposure can result in preterm delivery, fetal death, low birth weight, congenital malformation, and developmental disabilities (LeMasters, 1992, p. 153).

Research has shown increased birth defects among children born to female pharmaceutical workers and excessive spontaneous abortions and chromosomal alterations among health care personnel (NIOSH, 1988b, p. 1; USDHHS, 1987, p. 74). Ionizing radiation profoundly affects reproductive function in both men and women. It is estimated that 1.3 million persons are exposed to ionizing radiation at

**TABLE 21-6**

## Occupational Neurotoxins: Effects on the Peripheral Nervous System

| EFFECT | TOXIN* | COMMENTS |
|---|---|---|
| Motor neuropathy | Lead | Primarily wrist extensors |
| | | Wrist drop and ankle drop rare |
| Mixed sensorimotor neuropathy | Acrylamide | Ataxia common |
| | | Desquamation of hands and soles |
| | | Sweating of palms |
| | Arsenic | Distal paresthesias earliest symptom |
| | | Painful limbs, especially in calves |
| | | Hyperpathia of feet |
| | | Weakness prominent in legs |
| | Carbon disulfide | Peripheral neuropathy rather mild |
| | | CNS effects more important |
| | Carbon monoxide | Only seen after severe intoxication |
| | DDT | Only seen with ingestion |
| | n-hexane and methyl n-butyl ketone | Distal parethesias and motor weakness |
| | | Weight loss, fatigue, and muscle cramps common |
| | Mercury | Predominantly distal sensory involvement |
| | | More common with alkyl mercury exposure |
| | Organophosphate insecticides (selected agents) | Delayed onset following single exposure (usually nonoccupational) |

*Includes most but not all of the neurotoxic substances associated with listed conditions.
Source: Baker EL: Disorders of the nervous system. In Levy BS, Wegman DH, editors: *Occupational health. Recognizing and preventing work-related disease and injury*, Philadelphia, 2000, Lippincott, Williams & Wilkins, 563-578.

work, and that 44% of these workers are in health care, including a disproportionate number of nurses (Barrett, Phillips, 1995, p. 43). Nurses are considered high risk for reproductive disorders caused by exposure to anesthetic gases, antineoplastic drugs, viruses, bacteria, and ionizing radiation (Paul, Frazier, 2000, p. 596).

Exposure to reproductive hazards for males can result in lower sperm counts, abnormal sperm shape, altered sperm transfer, and altered sexual performance (NIOSH, 1996). Research has shown impotence in workers exposed to specific neurotoxins (e.g., lead) and lowered sperm counts from exposure to excessive heat and radiation (NIOSH, 1996). The pesticide dibromochloropropane is a well-known spermatotoxin, as are glycol ethers (Paul, Frazier, 2000, p. 591).

The OHN needs to make workers aware of such hazards in the workplace. The nurse needs to give special attention to pregnant workers and provide counseling about good nutrition, proper rest, prenatal care, and hazards outside of the work environment such as fetal alcohol syndrome and drug abuse. The key to promoting the reproductive health of American workers is primary preventive education and counseling workers about reproductive hazards so that they can make informed decisions about their reproductive health (Barrett, Phillips, 1995, p. 48).

## Neurotoxic Disorders

Disorders of the nervous system that result from toxic exposures in the workplace have been recorded throughout history. As early as the first century, palsy in workers exposed to lead dust was noted (NIOSH, 1988b, p. 1). The Mad Hatter of Lewis Carroll's *Alice in Wonderland* was not a figment of Carroll's imagination. In Carroll's time, hatters used mercury in hat making; mercury is a neurotoxin, and many hatters went mad as a result of mercury poisoning.

**Neurotoxic disorders** occur when people are exposed to neurotoxins. The number of American workers exposed to *neurotoxins*, chemicals toxic to the central nervous system, has been estimated in the millions. Chemicals well known for causing neurotoxic symptoms include lead, mercury, arsenic, carbon monoxide, carbon disulfide, ketone, and manganese. More than 100 chemicals, including almost all solvents, can cause central nervous system depression and several neurotoxins can cause peripheral neuropathy (Levy, Wegman, Halperin, 2000, p. 107). Almost all industrial toxins that affect the peripheral nervous system have a mixed sensorimotor peripheral neuropathy (Baker, 2000, p. 567). Peripheral neuropathy results in sensory loss in relation to pain and temperature discrimination, impaired vibratory sense, and decreased touch sensation. It is often characterized by numbness and tingling in the feet or hands followed by decreased coordination (Baker, 2000, p. 567). The effects can be temporary or permanent. Behavioral neurotoxicity, changes in behavior resulting from chemical exposure, can also occur. See Table 21-6 for the peripheral nervous system effects of selected occupational neurotoxins.

Recent research showed that the use of a mercury-containing (mercurous chloride) cosmetic cream manufactured in Mexico by residents of a Texas border town resulted in elevated mercury levels in cream users. Workers and consumers need to be aware of the possible effects of such substances on health (McRill, Boyer, Flood, Ortega, 2000).

Lead poisoning remains a national concern, and *Healthy People 2010* has a specific objective to reduce the number of persons who have elevated blood lead concentrations from work exposures. Thousands of American workers have elevated blood lead levels (USDHHS, 2000, p. 20-14). Industries in which workers are at high risk of lead exposure include battery manufacturing, foundries, potters, ammunition casting, radiator repair, lead smelters, construction and demolition, and firing ranges. Lead taken home from the workplace on clothing and other items can harm family members.

Nursing interventions should include surveillance of the workplace for neurotoxins, screening workers for exposure to neurotoxic agents to detect the early symptoms of central nervous system damage, and education on neurotoxins in the workplace.

## Psychological Disorders

**Psychological disorders** cover a broad range of conditions and occurrences. Disorders seen in the workplace commonly include stress, anxiety, depression, maladaptive lifestyle behaviors, and substance abuse (NIOSH, 1988c, p. 2). They are heavily concentrated among workers with lower income, lower education, fewer skills, and less prestigious jobs (NIOSH, 1988c, p. 4).

Psychological disorders can be job related and psychological stressors are present in all job settings (Baker, Karasek, 2000). Job stress has been identified as a significant risk factor for many health problems including cardiovascular disease, musculoskeletal disorders, psychological disorders, ulcers, and impaired immune function (Baker, Karasek, 2000; NIOSH, 1999c, USDHHS, 2000, p. 20-16). Job stress is defined as "the harmful physical and emotional responses that occur when the requirements of the job do not match the capabilities, resources, or needs of the worker" (NIOSH, 1999c, p. 6). Workers who are balancing multiple responsibilities that combine employment, school, and caring for dependent children and/or dependent parents are at high risk for experiencing psychological stress. Stress can lead to injury and is a leading cause of worker disability in the United States (Baker, Karasek, 2000; NIOSH 1999c; USDHHS, 2000, p. 20). Studies show that up to 40% of workers report their job is extremely stressful (NIOSH, 1999c). Job stress needs to be minimized (USDHHS, 2000 p. 20-16).

Depression has been discussed in Chapter 17. It is the leading mental health problem in the United States, has the highest medical benefit cost of all work-related behavioral health conditions, and is the most common Employee

Assistance Program diagnosis (Williams, Strasser, 1999). Depression is a very treatable illness.

Research has documented psychological symptoms in response to occupational exposures to neurotoxins such as lead, arsenic, mercury, styrene, carbon monoxide, and organic solvents (Baker, 2000, p. 571). Acute and chronic lead exposure can result in symptoms such as fatigue, decreased libido, restlessness, and depression (Fielder, Caccappolo, 2000, p. 581).

An interesting work-related psychological phenomenon is *mass psychogenic illness*. Mass psychogenic illness occurs when a number of workers simultaneously experience similar symptoms seemingly contagious but whose etiology can only be linked to a psychological stressor. Symptoms of mass psychogenic illness include headaches, nausea, chills, blurred vision, muscular weakness, and difficulty breathing (Colligan, Stockton, 1978; Moss, 1992, p. 671); the illness is frequently linked with workers being overcome by strange odors (Colligan, Murphy, 1979; Moss, 1992, p. 671). Epidemics of mass psychogenic illness typically occur in settings such as factory assembly lines (Moss, 1992, p. 671), and it has been routinely linked with stressful job situations.

If outbreaks of mass psychogenic illness occur, it is recommended that symptomatic persons be removed to an out-of-the-way area and the situation be handled as quietly as possible to prevent spread of the symptoms (CDC, 1983b). It is important to remember that the symptoms are real to those who are experiencing them. *The nurse must evaluate such situations carefully because there may actually be an occupational hazard present.*

Nursing interventions in relation to work-related psychological disorders can address improving working conditions to minimize stress, casefinding, anticipatory guidance, education, referral to community agencies, and advocating for increased mental health services for workers. Nursing interventions such as group sessions on stress awareness and management may be especially helpful. The OHN should be sensitive to the fact that family members are often the victims of the effects of work stress and psychological disturbance. OHNs need to assess workers for psychological disorders and help remove the stigma attached to mental health conditions. Many workplaces have Employee Assistance Programs (EAPs) that provide mental health services to employees. The nurse frequently refers employees to these programs.

## Hearing Loss

**Hearing loss** can be mechanical or sensory. Occupational noise exposure is a significant problem in industry and often results in hearing loss. *Healthy People 2010* has a specific objective to reduce the incidence of work-related noise-induced hearing loss (USDHHS, 2000, p. 20-18). Approximately 30 million American workers are exposed to hazardous noise levels on the job and another 9 million are at risk for hearing loss from ototoxic solvents and metals

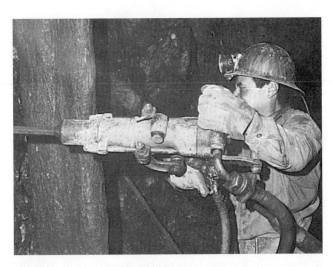

**FIGURE 21-3** Many American workers are exposed to dangerous levels of noise. (Courtesy World Health Organization.)

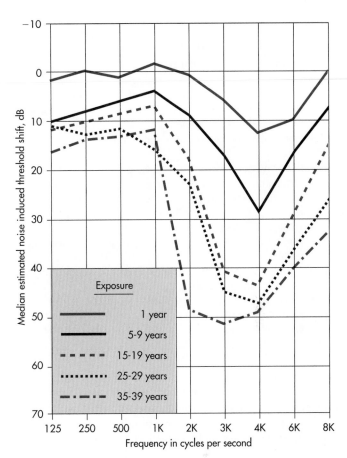

**FIGURE 21-4** Median permanent threshold shifts in hearing levels as a function of exposure years to jute weaving noise. (Data from Taylor WA, Mair A, Burns W: Study of noise and hearing in jute weaving, *Acoustical Society of America* 48:524-530, 1965, as cited in USDHHS: *NIOSH publication on noise and hearing: criteria for a recommended standard—occupational exposure to noise*, Cincinnati, Ohio, 1991b, NIOSH, p. 511.)

(NIOSH, 2000d) (Figure 21-3). Noise-induced hearing loss usually develops gradually as a result of damage to the sensory hair cells in the cochlea. Noise-induced hearing loss is preventable, but once it occurs it is often permanent and irreversible (NIOSH, 2000d). Thousands of American workers experience work-related hearing loss each year.

Noise-induced hearing loss in the workplace was recognized in the early 1700s by Bernardo Ramazzini in his writings on the diseases of occupations. By the early twentieth century boilermakers' deafness, caused by riveting inside metal boilers, was an occupational hazard of considerable magnitude (NIOSH, 1988c, p. 1). Industries with high numbers of workers exposed to hazardous noise levels include agriculture, mining, construction, manufacturing, utilities, transportation, and military (Dunn, 2000; NIOSH, 2000d). Ninety percent of coal miners have a hearing impairment by age 52 (NIOSH, 2000d). Regardless of its characteristics, noise can be contained or absorbed and hearing loss prevented (Lowey, 2000, p. 95). When noise cannot be controlled at the source, the employee should use personal protective equipment such as muffs and plugs (Stearns, 2000, p. 99).

Many research studies indicate that worker hearing loss is directly related to worker noise exposure levels and increases with the noise level and duration (McGuire, 1994; 2001). Hearing loss caused by industrial noise is often represented on audiograms by a descending slope with a "notch" at 3000 Hz to 4000 Hz, which is often referred to as the industrial noise trauma notch (Figure 21-4). The person suffering from industrial hearing loss may initially notice *tinnitus,* which is a ringing or hissing sound in the ear (Griest, Bishop, 1998). The onset of hearing loss is usually gradual and painless, and the individual may not be aware of the hearing loss until the damage is permanent or communication is affected (McGuire, 2001).

The OHN plays a key role in an industrial hearing conservation program and frequently has primary responsibility for the implementation, administration, coordination, and evaluation of the hearing conservation program (McGuire, 1991, pp. 233, 239; McGuire, 2001). A successful industrial hearing conservation program complies with or exceeds the OSHA hearing conservation regulations. Some activities implemented by the nurse in these programs are given in Box 21-10.

Nursing interventions include obtaining the workers' medical and occupational histories, audiometric testing, referring employees with hearing complaints or questionable audiograms to a physician, educating and counseling employees about industrial noise, supplying employees with hearing protection muffs or plugs, and encouraging employees to wear the protection in and outside the work environment as appropriate. Other activities to prevent work-related hearing loss include the development of noise abatement methods and plant design to make work

### BOX 21-10

*Nursing Activities in Hearing Conservation Programs*

- Assesses the workers' environment for noise exposure and coordinates with management work areas where hearing protection should be worn
- Determines employees who may be predisposed to hearing loss
- Performs audiometric testing on prospective employees, continues to measure employees' hearing periodically, and examines audiometric data for accuracy and reliability
- Provides effective hearing protection for employees, including individually fitting employees for such hearing protection
- Provides ongoing educational programs on hearing conservation and noise abatement in the workplace
- Assists in implementing administrative and engineering controls to reduce noise levels and prevent noise in the workplace

processes quieter, attenuating workplace noise sources, implementing effective hearing conservation programs (including the use of hearing protection by workers), and research on noise-induced hearing loss.

### Occupational Skin Disorders

An **occupational skin disorder (OSD)** is "an immediate adverse effect on the skin that results from instantaneous trauma or brief exposure to toxic agents...in the work environment" (Bigby, Arndt, Coopman, 2000, p. 537). Occupational skin disorders amount to more than 13% of all occupational illnesses reported each year, making them the most common nontrauma-related occupational illness (Bigby, Arndt, Coopman, 2000, p. 537; USDHHS, 2000, p. 20-15). It is actually estimated that OSDs are 10 to 50 times higher than those reported (USDHHS, 2000, p. 20-15). It also is estimated that at least 200,000 workdays are lost each year due to OSDs (Bigby, Arndt, Coopman, 2000, p. 537).

The skin is often directly exposed, making this organ especially vulnerable to occupational diseases, and dermal absorption of some chemicals may be more serious than absorption by inhalation (NIOSH, 1988d, p. 1). Occupational dermatoses can be (1) *mechanical*—friction, pressure, vibration; (2) *chemical*—oils, resins, solvents, nickel compounds; (3) *physical*—heat, cold, wind, sunlight, radiation; and (4) *biological*—viruses, bacteria, fungi, parasites, plant and wood substances (Bigby, Arndt, Coopman, 2000, p. 540).

OSDs are a national occupational health research priority and *Healthy People 2010* has a national occupational health objective to reduce incidence of OSDs. Contact dermatitis accounts for about 90% of all OSDs (Levy, Wegman, Halperin, 2000, p. 106). Other OSDs include infections, pi-

losebaceous abnormalities (e.g., acne), pigment disorders, neoplasms, and disorders of the hair and nails. OSDs are preventable. Unfortunately, they are on the rise and are a frequent cause of lost time from work (USDHHS, 1995, p. 75). Fortunately, dermatological conditions usually respond well to early diagnosis and treatment.

Preventive measures to decrease the incidence of OSDs include identifying allergens and irritants, substituting less irritating chemicals, engineering controls that eliminate or reduce skin exposure, containment or redesign of industrial processes, use of personal protective clothing, using barrier creams, emphasizing personal and occupational hygiene, establishing educational programs to increase awareness in the workplace, and providing health screening (USDHHS, 2000, pp. 20-15, 20-16). A combination of several of these interventions has proved beneficial to workers in reducing OSDs (USDHHS, 2000, p. 20-16).

## OTHER CONCERNS IN THE WORKPLACE

In addition to the work-related diseases and conditions already discussed, *Healthy People 2010* notes a number of additional conditions that also need attention, including hepatitis B, AIDS, tuberculosis, smoking in the workplace, substance abuse, and violence in the workplace.

### Acquired Immunodeficiency Syndrome

Almost 40,000 people become infected with the AIDS virus each year (Gantz, 2000, p. 402), and a separate focus area in *Healthy People 2010* is devoted to HIV infection. There is no known cure for AIDS and no vaccine to prevent it. Public health measures to control the disease focus on primary prevention. AIDS was highlighted in Chapter 13; the role of the occupational health nurse in AIDS treatment and prevention is discussed here.

Employees potentially exposed to the HIV virus need to report the incident immediately for evaluation, counseling, and appropriate treatment (Stone, 2000, p. 74). CDC's postexposure prophylaxis guidelines call for treatment with antiviral medications within a few hours following a needlestick injury, and current recommendations for post-HIV exposure include blood testing immediately following exposure and at 3 and 6 months after the exposure (CDC, 1998; Stone, 2000, p. 74).

The AAOHN has the following recommendations for AIDS: (1) workers with AIDS should be employed for as long as possible, (2) confidentiality of HIV testing results and records should be maintained, (3) management should take aggressive action to establish an AIDS policy and education at the workplace, and (4) discrimination against the HIV-positive employee should be discouraged (AAOHN, 1989). There is no indication that people who test HIV-positive and are asymptomatic are any less capable of performing on the job than noninfected workers (Jaffe, Schmitt, 1992, p. 693).

Research has consistently shown that many workers hold negative attitudes and myths about HIV-positive coworkers. There is a great need for health education programs to educate workers and employers about AIDS and to dispel myths. Significant improvements in AIDS knowledge can result following an AIDS education program.

The OHN plays a key role in AIDS policy development and education at the workplace and this requires that the nurse keep up to date with rapidly changing AIDS research, information, and treatment. Nursing intervention frequently involves implementing AIDS education in the workplace and referring workers to community resources for confidential testing and follow-up. In the workplace the risk of HIV infection is directly related to potential exposures to blood or body fluids from coworkers or clients (Jaffe, Schmitt, 1992, p. 693). Nurses play a significant role in reducing exposure by educating employers and employees about OSHA's regulation of bloodborne pathogens.

## Hepatitis B and Other Bloodborne Pathogens

As previously discussed, AIDS is a bloodborne pathogen. Other bloodborne pathogens in the workplace include hepatitis B, hepatitis C, and cytomegalovirus. The occupational risks from bloodborne pathogens is a serious and worsening problem, especially in health care environments (Corser, 1998). Each year thousands of health care workers in the United States are exposed to infectious body fluids on the job, and the majority of the resulting clinical infections are attributable to bloodborne pathogens (Corser, 1998, p. 246). Hepatitis B is a serious workplace concern and is a bloodborne pathogen often associated with incidents of health care worker exposures (Corser, 1998, p. 246; Hershey, Martin, 1994).

Each year hundreds of health care workers continue to become infected with hepatitis B. However, this is a great decline from 1990 when more than 12,000 became infected. National health objectives have been effective in reducing the incidence of hepatitis B in the workplace and increasing the rate of immunization among occupationally exposed workers. Up to 10% of persons infected with hepatitis B will become chronic carriers (Gantz, 2000, p. 404). Needlestick injuries are responsible for approximately 80% of all environmental exposures to hepatitis B blood (Corser, 1998, p. 247; Hibberd, 1995). *Healthy People 2010* has a specific objective to reduce needlestick injury in the workplace. Hepatitis B can survive in dried blood at room temperature on an environmental surface for over 7 days (Corser, 1998, p. 247; O'Neal, 1996).

Employers must provide hepatitis B vaccine free of charge to employees who are occupationally at risk for the disease. Vaccination of workers who already have antibodies to hepatitis B has not shown to cause adverse effects (CDC, 1995). Nurses and other health care workers are considered to be at high risk. Nursing interventions to prevent hepatitis B include encouraging safe work practices such as the use of gloves, masks, protective clothing, and universal precautions; vaccinating workers against hepatitis B; and health education activities, such as teaching workers about the infective nature of these diseases, proper handling of blood products, and disposal of contaminated waste.

## Tuberculosis

Millions of people in the United States are infected with M. *tuberculosis*, but infection with the bacilli does not mean that a person has active disease. The OSHA estimates that more than 5 million health care workers in the United States are exposed to tuberculosis (TB) at work (Stone, 2000, p. 76).

The epidemiology of TB was discussed in Chapter 11. Although there has been a recent decline in the annual incidence of TB after an extensive period of moving upward, TB continues to remain a significant health problem in the United States. There was a resurgence of TB in the United States with the AIDS epidemic.

A low index of suspicion of tuberculosis with primary care providers can lead to missed diagnosis. All health care workers are a significant risk group for TB. Employees in nursing homes, mental hospitals, and prisons are also at increased risk (Gantz, 2000, p. 408).

TB is transmitted by airborne, droplet nuclei that disperse throughout the air and can be carried on air currents throughout a building; transmission of disease is facilitated by prolonged exposure in relatively small, enclosed spaces with inadequate ventilation. Hundreds of workplace-originated cases of TB have occurred in the United States (USDHHS, 1993).

Nursing intervention in preventing workplace exposure to TB combines health education and disease prevention activities, early detection (TB skin tests and radiographs), case tracking, prophylactic treatment of converters, and follow-up on treatment plans. OSHA is developing a standard and protocols for controlling TB exposure in the workplace (Stone, 2000, p. 76). Frequency of testing is based on the risk of exposure. Health care workers at high risk with negative skin tests should be tested every 3 to 6 months, others can be tested annually (Stone, 2000, p. 76). Criteria for interpretation of a positive tuberculin skin test depend on the health status of the host. For example a test is considered positive for TB in an HIV-infected person with an induration of 5 mm or more; other immunosuppressed people, 10 mm or more; and for normal hosts, an induration of 15 mm or more (Gantz, 2000, p. 409). The OHN must be involved in prevention and surveillance interventions that can help prevent the spread of this disease.

## Smoking

Smoking is a leading cause of morbidity and mortality. Smoking and health is discussed in Chapter 17. Smoking in the workplace is a serious health problem for smokers and nonsmokers alike. Research has shown that passive inhalation of smoke is also damaging to health. *Healthy People*

2010 has objectives in relation to smoking cessation. Relatively small, enclosed work spaces with inadequate ventilation in many workplaces adds to the risk of developing smoking-related diseases. If the work environment is not smoke free, other workers can suffer the effects of passive inhalation of smoke. The benefits of a smoke-free work force include better health, reduced absenteeism, and increased worker productivity.

To effectively intervene with workers who smoke, the nurse must understand the physiological, behavioral, social, and addictive aspects of smoking (Caplan, 1995, p. 634). Nursing intervention involves providing smoking cessation programs at the worksite, individual counseling on smoking and health, and referring workers to community smoking cessation resources.

## Violence

Violence in the American workplace takes many forms and is on the rise. It includes harassment, assaults, and threats, as well as injury and death. Risk factors for being a victim of violence in the workplace include interacting with the public, exchanging money, delivery of services or goods, working late at night or during early morning hours, working alone, guarding valuable goods or property, and dealing with violent people or volatile situations (NIOSH, 1997c).

An average of 20 American workers are murdered at the workplace each week (NIOSH, 1997c), and an estimated 1 million workers are victims of nonfatal workplace assaults each year (NIOSH, 1997c; USDL, 1996). Homicide is the second leading cause of fatal injury for all workers and the leading cause of fatal injury in the workplace for women (Gates, 1996, p. 171; NIOSH 1997b). The majority of workplace homicides are robbery-related, and less than 10% are committed by coworkers or former workers (NIOSH, 1997c). The highest risk of robbery is in occupations where money is exchanged (Levin, Hewitt, Misner, 1996, p. 327).

The majority of nonfatal workplace assaults occur in service settings such as hospitals, nursing homes, and social service agencies, and almost half of nonfatal assaults are committed by a health care client (NIOSH, 1997c). Health care workers are at risk for verbal and physical aggression, and violence toward health care workers is an important emerging issue (DiBenedetto, 1995, p. 134; Felton, 1993).

There are thousands of incidents of domestic violence each year in American workplaces. Domestic violence is a significant workplace health problem and places all employees at risk (Fitzgerald, Dienemann, Cadorette, 1998). In addition, domestic violence at home impacts on workplace productivity and attendance and increases insurance and health care costs (USDL, 1994). Many women in domestic violence relationships report being harassed by their abuser at work, either by telephone or in person (Fitzgerald, Dienemann, Cadorette, 1998).

Violence prevention research is needed and will facilitate development of appropriate nursing interventions,

policies, procedures, security measures, and prevention strategies in relation to workplace violence (Gates, 1996, p. 175). According to NIOSH (1997c), prevention strategies should include good visibility within and outside the workplace, good lighting, safe cash-handling policies, physical separation of workers from customers or clients, security devices and precautions, escort services, and employee training. Workplaces need to document incidents of violence, have specific procedures in place in the event of incidents and keep lines of communication open between employers and employees.

A study by Gates (1996) found that many OHNs believe their companies are at risk for violence and that their job responsibilities place them at an increased risk for violence. In the study 70% of the OHNs considered their companies at risk for violence, 58% said they had been harassed at their current workplaces, 15% had been threatened, and almost 5% had been physically assaulted. Almost 40% of the nurses in the study stated that their companies had conducted some type of violence prevention program in the last year.

Stress-producing incidents need to be minimized and neutralized, and employees need to be referred to appropriate social service and mental health resources in the community. Nurses need to work with employers to focus on domestic violence as it relates to worker safety and help companies develop policies related to domestic violence (Fitzgerald, Dienemann, Cadorette, 1998, p. 345). Employers need to take steps to ensure a safe workplace. Nurses need to work to maintain and create nonviolent workplaces and educate workers about safety.

## Substance Abuse

Substance abuse with alcohol and other drugs is a national concern and has a significant impact on the workplace. In the workplace it contributes to decreased productivity, accidents, absenteeism, and increased health care costs (Conrad, Furner, Qian, 1999; McAndrew, McAndrew, 2000). It is estimated that 70% of illegal drug users are employed, and drug use is a major reason for the rise in workplace violence (McAndrew, McAndrew, 2000, p. 32). *Healthy People 2010* has a focus area that addresses substance abuse.

The nurse encounters substance abuse problems in the workplace. If an employee comes to work under the influence of drugs and/or alcohol and the employer allows the individual to remain in the worksite, workers' compensation laws in many states rule in favor of the worker in the event of occupational injury. OHNs often evaluate workers thought to be impaired. Impairment due to substance abuse is often detected through behavior that raises concern about the employee's ability to do job duties without jeopardizing their safety and the safety of others (AAOHN, 1999c; McAndrew, McAndrew, 2000, p. 32). Signs of impairment in relation to substance abuse are given in Chapter 13.

For the safety of the workers, and to protect the employer from liability, employees who are unfit to work should not be permitted at the worksite. In some cases the workers' supervisor will make the decision regarding fitness for work, and in other cases the nurse will. The challenge for the OHN is to influence management to initiate effective interventions and treatment programs. Employee assistance counseling is an integral component of the occupational health service (Rogers, 1994a, p.256).

## MINORITY WORKERS AND OCCUPATIONAL HEALTH

**Minority health** is a rising workplace concern. In general, minority workers often have less education, lower income levels, inferior housing, worse health status, and less access to health care and community resources (Taylor, Murray, 2000, p. 679). The wages of minority workers have not kept up with their white counterparts, and they often work in the more hazardous jobs (Taylor, Murray, 2000, pp. 679-680).

Employment in hazardous occupations is much more common among minority workers and results in a disproportionate number of occupational diseases, injuries, and deaths within these population groups. Minority workers are more likely to receive inadequate health care and to become disabled from occupational injuries. Nurses need to consider this in their plans of care and implementation of health education and safety programs.

More than 50% of the laborers in the hazardous lead smelting industry are African American or Hispanic (Taylor, Murray, 2000, p. 680). Eighty-five percent of the migrant and seasonal farmworker populations are composed of minorities (Fact sheet, 1993). Minorities are at particular risk for agricultural work-related fatal injury: the risk for work-related death among Hispanic and African-American agricultural workers is almost 30% greater than among whites, and for all other minorities, the risk is twice as great as for whites (CDC, 1992b, p. 11). Farm work has one of the highest occupational fatality rates in the United States, and many of these deaths and injuries occur among seasonal migrant farm workers. For such reasons agricultural workers are addressed more extensively.

## AGRICULTURAL WORKERS

Agriculture is the world's largest economic activity and involves more than 60% of the population in developing countries (Fenske, Simcox, 2000, p. 729). **Agricultural workers** in the United States encompass more than 4 million people, composed of primarily African Americans; Native Americans; and immigrants from Mexico, Puerto Rico, Haiti, Jamaica, and Central America (Fenske, Simcox, 2000). Additionally, 6 million persons are considered members of farm families (Olson, Bark, 1996).

Health risks and disparities in rural, American communities are discussed in Chapter 3.

Agricultural workers encompass several groups, including farm owners and their families; migrant and seasonal workers; and agricultural service workers. Major differences in the agricultural work force, compared with workforces in general industry, are that the workplace is often the farmer's home (Connon, Freund, Ehlers, 1993), and occupational exposures change as the production process, equipment, weather, and conditions change (Olson, Bark, 1996).

Historically, farm workers have not been protected well by federal laws, placing their health and well-being at risk (Fenske, Simcox, 2000, pp. 729-730; Kelsey, 1994; Pollack, Rubenstein, Landrigan, 1994). It is difficult to monitor the safety, environmental health, and labor practices of farmers.

### OHNs in Agricultural Communities Program

To prevent illness, injury, and death with agricultural workers, NIOSH started the "agricultural initiative" that includes the OHN in Agricultural Communities (OHNAC) program, the Farm Family Health and Hazard Survey, Agricultural Health Promotion System, Cancer Screening in Farmers, and Agricultural Research Centers (Connon, Freund, Ehlers, 1993). The OHNAC Program created a new role for OHNs. This program is carried out in 10 states by nurses with the cooperation of local health departments, rural hospitals, migrant health centers, county cooperative extension offices, and clinics (Randolph, Migliozzi, 1993). Using an epidemiological framework, the nurse draws on knowledge from both community health and occupational health nursing (Randolph, Migliozzi, 1993).

The OHNAC Program goals are to conduct active surveillance of injuries and illness affecting agricultural workers and their families; identify preventable health events; and develop interventions directed at reducing or eliminating these events (Dobler, 1995). Nursing interventions include collecting data; writing prevention-oriented articles; making presentations to farm groups, schools, and individuals; addressing the sociocultural aspects of health; and conducting farm safety programs that include educating workers about farm hazards, agricultural respiratory conditions, and hearing conservation (Dobler, 1995). OHNAC nurses must know the communities in which they work and develop community partnerships (see Chapters 3 and 14). The nurse is in a unique position to teach about risk awareness, safety principles, and community resources (Olson, Bark, 1996).

### Some Health Concerns of Agricultural Workers

Agriculture is one of the most hazardous occupations in the United States (Fenske, Simcox, 2000, p. 732). Farming injuries and fatalities have become so frequent that they are sometimes accepted by the farming community as unavoidable (Lexau, Kingsbury, Lenz, et al., 1993). Nurses must work to prevent injuries and change attitudes about prevention.

Workers in agriculture have the second highest rate of occupational illnesses (Fenske, Simcox, 2000, p. 733). Agricultural workers have an injury rate four times the number of all other occupations (Dobler, 1995). Injury and disease associated with physical, chemical, and biological hazards occur disproportionately among agricultural workers and their families. Agricultural machinery, especially farm tractors, is a major cause of work-related deaths among farm workers.

SKIN DISORDERS. Skin disorders were discussed previously in this chapter. They are the most frequently reported agricultural disease, and agricultural workers have the highest rate of these disorders in the nation (Fenske, Simcox, 2000, p. 733). The high incidence of occupational skin disorders is largely a result of exposure to pesticides and agricultural chemicals that results in contact dermatitis and other skin conditions.

MUSCULOSKELETAL DISORDERS. Musculoskeletal disorders were discussed previously in this chapter. With agricultural workers, musculoskeletal conditions and injuries are common occurrences. They often occur from heavy lifting and carrying, bending, kneeling, and fast-paced work. Farm workers have a higher prevalence of arthritis than do all workers combined (Fenske, Simcox, 2000, p. 734).

RESPIRATORY ILLNESS. Agricultural workers have a high incidence of respiratory illnesses including (1) airway inflammatory responses to organic dust exposure (e.g., rhinitis, pharyngitis, laryngitis, bronchitis, asthma, toxic organic dust syndrome), (2) airway immunological responses to organic dust exposures (e.g., allergic rhinitis, extrinsic asthma), (3) interstitial immunological responses to certain fungi and bacteria (e.g., hypersensitivity pneumonitis or "farmer's lung" and pneumonia), and (4) respiratory injury responses to chemical exposures (e.g., laryngeal edema, pharyngitis, pulmonary edema, interstitial fibrosis, bronchitis, and respiratory depression or arrest (American Lung Association of Iowa, 1986, p. 2).

Frequently, respiratory illnesses are diagnosed incorrectly, and farmers return to a work setting that further induces or aggravates the condition (American Lung Association of Iowa, 1986, p. 1). Permanent lung damage can be prevented by eliminating the exposures. Farm management and engineering changes that reduce exposure to dusts are advisable for all farmers (American Lung Association of Iowa, 1986, p. 1). "Farmer's lung" is a respiratory condition that is gaining increased attention.

*Farmer's lung.* *Farmer's lung* is one of many respiratory conditions to which agricultural workers are susceptible. Farmers tend to inhale a significant amount of bacterial and fungal spores that can lead to a condition called "farmer's lung," or hypersensitivity pneumonitis. Farmer's lung was first described in the literature more than 40 years ago (Dickie, Rankin, 1958; Totten, Reid, Davies, Moran, 1958)

and is a form of allergic alveolitis. Like coal miner's black lung and textile worker's brown lung, it is an occupationally related disease; unlike these diseases there is often an immediate recovery when the person is removed from the causative environment (Reyes, Wenzel, Lawton, Emanuel, 1982). Residual lung damage in the form of pulmonary fibrosis can occur (American Lung Association, 1989, p. 4).

Symptoms of an acute attack are similar to those of the flu and appear some 4 to 6 hours after the person breathes the offending dust; they may persist for as little as 12 hours or as long as 10 days (American Lung Association, 1989, p. 1). After repeated exposure to the dust, chronic cough may develop with excessive sputum production, cough, dyspnea, myalgia, and malaise (American Lung Association, 1989, p. 1). The changes are those of hypersensitivity pneumonitis, and the disease is characterized by unresolved pneumonia, interstitial pneumonitis, pleural fibrosis, and granuloma and edema (Reyes, Wenzel, Lawton, Emanuel, 1982). Most drugs are of limited value in the treatment of the disease. Avoidance of the offending dust is the most important treatment and control measure.

CHILDREN AND AGRICULTURE. Almost 2 million children live or work on farms in the United States and each year approximately 100,000 of them are injured and 100 are killed (NIOSH, 1997d). Even young children are frequently involved in aspects of operating the farm. Children are often exposed to farm chemicals and other hazards. Nurses need to promote childhood farm safety and protection (Lexau, Kingsbury, Lenz, et al., 1993). Until recently, there was no national coordinated effort to protect children in the agricultural industry. However, NIOSH now receives funding from the federal government to prevent agriculture injury and death among children (NIOSH, 1997d).

## Migrant Farm Workers

**Migrant farm workers** are a special group of agricultural workers. There are approximately 4 million migrant farm workers and their dependents in the United States (Fenske, Simcox, 2000, p. 729). They face numerous health hazards (Figure 21-5) and are not protected by many of the laws that govern the health and welfare of other workers. Migrant farm workers encounter problems that include financial instability, child labor, poor housing, lack of education, and impaired access to health and social services.

Migrant farm work is one of the most hazardous occupations in the United States. A major problem with estimating occupational injury among migrant farm workers is that few reliable statistics are kept. Two well-documented occupational health hazards for the migrant farm worker are injuries from farm machinery and exposure to agricultural chemicals such as pesticides.

The stresses the migrant worker must face, such as poor working conditions, problems with access to health services, decreased educational opportunities for themselves and their children, and low wages, all contribute to poverty

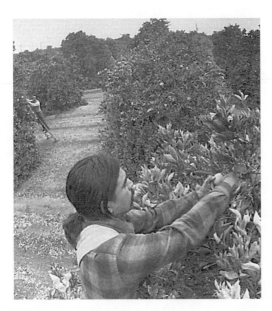

**FIGURE 21-5** Migrant farm workers are exposed to many health risks. (Courtesy of U.S. Department of Agriculture.)

and poor health beyond what most Americans will ever experience. Because the migrant worker is often concerned with immediate, day-to-day survival, planning for the future is difficult. The nurse working with migrant families can facilitate their efforts in obtaining health care and improve their quality of life. The nurse often needs to assume the role of client advocate. Helping to ensure the health of migrant workers is a challenging endeavor, as well as a social and professional responsibility that cannot be ignored.

**FINANCIAL STABILITY.** Migrant farm workers represent a large, mobile supply of cheap labor. Their work is characterized by low wages, long hours, few benefits, and poor working conditions. They are the working poor, without many of the health and welfare benefits that other workers have. Many migrant farm families have incomes below the poverty level and live in chronic poverty. Many migrant families have incomes of less than $7500 a year (Migrant health, 1993).

**CHILD LABOR.** Child labor has all but disappeared from U.S. industry except in the agricultural sector. Generally, in the United States a child must be 16 to work and 18 to take part in hazardous work. The Fair Labor Standards Act allows children as young as 12 years old to work as agricultural laborers, and children as young as 16 can take part in hazardous agricultural activities (Fenske, Simcox, 2000, p. 731). Many migrant children work to supplement the family income. Employers use child labor because it is inexpensive and available. Children who work are subjected to the same agricultural hazards and health risks as adults, including long hours, hazardous or faulty equipment, exposure to the elements, and toxic chemicals. Working children have a high rate of accidental injury on the job. The use of children as agricultural laborers can jeopardize their educa-

tional and developmental opportunities and place them at increased risk for injury, illness, disability, and death (Fenske, Simcox, 2000, p. 730). As previously mentioned, 100,000 children have agriculture-related injuries each year.

**HOUSING.** Migrant farm workers often live in substandard housing that is crowded, inadequate, and unsanitary (Fact sheet, 1993; Watkins, Larson, Harlan, Young, 1990, p. 567). Migrant housing is continually described as horrible and dehumanizing, without adequate heat, light, or ventilation, and often without plumbing or refrigeration (Fact sheet, 1993; Goldfarb, 1981, p. 42). In eight major agricultural states, more than 35% of this housing lacked inside running water, and few employers provided even minimal toilet facilities in the field for farm workers (Fact sheet, 1993). These unsanitary and unsafe housing conditions are breeding grounds for diseases, disability, hopelessness, and death.

**EDUCATION.** Many migrant children never enter high school and, of those who do, few graduate. It is not that migrant families do not want an education for their children; they just have great difficulty obtaining it. Their mobility and the seasonal nature of farm work necessitate frequent school changes and absences. School officials are often lax in enforcing attendance and other regulations for migrant children. Migrant children may be labeled slow, retarded, uncooperative, or uninterested when actually the situation is more a social problem than a question of educational ability. The aspirations of migrant families for their children to receive a good education often go unfulfilled. As long as migrant children are poorly educated, it will be difficult for them to escape their present living conditions.

**ACCESS TO SERVICES.** Migrant families face language, cultural, financial, immigration, educational, and other barriers to obtaining health and welfare services. Communities may be indifferent to issues of migrant health and welfare. Migrant workers generally have no voice in community planning and decision making and often do not feel a sense of belonging to the communities in which they work. Although migrant families may qualify for federal aid programs and services, they may not be aware of them. In 1969 a Supreme Court decision (Shapiro v. Thompson, 394 U.S. 618) ruled that a state could not exclude persons from welfare benefits because they were not residents of that state. As a result of this ruling, many migrant families are eligible for services such as Temporary Assistance to Needy Families, food stamps, and Medicaid. However, the 1996 welfare reform law allows states the option to bar or limit current residents and new immigrants from several welfare benefits (National Immigrant Law Center, 1996).

**HEALTH.** The transient nature of their work makes it difficult to provide continuous, comprehensive health services. Many migrant families are uninsured and are not aware of the health care services available to them. They often do not have a regular source of primary health care, have numerous and complex health problems, and evidence higher rates of diseases and conditions than other Americans. Migrant farm workers suffer as much as twenty times the rate of diarrhea found among the urban poor, and up to 78% suffer from parasitic infection, as compared with 2% to 3% of the general population (Fact sheet, 1993). They suffer and die from heat stress and dehydration, and more than 40% have positive TB skin test results (Fact sheet, 1993). In addition, in relation to the general population, migrant farm workers have higher incidence of diabetes, digestive diseases, hypertension, malnutrition, high-risk pregnancies, infant mortality, and dental disease (CDC, 1992a, p. 2). They are six times more likely to develop tuberculosis than other employed adults (CDC, 1992a, p. 1).

Although they have a higher incidence of high-risk pregnancies, migrant women are less likely to have adequate prenatal care than their white counterparts. The majority of preschool farm children are not adequately vaccinated for their age level (Fact sheet, 1993). Migrant children have a high incidence of hospitalization and chronic illness (Watkins, Larson, Harlan, Young, 1990, p. 568). Research has shown that migrant workers are at high risk for developing malignant lymphoma, leukemia, multiple myeloma, testicular cancer, and cancer of the gastrointestinal tract (Moses, 1989, pp. 121-122). Goldfarb (1981) found that the average life expectancy for the migrant worker was 49 years, while the average life expectancy for the nation as a whole was 74 years. This figure is statistically and *morally* significant. Migrant health is an important area that needs to be addressed in the United States.

Thousands of farm workers are affected each year from exposure to pesticides. Acute health effects from exposure to pesticides range from contact dermatitis to systemic poisoning and death. The primary route of exposure to pesticides, except for fumigants, is through the skin, and they may persist on the skin for several months (Moses, 1989, p. 116). Few studies have been done on the chronic health problems related to pesticide exposure, and surveillance and record keeping on these exposures is lacking.

MIGRANT HEALTH CENTERS. With the passage of the Migrant Health Act in 1962, **migrant health centers** were established. These centers are an important source of heath care for migrant workers and their families. Services provided by these centers include mental health, substance abuse, transportation, pharmacy, dental, emergency, environmental health, prenatal, pediatric, and social services (National Association of Community Health Centers, Inc., 1991, p. 19). Preventive services provided by these centers include health education and counseling, immunizations, blood lead screening, antepartal care, developmental and physical assessments, hearing examinations, and the Supplemental Food Program for Women, Infants, and Children (WIC) (National Association of Community Health Centers, Inc., 1991, p. 19). Thousands of migrant workers are served by these centers each year (CDC, 1992a, p. 2). The

nurse plays a major role in service provision in these centers, and many services are provided by advanced practice nurses.

## OCCUPATIONAL SAFETY AND HEALTH: A LOOK TO THE FUTURE

As a priority area in *Healthy People 2010*, occupational health will remain at the forefront of the nation's health agenda. AAOHN was instrumental in the development of the national occupational health objectives and continues to play an active role in promoting occupational health. More than any other health profession, the nurse has been at the forefront of occupational health in the United States.

Our national health agenda is now emphasizing community-based care and preventive health services. The OHN has historically been involved in these activities. Nurses will be called on to develop, implement, and evaluate worksite health promotion programs. The occupational health programs of the future must integrate occupational health research into program and service planning, work in partnership with communities to support worker health and utilize resources, include employees in planning and implementing occupational health programs, recognize the importance of prevention versus treatment, use state-of-the-art surveillance and treatment, promote continuing education for occupational health staff, continuously evaluate programs, and provide quality care.

AAOHN has made a firm commitment to research, and OHNs will expand their research agendas. Educational opportunities will increase in occupational health nursing, and more OHNs will obtain graduate education. In addition, they will be involved in educating school children and the general public about occupational health.

Ethical issues will increase in scope and individual nurses, as well as their professional organizations, will need to monitor them closely. Workplace issues such as communicable disease, violence, confidentiality, legal/ethical dilemmas, and right-to-know about occupational hazards will continue to need to be addressed. Case management techniques will be used increasingly, and cost containment and efficiency of service will remain important issues. Standards of care will be updated and revised and continue to guide the profession.

International occupational health concerns will increasingly emerge. Rapid industrialization, lack of occupational safety and health legislation, inadequate control measures for communicable disease, and inadequate health care systems place many countries at risk for worker health problems (Levy, 1996). Levy noted that in some countries where workers are unprotected and plentiful, managers know that for every worker who cannot work because of illness or injury incurred at work, several people are waiting to be hired for the same job. Nurses need to be proactive in national and international occupational health issues and advocate for better occupational health policies. Nurses need to remain politically and socially active, advocate for effective occupational health legislation and services, and help shape national and international health objectives reflective of current occupational health issues.

## SUMMARY

Occupational health influences not only the status of the individual worker but also the health of society as a whole. Maintaining the health of the working population is an important task for all health professionals. Historically, nursing has been at the forefront of occupational health activities and has served as a role model to other professions in the field.

This chapter has addressed many occupational health concerns of workers, their families, and the community, illustrating that occupational health is a rapidly emerging and changing field. It is notable that there have been more advances in the protection of workers from occupational health hazards in the United States in the last 25 years than in the entire history of the nation. Our country now has federal and state legislation to protect the health and safety of the worker, occupational health is a national health priority, and national occupational health objectives are being implemented. Occupational health nursing will provide many opportunities for future practitioners and advanced practice nurses will be increasingly used in the workplace. Increasingly, community-based initiatives for health promotion will be directed toward workers in the occupational health setting. Occupational health nursing will be an important part of the nursing of the future; it is an exciting, challenging field with unlimited potential.

## CRITICAL THINKING
*exercise*

Taking into consideration that nurses are workers, analyze some of the occupational stressors that nurses are exposed to in the workplace and identify primary prevention activities to protect nurses from their effects. What are some of the occupational stressors you are concerned about encountering in your nursing careers?

## REFERENCES

Adams J, Mackey T, Lindenberg J, Baden T: Primary care at the worksite: the use of health risk appraisal in a nursing center, *AAOHN J* 43(1):17-22, 1995.

American Association of Industrial Nurses (AAIN): *The nurse in industry*, New York, 1976, AAIN.

American Association of Occupational Health Nurses (AAOHN): A year of progress...American Association of Occupational Health Nurses Annual Report, *AAOHN J* 37(4), 1989.

American Association of Occupational Health Nurses (AAOHN): *Occupational health nursing: the answer to health care cost containment*, Atlanta, 1991, AAOHN.

American Association of Occupational Health Nurses (AAOHN): *Educational preparation for entry into professional practice*, Atlanta, 1996a, AAOHN.

American Association of Occupational Health Nurses (AAOHN): *Employee health records: requirements, retention, and access*, Atlanta, 1996b, AAOHN.

American Association of Occupational Health Nurses (AAOHN): *Position Statement. Occupational health surveillance*, Atlanta, 1996c, AAOHN.

American Association of Occupational Health Nurses (AAOHN): *Position Statement. The occupational health nurse as a case manager*, Atlanta, 1996d, AAOHN.

American Association of Occupational Health Nurses (AAOHN): *Occupational and environmental health nursing. Your key to health care cost containment*, Atlanta, 1998a, AAOHN.

American Association of Occupational Health Nurses (AAOHN): *AAOHN research priorities in occupational and environmental health nursing*, Atlanta, 1998b, AAOHN.

American Association of Occupational Health Nurses (AAOHN): *Code of ethics and interpretive statements*, Atlanta, 1998c, AAOHN.

American Association of Occupational Health Nurses (AAOHN): *Position Statement. Confidentiality of health information*, Atlanta, 1998d, AAOHN.

American Association of Occupational Health Nurses (AAOHN): *Standards of occupational and environmental health nursing*, Atlanta, 1999a, AAOHN.

American Association of Occupational Health Nurses (AAOHN): *Advisory. Nurse practitioners in occupational and environmental health*, Atlanta, 1999b, AAOHN.

American Association of Occupational Health Nurses (AAOHN): *Advisory. Work fitness impairment evaluation in occupational and environmental health*, Atlanta, 1999c, AAOHN.

American Lung Association: *Facts about...hypersensitivity pneumonitis: lung hazards on the job*, Washington, DC, 1989, The Association.

American Lung Association of Iowa: *Agricultural respiratory hazards: education series for the health professional*, Des Moines, Iowa, 1986, The Association.

Ashford N: Government regulation. In Levy BS, Wegman DH, editors: *Occupational health. Recognizing and preventing work-related disease and injury*, Philadelphia, 2000, Lippincott, Williams & Wilkins.

Baker DB, Karasek RA: Stress. In Levy BS, Wegman DH, editors: *Occupational health. Recognizing and preventing work-related disease and injury*, Philadelphia, 2000, Lippincott, Williams & Wilkins.

Baker EL: Disorders of the nervous system. In Levy BS, Wegman DH, editors: *Occupational health. Recognizing and preventing work-related disease and injury*, Philadelphia, 2000, Lippincott, Williams & Wilkins.

Bale A: Assuming the risks: occupational disease in the years before workers' compensation, *Am J Indus Med* 13:449-514, 1988.

Barlow R: Role of the occupational health nurse in the year 2000, *AAOHN J* 40:463-467, 1992.

Barrett V, Phillips JA: Reproductive health in the American workplace, *AAOHN J* 43:40-51, 1995.

Bigby ME, Arndt KA, Coopman SA: Skin disorders. In Levy BS, Wegman DH, editors: *Occupational health. Recognizing and preventing work-related disease and injury*, Philadelphia, 2000, Lippincott, Williams & Wilkins.

Breckon DJ, Harvey JR, Lancaster RB: *Community health education. Settings, roles and skills for the 21st century*, ed 4, Gaithersburg, Mass, 1998, Aspen Publishers.

Brown ML: *Occupational health nursing*, New York, 1956, Springer.

Brown ML: An historical perspective: one hundred years of industrial or occupational health nursing in the United States, *AAOHN J* 36:433-435, 1988.

Caplan D: Smoking: issues and interventions for occupational health nurses, *AAOHN J* 43:633-645, 1995.

Caplan LS, Coughlin SS: Worksite breast cancer screening programs, *AAOHN J* 46:443-451, 1998.

Centers for Disease Control (CDC): Leading work-related diseases and injuries—U.S. (occupational lung diseases), *MMWR* 32:24-27, January 21, 1983a.

Centers for Disease Control (CDC): Epidemic psychogenic illness in an industrial setting—Pennsylvania, *MMWR* 32:189-190, 1983b.

Centers for Disease Control and Prevention (CDC): Leading work-related diseases and injuries: U.S. (occupational cancers other than lung), *MMWR* 33:126, 1984.

Centers for Disease Control and Prevention (CDC): Prevention and control of tuberculosis in migrant farm workers, *MMWR* 41:1-15, June 5, 1992a.

Centers for Disease Control and Prevention (CDC): Surgeon General's Conference on Agricultural Safety and Health, 1991, *MMWR* 41:5, 11-12, 1992b.

Centers for Disease Control and Prevention (CDC): Recommendations to prevent hepatitis B virus transmission—United States, *MMWR* 44:574-575, 1995.

Centers for Disease Control and Prevention (CDC): Public Health Service guidelines for the management of health-care worker exposure to HIV and recommendations for postexposure prophylaxis, *MMWR* 47(RR-7):1-175, 1998.

Christiani DC, Wegman DH: Respiratory disorders. In Levy BS, Wegman DH, editors: *Occupational health. Recognizing and preventing work-related disease and injury*, Philadelphia, 2000, Lippincott, Williams & Wilkins.

Colligan MJ, Murphy LA: Mass psychogenic illness in organizations: an overview, *J Occup Psychol* 52:77-90, 1979.

Colligan MJ, Stockton W: The mystery of assembly-line hysteria, *Psychology Today*, June 1978, pp. 93-99, 114-116.

Connon CL, Freund E, Ehlers JK: The occupational health nurses in agricultural communities program: identifying and preventing agriculturally related illnesses and injuries, *AAOHN J* 41:422-428, 1993.

Conrad KM, Furner SE, Qian Y: Occupational hazard exposure and at risk drinking, *AAOHN J* 47:9-16, 1999.

Corser WD: Occupational exposure of health care workers to blood-borne pathogens; a proposal for a systematic intervention approach. *AAOHN J* 46:246-252, 1998.

Cullen MR: Personal reflections on occupational health in the twentieth century: spiraling to the future. In Fielding JE, Lave LB, Starfield B, editors: *Annu Rev Public Health* 20:1-13, 1999.

Davidhoff F: New disease, old story, *Ann Intern Med* 129:327-328, 1998 (editorial).

DiBenedetto DV: Occupational hazards of the health care industry, *AAOHN J* 43:131-137, 1995.

Dickie HA, Rankin J: Farmer's lung: an acute granulomatous interstitial pneumonitis occurring in agricultural workers, *JAMA* 167:1069-1078, 1958.

Dobler LK: Occupational health nurses in agricultural communities, *Prairie Rose* June, July, August:11-12, 1995.

Dunn AC: Noise. In Levy BS, Wegman DH, editors: *Occupational health. Recognizing and preventing work-related disease and injury*, Philadelphia, 2000, Lippincott, Williams & Wilkins.

Duvall EM, Miller BC: *Marriage and family development*, ed 6, New York, 1985, Harper & Row.

Fact Sheet: *Basic health*, Austin, Tex, 1993, National Migrant Resource Program.

Felton JS: 200 years of occupational medicine in the U.S., *J Occup Med* 28:809-814, 1976.

Felton JS: The genesis of American occupational health nursing: part II, *AAOHN J* 34:31-35, 1988.

Felton JS: Occupational violence—an intensified work concomitant, *OEM Report* 7(12):101-103, 1993.

Fenske RA, Simcox NJ: Agricultural workers. In Levy BS, Wegman DH, editors: *Occupational health. Recognizing and preventing work-related disease and injury*, Philadelphia, 2000, Lippincott, Williams & Wilkins.

Fielder NF, Caccappolo E: Psychiatric disorders. In Levy BS, Wegman DH, editors: *Occupational health. Recognizing and preventing work-related disease and injury*, Philadelphia, 2000, Lippincott, Williams & Wilkins.

Fincham SM, Ugnat AM, Hill GB, et al.: Is occupation a risk factor for thyroid cancer? *J Occup Indus Med* 42:318-322, 2000.

Fitzgerald S, Dienemann J, Cadorette MF: Domestic violence in the workplace, *AAOHN J* 46:345-353,1998.

Frumkin J, Thun M: Carcinogens. In Levy BS, Wegman DH, editors: *Occupational health. Recognizing and preventing work-related disease and injury*, Philadelphia, 2000, Lippincott, Williams & Wilkins.

Gantz NM: Infectious agents. In Levy BS, Wegman DH, editors: *Occupational health. Recognizing and preventing work-related disease and injury*, Philadelphia, 2000, Lippincott, Williams & Wilkins.

Gardner MS: *Public health nursing*, New York, 1916, MacMillan.

Gates DM: Workplace violence: occupational health nurses: beliefs and experiences, *AAOHN J* 44:171-176, 1996.

Goldfarb RL: *Caste of despair*, Ames, Iowa, 1981, Iowa University Press.

Goldstein BD, Kipen HM: Hematologic disorders. In Levy BS, Wegman DH, editors: *Occupational health. Recognizing and preventing work-related disease and injury*, Philadelphia, 2000, Lippincott, Williams & Wilkins.

Griest SE, Bishop PM: Tinnitus as an early indicator of permanent hearing loss, *AAOHN J* 46:325-329, 1998.

Gross GM, Fuchs A: Reduce musculoskeletal injuries with corporate ergonomics programs, *Occup Health Safety* 59(1): 28-29, 1990.

Guzik A: Workers' Compensation, FMLA, and ADA, *AAOHN J* 47:261-274, 1999.

Haag AB, Glazner LK: A remembrance of the past, an investment for the future, *AAOHN J* 40:56-60, 1992.

Hamilton A: *Industrial poisons in the United States*, New York, 1925, MacMillan.

Hamilton A: *Exploring the dangerous trades: the autobiography of Alice Hamilton, M.D.*, Boston, 1943, Little, Brown.

Hershey JC, Martin LS: Use of infection control guidelines by workers in healthcare facilities to prevent occupational transmission of HBV and HIV: results from a national survey, *Infect Control Hosp Epidemiology*, 15:243-252, 1994.

Hibberd PL: Clients, workers, and health care workers, *J Intravenous Nurs* 18:65-76, 1995.

Jaffe HA, Schmitt J: AIDS in the workplace. In Rom WR: *Environmental and occupational medicine*, ed 2, Boston, 1992, Little, Brown.

Karas BE, Conrad R: Back injury prevention interventions in the workplace, *AAOHN J* 44:189-196, 1996.

Keim K: Application of the ADA in the workplace. Employment issues, *AAOHN J* 47:213-216, 1999.

Kelsey TW: The agrarian myth and policy responses to farm safety, *Am J Public Health* 84:1, 171, 177, 1994.

Kern DG, Crausman RS, Durand KTH, et al.: Flock worker's lung: chronic interstitial lung disease in the nylon flocking industry, *Ann Intern Med* 129:261-272, 1998.

Killien MG: Women's work, women's health. In Hinshaw AS, Feetham SL, Shaver JLF: *Handbook of clinical nursing research*, Thousand Oaks, Calif, 1999, Sage.

Kosinski M: Effective outcomes management in occupational and environmental health, *AAOHN J* 46:500-509, 1999.

LeMasters G: Occupational exposures and effects on male and female reproduction. In Rom WR: *Environmental and occupational medicine*, ed 2, Boston, 1992, Little, Brown.

Levin PF, Hewitt JB, Misner ST: Workplace violence: female occupational homicides in metropolitan Chicago, *AAOHN J* 44:326-331, 1996.

Levy BS: Global occupational health issues, *AAOHN J* 44:244-248, 1996.

Levy BS, Wegman DH: Occupational health: an overview. In Levy BS, Wegman DH, editors: *Occupational health. Recognizing and preventing work-related disease and injury*, Philadelphia, 2000, Lippincott, Williams & Wilkins.

Levy BS, Wegman DH, Halperin WE: Recognizing occupational disease and injury. In Levy BS, Wegman DH, editors: *Occupational health. Recognizing and preventing work-related disease and injury*, Philadelphia, 2000, Lippincott, Williams & Wilkins.

Lexau C, Kingsbury L, Lenz B, et al.: Building coalitions: a community wide approach for promoting farming health and safety, *AAOHN J* 41:440-449, 1993.

Lowey B: Noise know how, *Occup Health Safety* 69(6):95-100, 2000.

Lukes E, Johnson M: Hearing conversation: community outreach program for high school students, *AAOHN J* 46: 340-343, 1998.

Lusk SL: Corporate expectations for occupational health nurses' activities, *AAOHN J* 38:368-374, 1990.

Lusk SL: Linking practice and research, *AAOHN J* 41:153-157, 1993.

Maddux J: OSHA gears up for more streamlined, user-friendly record keeping standard, *Occup Safety Health* 64(1):34-36, 1995.

Markolf AS: Industrial nursing begins in Vermont, *Public Health Nurs* 37:125-129, 1945.

Martin C, Andrew-Tuthill DM: Office ergonomics. Measurements for success, *AAOHN J* 47:479-491, 1999.

Martin G: New roles for the occupational health nurse, *Job Safety and Health* 5(4):9-15, 1977.

McAndrew KG, McAndrew SJ: Workplace substance abuse impairment, *AAOHN J* 48:32-44, 2000.

McCall B: How West Germany protects its workers, *Job Safety and Health* 5(7):21-25, 1977.

McGrath BJ: Fifty years of industrial nursing in the United States, *Public Health Nurs* 37:119-124, 1945.

McGrath BJ: *Nursing in commerce and industry*, New York, 1946, The Commonwealth Fund.

McGuire JL: Hearing conservation and employee conservation. In Hansen DJ, editor: *The work environment: occupational health fundamentals*, vol I, Chelsea, Mich, 1991, Lewis.

McGuire JL: Nuisance noise in the office. In Hansen DJ, editor: *The work environment: occupational health fundamentals*, vol III, Ann Arbor, Mich, 1994, Lewis.

McGuire JL: *Conversation with author: worker hearing conversation*, Jan 28, 2001.

McNeely E: Tracking the future of OSHA, *AAOHN J* 40:17-23, 1992.

McRill C, Boyer LV, Flood TJ, Ortega L: Mercury toxicity due to use of a cosmetic cream, *J Occup Envir Med* 42(1):4-7, 2000.

Migrant health status: profile of a population with complex health problems, Austin, Tex, 1993, National Migrant Resource Program.

Mitchell R, Leanna JC, Hyde R: Client satisfaction with nursing services, *AAOHN J* 47:74-79, 1999.

Merservy D, Bass J, Toth W: Health Surveillance. Effective components of a successful program, *AAOHN J* 45:500-510, 1997.

Morris R: *The American worker*, Washington, DC, 1976, US Government Printing Office.

Moses M: Pesticide related health problems and farm workers, *AAOHN J* 37:115-130, 1989.

Moss L: Mental health and the changing workplace environment. In Rom WR, et al.: *Environmental and occupational medicine*, ed 2, Boston, 1992, Little, Brown.

Mueller JL: Returning to work through job accommodation, *AAOHN J* 47:120-129, 1999.

National Association of Community Health Centers, Inc.: *Community and migrant health centers: a key component of the U.S. health care system—overview and status report 1991*, Washington, DC, 1991, The Association.

National Immigration Law Center: *Overview of benefit restrictions to immigrants in 1996 welfare and immigration laws*, Washington, DC, 1996, The Center.

National Institute for Occupational Safety and Health (NIOSH): *Proposed national strategies for the prevention of leading work-related diseases and injuries: musculoskeletal injuries* (NIOSH Pub No 89-129), Cincinnati, Ohio, 1986, NIOSH.

National Institute for Occupational Safety and Health (NIOSH): *List of ten leading work-related diseases and injuries*, Cincinnati, Ohio, 1988a, NIOSH.

National Institute for Occupational Safety and Health (NIOSH): *Proposed national strategies for the prevention of leading work-related diseases and injuries: disorders of reproduction* (NIOSH Pub No 89-133), Cincinnati, Ohio, 1988b, NIOSH.

National Institute for Occupational Safety and Health (NIOSH): *Proposed national strategies for the prevention of leading work-related diseases and injuries: psychological disorders* (NIOSH Pub No 89-137), Cincinnati, Ohio, 1988c, NIOSH.

National Institute for Occupational Safety and Health (NIOSH): *Proposed national strategies for the prevention of leading work-related diseases and injuries: dermatological conditions* (NIOSH Pub No 89-136), Cincinnati, Ohio, 1988d, NIOSH.

National Institute for Occupational Safety and Health (NIOSH): *New directions at NIOSH*, Cincinnati, Ohio, 1995, NIOSH.

National Institute for Occupational Safety and Health (NIOSH): *The effects of workplace hazards on male reproductive health*, Cincinnati, Ohio, 1996, NIOSH.

National Institute for Occupational Safety and Health (NIOSH): *Work-related musculoskeletal disorders*, Cincinnati, Ohio, 1997a, NIOSH.

National Institute for Occupational Safety and Health (NIOSH): *Breast cancer research at NIOSH*, Cincinnati, Ohio, 1997b, NIOSH.

National Institute for Occupational Safety and Health (NIOSH): *Violence in the workplace*, Cincinnati, Ohio, 1997c, NIOSH.

National Institute for Occupational Safety and Health (NIOSH): *Health and safety for kids on the farm*, Cincinnati, Ohio, 1997d, NIOSH.

National Institute for Occupational Safety and Health (NIOSH): *National occupational research agenda*, Publication No. 99-108, Cincinnati, Ohio, 1999a, NIOSH.

National Institute for Occupational Safety and Health (NIOSH): *The effects of workplace hazards on female reproductive health*, Cincinnati, Ohio, 1999b, NIOSH.

National Institute for Occupational Safety and Health (NIOSH): *Stress at work*, No. 99-101, Cincinnati, Ohio, 1999c, NIOSH.

National Institute for Occupational Safety and Health (NIOSH): *Worker health chartbook, 2000*, Washington, DC, 2000a, USDHHS.

National Institute for Occupational Safety and Health (NIOSH): *Alice Hamilton, M.D.*, Cincinnati, Ohio, 2000b, NIOSH. *http://www.cdc.gov/niosh/hamhist.html*

National Institute for Occupational Safety and Health (NIOSH): *National occupational research agenda. Update May 2000*, Cincinnati, Ohio, 2000c, NIOSH.

National Institute for Occupational Safety and Health (NIOSH): *Work-related hearing loss*, Cincinnati, Ohio, 2000d, NIOSH.

National Institute for Occupational Safety and Health (NIOSH): *NIOSH Education and Research Center Grants (ERC's)*. *http://www.cdc.gov/niosh/centers.html*

National Research Council: *Work-related musculoskeletal disorders: a review of the evidence*, Washington, DC, 1998, National Academy Press.

Office of Management and Budget: *Budget of the United States government FY 2000*, Washington, DC, 2000, US Government Printing Office.

Olson DK, Bark SM: Health hazards affecting the animal confinement farm worker, *AAOHN J* 44:198-206, 1996.

Olson DK, Kochevar L: Occupational health and safety content in baccalaureate nursing programs, *AAOHN J* 37:33-38, 1989.

O'Neal J: *The bloodborne pathogens standard*, New York, 1996, Norstrand Reinhold.

Ostendorf JS, Rogers B, Bertsche PK: Ergonomics. CTD management evaluation tool, *AAOHN J* 48:17-24, 2000.

Parker-Conrad J: A century of practice: occupational health nursing, *AAOHN J* 36:156-161, 1988.

Parrish RS, Allred RH: Theories and trends in occupational health nursing, *AAOHN J* 43:514-521, 1995.

Paul M, Frazier L: Reproductive disorders. In Levy BS, Wegman DH, editors: *Occupational health. Recognizing and preventing work-related disease and injury*, Philadelphia, 2000, Lippincott, Williams & Wilkins.

Pinkham J: 100 years of industrial nursing has vastly improved workplace safety, *Occup Safety Health* 57(4):20-23, 1988.

Pollack S, Rubenstein H, Landrigan P: Child labor. In Last J, Wallace R, editors: *Public health and preventive medicine*, Norwalk, Conn, 1994, Appleton-Lange.

Pravikoff DS: General nursing and occupational health nursing, *AAOHN J* 40:531-537, 1992.

Randolph SA: Occupational health nursing: a commitment to excellence, *AAOHN J* 36:166-169, 1988.

Randolph SA, Migliozzi AA: The role of the agricultural health nurse: bringing together community and occupational health, *AAOHN J* 41(9):429-433, 1993.

Rest KM: Ethics in occupational and environmental health. In Levy BS, Wegman DH, editors: *Occupational health. Recognizing and preventing work-related disease and injury*, Philadelphia, 2000, Lippincott, Williams & Wilkins.

Reyes CN, Wenzel FJ, Lawton BR, Emanuel DA: The pulmonary pathology of farmer's lung disease, *Chest* 81(2):142-146, 1982.

Rogers B: Occupational health nursing education: curricular content in baccalaureate programs, *AAOHN J* 39:101-108, 1991.

Rogers B: *Occupational health nursing: concepts and practice*, Philadelphia, 1994a, WB Saunders.

Rogers B: Research, prevention and practice, *AAOHN J* 42:190-191, 1994b.

Rogers B: Occupational health nursing expertise, *AAOHN J* 46:477-483, 1998.

Rogers B, Cox AR: Advancing the profession of occupational health nursing, *AAOHN J* 42:158-163, 1994.

Rogers B, Livsey K: Occupational health surveillance, screening, and prevention activities in occupational health nursing practice, *AAOHN J* 48:92-99, 2000.

Rogers B, Winslow B, Higgins S: Employee satisfaction with occupational health services, *AAOHN J* 41:58-65, 1993.

Rosenstock L, Landrigan PJ: Occupational health: the intersection between clinical medicine and public health. In Breslow L, Fielding JE, Lave LB, editors: *Annu Rev Public Health*, 7:337-356, 1986.

Rutstein DD, Mullan RJ, Frazier TM, et al.: Sentinel health events (occupational): a basis for physician recognition and public health surveillance, *Am J Public Health* 73:1054-1062, 1984.

Salazar MK, editor: *AAOHN core curriculum for occupational health nursing*, Philadelphia, 1997, WB Saunders.

Sattler B: Occupational and environmental health: from the back roads to the highways, *AAOHN J* 44:233-237, 1996.

Serafini P: Nursing assessment in industry, *Am J Public Health* 66(8):755-760, 1976.

Sophie JK: Creating a successful occupational health and safety program. Using workers' perceptions, *AAOHN J* 48(3):125-130, 2000.

Stearns M: Hearing protection. Recognition, evaluation and control, *Occup Safety Health* 69(6):97-100, 2000.

Stellman JM, Daum DM: *Work is dangerous to your health*, New York, 1973, Vintage Books.

Stevenson JS: *Issues and crisis during middlescence*, New York, 1977, Appleton-Century-Crofts.

Stone DS: Health surveillance for health care workers, *AAOHN J* 48:73-79, 2000.

Taylor AK, Murray LR: Minority workers. In Levy BS, Wegman DH, editors: *Occupational health. Recognizing and preventing work-related disease and injury*, Philadelphia, 2000, Lippincott, Williams & Wilkins.

Taylor WA, Mair A, Burns W: Study of noise and hearing in jute weaving, *Acoustical Society of America* 48:524-530, 1965.

Theriault G, Amre D: Cardiovascular disorders. In Levy BS, Wegman DH, editors: *Occupational health. Recognizing and preventing work-related disease and injury*, Philadelphia, 2000, Lippincott, Williams & Wilkins.

Thomas PA: Preparing nursing students for practice: successful implementation of a clinical practicum in occupational health nursing, *AAOHN J* 43:412-415, 1995.

Totten RS, Reid DS, Davies HO, Moran JJ: Farmers' lung, *Am J Med* 25:803-810, 1958.

US Department of Health and Human Services (USDHHS): *Promoting health, preventing disease: objectives for the nation*, Washington, DC, 1980, US Government Printing Office.

US Department of Health and Human Services (USDHHS): *The national health survey of workplace health promotion activities*, Washington, DC, 1987, US Government Printing Office.

US Department of Health and Human Services (USDHHS): *Healthy people 2000: health promotion and disease prevention objectives for the nation, full report, with commentary*, Washington, DC, 1991a, US Government Printing Office.

US Department of Health and Human Services (USDHHS): *NIOSH publication on noise and hearing: criteria for a recommended standard—occupational exposure to noise*, Cincinnati, Ohio, 1991b, NIOSH.

US Department of Health and Human Services (USDHHS): Initial therapy for tuberculosis in the era of multidrug resistance: recommendations for the Advisory Council for the elimination of tuberculosis, *MMWR* 42(RR7):1-8, 1993.

US Department of Health and Human Services (USDHHS): *Healthy people 2000: midcourse review and 1995 revisions*, Washington, DC, 1995, US Government Printing Office.

US Department of Health and Human Services (USDHHS): *Healthy people 2010: conference edition*, Washington, DC, 2000, US Government Printing Office.

US Department of Labor (USDL): *Labor firsts in America*, Washington, DC, 1977, US Government Printing Office.

US Department of Labor (USDL): *Working women count! A report to the nation*, Washington, DC, 1994, Women's Bureau, USDL.

US Department of Labor (USDL): *Fatal workplace injuries in 1994: a collection of data and analysis*, Washington, DC, 1996, USDL.

US Department of Labor (USDL), Bureau of Labor Statistics: *Occupational injuries and illnesses in the U.S. by industry* (Bulletin 98-494, December 17, 1998), Washington, DC, 1998a, US Government Printing Office.

US Department of Labor (USDL), Bureau of Labor Statistics: *Issues in labor statistics: repetitive tasks loosen some workers' grip on safety and health industry*, Washington, DC, 1998b, US Government Printing Office.

Vaught W, Paranzino GK: Confidentiality in occupational health care, *AAOHN J* 48:243-252, 2000.

Walton C, Timms J: Providing worksite health promotion through university-community partnerships. The South Carolina DOT project, *AAOHN J* 47:449-455, 1999.

Waters Y: Industrial nursing, *Public Health Nurs* 11:728-731, 1919.

Watkins EL, Larson K, Harlan C, Young S: A model program for providing health services for migrant farmworker mothers and children, *Public Health Rep* 105(6):567-576, 1990.

Williams RA, Strasser PB: Depression in the workplace. Impact on employees, *AAOHN J* 47:526-537, 1999.

Wright FS: *Industrial nursing,* New York, 1919, MacMillan.


## SELECTED BIBLIOGRAPHY

American Association of Occupational Health Nurses (AAOHN): Position Statement. The occupational health nurse's role in preventing and reducing workplace violence, *AAOHN J* 49:8, 2001.

American Association of Occupational Health Nurses (AAOHN): Advisory: Over-the-counter medications, *AAOHN J* 49:9-10, 2001.

Bain EI: Assessing occupational hazards, *Am J Nurs* 100:96, 2000.

Brown ML: *Occupational health nursing: principles and practice,* New York, 1981, Springer.

Burgel BJ: Primary care at the worksite: policy issues, *AAOHN J* 44:238-243, 1996.

Felton JS: Teaching occupational health at the secondary level, *J Occup Med* 23:27-29, 1981.

Finn PL: Occupational safety and health education in the public schools: rationale, goals, and implementation, *Preventive Med* 7(3):245-249, 1978.

Kerr M, Struthers R, Huynh WC: Work force diversity. Implications for occupational health nursing, *AAOHN J* 49:14-20, 2001.

Lusk SL: Health promotion and disease prevention intervention in worksites. In Hinshaw AS, Feetham SL, Shaver JLF, *Handbook of clinical nursing research,* Thousand Oaks, Calif, 1999, Sage.

National Academy on an Aging Society: Workers and chronic conditions. Opportunities to improve productivity, Washington, DC, 2000, The Academy.

Rogers B: Why a Code of Ethics? *AAOHN J* 49:11-12, 2001.

Theriault G, Kipen HM: Hematologic disorders. In Levy BS, Wegman DH, editors: *Occupational health. Recognizing and preventing work-related disease and injury,* Philadelphia, 2000, Lippincott, Williams & Wilkins.

# NIOSH Education and Research Centers

ALABAMA EDUCATION AND RESEARCH CENTER
University of Alabama at Birmingham
School of Public Health
1530 3rd Avenue South
Birmingham, AL 32594-0022
205-934-6208
Dr. R. Kent Oestenstad, Director

CALIFORNIA EDUCATION AND RESEARCH
  CENTER—NORTHERN
University of California, Berkeley
School of Public Health
140 Warren
Berkeley, CA 94720-7360
510-642-0761
Dr. Robert C. Spear, Director

CALIFORNIA EDUCATION AND RESEARCH
  CENTER—SOUTHERN
University of California
School of Public Health
10833 Le Conte Avenue
Los Angeles, CA 90095-1772
310-825-7152
Dr. William Hinds, Director

CINCINNATI EDUCATION AND RESEARCH
  CENTER
University of Cincinnati
Department of Environmental Health
PO Box 670056
Cincinnati, OH 45267-0056
513-558-1749
Dr. C. Scott Clark, Director

HARVARD EDUCATION AND RESEARCH CENTER
Harvard School of Public Health
Department of Environmental Health
665 Huntington Avenue
Boston, MA 02115
617-432-3323
Dr. David C. Christiani, Director

ILLINOIS EDUCATION AND RESEARCH CENTER
University of Illinois at Chicago
School of Public Health
2121 West Taylor Street, Rm. 215
Chicago, IL 60612-7260
312-996-7469
Dr. Lorraine M. Conroy, Director

IOWA EDUCATION AND RESEARCH CENTER
University of Iowa
College of Public Health
Department of Occupational and Environmental Health
100 Oakdale Campus - 108 IREH
Iowa City, IA 52242-5000
319-335-4429
Dr. Nancy L. Sprince, Director

JOHN HOPKNS EDUCATION AND RESARCH
  CENTER
Johns Hopkins University
School of Hygiene and Public Health
615 North Wolfe Street
Baltimore, MD 21205
410-955-4037
Dr. Jacqueline Agnew, Director

MICHIGAN EDUCATION AND RESEARCH CENTER
University of Michigan
School of Public Health
1420 Washington Heights
Ann Arbor, MI 48109-2029
734-936-0758
Dr. Thomas Robins, Director

MINNESOTA EDUCATION AND RESEARCH
  CENTER
University of Minnesota
School of Public Health
Box 807 Mayo Memorial Building
Minneapolis, MN 55455
612-676-5220
Dr. Ian A. Greaves, Director

From National Institute for Occupational Safety and Health: *NIOSH Education and Research Center Grants (ERC's)*. Retrieved from the internet July 23, 2000. Available from: *http://www.cdc.gov/niosh/centers.html*

# NIOSH Education and Research Centers (cont'd)

NEW YORK/NEW JERSEY EDUCATION AND
　RESEARCH CENTER
Mt. Sinai School of Medicine
Department of Community and Preventive Medicine
PO Box 1057
One Gustave L. Levy Pl.
New York, NY 10029-6574
212-241-4804
Dr. Philip J. Landrigan, Director

NORTH CAROLINA EDUCATION AND RESEARCH
　CENTER
University of North Carolina
School of Public Health
Rosenau Hall, CB# 7400
Chapel Hill, NC 27599-7410
919-966-3473
Dr. Michael Flynn, Director

SOUTH FLORIDA EDUCATION AND RESEARCH
　CENTER
University of South Florida
College of Public Health
13201 Bruce B. Downs Blvd., MDC Box 56
Tampa, FL 33612-3805
813-974-6626
Dr. Stuart M. Brooks, Director

TEXAS EDUCATION AND RESEARCH CENTER
The University of Texas Health Science Center at
　Houston
School of Public Health
PO Box 20186
Houston, TX 77225-0186
713-500-9459
Dr. George L. Delclos, Director

UTAH EDUCATION AND RESEARCH CENTER
University of Utah
Rocky Mountain Center for Occupational and
　Environmental Health
75 South 2000 East
Salt Lake City, UT 84112-5120
801-581-8719
Dr. Royce Moser, Jr., Director

WASHINGTON EDUCATION AND RESEARCH
　CENTER
University of Washington
Department of Environmental Health
P.O. Box 357234
Seattle, WA 98195-7234
206-685-3221
Dr. Michael S. Morgan, Director

# Assessment Guide for Nursing in Industry

1. Community in which industry is located

   a. Description of the community
      1. Size in area and population

      2. Climate, altitude, rainfall

      3. Pollution (noise, radiation, etc.)

      4. Housing

      5. Transportation

      6. Schools

      7. Sanitation
      8. Protection: fire, police, etc.
      9. Trends

   b. Population

      1. Age distribution
      2. Sex distribution
      3. Ethnic and religious composition

      4. Socioeconomic characteristics

   c. Health information
      1. Vital statistics

      2. *Disease incidence and prevalence*
      3. *Health facilities available*
      4. Community resources

2. The company
   a. Historical development

   b. Organizational chart

   c. *Policies*

      1. Length of the work week
      2. Length of work time

1. Just as industry affects the community, so the community affects industry.
   a. Use three or four key descriptive words.
      1. How far do the employees travel to work and are the workers neighbors?
      2. Are there times or seasons that are more hazardous than others?
      3. Can the workers' dermatitis or hearing loss be attributed to the community or is it work related?
      4. Is there adequate, safe housing in the area? Must the worker spend too great a percentage of his or her salary on housing?
      5. Is there safe, adequate transportation to work as well as to a hospital or school?
      6. Do children have to be bused to school or attend overcrowded classes?
      7. Are roaches and rats common to the area?
      8. Are the workers and the industry protected?
      9. Is the area becoming more urban? Residential? Rundown? Deserted?
   b. How alike or different is the population of the industry from that of the community?
      1. Are the families of child-rearing age or of retirement age?
      2. Are there more men or more women?
      3. Are there certain customs or languages that are predominant in the community?
      4. What is the level of education of the community? What is the mean community income?
   c. Is it an ill or well community?
      1. What is the infant mortality rate, birth rate, average life expectancy? Usually the local health department has this information.
      2. *What are the leading causes of morbidity and mortality?*
      3. *What physical facilities and professional services are available?*
      4. Are there day-care centers, drug rehabilitation facilities, Alcoholics Anonymous groups, etc.?

2. The official name and address of the company.
   a. Get a perspective on how, why, and by whom the company was founded and compare it with the present situation.
   b. What is the formal order of the system and to whom will the nurse be responsible?
   c. *If there is a policy manual, try to obtain a copy. Are the workers aware of the manual?*
      1. How many days a week does the industry operate?
      2. Are there several shifts? Breaks? Is there paid vacation?

From Serafini P: Nursing assessment in industry, *Am J Public Health* 66(8):755-760, 1976. (Author's name is now P. Serafini Blanco.)

# Assessment Guide for Nursing in Industry (cont'd)

2. The company—cont'd
   c. *Policies*—cont'd
      3. *Sick leave*
      4. *Safety and fire provisions*

   d. Support services (benefits)
      1. Insurance programs

      2. Retirement program
      3. Educational support

      4. Safety committee

      5. Recreation committee

   e. Relations between worker and management
   f. Projection for the future

3. The plant

   a. General physical setting
      1. The construction

      2. Parking facilities and public transportation stops
      3. Entrances and exits
      4. Physical environment
      5. Communication facilities
      6. Housekeeping
      7. Interior decoration
   b. The work areas

      1. Space
      2. Heights: workplace and supply areas
      3. Stimulation
      4. Safety signs and markings
      5. Standing and sitting facilities

3. Is there a clear policy, and do the workers know it?
4. Is management aware of situations or substances in the plant that represent danger? Are there organized fire drills? *The Federal Register* is the source of information for federal standards and serves as a helpful guide.

   d. What is the attitude of management concerning worker benefits?
      1. *Is there a system for health insurance and life insurance, and is it compulsory?* Does the company pay all or part? *Who fills out the necessary forms?*
      2. Are the benefits realistic?
      3. Can the worker further his or her education? Will the company help financially?
      4. The programmed Red Cross First Aid course is excellent. For information consult your Red Cross. *If there is no committee, do certain people routinely handle emergencies?*
      5. Do the workers have any communication with or interest in each other outside the work setting?
   e. This is difficult information to get, but it is important to know how each perceives the other.
   f. If the company is growing, workers may see themselves as having a secure future; if not, they may be worried about their job security. How will plant expansion affect the need for nursing services?

3. Draw a small map to scale, labeling the areas. When an accident occurs, place a pin in the exact location on your map. Different-color pinheads can be used for keeping statistics.
   a. What is the gross appearance?
      1. What is the size and general condition of buildings and grounds?
      2. How far does the worker have to walk to get inside?

      3. How many people must use them? How accessible are they?
      4. Comment on heating, air conditioning, lighting glare, drafts, etc.
      5. Are there bulletin boards, newsletters?
      6. Is the physical setting maintained adequately?
      7. Are the surroundings conducive to work? Are they pleasing?
   b. Get permission to examine them. Use *The Federal Register* as a guide.
      1. Are workers isolated or crowded?
      2. *Falls and falling objects are dangerous and costly to industry.*
      3. Is the worker too bored to pay attention?
      4. Is danger well marked?
      5. Are chairs safe and comfortable? Are there platforms to stand on, especially for wet processes?

# Assessment Guide for Nursing in Industry (cont'd)

3. The plant—cont'd
  b. The work areas—cont'd
    6. Safety equipment

  c. Nonwork areas
    1. Lockers

    2. Hand-washing facilities

    3. Rest rooms
    4. Drinking water

    5. Recreation and rest facilities

    6. Telephones

    7. Ashtrays
4. The working population
  a. General characteristics
    1. *Total number of employees*

    2. General appearances
    3. *Age and sex distribution*

    4. Race distribution

    5. Socioeconomic distribution

    6. Religious distribution

    7. Ethnic distribution
    8. Marital status
    9. *Educational backgrounds*
    10. Lifestyles practiced
  b. Type of employment offered

    1. Background necessary
    2. Work demands on physical condition
    3. Work status

6. Do the workers make use of hard hats, safety glasses, face masks, radiation badges, etc.? Do they know the safety devices the OSHA regulations require?
  c. Where are they located? Is there easy access?
    1. If the work is dirty, workers should be able to change clothes. Are they taking toxic substances home?
    2. If facilities and supplies are available, do workers know how and when to wash their hands?
    3. How accessible are they and what condition are they in?
    4. Can a worker leave the job long enough to get a drink of water when he or she wants to?
    5. Can a worker who is not feeling well lie down? Do workers feel free to use the facilities?
    6. Can a worker receive or make a call? Does a working mother have to stay home because she can't be reached at work?
    7. Are people allowed to smoke in designated areas? Is it safe?
4. Include worker and management, but separate data for comparison.
  a. Be as accurate as possible, but estimate when necessary.
    1. Usually, if an industry has 500 or more employees, full-time nursing services are necessary.
    2. Heights, weights, cleanliness, etc.
    3. Certain screening programs are specific for young adults whereas others are more for the elderly. Some programs are more for women; others are more for men. Is there any difference between the day and evening shift? Are the problems of the minority sex unattended?
    4. Does one race predominate? How does this compare with the general community?
    5. Great differences in worker salaries can sometimes cause problems.
    6. Does one religion predominate? Are religious holidays observed?
    7. Is there a language barrier?
    8. Widowed, single, divorced people often have different needs.
    9. *Can all teaching be done at approximately the same level?*
    10. Are certain lifestyles frowned upon?
  b. What percentage of the work force is blue-collar and what percentage is white-collar?
    1. What educational level is required? Skilled vs. unskilled?
    2. Strength needed: sedentary vs. active.
    3. Part-time vs. full-time; overtime?

# Assessment Guide for Nursing in Industry (cont'd)

4. The working population—cont'd
   c. Absenteeism
      1. *Causes*
      2. Length

   d. Physically disabled
      1. Number employed
      2. *Extent of disabilities*

   e. Personnel on medication
   f. Personnel with chronic illness

5. The industrial process
   a. Equipment used
      1. General description of placement
      2. Type of equipment
   b. Nature of the operation


      1. *Raw materials used*

      2. Nature of the final product

      3. Description of the jobs
      4. Waste products produced

   c. *Exposure to toxic substances*




   d. Faculties required throughout the
      industrial process

   c. Is there a record kept? By whom? Why?
      1. *What are the five most common reasons for absence?*
      2. Absenteeism is costly to the employer. There is some differ-ence between one 10-day absence and ten 1-day absences by the same person.
   d. Does the company have a policy about hiring the disabled?
      1. Where do they work? What do they do?
      2. Are they specially trained? Are they in a special program? Do they use prosthetic devices?
   e. Know what medication and where the employee works.
   f. At what stage of illness is the employee? Where does the em-ployee work? Will he or she be able to continue at this job?
5. What does the company produce and how?
   a. Portable vs. fixed; light vs. heavy.
      1. Mark each piece of large equipment on the scale map.
      2. Fans, blowers, fast moving, wet or dry.
   b. Get a brief description of each state of the process so that you can compare the needs and abilities of the workers with the needs of the job.
      1. *What are they and how dangerous are they? Are they properly stored?* Check *The Federal Register* for guidelines on storage.
      2. Can the workers take pride in the final product or do they make parts?
      3. Who does what? Where? Label the map.
      4. What is the system for waste disposal? Are the pollution con-trol devices in place and functioning?
   c. *Describe the toxins to which the worker is exposed and the ex-tent of exposure.* Include physical and emotional hazards. Re-member that chronic effects of industrial exposure are subtle; a person often gets used to having mild symptoms and won't re-port them. *The Federal Register* contains specifications for expo-sure to toxins and some states issue state standards.
   d. The need for speed, hearing, color vision, etc., can help deter-mine the types of screening programs necessary.

# Assessment Guide for Nursing in Industry (cont'd)

6. The health program

a. Existing polices
   1. Objectives of the program
   2. *Preemployment physicals*

   3. First-aid facilities
   4. *Standard orders*

   5. *Job descriptions for health personnel*
b. Existing facilities and resources

   1. Trained personnel
   2. Space

   3. *Supplies*
   4. *Records and reports*

c. *Services rendered in the past year*
   1. Care needed
   2. Screening done
   3. Referrals made
   4. Counseling done
   5. Health education

d. *Accidents in the past year*

e. Reasons employees sought health care

6. Outline what is actually in existence as well as what employees perceive to be in existence.
a. Are there informal, unwritten policies?
   1. Are they clear?
   2. Are they required? Are they paid for by the company? Is the information used to deselect?
   3. What is available? What is not available?
   4. Is there a company physician who is responsible for first aid or emergency policy? If so, work closely with him or her in planning nursing services.
   5. If there are no guidelines to be followed, write some.
b. Sometimes an industry that denies having a health program has more of a system than it realizes.
   1. *Who responds in an emergency?*
   2. Where is the sick worker taken? Where is the emergency equipment kept?
   3. *Make a list and describe the condition* of each item.
   4. What exists? The Occupational Safety and Health Act requires that employers keep three types of records: a log of occupational injuries and illnesses, a supplemental record of certain illnesses or injuries, and an annual summary (forms 100, 101, and 102 are provided under the act). Good records provide data for good planning.
c. Describe as specifically as possible.
   1. Chronic or acute? Why?
   2. Where? By whom? Why?
   3. By whom? To whom? Why?
   4. Often informal counseling goes unnoticed.
   5. What individual or group education was offered by the company?
d. Including those occurring after work hours, as some of these accidents may be directly or indirectly work related.
e. List the five major reasons.

# 22

# Clients with Long-Term Care Needs

*Debra C. Wallace*

## OBJECTIVES

*Upon completion of this chapter, the reader should be able to:*

1. Define long-term care.
2. Identify the factors influencing the need for long-term care.
3. Describe population groups requiring long-term care.
4. Differentiate care and services offered by hospice, home care, nursing home, assisted living, families, and other community agencies and groups.
5. Explain legislation and financing influencing long-term care.
6. Discuss facilitators and barriers to the provision of both formal and informal long-term care.
7. Analyze the role of the community health nurse in assisting persons with long-term care needs.
8. Discuss the ethical issues in long-term care.

## KEY TERMS

Activities of daily living (ADL)
Adult day care
Adult foster care
Assisted living
Board and care homes
Continuing care retirement
    communities

Home- and community-based services
    (HCBS)
Home-sharing arrangements
Hospice
Instrumental activities of daily living
    (IADL)
Long-term care

Nursing homes
Older Americans Act of 1965 (OAA)
Respite care
Skilled nursing facility (SNF)
Social Services Block Grants to States
Special care units (SCUs)

Perhaps no group is growing more rapidly than the population that requires long-term care, which includes the elderly, the chronically ill, children and adults with disabilities, people with mental illness, acquired immunodeficiency syndrome (AIDS) sufferers, and trauma victims. Traditionally, members of this group have been ignored by society because their productivity and worth were often not recognized. Attempts to meet the health and social needs of this segment of society are changing as we move from a primarily acute care system to one dealing with persons with chronic and noninstitutional health needs. Health professionals, the government, and the private sector are developing new markets, housing options, clinical practice guidelines and care provision strategies to meet the needs of individuals and families with long-term care needs.

Because demand for long-term care is growing, the focus of this chapter is on examining how nurses can assist indi-

viduals, families, and communities with long-term care needs. Emphasis is placed on assessing and prioritizing those needs, accessing resources, and developing, implementing, and evaluating delivery models, levels of care, financing, collaboration, and outcomes.

Funding for long-term care accounts for more than 12% of public health care dollars (Agency for Healthcare Research and Quality [AHRQ], 2001a, 2001b; National Center for Health Statistics [NCHS], 2000). More than half of the expenditures have been used for nursing home care and were paid from Medicaid and Medicare. In addition, much private and out-of-pocket money is spent on long-term care. Managed care has not decreased these costs, and prices are escalating. At the same time, traditional providers of long-term care services (families and nursing homes) are becoming unable to meet the demand. Families are having difficulty providing these services because often all of the primary caregivers in the home need to be employed to meet the basic family needs. Additionally, nursing homes face overcrowding and employ many unlicensed and non-professional workers, which frequently leads to consumer dissatisfaction and ineffective care. Also, partially because of the increased need for long-term care and the caregiver difficulties noted, abuse and neglect of elders and disabled persons are reported more and more frequently (Administration on Aging [AoA], 2001e; National Center on Elder Abuse, 2001).

## DEFINING LONG-TERM CARE

Long-term care traditionally has been equated to nursing home care. Currently, many types of agencies and services provide long-term care. Nursing homes, home health, adult day care, hospice, case management/care coordination, personal care, transitional care, rehabilitation, and assisted living are modes of formal service delivery, and caregiving is the primary informal mode of delivery.

Long-term care is a continuum of services, "beginning with respite for the caregiver" (AHRQ, 2001a), that provides physical, psychological, spiritual, social, and economic services (American Nurses Association [ANA], 1995; Lutsky, Corea, Alecxih, 2000). Services can include housing, medications, health care, social services, transportation, assistive devices, and other supportive services needed by persons with physical, mental, or cognitive limitations, regardless of age or diagnosis, that are severe enough to compromise independent or healthy living. Long-term care services can be needed on a regular or intermittent basis. How monies are spent for long-term care services in the United States is given in Figure 22-1. Sources of long-term care financing are shown in

Figure 22-2. The need for long-term care is determined in several ways.

## Assessing the Need for Long-Term Care

First, a person's ability to independently carry out activities and routines of daily living is assessed. Activity limitation is defined by *Healthy People 2010* as "problems in a person's performance of everyday functions such as communication, self-care, mobility, learning, and behavior" (U.S. Department of Health and Human Services [USDHHS], 2001c, p. 6-19).

One of the more common ways to assess persons' limitations are to measure their ability to perform self-care tasks such as **activities of daily living (ADL)** and **instrumental activities of daily living (IADL)** (see Chapter 18). ADLs include eating, bathing, dressing, getting to and using the bathroom, and getting in or out a bed and/or chair. ADLs are greater among minorities than whites and for the very poor as compared with other income status groups (NCHS, 2000). IADLs indicate the ability of the person to perform household chores and social tasks. These tasks include activities such as shopping, doing light housework, keeping track of money, using the telephone, and preparing meals. Assessing tasks such as the ability to attend school, be educated, be employed, behavioral problems, and appropriate orientation and cognition also are used.

These needs reflect emotional and psychosocial capabilities and may be found in conjunction with impaired physical function. A more recent determination that has emerged is that of needing assistance with regular management of health care needs. An example of this is the need for knowledge, skills, and actual assistance with activities related to blood glucose monitoring, dependence on life-sustaining technology, peritoneal dialysis, medication administration, and management or personal safety. Depending on what needs a client has, various settings for care are considered.

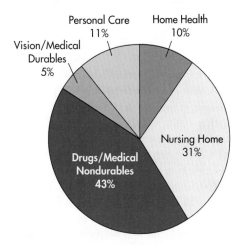

**FIGURE 22-1** National health expenditures for long-term care, 1998. (From HCFA, Office of the Actuary: *National health expenditures, by source of fund and type of expenditure: selected calendar years 1994-1999,* June 2001, HCFA. Retrieved from the internet June, 2001. *http://www.hcfa.gov/stats/nhe-oact/tables/t3.htm*)

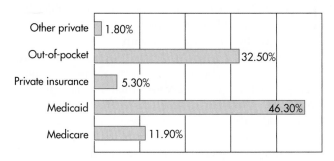

**FIGURE 22-2** Nursing home expenditures by source of funds, 1998. (From National Center for Health Statistics [NCHS]: *Health, United States, 2000 with adolescent health chartbook,* Table 119, Hyattsville, Md, 2000, NCHS.)

## *HEALTHY PEOPLE 2010* AND LONG-TERM CARE

Many of the focus areas in *Healthy People 2010* have implications for long-term care. The *Healthy People 2010* focus area, *Disability and Secondary Conditions*, has many long-term care implications and is presented in Chapter 18. This focus area has numerous objectives that address improving the quality of life for people with long-term care needs such as moving children and adults from long-term, institutional settings to community settings, increasing the proportion of people with long-term care needs who have access to assistive or technological devices, decreasing environmental barriers to care, and increased social activity. Other focus areas such as diabetes, cancer, and heart disease and stroke all have implications for long-term care.

A new program to address the *Healthy People 2010* objectives is the *Real Choice Systems Grants* that help states expand services and opportunities to help people with long-term care needs avoid institutionalization and to lead as normal a life in their communities as possible. Housing, personal care, education and training, and innovations for new or revised services and increased consumer control are the efforts and outcomes expected (USDHHS, 2001b).

## INSTITUTIONAL AND NONINSTITUTIONAL CARE SETTINGS

Usually, a distinction is made between institutional long-term care and home- and community-based long-term care. Institutional care is provided at nursing homes, mental health facilities, and developmental and rehabilitation centers. Developmental centers, especially for children and adolescents, started in the 1950s for children with polio, cerebral palsy, and other mobility problems. In 2001, centers provide not only for those with orthopedic and nervous system conditions but children and adolescents with other health needs such as oncology, substance abuse, and behavioral needs. Rehabilitation centers facilities began in the 1970s and 1980s with the advent of 911 service, trauma survivorship, prosthetic technology, innovations in spinal cord surgery and neonatology, and post-stroke expectations.

Noninstitutional long-term care flourished in the1980s and 1990s. With the majority of persons with long-term care needs living in private or congregate residences in the community, the development of services that could be delivered in those settings were necessitated. Home health, personal care, hospice, and home delivered meals were services that grew out of the need for home care. Day care, transitional care, congregate meals, and social interaction child and senior centers were developed for episodic care in the community.

## FACTORS INFLUENCING THE GROWTH OF LONG-TERM CARE SERVICES

Several factors have influenced the need for increasing organized long-term care services: epidemiologic trends, demographic trends, health conditions, employment and mobility, sociocultural changes, consumer preferences, and increasingly sophisticated medical technology. The 1965 passage of Medicare and Medicaid had a powerful effect on these factors and long-term care. Originally designed as a safety net for a small elder segment, Medicare entitlement is now the health plan for 39 million elderly and disabled Americans. Medicaid, a means tested health plan, covers 41 million children and adults with varying health needs (NCHS, 2000). Factors influencing the growth of long-term care services include an aging population, increased incidence of chronic and disabling health conditions, employment and mobility patterns, sociocultural changes, consumer preference, medical technology, and Medicare.

### An Aging Society

The nurse's role with elderly clients in the community has been discussed in Chapter 19. America is aging. The world is aging. Americans are living longer than ever before, and the gap between male and female longevity is widening. The elderly population has increased 20% in the past two decades and is expected to increase dramatically in size in this century. In the United States, persons 85 and older are increasing in number the most rapidly (AoA, 2001f; Federal Interagency Forum on Aging-Related Statistics, 2000).

The incidence of chronic and disabling conditions increases with age, and elders are more likely to have limitations in the ADLs and IADLs discussed previously in this chapter. Table 22-1 gives information on the incidence of ADL limitations with community-dwelling elders.

Although not all elderly require long-term care services, they have the greatest likelihood of needing this care. The need for long-term care increases significantly after the age of 85. Projections for the number of elderly needing long-term care will reach 10 to 14 million by 2020, compared with 7 million today. This increase has great implications for nursing practice.

### Health Conditions

Infectious diseases largely have been irradicated by the use of early diagnosis and pharmacological advances. Chronic illnesses (e.g., cardiovascular disease, diabetes, cancer) are the most frequent causes of death and disability for adults in the United States. Cerebral palsy, cystic fibrosis, fetal alcohol syndrome, Down syndrome, and asthma have increased in prevalence and have presented numerous long-term care needs for clients and families. Violence and trauma also increased drastically during the 1990s and show little signs of slowing in the next decade. Much progress has been made with AIDS, which means that persons with the condition

**TABLE 22-1**

*Projections of the Noninstitutional Population 65 Years and Over with ADL Limitations: 1990 to 2040*

(Number in thousands. Based on sample data for past years.)

| | NUMBER | | PERCENT OF POPULATION* | |
|---|---|---|---|---|
| YEAR | TOTAL WITH ADL LIMITATIONS | SEVERELY DISABLED | TOTAL WITH ADL LIMITATIONS | SEVERELY DISABLED |
| 1990 | 6,029 | 1,123 | 18.8 | 3.5 |
| 1995 | 6,712 | 1,265 | 19.3 | 3.6 |
| 2000 | 7,262 | 1,384 | 20.0 | 3.8 |
| 2020 | 10,118 | 1,927 | 19.2 | 3.7 |
| 2040 | 14,416 | 2,806 | 21.4 | 4.2 |

From Administration on Aging (AoA): *Aging into the 21st century,* 1997, AoA. *Retrieved from the internet February 2001. http://www.aoa.dhhs. gov/aoa/stats/aging21/health.html#disability*
Calculated on the basis of projections of the U.S. population prepared by the U.S. Social Security Administration and preliminary data from the 1982 National Long-Term Care Survery. See K. Manton and K. Liu (1984).
*Base includes the institutional population.
Table compiled by the National Aging Information Center.

live longer and continue to have health care needs. All of these health conditions exacerbate the requirement for long-term health care programs and services that focus on adults and younger adolescents and children that are racially and ethnically diverse.

People in need of long-term care are not just elderly; many children, adolescents, and young adults also require long-term care. Among children and young adults, accidents and injury and violence are the leading causes of death and disability and continue to increase (NCHS, 2000). Years ago, diving accidents were a major cause of paraplegia and quadriplegia in young men; now gunshots wounds and motor vehicles are a close second. Emotional difficulties, such as depression, anxiety, and sleeplessness, are higher among children and adults with disabilities than those not experiencing disabilities, and differences are found among racial and ethnic groups (USDHHS, 2001c, 2001d). Increases in the number of persons with long-term care needs require an increase in the number and type of services for children and adults.

The emergency management system and improved trauma care provide high rates of survivorship. Resulting quality and quantity of life, however, often requires technological, material, or human assistance. The increase in trauma in society has resulted in increased emphasis in health care practice on rehabilitation.

In addition to the conditions mentioned, there has been increased incidence in cognitive and mental health conditions. Causes of cognitive impairment include dementia; delirium; toxic effects of medications, drugs, or other substances; trauma; and psychiatric illness. Alzheimer's disease, cardiovascular disease, and strokes have placed increased demands on long-term care resources.

Another cause of cognitive impairment is that of substance abuse, especially among adolescents and young adults. Cocaine or "crack" usage has skyrocketed and resulted in the increase of prevention and treatment centers, mental health services, and massive public outcry. Substance abuse often results in gun violence and trauma to persons of all ages. Alcohol abuse has resulted in direct neural impairment and is a leading cause of motor vehicle accidents. Increasing complexity and stress of life in the American society has resulted in increases in diagnosis of specific mental health conditions: posttraumatic stress syndrome, "character assassination" syndromes, and attention deficit disorder. The use of behavioral modification and pharmacological treatment has increased, especially in home and community settings.

## Employment and Mobility Patterns

Industrialization, geographical mobility, rising incomes, urbanization, and women in the workplace are changing the ability of families to provide informal care and support. Although the mobility rate has been declining in the past several decades, a large number of people move from one residence to another, and many move significant distances. Rising incomes allow people to live apart and to negate the physical or financial dependence among families and loved ones. Industrialization has made it both possible and necessary for women to take on a career outside the home. During recent decades females have increasingly joined the paid labor force, making it more difficult for them to provide home care for family members. It is anticipated that work obligations may conflict with caregiving responsibilities to a greater extent in the future than they do now.

## Sociocultural Changes

Other factors that influence the increasing need for long-term care services are the decline in the number of children a family chooses to have, different choices for partners and lifestyle, the aging of care providers, and the increasing rates of divorce and remarriage. Divorce often changes the bonds of affection and obligation, and children, stepchildren, and in-laws face difficult decisions about whom they should care for.

Women or men are not available to care for a loved one, and often reproduction does not take place or is at a lower rate than previous generations. Simply summarized, there are fewer children and younger persons to care for parents or significant others who face disability or longer lives. Also, persons providing information or care are becoming older when they choose to care for parents, siblings, and partners. Aged persons may be alone as the result of having no children, experiencing a divorce, or partner and sibling death.

## Consumer Preference

Many people want to be treated and cared for at home rather than in institutional settings. Home has the advantage of providing security and familiarity, and it also reduces exposure to the iatrogenically induced problems of hospitals and nursing homes. At home there is less constraint on who can assist with care and support, and there can be less financial burden.

Care levels can range from personal hygiene to critical care in nonhospital settings. Perhaps, most importantly, the individual and family are able to more fully be involved in making decisions regarding care. The issue of autonomy and self-responsibility for our life and health has been especially desired at the end of the twentieth century. The passage of the *Patient Self-Determination Act* and many state *advanced directives laws* are a reflection of that desire.

## Medical Technology

Apnea monitors, dialysis machines, ventilators, and other high tech equipment have been in nonhospital settings for two decades, although not to the extent that now is true. With every new diagnostic, lifesaving, and genetic examination, more and more persons are surviving illnesses and conditions previously undetected, untreatable, or unknown. Gastrointestinal feeding tubes, skin care alternatives, intravenous (IV) vasopressors, pain management, chemotherapy, and AIDS-related treatments are common in community-based settings, including the home. Family and professionals are providing these services, treatments, and care management. This is possible because of new monitoring methods, infusion pumps, communication avenues, and synthetic materials developed and tested for effectiveness through medical, engineering, physical therapy, and nursing research.

At the beginning of the twenty-first century, no area of medical technology is as exciting and concerning as that of genetics. First, there was the use of fetal tissue for stem cell research to regenerate nerve or brain tissue and to fight cancer. Then a sheep and calf were cloned in different parts of the world. Just as society was dealing with the profound human genome mapping, another group of scientists reported the successful addition of disease-preventing genetic material in a monkey. Telehealth is discussed in Chapter 24.

## Medicare

Home care agencies of various types have been providing high-quality services for more than 100 years (see Chapter 1). However, the enactment of Medicare in 1965 greatly spurred the growth of this industry. Medicare made home care services, primarily skilled nursing and therapy of a curative or restorative nature, available. After the passage of Medicare the number of agencies certified to participate in Medicare went from approximately 1800 in 1967 to almost 3000 in 1980 (National Association for Home Care [NAHC], 1995). There are almost 8000 such agencies today (Health Care Financing Administration [HCFA], 2000a).

Hospital-based and proprietary agencies have grown faster than other types of certified agencies; proprietary agencies make up about 40%, and hospital-based agencies about 25%, of all certified agencies. Table 22-2 depicts the growth in the number and kinds of Medicare-certified agencies from 1967 to 1999. The decreases noted in 1999 were primarily the result of the *Balanced Budget Act of 1997* that placed restrictions on nursing home, home health, and other long-term care services.

## AGGREGATES WITH LONG-TERM CARE NEEDS

The long-term care population includes people of all ages with a wide array of disabling conditions and assistance needs. Chapter 16 presents information on children with disabilities, and Chapter 18 looks at services for adults with disabilities. This chapter looks at disabling conditions in relation to long-term care needs.

An estimated 54 million persons with disabilities live in the United States. Thus a full 20% of the population needs some form of long-term assistance with environmental, medical, social, emotional, or physical function. Disabilities are classified according to categories by communication, mobility, learning, and personal-care limitations by the Disability and Health Branch of the Centers for Disease Control and Prevention (CDC, 2001c). The *Center on Disability and Health* of the United States Department of Health and Human Services (USDHHS) identifies four major areas of disability and thus needs for long-term care: sensory impairment, physical impairment, cognitive impairment, and communication needs. These limitations include limb loss, sensory impairment, developmental or cognitive loss, fetal or birth defects, physical impairment, and chronic illness progression. Individuals with these limitations often require

**TABLE 22-2**

*Number of Medicare-Certified Home Care Agencies, by Type of Agency*

| YEAR | FREESTANDING AGENCIES | | | | | | FACILITY-BASED AGENCIES | | | TOTAL |
|---|---|---|---|---|---|---|---|---|---|---|
| | VNA | COMB | PUB | PROP | PNP | OTH | HOSP | REHAB | SNF | |
| 1967 | 549 | 93 | 939 | 0 | 0 | 39 | 133 | 0 | 0 | 1753 |
| 1975 | 525 | 46 | 1228 | 47 | 0 | 109 | 273 | 9 | 5 | 2242 |
| 1980 | 515 | 63 | 1260 | 186 | 484 | 40 | 359 | 8 | 9 | 2924 |
| 1985 | 514 | 59 | 1205 | 1943 | 832 | 4 | 1277 | 20 | 129 | 5983 |
| 1986 | 510 | 62 | 1192 | 1915 | 826 | 4 | 1341 | 17 | 117 | 5984 |
| 1987 | 500 | 61 | 1172 | 1882 | 803 | 1 | 1382 | 14 | 108 | 5923 |
| 1988 | 496 | 55 | 1073 | 1846 | 766 | 1 | 1439 | 12 | 97 | 5785 |
| 1989 | 491 | 51 | 1011 | 1818 | 727 | 1 | 1465 | 10 | 102 | 5676 |
| 1990 | 474 | 47 | 985 | 1884 | 710 | 0 | 1486 | 8 | 101 | 5695 |
| 1991 | 476 | 41 | 941 | 1970 | 701 | 0 | 1537 | 9 | 105 | 5780 |
| 1992 | 530 | 52 | 1083 | 1962 | 637 | 28 | 1623 | 3 | 86 | 6004 |
| 1993 | 594 | 46 | 1196 | 2146 | 558 | 41 | 1809 | 1 | 106 | 6497 |
| 1994 | 586 | 45 | 1146 | 2892 | 597 | 48 | 2081 | 3 | 123 | 7521 |
| 1995 | 579 | 38 | 1161 | 3730 | 667 | 59 | 2357 | 3 | 153 | 8747 |
| 1999 | 452 | 35 | 918 | 3192 | 621 | 65 | 2300 | 1 | 163 | 7747 |

From National Association for Home Care (NAHC): Basic statistics about home health care, Washington, DC, 2000, NAHC. Retrieved from the internet January, 2001. *http:www.nahc.org/consumer/hcstats.html*

VNA: Visiting Nurse Associations are freestanding, voluntary, nonprofit organizations governed by a board of directors and usually financed by tax-deductible contributions as well as by earnings.

COMB: Combination agencies are combined government and voluntary agencies. These agencies are sometimes included with counts for VNAs.

PUB: Public agencies are government agencies operated by a state, county, city, or other unit of local government having a major responsibility for preventing disease and for community health education.

PROP: Propietary agencies are freestanding, for-profit home care agencies.

PNP: Private not-for-profit agencies are freestanding and privately developed, governed, and owned nonprofit home care agencies.

OTH: Other freestanding agencies are agencies that do not fit one of the categories for freestanding agencies listed above.

HOSP: Hospital-based agencies are operating units or departments of a hospital. Agencies that have working arrangements with a hospital, or perhaps are even owned by a hospital but operated as separate entities, are classified as freestanding agencies under one of the categories listed above.

REHAB: Refers to agencies based in rehabilitation facilities.

SNF: Refers to agencies based in skilled nursing facilities.

long-term care services. Annual costs for disability in the United States are estimated at more than $300 billion dollars, which is split evenly among medical expenditures and lost productivity (USDHHS, 2001c). The *International Classification of Functioning, Disability, and Health* (ICIDH-2) provides a framework for determining social, emotional, and physical functioning; health; and disability status. Racial, ethnic, and gender disparities occur, as with most health issues.

Disability can result from mental disabilities such as traumatic brain injuries, mental retardation, or Alzheimer's dementia. Physical limitations can be the result of paraplegia, heart disease and stroke, asthma, and arthritis. AIDS sufferers can experience both types of limitations necessitating long-term care. Among both elderly and nonelderly persons, arthritis, heart disease, and mental health conditions are common reasons for long-term care services.

The range of services needed by clients and their families from the long-term care system varies greatly. Persons with mental disabilities often require supervision and protection

as opposed to hands-on care. Not everyone with the same diagnosis needs the same level of care, and that level of care can change for the same person over time. Further, the needs of the elderly, working adults, adolescents, and children vary over time because of the developmental life stage of each of these aggregates.

As previously noted, long-term care needs are not limited to the elderly; many children, adolescents, and young adults also need long-term care, in large part because of accidents and injuries. In addition, advances in technology have made saving lives more of a reality.

## Children

Although elderly persons have traditionally been the primary users of long-term care, the 1980s and 1990s saw a dramatic increase in the number of children with complex health needs or "special needs" that required care in facilities or at home. Seventeen percent of U.S. children under 18 have a developmental disability that is caused by physical, cognitive, sensory, speech, or psychological impairments (CDC, 2001b, 2001e). This includes technology-dependent children on ventilators and those with sensory deficits, physical limitations, behavioral problems, and emotional needs. Often these children fall into more than one category of need. Figure 22-3 shows disability rates for children and youth; note that lower rates of disabilities are reported for girls.

Limitations in activity caused by chronic conditions are experienced by 6.6% of children under age 18. The rate is half (3.5%) that for children under 5 years of age. For children less than 1 year of age, congenital anomalies and low birth weight or early gestation are often related to these limitations. Children 1 to 4 years of age experience anomalies, but unintentional injuries, violence, and cancer are also major etiologies. When a child reaches 5 years of age, injuries remain a major health concern rivaled primarily by cancer (NCHS, 2000).

Birth defects contribute to the increased number of children needing long-term care. Advances in *technology* have resulted in more infants with birth defects surviving. With rapid development of life-sustaining, surgical and diagnostic equipment, techniques, and practices, babies who would have died now survive many birth defects, low birth weight, early gestational age, and mothers' risk behaviors. Children experiencing drowning, injury, and accidents now survive and can be technology dependent into adulthood. While these children have medical needs similar to adults, the developmental and family tasks are quite different.

## Stop and Think About It
What medical, social, and educational resources in your community provide services for children who have disabilities?

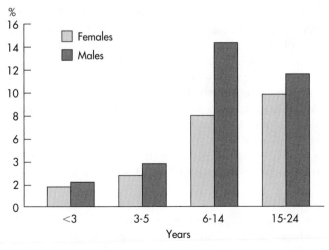

**FIGURE 22-3** Disabilities among children and youth by age and gender group. (From US Census Bureau: *Americans with Disabilities, 1997: household economic studies,* 2001, US Census Bureau. Retrieved from the internet March, 2001. *http://www.census.gov/hhes/www/disability.htm*

Yearly, almost 110,000 children born with birth defects survive past the first year of life in the United States (CDC, 2001a). Ethical and legal issues have resulted as babies who would not otherwise have survived are kept alive (e.g., anacephalic babies). Fetal alcohol syndrome (FAS) and crack cocaine also contribute to the number of children requiring long-term care, with FAS alone estimated to cost more than $1.9 billion annually (CDC, 2001d). As many as 8000 children are born with FAS each year in the United States (CDC, 2001a, 2001d). Many of these infants go on to have long-term care needs.

States and federal education departments spend approximately $36 billion dollars each year on education programs for persons with developmental disabilities who are less than 21 years of age (CDC, 2001b). This can be in the form of special education classes or teachers and individualized education in the home. Schools for the deaf and blind are available in most states, although this usually necessitates children living away from home during the week. State and federal dollars support long-term care facilities for diagnosing, treating, and researching developmental disabilities.

The *consumerism movement* has affected long-term care for children. Parents want "everything" humanly and technologically possible to be used to save the lives of their babies and children. Second, parents wanted to be actively involved in the care of their babies and children and demanded a family approach.

A significant problem for families with children with long-term care needs is the financial stress the care places on the family. Even when third-party insurance covers health needs, these children reach lifetime maximum "payout" before young adulthood. Most are placed on Medicare or Medicaid. Children with special needs have varying coverage across states. This coverage has increased with the 1998 establishment of the *Children's Health Insurance Program* (CHIP), coverage for children who would otherwise be without coverage. As of January 2001, 3.3 million children were enrolled and all 50 states and the District of Columbia had programs approved by USDHHS (HCFA, 2001b; USDHHS, 2001a). However, all states have not fully implemented the program or enrolled all eligible children (USDHHS, 2001a). Most programs are run as either Medicaid programs or as combined state- and employer-based plans.

Home health nurses provide acute care for babies and children in the home. Apnea monitors, ventilators, and feeding tubes are common components of a premature infant's home care regimen. Treatments for children's cancer also have increased. Much of the chemotherapy is administered outpatient, necessitating caregiving by parents. In addition to emotional support, teaching parents to care for a central line has become standard nursing practice in the community. Another role of community nurses has been client education and initiation and participation in support groups for parents of children with asthma, cancer, diabetes, technology dependence, and developmental or behavioral difficulties.

All of these children have long-term care needs that require family and culturally appropriate strategies and services (HRSA, 2001a). Community nurses play an important role in assisting these children and their families to meet those tasks, as noted in the *National Agenda for Children with Special Health Care Needs* (HRSA, 2001b).

## Adolescents

The adolescent population exhibits risk behaviors, many of which are dramatically increasing in number and complexity (Table 22-3). The consequences of those behaviors are resulting in more need for long-term care in home health, rehabilitation, mental health, and caregiving.

Risk behaviors include alcohol and drug abuse, smoking, driving fast and while impaired, a lack of safe sex, low physical activity, and violence. The Youth Risk Behavior Surveillance System (CDC, 2001e) is a survey of high school students conducted every 2 years to ascertain health risks for this age group. From 1970 to 1994, activity limitations among persons under age 18 increased 33% among girls and 40% among boys.

In 1997, 8% of adolescents had some form of activity limitation due to physical, emotional, or mental problems.

### TABLE 22-3

*Youth Health Behaviors with Consequences for Long-Term Care*

| HEALTH BEHAVIOR | 1991 | 1993 | 1995 | 1997 | 1999 |
|---|---|---|---|---|---|
| Carried a gun | NA | 7.9 | 7.6 | 5.9 | 4.9 |
| Seriously considered suicide | 29.0 | 24.1 | 24.1 | 20.5 | 19.3 |
| Attempted suicide | 7.3 | 8.6 | 8.7 | 7.7 | 8.3 |
| Current alcohol use | 50.8 | 48.0 | 51.6 | 50.8 | 50.0 |
| Episodic heavy drinking | 31.3 | 30.0 | 32.6 | 33.4 | 31.5 |
| Lifetime marijuana use | 31.3 | 32.8 | 42.4 | 47.1 | 47.2 |
| Current cocaine use | 1.7 | 1.9 | 3.1 | 3.3 | 4.0 |
| Lifetime illegal steroid use | 2.7 | 2.2 | 3.7 | 3.1 | 3.7 |
| Never or rarely wore a seat belt | 25.9 | 19.1 | 21.7 | 19.3 | 16.4 |
| Rode with a drunk driver | 39.9 | 35.3 | 38.8 | 36.6 | 33.1 |
| Had 4 or more sexual partners | 18.7 | 18.7 | 17.8 | 16.0 | 16.2 |
| Currently sexually active | 37.5 | 37.5 | 37.9 | 34.8 | 36.3 |

From Centers for Disease Control and Prevention (CDC): *Fact sheet: youth risk behavior trends,* 2001e, CDC. Retrieved from the internet February, 2001. *www.cdc.gov/nccdphp/dash/yrbs/trend.htm*
NOTE: Numbers are percentages of behavior.

Such limitations can lead to long-term care needs. Almost half of those adolescents had more than one limitation, and 5% had limitations related to school. Limitations include both special education and other types of health needs. Rates are higher among females 16 to 17 years old and males when compared with 10 to 12 and 13 to 15 year olds. Males have higher rates of limitation in all of the age groups. Whites and African Americans experience limitations more often than Hispanics, and those with the highest poverty status experience 50% more limitations than persons with better incomes (NCHS, 2000). Of children eligible for Medicaid or CHIP, about 7% or 530,000 have a disability (Office of Disability, Aging, and Long-Term Care Policy, 2000).

## Adults and the Elderly

Young adults also have long-term care needs. Disability caused by chronic conditions in the 18-to-44 age group is 7%, with increased prevalence after age 25 (Figure 22-4). The rate doubles for persons 45 to 54 years of age and increases again for persons 55 to 64. Men experience more activity limitations in young adulthood, and women experience more activity limitations in old age (Figure 22-5) (InfoUse, 2001).

Adults aged 65 and older are the traditional users of long-term care. For decades, families and institutions have provided care for elderly persons. For all persons aged 65 and older, the rate of disability is 39%, with more prevalence in those older than 75. Elders also have higher rates of activity limitations, acute and chronic diseases, comorbidity, and mental illnesses than other aggregates. Retirement, poverty, distance from family, spousal death, urbanization, crime, and abuse serve as exacerbating factors to many of their assistance needs. This group uses more total and individual health care resources than any population subgroup, except the premature and infants (Federal Interagency Forum on Aging-Related Statistics, 2000; NCHS, 2000). As the elderly population continues to increase in size, proportion, and diversity, needs will necessitate additional and new long-term care services, payment, and foci. Dementia as a long-term care need is discussed later in this chapter.

Memory impairment also can cause disability. In the elderly, 5% of those 65 to 69 but 36% of those 85 and older suffer from a moderate-to-severe memory impairment. Severe depressive symptoms are found in more than 14% of all aged elderly, with increases as the elderly age (Federal Interagency Forum on Aging-Related Statistics, 2000).

## Homeless

The homeless population is discussed in Chapter 13. This aggregate presents many needs for long-term care, including housing, nutrition, mental health, and substance abuse treatment. Traditionally, many of these persons were adult males and many of these men were veterans. The 1990s resulted in an increase in the number of homeless women and children, partially because of domestic violence.

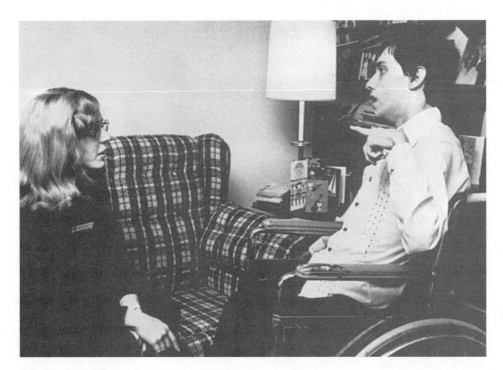

**FIGURE 22-4** Young adults who are physically disabled frequently have extended health care needs that need to be considered when plans for long-term care are developed. These young adults can become productive members of society whey they have social and community supports that help them handle their disabling conditions. (From Gennessee Region Home Care Association, Rochester, NY.)

Although the *Stewart B. McKinney Homeless Act* (see Chapter 4) has increased federal involvement in providing care for homeless persons, most of the provision still resides at the local level. Much of the funding is through private donations and contributions. Many towns and cities have homeless shelters and soup kitchens that provide services to this aggregate. Some of these sites provide mental health and substance abuse counseling, or they refer to local community agencies that provide this service. Nurse-run clinics at homeless shelters often provide services such as blood pressure monitoring, foot care, vision and hearing screenings, skin assessment, and some may provide primary care.

Overnight and long-term housing is provided by many homeless shelters and is partially funded by the federal government. Much of the effort is to meet immediate, short-term needs for safety, clothing, food and shelter, including referrals and consultations with other agencies. Although this aggregate does not provide the traditional formal setting, care plan, or role for nursing, it is one of the most in need of acute and long-term care services.

## Veterans

Another population requiring long-term care is that of veterans. This group provides many opportunities for nursing care in both long-term and community settings. Men and women who served as members of the U.S. Armed Forces are eligible for much of their health care through TRI-

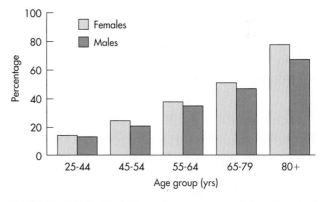

**FIGURE 22-5** Disability rates among adult men and women. (From US Census Bureau: *Americans with Disabilities, 1997: household economic studies,* 2001, US Census Bureau. Retrieved from the internet March, 2001. *http://www. census.gov/hhes/www/disability.htm*)

CARE (United States Department of Defense [USDOD], 2001) or the Veterans Health Administration (VHA). The VHA has a budget of more than $20 billion, 173 medical centers, over 200 counseling centers, 134 nursing homes, more than 700 clinics, and other facilities (VHA, 2000, 2001). Much of the long-term care for veterans was established after World War II. In the 1960s and 1970s, an increase in long-term psychiatric and rehabilitation hospitals occurred as a result of posttraumatic stress syndrome, amputations, and drug or alcohol abuse among veterans. Old Soldier's homes, which began in the previous century, started as rest homes but more recently provide more skilled care.

The *Veterans' Millennium Health Care and Benefits Act* (PL 106-117) extended long-term care services and requires pilot projects on specific long-term care services. Nursing home care is available for persons with a service-connected disability or for veterans who need this type of care and have at least a 70% service-related disability. This act also defined medical service as including noninstitutional extended care services, specified as geriatric evaluation, adult day care, and respite care. Pilot programs have been designed to determine effectiveness of "all-inclusive" care delivery to avoid or reduce hospital and nursing home care. Medical, adult day health, transportation, coordination of care, home care, assisted living, and use of respite services to decrease the need for long-term care will be evaluated (Veterans' Millennium Health Care and Benefits Act, 1999).

Nurses are employed by hospitals, clinics, and counseling, and long-term care facilities in the VHA system. Nursing roles include staff nurse, nurse practitioner, clinical specialist, mental health specialist, nurse anesthetist, administrator, researcher, and educator. Responsibilities for nurses can range from client teaching, acute care, primary care, and chronic care to mental health therapy and counseling, rehabilitation, substance abuse work, skilled care, and care management. Development, research, and evaluation of care models, quality of care, and client and system outcomes are conducted by nurses providing long-term care to this aggregate. Emotional support and coping with chronic health needs are major foci for beginning professional nurses working with veterans.

### Persons with Mental Health Needs

People with mental health needs are discussed separately because of the immense long-term care implications for this aggregate. Mental health conditions and impairments exist across the life span. More than 51 million persons are diagnosed with depression, bipolar disorders, schizophrenia, anxiety disorders, eating disorders, and other problems each year in the United States (USDHHS, 1999a). More than 6.5 million Americans are disabled by mental illness, with 4 million of those persons children and adolescents. However, it is estimated that only 1 in 3 children or adolescents or 1 in 4 adults that need mental health services receive the same (USDHHS, 1999b). Mental health conditions also have been linked with violence and substance abuse among adolescents. Lifetime prevalence of certain mental health conditions is given in Figure 22-6.

The first White House Conference on Mental Health was held in June 1999 under the direction of the Secretary of the USDHHS and had a major impact on the release of

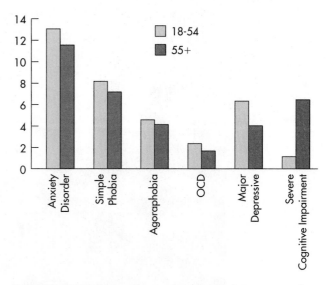

**FIGURE 22-6** Best estimate 1 year prevalence rates of selected mental disorders based on Epidemiological Catachment Area, ages 18-54 and 55+. (From US Department of Health and Human Services: *Mental health: a report of the Surgeon General—executive summary*, 1999b, USDHHS. Retrieved from the internet March, 2001. http://www.surgeongeneral.gov/library/mentalhealth

the first *Surgeon General's Report on Mental Health*. This report identified areas of concern and need, as well as opportunities for making mental health less of a public health problem. Recommendations for efforts by health professionals and lay persons included conducting research into the etiology and prevention of mental illness, determining the most effective treatments, and reducing financial burdens to care (USDHHS, 1999b).

The National Institute of Mental Health (NIMH) and the Substance Abuse and Mental Health Services Administration (SAMHSA) are major federal programs to develop and evaluate mental health needs and services. In fiscal year 2000, $1.6 billion were allocated to mental health prevention, diagnosis, and treatment through USDHHS. The 2500 Community Mental Health Centers partially supported by USDHHS are intended to provide mental health and substance abuse care for uninsured and underinsured persons, primarily in underserved areas. Medicare and Medicaid, as well as private insurance plans cover mental health services. A major change in coverage for mental health care occurred with the 1996 *Mental Health Parity Act*, which provided increased insurance coverage for mental health services. Before this act, many insurers capped mental health coverage at levels much lower than medical or surgical coverage.

There has been a rise in *eating disorders* among children and adolescents. In addition, much attention was focused on *attention deficit hyperactivity disorder* during the 1990s, with Ritalin the treatment of choice. Depression is a significant problem in this age group.

Family therapists, marriage therapists, psychiatric nurse specialists, sex therapists, substance abuse specialists, social workers, psychologists, and psychiatrists provide mental health services. Community mental health centers offer numerous mental health services. Private care is often expensive, and insurance plans usually require preauthorization and reauthorization for mental health services.

Implications for community nurses include working to remove the stigma associated with mental illness; recognition of the disease and disability burden; providing age, gender, and culturally sensitive and appropriate care; and facilitating and encouraging individuals and families to seek treatment early. Nurse's responsibility with clients includes assisting them to acknowledge or identify mental health needs and access the appropriate services. Nurses often realize the problem is a mental health one before the family does. Dealing with the stigma of having a mental health need requires education and support. In many situations, the nurse must educate teachers, coworkers, neighbors, and the community at large, in addition to the family.

With mental health conditions requiring inpatient care, nurses must be diligent to establish, implement, and evaluate a plan of care. Since most payment forms have some limits on daily therapy or length of stay, it is imperative to use each visit, each group session, or each day of inpatient therapy to the fullest. Keeping informed of the nature and requirements of payment or insurance coverage by Medicare, Medicaid, or a third party payer can avoid premature discharge and client reluctance to return because of denied services.

Nurses and clients can contact the local mental health provider or center or the National Mental Health Services Knowledge Exchange Network to find information and resources for families and providers (1-800-799-2967 or *www.mentalhealth.org*). Two mental health conditions, depression and Alzheimer's disease, have major implications for long-term care.

## Depression

Depression is discussed in Chapter 13. It is the most frequently occurring mental health condition in the United States. Unfortunately, depression often goes undiagnosed and untreated. As a long-term condition it greatly decreases a person's quality of life. Antisocial and other behavior problems also are associated with depression (USDHHS, 1999b). Suicide is the third leading cause of death among adolescents and is linked to mood conditions such as depression 90% of the time.

For older adults, depression is a pressing mental illness (AoA, 2001a). Older males have the highest rate of suicide in the nation. NIMH estimates that over 2 million elders each year are diagnosed with depression (USDHHS, 1999a). This depression can be related to relocation, spouse loss, dealing with chronic illness, low income, changes in physical function, a decrease in social interaction, and many other changes in older age. The use of newer pharmacological treatments, caregiver support, senior center access, transportation services, congregate living facilities, and various individual therapies and counseling are major modes of prevention and treatment.

## Alzheimer's Disease

Alzheimer's disease (AD) is a degenerative brain disease marked by changes in behavior and personality and an irreversible decline in intellectual abilities. In AD the death of neurons in key parts of the brain impairs thinking, memory, and judgment, and the deterioration advances in several stages that range from mild forgetfulness to severe dementia. The disease presents a recent public health problem and emerging pubic health epidemic and is a major reason for long-term care.

Today, 4 million Americans, 1 in 10 persons over 65 and nearly half of those over 85 years of age, have AD. Unless a cure or prevention is found, that number will jump to 14 million by the year 2050. Worldwide it is estimated that 22 million individuals will develop AD in the next 3 decades. Of the 3 million Americans who report they know someone with AD, 19 million have a family member with AD (Alzheimer's Association, 2001).

Most persons with AD are cared for at home for years before they are placed in a nursing home. AD causes mental anguish for the affected person and for the significant others. Caring for the individual places a constant burden on families and taxes their resources. A valuable resource for clients, families, and health professionals is the Alzheimer's Association (1-800-272-3900 or *www.alz.org*) for support, educational, and research information.

Lay persons and professionals work together in the Alzheimer's Association to provide education, support, information, and funds for AD research. It provides resource materials that help families establish an effective home management program.

Various other social and aging services are available in the community to assist families of people with AD. Some care services for individuals with dementia that help them to remain in their homes and communities are given in Box 22-1. Community health nurses are in a unique position to help families obtain needed services.

---

### Stop and Think About It

You are working with an elderly man in the hospital who was recently diagnosed with diabetes and hypertension. He has expressed an interest in home health care upon hospital discharge, because he has a limited understanding of his condition. Considering the resources in your community, where would you refer him for follow-up care?

**BOX 22-1**

*Selected Services for Individuals with Long-term Care Needs*

| | | | |
|---|---|---|---|
| Adult day care | Home health | Client assessment | Respite care |
| Care coordination | Homemaker services | Personal care | Skilled nursing |
| Caregiver training | Hospice services | Pet therapy | Social services |
| Case management | Housekeeping services | Physical therapy | Speech therapy |
| Chore services | Information and referral | Physician services | Telehealth |
| Congregate meals | services | Protective services | Telephone reassurance |
| Dental services | Legal services | Recreation services | Transportation |
| Emergency response | Mental health services | Rehabilitation | Volunteer companion |
| services | Occupational therapy | Reminiscence therapy | |
| Home-delivered meals | Paid sitters | | |

## SETTINGS, TYPE OF CARE, AND NURSING ROLE

In 1997 more than 24,000 persons with disabilities under age 21 were in long-term, congregate care facilities, and persons age 22 and older accounted for more than 90,000 such placements (USDHHS, 2000a). *Healthy People 2010* goals are to eliminate the child and adolescent population in such settings and cut the adult number in half (USDHHS, 2000a). Much of this effort is anticipated to be through the *Medicaid Home and Community-Based Services* waiver program of the Social Security Act. Services under this program increased an average of 24% from 1990 to 1997, but still less than 5% of Medicaid expenditures are for community-based care (USDHHS, 2001c). A number of settings for long-term care exist, including the home, hospice facilities, transitional care, and residential housing options.

### Home Health Care

The founder of modern community health nursing, Lillian Wald, was introduced in Chapter 1. Wald and her contemporaries nursed the sick of all ages in their homes and also provided instructions to reduce illness and to promote health. The goals of these early home health care visits were to care for the sick, to teach the family how to care for the ill person, and above all to protect the public from the spread of disease (Buhler-Wilkerson, 1991, p. 7).

Wald's work with the Metropolitan Life Insurance Company to provide home health services was also a significant event in the history of home health care. She was instrumental in developing a plan to extend nursing care to the company's policyholders during illness. The experiment was tremendously successful because the nurses, at a cost of 5¢ per policy, reduced the number of death benefits paid and also created the public image of a concerned humanitarian institution for the company.

To provide this care across the country, the organization used both existing visiting nurse associations and their own nurses. For many visiting nurse associations, this new business partnership meant that without additional fund-raising, they could extend their services to more of the working class. Only 3 years later, Metropolitan Life Insurance Company was paying for 1 million nursing visits each year at a cost of roughly $500,000 per year. By 1916, the Metropolitan visiting nurse service was available to 90% of its 10.5 million policyholders living in 2000 United States and Canadian cities (Buhler-Wilkerson, 1991, pp. 7-8) (Figure 22-7).

By the 1920s, 20 years later, care of ill people in their homes by nurses had declined. Infectious diseases such as smallpox and yellow fever were no longer the leading causes of death, and chronic diseases, much less dramatic in their impact, generated public concern. Further, clients of all classes began to seek hospital-based care because practitioners in this setting were better prepared than previously. Despite these changes, home care has been reaffirmed as an essential community service from a public health perspective throughout this century (Administration of Home Health Nursing, 1945; ANA, 1992, 1993; Bedside nursing care, 1945; Haupt, 1953; Olson, 1986; Stulginsky, 1993a).

In the 1990s, home health care was the fastest growing industry in the United States. A primary reason was that diagnostic related group (DRG) payment, especially for disabled and elders on Medicare, resulted in early discharge. Also, hospitalized clients were sicker and consumers demanded care in the home. Including certified and noncertified agencies, total numbers of home care agencies grew from 11,765 in 1990 to 15,027 in 1994. However, the growth slowed dramatically by 1999.

In 1992 the ANA refined the concept of home health nursing in its document *A Statement on the Scope of Home Health Nursing Practice*. This document defined home health nursing as a "synthesis of community health nursing and selected technical skills from other specialty nursing practices" (ANA, 1992, p. 5), such as medical-surgical nursing, gerontological nursing, and parent-child nursing. The health care deficits of the client determine the appropriate augmentation of other specialty skills with community

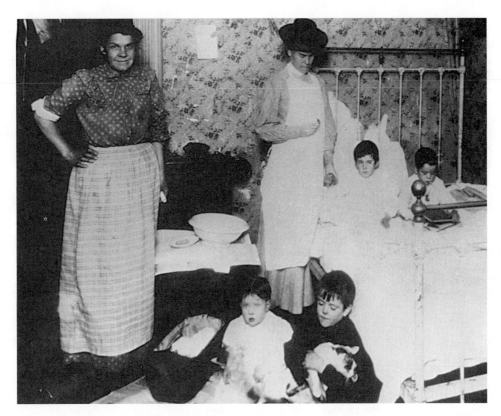

**FIGURE 22-7** The emphasis being placed on home health care is not new. Public health nurses in the United States have provided home health care services since the late 1800s. Individuals across the life span benefit from these services. (Courtesy Metropolitan Life Insurance.)

health nursing practice. As discussed in Chapter 2, the home health nurse who practices within a community health nursing framework provides specialty focused skilled care beyond the individual and family. Nursing care from this perspective directs attention to aggregate needs, "with the predominate responsibility for care to the population as a whole" (ANA, 1992, p. 5). In line with this philosophy, the home health nurse's role as a multidisciplinary care coordinator is important in facilitating the goal of care (ANA, 1992, p. 6). Chapter 10 illustrated the importance of the community health nurses' care coordinator role in facilitating the goal of care beyond the individual family.

Home care includes a broad range of home-based health and social services such as home management assistance, personal care, consumer education, and financial counseling services. Social home care services are covered under Title XX of the Social Security Act for clients who qualify (Title XX is discussed later in this chapter). These services are provided by numerous community agencies such as local departments of social service, family service organizations, and councils on agencies.

Home care visits at one time centered around visits to mothers and children, care of the chronically ill person, and had an emphasis on health promotion. Today this specialty area of nursing is increasingly involved with intensive at-

home care. Home health nurses are no longer exclusively generalists: advanced practice nurses are used to address the complexity and acuity found in the home setting.

The Balanced Budget Act of 1997 (PL 105-33) established payment for clinical nurse specialists and nurse practitioners to provide home health care. Several levels of nursing expertise are needed from both a generalist and specialist perspective to provide care in the home for clients across the life span with a variety of needs.

Although both hospital-based nurses and home health nurses use acute care and high technology skills, the home visit requires nursing practice that is very different from the hospital setting. This can even include integration of interactive technology such as telehealth visiting, heart monitoring, email communication follow-up, and client computers for medication administration (Keener, 2000). The competencies needed by nurses in home health have been developed more fully in the past decade (Benefield, 1998; Stulginsky, 1993b). Some of those competencies are reflected in the comments shared by expert home care nurses (Box 22-2).

Multiple types of agencies (Table 22-4) provide services in home settings. Both the government and private sectors of the health care delivery system are active in delivering home health services. The proliferation of home health care

## BOX 22-2

### The Practical Wisdom of Expert Home Care Nurses

*Build trust and rapport:* Enter the home as a guest; sense "where people are"; do not enter the family's "space"; note the family's customs; negotiate visit times around family needs; honor time commitments

*The first contact sets the tone:* Because few people understand what home care is, the first visit is crucial to developing a lasting helpful relationship; define what nursing can and cannot do; work on mutually acceptable goals; speak slowly and allow processing; ascertain that families know where to call in emergencies

*Assessing the home involves common sense and imagination:* There is no baseline from home to home; listen, look, smell, look for patterns, space, touch, availability of supports; develop giant antennae

*Setting limits to encourage self-care:* Help people solve their own problems, help them look to the past to find their own strengths

*Priorities remain fluid:* Base priorities for visits on (1) potential threats to health, (2) degree of concern to the client, (3) ease of solution

*Suspend one's own values:* Accept things where they are and find common ground; communicate trust and respect in the family's ability to make good decisions

*Teach survival to clients:* Teach information that will keep the client safe until the next visit; understand learner readiness; teaching while doing; enable and empower clients to do for themselves

*Professional boundaries are rarely secure:* With the familiarity of home visits, self-disclosure, accepting gifts and hospitality, and maintaining therapeutic distance are all boundaries one struggles with to find a place of comfort; rarely are those boundaries secure

*Homes can be more distracting than clinical settings:* There may be environmental (clutter, noise), behavioral (drug seeking, avoidance), or nurse initiated (fears of harm, reaction to lifestyle) distractions to providing care. Deal with them directly whenever possible

*Nurses need to protect themselves:* Threats to safety must be handled realistically; heed subtle and not-so-subtle messages from families

*Making do is an essential skill:* Equipment and supplies are not always available; adapting can be a challenge for both nurse and family

*Time is the nurse's most precious resource:* As a result of third-party reimbursement, paperwork is a home health nurse's biggest complaint; develop your own techniques for keeping this at a minimum

From Stulginsky MM: Nurses' home health experience. Part II: the unique demands of home visits, *Nurs Health Care* 14(9):476-485, 1993b.

agencies provided an impetus for the development of *Standards of Home Health Nursing Practice* by the ANA in 1986. Reflective of the changes in health care, the 1999 revision added the focus on quality of care and appropriate resource utilization (ANA, 1999). These standards guide agencies and nurses in providing care of the highest quality for home health care clients.

Presented in the View from the Field are four case histories that represent the type of care offered by home health agencies. The case situations illustrate the direct service role, as well as the care coordinator role, of the home health care nurse. Case histories reflect current practice and clearly illustrate that individuals across the life span need community-based home care services. They also reflect the increasing acuity of client care demands and the need for coordinated, multidisciplinary home health services. Most importantly, they show that skilled home-based nursing services can make a difference. They help families strengthen their coping abilities, and they assist disabled children and adults to improve their functional capabilities and avoid unnecessary institutionalization.

MANAGED CARE AND HOME HEALTH. Increasing numbers of clients seen by home health nurses are part of managed care organizations (see Chapter 4). The number of Americans on managed care plans has increased steadily dur-

ing the 1990s. In 1998 approximately 80% of Americans with employer-sponsored health insurance had managed care plans. This is continually changing and future delivery models may be very different from those presently guiding care.

As of November 2000, more than half of the states had gained approvals for and were operating statewide Medicaid managed care programs. Medicaid managed care covers 16.5 million persons or 54% of recipients; California and Tennessee have the largest number of recipients. Medicare beneficiaries originally had health maintenance organization (HMO) options, beginning in 1997, but now have *Medicare +Choice*, which includes HMO, point of service (POS), and preferred provider organization (PPO) options. Six million persons (14%) are in Medicare managed plans, which receive 18% of the payments (HCFA, 2000b). Additionally, the prospective payment system (PPS) for Medicare changes the services, care, and clients associated with home care (Gundling, 2000; Levy, 2000; St. Pierre, 1999). In other words, the payment for a specific type of visit or service is predetermined by the payer rather than by the provider. There is often disagreement on whether reimbursement is at the appropriate level to compensate providers for services and care.

The significance of managed care on home health cannot be understated. Managed care companies face incentives to

**TABLE 22-4**

*Types of Home Health Care Agencies in the United States\**

| TYPE OF AGENCY | DESCRIPTION OF AGENCY |
| --- | --- |
| Official | A governmental or public agency, usually a local health department, that is supported by state and local taxes. Official agencies are mandated by law to provide certain specific services, such as communicable disease follow-up. They provide health promotion and disease prevention services as well as home health care. |
| Voluntary | A private, nonprofit agency whose operating funds come largely from individual contributions, fees-for-service, united community funds, contracts for service, grants, and other nonofficial sources of funding. Voluntary agencies are governed by a board of directors. These agencies are not required by law to provide specific types of services; they primarily, but not exclusively, provide home health care services. The visiting nurse associations traditionally have been the major voluntary organizations that provide home health care services in a local community. |
| Combination | A combined governmental (a local health department) and voluntary agency (a VNA), whose operating funds came from both official and nonofficial sources. This organizational structure was promoted for the purposes of preventing duplication of services, decreasing continuity of care difficulties and reducing the cost of delivering local health care services. A combination agency provides both health promotion/disease prevention and home health care services. |
| Private, nonprofit | A privately owned agency that is tax exempt because of its nonprofit status. Unlike voluntary agencies, these agencies are governed by the owner(s) of the organization. Their major source of revenue is fee-for-service. Private nonprofit agencies are usually established to provide home health care services only. |
| Proprietary | A private agency established to make a profit. These agencies are not eligible for tax exemption. They are governed by their owner(s), who are increasingly large corporations. Their major source of revenue is a fee for service. Like the private, nonprofit agencies, proprietary agencies are usually established to provide home health care services only. |
| Hospital-based | A home health care agency run and governed by a hospital. Sources of revenue and tax status vary depending on the type of hospital (governmental, voluntary, private, nonprofit, or proprietary) that has established the home health care agency. It is predicted that the numbers of hospital-based home health care agencies will increase dramatically in the next decade. |

Modified from Health Care Financing Administration: *Medicare program: home health agencies—conditions of participation and reductions in recordkeeping requirements,* 42 CFR, Part 484, Sections 484.1 through 484.52, Washington, DC, October, 1994, U.S. Department of Health and Human Services; and Hirsh L, Klein M, Marlowe G: *Combining public health nursing agencies: a case study in Philadelphia,* New York, 1967, Department of PHN, NLN, p. 3.

*\*See Chapter 5 for further discussion of official and voluntary agencies.*

lower costs. It is anticipated that the use of advanced practice nurses to complement or replace physicians under these plans will expand. Nursing interventions need to be documented and their cost-effectiveness determined. These interventions can then be related to client satisfaction and other outcomes.

McCloskey and Bulechek's (2000) work with the Iowa Intervention Projection is a sound step in this direction. Their research work established 486 interventions, each having a name, a definition, and a list of activities that a nurse does to implement the intervention. The interventions are linked to the diagnoses of the North American Nursing Diagnosis Association (NANDA) (see Chapter 9).

Another example of documenting nursing effectiveness is work by Naylor and McCauley (1999) that showed collaborative and coordinated discharge planning and advanced practice nurse follow-up for elders resulted in fewer hospital days and re-admissions. Future research with the

intervention structure will enable nurses to begin to objectively identify the work that is done by nurses assisting clients to improve health with the possibility of costing out care by intervention.

Nurses in home care must understand that they are part of an industry, that the time spent and the outcomes achieved with clients and their families are carried out within the framework of the managed care setting. Case managers authorize the kinds of services that the home care nurse can provide for clients, and those services need to lead to planned outcomes within a specific time frame. Effective nurses have communication skills that appropriately convey the client needs to the case manager and other disciplines involved in the care. The nurse's approach to client care needs to change from a focus on "caring for the client" to a mindset that assists the individual, family, and/or caregiver in providing care for the client. Nurses also need the skills to delegate to other levels of caregivers (see Chapter 24).

*A view from the field*

## VNS CARING IN TOLEDO, OHIO: FOUR CASE EXAMPLES

### Case Example One

Sixteen-year-old boy run over by train, which inflicted massive trauma resulting in amputation of left hindquarter, amputation of arm, multiple pelvic fractures, fracture of transverse process, avulsion of urethra-prostate-testes and L-sileium exposing peritoneal sac, laceration L. ureter and L. iliac arteries, resulted in colostomy, suprapubic cystotomy, hemipelvectomy, bilateral orchiectomy, skin grafts to hip sockets, etc.

After only five weeks in the hospital, client was allowed to go home (on Coordinated Home Care, saving over 30 hospital days) with a 24" × 24" graft in L pelvic area with open draining area. The VNS Home Care Coordinator managed this complex referral, coordinated arrangements for special dressing supplies and equipment, and facilitated care throughout the period of need. The case nurse said, "The coordinator made it all come together and work." Clearly, the value of the coordinator having home care experience and familiarity with agency operations was evident.

Nursing visits were daily for two weeks, then reduced to three times a week as the family became more confident in care. Nursing activities included aseptic wound care, supervision of colostomy care, suprapubic catheter care, observation for complications with prompt intervention, instruction of family in all aspects of care, and encouraging this adolescent to become independent in ADLs. To promote usual family activities, the nurse supported their decision to go on a weekend camping trip within the first two weeks and arranged to make visits at the local campsite.

Physical and occupational therapy services were provided for ADLs, gait training, transfers, strengthening, and stump wrapping. Because this boy was left-dominant, he had to relearn all activities one-handed with the non-dominant side. When a left arm prosthesis was secured, the OT (who herself has an upper extremity prosthesis) resumed visits to aid in learning its use.

A total of 129 home health visits were provided over a nine-month period to aid in his excellent recovery, and he has now returned to school.

Although several intervening hospitalizations were required for re-evaluations and surgical revisions, none were necessary for complications (e.g., infection).

This example of teamwork included various surgery specialists, numerous VNS staff, and, of course, the family.

### Case Example Two

A 70-year-old client who had transhepatic biliary disease, probably cancer of head of pancreas, and a history of cancer of gallbladder was admitted to service after insertion of a transhepatic ring catheter that allows bile to drain from the common duct to the duodenum.

The client and family were quite anxious regarding involved procedures. The visiting nurse instructed the family in home care including such things as withdrawing of bile, irrigating ring catheter technique, dressing changes using aseptic technique, changing catheter plug, and teaching of signs of complications, in addition to monitoring hypertension status, nutrition/hydration, reactions to radiograph treatment, medications, and pain control.

After verbal and demonstrative teaching, the family was able to provide the necessary care and the client was discharged in stabilized condition.

### Case Example Three

A 5-month-old infant who had been normal at birth developed pneumococcal meningitis with resulting hydrocephalus, severe neurologic deficits, and seizure disorders. The mother, who was single and 16 years old, wanted to care for the child at home as long as possible so a referral was made to VNS.

At the time of hospital discharge, the child was totally unresponsive and had no purposeful movements, was on continuous gastric tube feedings with a Kangaroo pump, and required a suction machine and vaporizer. Nursing care consisted of providing and teaching regarding dressing changes around the G-tube, tube irrigation, frequent repositioning, range of motion, skin care and hygiene, relaxation and stimulation techniques, and use of Kangaroo pump. Additionally, the home care nurse assessed neurological and respiratory status and provided frequent intervention related to medication regimen, irritability, and seizure control. A home health aide assisted the mother with care, bathing, and stimulation techniques. A total of 54 home health visits were provided over a five-month period.

The Maternal Child Health nurse supported this young mother in her difficult decision to place the child in an extended care unit for the developmentally disabled at one year of age (where she visits frequently and takes her home every other weekend) so she could return to school.

From Visiting Nurse Service (VNS) of Toledo: Eighty-three years of caring, *Caring* 3:61, 1984. Case examples were written by Janet Blaufuss, RN, former executive director of the Visiting Nurse Service of the Toledo District Nurse Association, Toledo, Ohio, 1984.

*Continued*

*A view from the field*

At the time of discharge from VNS, this young child could take water orally, respond to the mother, and had some purposeful movement.

*Case Example Four*

A 76-year-old client had a long history of Crohn's disease and malabsorption syndrome, and after multiple admissions for weight loss, malnutrition, and dehydration, a permanent subclavian line was inserted in early summer of 1981 for total parenteral nutrition. It became apparent that adequate nutrition could only be attained through TPN and she would need regular infusions of amino acids, electrolytes, minerals, and, eventually, fatty acids through this subclavian line. VNS nurses worked closely with physicians, hospital nurses, nutritionists, pharmacists, social workers, and client's family in planning for adequate predischarge teaching and adequate home support for this client. Through a joint effort between VNS and the community hospital, the client's elderly brother has been successfully managing her four-times-a-week home TPN infusion and once-a-week lipid infusion. This client has the original subclavian line in place (for over two years) and it has remained free of any signs and symptoms of infection for over two years. In addition to care for the subclavian line and TPN infusions, VNS has helped the brother learn to care for the client's permanent colostomy and chronic abdominal fistula.

Client's condition has deteriorated gradually over the last two years; she now has an indwelling foley catheter and is essentially bed bound, requiring the services of a home health aide. Client appears to have suffered at least one CVA and has been hospitalized for erratic blood sugars and abnormal blood values which reflects the necessary and frequent nursing intervention. Nutritionally she has remained stable, demonstrating a weight gain of sixteen pounds over two years (originally weight was 88 pounds and now is 104 pounds).

Through the joint efforts of VNS, the community hospital, and the family, this client has been able to go home and remain at home, without serious nutritional compromise, over the last two years.

In managed care, focus is on both outcomes achieved and quality of care given. Clients have a major role in determining both what that quality is and what the outcomes will be. Nurses must be leaders and managers of their own caseloads to achieve the highest quality in the shortest amount of time (see Chapter 24). Nurses will use progressive technologies, work with disciplines in collaborative efforts, and provide primary and not specialty care (note the *Competencies Needed for Health Professionals* listed by the Pew Health Professions Commission and presented in Chapter 26).

## Hospice

Hospice is a long-term care service that is intended to provide assistance and palliative care rather than the curative care that the traditional medical system offers. The hospice movement developed from the work of Cicely Saunders, a physician from England. She founded St. Christopher's Hospice in 1960, which became a model for similar programs in the United States. In the early 1970s the first American hospice was organized in New Haven, Connecticut.

The development of the hospice movement in the United States is relatively recent, beginning about 25 years ago. The authorization of the Medicare hospice benefit under the *Tax Equity and Fiscal Responsibility Act of 1982* spurred the growth of this industry and has increased to 2287 Medicare program hospices in the United States in 1998.

Also, there are hundreds of volunteer hospices provided by religious, lay, civic, and professional organizations (NAHC, 1999). Hospices can be associated with hospitals, home health agencies, and nursing home facilities, or the facilities and services can be freestanding. Hospice is a movement that emphasizes the following ideals (ANA, 1987):

- Help in dealing with emotional, spiritual, and medical problems
- Support for the entire family
- Keeping the client in his or her home for as long as appropriate and making his or her remaining life as comfortable and as meaningful as possible
- Centrally coordinated home care; inpatient, acute, and respite care; and bereavement services
- Professional services from a health care team supplemented by volunteer services, as appropriate to individual circumstances
- Relief of pain and other symptoms

*Hospice Medicare* began with PL 97-248 in 1982, which covered persons with terminal illness to receive care at home. Originally the benefit was basically unlimited as long as the person was terminally ill. Today hospice benefits under Medicare or Medicaid are specifically designed for persons expected to live less than 6 months (HCFA 2001c, 2001e). In 1996, over 8 million persons were served by hospice agencies, a 400% increase from 1992. About 85% of hospice clients are being served by voluntary nonprofit agencies, while only 11% are served by proprietary agencies (Haupt, 1998).

The *Balanced Budget Act of 1997* clarified hospice coverage. The benefit under Medicare is based on time periods of recertification of terminal illness and eligibility. Two 90-day periods can be followed by an unlimited number of subsequent 60-day periods, as long as a person remains eligible (HCFA, 2001a). Although states are not required to use this for Medicaid hospice, most use the same payment as Medicare. In 1997, 50 days was the average period of service among Medicare agencies (Haupt, 1998), indicating appropriate use of the service.

Four levels of service are provided by Medicare payment: *routine home care day* ($106.93); *continuous home care day* ($624.13 for 24 hours or $26.01/hour); *inpatient respite care* ($110.62); and *general inpatient care day* ($475.69) (HCFA, 2001a). Medicare payment (Part A) for hospice increased from $325 million (0.5%) in 1990 to $2.1 billion (1.6%) in 1998, a 300% increase in the proportion of expenditures but a sixfold increase in terms of actual dollars (NCHS, 2000).

While Medicare continues to be the largest source of documentable payment for hospice services, private insurance and philanthropic organizations continue to outpace Medicaid payment. Medicaid payments totaled $327 million in 1997 (NAHC, 1999), with 44 states having some form of hospice benefit.

Original hospice users were adults with cancer. As the AIDS epidemic spread, trauma survivorship and children with special needs have increased, and the use of hospice by persons other than elderly has increased. The most frequent diagnoses for hospice users are provided in Table 22-5. Also, diagnostic and surgical procedures are commonly related to admission for the hospice client. The most frequent users of hospice continue to be the elderly, with 8% of users under age 45 years. Most are white, but use by gender is generally equal (Haupt, 1998; NAHC, 1999, 2000).

Services that can be provided include nursing care, coordination and referral by a medical social worker, medical care by a physician, a home care aide, and specified homemaker services. Some Medicaid clients can receive short-term inpatient, nursing home, and respite hospice services. Symptom and pain management, ADL and IADL assistance, medical equipment, and medications are provided if included on the established plan of care (HCFA, 2001c, 2001e). Therapies for muscle strength and mobility, hand dexterity, and cognitive function can be provided if deemed necessary. A plan of care is usually required to be established before payment or services can begin.

Two holistic provisions of hospice are the counseling provided to the client and significant others and the bereavement care for family members that can last up to 13 months. This type of care often is provided in the form of support groups before and after death. Nurses are especially involved in providing emotional support, education, and pain and symptom management to clients and their families. Nurses often become close to the hospice families they work with. Hospice

**TABLE 22-5**

## Top Ten Primary Diagnoses in Hospice

| PRIMARY DIAGNOSIS | PERCENT OF USERS |
| --- | --- |
| Lung cancer | 16.5% |
| Congestive heart failure | 5.7% |
| Prostate cancer | 5.3% |
| Breast cancer | 4.0% |
| Chronic airway obstruction | 4.0% |
| Colon cancer | 3.4% |
| Pancreas cancer | 3.2% |
| Acute cerebrovascular disease | 2.9% |
| Rectosigmoid cancer | 2.3% |
| Alzheimer's disease | 2.3% |

SOURCE: Analysis of Medicare Standard Analytic file, 1996 US Department of Health and Human Services (USDHHS), Office of Disability, Aging, and Long-Term Care Policy and the Urban Institute: *Medicare's hospice benefit: use and expenditures,* 2000b, USDHHS. Retrieved from the internet March, 2001. *http://aspe.hhs.gov.daltcp/reports/96useexp.htm*

nurses often attend the funerals of clients, which is not the traditional expectation of nurses providing other types of care.

## Special or Transitional Care

A model of care that can be institutional or community based is special and transitional care. Institutional **special care units (SCU)** are programs designed specifically for persons with Alzheimer's or other dementias, physical disabilities, and short-term care for acute or exacerbations of chronic illnesses, primarily for adults. These also are called subacute care (Griffin, 1998).

Programs vary widely from freestanding facilities that are specifically designed with highly trained staff members to hospital and nursing home units that segregate persons with specific diagnoses from others. There has been some lack of standardization of what constitutes a SCU and the purposes and foci of care. Units differ in size and by age and health status of clients, services provided, staff numbers and qualifications, insurance coverage, cost, quality, and regulation. Many SCUs are for clients with AD and other cognitive impairments and can be found in nursing homes, mental health facilities, hospitals, adult day cares, and assisted living centers. The original purpose was to isolate the clients from others in the facilities. Consumer demand recently has been for respite care and assistance in dealing with these clients or the inability to deal with them in a home setting. Also, regulation and licensing have changed the foci to personal safety and health promotion and maintenance activities and interventions.

Transitional care or rehabilitation SCUs were added in hospital and nursing homes in the 1980s, primarily for care following hip surgery or stroke. While that use has continued, the addition of recuperation and physical therapy, wound and ostomy care, medication administration, and client and family education have provided no lack of clients. Most patients are still adults and Medicare and private pay reimburse for care with limits of 7 to 10 days for most clients for episodic or recuperative care.

For those SCUs that house clients for longer, such as those for ventilator-dependent clients, certificates of need must be filed with state and federal agencies for licensing that includes bed and client limitation, quality initiatives, and payment. Many hospital and assisted living centers with these units actually obtain **skilled nursing facility (SNF)** or intermediate SNF classification and payment for those services. Such classifications are based on a required specific level of skilled nursing care. Research continues on comparing and evaluating these SCUs regarding their effectiveness and efficiency in meeting client, family, community, and societal needs.

Another type of transitional nursing care service that includes both hospital and community care is that described in the project conducted by nurses at the University of Pennsylvania and directed by Dr. Mary Naylor. This project involved determining whether providing special transitional care for older persons with common medical and surgical problems would increase positive health outcomes. Advanced practice nurses provided the hospitalized clients comprehensive discharge care and follow-up home care. Dr. Naylor and her colleagues found that these clients had lower rates of readmission to hospitals, and that hospital days were fewer than persons in the group that did not receive the specialized intervention (Naylor, McCauley, 1999). This collaborative nursing model of care was positive for the client and family and reduced costs. Research on nursing care such as this shows that when care includes holistic assessment of client needs and resources, education, and caregiver assistance, self-care management skills can result in positive outcomes for the client, family, and health system.

Medicare payment for special or transitional care was altered with the Balanced Budget Act of 1997. Specifying auspices of care and payment, the federal government and the Joint Commission on Accreditation of Health Care Organizations (JCAHO) defined and legitimized this type of care; the settings in which it could be provided; and the spectrum of care, services, and professionals that should be involved (Griffin, 1998). Managed care also has increased the need for care specific to the type and level of care that matches a client's health needs. Rather than hospital or nursing home care, this type of care may be in a variety of long-term care settings in the community. The anticipated outcomes are improved health for the client and lower costs for the system. Development of innovative models of care and evaluation (research) of their effectiveness is underway. Specific regulation of this type of care is not fully developed across all states.

## Residential and Housing Options

Several residential options are available to people who either cannot or do not want to maintain an independent household and who have varying needs for long-term care. They include nursing homes, board and care homes, continuing care retirement communities, home sharing arrangements, respite care, adult day care, adult foster care, and assisted living.

These options vary in price from those who serve people on Supplemental Security Income (SSI) (see Chapter 5) to those that advertise for the affluent. Residential options for people with disabilities are presented in Chapter 18. Community health nurses play a crucial role in assessing the level of care needed by clients who require long-term care services. Unfortunately few funds are available to assist clients with their greatest needs: personal care, housekeeping, meal preparation, and home chore service.

**NURSING HOMES.** **Nursing homes** have long been the mainstay of long-term care in the United States and is often what is thought of in terms of an institutional, residential long-term placement. Nursing homes can be for profit or nonprofit and offer skilled, intermediate, or basic nursing care. Nursing homes have historically housed people who were elderly, but all age groups currently reside in nursing homes.

When visiting clients in the home, community health nurses assess characteristics that place them at risk for nursing home placement. Reducing inappropriate use of nursing home beds by people who are capable of living at home is a gatekeeping mechanism that can save costly and scarce health care resources and can better meet clients' physical, emotional, and social needs. Nurses should work with the client and family to explore other options to long-term care.

**BOARD AND CARE HOMES.** **Board and care homes** usually provide housekeeping and congregate meals and may include some oversight from staff members. Typically they do not provide a comprehensive range of services and do not claim to meet unscheduled needs. Every state has adopted a form of licensure for these facilities, but many states have unlicensed facilities (Hawes, Rose, Phillips, 1999; Kane, Wilson, 1993).

**CONTINUING CARE RETIREMENT COMMUNITIES.** **Continuing care retirement communities** usually have three levels of care. The level of care between independent living and a nursing home is a form of assisted living. Independent and assisted living homes tend to be available only to aggregates that can afford the high fees.

**ADULT FOSTER CARE HOMES.** **Adult foster care** homes generally serve the mentally and developmentally disabled rather than those with physical disabilities. Placements in these homes are provided in many states for people over 18 who are socially, mentally, or physically handicapped. The purpose is to provide the opportunity for normal family and community life and help with problems. A foster home for adults is usually operated by individuals in their own homes and provides room, board, housekeeping, personal care, and supervision to four or fewer adults on a 24-hour basis. Those eligible for the program include people who receive Temporary Assistance to Needy Families (TANF) or SSI.

HOME-SHARING ARRANGEMENTS. **Home-sharing arrangements,** several individuals or families living together in a single family home, can work very well in some instances. Intergenerational families, with grandparents and grandchildren living in one home and sibling cohabitation, have again become prevalent.

ADULT DAY CARE. **Adult day care** provides assistance for adults who cannot be left alone during the day yet do not require 24-hour nursing care in an institution. A wide variety of services, including nutritious lunches; medical and social services; occupational, speech, and physical therapy; and health screening are often available to clients. Those who use this kind of service are persons with AD, the physically impaired with diagnoses such as arthritis or stroke, the mentally impaired, and the socially impaired or isolated individual. Candidates are evaluated in their homes before enrollment, and the daily attendance fee is usually based on a sliding scale fee schedule. This service allows many people with dementia and other long-term disabling conditions to remain living with their family and avoid or delay institutional placement. These placements have started developing in recent years, although not as fully as would be helpful. Many of these placements are on a private pay basis.

RESPITE CARE. **Respite care** is discussed in Chapter 18 and is the temporary care of a person who has a disability to give caregiver relief. This may involve a temporary caregiver providing in- or out-of-home care. Again, placements are usually on a private pay basis, especially for adult clients with disabilities, and often are not widely available. Respite services include a wide range of services intended to give temporary relief for families caring for members with special needs and disabilities. Recognition of the need of formal respite services has not been widely present in the United States until the late 1990s.

ASSISTED LIVING. **Assisted living** is the most rapidly growing industry for long-term elder care. This setting involves the person being able to live independently in the community with assistance. This assistance can take many forms such as provision of housekeeping services, meal preparation, or personal care.

The trend toward assisted living is expected to continue through 2025 (National Center for Assisted Living, 2001). There are differences in the designation of assisted living, often including board and care homes, special units in nursing homes, congregate housing, retirement living, independent living, and residential care. This discussion focuses on the community-based residential arrangement that offers a mix of personal care, ADL/IADL assistance, meal preparation, housekeeping, and medication administration for a monthly fee. This discussion does not include those retirement centers where an individual pays for the apartment or "turns over their estate" to a facility in exchange for lifetime care. However, those facilities may actually include an assisted living level of care. Regardless, one of the positive aspects of assisted living is that of personal security and safety.

Social interaction is also a positive effect of such a congregate living facility (Rose, Pruchno, 1999). Maintaining independence in having an apartment, paying one's own bills; continuing driving and car ownership; and perhaps most importantly, autonomy, are major benefits for the individual client.

Designed to assist and respond to regular and unexpected needs for older adults, it was not health care professionals or providers who initiated assisted living. Business managers and construction companies in the private sector have built facilities in response to consumer demand. Although assisted living could provide residential long-term care for disabled and older people with public support, this type of long-term care has remained a private pay or an out-of-pocket expenditure. There is essentially no federal funding for assisted living, and rarely state funding. Lack of government funding has resulted in little standardization, regulation, or oversight of long-term care in these facilities. Also, there remain varying levels and types of services provided (Bectel, Tucker, 1998). Some facilities are residential only (independent living), similar to a condominium or apartment, with no yard or maintenance responsibilities. Other facilities offer personal care, meal, social, nursing, transportation, and psychological services.

Standardization is becoming more prevalent primarily because of the dramatic increase in state regulation during 1997 to 2000 (National Center for Assisted Living, 2001). The different policies for licensing and reimbursement have been compiled through the *National Study of Assisted Living for the Frail Elderly* conducted by the Office of Disability, Aging, and Long-term Care Policy (Hawes, Rose, Phillips, 1999; USDHHS, 1998).

Most clients utilizing assisted living services are white, middle and upper class elderly men and women who are ambulatory and cognitively intact. Costs are dependent on the spectrum of services and amenities available but can range from a low of $1000 per month to more than $3000 per month. Of course the charge in Los Angeles will be different from the charge in Charlotte, North Carolina, because of market share, property value, salaries, ownership, size, and cost of living. As regulations increase, an expected cost increase should be anticipated. In addition, most state regulations require administrators to include families in decision making.

When nurses work in an assisted living facility or are assisting an individual or family to decide upon using this type of long-term care, several issues should be examined: number and qualifications of staff, professional dietary consultation, opportunity for physical activity and social gatherings, available parking and transportation, visitation policies, rooms or apartments, single versus shared rooms or bathrooms, emergency pull cords in all rooms, environmental safety, fire or emergency egress, educational facilities such as a library and reading or computer room, use of one's own furniture, appliances in rooms, and nonsmoking areas.

Nurses and families also should consider the specific requirements of the client and available assistance with medications, hygiene, eating, dressing, bathing, and toileting. Can the facility or staff meet the special needs of the client? For example, how well can a facility address clients who have a colostomy or prosthesis, are deaf or blind, or exhibit wandering behaviors? Most facilities will not assume responsibility for adults with special needs; those adults must often use traditional personal care homes (Quinn, Johnson, Andress, et al., 1999). Additionally, few assisted living sites will accept children or adolescent residents.

Individuals, families, and staff should ask to review and become familiar with quality of care, accountability, client/family rights policies, and elder abuse laws. State ombudsmen, commissions on aging, insurance commissioners, division of facilities services, departments of health, attorneys general offices, and state statutes provide regulatory and legal licensure requirements. Also, many state regulatory boards keep consumer information on complaints filed and compliances of the facility and owners. It is anticipated that because of the demographic and epidemiological trends discussed earlier, assisted living care will continue to grow and evolve over the next three decades.

## Informal Care: Caregiving

More than half of adults expect to care for a loved one at some time in their lives. While the majority of care recipients are parents, there is an increasing number of siblings, in-laws, children, grandchildren, and significant others. In a study conducted during 2000, it was estimated that 54 million persons provide care for a family member or friend. Most of these caregivers are middle-aged adults, with women outnumbering men. One third (37%) of the caregivers live in the same residence as the care recipient, and almost half of these households have incomes less than $30,000. ADL assistance is provided by more than half, and almost half (46%) provide care such as medications or wound care (National Family Caregivers Association [NFCA], 2001).

Care provided by family and friends has been estimated at over $196 billion per year (NFCA, 2001). Although such efforts are unpaid, they are associated with burdens and costs. Caregiving often means a loss of income for the caregiver and losses in productivity for employers. *The Family and Medical Leave Act* (PL 103-3) allows persons to take unpaid time from work to care for family members, either elders or children. However, many persons cannot afford to take unpaid leave for jobs or they lose their own health benefits. Also, some caregivers may work in companies or part-time positions that are not covered by the act.

The importance of informal support networks in preventing institutionalization cannot be overestimated. As previously discussed, about 75% of the dependent elderly are cared for in their homes. Most families want to care for their disabled family members and keep them at home as long as possible. Often in doing so, these families experience extreme financial costs and stress, placing them at risk for experiencing health problems. Families usually opt for institutional care as a solution for dealing with their stress

only after their personal resources for coping have become exhausted. Being able to be maintained in a community setting enhances quality of life (Figure 22-8).

Often caregiving includes moving a loved one into a home that is multigenerational in nature. This can be a positive experience but that depends on the nature of the relationships between the care recipient and caregiver(s), the type of care needed, the number of hours of care, financial resources, health of the care recipient and caregiver(s), and available assistance or respite.

Cultural beliefs also are important with respect to the positive or negative nature of the caregiving situation (Kaye, 2000; Tennstedt, Chang, Delgado, 1998). Several studies document the burden of caregiving (Cain, Wicks, 2000; Calderon, Tennstedt, 1998; Teel, Press, 1999; Witucki, 2000; Yates, Tennstedt, Chang, 1999). One major concern for nursing is the declining health of caregivers, especially among older caregivers, those who provide medical care or treatments, and those who provide more than 21 hours per week or "intense" caregiving. Another concern is whether the child, elder, or adult is being abused or neglected. This may occur both with intent and as a result of knowledge deficits, fatigue, and declining health on the part of the caregiver.

Nursing care, then, should provide periodic monitoring of the caregiving situation and the health of care recipients and caregivers. Client education is one avenue to provide knowledge and technical skills to caregivers. Emotional support and clear communication about expectations can help the caregiver and care recipient work together, make health decisions, understand their roles and contributions, and know when to ask for help. Accessing resources (e.g., human, material, financial, emotional) from social services, churches, family

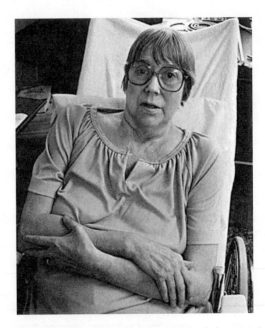

**FIGURE 22-8** Jane Richards, who lost both legs to circulatory disease, lives at home rather than in a nursing home. (Courtesy Anne Lennox/*Times-Union*.)

members and neighbors, councils on aging, civic groups, support groups, community services, and mental health and children's providers and institutions is another strategy long used by public health nurses and nurses providing discharge planning activities, as has been documented in studies (Chang, Noonan, Tennstedt, 1998; Tuck, Wallace, 2000).

All of these efforts should be through culturally competent practice that considers and respects racial/ethnic, religious, social, and developmental beliefs and values. The importance, needs, burden, and effectiveness of caregiving are varied among cultural and gender groups (Calderon, Tennstedt, 1998; Coe, Neufield, 1999; Kim, Theis, 2000; Porter, Ganong, Armer, 2000; Tennstedt, Chang, 1998; Wallace, Witucki, Boland, Tuck, 1998). Box 22-3 has tips for caregivers in establishing a caregiving routine. Box 22-4 identifies questions that help caregivers determine what they need to know. The

---

**Teaching TIPS BOX 22-3**
### Establish a Caregiving Routine

1. Put yourself in control
   a. Plan a caregiving schedule that fits your own routine and activities.
   b. Plan your routine in partnership with: home care nurse, family members, and others.
   c. Use a calendar to write down the things you need to do. Include doctor appointments and ordering supplies.
   d. Get a spiral notebook and make a chart. Write down important information in the spaces, such as daily weights or blood sugars.
   e. Use your notebook for reminders you want to discuss with the physician or nurse. Take the notebook to the physician's office.
2. Ask for help
   a. Think about how much help you need. You will often need more help in the beginning. It is helpful to have someone to call every day.
   b. It is okay to ask others for help. It is best to have someone to help you in case something unexpected happens.
3. Control supplies and medicines
   a. Start a list of all needed supplies.
   b. Keep supplies in a separate cabinet, closet, or room. Keep this place clean and organized.
   c. Sterility and cleanliness are the most important factors to help in avoiding infections.
4. Know what to tell the doctor or nurse
   a. Record daily information as instructed by your nurse, such as blood sugars or urine output.
   b. Write any progress or changes in symptoms in your spiral notebook.
   c. Tell your physician or nurse about changes they have asked you to record. Examples are fever or weight changes.

**Remember—everyone has good and bad days!** Do not worry about one bad day. There are times when you may need professional support from a minister or counselor. Signs of depression include a loss of self-worth, frequent crying spells, loss of interest in family life, and difficulty concentrating or sleeping. Tell the physician or nurse about these signs if they occur. You can get help for depression.

Modified from Martin KS, Larson BJ, Gorski LA, Hayko DM, editors: *Mosby's home health client teaching guides: R*x *for teaching,* St Louis, 1997, Mosby, p. III-F-1-6.

---

**Teaching TIPS BOX 22-4**
### Caregiving: What Do I Need to Know?

1. Illness and treatment
   a. What do I need to know about the illness and the treatment?
   b. How does the treatment work?
   c. How much will this cost?
   d. Will my insurance pay for this?
2. Emergency care
   a. When should we call for help?
   b. Who should we call for help?
   c. Is fever an emergency?
3. Daily activities
   a. How will this illness and treatment affect everyday life?
   b. Can we still do "normal" things?
   c. Will we still be able to have sexual relations?
4. Treatments and procedures
   a. How do we keep the treatments sterile?
   b. What is the best way to sleep with tubing hooked up?
   c. How do we use the machine (e.g., hook it up, keep it clean, and set the volume)?
5. Medicine and supplies
   a. How do we know if the medicine or treatment is not working?
   b. What do we do if the medicine does not seem to work?
   c. When should we order supplies?
   d. How can we cut costs on supplies and medicines?
6. Food and beverages
   a. What kinds of supplements are required?
   b. Should the diet for the rest of the family change?
7. Emotional reactions to illness
   a. What if the doctors do not seem to understand?
   b. How do we cope with loneliness, sadness, or depression?
   c. If our relationships with friends change, how do we handle the changes?
8. Home care services
   a. What type of help will home care provide?
   b. When do we call the home care nurse?
   c. Will insurance pay for home care?

From Martin KS, Larson BJ, Gorski LA, Hayko DM, editors: *Mosby's home health client teaching guides: R*x *for teaching,* St Louis, 1997, Mosby, p. III-F-1-6.

*National Family Caregiving Association* provides tips for family caregivers (*http://www.nfcacares.org/tentipsf.html*).

A new avenue of assistance for persons caring for older loved ones is the National Family Caregiver Support Program (PL 106-501). States receive funds through the State Agencies on Aging to develop caregiver services such as counseling, support, training, respite, and education (AoA, 2001a, 2001c, 2001d). At the present time, there is no provision for caregivers of special needs children or younger disabled adults, although some states have provided tax credits.

## LONG-TERM CARE FINANCING

The federal government's Centers for Medicare and Medicaid Services (CMS), formerly named the Health Care Financing Administration (HCFA), is the primary source of funding for long-term care. Payment sources for long-term payment from the government include monies from the Older Americans Act, Social Services Block Grants, Children's Health Insurance Program (CHIP), Medicare, and Medicaid.

The major portion of public expenditures for long-term care goes to institutional care, with the Medicaid program being the principal payer. The Medicaid program pays for over half of all nursing home expenditures. The Medicare program provides payment for home health aide and nursing services, care in skilled nursing facilities, selected mental health care, and hospice.

Different from Medicaid, Medicare covers clients according to the type of plan they select (e.g., fee for service, HMO) and entitlement and eligibility criteria. Publicly funded noninstitutional long-term care, specifically home care, is funded by Social Security Act programs, including Medicare, Medicaid, block grants to states for social services, and the Children's Health Program and through provisions of the Older Americans Act. This legislation and the basic characteristics of these programs are discussed in Chapters 4 and 5. Current coverage for selected Medicare long-term care is shown in Table 22-6.

### Medicare

Medicare provides the largest governmental expenditures for home health care and hospice services. Both part A (hospital insurance) and Part B (supplemental medical insurance) of Medicare include provisions for home health care and hospice. The newer managed care plans cover long-term care services in varying ways. Historically, Medicare reimbursed a home health care agency for:

- *Intermittent* skilled nursing services provided by or under the supervision of a registered nurse
- *Intermittent* physical, occupational, or speech therapy provided by or under the supervision of a qualified therapist

**TABLE 22-6**

*Long-Term Care Benefits Under Medicare*

| MEDICARE A | MEDICARE B |
|---|---|
| *Skilled Nursing Facility (SNF) Care\** Semiprivate room, meals, skilled nursing and rehabilitative services (after a 3-day hospital stay). | *Medical and Other Services:* Doctors' services (except for routine physical examinations), outpatient medical and surgical services and supplies, diagnostic tests, ambulatory surgery center facility fees for approved procedures, and durable medical equipment (such as wheelchairs, hospital beds, oxygen, and walkers). |
| *Home Health Care\** Part-time skilled nursing care, physical therapy, speech-language therapy, home health aid services, durable medical equipment (e.g., wheelchairs, hospital beds, oxygen, and walkers) and supplies, and other services | *Home Health Care\** Part-time skilled care, home health aide services, durable medical equipment when supplied by a home health agency while getting Medicare-covered home health care, and other supplies and services. |
| *Hospice Care\** Medical and support services from a Medicare-approved hospice, drugs for symptom control and pain relief, short-term respite care, care in a hospice facility, hospital, or nursing home when necessary, other services not otherwise covered by Medicare. Home care also is covered. | *Outpatient Hospital Services* Services for the diagnosis or treatment of an illness or injury. |

\*The person must meet certain conditions in order for Medicare to cover these services.
From Health Care Financing Administration (HCFA): *Medicare and you 2001: your Medicare benefits,* 2001f, HCFA. Retrieved from the internet January, 2001. *http://www.medicare.gov*

- *Intermittent* medical social services provided by or under the supervision of a qualified social worker
- *Intermittent* home health services provided by a home health aide who has completed a competency evaluation program and is supervised by a registered nurse who possesses a minimum of 2 years of nursing experience, at least 1 year of which must be in the provision of home health care, and who has a performance review of 12 hours of in-service and training annually.
- Medical supplies (other than drugs and medications) and the use of medical appliances
- Hospice services including short-term inpatient care, nursing care, therapy services, medical social services, home health aide services, physician services, and counseling

Provisions of the *Omnibus Budget Reconciliation Act of 1980* (Public Law 96-499) expanded the home health benefits offered by Medicare so that beneficiaries were permitted unlimited home health visits without the requirement for a prior hospital stay or payment of a deductible amount. To qualify for these benefits, beneficiaries must be *homebound;* the services must be prescribed and periodically reviewed by a physician; and the client must need part-time or *intermittent, skilled* nursing care and/or therapy services (e.g., physical, occupational, or speech therapy). When home health aide services are needed an appropriate professional staff member must make supervisory visits to the client's residence on a regular basis (HCFA, 1991).

Landmark changes in the Medicare program have occurred as a result of a lawsuit brought against Medicare by the National Association for Home Care (NAHC) in the late 1980s. The suit contained two essential claims: (1) the challenge to the part-time or intermittent policy for length of care allowed clients, and (2) how "medical necessity" is interpreted to qualify a client for care. The successful conclusion to the lawsuit did not change Medicare regulations but did change HCFA's interpretation of them, so that more services could be provided. Several of these changes are noteworthy (Staggers' Lawsuit, 1988, pp. 1-3):

- Clients are considered homebound if they attend adult day care centers, renal dialysis clinics, or outpatient radiation or chemotherapy facilities when the purpose is to receive medical care. Regarding adult day care clients, it is the agency's responsibility to demonstrate that attendance at the day center is for the purpose of receiving medical care.
- A new skilled service is described "skilled nursing management and evaluation of a client care plan" that allows coverage for nurses who need to manage certain complex unskilled care cases.
- Specific coverage standards are set out for venipuncture in stable and unstable clients. For example, a client receiving prothrombin whose blood test results indicate stability within the therapeutic range will qualify for a skilled nursing visit once a month to continue appropriate monitoring.

- A client cannot be denied solely on the basis of having a chronic disease or terminal illness.
- An order for personal care of a home health aide is allowed, with the boundaries of that personal care to be determined by the nurse following a care plan rather than by a physician.
- Coverage of family counseling is specifically recognized as part of the function of a medical social services visit, in which family counseling is incidental to beneficiary counseling and designed to remove an impediment to the delivery of safe and effective care.

The skilled nursing management change under Medicare generated a model for nurses to provide case management for persons at risk for rehospitalization. It is significant because for the first time Medicare eligibility rules do the following (Allen, 1994): (1) recognize and reimburse nurses as case managers in the home, (2) reimburse for prevention and health promotion in the home, and (3) acknowledge and reimburse chronic rather than exclusively acute care for its recipients. *The Medicare Home Health Agency Manual* was rewritten to address the changes noted in the Staggers' Lawsuit. It contains case examples clarifying coverage criteria and is useful on a daily basis for the staff nurse. Failure to comply with the conditions of participation results in an agency's loss of certification by Medicare and the ability to receive Medicare reimbursement.

Medicare monies providing for long-term care decreased dramatically with the *Balanced Budget Act of 1997.* This federal legislation required establishment of a prospective payment system for home health care to cut costs and prevent abuse of services. One major change was the denial of Medicare coverage for a home health visit if venipuncture was the only medically necessary reason. The outcome of that decision was that many persons were dropped from receiving services and 14% of Medicare-certified home health agencies closed during the first year following the legislative change (Magruder, Legeay 1999; Turnbull, 2000).

Another major change was that a case-mix formula with *Resource Utilization Group* (RUG) reimbursement also came into effect for skilled and subacute nursing facilities (Randall, 1999). Thus rather than traditional actual costs reimbursement by a daily bed fee and additional charges for physical therapy and medications, payment is for a fixed per diem rate based on RUGs, similar to DRGs in hospitals.

The third major change was the initiation of a systematic database and outcomes management using the OASIS system (HCFA, 2000a; NAHC, 2000). This requires tracking and regular documentation of patient assessment, visits, personnel use, and outcomes achieved. While the industry has been unhappy with these changes, it was seen as necessary by those outside the industry because of an increase in Medicare costs of 28% each year for 7 consecutive years (Grimaldi, 1999).

## Medicaid

The current Medicaid statute provides states with the authority to include a variety of home- and community-based services in their Medicaid programs. Because Medicaid is a state-administered program, the range of home care benefits offered varies from state to state. States also have the freedom to determine eligibility requirements and the amount of service they will reimburse under Medicaid. However, in order to be federally subsidized under Medicaid, a state must provide at least home health services. Some states extend home care benefits to the medically needy or those persons who do not qualify for regular Medicaid benefits but who have inadequate financial resources to meet health care costs.

Originally, the *Omnibus Budget Reconciliation Act of 1981* (PL 97-35) expanded the range of long-term services that can be offered by the Medicaid program. This act established the Medicaid Waiver Authority to implement home- and community-based care programs. Under these programs, states could provide a comprehensive array of medical and social services including case management, homemaker and home health aides, personal care, adult day care, habilitation care, and respite care to avoid more costly institutional care. These programs serve individuals in the community who would require the level of care provided in a SNF or intermediate care facility if they did not receive waiver services. The costs of the community-based waiver services could not exceed the cost of institutional care.

More recent waivers include demonstration programs, where states can develop alternative systems to traditional Medicaid reimbursement for primarily physician and hospital care. Oregon had the first such demonstration program. Two states with the largest Medicaid enrollees in 2000 (California "MediCAL" and Tennessee "TennCare") extended coverage to persons either uninsurable or uninsured. Because of the underestimations of persons eligible and enrolling in the programs, both states are experiencing difficulty in paying for coverage and maintaining insurers that provide coverage.

The newest Medicaid waiver allows for *Home- and Community-Based Services* to be used in creative ways as alternatives to hospital, nursing home, or intermediate facilities for persons suffering from mental retardation. Seven services are required to meet waiver approval and payment: case management, homemaker/home health aide, personal care, adult day health, respite, and habilitation. States also can apply to use funds for transportation, adult day care, communications equipment (e.g., computer for disabled or child), and day or partial hospitalization (HCFA, 2001d).

Medicaid continues to cover selected rehabilitation; hospice; personal care; physical therapy; occupational therapy; speech, language, and hearing; and home health services for clients or agencies meeting eligibility criteria if that service is offered in the state of residence. Institutions for mental diseases also can seek reimbursement for care provided. For clients to qualify for home health services under Medicaid, they must receive services in their place of residence and have the services ordered by a physician that reviews the established plan of care every 60 days. Clients do not need to be homebound to receive Medicaid benefits. Care can be on a part time or intermittent basis but must include nursing services as defined by each state's nursing statutes. Agencies and facilities also must follow guidelines for care. Nursing homes under Medicaid long-term care coverage must provide comprehensive services for clients including nursing, rehabilitation, medically related social services, pharmaceutical, dietary, dental, activity, and mental health services. Each facility also must abide by the resident rights' document and have in place a process for dealing with injury, failure to meet client rights, and transfer or discharge from the facility (HCFA, 2001e).

As is the case with Medicare, home health services are only a small percentage of the total Medicaid expenditures. Of the almost $160 billion spent on Medicaid payments more than 64% of the expenditures went to hospital and SNF services and less than 4% as home health care payment (HCFA, 2001h). This trend is expected to continue until at least 2003. The major alterations are anticipated to be shifts to long-term care in the Veteran's Health Administration, CHIP, and waiver programs.

Medicaid costs for health care are rising rapidly, and legislators are looking for ways to increase revenues and cut costs. There is continual monitoring of a number of issues under debate by legislators at every level of government that could affect the aggregate of low-income persons needing long-term care, as well as access and payment to their providers. Concerned professionals will need to remain keenly aware of legislative debates, proposals, and allocation decisions.

## Social Services Block Grants to States

The **Social Services Block Grants to States** program (Title XX of the Social Security Act) was established in 1975. The Omnibus Budget Reconciliation Act of 1981 (PL 97-35) altered the program and reformulated it as a federally funded Social Services Block Grant. The Social Services Block Grant, like other block grants, provides the states freedom in determining the populations to be served and the types of services to be offered. This grant program provides funding for a comprehensive array of social services directed toward the following goals:

- Achieving or maintaining economic self-support to prevent, reduce, or eliminate financial dependency
- Achieving or maintaining self-sufficiency, including reduction or prevention of dependency for daily care
- Preventing or remedying neglect, abuse, or exploitation of children and adults unable to protect their own interests, or preserving, rehabilitating, or reuniting families
- Preventing or reducing inappropriate institutional care by providing for community-based care, home-based care, or other forms of less intensive care

- Securing referral or admission for institutional care when other forms of care are not appropriate, or providing services to individuals in institutions

A broad range of home-based services can be provided by the states under the program, including homemaker, home health aide, home management, personal care, consumer education, and financial counseling services. As with Medicaid, the benefits offered under this program vary from state to state. To qualify for services, clients must meet income eligibility requirements.

For states to participate in the program they must establish a Comprehensive Annual Service Program plan that outlines the services they will provide to whom and by what methods. Federal spending under the program is capped, and funds are allocated among states on the basis of their populations. Social Services Block Grant funds aid states in meeting local needs not met by other social service agencies in the community. However, the limited funding for this program does not allow states to expand home care services significantly.

## Older Americans Act

The Older Americans Act (OAA) of 1965 (see Chapter 19) established the Administration on Aging in the Department of Health, Education, and Welfare and authorized a variety of health and social services projects for aging citizens (see Chapters 5 and 19). In 1978 amendments to the act consolidated several existing titles and revised and expanded provisions of the act. Under Title III of the act a broad range of social services are mandated for the elderly, including home health, home health aide, homemaker, and nutritional services. The only eligibility requirement for participation in these services is that clients must be at least age 60. Unlike Medicare, clients do not need to be homebound and do not need skilled nursing care to qualify for home health benefits.

The Older Americans Act Amendments of 2000 increased funds and authorization for long-term care services, including the establishment of the caregiver support program. Funding exceeds $1 billion for Title III for fiscal year 2001 (AoA, 2001c, 2001d, 2001g).

## Other Programs Funding Long-term Care

Other programs that pay for long-term care, primarily home health services, include the following:
- *Private health insurance:* This is generally limited to physician-directed medical services, courses of therapy, and equipment. For the elderly, coverage under long-term care insurance is increasing.
- *Veterans Health Administration:* Veterans with a disability are eligible for home health care coverage and other long-term care services, with many new ones added in 2001. Services must be authorized by a physician and are provided through the VHA network of providers.
- *TRICARE (was CHAMPUS):* Managed care for 5 million military service personnel and family members. This program covers noncustodial skilled care and other long-term care, depending on the plan selected. Options of coverage are Prime, Extended, Standard, and Senior Prime. There is also a Program for Persons with Disabilities option (VHA, 2000).
- *Social service organizations:* Organizations that operate with private charitable funding, such as the United Way, may offer a wide range of services, including most of the health and supportive home care services needed by clients. Depending on eligibility, agencies may require sliding scale payments, donations, or services without charge.
- *Private pay:* In spite of the many methods of reimbursing home care providers, when formal and informal health care services are considered, the majority of home care expenses are still paid for out-of-pocket (see Chapter 5) because of the limitations of coverage under both public and private financing programs.

## Problems with Government Funding

The Medicare Trust Fund could go bankrupt in 2010 if expenditures continue to grow at their current rate and the baby boomers become full Medicare recipients. Efforts to revise Medicare and avoid this problem, as well as to "lock box" funds from payroll deductions, have failed in Congress. In 2001, the beginning sessions of Congress are anticipating that the major changes to Medicare will be the addition of a prescription drug benefit, which will further bankrupt the system unless substantial changes are made and Congress leaves the trust fund alone. The solvency of the Trust Fund is especially uncertain after the terrorism events of September 11, 2001, and the corresponding congressional actions.

The first sections of this chapter discussed the factors that have influenced the needs for long-term care services in this country. With the concomitant costs and needs associated with those services, there have been almost yearly amendments to the Social Security Act to both restrict and expand long-term care services. For example, in 1993 there was a reduction in payment to agencies providing hospice services, a repeal of the mandate requiring personal care services to be covered under state Medicaid programs, an extension of social HMO demonstrations (discussed in the next section of this chapter), and an extension of monies for AD demonstration projects (NAHC, 1995). In the 1990s the Health Security Bill was developed as part of the President's agenda for a national health plan. The future Senator Hillary Clinton chaired that task force, but the legislation was not passed. *The Balanced Budget Act of 1995*, which contained sweeping changes in both Medicare and Medicaid, was vetoed by President Clinton. However, the *Balanced Budget Act of 1997* was passed by Congress and signed into law by the President. Under this act several health coverages changed, including home health, hospital, and nursing home care.

With traditional statutory emphases on part-time acute and postacute treatment of illness, government programs only recently have begun to seriously address the increasing long-term care needs of the nation. The homebound and the part-time or intermittent skilled nursing criteria for eligibility make it impossible for many chronically ill or disabled aging persons to qualify for Medicare home health care benefits. With respect to Medicaid, the state run health program, many eligibility criteria are similar to Medicare. However, states often have placed caps on Medicaid long-term care services. These caps resulted in a 1999 lawsuit by Olmstead to remove state mandated caps for long-term care, which often resulted in the client having to be institutionalized for payment purposes. This is especially important for persons with disabilities of all ages. However, this lawsuit does not require states to provide any additional long-term care services (Rosenbaum, 2000).

The ANA (*http://www.ana.org*), the American Public Health Association (APHA) (*http://www.apha.org*), and the NAHC (*http://www.nahc.org*) employ lobbyists to work with state and federal legislators to enhance long-term care priorities and funding. Professions from across the nation provide input to these organizations to help influence health policy.

## Costs of Care

Although the home is the site of care for the majority of people needing long-term care services, care in institutional settings constitutes about 75% of Medicaid expenditures for long-term care. In this country expenditures for

nursing facilities are financed about equally by Medicaid and private out-of-pocket payments. In 1998 Medicaid provided $36.3 billion (46.3%) of the $87.8 billion spent on nursing home care, including care in intermediate care facilities for the mentally retarded. Private individuals paid $28.5 billion (32.5%) out of pocket. The remainder was covered by Medicare (11.9%), private insurance (5.3%), and other sources (NCHS, 2000). Another 9% of Medicaid dollars were for home health, personal care and home- and community-based waiver programs. In 1998, home care costs averaged $93 per visit, skilled facilities charged on average $523 per day, and hospital charges averaged $2401 per day for Medicare charges (NAHC, 2000).

## Personal Health Expenditures

As shown in Table 22-7, approximately 37% of all long-term care costs in 1998 were paid out-of-pocket by consumers. Total personal care expenditures increased from two thirds of a million dollars in 1991 to over a trillion dollars in 1998. Out-of-pocket costs increased a similar 30% during that time. Drugs and other medical nondurables have continued to be the largest cost, with $55.4 billion spent in 1998 for these items. Nursing home payments continued to increase over the 8-year period, as did home health care (HCFA, 2001h).

Among the elderly, community residing Americans aged 65 and over were projected to spend on average $2430 or 19% of their income on out-of-pocket health care expenses in 1999

**TABLE 22-7**

*Selected Expenditures for Long-term Care by Type and Source of Fund*

| SOURCE OF FUNDS | HOME HEALTH CARE | DRUGS AND MEDICAL NONDURABLES | VISION PRODUCTS/ MEDICAL DURABLES | NURSING HOME CARE | OTHER PERSONAL CARE |
|---|---|---|---|---|---|
| **1991** | | | | | |
| Out of pocket | 4.3 | 42.7 | 6.9 | 23.1 | — |
| Private insurance | 2.5 | 15.2 | 0.8 | 2.4 | — |
| Medicaid | 2.5 | 6.2 | — | 27.5 | 5.1 |
| Medicare | 4.2 | 0.1 | 3.1 | 1.9 | — |
| **1995** | | | | | |
| Out of pocket | 5.9 | 48.3 | 7.2 | 26.5 | — |
| Private insurance | 3.7 | 28.6 | 0.7 | 3.4 | — |
| Medicaid | 3.9 | 9.7 | — | 35.5 | 13.9 |
| Medicare | 11.9 | 0.4 | 5.0 | 6.9 | — |
| **1998** | | | | | |
| Out of pocket | 6.0 | 55.4 | 8.2 | 28.5 | — |
| Private insurance | 4.0 | 47.8 | 0.8 | 4.7 | — |
| Medicaid | 5.0 | 15.5 | — | 40.7 | 19.0 |
| Medicare | 10.4 | 1.2 | 5.9 | 10.4 | — |

From HCFA, Office of the Actuary: Personal health care expenditures, by type of expenditure and source of funds: calendar years 1991-98, 2001h, HCFA. Retrieved from the internet January, 2001. http://*www.hcfa.gov/stats/nhe-oact/tables/t9.htm*

*Numbers denote billions of dollars.

(not counting home care and nursing home costs). More than half (54%) of this amount was to pay for direct goods and services. Included in this expenditure is 17% for prescription drugs and 6% for hospital inpatient and outpatient services. The other large portion of costs (46%) was expended for premiums on Medicare B, private insurance, or *Medicare +Choice* coverage. These premiums, however, did not result in *not* acquiring additional charges. Even persons with *Medigap* insurance and other supplemental insurance could expect to spend more than $2500 on health care (Gross, Brangan, 1999).

Regardless of the source of payment, clients, agencies, and providers must face the reality of managed care, prospective payment (Gundling, 2000; Levy, 2000; St. Pierre, 1999), increased costs, and accountability. Complacency and inflexibility will need to be replaced by creative innovation and collaborative practice to meet the needs of clients with long-term care needs. Outcomes intervention and research to document appropriate use of services (Madigan, Fortinsky, 1999) identify clients likely to be high users of services (Lee, Mills, 2000) and effectiveness of services (Bishop, 1999). Dialogue and clear communication among policy makers, payers, consumers, and providers will be necessary to ensure the quality and quantity of care Americans expect.

## BARRIERS TO ADEQUATE COMMUNITY-BASED LONG-TERM CARE

Various problems in the community and in the health care delivery system make it difficult for clients who have long-term care needs to avoid unnecessary institutionalization. These problems can be summarized under five categories: (1) lack of community resources, (2) acute-focused reimbursement mechanisms, (3) fragmentation and lack of coordination, (4) family burnout, and (5) a lack of political activism among providers and professionals.

### Lack of Community Resources

A significant factor preventing many of the chronically ill, disabled, and elderly from obtaining adequate long-term care is the scarcity of formal alternatives to institutionalization. Staying in the home or community depends on social support, financial resources, and the availability of health and social services.

Many children and older adults, especially those older than 75, with chronic illness and disabilities, have characteristics that place them at risk for being institutionalized. Unfortunately, the very dependent find it difficult to obtain needed services in the home. Expensive medical equipment and assistive devices are not available in all areas and under all payers. Respite care has not been formalized into the health delivery system. Although it is made available in the community by lay, civic, and religious organizations, it is primarily on a one-to-one or immediate need basis.

Schools are not prepared for children and adolescents with disabilities, and universities are not overwhelmingly prepared to meet the needs of adult disabled persons. Most of the allowances have been those required by the Americans with Disabilities Act (ADA) for physical access, not emotional, sensory, or communication difficulties. These are available, but like previously noted services, not in an organized or comprehensive fashion. In addition, stigma associated with need for services often deters persons from requesting assistance when it may in fact be available.

The lack of adequate housing (and especially supportive congregate or domiciliary housing for people who live alone) for the frail elderly and disabled is a major barrier to community long-term care services. One problem with current housing arrangements is affordability: fuel prices, interest rates, and construction costs have all made housing costs difficult to manage on a limited income.

Another problem is that households are becoming smaller; although rents are increasing, the number of people paying rent in a household is decreasing as a result of increasing divorce rates and increasing numbers of aged and deinstitutionalized people living alone. In large cities, single room occupancy hotels, formerly a source of housing for many, are being converted into condominiums.

In some communities innovative housing programs sponsored by the Department of Housing and Urban Development have provided suitable alternatives to institutionalization. The National Housing Act, Section 202, provides a direct loan program based on the current securities marketed by the Treasury Department. The level of these interest rates makes housing projects attractive to builders. Section 8 of the same act provides for direct subsidies to individuals who occupy Section 8 housing. The sponsors of such housing, usually nonprofit organizations, receive full market rent. However, the federal government pays a portion of the rent.

Often, caregivers of children and adolescents with disabilities at home receive no housing assistance from the formal system. Some community-based organizations and personal contacts do build wheelchair ramps, install additional electric outlets, and assist with obtaining special furniture. Churches and disease specific organizations, such as the Multiple Sclerosis Association, often help with this type of need.

### Acute-Focused Reimbursement Mechanisms

Another barrier to effective long-term care is inadequate financial coverage for long-term care. The Medicare program was specifically designed to provide protection for acute care. Once a client's condition becomes stable or once skilled services such as nursing, speech, or physical therapy are no longer needed, Medicare coverage for home health care ceases. Medicare specifically prohibits payment for custodial care. Care is considered custodial when it is for the purpose of meeting personal needs and could be provided by persons without professional skill or training. For example, help in walking, getting in and out of bed, bathing, eating, dressing, and taking medicine is considered custodial care. These are precisely the functions needed by many clients with long-term care needs. Personal care is another area where unlicensed but often trained persons provide care in the home for such things as dressing changes, tube feedings, hair care, and physical and social activity.

Often services such as housekeeping and food preparation are the services that can assist a person to remain in the home. However, most insurances and governmental payment forms do not cover these services. One of the most serious problems is that services must be *intermittent* to be covered. For example, home health aides, in conjunction with other services and for a finite period of time, may work only a few hours a day, several days a week, and their hours may not exceed 32 per week. This type of care is often inadequate when a client needs help with ADLs on a constant basis. With the addition of more strict home health regulations in 1998, this type of care is often no longer completed by home health aides.

Medicaid, the assistance program for the very poor, does cover long-term care, but clients must deplete their own resources to qualify as medically needy to receive these funds. However, for persons who meet the eligibility requirements, the Medicaid program more effectively meets the long-term care needs of clients than does Medicare. Primarily these needs are met by skilled and limited ADL services. Medicaid expenditures for home care remain small. Because Medicaid is a state-administered program and long-term care is an optional provision, services and eligibility vary considerably from state to state. Limited in-home and community-based services have occurred because these states viewed the services as (1) costly, (2) difficult to manage, (3) difficult to maintain a definitive assessment of eligibility, and (4) diverting funds from necessary nursing home payment. Two major external reasons for hesitancy by states to embrace alternatives to institutionalization are the strong lobbying by the nursing home industry and a lack of evidence on which alternatives are most effective, efficient, and appropriate for client need.

The trends are beginning to change as states have established long-term care offices and clear definitions of home- and community-based services. The **Home- and Community-Based Services (HCBS)** waivers afford additional funds and strategies to provide long-term care. Client, family, and nurses and other professional efforts to educate state and federal legislators on the need and effect of HCBS have resulted in changes.

More states are applying for waivers, and the AHRQ, National Institutes of Health (NIH), and private foundations are funding research studies to evaluate the appropriateness and effectiveness of HCBS (AHRQ, 1999, 2001a;

Coleman, 2000). Oregon, North Carolina, and several other states have increased the proportion of Medicaid dollars allocated to alternatives to nursing homes, even up to 50% in some areas. Other states, such as Tennessee, have chosen to put any additional out-year Medicaid funding increases into long-term care community alternatives. However, when only 5% of $90 million is used for home and community-based services, there is a limitation in what and how many services can be offered.

## Fragmentation and Lack of Coordination

It has consistently been documented that the "piecemeal" fragmentation and lack of coordination in the long-term care system make it extremely difficult for clients to obtain appropriate and adequate services. Consequently, a significant number of noninstitutionalized clients do not receive necessary long-term care. Existing formal long-term care services are provided by an array of state and local agencies that have differing eligibility requirements and finance mechanisms. Clients who have multifaceted needs find it difficult, if not impossible, to identify the appropriate service provider. Many communities have no central organization or professional that assists the client in locating and coordinating needed long-term care services.

Thus accessing and obtaining long-term care services often places unnecessary hardships on the client. It is not unusual for clients to have to make separate trips to several agencies in order to arrange a comprehensive package of services. An aged client, for example, may have to apply separately for Medicaid, Meals-on-Wheels, transportation services, Title XX homemaker services, and home nursing services. It is not unusual for a parent to make 25 to 30 phone calls to obtain medical equipment for their technologically dependent child while providing care for that child and other children in the home. Fragmentation and lack of coordination have left many gaps in the long-term care delivery systems. Unnecessary institutionalization among high-risk groups continues, and the costs for long-term care services are rising dramatically. Efforts to develop comprehensive, coordinated systems for delivering community-based services must be expanded.

## Family Burnout

An estimated 60% to 85% of all people who are disabled are helped by the family in a significant way. It has been demonstrated over the years that the family is the primary source of care for many persons in the community. Some family members and friends provide this care out of a sense of responsibility, but most do so primarily because they care.

Family caretakers play a pivotal role in helping chronically disabled family members avoid institutionalization. Caring for impaired family members, however, can place a heavy and expensive burden on the family, especially when care is required for an extended period of time. Many chronically impaired persons have been placed in nursing homes because their families are unable to bear the emotional, physical, and financial strain of providing home care in the absence of support from community programs.

For long-term care programs to be effective, the needs of family caregivers, as well as dependent family members, must be addressed. As discussed previously, caregivers of the dependent disabled need respite care, information about services, a broad array of community- and home-based health and social services, and knowledge about health conditions and care methods. The *ElderCare Locator* and local *Councils on Aging* provide the most frequently funded assistance. Church and civic volunteer groups are becoming more involved in many areas. Nonprofit agencies provide respite and personal care services.

## Funding

Although much long-term care is paid by the federal government through Medicare, Medicaid, and Social Security titles, estimates from the General Accounting Office are that the Social Security trust fund will be unable to meet these obligations starting in the year 2010. In fact, to continue funding Social Security and Medicare would require double digit increases in payroll taxes of 17% and 50%, respectively (Walker, 2000). Also, because much of the newer alternatives to nursing home and home health are not covered, persons should consider long-term care savings or insurance plans. Few persons have long-term care insurance through private or employer-based plans (Lutsky, Corea, Alecxih, 2000). Policies that are purchased often have "term limits" of payment, often 2 years. Individual retirement accounts, Keogh plans, and 401(k) are strategies to increase funds for aging needs. For persons with children and young adults needing long-term care, reverse mortgages and life insurance loans provide some of the few options to pay for the prolonged expenses incurred.

Nurses must assist clients and families to understand which private or public coverage provides for their long-term care needs, regardless of age, health condition, or disability status. CMS maintains a website that allows individuals to compare costs and benefits of Medicare plans in each state or by zip code (*http://www.medicare.gov/mphcompare/home.asp*).

Unfortunately, state offices are not consistent in providing similar information on plans, payers, and providers of Medicaid. Long-term care insurance plans should be gathered from companies and discussions should occur with client, family, primary provider, attorney, and investment officer, or accountant participation.

## FACILITATORS OF LONG-TERM CARE

While there are many barriers and problems with long-term care, several efforts have the potential to enhance long-term care. New initiatives to measure quality of care and health outcomes from the client, family, provider, and sys-

tem perspective will provide evidence to substantiate the effectiveness and appropriateness of long-term care.

### Initiatives to Measure Quality

The focus on quality assessment has moved from *structure* and *process* to the *outcomes* of care. Although all three are essential, in managed care the outcomes of care are the focus as the twenty-first century begins.

A major long-term care outcomes focus was developed from Shaughnessy's research (1996), which resulted in the Medicare's *Standardized Outcome and Assessment Information Set for Home Health Care* (OASIS). OASIS is a data set with the following categories of items: demographics and client history, living arrangements, supportive assistance, body systems, ADL/IADL, medications, equipment management, and emergent care. The data are assessed on admission to a home health agency, at a point in time during care, and then upon discharge. OASIS is used for measuring outcomes defined as a change in health status between two or more time points. The database system was mandated by the Balanced Budget Act of 1997 (PL 105-33) and regulations by HCFA to monitor outcomes of the care provided by Medicare-certified agencies. Because Medicare benefits typically account for the majority of home health agencies' revenues, OASIS will provide a national database and evaluation of the outcomes of home health care.

AHRQ (1999, 2001a) and the American Association of Retired Persons (Coleman, 2000) have research initiatives in place to determine and measure outcomes in nursing homes, home care, and assisted living. Additionally, the National Institute of Nursing Research (NINR) and several foundations are working with end-of-life care in home health and hospice. Acceptance of professional standards and scope of practice, especially through ANA (1999), the Community Health Accreditation Program (CHAP) (2000), and the Joint Commission on Accreditation for Healthcare Organizations (JCAHO) (2001) could provide the basis for establishment of outcome criteria to measure quality. Development of standards of care (AHCPR, 1995) and evidenced-based practice (Bergstrom, Braden, Kemp, et al., 1996, 1998; Jirovec, Wyman, Wells, 1998; McClish, Wyman, Sale, et al., 1999; Sampselle, Burns, Dougherty, et al., 1997) guide professionals in providing quality and cost-effective care (Lobianco, Mills, Moore, 1996; Naylor, McCauley, 1999). Involvement of families and communities in the development of interventions to achieve outcomes desired (Dumont, 1999) also helps increase the belief in long-term care services that are culturally appropriate.

### Demographics, Consumerism, and Technology

Other facilitators are factors noted at the beginning of this chapter: demographics, consumerism, and advancing medical technology. Sheer number of persons with needs for long-term care necessitate that these types of services be available and accessible. Home health grew out of this demand in the 1980s. The growth of the aged, disabled, and special needs children groups provide a large population with similar long-term care needs. The organizations that help these populations of interest can work together on innovative strategies to develop, implement, and evaluate care. When large numbers of persons and organizations lobby congressional members, state legislators, county health officials, and health system officers to make long-term care a priority that requires federal emphasis and funding, it is more likely to occur.

*Healthy People 2010* validates the need for long-term care services. It is difficult to dispute the need when issues such as disability are major focus areas for national health. Achievement of these objectives should help reduce the need for long-term care and improve the lives of those who need it. Efforts for educating professionals and communities, determining funding modes and levels, and evaluation of care should address these national health priorities and objectives.

Consumerism and the move for self-responsibility in health both enhance the possibility for long-term care growth. As clients, families, and providers are held accountable for outcomes, the social expectations of these services will grow. The collaborative nature of long-term care to engage client and family in decision making provides an ownership not often seen in traditional health care settings. This engagement can serve to increase self-esteem, decrease loss of control, and lead to more effective and appropriate use of services according to the outcomes desired.

Advancing technology will continue to allow clients, families, and providers access to nontraditional settings of care. Telehealth, electronic communication, Lifeline systems, assistive devices, and new modes of care provide unlimited opportunities for alternate methods of care, for participation by persons other than providers, and for developing innovative delivery settings.

## Increased Funding

Although funding is not always as large or as rapid as long-term care providers would like, there have been increases in the dollars allocated to mental health, community centers, quality initiatives, and demonstration projects for disabled and other groups requiring long-term care. In addition to the federal government, it will be important to ensure that state legislators participate in funding programs and services for long-term care. Creative strategies for more formal involvement of religious and civic organizations in communities and foundations and companies in the private sector will be necessary to maximize the potential of long-term care.

## Expansion of Noninstitutional Alternatives

A number of settings and types of long-term care have been discussed previously in this chapter. Some new and innovative ideas are presented here. Demonstration projects have been funded at the state and federal level to evaluate the appropriateness of HCBS alternatives and more efficient use of institutional facilities. In the state of New York, for example, the *Nursing Home Without Walls* program was initiated in 1978 to encourage noninstitutional alternatives as an appropriate cost-effective policy for long-term care of the elderly. Four components of the program include (1) intervention in the actual process of nursing home placement so that clients are exposed to home care before a nursing home placement decision is made, (2) cost containment with a limit set on the per capita cost of services, (3) case management of services so that social and medical services are integrated into the system, and (4) waivered services so that services not included in the Medicaid law, such as respiratory therapy and home improvement, can be offered to those needing them.

Another demonstration of the expansion of noninstitutional forms of long-term care is *enriched housing*. Enriched housing serves that portion of the population who is able to live independently but needs some help with personal care, meal preparation, housekeeping, shopping, laundry, heavy cleaning, transportation, and 24-hour emergency coverage. The typical person entering this program does not have an informal support network to help him or her to live independently. The program differs from the Nursing Home Without Walls program in that the client must also need housing. In this program the person enters the housing secured by the program, usually a portion of a rent-subsidized building. Economical shared housing for the elderly has begun, although most is in the private and for-profit sector. During the 1990s personal care organizations and care management services saw increases in demand. The care provided is personal assistance with ADL; some light housekeeping; and a combination respite, hair care, and transportation assistance. Most of these are private pay or philanthropic or community funded, such as funding by United Way and county or city councils.

## Developing Effective Gatekeeping Mechanisms

Developing models, such as local area management organizations (LAMOs) and social health maintenance organizations (S/HMOs), are another solution for dealing with the problems in the long-term care system. (Both are methods of financing and organizing health care for the elderly and are variations of the HMOs described in Chapters 5). Funding for LAMOs and S/HMOs comes from all public monies currently designated for short-term and long-term medical care, rehabilitation, and custodial services. The LAMO enrolls all people with functional deficits and provides the services necessary to help them at home, using informal supports whenever possible. The S/HMO enrolls all elderly people, anticipating that low use of services by the relatively well elderly compensates for extensive use by the vulnerable severely ill. Both models function as gatekeepers into the long-term care system. Case managers function as brokers for the services needed by the elderly population served, and they also certify the level of care needed.

## Other Methods for Improving the Long-Term Care System

With population estimates that project dramatic changes in people who are disabled, chronically ill, mentally ill, and over age 75, and with health care costs expanding, it is obvious that the present system is not meeting and will not meet the future need for long-term care services. Additional methods for improving the system have been suggested and some are being implemented, including the following:

- Emphasis on appropriate discharge planning and transitional care from hospital, rehabilitation facilities, and nursing homes
- Targeting home care services to the people to help them remain independent in their homes and communities
- Developing alternative home and community-based services to meet client needs, with developmental and health needs considered

## FACTORS INFLUENCING ETHICAL DECISION MAKING IN LONG-TERM CARE

A number of factors influence ethical decision making in long-term care, such as client competence, available resources, presence of multiple caregivers, cultural competence, client priorities versus professional or system priorities, personal and professional values, and case-mix and case-load. With any dilemma, consultation with other professionals, clients, and legal counsel provide additional viewpoints, a better understanding of alternatives and consequences, and methods to make decisions. Ombudsmen (AoA, 2001e), ethics committees, and ethicists are available in most areas to assist the client, family, and professionals with ethical situations. A frequently encountered ethical dilemma is the conflict between health providers' desires to provide quality care that meets needs and the demands of third party payers.

For example, Medicare pays for skilled intermittent care, but at times a client only needs an aide to be with him or her 24 hours a day for a few days to ensure his or her independence and safety. How do providers order and obtain payment for this type service without fraudulent filing? More importantly, what is the most appropriate level of care for this client? Another ethical dilemma experienced in long-term care is the implementation of the Patient Self-Determination Act of 1990. This legislation mandates that agencies that participate in Medicare and Medicaid provide information and education about advanced directives to clients so that they have the right to control their own health care decisions. With the medical technology that is available, advanced directives can help minimize people's fears of being kept on artificial life support after meaningful

life for them has ceased. While there is little disagreement with the legislation, health providers may see conflicts between the decision a client makes and that made by his or her family. Nurses also may question the cognitive ability of a client to make a decision.

*Advanced directives* are written documents by which competent persons can seek to influence their medical treatment in the event of serious illness and subsequent loss of consciousness. The Living Will is often referred to as a type of advanced directive, but it needs to be properly executed to be legally binding. The Durable Power of Attorney for Health Care is a more effective instrument as a proxy directive, because a specific person is legally designated to make treatment decisions on behalf of another person. Nurses working in the home health care environment deal with the concept of advanced directives on a daily basis. One of the conditions of participation in the Medicare program and a part of the JCAHO accreditation criteria is the mandate of an advanced directive program.

The increasing number of persons that require long-term care is another area of concern. How is a client's worth determined? How do we provide care to one person and not another? There will continue to be discussions in this country about how to distribute the enormous resources available so that justice, equality, and beneficence are applied across the life span. Increasingly, state home health organizations are focusing on developing guidelines to facilitate ethical decision making in practice. The ANA also assists practitioners and administrators in dealing with ethical issues encountered in the clinical setting. The ANA can be reached by phone at 1-800-274-4ANA.

## THE ROLE OF THE COMMUNITY HEALTH NURSE IN LONG-TERM CARE

Nurses are increasing their involvement with the growing at-risk long-term care population and are becoming leaders in caring for persons with long-term needs. Long-term care is a growing area of opportunity in professional nursing.

Nurses already represent the largest number and proportion of professional workers involved in long-term care. However, estimates suggest that there is a growing shortage of nurses in the areas of long-term care and gerontology.

Community health nurses should focus on six areas to provide more adequate long-term care. These areas are health prevention across the life span; functional independence for clients; enhancing provider and families' caregiving knowledge and abilities; collaboration with lay, professional, public, and private agencies and organizations; evaluation of services; and participation in public policy; and resource allocation decision making.

### Prevention

Throughout this text the concepts of disease prevention and health promotion have been stressed. The importance of these concepts cannot be overemphasized, especially when one examines the problems encountered by long-term care population groups. To decrease the number of people needing long-term care, it is essential to concentrate our efforts on the primary prevention of chronic problems and the exacerbations or complications of these conditions. Since the prepathogenesis period of disease (see Chapter 11) begins early in life, primary prevention and health promotion interventions that address many problems encountered by chronically disabled persons and the aged must be introduced when working with young people. Health education programs that address such matters as lifestyle modification, stress management, retirement planning, and counseling services that help individuals to develop a risk profile are examples of such interventions. Other examples are integrated throughout Chapters 16 to 22.

Community health nurses are uniquely able to apply the concepts of prevention as they work with clients who need long-term care. Primary, secondary, and tertiary preventive interventions are commonly implemented by nurses who provide home health care services. Examples of primary prevention interventions include accident prevention education and teaching about infection control. Helping a client with diabetes learn how to self-administer insulin injections and handle postsurgical wound care are examples of secondary prevention interventions. Tertiary prevention, continuing care, and rehabilitation frequently are carried out with people who need long-term care. These persons often need help with physical, occupational, and/or speech therapy to return to or maintain their optimal level of functioning. The challenge facing the community health nurse at the tertiary level of prevention is how to maintain an ongoing working relationship with clients so that the plan of action can be adjusted in response to the client's and family's changing circumstances, conditions, and desires. Strategies that community health nurses can use to help clients manage disabilities and chronic diseases include medical record coauthoring; self-monitoring; educational support groups; family involvement; and telephone, email, or postcard contact with clients.

## Formal and Informal Caregiving

As discussed previously, 8 of 10 long-term care clients in the United States receive unpaid care from relatives and friends. Community health nurses should not expect families and other informal supports to provide care with no education, respite, or validation. It is important to establish clear lines of effective and regular communication; provide emotional support and education; assist clients and families in identifying their needs, outcomes, and priorities; and access the resources most appropriate for the client.

Formal and informal caregivers share the responsibility for meeting the long-term care needs of clients. Often the family caregiver wants the following from the formal caregivers, nurse, and home health agency (Nottingham, 1995):

- Close involvement with a competent and caring professional who is part of an integrated health or social service delivery system
- Professionals who can relate easily and comfortably with families
- Cooperation, understanding, and support among formal and informal caregivers
- Families working with the professional who represents the formal service delivery system and both working jointly on what needs to be done
- Having their own knowledge and skills valued

Health care professionals have made the choice of careers that involves helping others cope with difficult situations. Informal caregivers have often not consciously made this choice, but both groups of caregivers need to take care of themselves. Health professionals should know the symptoms of burnout or emotional exhaustion that come from excessive demands on one's energy, strength, or resources. Prevention of excessive demands for long periods without asking for help is imperative in long-term care. The healthiest way to take care of another is to take care of you.

Because the vast majority of caregivers are women (wives, daughters, and daughters-in-law), society needs the message that the obligation of caregiving should be met by all adult children who have such responsibilities and not just daughters. This would have the effect of reshaping societal expectations about women as well as the discussion about the implications of obligations of gratitude for caregiving throughout the life cycle. Society needs to hear the message that caregivers often need support and the state should support families who are caregivers of their adult members by providing financial subsidies for those who cannot afford to quit working.

The *Family and Medical Leave Act* provides job protection for caregivers of children, spouses, and parents, but the leave is without pay for a limited time. The establishment of a caregiver program and the reauthorization of the Older Americans Act, both in 2000, should provide support to the most needy families. However, development of creative avenues to meet these needs should be continued by religious, civic, and lay and professional organizations. Efforts by the *National Association of Home Care and the National Family Caregivers Association* (*http://www.nfcacares.org*) have been invaluable in encouraging assistance to families.

## Focus on Functional Independence

Clients with long-term care needs often have conditions that cannot be cured. The goal for care is to assist clients and families to maintain or achieve quality in their lives and continue to function at the highest possible level. With the cure orientation that pervades our health care system, this can be a difficult orientation for a community health nurse to develop and maintain. This orientation becomes easier to handle as one sees through practice that clients can live satisfying lives even when they have not been cured. Community health nurses play a significant role in assisting clients to achieve greater functional independence. In addition to client priorities, a major guide to care can be the *Healthy People 2010* focus areas and objectives.

## Collaboration

No one discipline can address the array of needs experienced by long-term care clients. The problems involved with long-term care demand that all members and levels of health care providers as well as clients and families participate. The community health nurse must learn to use the health care team's experience and expertise and the client and family resources. Often functioning as the coordinator of the health care team, the nurse must maintain good communication and respect for the contributions of all team members. The client can easily feel that care is fragmented if no one person has overall responsibility for complete care. Understanding the roles of each team member can facilitate planning and coordination. The role definitions presented in Table 22-8 should be regarded only as a starting point for developing effective team relationships. When entering any new client situation, assess who is involved in care; the traditional communication modes; decision-making processes; and human, material, and financial resources available.

The central figures on any long-term health care team must be the client and his or her family. To achieve the highest level of functioning possible for the client, the client must be actively involved in establishing a plan of care appropriate to his or her needs and priorities. Engaging families in the therapeutic process is essential because often they have needs of their own that must be addressed. In addition, families are frequently participants in the caregiving and rehabilitation process and provide support for disabled family members when formal health care providers are not present.

## Evaluate Services

An integral part of future health care is evaluation. The evaluation process helps health care professionals determine whether they are providing appropriate, effective, and quality services. In this era of decreasing resources it is essential for community nurses to carefully monitor resources. The needs of at-risk aggregates, such as those comprising the long-term care population, can only be met if resources are allocated and used in a responsible manner. Community health nurses at all levels must assume responsibility for evaluating the way in which nursing services are delivered. Although nursing administrators have the overall task of seeing that evaluation is done, staff-level professionals must be accountable for assessing their own competence, practice, and effectiveness. Nurses also supervise care that they delegate to others, such as home health aides and homemakers. When community health nurses delegate or assign

tasks to others, they are responsible for ensuring that the care is performed in an acceptable way (see Chapter 24).

A variety of direct and indirect measures currently are used by community health nurses to evaluate the delivery and outcomes of nursing services, such as direct observation of care, case management conferences, annual performance evaluations, client health status changes, number of hospitalizations and emergency room visits, and record reviews. Client health status outcomes are a primary part of evaluation. Thus it is necessary to set goals, establish outcomes desired, and assess health status upon initiation of the therapeutic relationship. Discussions with clients and families of what they expect from the care provided, the condition or illness they experience, the formal health care system, and the community can provide clear direction for establishing priorities and health outcomes.

## Professional Competence and Accountability

The *Standards of Home Health Nursing Practice* and *Standards of Community Health Nursing* (ANA, 1999) referred to earlier in this chapter should guide the development of quality care and evaluation that includes criteria for measuring quality and methods for ensuring that care is consistent with professional standards of care and performance (see Chapter 24). Understanding reimbursement sources must be integrated into care delivery and evaluation. Community health nurses in all settings and agencies must participate in the assessment, planning, implementation, and evaluation of long-term care services to meet clients' needs. Examples of activities and strategies are:

1. Complete a needs assessment for long-term care in the community
2. Participate in research to develop evidenced-based practice pathways
3. Deliver evidence-based practice
4. Obtain certification in an area of specialty
5. Develop client, provider, and system outcome measures and strategies
6. Serve on boards and provide consultation to long-term care agencies
7. Maintain and increase professional competence for practice through continuing education and other professional activities
8. Engage families, communities, agencies, payors, and providers in dialogue
9. Implement quality improvement strategies, including outcome measures

Staff-level community health nurses play a very important role in all quality of care and evaluation review procedures. Staff involvement in evaluation processes helps administrators obtain a clearer picture about service delivery issues. As case managers, staff-level nurses are in a unique position to identify gaps or omissions in service, overuse of resources, quality of care, and outcomes achieved. Nurses are held responsible for quality care and the utilization of

**TABLE 22-8**

*Descriptions for Select Members of the Long-Term Health Care Team\**

| DISCIPLINE | ROLE DESCRIPTION |
|---|---|
| Advanced practice nurse | Professional member of the team who provides expert clinical decision making, treatment decisions, and referrals—The primary responsibility is to assist clients and families in meeting their health needs. These needs can be emotional, educational, physical, financial, social, adaptation, coping, or related to dealing with loss and death. Advanced practice nurses also coordinate team efforts to achieve positive health outcomes. Consultative and collaborative efforts with other team members, especially the client, physician, and social worker, provide a focus to the implemented plan of care. Continual assessment and evaluation of the client's status and progress, as well as appropriate use of resources, are important responsibilities. |
| Community health nurse† | *An essential professional member of the health care team*—The professional nurse uses the nursing process to determine client needs, to establish a plan of care in conjunction with the client, to provide skilled nursing services, and to evaluate care delivered by the nursing team. Traditionally, the professional nurse has assumed a case management role on the health care team. As a care manager, the community health nurse focuses on determining the comprehensive needs of the client and the client's family, makes referrals to appropriate community resources as needed, and coordinates care among the multiple agencies providing services to a family. |
| Homemaker–health aide | *A paraprofessional who is trained to assist clients with personal care and light household tasks*—According to the Medicare conditions of participation for home health agencies, a home health aide's "duties include the performance of simple procedures as an extension of therapy services, personal care, ambulation and exercise, household services essential to health care at home, assistance with medications that are ordinarily self-administered, reporting changes in the patient's condition and needs, and completing appropriate records" (HCFA, 1989). Home health aides providing only personal care must be supervised by professional nurses via supervisory visits to the client's home at least every *2 weeks* if skilled nursing or therapy service is also needed by the client. If the client needs only custodial care, home health aide supervisory visits must be made once every 62 days (HCFA, 1994). |
| Nutritionist | *A professional team member who assists clients in meeting their basic nutritional needs*—The nutritionist assesses a client's nutritional status, helps the client plan an adequate and appropriate dietary intake, suggests ways to plan economical nutritious meals, helps clients learn about therapeutic diets, and teaches about food purchasing and preparation. These professionals are often used as resource persons by other members of the health care team. |
| Physician | *A professional team member who is either a doctor of medicine or osteopathy*—The Medicare conditions of participation for home health agencies specify that the physician must establish and authorize the client's plan of treatment in writing and must review this treatment plan at least once *every 62 days* to determine if care is appropriate and necessary (HCFA, 1994). In addition to establishing a plan of treatment, the physician evaluates the client's medical status and provides medical care as needed. A physician also serves on a home health agency's professional advisory committee. |
| Social worker, medical | *A professional member of the home health care team who works with clients who are experiencing significant psychosocial, financial, or environmental difficulties*—Medical social workers apply the principles of social case work to help clients enhance their emotional and social adjustment and adapt to change. The primary purpose of their intervention is to reduce psychosocial, financial, and environmental barriers that are adversely affecting a client's health status or response to health care. Medical social workers provide direct counseling services, refer clients to community resources, assist clients in attaining needed social and health care services, and help plan for institutional community placements such as nursing home or extended-care facility placements. They also serve as resource persons for other members of the health care team who are dealing with difficult psychosocial, financial, or environmental problems. |

Modified from Health Care Financing Administration (HCFA): *Medicare program: home health agencies—conditions of participation and reductions in record keeping requirements,* 42 CFR, Part 484, Sections 484.1 through 484.52, Washington, DC, October 1989, US Department of Health and Human Services; and HCFA: *Medicare program: home health agencies—conditions of participation and reduction in record-keeping requirements,* 42 CFR, Part 484, Section 484.1 through 484.52, Washington, DC, October 1994, USDHHS.

\*The central figures on any long-term health care team must be the client and his or her family.

†To be certified for Medicare and Medicaid funding, a home health agency must provide nursing services.

*Continued*

**TABLE 22-8**

*Descriptions for Select Members of the Long-Term Health Care Team\*—cont'd*

| DISCIPLINE | ROLE DESCRIPTION |
|---|---|
| Therapists, occupational | *Professional members of the team who work with clients that have difficulty carrying out activities of daily living*—After determining the self-care activities most important to the client, the occupational therapist assesses the environment to identify safety hazards and barriers to self-care, recommends environmental modifications that would help the client increase independence and prevent accidents, and assists the client in learning techniques, such as the use of simple eating and dressing devices, that promote effective and efficient client functioning. The occupational therapist focuses on helping the client improve motor coordination and muscle strength so that the client can reach his or her maximum level of functioning. |
| Therapists, physical | *Professional members of the team who work with clients who have functional impairments related to neuromuscular problems*—After assessing the client's functional abilities, physical therapists help clients preserve, restore, and improve neuromuscular functioning and increase their self-care capabilities. Physical therapists carry out a broad range of activities to help clients reach their maximum level of functioning. Performing needed range-of-motion, strengthening, and coordination exercises; recommending the use of appropriate orthopedic and prosthetic devices; and teaching clients ambulation techniques and how to use assistive appliances are a few examples of the activities performed by physical therapists. |
| Therapists, speech-language | *Professional members of the team who work with clients who have communication problems*—After assessing the client's speech, language, and hearing abilities, speech therapists concentrate on helping clients increase their functional communication skills. Based on client needs, the speech therapist may initiate exercises to increase functional speaking skills, teach esophageal speech, recommend the use of communication appliances such as intraoral devices or hearing aids, identify barriers in the environment that inhibit effective communication, and teach significant others in the environment how to communicate with the client. |

resources by practice standards, employers, or clients. Developing a documentation system for quality, outcomes, and evaluation is imperative.

## Work Toward Responsible Public Policy

Thus far in this chapter, ample evidence has been presented to demonstrate that public policy for long-term care in this country is inadequate. Involvement in development, implementation and evaluation, and regulation of public policy occurs at several levels and through many activities. These levels range from voting to holding public office. Knowledge of the issues, involvement in the political arena, and working through professional organizations such as the National Association for Home Care and the American Public Health Association are other avenues for involvement. These organizations are making a concerted effort to analyze key health care issues; promote strategies to resolve health care problems; and educate legislators of priority health, allocation, and policy needs.

## SUMMARY

Increasing numbers of people across the life span have long-term care needs that must be addressed by local communities throughout our nation. Elderly persons, who constitute the most rapidly growing population group in America, are particularly at risk for needing long-term care services. Although most elderly people experience good health, certain chronic, disabling illnesses do increase with aging.

The fastest-growing component of the United States health care delivery system is long-term care. Diverse and multiple social, health-related, and health care organizations deliver a variety of long-term care services to people in need. Despite the dramatic growth in the long-term care industry, many chronically disabled persons do not receive the services they need. Developing strategies to eliminate barriers to effective and appropriate long-term care must receive greater attention by health care providers; citizens, lay, and professional organizations; and communities, lawmakers, and bureaucrats. Research, education, policy development, and evaluation and effective delivery systems and management of resources, as well as ethical guidelines, are required to meet the increasing demand for long-term care in the United States.

Long-term care presents challenges and opportunities for the community health nurse. Developing solutions to overcome the deficiencies and to fill the gaps in the long-term care system will require major policy changes at all three levels of government. However, community health nurses at all levels of practice can be instrumental in effecting change in the health care delivery system.

# CRITICAL THINKING
*exercise*

Three case situations are provided for clients with long-term care needs. As the professional nurse you must consider many issues related to the care to be provided. Answer the following questions for each case situation.

1. How will you determine the client's priority health needs?
2. What additional information do you need?
3. With whom will you collaborate?
4. What types of services might be needed by the client and his or her family?
5. How will you evaluate the client and family outcomes?
6. What role and responsibility do you have in the client's care?
7. What ethical, legal, cultural, and economic issues might need to be considered?

A. John is 21 years old; he was shot at school 4 years ago and is paralyzed from the waist down. He has had numerous surgeries to repair internal injuries. His colostomy is permanent and he must catheterize himself to empty his bladder. John has been put on medications to alleviate bowel and bladder spasms. He lives with his parents and two younger brothers. John did not finish high school and he cannot drive. John has just arrived home from a recent hospitalization for a urinary tract infection (UTI).

B. Hospice: Mrs. Jones recently has been admitted to the hospice service where you work. She is a diabetic and has had lung cancer for 6 years. She is on insulin every morning and does her urine checks independently. Her physician has not yet ordered any pain medication, but provided a sleeping pill for Mrs. Jones. She uses oxygen 2 L/min by cannula. Mrs. Jones' husband died last year and she now lives alone. Her daughter works in a town nearby. Mrs. Jones was active in her church until her husband's death and her recent illnesses.

C. Mental Health: Suzy is an active 8-year-old third grader at a local school. The school nurse refers her case to you as the local case manager for the school system. Suzy's mother and father divorced last year; she lives with her mother and older brother. She is mad at her father and refuses to see him every weekend. Suzy recently was brought to the emergency room with dehydration and weight loss. The pediatric nurse practitioner is concerned that Suzy is depressed, although her teachers say she is *very* active in the classroom.

# REFERENCES

Administration on Aging (AoA): *Aging into the 21st century,* Nov 1997, AoA. Retrieved from the internet December, 2000. *http://www.aoa.dhhs.gov/aoa/stats/aging21/health.html*

Administration on Aging (AoA): *The National Elder Abuse Incidence Study: Final Report,* Sept 1998, AoA. Retrieved from the internet January, 2001. *http://www.aoa.dhhs.gov/abuse/report*

Administration on Aging (AoA): *AoA to release funds to support family caregivers,* 2001a, AoA. Retrieved from the internet January, 2001. *http://www.aoa.gov/pr/Pr2000/nfcsp011101.html*

Administration on Aging (AoA): *Older adults and mental health: Issues and opportunities,* 2001b, AoA. Retrieved from the internet January, 2001. *http://www.aoa.dhhs.gov/mh/report2001/default.htm*

Administration on Aging (AoA): *Older Americans Act Amendments of 2000,* 2001c, AoA. Retrieved from the internet January, 2001. *http://www.aoa.gov/oaa/status/summary.html*

Administration on Aging (AoA): *Older Americans Act appropriations information,* 2001d, AoA. Retrieved from the internet January, 2001. *http://www.aoa.gov/oaa/oaaapp.html*

Administration on Aging (AoA): *Ombudsmen protect lives, rights, and health of long-term care residents,* 2001e, AoA. Retrieved from the internet January, 2001. *http://www.aoa.gov/pr/Pr2000/ltcombudsman.html*

Administration on Aging (AoA): *Profile of older Americans: 2000,* 2001f, AoA. Retrieved from the internet January, 2001. *http://www.aoa.gov/aoa/STATS/profile/default.htm*

Administration on Aging (AoA): *Side by side comparison of OAA as amended in 1992 with OAA as amended in 2000,* 2001g, AoA. Retrieved from the internet January, 2001. *http://www.aoa.gov/oaa/2000/side-by-side-fin.html*

Administration of Home Health Nursing: Care of the sick by health departments, *Public Health Nurs* 37:339-342, 1945.

Agency for Health Care Policy and Research: *AMDA adapting AHCPR clinical practice guidelines for use in long-term care facilities,* 1995, AHCPR. Retrieved from the internet January, 2001. *http://www.ahrq.gov/news/press/adapting.htm*

Agency for Healthcare Research and Quality: *Quality of care most important nursing home measure,* 1999, AHRQ. Retrieved from the internet January, 2001. *http://www.ahrq.gov/news/press/pr1999/homeqoc.htm*

Agency for Healthcare Research and Quality: *Research on long-term care,* 2001a, AHRQ. Retrieved from the internet January, 2001. *http://www.ahrq.gov/research/longtrm1.htm*

Agency for Healthcare Research and Quality: *AHRQ research on long-term care,* 2001b, AHRQ. Retrieved from the internet January, 2001. *http://www.ahrq.gov/research/longtrm.htm*

Allen SA: Medicare case management, *Home Healthc Nurse* 12(3):21-27, 1994.

Alzheimer's Association: *Frequently asked questions,* 2001, Alzheimer's Association. Retrieved from the internet January, 2001. *http://www.alz.org/people.faq.htm#howmany*

American Association of Health Plans: 2001, American Association of Health Plans.

American Nurses Association (ANA): *Standards of clinical nursing practice,* Washington, DC, 1986, ANA.

American Nurses Association (ANA): *Standards of home health nursing practice,* Kansas City, Mo, 1986, ANA.

American Nurses Association (ANA): *Standards of scope and hospice nursing practice,* Kansas City, Mo, 1987, ANA.

American Nurses Association (ANA): *A statement on the scope of home health,* Kansas City, Mo, 1992, ANA.

American Nurses Association: *Position statement on the health care service system and linkage of primary care, substance abuse, mental health, and HIV/AIDS related services,* 1993, ANA. Retrieved from the internet January, 2001. *http://www.nursingworld.org/readroom/position/blood/blcare.htm*

American Nurses Association: *Position statement on long-term care,* 1995, ANA. Retrieved from the internet January, 2001. *http://www.nursingworld.org/readroom/position/social/scltcr.htm*

American Nurses Association (ANA): *ANA response to the Pew Commission Report,* 1997, ANA. Retrieved from the internet January, 2001. *http://www.nursingworld.org/readroom/pew.htm*

American Nurses Association (ANA): *Scope and standards of home health nursing practice,* Washington, DC, 1999, ANA.

Bectel RW, Tucker NG: *Across the States 1998: profiles of long-term care systems,* 1998, AARP. Retrieved from the internet *January, 2001. http://research.aarp.org/health/d16550_states_1.html*

Bedside nursing care by official agencies, *Public Health Nurs* 37:333-334, 1945.

Benefield, LE: Competencies of effective and efficient home care nurses, *Home Care Manager* 2(3):25-28, 1998.

Bergstrom N, Braden B, Kemp M, et al.: Multisite study of incidence of pressure ulcers and the relationship between risk level, demographic, characteristics, diagnoses, and prescription of preventive interventions, *J Am Ger Soc* 44:22-30, 1996.

Bergstrom N, Braden B, Kemp M, et al.: Predicting pressure ulcer risk: a multisite study of the predictive validity of the Braden Scale, *Nurs Research* 47:261-269, 1998.

Bishop CE: Efficiency of home care: notes for an economic approach to resource allocation, *J Aging and Health* 11(3):277-298, 1999.

Buhler-Wilkerson K: Home care the American way: an historical analysis, *Home Healthc Serv Q* 12(3):5-17, 1991.

Cain CJ, Wicks MN: Caregiver attributes as correlates of burden in family caregivers coping with chronic obstructive pulmonary disease, *J Fam Nurs* 6:46-68, 2000.

Calderon V, Tennstedt SL: Ethnic differences in the expression of caregiver burden: results of a qualitative study, *J Gerontological Social Work* 30:159-178, 1998.

Centers for Disease Control and Prevention (CDC): *Birth defects and pediatric genetics,* 2001a, CDC. Retrieved from the internet January, 2001.

Centers for Disease Control and Prevention (CDC): *Developmental disabilities,* 2001b, CDC. Retrieved from the internet January, 2001.

Centers for Disease Control and Prevention (CDC): *Disability and health,* 2001c, CDC. Retrieved from the internet January, 2001.

Centers for Disease Control and Prevention (CDC): *Fetal alcohol syndrome,* 2001d, CDC. Retrieved from the internet January, 2001.

Centers for Disease Control and Prevention (CDC): *Fact sheet: youth risk behavior trends,* 2001e, CDC. Retrieved from the internet February, 2001. *http://www.cdc.gov/nccdphp/dash/yrbs/trend.htm*

Chang B, Noonan AE, Tennstedt SL: The role of religion/spirituality in coping with caregiving for disabled elders, *Gerontologist* 38:463-470, 1998.

Coe M, Neufield A: Male caregivers' use of formal support, *Western J Nurs Research* 21:568-588, 1999.

Coleman B: *Assuring the quality of home care: the challenge of involving the consumer,* 2000, AARP. Retrieved from the internet January, 2001. *http://research.aarp.org/health/ib43_quality_1.html*

Community Health Accreditation Program (CHAP): *Care standards,* New York, 2000, CHAP.

Dumont P: *Family strengthening program.* Substance Abuse and Mental Health Services Administration Grant, 09/99-9/01, 1999, SAMHSA.

Federal Interagency Forum on Aging-Related Statistics: *Older Americans 2000: key indicators of well-being,* Washington, DC, 2000, US Government Printing Office.

Griffin KM: Evolution of transitional care settings: Past, present, future, *AACN Clinical Issues* 9:398-408, 1998.

Grimaldi PL: New skilled nursing facility payment scheme boosts Medicare risk, *Health Care Finance* 25(3):1-9, 1999.

Gross D, Brangan N: *Out of pocket health spending by Medicare beneficiaries age 65 and older: 1999 Projections,* 1999, AARP. Retrieved from the internet January, 2001. *http://research.aarp.org/health/inb14_spend.html*

Gundling R: Home health agencies should prepare for prospective payment, *Healthc Financial Management* 2:72-73, 2000.

Haupt AC: Forty years of teamwork in public health nursing, *Am J Nurs* 1:53, 1953.

Haupt BJ: *An overview of home health and hospice care patients in the 1996 National Home and Hospice Care Survey,* DHHS (PHS) 98-1250, Hyattsville, Md, 1998, National Center for Health Statistics.

Hawes C, Rose M, Phillips CD: *A national study of assisted living for the frail elderly,* 1999, Myers Research Institute. Retrieved from the internet January, 2001. *http://aspe.hhs.gov/daltcp/reports/facreses.htm*

Health Care Financing Administration (HCFA): *Medicare program: home health agencies conditions of participation and reductions in record keeping requirements,* 42 CFR, Part 484, Sections 484.1 through 484.52, Washington, DC, 1989, USDHHS.

Health Care Financing Administration (HCFA): Medicare program: home health agencies conditions of participation, 42CFR, Part 484, *Federal Register* 56:32967-32975, 1991.

Health Care Financing Administration (HCFA): *Medicare program: home health agencies—conditions of participation and reduction in record-keeping requirements,* 42 CFR, Part 484, Sections 484.1 through 484.52, Washington, DC, 1994, USDHHS.

Health Care Financing Administration (HCFA), Office of the Actuary: *National health expeditures by source of fund and type of expenditure: selected calendar years 1993-1998.* Retrieved from the internet January, 2001. *http://www.hcfa.gov/stats/nhe-oact/tables/t3.htm*

Health Care Financing Administration (HCFA): *Basic statistics about home health care,* Washington, DC, 2000a, NAHC.

Health Care Financing Administration (HCFA): *Trends 1998,* Washington, DC, 2000b, HCFA.

Health Care Financing Administration (HCFA): *Change in hospice payment rates as required by the Benefits Improvement and Protection Act,* 2001a, HCFA. Retrieved from the internet January, 2001. *http://www.hcfa.gov/pubforms/transmit/a0104.pdf*

Health Care Financing Administration (HCFA): *Children's Health Insurance Program* 2001b, HCFA. Retrieved from the internet January, 2001. *http://www.hcfa.gov/init/children.htm*

Health Care Financing Administration (HCFA): *Hospice manual: chapter IV reimbursement for hospice care,* 2001c, HCFA. Retrieved from the internet January, 2001. *http://www.hcfa.gov/pubforms/21%5Fhospice/hs401.htm*

Health Care Financing Administration (HCFA): *Home and community-based services 1915(c) waivers,* 2001d, HCFA. Retrieved from the internet January, 2001. *http://www.hcfa.gov/medicaid/hpg4.htm*

Health Care Financing Administration (HCFA): *Medicaid long-term care services,* 2001e, HCFA. Retrieved from the internet January, 2001. *http://www.hcfa.gov/medicaid/ltchomep.htm*

Health Care Financing Administration (HCFA): *Medicare and you 2001: your Medicare benefits,* 2001f, HCFA. Retrieved from the internet January, 2001. *http://www.medicare.gov*

Health Care Financing Administration (HCFA): *Personal health care expenditures by type of expenditure and source of funds: calendar years 1991-98,* Jan 2001g, HCFA. Retrieved from the internet March, 2001. *http://www.hcfa.gov/stats/nhe-oact/tables/t9.htm*

Health Resources and Services Administration, Division of Services for Children with Special Healthcare Needs: *Family perspectives: cultural/ethnic issues affecting children with special health care needs,* 2001a, HRSA. Retrieved from the internet January, 2001. *http://www.mchb.hrsa.gov/html/dscshn.html*

Health Resources and Services Administration, Division of Services for Children with Special Healthcare Needs: *National agenda for children with special health care needs: achieving the goals 2000,* 2001b, HRSA. Retrieved from the internet January, 2001. *http://www.mchb.hrsa.gov/html/dscshn.html*

Hirsh L, Klein M, Marlowe G: *Combining public health nursing agencies: a case study in Philadelphia,* New York, 1967, Department of PHN, NLN.

InfoUse: *Chartbook on women and disability,* 2001, National Institute on Disability and Rehabilitation Research. Retrieved from the internet January, 2001. *http://www.infouse.com/disabilitydata/womendisability.html*

Jirovec MM, Wyman JF, Wells TF: Addressing urinary incontinence with educational continence-care competencies, *Image: J Nurs Scholars* 30:375-378, 1998.

Joint Commission on Accreditation of Healthcare Organizations (JCAHO): *2000-2001: Comprehensive accreditation manual for home care*, Oakbrook Terrace, Ill, 2001, JCAHO.

Kane RA, Wilson KB: *Assisted living in the United States: a new paradigm for residential care for frail older persons*, Washington, DC, 1993, AARP.

Kaye J: *Spirituality and the emotional and physical health of black and white southern caregivers of persons with Alzheimer's disease and other dementias*, Medical College of Georgia, Augusta, Ga, 2000, Dissertation.

Keener RE: Home care looks toward technology, *Health Management Technology* 9:44-46, 2000.

Kim JH, Theis SL: Korean American caregivers: who are they? *J Transcultural Nursing* 11:264-273, 2000.

Lee TT, Mills ME: Analysis of patient profile in predicting home care resource utilization and outcomes, *J Nurs Admin* 30(2):67-75, 2000.

Levy S: Prospective payment system for home health set to start, *Drug Topics*, 71-72, 2000.

Lobianco MS, Mills ME, Moore HW: A model for case management of high costs Medicaid users, *Nurs Economics* 14:303-307, 314, 1996.

Lutsky S, Corea J, Alecxih L: *A survey of employers offering group long-term care insurance to their employees*, 2000, USDHHS, Office on Disability, Aging, and Long-Term Care Policy. Retrieved from the internet January, 2001. *http://aspe.hhs.gov/daltcp/reports/ltinfres.htm*

Madigan EA, Fortinsky RH: Alternative measures of resource consumption in home care episodes, *Public Health Nurs* 16:198-204, 1999.

Magruder J, Legeay S: When patients lose the Medicare venipuncture benefit: one agency's story, *Caring* 50-52, Sept 1999.

Martin KS, Larson BJ, Gorski LA, Hayko DM, editors: *Mosby's home health client teaching guides: R$_x$ for teaching*, St Louis, 1997, Mosby.

McClish DK, Wyman JF, Sale PG, et al.: Use and costs of incontinence pads in female study volunteers, *J Wound, Ostomy Continence Nurs* 26:207-13, 1999.

McCloskey JC, Bulechek GM, editors: *Nursing interventions classification (NIC)*, ed 3, St Louis, 2000, Mosby.

National Association for Home Care (NAHC): *Basic statistics about home health care 1995*, Washington, DC, 1995, NAHC.

National Association for Home Care (NAHC): *Basic statistics about hospice*, 1999, NAHC. Retrieved from the internet January, 2001. *http://www.nahc.org/Consumer/hpcstats.html*

National Association for Home Care (NAHC): *Basic statistics about home health care*, 2000, NAHC. Retrieved from the internet January, 2001. *http://www.nahc.org/Consumer/hcstats.html*

National Center for Assisted Living: *A consumer's guide to assisted living and residential care*, Jan 2001. Retrieved from the internet January, 2001. *http://www.ncal.org/consumer/thinking.htm*

National Center on Elder Abuse: *What is elder abuse?* 2001, National Center on Elder Abuse. Retrieved from the internet January, 2001. *http://www.elderabuse.org*

National Center for Health Statistics (NCHS): *Health, United States, 2000 with adolescent health chartbook*, Hyattsville, Md, 2000, NCHS.

National Family Caregivers Association (NFCA): *Family caregiving statistics*, 2001, National Family Caregivers Association. Retrieved from the internet January, 2001. *http://www.nfcacares.org/NFC1998_stats.html*

Naylor MD, McCauley KM: The effects of a discharge planning and home follow-up intervention on elders hospitalized with common medical and surgical cardiac conditions, *J Cardiovascular Nurs* 14(1):44-54, 1999.

Nottingham JA: Navigating the seas of caregiving: allies and ideas for success, *Caring* 14(4):16-20, 1995.

Office of Disability, Aging, and Long-Term Care Policy: *Considering children with disabilities and the State Children's Health Insurance Program*, Washington, DC, 2000, The Office.

Olson HH: Home health nursing, *Caring* 5(8):53-61, 1986.

Porter EJ, Ganong LH, Armer JM: The church family and kin: an older rural Black woman's support network and preferences for care providers, *Qualitative Health Research* 10:452-470, 2000.

Quinn ME, Johnson MA, Andress EL, et al: Health characteristics of elderly personal care home residents, *J Adv Nurs* 30:410-417, 1999.

Randall D: PPS's effect on subacute providers has produced a timely example of its limiting potential and how providers can fight back, *Rehab Management* 44-45, 1999.

Rose MS, Pruchno RA: Behavior sequences of long-term care residents and their social partners, *J Gerontology* 54B:S75-S83, 1999.

Rosenbaum S, *Olmstead v LC: implications for older persons with mental and physical disabilities*, 2000, AARP Public Policy Institute. Retrieved from the internet January, 2001. *http://research.aarp.org/health/inb30_disabilities.html*

Sampselle CM, Burns PA, Dougherty MC, et al: Continence for women: evidenced-based practice, *J Obstetric, Gynecologic, Neonatal Nurs* 26:375-389, 1997.

Sanger AD: *Planning home care with the elderly patient, family, and professional views of an alternative to institutionalization*, Cambridge, Mass, 1983, Ballinger.

Shaughnessy PW: *Using outcomes to build a continuous quality improvement program for home care*, 11th National Nursing Symposium on Home Health Care, Ann Arbor, Mich, 1996, University of Michigan School of Nursing.

Staggers' Lawsuit: *Part II, NAHC Report*, No. 275, Washington, DC, 1988, NAHC, pp. 1-3.

Stulginsky MM: Nurses' home health experience. Part I: the practice setting, *Nurs Health Care* 14(8):402-407, 1993a.

Stulginsky MM: Nurses' home health experience. Part II: the unique demands of home visits, *Nurs Health Care* 14(9):476-485, 1993b.

St. Pierre M: Home health PPS, *Caring* 18:16-19, 1999.

Teel CS, Press AN: Fatigue among elders in caregiving and noncaregiving roles, *West J Nurs Research* 21:498-520, 1999.

Tennstedt S, Chang B: The relative contribution of ethnicity versus socioeconomic status in explaining differences in disability and receipt of informal care, *J Gerontology* 53B:S61-70, 1998.

Tennstedt SL, Chang B, Delgado M: Patterns of long-term care: a comparison of Puerto Rican, African-American and non-Latino white elders, *J Gerontological Social Work* 30:179-199, 1998.

Tuck I, Wallace DC: Exploring parish nursing from an ethnographic perspective, *J Transcultural Nurs* 11:290-299, 2000.

Turnbull GB: Thriving and surviving in home care and skilled nursing facilities under the Balanced Budget Act of 1997, *J Wound, Ostomy Continence Nurses* 27:79-82, 2000.

US Census Bureau: *Americans with Disabilities, 1997: household economic studies*, 2001, US Census Bureau. Retrieved from the internet March, 2001. *http://www.census.gov/hhes/www/disability.htm*

US Department of Defense: *TRICARE fact sheets*, 2001, US Department of Defense. Retrieved from the internet February, 2001. *http://www.tricare.osd.mil/Factsheets/*

US Department of Health and Human Services (USDHHS): *State assisted living policy 1998*, Washington, DC, 1998, Office on Disability, Aging, and Long Term Care Policy.

US Department of Health and Human Services (USDHHS): *HHS fact sheet: the Department of Health and Human Service on mental health issues*, 1999a, USDHHS. Retrieved from the internet March, 2001. *http://www.hhs.gov/news/press/2001pres/01fsmentalhlth.html*

US Department of Health and Human Services (USDHHS): *Mental health: a report of the Surgeon General-executive summary*, 1999b. Retrieved from the internet March, 2001. *http://www.surgeongeneral.gov/library/mentalhealth*

US Department of Health and Human Services (USDHHS): *Healthy People 2010*, conference edition, Washington, DC, 2000a, USDHHS.

US Department of Health and Human Services (USDHHS), Office of Disability: *Aging and long-term care policy and the Urban Institute,* 2000b, USDHHS. Medicare's Hospice Benefit: Use and Expenditures. Retrieved from the internet January, 2001. *http://aspe.hhs.gov/daltcp/reports/96useexp.htm*

US Department of Health and Human Services (USDHHS): *HHS fact sheet: CHIP enrollment reaches 3.3 million, final regulation published,* 2001a, USDHHS. Retrieved from the internet March, 2001. *http://www.hhs.gov/news/press/2001pres/20010106.html*

US Department of Health and Human Services (USDHHS): *HHS news: HHS announces new grants, new opportunities for people with disabilities,* 2001b, USDHHS. Retrieved from the internet January, 2001. *http://www.hhs.gov/news/press/2001pres/20010110.html*

US Department of Health and Human Services (USDHHS): *Healthy People 2010,* 2001c, USDHHS. Retrieved from the internet January, 2001. *http://www.health.gov/healthypeople*

US Department of Health and Human Services (USDHHS): *The initiative to eliminate racial and ethnic disparities in health,* 2001d, USDHHS. Retrieved from the internet February, 2001. *http://raceandhealth.hhs.gov*

Veterans Health Administration: *Gateway to health programs and initiatives,* 2000, VHA. Retrieved from the internet January, 2001. *http://www.va.gov/About_VA/Orgs/VHA/VHAProg.htm*

Veterans Health Administration: *Department of Veterans Affairs,* 2001, VHA. Retrieved from the internet January, 2001. *http://www.va.gov*

*Veterans' Millenium Health Care and Benefits Act, PL 106-117,* (38 US CODE 101, 113 STAT 1545) (Nov 1999).

Visiting Nurse Service of Toledo: Eighty-three years of caring, *Caring* 3:57-61, 1984.

Walker DM: *Medicare reform: leading proposals lay groundwork, while design decisions lie ahead.* Testimony before the US Senate Committee on Finance. GAO/T-HEHS/AIMD-00-103, 2000, General Accounting Office. Retrieved from the internet January, 2001. http://www.gao.gov

Wallace DC, Witucki J, Boland C, Tuck I: Cultural context of caregiving with elders, *J Multicultural Nurs Health* 4(3):42-48, 1998.

Witucki J: *Help-seeking by older wife caregivers of demented husbands: a grounded theory approach.* University of Tennessee, Knoxville, Tenn, 2000, Dissertation.

Yates ME, Tennstedt SL, Chang B: Contributors to and mediators of psychological well-being for informal caregivers, *J Gerontol* 54B:P12-22, 1999.

## SELECTED BIBLIOGRAPHY

de Savorgnani A, Haring R: The impact of cultural issues on home care personnel and patients, *Caring* 17(4), 22-27, 1999.

Drane J: *Caring to the end: policy suggestions and ethical education for hospice and home health care agencies,* Erie, Penn, 1997, Lake Area Health Education Center.

Maier F: Ethics in home care agencies, *Caring* 18(8), 6-13, 2000.

Rice R: *Handbook of home health nursing procedures,* ed 2, St Louis, 2000, Mosby.

# 23

# Population-Focused Intervention in Clinics, Nontraditional Settings, and Through Group Process

*Susan Clemen-Stone*

## OBJECTIVES

*Upon completion of this chapter, the reader should be able to:*

1. Discuss how population- or aggregate-focused interventions can promote the health of the community.
2. Describe the differences between psychoeducational, task, and supportive groups.
3. Understand how community health nurses use the group process to target population-focused, preventive health services.
4. Summarize the phases in the life of a group and leadership interventions that facilitate movement from one phase to the next.

5. Discuss how societal trends have contributed to the development of population-focused clinic and nursing center services.
6. Articulate factors community health nurses consider when establishing and maintaining population-focused clinic and nursing center services.
7. Describe how parish nursing and block nursing can meet the needs of targeted populations in the community.

## KEY TERMS

Ambulatory health services
Block nursing
Clinics
Community health centers (CHCs)
Contract
Group
Group cohesiveness

Group culture
Group norms
Group phases
Group process
Group work
Nursing centers
Outreach activities

Parish nurse
Parish nursing
Parish nursing practice models
Psychoeducational group
Supportive or counseling groups
Target population
Task groups

---

*Even if you are on the right track, you will get run over if you just sit there.*

WILL ROGERS

Just as a map provides alternative roads to a destination, various community health nursing interventions and settings provide alternatives for addressing the health needs of clients in the community. Historically, community health nurses have recognized that multiple methods must be used to resolve the complex problems existing in society

and that they must be proactive in developing interventions that will meet the needs of diverse client groups. Community health nurses have initiated collaborative working relationships with professionals from other disciplines and community residents to reach underserved clients in unique ways. National data concerning health disparities among Americans, health care access issues, and changing demographics (Health Resources and Services Administration [HRSA], 2000; U.S. Department of Health and Human Services [USDHHS], 2000) urgently propel community health nurses to continue to develop effective alternatives for

**BOX 23-1**

## *A Population-Based, Community-Focused Intervention in Action*

The Crystal Bartlett Neighborhood Health Center has served infants, children, and young adults through the age of 25 for over 20 years. Concerned about the increased incidence of illegal drug abuse among its teen clientele, clinic staff obtained funding to establish a teen theater troop to address this issue. Working in collaboration with clinic staff and local organizations addressing substance abuse problems, the theater troop developed an action-oriented skit aimed at addressing the consequences of all types of substance abuse. The theater troop is invited by schools, churches, social service clubs, and numerous other organizations to educate children, teens, and adults about substance abuse, including where to get help to deal with this problem. Recently, a citizens group in one local neighborhood set up a crime watch program to report drug dealings to the police after actively participating in the skit with the theater troop.

intervening with diverse clients at risk, including individuals, families, populations, and communities.

From both a cost containment and a quality perspective, it is important for community health nurses to consider population-focused as well as individual- and family-focused interventions that take into account the client's unique environment. There is a growing recognition that health behavior is significantly influenced by environmental factors and that health promotion interventions that focus only on changing individual behavior neglect important influences in the social cultural environment (Bracht, 1999; Glanz, Rimer, 1997; Steckler, Allegrante, Altman, et al., 1995). "To have enduring effects, interventions must have an impact on social norms and accepted ways of functioning that may be deleterious to health" (Clark, McLeroy, 1995, p. 277).

Population-based, community-focused interventions emphasize creating changes in community norms, attitudes, awareness, and standards of practices for the purpose of improving the population's health status and capacity (Minnesota Department of Health, 1997). Illustrative of this type of intervention is a teen theater troupe, established by the Crystal Bartlett Neighborhood Health Center, that educates peers and adults about the consequences of illegal substance abuse and other social issues (Box 23-1). This theater troupe has helped raise community awareness and attitudes about substance abuse, which has resulted in the community taking action to stop illegal drug trafficking in local neighborhoods.

Although population-based nursing roles and interventions have been addressed throughout this text, this chapter broadens discussion about the roles community health

nurses assume and interventions they use when working with small groups and populations in select community sites. The emphasis is on examining how community health nurses use the group process to provide targeted preventive services and how they function in clinic, nursing center, parish, and neighborhood settings to address the needs of populations across the life span. Increasing evidence supports the fact that targeted, group-specific interventions and nontraditional as well as traditional approaches are needed to effectively work with the diverse populations in the community (Clark, McLeroy, 1995; Freudenberg, Eng, Flay, et al., 1995; Glanz, Rimer, 1997; Marín, Burhansstipanov, Connell, et al., 1995). The settings in which health care professionals function provide channels for reaching targeted groups (Mullen, Evans, Forster, et al., 1995).

## INTERVENING WITH POPULATIONS THROUGH GROUP PROCESS

Community health nurses have long worked with groups of people to meet health care needs effectively. In this context, **group** is defined as a gathering of people who are working together for a specific reason. An example of the use of group work in community health nursing practice is a parent education and support class. Parents in this situation come together to achieve a specific goal. That is, to collectively discuss ways to rear children effectively. A gathering of strangers waiting at a bus stop does not meet the definition of a group.

**Group work** is a goal-directed activity used to meet a variety of client needs or to accomplish specific tasks. This activity is directed to individual members of a group and to the group as a whole within a system of service delivery (Toseland, Rivas, 2001, p. 12). Toseland and Rivas contend that a group worker should have a dual focus: goal-directed activities with individual participants and with the group as a whole.

Group work is an effective population-focused intervention. Through group work, community health nurses are able to assist people with common needs to learn new knowledge and skills, to support group members during stressful times, or to problem solve. Community assessment and caseload analysis data help community health nurses identify populations, within the community and the nurse's work area, that have common needs and that might benefit from group intervention. Displayed in Box 23-2 are examples how community health nurses use these data to promote the health of vulnerable populations through group work.

### Brief Historical Perspective on Group Work

Group work in the United States began mainly in settlement houses around the turn of the twentieth century. The settlement houses offered group experiences to assist their clients with education, recreation, socialization and community involvement (Toseland, Rivas, 2001). The settlement houses saw the group approach as an effective way "for citizens to gather to share their views, gain mutual support, and exercise the power derived from their association for social change" (Toseland, Rivas, 2001, p. 48). Early group work efforts placed a heavy emphasis on group activities such as camping, community services, cooking, and education.

Group psychotherapy was another development in the group approach to health. Therapy groups became a part of the treatment plan of psychologists and psychiatrists during the early part of the twentieth century and became quite prevalent during the 1940s and 1950s (Toseland, Rivas, 2001). During the 1960s, group work and group psychotherapy came together (Loomis, 1979). At this time the encounter group movement proliferated, and it was realized that everyone, not just *sick* people, could benefit from the group process.

Kurt Lewin's study of group dynamics during the 1940s was instrumental in demonstrating the benefits of group work in a variety of situations. His research during World War II was aimed at increasing work production and changing food consumption patterns. Lewin found that group discussion and decision making helped people change their behavior much more effectively than lectures or even individual instruction (Lewin, 1947). Giving people information alone did not motivate them to change personal attitudes and behavior. Rather, discussion in groups helped persons become involved, conceptualize ideas, and take health action. Group participants learned something about their own behavior in group settings, and the information gained was relevant to their personal lives.

"During the 1960s and 1970s, groups reached their zenith; then the group fever declined for a decade" (Corey, Corey, 1997, p. 5). In the 1990s, another surge of interest in the use of group work emerged. Some see the group approach to care as a cost-effective and a quality way to address client needs in a managed care environment (MacKenzie, 1995; Sleek, 1995). Corey and Corey (2002) believe that groups are the treatment of choice for many situations, not a second-rate cost containment approach to helping people change. "Groups have immense power to move people in creative and more life-giving directions" (Corey, Corey, 1997, p. 5).

Clearly group work is an integral part of life in the United States. Groups are formed for a variety of psychological, social, and educational purposes such as losing weight; controlling drug usage and smoking; and giving support during divorce, death, and other transitional periods in the life of clients. Nurses are members of multiple groups. They are part of a group on the health team and in professional associations and are also a part of many community groups such as parent-teacher organizations, League of Women Voters, and faith-related groups at their local church. Nurses help develop and maintain many of these groups.

**BOX 23-2**

## *Group Interventions Promote the Health of Populations*

### *Community Health Nurses Take Action to Address Needs of Vulnerable Groups....*

Sue Talbert, a staff nurse at a local health department, formed a parent support group for families with children who had developmental delays. An analysis of referral and caseload data helped Sue to recognize the long-term, complex needs of these families. Sue believed that a support group could better assist the parents in identifying and using appropriate community resources and in addressing their long-term primary and secondary preventive health needs.

The nursing administrator of a local health department established a Child Death Review Team, a formal community coalition, when analysis of community assessment data revealed that the county's sudden infant death syndrome (SIDS) and childhood death rates were significantly higher than state and national rates. Representing many community agencies, such as local hospitals, schools, the police department, the domestic violence center, and the health department, this coalition was charged with the task of comprehensively analyzing all county deaths among children age 18 years and younger and identifying interventions for reducing childhood mortality rates.

A higher than average elderly population in her faith community prompted the parish nurse from a large urban congregation to establish a psychoeducational group for caregivers of elderly family members. This nurse used assessment data from the church's wellness team to support the need for such a group.

## Advantages and Disadvantages of Group Work

Promoting and preserving the health of populations is a major focus of community health nursing practice. To carry out this responsibility, nurses are constantly viewing ways of helping people look critically at their own behavior for the purpose of promoting healthy lifestyle changes. Clinical and empirical evidence suggests that group work is one approach for achieving lifestyle changes and other health promotion goals (Toseland, Rivas, 2001). Groups can provide a supportive environment that helps people with similar concerns work together on these goals.

When carefully planned, groups can have several advantages. Frequently cited benefits of group intervention are displayed in Box 23-3. In general, group work is being used to enhance effective problem solving and decision making, help people learn new knowledge, promote commitment to common goals, and address psychosocial concerns. For example, the use of focus groups has helped practitioners promote commitment to specific goals and obtain data that address health issues from multiple perspectives. These type of

**BOX 23-3**

*Select Potential Benefits of Group Intervention*

- Provides a stimulus for creative and productive problem solving and decision making
- Promotes a shared vision regarding goals and outcomes common to participants
- Brings together the assets of many for complex problem solving
- Brings together a wide variety of skills and resources for collective action
- Helps participants focus on priority concerns
- Helps group members complete tasks effectively and efficiently
- Provides a supportive environment for addressing individual as well as group concerns

data help professionals and consumers to more effectively identify and solve health problems. The use of focus groups to assess client strengths and needs has been a common practice in recent years and has strengthened client assessment processes.

Group work has the potential to strengthen many decision-making and change processes. It has been found that group work can be helpful in ameliorating personal problems (DeLucia-Waack, 2000), can produce positive social and health-related outcomes among group participants (Humphreys, Ribisl, 1999), can increase intergenerational understanding (Vacha-Haase, Ness, Dannison, Smith, 2000), and can enhance completion of complex tasks (Hare, Blumberg, Davies, Kent, 1995). Group work can also help people alter ineffective patterns of functioning through observation of how other group members handle stressful situations; help group participants validate thoughts, feelings, and experiences; and facilitate the development of a social network (Corey, Corey, 1997, 2002). Currently online internet support groups are allowing people in geographically remote areas or people who have other health care access issues to participate in support groups (Page, Delmonico, Walsh, et al., 2000).

Group intervention will not meet the needs of all clients. Some people will not feel secure enough to leave their own familiar surroundings, to find transportation, to have the needed energy and skill, or even to want to become part of a group. There are other people who lack the social expertise, experience, and motivation required to become involved in a group. This behavior can be learned, but it requires patience and skill on the part of the nurse to help some clients participate in the group process. An overwhelmed 17-year-old single mother of two children under 2 years of age, who has exhibited poor bonding behaviors with her newborn, probably needs an intense one-on-one

relationship with a nurse before she can profit from a group discussion about parenting.

Some people like to function in groups while others do not. These differences need to be respected because an individual's attitude and beliefs regarding the group experience will have an effect on group learning and outcomes. Successful group outcomes have been limited in situations where the group's culture is not amenable to sharing problems with strangers or where the social conditions (e.g., lack of child care, long working hours, or dangerousness of neighborhood) make participation in groups less likely (Marín, Burhansstipanov, Connell, et al., 1995, p. 353). However, successful group outcomes have been achieved among underserved groups, especially when targeted group strategies are planned (Clark, Janz, Dodge, Sharpe, 1992; Marín, Burhansstipanov, Connell, et al., 1995).

Understanding the advantages and disadvantages of using group work to meet the needs of populations in the community assists nurses in identifying clients who may or may not be responsive to involvement in groups and outcomes that may or may not be achieved through the group process. Toseland and Rivas (2001) contend that the use of the group process needs to be evaluated within the context of the specific situation and in reference to the types of goals to be achieved. When clients are not responsive to group work, the professional needs to seek alternative interventions for meeting their needs.

## Types of Groups in the Community Setting

Nurses work in a variety of groups in the community setting. Many of the groups that community health professionals develop and implement on a regular basis can be classified under three major categories: task groups, psychoeducational groups, and supportive or counseling groups (Clark, 1994; Corey, Corey, 2002; Toseland, Rivas, 2001). Types of "groups differ with respect to goals, techniques used, the role of the leader, training requirements, and the kind of people involved" (Corey, Corey, 1997, p. 9). Training requirements vary, based on the type of strategies used by the group leader, the role of the leader, and the primary goal of the group. For example, a group leader guiding a psychoeducational group needs a firm understanding of the principles of teaching and learning, behavioral change theories, and health promotion and social marketing concepts. On the other hand, a leader conducting a supportive or counseling group needs strong counseling and problem-solving skills, while the leader working in a task group needs team-building, problem-solving, change-agent, and management skills. The task group leader also may need community organization and health planning skills if he or she is working in a group established to promote community capacity (Corey, Corey, 1997).

TASK GROUPS. **Task groups** usually are developed to accomplish a specific task or goal and often within specified time limits. Task groups are commonly used in organizations to find solutions to problems, generate new ideas, and guide decision making (Toseland, Rivas, 2001). Groups can be more effective then individuals in addressing large, complex tasks requiring high levels of creativity (Hare, Blumberg, Davies, Kent, 1995). In the community setting it is not usual to work with an interdisciplinary team when addressing complex client and organizational issues. The multidisciplinary team in the community health setting may include nurses, physicians, environmentalists, physical and occupational therapists, nutritionists, social workers, and other professional consultants meeting as a group to address the needs of populations at risk. Future health care providers will increasingly work in interdisciplinary groups in more focused ways to ensure effective and efficient coordination of care (O'Neil, Pew Health Professions Commission, 1998).

Within community health nursing practice, numerous task groups are continuously formed to achieve specified goals and objectives. An example of a large-scale, population-focused group effort designed to accomplish a specific task is the work done by groups established to develop the *Healthy People 2010* national health objectives. These work groups focused on developing goals for improving the health status among Americans and objectives for achieving these goals. The *Healthy People 2010* work groups had representation from an extensive list of national organizations from around the country.

Task groups exist at all levels of community health nursing practice. Nursing organizations have local, state, and national political action groups that address legislative concerns regarding the health of the people within given states. Community action groups, such as Mothers Against Drunk Driving (MADD), also exist on national, state, and local levels and are becoming a powerful force in influencing the health care delivery system. Professional and community action groups are involved in areas such as fundraising for innovative health planning activities, informing the public about major health problems, and influencing public policy through interactions with legislators and other public officials.

It has been stressed throughout this text that working in active partnership with clients is a significant way to accomplish tasks and reach desired goals. Group work can facilitate partnership formation and task completion. For example, one large senior citizen's center uses group work to bring together retired volunteer nurses, physicians, laypersons, and residents of the center to plan and implement a monthly health screening program. The retired workers and clients involved in this task feel needed, and the clients screened feel they are helped "by people who understand them." Other examples of task groups involving clients and providers are healthy community planning groups, coalition groups established to address a specific issue such as domestic violence or asthma among adults and children, and client care conference groups.

**PSYCHOEDUCATIONAL GROUPS.** The term **psychoeducational group** is used to reflect both the support and learning aspects of educational groups that help group members obtain new knowledge and skills. Psychoeducational groups are formed to work with relatively healthy individuals who have information deficits. These types of groups are designed to address educational deficits and prevent psychological problems that could be associated with these deficits (Corey, Corey, 2002).

Educating implies that someone wants to learn, and as an outcome of the educative intervention, there is an expected learning-behavior change. For group education to be effective it must be determined that the group participants have need for the information being shared and are ready or motivated to learn the information. Chapter 12 discusses assessment of learning needs and learner readiness and examines how to select appropriate educational objectives and teaching methods.

There are numerous psychoeducational groups in the community setting. For example, these types of groups are assisting clients to deal with a new diagnosis of an illness such as diabetes, hypertension, multiple sclerosis, or asthma, or transitional issues such as parenting, career changes, or retirement. Clients in educational groups often must learn new methods of functioning and ways to cope with changes in their lifestyle. Numerous topics can be dealt with in educational groups such as parenting, childbirth, breastfeeding, weight loss, care of a new colostomy, and managing stress. Groups composed of clients with common problems often provide support in addition to helping participants increase their knowledge of a disease process and treatment options.

Community health nurses assume a variety of roles in educational groups. They may focus on providing information unknown to group participants, such as when the nurse is working with a group of expectant parents who want to learn about labor and delivery processes. At other times community health nurses focus on the facilitator role, especially when group members are learning how to cope with normative and nonnormative stresses. As was explained in Chapter 8, anticipatory education can help persons address more effectively these types of stresses.

Educational groups should be carefully planned and related to the purpose of the group experience so that the desired outcome can be achieved. A fundamental premise when planning any type of an educational or health communication program is that to be viable, the program must be based on an understanding of the needs and perceptions of the target audience (National Institutes of Health [NIH], 1995). This understanding can help the nurse select appropriate content, educational materials, and educational objectives and strategies.

The Stages of the Health Communication Wheel is a useful tool for facilitating the development, implementation, and evaluation of appropriate educational interventions.

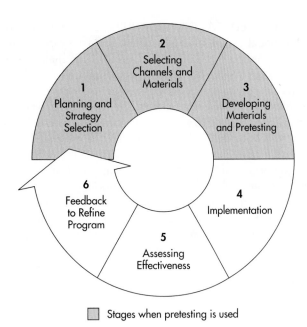

Stages when pretesting is used

**FIGURE 23-1** Stages in the health communication process. (From National Institutes of Health (NIH): *Making health communication programs work: a planner's guide,* Atlanta, 1995, USDHHS. Retrieved from the internet April 1, 2001. *http://rex.nci.nih.gov/NCI_Pub_Interface/HCPW/OVER.HTM*)

This wheel (Figure 23-1) is based on social marketing concepts and was designed to help professions plan effective health education or health communication programs. Social marketing concepts concentrate on tailoring health and other types of programs to serve a defined target group (Glanz, Rimer, 1997). A **target population** may be all the persons in a local community or only the persons in a small educational group. The stages of the health communication wheel provide a framework for planning, implementing, and evaluating health education interventions, regardless of the setting or targeted group. The issues to be considered during each stage of the health communication process are displayed in Box 23-4.

SUPPORTIVE OR COUNSELING GROUPS. The primary purposes of **supportive or counseling groups** are to help participants deal with emotions associated with normative and nonnormative stressors that could lead to crises and to revitalize existing coping abilities (Clark, 1994; Corey, Corey, 2002; Toseland, Rivas, 2001). Supportive or counseling groups differ from therapy groups in that they are designed to address specific short-term issues that are not aimed at major personality changes or the treatment of severe psychological and behavioral disorders (Corey, Corey, 2002). These types of groups help persons deal with the usual stressful life events.

Community health nurses work with clients across the life span who are experiencing stressful events. Most of these people are healthy, but during periods of rapid development and change, they may need help to manage stress and develop effective coping strategies. Examples of groups that help individuals deal with stressful events are widow-to-widow programs, educational groups for lay caregivers, parenting groups for grandparents, and groups for parents who have disabled children. The thrust of these types of groups is to *prevent* future upsets by helping participants learn ways to effectively express their emotions and methods of coping in potentially difficult situations (Clark, 1994). These groups also help participants anticipate and prepare for the normative stressors discussed in Chapter 8.

Community health nurses frequently initiate support groups for at-risk clients. Support groups are established in a variety of settings including schools, clinics, industries, neighborhood centers, and other community facilities. They are developed for multiple purposes and have been used effectively with persons of all ages. For example, support groups have been used with all ages to deal with death and dying issues. They also have been used with the elderly to address reality orientation for persons with dementia, remotivation for daily living, and reminiscence and life review (Corey, Corey, 2002; Murray, Zentner, 2001); and the young to address living with a disability. Supportive or counseling groups can be an effective intervention for meeting the needs of populations experiencing a variety of stresses. These types of groups can help individuals learn about different problem-solving techniques and expand their social network. This, in turn, can assist them in dealing more effectively with normative and nonnormative stressors.

*Stop and Think About It*
Taking into consideration the current clients you are serving, think about what types of groups might benefit these clients or why the group process might not be helpful for them. How would you go about finding group experiences in your local community that would benefit your clients?

## Developing a Group
When nurses begin to think about forming a group, they take into consideration the characteristics and needs of the clients they are serving, the goals they hope to achieve through the group process, and workload responsibilities. From a workload perspective, nurses examine if the proposed group work would increase or decrease workload demands. If it increases work responsibilities, can they handle the added demands? Use of the workload management concepts addressed in Chapter 24 helps nurses analyze workload management issues such as these in an organized and realistic manner.

Because community health nurses work with populations within a county, a city, or a township, common needs that can be met by group work may be expressed by clients, staff nurses, or other stakeholders in the community, such as school officials. If the client and the nurse are so inclined, almost any health need can be met by the group process, except those for which clients need one-to-one relationships.

**Teaching TIPS** | **BOX 23-4**

## Issues to Address During the Six Stages of the Health Communication Process*

### Stage 1: Planning and Strategy

The planning stage of a program provides the foundation for the entire health communication process. Faulty decision making at this point can lead to the development of a program that is "off the mark." Careful assessment of a problem in the beginning can reduce the need for costly midcourse corrections.

**KEY ISSUES**

- What is already known about the health problem? (Analyze existing data.)
- What new information will be needed before planning the program? (Generate new data if needed.)
- Who is (are) the target audience(s)? What is known about it (them)?
- Overall, what change is planned to solve or lessen the problem? (Establish goals.)
- What measurable objectives can be established to define success?
- How can progress be measured? (Plan evaluation strategies.)
- What should the target audience be told? (Draft communication strategies.)

### Stage 2: Selecting Channels and Materials

The decisions you make in Stage 1 will guide you in selecting the appropriate communication channel(s) and producing effective materials. Without clear objectives and knowledge of your target audience, you risk producing materials that are inappropriate for the target audience or the issue being addressed.

**KEY ISSUES**

- Are there any existing materials that could be adapted for the program?
- Which channels are most appropriate for reaching the target audience (e.g., worksite, mass media, face-to-face)?
- What formats will best suit the channels and the messages (e.g., booklets, videotapes, curricula)?

### Stage 3: Developing Materials and Pretesting

In Stages 1 and 2, most program planning is completed, providing the basis for developing messages and materials. Often, several different concepts are developed and tested with target audiences. Feedback from the intended audience is critical in Stage 3.

**KEY ISSUES**

- What are the different ways that the message can be presented?
- How does the target audience react to the message concept(s)?
- Does the audience:
  - understand the message?
  - recall it?

- accept its importance?
- agree with the value of the solution?
- How does the audience respond to the message format?
- Based on responses from the target audience, do changes need to be made in the message or its format?
- How could the message be promoted, the materials distributed, and progress tracked?

### Stage 4: Implementation

The fully developed program is introduced to the target audience; promotion and distribution begin through all channels. Program components are periodically reviewed and revised if necessary. Audience exposure and reaction are tracked to permit alterations if needed.

**KEY ISSUES**

- Is the message making it through the intended channels of communication?
- Is the target audience paying attention and reacting?
- Do any existing channels need to be replaced or new channels added?
- Which aspects of the program are having the strongest effect?
- Do changes need to be made to improve program effect?

### Stage 5: Assessing Effectiveness

The program should be assessed by analyzing the results of measurements planned in Stage 1 and used throughout the program's life span.

**KEY ISSUES**

- Were the program objectives met?
- Were the changes that took place the result of the program, other factors, or both?
- How well was each stage of program planning, implementation, and assessment handled?

### Stage 6: Feedback to Refine Program

At each stage useful information is gathered about the audience, the message, the channels of communication, and the program's intended effect. All of this information helps prepare for a new cycle of program development. The more information that can be reviewed at the end of the first program phase, the more likely it is that these questions can be answered.

**KEY ISSUES**

- Why did the program work or not work?
- Should program changes or improvements be made to increase the likelihood of success or to address change in the audience or problem situations?
- Were lessons learned that could help make future programs more successful?

From National Institutes of Health: *Making health communication programs work: a planner's guide,* Atlanta, 1995, USDHHS. Retrieved from the internet April 1, 2001. *http://rex.nci.nih.gov/NCI_Pub_Interface/HCPW/OVER.HTM*
*The Health Communication Process is displayed in Figure 23-1.

The very young single mother referred to earlier is a client whose needs may not be met by the group process. However, at times it can be helpful to combine the use of group and individual intervention strategies. For example, one nurse had a family in her caseload that had a child with spina bifida and resultant paraplegia. The nurse visited the home to assess family functioning and environmental factors influencing the child's development. During these visits, the nurse also helped the parents deal with the child's daily routine. In addition, the nurse referred the parents to a support group held at a local school, where they received support from families with similar problems.

Once a need common to a number of people has been established, it is important to develop a clear implementation plan with specific goals. When working in an organization, good ideas for groups are frequently not put into practice because they have not been developed into a convincing plan or proposal (Corey, Corey, 2002). A proposal for a group addresses issues related to the group's purposes, group composition, selection of group members, the setting for the group, group implementation and evaluation activities, and financial resources needed for group activities (Corey, Corey, 2002; Toseland, Rivas, 2001). It is important to realize that financial resources may be needed to cover personnel time, the rent of an appropriate facility, and group activities. Funds also may be needed for such things as travel costs for group participants and child care assistance. It is not uncommon to underestimate the cost of group intervention.

## Practical Tips for Developing a Group

When developing a group, a health care professional needs to address a number of variables related to group membership, the setting for the group, the group's purpose(s), and where the group is to be held. Decisions about group composition are significant. "In general, for a specific target population with given needs, a group composed entirely of members of that population (e.g., Parents Without Partners, clients who abuse drugs, or persons with memory loses) is more appropriate than a heterogeneous group" (Corey, Corey, 2002, p. 107).

Toseland and Rivas (2001) confirm the importance of homogeneity in relation to group members' characteristics and purposes for group involvement. Other important principles of group composition shared by these authors are displayed in Box 23-5. These principles highlight the need for group members with similar characteristics and interest but also the value of having varying strengths and assets in the group. Group composition principles, when followed, promote a group structure or membership that can facilitate learning among group members. Diversity among group participants provides differing opportunities for support, validation, mutual aid, and learning, and a range of resources for problem solving (Toseland, Rivas, 2001).

**BOX 23-5**

## *Group Composition Principles*

- A homogeneity of members' purposes and certain personal characteristics
- A heterogeneity of members' coping skills, life experiences, and expertise
- An overall structure that includes a range of members' qualities, skills, and expertise

From Toseland RW, Rivas RF: *An introduction to group work practice,* ed 4, Boston, 2001, Allyn and Bacon, p. 167.

When potential group members are identified, the nurse should discuss with them the purposes of the group and objectives that can be accomplished. The important principle involved is that the nurse must have expected outcomes for the group that are consistent with the client's needs and interests. This principle is also important to consider when referring a client to an already established group. The group experience must meet the needs of the referred client. For example, a support group for new parents may not be helpful for a client with severe postpartum depression, but it could be very beneficial for a couple that has recently moved and has a limited support network in the community.

Contracting is used to determine congruency between individual participant's goals and group goals. As was explained in Chapter 9, a **contract** is a statement of the mutual expectations that both the client and the nurse have for each other. In general these contracts are usually verbal agreements when working with groups, such as "yes I am interested in learning about hypertension and ways to control this condition." Client contracting is a negotiated agreement with a client that reinforces a specific behavior change (Bulechek, McCloskey, 1999). Contracts provide a basis for evaluation of the progress that takes place and helps group members determine if the outcomes were achieved.

The setting plays a crucial role in groups. Several questions, such as those identified in Box 23-6, should be asked to determine whether a particular setting is appropriate. Potential group members can play a significant role in helping the professional select an appropriate meeting site.

Besides the setting, there are many other factors to consider when developing a group. The size of the group is a major consideration. The size of the group "depends on several factors: the age of the clients, the experience of the leader, the type of group, and the problems to be explored. For example, a group composed of elementary school children might be kept to three or four, whereas a group of adolescents might be made of six to eight people" (Corey, Corey, 2002, p. 102). Although there are no clear rules about group size, it is important to remember that **group cohesiveness** decreases as groups become larger (Clark, 1994).

**BOX 23-6**

*Obtaining an Appropriate Group Setting: Select Questions to Consider*

- Is the group meeting in a place that is easily accessible, that can be reached by public transportation or personal cars easily?
- Is the meeting place near the population being served?
- Is the setting acceptable to the population being served?
- Is the location of the meeting place safe after dark?
- Does the meeting room provide privacy and warmth?
- Do seating arrangements facilitate group interaction?
- Will the facility be consistently available?

"Cohesiveness is the attraction of the group members for each other" (Clark, 1994, p. 49). Group cohesion can help keep groups together until desired goals are achieved. Cohesive groups promote positive relationships and support within the group and a sense of trust and satisfaction among group participants.

Another important variable to consider when developing a group is when the group should meet. If the group is composed of retired persons, daytime hours may be fine. On the other hand, wage earners who work during the day are likely to be free only in the evenings. The frequency and length of meetings and childcare arrangements are other issues that need to be decided by the nurse and clients. If small children are to be brought along with clients, there needs to be a place with play equipment and a caretaker provided. None of these details have "right" and "wrong" answers, but it is essential that clients know them and help plan to address them. It is important to take into consideration the characteristics and needs of group participants.

Many nurses are hesitant to use the group process because they lack experience with this intervention strategy. Careful planning, staff development activities that facilitate the understanding of group dynamics, and guidance from professionals comfortable with group work reduce fear.

## The Life of a Group

It is important for nurses who lead groups to understand that a group goes through **group phases.** These phases have been labeled differently by authors but in general include an orientation or beginning phase, a transitional phase, a working phase, and a termination or ending phase. During the orientation phase the group is introduced to its goals, purposes, and group norms. Included also in this phase are discussions about group processes and common concerns of group participants. The group leader focuses on using strategies for creating a trusting environment and helping members to feel part of the group (Corey, Corey, 2002; Toseland,

Rivas, 2001). One such strategy might be to point out the commonalities between group members.

The transitional phase is a trust building phase in which anxieties and fears related to the group process are dealt with and conflicts are addressed. It is not uncommon for the group leader to be challenged during this phase (Corey, Corey, 2002). The working phase encourages problem solving through intense discussion and sharing between members and work toward achieving group goals. During this phase, group members become more involved in the group process and are encouraged to build upon their assets to solve problems or to learn new coping behaviors.

During the termination or ending phase of a group, members are encouraged to review what has been accomplished and their satisfaction with the group process. They also are asked to express their emotions, thoughts, and feelings related to separating from the group. In support and counseling groups termination can provoke anxiety. This happens less frequently in educational groups. The leader must be prepared to help group members deal with feelings about separation so that they do not leave feeling dejected (Clark, 1994).

## Group Process

Group process influences progression through the phases of a group and goal achievement. "**Group process** pertains to dynamics such as the norms that govern a group, the level of cohesion in groups, how trust is generated, how resistance is manifested, how conflict emerges and is dealt with, the forces that bring about healing, intermember reactions, and the various stages in a group's development" (Corey, Corey, 2002, p. 7). A group's culture is also an important dimension of group process. **Group culture** is derived from the group environment as well as from the beliefs, customs, and values of its members. Group culture can influence group goals, priorities, and process (Toseland, Rivas, 2001).

As a group evolves, it develops **group norms** or rules of conduct that define acceptable and nonacceptable behavior. It is helpful to explicitly identify these norms early in the group process. When doing so it is important to consider that norms of social control can inhibit as well as facilitate group process. Norms that are facilitative promote trust, respect for the rights of others, and effective group communication and interaction processes. Norms that provide too much structure can inhibit communication and interaction processes and restrict critical thinking and problem solving. This, in turn, can affect group cohesion and goal accomplishment.

As mentioned earlier in this chapter, group cohesion involves all the factors that foster group stability and participant attraction to the group. One key factor influencing the attractiveness of the group to its members is the group's norms. Facilitative group norms can provide security for group participants and promote an environment that advances goal

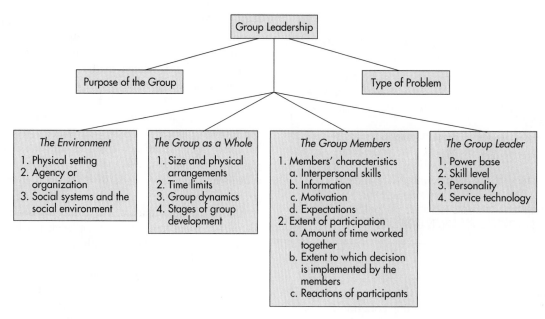

**FIGURE 23-2** An interactional model of group leadership. (From Toseland RW, Rivas RF: *An introduction to group work practice*, ed 4, Boston, 2001, Allyn and Bacon, p. 103. Reprinted with permission.)

achievement. It is important for a group leader to help group members establish and maintain an environment that assists its members to accomplish positive outcomes.

## Group Leadership

Effective leadership is fundamental to a positive group experience and involves leadership interventions that promote group movement toward defined goals. Group leadership is a complex phenomena influenced by multiple factors. Toseland and Rivas (2001) have developed an interactional model (Figure 23-2) to reflect the variables that impact group leadership. This model portrays leadership as a shared function and shows that leadership emerges from several interacting forces as the group develops and maintains itself (Toseland, Rivas, 2001). Both the designated group leader and group participants use leadership skills to move the group toward goal achievement.

Group leaders perform several important functions throughout the life of the group. During early group sessions they facilitate the development of a sense of cohesion and connectedness among group members, provide sufficient structure to maintain a secure group atmosphere, and help group participants identify group norms. During the later phases of the group, leadership functions focus on facilitating group processes, directing action toward realizing goal achievement, and evaluating the effectiveness and efficiency of the group process.

Group leaders use a variety of leadership skills to promote group movement toward defined goals. Examples of group leadership skills include focusing group discussion on substantive issues, clarifying content, thoughts, feelings, and behaviors, supporting expression of ideas and opinions, modeling effective communication and interaction patterns, and providing a structure for goal achievement. The Nursing Intervention Classification (NIC) System (McCloskey, Bulechek, 2000) further identifies activities nurses would implement when developing, implementing, and evaluating teaching and therapy groups. NIC is a valuable resource for identifying nursing activities that facilitate group process.

Community health nurses and community citizens are making a significant contribution to the public's health through group work. At times group intervention is focused on helping a small group of individuals with a defined need. At other times group efforts are focused on helping the community as a whole, such as the theater troupe at the Crystal Bartlett Neighborhood Health Center (see Box 23-1) that has been educating the community about substance abuse and ways to take back its streets. Groups like these also are helping communities provide alternative health and social services in local neighborhoods for individuals who have difficulty accessing care (Urban Health Institute for the Johns Hopkins University and the East Baltimore Community, 2001). Often these services are provided in neighborhood health centers, clinics, and community churches. These settings frequently provide a channel for reaching targeted, underserved populations.

## Stop and Think About It

Your local church has asked you to set up a health fair for their parishioners (Figure 23-3). It is anticipated that about 200 people consisting of all ages will attend. Using the stages in health communication process, think about how you would go about planning this educational event for this specific faith community.

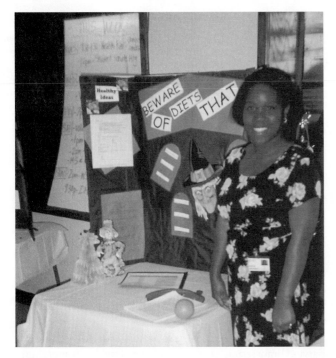

**FIGURE 23-3** Health fairs in malls, schools, churches, and other community settings are frequently conducted to educate the community as a whole about healthy lifestyle behaviors and community resources that provide health promotion services.

## POPULATION-FOCUSED CLINIC AND NURSING CENTER SERVICES

Community health nurses have long established clinics and nursing centers in local communities to reach targeted populations. Early efforts at the beginning of the century to improve maternal-child health and to control communicable disease frequently resulted in the development of clinic services for underserved populations. Between 1900 and 1930 many milk dispensaries evolved into preventive health centers.

In her history of the origins of nursing centers, Glass (1989) discusses how nursing centers were developed to serve populations at risk. She describes the work of Lillian Wald in milk dispensaries; the endeavors of Mary Breckinridge with the Frontier Nursing Service in Hyden, Kentucky; and the efforts of Margaret Sanger, the birth control activist in Europe and the United States. These three women were pioneer feminists who worked for the health of women, children, and families. Wald's extensive accomplishments are detailed in Chapter 1. In 1923 Breckinridge used the principles of program planning, described in Chapter 15, to determine where nursing services were needed in rural, mountainous Kentucky. After surveying a three-county area covering 1000 square miles, she concluded that a decentralized system of health care was essential. Based on her study, The Kentucky Committee for Mothers and Babies opened their

first nursing center in Hyden, Kentucky, in September 1925. By 1930 Breckinridge had established six nursing centers, each serving a 5-mile radius. The objectives for these centers were to provide skilled care for the sick of all ages and women in childbirth, health education for the population as a whole, and social services for vulnerable families. These nurses also promoted the advancement of economic independence (Glass, 1989).

Margaret Sanger (1870-1966) began her career as a visiting nurse in New York City. Her work with poor women and children stimulated her interest in birth control and women having control over their own bodies. Because the Comstock Act of 1873 declared birth control material obscene and prohibited the mailing of it, Sanger traveled to France to obtain information. She opened the first birth control clinic in America in 1916 in Brooklyn. The establishment of today's Planned Parenthood Federation is to her credit, and her contributions to the health of women are inestimable (Glass, 1989).

These are dramatic, wonderful examples of the beginnings of nursing centers as we know them today. Additionally, large-scale demonstration projects were sponsored by the Metropolitan Life Insurance Company to combat tuberculosis and other communicable diseases, and included programs of mass screening, health assessment, and community education activities (Kalisch, Kalisch, 1986). By the 1930s maternal and child health clinics were well established. These clinics provided safety net services for vulnerable populations in local communities throughout the twentieth century. During the later part of the twentieth century there was tremendous growth in ambulatory care or clinic services for populations across the lifespan. This trend will continue in the future.

## POPULATION-FOCUSED CLINIC SERVICES

**Clinics,** often called **ambulatory health services,** are centers that examine and treat clients on an outpatient basis. They are frequently operated under the auspices of a larger institution such as a hospital, neighborhood health center, group practice, health maintenance organization (HMO), health department, church, or community organization. Precisely identifying the services offered by clinics is difficult because they vary from one institution to another.

Clinic settings offer a wide range of preventive health services, often by an interdisciplinary team of professionals. Some clinics may provide only primary preventive interventions. This is usually the main focus in immunization clinics. Other clinics may provide screening, diagnosis, and treatment services, such as those provided by clinics treating sexually transmitted diseases (STDs). In these clinics STDs are identified, appropriate treatments are administered, and contacts of infected clients are located for screening.

Clinics may serve only a specific population. Well-baby clinics usually provide assessment services for children from birth to 5 years of age, and family planning clinics usually serve females of childbearing age. Or clinics may serve anyone who comes at any time with any problem, as do walk-in clinics of large teaching hospitals and neighborhood health centers. Emergency rooms function as ambulatory clinics in some towns where there are no other resources or when clients lack insurance.

The needs of populations at risk also have been addressed through the use of mobile clinics that target specific populations (McNeal, 1996; Therien, 2000). Communities are using mobile units to provide a wide array of health care, including dental services, multiphasic screenings, immunizations, family planning and pregnancy testing, and acute and chronic disease treatment services. Mobile health care units help professionals to outreach in underserved areas and are often the only source of care for some populations at risk. Through the use of these units, many of the primary and secondary preventive needs of at-risk populations in underserved areas can be addressed.

Many health, social service, and educational organizations are increasingly providing multiphasic diagnostic and primary health care services through clinics on an ongoing basis. Frequently, these services are targeted to specific population groups. For example, services for teens are increasingly being provided in settings, such as teen centers and school-based clinics, that are easily accessible, safe, and confidential (Blum, Beuhring, Wunderlich, et al., 1996; Ferretti, Verhey, Isham, 1996; Scott, 1996; Yawn, Yawn, 1997). The St. Paul Maternal and Child Health Program, one of the oldest school-based clinic projects, offers a wide range of services to students during school hours, such as immunizations, mental health counseling, prenatal care, family planning, and supportive group services (Maternal and Child Health Program, undated).

Significant community health need has provided the stimulus for the development of clinic services by private and official community health agencies. An example of this is how communities have responded to the needs of homeless populations by reaching out to them in a variety of nontraditional settings. In one inner-city community, a nursing clinic was established in a soup kitchen as a walk-in clinic for the homeless. Clinic hours coincided with the times that the soup kitchen was open. In this situation, nurses were able to provide health services in a familiar setting that met many of the physical and psychosocial needs of the homeless (Scholler-Jaquish, 1996).

**Community health centers (CHCs)** also have emerged to assist medically underserved populations. These centers, federally supported under Section 330 of the Public Health Service Act, are located throughout the nation. They exist in both urban and rural settings and serve persons with special needs, such as coal miners with respiratory and pulmonary impairments, the elderly, people who are confined to their homes, and migrant and seasonal farm workers.

Most migrant health centers are operated together with CHCs.

The type of care provided through clinics may be episodic, in which only the immediate needs of the clients are handled, or comprehensive, providing all levels of preventive services: primary preventive, diagnostic, therapeutic, and rehabilitative services. Primary preventive and diagnostic services (e.g., screening for infectious diseases or health risks such as high blood cholesterol) are frequently the focus in clinics sponsored by official health agencies.

## THE DEVELOPMENT OF NURSING CENTERS

A number of terms are used to refer to **nursing centers,** including *nurse-managed care, community nursing center* or *organization,* or *nurse-run clinic.* These terms refer to organizations in which nurses control practice and client care, and education and research are paramount (Riesch, 1992). Nurses do not always control practice in clinic or ambulatory care centers.

The American Nurses Association (ANA) (Aydelotte, Barger, Branstetter, et al., 1987) developed a comprehensive definition of nursing centers during the late 1980s. This definition highlights the significant responsibilities of nurses in these settings:

Nursing centers—sometimes referred to as nursing organizations, nurse-managed centers, nursing clinics, and community nursing centers—are organizations that give the client direct access to professional nursing services. Using nursing models of health, professional nurses in these centers diagnose and treat human responses to actual and potential health problems and promote health and optimal functioning among target populations and communities. The services provided in these centers are holistic and client centered and are reimbursable at a reasonable fee level. Accountability and responsibilities for client care and professional practice remain with the professional nurse. Overall accountability and responsibility remain with the nurse executive. Nursing centers may be freestanding businesses or may be affiliated with universities or other service institutions such as home health agencies and hospitals. The primary characteristic of the organization is responsiveness to the health needs of the population (Aydelotte, Barger, Branstetter, et al., 1987, p. 3).

As indicated previously in this chapter, nursing centers were developed at the turn of the twentieth century by Lillian Wald, Mary Breckenridge, and other pioneering public health nursing leaders. Contemporary nursing centers emerged as a significant force in the American health care system during the early 1970s. These centers were patterned on community health nursing models developed by nurse leaders in the early 1900s (Lundeen, 1999).

Nursing centers are being established in a variety of settings including housing projects (Anderson, 1996), homeless shelters (Gill, 2000), school-based settings (Krothe, Flynn, Ray, Goodwin, 2000; Lough, 1999), senior centers

(Shellman, 2000), and retirement communities (Arrington, 1997). Nursing centers provide a range of services based on the goals of the center and the populations being served. Some provide comprehensive primary care services while others provide only health promotion and referral services. The View from the Field at the end of the chapter showcases two academic nursing centers that demonstrate the variety of services delivered by these centers and gives some evidence of how students learn about models of care delivery that they can use in their own practice.

## Reimbursement of Nursing Center Services

Reimbursement for nursing center services is influenced by the type of care provided and the population served. Care offered by nursing centers may focus on health promotion and early casefinding services such as health education, health screening, and physical assessment or may span the entire range of primary care (Cole, Mackey, 1996; Ferretti, Verhey, Isham, 1996; Lundeen, 1999). Nursing centers may serve clients across the life span or a targeted population such as school-age children.

Care in nursing centers is reimbursed in several ways, including out-of-pocket fees, Medicare or Medicaid, and private insurance. Reimbursement also is provided through other financing mechanisms such as private foundation support, managed care contracts, worker compensation funding, and federal research and demonstration grants (Ferretti, Verhey, Isham, 1996; Starck, Mackey, Adams, 1995). Some funding sources only provide financial reimbursement for care to specific populations (e.g., veterans, migrants) or persons who meet specific criteria (e.g., poverty income to qualify for Medicaid). Criteria to obtain aid from several sources of funding are discussed in Chapter 4. A significant challenge for many nursing centers in the future will be how to financially survive in a changing health care environment. Some centers are forging relationships with managed care organizations or large organizational entities that can foster access to numbers of clients to strengthen their financial stability (Murphy, 1995). Other centers are also creatively developing relationships with other community organizations such as domestic violence centers and jails and are outsourcing their services to these agencies. Nursing centers are businesses established to meet unmet needs.

## ESTABLISHING POPULATION-FOCUSED CLINIC AND NURSING CENTER SERVICES

Community health nurses frequently assume a major role in planning, implementing, and evaluating services for populations with unmet health needs. When establishing new health care services, the nurse uses the health planning process described in Chapter 15. A discussion of some specific factors to consider when setting up clinic and nursing center services is addressed here.

Determining the need for clinic and nursing center services is the first responsibility of a health care professional interested in developing such services. Factors to consider during this process are the health status, lifestyle patterns, and demographic characteristics of the population being studied; community resources available to the population under consideration; health care utilization patterns; and health care access variables, such as location of resources and client referral processes. Chapter 14 describes how and where community health nurses obtain these data. When analyzing these data, it is important to examine trends over time and to identify strengths as well as limitations in the health care delivery system. The goal is to determine whether services are lacking or whether services are adequate but not used as a result of unique characteristics of the population being served or service delivery problems. For example, community health nurses have found that clients may not use clinic services because the location of these services makes them inaccessible or clients are unaware they exist. If a need is verified, careful planning should take place before starting a clinic or nursing center.

Several organizational activities need to be accomplished to ensure effective and efficient ambulatory care service delivery. Establishing specific objectives in collaboration with the targeted population helps the nurse determine what types of services to offer and resource needs. Resources needed to staff a center providing comprehensive primary care services would be significantly greater than those needed to staff a single purpose clinic such as an immunization clinic.

It is imperative that prospective clients and other stakeholders such as collaborative agencies are active members of the planning team. This involvement helps ensure that population-focused clinic or nursing center interventions address client needs. If interagency collaboration is needed to achieve proposed goals, responsibilities of each agency and financial arrangements should be clearly delineated. Identifying staff responsibilities helps the clinic staff to determine the resources needed to achieve desired outcomes.

Other organizational activities include determining the location for the clinic or center; securing necessary equipment and supplies; and organizing facilities to ensure client privacy and effective and efficient service delivery. These activities also involve establishing procedures such as follow-up policies that promote quality care, obtaining adequate professional staff with the skills needed to manage client health needs, securing and training volunteers, and developing marketing strategies. All of these activities require careful thought and planning and include several components. For example, securing necessary equipment and supplies involves such things as identifying what is needed, determining where to purchase it, and establishing appropriate storage procedures for vaccines, medications, and medical supplies.

Determining a site requires special attention because location of a clinic or a nursing center influences access of services and the way it will be used. Some clients are affected more than others by the location, namely, the poor and the aged. Difficulty and expense of access are important, so having knowledge of the possible transportation alternatives is important. Accessibility also involves appointment delay time, waiting time, clinic or nursing center hours, services offered, health care provided, and client/professional relationships.

Evaluation procedures should be established during the organizational phase of planning. An overall evaluation of operations should occur at least once a year, but evaluation is an ongoing process that needs attention regularly. Procedures need to be established to evaluate overall operations and usage patterns. Questions for planners to consider when evaluating services are shared in a later section of this chapter and in Chapter 15.

The importance of adequate planning when establishing a clinic or nursing center cannot be overstated. Neglecting significant details during the planning phase can result in poor use of services. For example, one local public agency decided to open a well-baby clinic because it was determined that a rural portion of a large county was underserved. The first decision made was to send a staff nurse to school for preparation as a pediatric nurse practitioner. However, steps of the planning process were not logically followed after preparing this staff nurse for new role responsibilities. Thus even though there were no other facilities for well-child care in the area, the clinic closed because of lack of clients. Many underserved clients could not use the service because there was no public transportation to the clinic.

## Role of the Community Health Nurse in Clinics and Nursing Centers

The community health nurse can function in various ways to meet the health needs of at-risk populations. Often agencies use an outreach approach to facilitate the identification of underserved clients who could benefit from clinic and nursing center services. **Outreach activities** are strategies designed to identify underserved populations who lack access to care. Nurses frequently are responsible for these activities. Outreach activities include such things as working with community leaders to advertise services, meeting with community agencies (e.g., domestic violence centers and homeless shelters) that normally work with underserved populations to identify potential clients, and using lay workers to survey families in their neighborhood about unmet needs.

The client populations being served in many clinics have complex needs. As the nurse practitioner movement evolved, nursing practice expanded to more adequately address the complex needs of people in clinics and nursing

centers. Nurses no longer serve as schedulers and receptionists. Their roles have enlarged to include case management services for clients with both acute and long-term care needs, handling of complex treatments and procedures, client counseling, and health education. Nurses are often the primary providers for many clients and their families. One study on elder client satisfaction with nursing services provided by a community-based nursing center found that access to services in the center "helped to increase the older adult's knowledge of healthy behaviors, prevented potential problems, and maintained or improved current level of health" (Scott, Moneyham, 1995, p. 186).

As mentioned previously, the range of activities implemented by a nurse in a clinic setting or nursing center varies, based on its objectives and the needs of clients. Common roles assumed by the nurse in many community health nursing centers or clinics are discussed in the following section.

**MANAGER.** The role of manager was the main nursing function in clinics for many years. Nurses attended to the many details necessary for clinics to run smoothly: distributing client caseload, following up on clients with problems, bringing needed reports to physicians, preparing clients physically for examinations, performing procedures, supervising aides and practical nurses, and carrying out clerical work. Although attention to these details is necessary, the nurse needs to also have time to perform essential nursing activities. The nurse should educate and supervise assistive personnel as described in Chapter 24, so that they can carry out the functions that do not require the professional skills of a registered nurse. This means that the nurse understands the different levels of functioning of team members and uses them appropriately. Clerks and aides, as well as volunteers, are valuable assets in the clinic. As they interact with clients these personnel can assist clients to become comfortable in the setting and can carry out several technical skills. They can weigh and measure babies, file and pull records, label and carry specimens to the laboratory, act as receptionists, and take temperatures. Smooth flow of clients from waiting to examining rooms is extremely important and can be facilitated by aides. As a manager, the community health nurse must understand that she or he is responsible for the care that these team members give. The nurse's supervision of team members is fundamental to the care given clients in the clinic setting.

In contemporary nursing centers nurses are assuming a broad range of advanced management responsibilities that focus on resource and personnel management issues. These responsibilities are discussed in Chapter 24. Nurse managers in nursing centers need to be particularly knowledgeable about system and community organizational concepts, financial management principles, and strategic planning processes. Nurse managers in these settings assume a major role in securing funds for developing, maintaining, and expanding center services. They also focus on the effective and efficient use of all levels of personnel to achieve defined outcomes.

GROUP LEADER AND EDUCATOR. An important function in many clinics and nursing centers is group education that is designed to promote healthy lifestyles. One example is a hypertension-screening clinic that uses the group process to disseminate information about lifestyle changes that can help clients prevent or cope with cardiac problems. Another example is a prenatal education program in a nursing center in which the community health nurse meets with clients before appointments to share information about pregnancy, childbirth, childcare, and role transition concerns. The concepts presented earlier in this chapter on developing and leading a group are applicable to the nurse's role in clinics as group leader and educator.

PRACTITIONER. The expanded role of the nurse has provided nurses with advanced physical assessment, diagnostic, and care management skills. Practitioners are able to identify the current health status of clients, including emotional and physical components, and to plan interventions that meet clients' needs. Practitioners carry out a variety of functions in both adult and child health clinics. They provide physical, mental, social, and emotional support, educate clients about their health conditions, diagnose and treat common health problems, and refer clients to needed community resources. Practitioners often work with an interdisciplinary team and actively participate in client care conferences. They provide a continuum of nursing services, especially for clients who have chronic health conditions or preventive health needs.

EVALUATOR. An integral part of working in population-focused settings is evaluation. This process was discussed in depth in Chapter 15. Examples of questions to ask when evaluating clinic or nursing center services include the following: Are the objectives of the clinic or nursing center being met? If this is the immunization clinic in Smith County, for example, are children completely immunized at age 2 and upon school entrance? Are the numbers of clients being served increasing or decreasing? If the number of clients being served is changing, is it because the health service area population is changing or because clients feel that they are not being served adequately? The way clients feel about the care they receive determines whether they will continue to use the health facility. Some formal method for obtaining client feedback on a regular basis, either questionnaire or interview, is needed to provide data concerning client satisfaction. Knowing who is served is also very important and means that a record system will be in operation so that number and kinds of visits can be tabulated easily. A good record system will help provide continuity of care from one visit to the next and analyze client needs and service outcomes. Information

technology is helping nurses in all settings to effectively and efficiently evaluate health outcomes.

## COMMUNITY HEALTH NURSING IN NONTRADITIONAL PRACTICE SETTINGS

In addition to clinic and nursing center services, community health nurses are increasingly working with a team of health care providers in nontraditional settings to provide services for underserved populations. An important role for community health nurses on these teams is to promote the philosophy of community health practice: orientation to wellness rather than illness, family-centered versus individual-centered care, continuous rather than episodic intervention, and population- and community-focused health planning. Regardless of where community health nurses function, these concepts should be central to their practice. As discussed in Chapter 2, it is *the nature of the practice*—not the setting—that distinguishes community health nursing from other specialty nursing areas. The concepts of community health nursing greatly enrich service delivery and nursing care in any setting.

Coordinated community-wide approaches targeted to specific populations are often needed to identify and help underserved groups in the community. Community health nurses have unique skills and knowledge to address this challenge and have diligently worked to expand services to these groups. The roles community health nurses have assumed in block nursing and parish nursing illustrate how nurses have used their skills to provide care for populations frequently not served by other professionals in the community and to expand health promotion services for specific groups of people in the community.

### Block Nursing and Parish Nursing

Block nursing and parish nursing are two creative, alternative ways for addressing the needs of specific populations in the community. Both provide a nontraditional setting for practice and are based on a holistic philosophy that addresses health promotion as well as curative health services. These settings provide an opportunity for nurses to use population-focused nursing interventions to assist clients in accessing health services. These interventions have prevented institutionalization for many people in the community. Both settings also provide opportunities for nurses to practice autonomous professional nursing and have helped clients obtain services lacking in other areas of the health care system (Armmer, Humbles, 1995; Jamieson, 1990).

Jamieson (1990) described block **nursing** as nursing on the block where the nurse lives, making services available based on need rather than reimbursement eligibility. Professional and volunteer community members; an informal network of family, friends, neighbors, church, and civic groups; service groups such as Boy and Girl Scouts; and people who are part of the neighborhood provide many of the services needed. These services include shopping, running errands, and providing respite care to relieve caregivers. Funding to pay for client assessments and direct care provided by aides/homemakers and nurses has come from sources such as grants, client fees, and demonstration projects. One block nurse program prevented hospitalization for 25% of its clientele. Referrals for block nursing services frequently come by word of mouth from the neighborhood. Block nursing "is reminiscent of earlier eras when a nurse was involved with a total community and all its citizens" (Jamieson, 1990, p. 251). Some nursing cen-

ters extend their services to the community in a similar way as block nursing.

**Parish nursing** meets many of the same needs as block nursing. However, churches and synagogues provide the system whereby the services are offered.

Churches and synagogues have been promoting health and wholeness for centuries through the ministries of worship, music, sharing and caring. A new dimension is the addition of the nurse to the ministry team. For the past dozen years, nurses across the state and across the country have been using their nursing skills to demonstrate religious witness. Some are volunteers; some are paid; some just get mileage. Some train volunteers; others actually staff the

---

### BOX 23-7

## *Standards of Parish Nurse Practice*

*Standards of Care*

**STANDARD I. ASSESSMENT**
The parish nurse collects client health data.

**STANDARD II. DIAGNOSIS**
The parish nurse analyzes the collected data about the client to determine the diagnosis.

**STANDARD III. OUTCOME IDENTIFICATION**
The parish nurse, with the client, identifies expected outcomes specific to the client's desired health outcomes.

**STANDARD IV. PLANNING**
The parish nurse assists the client in developing a plan for health promotion and other interventions that empowers the client to achieve desired health outcomes. The plan identifies the self-care activities to be done by the client, the interdependence with other systems, the interventions to be performed by the parish nurse, and the collaboration with and referral to other health care professionals and providers on the basis of the expected outcomes.

**STANDARD V. IMPLEMENTATION**
The parish nurse assists the client in implementing the interventions identified in the health promotion plan.

**STANDARD VI. EVALUATION**
The parish nurse continually evaluates client responses to interventions in order to determine the progress made toward desired outcomes.

*Standards of Professional Performance*

**STANDARD I. QUALITY OF CARE**
The parish nurse systematically participates in evaluation of the quality and effectiveness of his or her parish nursing practice.

**STANDARD II. PERFORMANCE APPRAISAL**
The parish nurse evaluates his or her own nursing practice in relation to professional standards, relevant statutes, and regulations.

**STANDARD III. EDUCATION**
The parish nurse acquires and maintains current knowledge in nursing practice and health promotion.

**STANDARD IV. COLLEGIALITY**
The parish nurse contributes to the professional development of peers, colleagues, and other health ministers.

**STANDARD V. ETHICS**
The parish nurse's decisions and actions reflect and are guided by client, personal, and professional ethical considerations.

**STANDARD VI. COLLABORATION**
The parish nurse collaborates with the client system, other health ministers, health care providers, and community agencies in promoting client health.

**STANDARD VII. RESEARCH**
The parish nurse uses research findings in practice.

**STANDARD VIII. RESOURCE UTILIZATION**
The parish nurse considers the effectiveness measures of appropriateness, accessibility, acceptability, and affordability of resources in the development and implementation of health promotion programs for clients.

Source: Health Ministries Association, American Nurses Association: *Scope and standards of parish nursing practice,* Washington, DC, 1998, American Nurses Publishing, American Nurses Foundation/American Nurses Association. Reprinted with permission.

program. Some minister to their congregations only; others reach out into their communities. *Parish nursing* takes many forms, depending on each congregation—its needs, visions, and resources (Parish nursing, 1993, p. 1).

"A **parish nurse,** sometimes known as a faith community nurse, is a registered professional nurse who is hired or recognized by a faith community to carry forward an intentional health promotion ministry" (Clark, Olson, 2000, p. 3). Faith communities are ideal settings for health promotion activities because these communities have health and healing missions that support their parishioners to achieve specific health goals (Buijs, Olson, 2001).

The role of the parish nurse is relatively new. The first institutionally based parish nurse program emerged in 1984 and, as a result, more parish nurse programs are continuing to develop throughout the United States (Djupe, 1996). Currently, four **parish nursing practice models** exist: (1) *hospital-sponsored,* in which the nurse works for the institution; (2) *parish-based,* in which the nurse is hired by the church; (3) *hospital-sponsored volunteer,* in which nurses associated with specific institutions volunteer to provide resource information to the parishioners in their congregation; and (4) *congregation-based,* which is a volunteer model in which the nurses from within a congregation volunteer to provide resources and services to the congregation (Armmer, Humbles, 1995, p. 66). Regardless of the model used, the parish nurse endeavors to provide holistic care by providing a variety of services through various roles.

The most common roles of the parish nurse include *health educator, health counselor, resource* and *referral agent, volunteer coordinator,* and *facilitator* or *troubleshooter.* The parish nurse helps bridge gaps between the parishioners and the health care system (Armmer, Humbles, 1995; Buijs, Olson, 2001; Djupe, 1996; Dunkle, 1996). The standards of practice in Box 23-7, developed by the Health Ministries Association (1998) and published by the ANA, guide nurses as they implement these roles. The accompanying "A View from the Field" box examines nursing interventions implemented by one parish nurse. The *International Parish Nurse Resource Center* in Park Ridge, Illinois (1-800-556-5368), is a valuable resource for persons interested in starting a health ministry.

Both block nursing and parish nursing are population- and community-focused interventions that meet needs that are not met by the traditional health care system. Both also build on the concept of nursing neighbors in one's community. Likely, not even the best national health care package will meet everyone's needs. Therefore, the idealism of these services should continue to be part of community health nursing. These nontraditional alternatives can serve as a guide for caring for others in unique and holistic ways.

## A view from the field

### PARISH NURSE CASE STUDY

An 82-year-old man had not been to church for 18 years. On my first two attempts to visit him at his home, I was not permitted to enter. When I finally obtained permission to enter the kitchen on my third try, I noticed a deck of cards on the table. I asked if he played cards. The answer was a resounding yes. For the next 2 hours we played cards. Not much dialogue was shared. I asked if I might return again the same time next week. A positive response was given. After 3 weeks of card playing, the man began to tell his story of life. The man had lost his wife to cancer 18 years ago and had been left with an 11-year-old daughter to raise. He was the postmaster of a small town, and the mail had to continue being delivered. Through his own reflection and discovery, he realized he had never cried. He was able to do so with me and thus began the grieving process. He realized that he had become paralyzed with fear and that in his living he was just trying to survive. Through our discussions he was able to accept a referral to a physician for treatment of depression.

After 2 months he began to come to church for the potlucks. He was welcomed back enthusiastically and rekindled two old friendships. After 4 months of telling his story, he was volunteering and coordinating the mailing of the church's newsletter. He also was coordinating a team of three other volunteers who were assisting him. As a parish nurse, I was able to be with this individual in his journey and was able to allow him to rediscover who he was and where he had been. This ultimately helped him to reclaim life with a quality he desired.

This example clearly shows what can happen when the practitioner utilizes the knowledge, skills, and values of an individual. It was through the values of self-awareness, appreciation of the client's whole person, respect for the mind/body/spirit unity, and the importance of being open and nonjudgmental that I was able to establish a relationship that allowed the individual to rediscover who he was and become a functioning human being and a contributing member of a community.

Cohen EL, De Back V: *The outcomes mandate: case management in health care today,* St Louis, 1999, Mosby, pp. 149, 150.

## NURSING CENTER MODELS: CASE STUDIES IN SUCCESS

### Southern Illinois University at Edwardsville Community Nursing Services

*By Barbara C. Martin, EdD, RNC; Jacalyn Ryberg, MA, RNC; and Jacquelyn Clement, PhD, RN*

The Southern Illinois University at Edwardsville (SIUE) Community Nursing Services provides an ideal setting for a community health experience. In this primarily black, inner city community, a clinical practicum for senior nursing students was developed with the local Head Start program in 1989.

Students were originally involved with case management for children with identified health problems. They worked with families to ensure that the children had access to appropriate care. Working with families provided an excellent community health experience for nursing students and resulted in faster, more comprehensive resolution of health problems for Head Start children.

The program later expanded to include health screening services. The nursing students set up screening sites, collect blood samples, operate the screening test machines, identify health problems, and keep records.

As the students and faculty identify health problems, there is an increased opportunity to speak with the teachers, and on occasion, parents. This dialogue facilitates information sharing and early intervention for the children.

In the summer of 1989, an elderly component was added to the practicum. In conjunction with the local housing authority, the students began to collect emergency data on a *Health Alert Form*. This form helps keep all pertinent data on the elderly residents of public housing in one accessible place.

The form is maintained in an opaque sleeve on the back of each apartment hall door. It is available to emergency teams, family members, and health care workers assuring continuity of care. Students visit the elderly in their homes, interview them, fill out the forms, and identify problems. In follow-up visits they do basic health education and medication teaching. They are also able to relate to problems of independent living that commonly occur upon hospital discharge.

Students appreciate the opportunity for practical application of the cultural concepts they learn in class as they are exposed to multigenerational families, elders in independent living settings, and accessing limited resources for those with limited financial assets.

As the nursing center grows, the educational experience opportunities for the students will expand. The potential benefits to clients, the community, the students, and the center are only limited by imagination.

### University of Texas Nursing Services—Houston

*By Glenda C. Walker, DSN, RN*

In February 1991, The University of Texas School of Nursing at the Health Science Center in Houston (UTNS-H) opened an ambulatory nursing service center. The purposes of the UTNS-H were to provide educational and research opportunities for students and faculty.

At UTNS-H categories or clinical services include: high risk screening, health education, well child care, and home infusion therapy. Other services currently under development include: geriatric nursing care, women's health care, and psychiatric health care. When deviations from normal are found, clients are referred to either their private physician or the UT Family Practice clinic. When the client needs follow-up monitoring and/or educational services, they are referred back to UTNS-H. This type of arrangement allows for cost-effective services delivered by the most appropriate provider with an emphasis on continuity of care.

UTNS-H also provides health education seminars on such topics as chronic disease, healthy lifestyles, stress management, and safety in the work place. In addition, ongoing health education classes are provided for clients who are referred to UTNS-H needing health education counseling, such as nutritional management of diabetes. UTNS-H encourages consumer/client responsibility and accountability for the management of their health care.

Well-child services provided by UTNS-H include: well-baby examinations (EPSDT), immunizations, TB skin tests, school physicals, and parenting classes. These services are provided at a variety of settings with an emphasis on easy access. For example, the UTNS-H pediatric nurse practitioner has provided EPSDT screenings at the City of Houston housing project apartments. In addition, a UTNS-H pediatric nurse practitioner provides well-child services at a community-based health clinic five mornings a week. A collaborative agreement with UT Department of Pediatrics allows for supervision of the medical protocols, consultation regarding cases, and referrals to the department for those clients needing more extensive care.

UTNS-H provides home IV infusion services for clients who need continuing care within the home environment. A case management approach is used to meet the physical and emotional needs of the family and clients. It is believed that this approach will strengthen the coping resources of the family thereby minimizing costly rehospitalization.

As nursing embraces and lobbies for *Nursing's Agenda for Health Care Reform*, it is important for nursing centers to analyze how their activities correlate with that agenda. An initial analysis of UTNS-H activities and the agenda has proven successful for our current path.

From National League for Nursing, Council for Nursing Centers: *Connections,* New York, Winter 1992, NLN, p. 2.

## SUMMARY

Community health nurses carry out numerous roles and functions in a variety of settings to meet the health care needs and goals of populations at risk in the community. Some roles implemented by nurses in the community setting are manager, health educator, health counselor, resource and referral agent, group leader, practitioner, and health planner. This chapter addresses how nurses implement these roles in clinic, nursing center, parish, and neighborhood or block settings to address the needs of populations across the life span. It also addresses how nurses use the group process to provide targeted preventive services. The emphasis is on working cooperatively with clients in identifying appropriate ways to deliver community health nursing services.

Increasingly, with a focus on cost containment, health care agencies are using creative ways to meet the needs of underserved populations in the community. It is important to remember that no one method will meet everyone's health needs. Nurses work in collaboration with clients to identify which interventions will effectively and efficiently assist them. This kind of choice contributes to the challenge, excitement, and creativity of community health nursing. It brings nurses closer to clients in the community and provides a stimulus for developing innovative nontraditional practice. Nurses' involvement in planning for the future will help them maintain a viable role for nursing in the evolving health care system.

## CRITICAL THINKING
### *exercises*

The accompanying View from the Field box contains descriptions of two academic nursing centers, demonstrating the variety of services offered by this segment of the health care delivery system. Think about the services offered and how they differ from the traditional clinic services that are part of many neighborhoods. Considering the characteristics of the community you are serving, identify populations at risk that could benefit from nursing center services. Additionally, identify potential locations for a nursing center and the type of services needed by at-risk groups in your community.

## REFERENCES

Anderson A: Nursing clinics in urban settings, *Home Health Nurse* 14(7):542-546, 1996.

Armmer FA, Humbles P: Parish nursing: extending health care to urban African-Americans, *Nurs Health Care* 16(2):64-68, 1995.

Arrington DT: Retirement communities as creative clinical opportunities, *Nurs Health Care Perspectives* 18:82-83, 1997.

Aydelotte MK, Barger SE, Branstetter E, Resnick M: *The nursing center: concept and design*, Kansas City, Mo, 1987, American Nurses Association.

Blum RW, Beuhring T, Wunderlich M, et al.: Don't ask, they won't tell: the quality of adolescent health screening in five practice settings, *Am J Public Health* 86(12):1767-1772, 1996.

Bracht N, editor: *Health promotion at the community level*, ed 2, Thousand Oaks, Calif, 1999, Sage.

Buijs R, Olson J: Parish nurses influencing determinants of health, *J Community Health Nurs* 18(1):13-23, 2001.

Bulechek G, McCloskey J: *Nursing interventions: effective nursing treatments*, ed 3, Philadelphia, 1999, WB Saunders.

Clark CC: *The nurse as group leader*, ed 3, New York, 1994, Springer Publishing Co.

Clark M, Olson J: *Nursing within a faith community: promoting health in times of transition*, Thousand Oaks, Calif, 2000, Sage.

Clark NM, Janz NK, Dodge JA, Sharpe PA: Self-regulation of health behavior: the "Take PRIDE" program, *Health Educ Q* 19:341-354, 1992.

Clark NM, McLeroy KR: Creating capacity through health education; what we know and what we don't, *Health Educ Q* 22:273-289, 1995.

Cohen EL, De Back V: *The outcomes mandate: case management in health care today*, St Louis, 1999, Mosby.

Cole FL, Mackey T: Utilization of an academic nursing center, *J Prof Nurs* 12:349-353, 1996.

Corey MS, Corey G: *Groups: process and practice*, ed 5, Pacific Grove, Calif, 1997, Brooks/Cole Publishing.

Corey MS, Corey G: *Groups: process and practice*, ed 6, Pacific Grove, Calif, 2002, Brooks/Cole Publishing.

DeLucia-Waack JL: The field of group work: past, present, and future, *Journal Specialists Group Work* 25(4):323-326, 2000.

Djupe AM: Parish nursing. In Cohen EL: *Nurse case management in the 21st century*, St Louis, 1996, Mosby.

Dunkle RM: Parish nurses help patients—body and soul, *RN* 59(5):55-57, 1996.

Ferretti CK, Verhey MP, Isham MM: Development of a nurse-managed, school-based health center, *Nurse Educ* 21:35-42, 1996.

Freudenberg N, Eng E, Flay B, et al.: Strengthening individual and community capacity to prevent disease and promote health: in search of relevant theories and principles, *Health Educ Q* 22(3):290-306, 1995.

Gill KM: My story: evolving a faculty-student practice in a homeless shelter, *Nurs Forum* 35(1):31-35, 2000.

Glanz K, Rimer B: *Theory at a glance: a guide for health promotion practice*, Washington DC, 1997, National Cancer Institute.

Glass LK: The historic origins of nursing centers. In *Nursing centers: meeting the demand for quality health care*, Pub No 21-2311, New York, 1989, National League for Nursing.

Hare A, Blumberg H, Davies M, Kent M: *Small group research: a handbook*, Norwood, NJ, 1995, Ablex.

Health Ministries Association: *Scope and standards of parish nursing practice*, Washington, DC, 1998, American Nurses Publishing.

Health Resources and Services Administration (HRSA): *Eliminating health disparities in the United States*, Rockville, Md, 2000, HRSA.

Humphreys K, Ribisl K: The case for a partnership with self-help groups, *Public Health Reports* 114(5):114-327, 1999.

Jamieson MK: Block nursing: practicing autonomous professional nursing in the community, *Nurs Health Care* 11(5):250-253, May 1990.

Kalisch PA, Kalisch BJ: *The advance of American nursing*, ed 2, Boston, 1986, Little, Brown.

Krothe JS, Flynn B, Ray D, Goodwin S: Community development through faculty practice in a rural nurse-managed clinic, *Public Health Nurs* 17(4):264-272, 2000.

Lewin K: Group decision and social change. In Newcomb TM, Hartley EL, editors: *Readings in social psychology*, New York, 1947, Holt.

Loomis ME: *Group process for nurses*, St Louis, 1979, Mosby.

Lough MA: An academic-community partnership: a model of service and education, *J Community Health Nurs* 16(3):137-149, 1999.

Lundeen S: An alternative paradigm for promoting health in communities: the Lundeen Community Nursing Center Model, *Fam Community Health* 21(4):15-28, 1999.

MacKenzie KR, editor: *Effective use of group therapy in managed care*, Washington, DC, 1995, American Psychiatric Press.

Marín G, Burhansstipanov L, Connell CM, et al.: A research agenda for health education among underserved populations, *Health Educ Q* 22(3):346-363, 1995.

Maternal and Child Health Program: *St. Paul Adolescent Health Services Project*, St Paul, Minn, undated, St. Paul-Ramsey Medical Center.

McCloskey JC, Bulechek GM, editors: *Nursing interventions classification* (NIC), ed 3, St Louis, 2000, Mosby.

McNeal GJ: Mobile health care for those at risk, *Nurs Health Care* 17(3):134-140, 1996.

Minnesota Department of Health (MDH): *Public health interventions: examples from public health nursing*, Minneapolis, Minn, 1997, MDH.

Mullen PD, Evans D, Forster J, et al.: Settings as an important dimension in health education/promotion policy, programs, and research, *Health Educ Q* 22(3):330-347, 1995.

Murphy B, editor: *Nursing centers: the time is now*, New York, 1995, National League for Nursing Press.

Murray R, Zentner J: *Health promotion strategies through the life span*, ed 7, Upper Saddle River, NJ, 2001, Prentice Hall.

National Institutes of Health (NIH): *Making health communication programs work: a planner's guide*, Atlanta, 1995, USDHHS. Retrieved from the internet April 1, 2001. *http://rex.nci.nih.gov/NCI_Pub_Interface/HCPW/OVER.HTM*

National League for Nursing (NLN), Council for Nursing Centers: *Connections*, New York, Winter 1992, NLN.

O'Neil EH, Pew Health Professions Commission: *Recreating health professional practice for a new century*, San Francisco, 1998, Pew Health Professions Commission.

Page BJ, Delmonico DL, Walsh J, et al.: Setting up on-line support groups using the palace software, *Journal for Specialists in Group Work* 25(2):133-145, 2000.

Parish nursing, *Penn Nurse* 48:1, July 1993, Pennsylvania State Nurses Association.

Riesch SK: Nursing centers. In Fitzpatrick JJ, Tauton RL, Jacox AK, editors: *Annu Rev Nurs Res*, vol 10, New York, 1992, Springer.

Scholler-Jaquish A: Walk-in health clinic for the homeless, *Nurs Health Care* 17(3):119-123, 1996.

Scott CB, Moneyham L: Perceptions of senior residents about a community-based nursing center, *Image J Nurs Sch* 27(3)181-186, 1995.

Scott MAK: Reducing the risks: adolescents and sexually transmitted diseases, *Nurse Pract Forum* 7(1):23-29, 1996.

Shellman J: Promoting elder wellness through a community-based blood pressure clinic, *Public Health Nurs* 17(4):257-263, 2000.

Sleek S: Group therapy: tapping the power of teamwork, *The APA Monitor* 26(7):1, 38-39, 1995.

Starck PL, Mackey TA, Adams J: Nurse-managed clinics: a blueprint for success using the Covey framework, *J Prof Nurs* 11:71-77, 1995.

Steckler A, Allegrante JP, Altman D, et al.: Health education intervention strategies: recommendations for future research, *Health Educ Q* 22:307-328, 1995.

Therien J: Establishing a mobile health and wellness program for rural veterans, *Nurs Clin North Am* 35(2):499-505, 2000.

Toseland RW, Rivas RF: *An introduction to group work practice*, ed 4, Boston, 2001, Allyn and Bacon.

US Department of Health and Human Services (USDHHS): *Healthy People 2010*, Washington, DC, 2000, US Government Printing Office.

Urban Health Institute for the John Hopkins University and the East Baltimore Community: Neighborhoods taking the lead in the fight against substance abuse, *Urban* 1(3):1, 2001.

Vacha-Haase T, Ness C, Dannison L, Smith A: Grandparents raising grandchildren: a psychoeducational group approach, *Journal for Specialists in Group Work* 25(1):67-78, 2000.

Yawn BP, Yawn RA: Adolescent pregnancy: a preventable consequence? *The Prevention Researcher* 4(1):1-4, Winter, 1997.

## SELECTED BIBLIOGRAPHY

Carletta J, Garrod S, Fraser-Krauss H: Placement of authority and communication patterns in workplace groups, *Small Group Research* 29(5):531-559, 1998.

Doyle E, Ward S: *The process of community health education and promotion*, Mountain View, Calif, 2001, Mayfield.

Furr SR: Structuring the group experience: a format for designing psychoeducational groups, *Journal for Specialists in Group Work*, 25(1):29-49, 2000.

Hays B, Sather L, Peters DA: Quantifying client needs for care in the community: a strategy for managed care, *Public Health Nurs* 16(4):246-253, 1999.

Johnson MO: Meeting health care needs of a vulnerable population: perceived barriers, *J Community Health Nurs* 18(1):35-52, 2001.

Keller LO, Strohschein S, Lia-Hoagberg B, et al.: Population-based public health nursing interventions: a model from practice, *Public Health Nurs* 15(3):207-215, 1998.

Kosidlak JG: The development and implementation of a population-based intervention model for public health nursing practice, *Public Health Nurs* 16(5):311-320, 1999.

Kreuter M, Lezin N, Kreuter M, et al.: *Community health promotion ideas that work: a field-book for practitioners*, Sudbury, Mass, 1998, Jones and Bartlett.

Merta RJ: Group work: multicultural perspectives: In Ponterotto J, Casus M, Suzuki A, et al., editors: *Handbook of multicultural counseling*, Newbury Park, Calif, 1995, Sage.

Morgan B, Hinsley L: Supporting working mothers through group work: a multimodel psychoeducational approach, *Journal for Specialists in Group Work* 23(3):298-316, 1998.

Novick LF, Mays GP: *Public health administration: principles for population-based management*, Gaithersburg, Md, 2001, Aspen.

Redman B: *The practice of patient education*, ed 8, St Louis, 1997, Mosby.

Selby ML, Riportella-Muller R, Sorenson JR, et al.: Improving EPSDT use: development and application of a practice-based model for public health nursing research, *Public Health Nurs* 6:174-181, 1989.

Solari-Twadell PA, McDermott MA, editors: *Parish nursing: promoting whole person health within faith communities*, Thousand Oaks, Calif, 1999, Sage.

Villa V: The demography, health and economic status of minority elderly populations: implication for aging programs and services, *J Geriatr Case Management* 18(2):5-8, 1999.

# 24

# Utilizing Management Concepts in Community Health Nursing

*Kathy Jo Ellison*

## OBJECTIVES

*Upon completion of this chapter, the reader should be able to:*

1. Explain how a staff-level community health nurse uses management and change concepts in the practice setting.
2. Analyze how the structure of an organization and the power relationships influence the nurse's role in decision making.
3. Describe the importance of the customer, change, and competition to health organizations.
4. Describe the five management functions used by community health nurses.
5. Discuss the elements involved in caseload analysis.
6. Describe the use of district, team, and case management care delivery models in community health nursing.
7. Describe the implications of managed care for priority determination and caseload management in community health nursing.
8. Describe factors to consider when scheduling community health nursing activities.
9. Identify selected ANA standards that can guide management practice in a community health nursing setting.
10. Describe outcomes assessment in community health.

## KEY TERMS

Administration
Case analysis
Case management nursing
Caseload analysis
Change model
Delegation

District nursing
Leadership
Leadership effectiveness model
Management
Management functions
Reengineering

Situational leadership
Team nursing
Teamwork
Technology
Telehealth

*We cannot direct the wind...*
*But we can adjust the sails.*

UNKNOWN

The community is an exciting setting that provides challenging opportunities for community health nurses. Community health nurses find themselves working in increasingly complex and diverse settings. An outstanding characteristic of community health nursing is the *independence* of its practice. In any one day, a community health nurse may decide what families to visit and in what order they will be visited. During that day the nurse may carry out nursing interventions without direct nursing supervision, without a doctor's order, or without even talking to another nurse. That day, the nurse may also receive new referrals and make decisions on their priority. Also, the nurse may be carrying out nursing care indirectly through delegation to licensed practical nurses, home health aides, or other assistive personnel. This independence and scope of community health nursing practice necessitates knowledge of management concepts. Available resources, such as finances and personnel, need to be managed so that maximum productivity, efficiency, and quality of care are achieved.

Managing the extensive amounts of data that community health nurses collect and use is increasingly complex. Computerized management information systems are crucial for today's community health nurse manager: these systems are being used by agencies across the country to facilitate effective and efficient resource management. Staff nurses use these systems as well to schedule and document client care and to communicate with members of the health care team.

Our knowledge base is rapidly expanding, technological advances are increasing the complexity of community-based care, and ethical dilemmas once reserved exclusively to the hospital have moved into the home and community. These increasing pressures coupled with rising costs and constrained resources are creating the need for more nurses in leadership roles. Good nursing managers who are able to tackle these challenges, as well as be proactive, are more important than ever before in guiding organizations and the profession toward positive outcomes and improved client care.

Whatever role a nurse assumes in the community setting, be it staff nurse, supervisor, or administrator, the nurse will participate in leadership and management functions. Community health nursing, like the management process, is a logical activity that helps clients, families, and aggregates make goal-directed changes. The nurse facilitates these changes through the work of others. Thus a conscious application of the management process to nursing care at any level can make the nurse more effective in arranging his or her own personal workload, as well as in functioning within a larger system.

This chapter looks at concepts of management for the community health nurse. The overall goal in discussing management concepts is to provide the information an individual needs to formulate a personal philosophy of management.

## THE HISTORICAL DEVELOPMENT OF MANAGEMENT CONCEPTS

Numerous leaders in the field of management contributed to its development. To list them all would be almost impossible. Modern concepts of management have evolved over time. Historically, emphasis was placed on analyzing the functions and processes of management tasks, without taking into consideration the needs of the worker (see Chapter 21). Later the trend was for managers to apply systems concepts in the work environment to determine how to maintain employee satisfaction and to increase productivity and efficiency. Today the emphasis is on the people and the processes in which they participate to make responsive and competitive organizations that create valued services for their customers (clients).

*Frederick Taylor* is the founder of the scientific management movement. His belief was that planning tasks should be separate from performing them. In relation to this thought, he felt that managers should be responsible for planning and controlling tasks and that employees should assume responsibility for production. He conducted *time-and-motion studies* to determine the best way to accomplish tasks, to develop work standards, and to identify how to divide the work between managers and employees. Taylor's book, *The Principles of Scientific Management*, was published in 1911.

*Henri Fayol* expanded on Taylor's thoughts by identifying a composite of well-defined functions and tasks for managers. In 1916 he published his ideas about management, which included the notion that managers have five basic functions: *planning, organizing, commanding, coordinating, and controlling*. With some minor changes, these functions are still used by most authorities on management. In a recent study of midmanagers in health care organizations, Timmreck (2000) found the classic management functions are in fact extensively used today. Managers in this study reported oral communication and problem solving as their top issues and organizing, coordinating, planning, and directing as the top four management functions used.

Significant criticism of management occurred during the first half of the twentieth century because managers emphasized task performance without looking at worker satisfaction. As a result of this criticism, modern management trends that focused on the importance of examining employee needs emerged. The classic Hawthorne experiment conducted by Elton Mayo clearly demonstrated to management the value of looking at employees as people.

The *Hawthorne Studies* of the Western Electric Company during the 1920s and 1930s applied the principles of psychology, social psychology, and sociology to the understanding of organizational behavior. The researchers of this study began by investigating the relationship between physical conditions of work and employee productivity. However, they found that social variables were much more important to productivity. The outgrowth of the Hawthorne study was the concept of human relations, or the study of human behavior for the purposes of attaining higher production levels and personal satisfaction. The human relations concept has expanded into the behavioral science approach to management. A trend toward emphasizing employee satisfaction to increase production on the job is still visible. Employee motivation, the workplace as a social system, leadership within the organization, communication within the system, and personal and professional employee development are major areas of concern to managers who use behavioral science methods and principles.

The *systems approach* was another development among management concepts. With the systems approach, both the structure and the processes of an organization are analyzed. Emphasis is placed on examining how all the parts of an organization interact and interrelate to achieve the goals of the organization. Systems managers recognize that a change in one part of the organizational system affects all the other parts, just as practitioners using a systems approach recognize that a change (illness) in the family unit affects all other members of the family system (see Chapter 7).

## Chaos Theory

Changing the manner in which systems are explored was described by Gleick (1987) in his book *Chaos,* which examined "the science of the global nature of systems" (p. 5). In contrast to Taylor's work and the work of others, Gleick examined systems holistically. Taylor and those who followed him used a *reductionistic approach:* complex phenomena could be understood by reducing them to their basic building blocks and looking at the mechanisms through which they interact. For example, a health care agency would be analyzed department by department for its effectiveness under the science of reductionism. The sum of how each department functioned would result in the effectiveness of the organization. The science of chaos examines the system holistically and focuses on the dynamics of the overall system and the order that comes from the interactions of the parts of the whole.

The importance of the science of chaos for managers, leaders, and all employees was discussed by Freedman (1992), who based his thoughts on the work of both Gleick (1987) and Senge (1990). Managers think that they know their organizations because they believe in the reductionistic theory of cause and effect. If the workers for whom they are responsible carry out their job descriptions, the objectives of the organization will be reached. However, the relationship between cause and effect is much more complicated than many people understand. People working in an organization, when asked what they do, describe the daily tasks that they do rather than the system in which they work. Frequently workers believe that they have little impact on this system. The science of chaos tells managers that their employees' tiniest thoughts and actions have a dramatic impact on the agency system. Senge (1990) reported that managers who master systems thinking have "learning organizations" (p. 37). Such organizations are highly decentralized, and decision making at the department level maintains order throughout to constantly adjust to change.

## A Leader Effectiveness Model

Hersey, Blanchard, and Johnson (2001) describe a leadership effectiveness model in which managers must use the appropriate leadership style in working with various people in different situations. This tridimensional theory is based on the relationships among the amount of direction (task behavior) and the socioemotional support (relationship behavior) the leader must provide and the level of task-relevant readiness of their followers. To be most effective, leaders must consider factors such as the expectations of their boss, their associates (peers), and the organization as well as job demands and time. Using this theory, leaders assess themselves, look at their followers' readiness, and assess the situation. Then, they select a leadership strategy such as telling, selling, participating, or delegating.

*Task behavior* is defined by Hersey, Blanchard, and Johnson (2001) as the extent to which leaders engage in one-way communication by directing what each follower is to do and specifying what, when, where, and how to do the task. *Relationship behavior* is the extent to which a leader engages in two-way communication by providing socioemotional support and facilitation behaviors. These two sets of leadership behaviors form a grid of low to high on each attribute (Figure 24-1).

Hersey, Blanchard, and Johnson (2001) emphasized that the leader must take into account where the followers are in terms of the task at hand in order to determine the leadership style to choose. Overlaid on the task and relationship grid is the concept of *readiness of followers.* Readiness is also on a continuum ranging from low to high and has two primary components, ability and willingness. Job ability is related to knowledge, past experience, problem-solving ability, and ability to take responsibility and meet deadlines. It represents the overall competence or ability to do a particular task. Readiness also includes the psychological motivation or willingness to do the particular task. It includes the willingness to take the responsibility as well as a confident attitude and wanting to do a good job.

According to Hersey, Blanchard, and Johnson (2001), there are four different levels of readiness combining ability and willingness that describe people in terms of accomplishing a specific task, all of which require a different leadership style: S1—low-follower readiness, S2—low ability–high motivation follower readiness, S3—high ability–low motivation follower, and S4—high-follower readiness. These levels of readiness are presented in Figure 24-1 and are briefly discussed in the following sections (Hersey, Blanchard, Johnson, 2001).

S1—LOW-FOLLOWER READINESS. When followers have low task ability and low motivations or willingness to do a task, the leader must define the roles for their followers and provide specific direction for the task. This is called the *"telling" style.* This may be useful when followers are new to a task or the group is new in working with each other. This style also may be useful when there are crucial time constraints to getting a job completed. Community health nurses may find this is their first role in working with a family or group in addressing a new long-term health problem. Because of a lack of knowledge about the illness and the interventions needed to address it and a resistance to changing their lifestyle, clients and/or their families may respond to "telling" or sharing of knowledge leadership at first. Nurses also may find this a useful strategy when faced with leadership of a new team that includes individuals who are not comfortable with the project or do not want to work together.

S2—LOW ABILITY–HIGH MOTIVATION FOLLOWER READINESS. When followers have low ability, leaders must

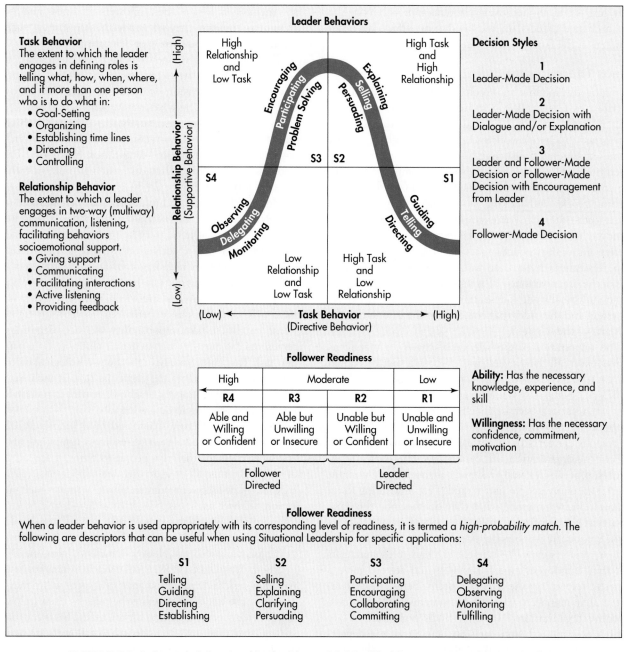

**Task Behavior**
The extent to which the leader engages in defining roles is telling what, how, when, where, and it more than one person who is to do what in:
• Goal-Setting
• Organizing
• Establishing time lines
• Directing
• Controlling

**Relationship Behavior**
The extent to which a leader engages in two-way (multiway) communication, listening, facilitating behaviors socioemotional support.
• Giving support
• Communicating
• Facilitating interactions
• Active listening
• Providing feedback

**Leader Behaviors**

High Relationship and Low Task

High Task and High Relationship

Encouraging · Participating · Problem Solving

Explaining · Selling · Persuading

S3 | S2

S4 | S1

Observing · Delegating · Monitoring

Guiding · Telling · Directing

Low Relationship and Low Task

High Task and Low Relationship

**Relationship Behavior** (Supportive Behavior) (High) ... (Low)

**(Low)** ◄──── **Task Behavior** ────► **(High)**
(Directive Behavior)

**Decision Styles**

**1**
Leader-Made Decision

**2**
Leader-Made Decision with Dialogue and/or Explanation

**3**
Leader and Follower-Made Decision or Follower-Made Decision with Encouragement from Leader

**4**
Follower-Made Decision

**Follower Readiness**

| High | Moderate | | Low |
|---|---|---|---|
| R4 | R3 | R2 | R1 |
| Able and Willing or Confident | Able but Unwilling or Insecure | Unable but Willing or Confident | Unable and Unwilling or Insecure |

Follower Directed | Leader Directed

**Ability:** Has the necessary knowledge, experience, and skill

**Willingness:** Has the necessary confidence, commitment, motivation

**Follower Readiness**
When a leader behavior is used appropriately with its corresponding level of readiness, it is termed a *high-probability match*. The following are descriptors that can be useful when using Situational Leadership for specific applications:

| S1 | S2 | S3 | S4 |
|---|---|---|---|
| Telling | Selling | Participating | Delegating |
| Guiding | Explaining | Encouraging | Observing |
| Directing | Clarifying | Collaborating | Monitoring |
| Establishing | Persuading | Committing | Fulfilling |

**FIGURE 24-1** Expanded situational leadership model. (Modified from Hersey P: *Situational selling*, Escondido, Calif, 1985, Center for Leadership Studies, 1985, p. 35. © 1998 Center for Leadership Studies. All rights reserved. Used with permission.)

still provide most of the direction in getting a task completed. However, when motivation to do the job is there, leaders can engage in more two-way communication and provide socioemotional support behavior to get followers to accept decisions that have to be made and the directions that must be given. The model terms this the *"selling"* style. Newly formed interdisciplinary care teams not yet cognizant of each other's roles and abilities may find this an effective leader style. Community advocacy and support groups for which motivation may be higher than knowledge and/or ability can benefit from this style of leadership. Also,

nurses working with clients and families highly motivated to make health changes and address health concerns yet without the knowledge and ability to do so may respond best to a "selling" leader.

S3—HIGH ABILITY–LOW MOTIVATION FOLLOWER READINESS. These followers have the ability to do a particular task but seem to lack the motivation. The initial leadership style that tends to be the most effective in this situation would be high-relationship, low-task behavior. Leaders in this situation need not provide much direction because of the followers' ability but need to share in the decision making through two-way communication or provide facilitating behaviors that will stimulate follower motivation and decision making. This style is termed the *"participatory" style* of leadership. Nurses may find themselves working with clients or client groups in this style when the knowledge is present for adequate health management, but a relapse in the motivation or desire to engage in positive health behavior has occurred. This style also is useful when groups who were functioning well begin to decline in performance and may serve to "get them back on track."

S4—HIGH-FOLLOWER READINESS. In this situation the followers have both the ability and the motivation to do a task. The leadership style with the highest probability of success would then be the *"delegating" style,* in which the leader uses both low-task and low-relationship behaviors. The leader demonstrates confidence and trust in the group by providing them with opportunities to "run the show." This style is needed with well-developed groups who have been nurtured and have gained the expertise for the task at hand and who work well together. In this situation, leaders use their time most wisely by reserving it for those activities that require more leader involvement and by appropriately recognizing their followers for their abilities. Well-established care teams and clients and families in the maintenance and follow-up stages of care benefit from this style.

**Situational leadership** in the model focuses on the appropriateness of the leadership style for the task-relevant readiness of the followers. In the developmental stages, the leader provides more task and relationship behaviors. As the group matures, they need less direction in relation to the task and provide their own reinforcements, thus needing less socioemotional support from the leader. The most well-developed group for a task needs little supervision from the leader. The cycle is illustrated in the bell-shaped curve going through the four leadership quadrants (see Figure 24-1). Many leaders have one or two "usual" styles and would be characterized as effective or ineffective based on the types of groups they usually lead. A leader who mostly employed involvement and participation behaviors with followers would be very effective with a knowledgeable group getting started on a task but could degenerate to "the blind leading the blind" with low-ability followers. Alternatively, a highly directive leader would be most successful with new low-ability groups and would greatly frustrate more mature followers. The leadership behavior with the highest probability of success in any given situation is based on a careful assessment of the task and the followers. The most effective leader has both good situation diagnostic skills and the ability to adapt his or her leadership style to fit the situation (Hersey, Blanchard, Johnson, 2001).

## THE THREE Cs: CUSTOMERS, COMPETITION, AND CHANGE

The successful community health nurse understands the three primary forces that, separately and in combination, shape health care organizations. These three forces, the three Cs, are customers, competition, and change (Hammer, Champy, 1993, p. 16).

*Customers,* commonly called clients or patients in the health care industry, want to be treated as individuals. They want care that matches their unique needs and schedules. They tell providers what they want and how they want it delivered. They demand appropriate, quality service and define what quality means for them. They are increasingly sophisticated and knowledgeable about the possibilities available to them.

*Competition* is the name of the game in the health care industry, driven by the costs of care. These costs have mandated a change in where care is delivered, resulting in the downsizing and/or closing of hospitals nationwide and the expansion of services delivered in the home and other community-based settings. Since 1988 the home health care sector of the health care industry has had the largest relative employment increase of any industry (Dittbrenner, 1996, p. 11). In this kind of climate, excellent agencies drive out those that are less than excellent because the lowest price, the highest quality, and the best service available from any of them quickly become the standard for all competitors. "Adequate is no longer good enough. If a company can't stand shoulder to shoulder with the world's best in a competitive category, it soon has no place to stand at all" (Hammer, Champy, 1993, p. 21).

The last C is *change.* Change today is pervasive, persistent, rapid, and normal. Although change may not be comfortable, it can be what we make it: an opportunity or a crisis. It can be a catalyst to make us think about what we are doing in different ways. Effective community health nurses are comfortable with change because it is part of daily life. Thus lifelong professional and personal development is their personal paradigm, the way they "see" the world.

## MANAGEMENT FOR THE TWENTY-FIRST CENTURY

The health care organizations of the past decades were well-suited to the growth that was occurring in this industry. The passage of Medicare and Medicaid in 1965 (see Chapter 5) and the development of private insurance plans, along with the increasing expectations of consumers for both quantity and quality in sickness care, brought about unprecedented growth in all sectors of the health care field.

The standard pyramidal organizational structure fit this high-growth environment because it could be enlarged easily. Nurses could be added at the bottom of the chart and management layers could be added above. It also was well suited to control and planning. By breaking work into small units, supervisors could ensure consistent and accurate performance. Budgets were easily approved and monitored, department by department, and planning was done in the same manner.

However, this kind of structure made delivery of a product—client care—increasingly complicated, and managing it became more difficult. The growing numbers of people in the middle of the chart—supervisors, assistant directors, and administrators—added greatly to the cost of the direct care given to people. Further, distance increased between the persons who delivered client care—staff nurses—and the agency administrators who planned and designed the care to be delivered. This all-too-common occurrence resulted in dissatisfied customers (clients), unhappy caregivers, and high costs.

Leaders influence how the nursing staff feel about themselves and their work accomplishments. In this way, organizational outcomes also are influenced. If nurses feel goal directed and their contributions are valued, they are more motivated to do a good job. Overall, the job satisfaction of nurses is one outcome of good leadership that has great importance to the organization. It is associated with the retention and recruitment of good nurses and overall individual and organizational work environment productivity.

Contemporary community health nurses are working in a challenging environment and confront daily the realization that the work world is a different place: old ways of doing things simply do not work any more. The economic crises facing all sectors of the global economy are not going to go away. "In today's environment, nothing is constant or predictable—not market growth, customer demand, product life cycles, the rate of technological change, or the nature of competition" (Hammer, Champy, 1993, p. 17). Leaders for the twenty-first century can help create an environment that will meet these challenges. Effective leaders will coach, encourage, and question in order to develop followers that utilize innovation, creativity, and collective problem solving (Anderson, 1997).

## Reengineering

How does an agency meet the many needs of its customers in an era of unprecedented competition and change? One answer used by corporations all over the United States is a process called reengineering. **Reengineering** is defined as the "fundamental rethinking and radical redesign of business processes to achieve dramatic improvements in critical, contemporary measures of performance, such as cost, quality, service, and speed" (Hammer, Champy, 1993, p. 32). Reengineering has five key concepts: process, teamwork, technology, leadership, and time (Boston Consulting Group, 1993, pp. 4-5). Each of these concepts is discussed in the following list:

1. *Process*. Although the concept of quality processes has been discussed for many years, with reengineering *complete* processes are designed end-to-end to service the customer (client). Rather than breaking down work into tasks and assigning them to different people, the emphasis is on the larger objective of the outcome(s) that needs to be accomplished. For example, in one large home health agency the desired result is quality care that assists clients in meeting their health outcomes in the shortest time possible. Every nurse in the agency knows how to take client admission calls, make initial admission assessment visits, contact the insurance company to receive clearance to make visits and preauthorization, and take care of all of the billing and paperwork. No longer do different individuals perform these separate tasks to admit new clients to care. The outcome is clients and families who are happier and a smoother care process from beginning to end.

2. *Teamwork*. In reengineering, teamwork is encouraged to find innovative approaches to health care issues. Teams have been a part of nursing for years, but under reengineering, teams are given the authority to make decisions and the power to carry them out.

3. *Technology*. Technology provides new possibilities for creativity and reduces time and cost. Health care organizations have increasingly become full-fledged partners in using technology, and the nurse increasingly uses health care technology, communication, and information technology. Many community health nurses use laptop computers as part of client care. Software may even be specifically designed to address the needs of the nursing organization and gives the nurse the ability to provide a comprehensive, up-to-date, individualized nursing care plan. Through the use of computers documentation can take place at the client's bedside and be transmitted to the agency's main computer. The use of email often makes it easier for nurses to communicate with families, community agencies, and the office. Computers have allowed almost immediate feedback about the clients being visited. Documentation of services can be automatically handled by the system and the nurse can be prompted for any additional data needed.

4. *Leadership*. In reengineering, managers become leaders—persons who harness the learning and creative power of organizations and generate results. Each person working in the organization is viewed as a leader and a manager: everyone has the responsibility to be visionary and to create possibilities, and each person also has the responsibility, power, and authority to get things done.

5. *Time*. Nurses must understand that "time is money" and that it is not possible to justify caring for clients without thinking in terms of the time required to achieve what needs to be done. Many home visits are reimbursed through the Medicare prospective payment system or managed care companies. The number of visits that a nurse can make and be reimbursed for in relation to a given diagnosis is often predetermined by these payment mechanisms. Successful nurses learn to accomplish quickly what needs to be accomplished within the specified time frames while maintaining quality service delivery.

Reengineering can present new ways of thinking for health care professionals. It is crucial to understand that quality care for clients is provided in the context of a business organization. Quality care must be paid for; health care providers, rightfully so, want appropriate reimbursement for their services. Unwillingness to learn the business of health care will make health care organizations increasingly noncompetitive in a world that is highly competitive.

## THE ORGANIZATIONAL STRUCTURE OF HEALTH CARE DELIVERY

The number of health care delivery organizations in which community health nurses work is increasing. The diverse organizations in which they work have differing missions, philosophies, organizational structures, and ways of delivering nursing services.

Nurses must know the organizational structure of their employing agencies so that they can determine how to use agency resources and identify appropriate ways to effect change within the organization. Organizational structure encompasses formal and informal patterns of behavior and relationships in an organization. This includes formal and informal position allocations, as well as the chain of command and the channels of communication.

### The Informal Organizational Structure

The informal organizational structure refers to the personal and social relationships of people who work together. Informal relationships have no formal power. However, they can have a major impact on the organization and its management. The way in which a manager is viewed by the staff does influence the manner and effectiveness of his or her management.

### The Formal Organizational Structure

Formal organizational structure defines which people will do which tasks so that the objectives of the organization can be accomplished. It is the power structure of the organization. The rules, policies, procedures, control mechanisms, and financial arrangements of the organization are all part of the formal structure. The schematic organization is part of this formal structure and can be seen in an organizational chart.

ORGANIZATIONAL CHART. An organizational chart diagrams the relationship among members of the organization and indicates the structure of authority, formal lines of communication, and levels of management and delegation. These all interrelate to accomplish the goals of the organization.

An organizational manual supplements an organizational chart by supplying information about the requirements of the various job positions represented on the chart. Organizational charts and manuals are useful tools that describe the formal relationships in a particular organization. Charts and manuals do not show the informal relationships that exist.

POWER RELATIONSHIPS. In any health care organizational structure a manager must have a basic understanding of organizational power relationships to manage effectively. Four types of power relationships evolve in any organization:

1. *Authority:* the power to direct the actions of others
2. *Responsibility:* the obligation to carry out or perform tasks in an acceptable way
3. *Accountability:* the obligation to answer for one's actions
4. *Delegation:* assigning and empowering one person to act for another with the responsibility for the act remaining with the person who assigned it

Organizational structure and resulting power relationships in a health care agency assist personnel in all positions to carry out effectively the functions of management. Regardless of the type of structure, it would be impossible to manage if such a structure did not exist. Effective and efficient management can occur only when personnel understand what they are responsible for and to whom they are accountable. Ignoring the power relationships in an organization can create real difficulties. Illustrative of this are the actions taken by the community health nurse in the following scenario.

**CASE** *Scenario*    A community health nurse identified a need for a family planning program in two of the census tracts she served. Knowing that the county health department did not include these services, she independently arranged a group meeting in the clubhouse at a local park to discuss the need for these services with the people of the community. This was done without discussing the action with her supervisor.

Twenty community members attended the meeting. They quickly became emotionally involved in the issue and wanted immediate action taken by the health department to initiate such a service. The nurse became uncomfortable because she recognized that she did not have the power to make a definite commitment regarding the establishment of a new program. The community members became frustrated with the nurse's lack of action.

Had proper channels within the agency power structure been considered, this situation would have been handled differently. While examining this situation, the following questions quickly become obvious: Did the nurse have the authority to organize this meeting? Was she acting in a responsible and accountable manner? What were her objectives for the meeting, and did she clarify them for herself and the group?

When planning a meeting with a group such as the one just described, it is crucial to seek the advice of individuals within the organization who have the authority to make decisions. When this is not done, it can result in stress and frustration for all parties involved. If the nurse had gone to her supervisor before the meeting, she would have been aware of the types of commitments she could make during the meeting. If, for instance, the health department did not have adequate resources to staff a family planning clinic, the group goal might have been to look at alternative ways to obtain funding for family planning services in the community, rather than discussing only how the health department might provide these services.

ORGANIZATIONAL POLICIES. Another component of the formal organization structure that maximizes functioning is organizational policies. Policies define the limits of acceptable activities and provide structure and guidelines for employee decision making. They are generally developed to handle situations that occur consistently in daily practice. Policies that address how to handle referrals (see Chapter 10), when and how to conduct nursing audits (see Chapter 25), and staff benefits such as travel allowances are a few examples of policies commonly found in a community health agency. These types of policies provide direction for decision making.

When policies are absolute, with no flexibility, they are considered *rules*. Rules are usually established to ensure client and staff safety and quality of care. The following are examples of rules:

- "No home visits are to be made at night in census tract 3 without an escort."
- "No immunizations are to be given until an allergy history has been taken."
- "Every fifth record closed to service must be audited."

When nurses accept employment within a health setting, it is assumed that they accept responsibility for following, enforcing, and informing others about agency policies. This means that the conditions of employment should be clearly understood before the nurse accepts a position within an organization. Otherwise the nurse may end up in a situation where it is necessary to follow certain policies that are inconsistent with his or her philosophy of practice. Nursing personnel at all levels may be involved in writing policies. Policy statements should include several important items (Box 24-1).

If used effectively, policies can increase the efficiency and ease with which individuals carry out their functions within an organization. Difficulties with implementing a policy will occur if employees do not understand the reason for the policy or their input is not obtained when the policy is formulated, if the policy is not clearly written, or if there are too many policies that prevent necessary flexibility for nursing practice.

**BOX 24-1**

*Select Factors to Consider When Writing a Policy*

1. Reason for establishing the policy (philosophy behind the policy)
2. Actual policy statement
3. Guidelines for implementing the policy
4. Lead persons or department implementing the policy
5. Persons affected by the policy

## PROFESSIONAL STANDARDS

The American Nurses Association (ANA) (1995) has developed *Scope and Standards for Nurse Administrators*. The standards provide guidance to nurse administrators in addressing the rapid changes sweeping all settings where nursing care is delivered. Each of the standards has criteria or measurable indicators identified. Agencies that follow these standards or similar ones are likely to promote organizational and staff growth and provide direction for the delivery of quality nursing services as well. This helps neophyte and experienced nurses who use the standards to make decisions about the most effective employment opportunities. Both experienced and inexperienced students and nurses need guidance in using standards in the practice setting.

## DEFINING MANAGEMENT LANGUAGE

**Management** is the planning, organizing, directing, coordinating, and controlling of activities in a system so that the objectives of that system are met. For community health nurses, that system may be represented by any number of settings in which the nurse practices, such as a public health agency, an ambulatory care setting, a school, an industrial plant, or a home care organization. Managers use leadership skills and manipulate the environment to achieve planned system goals and objectives. The work of nursing management could then be defined as those discrete and important functions that provide an environment facilitating delivery of appropriate client services. Management is a logical process based on problem-solving principles. Managers develop plans to enable people to achieve specific goals. Then the manager directs and coordinates the work as it is occurring, making adjustments and corrections as needed to control the outcome.

**Administration** is a term that is often mistakenly used interchangeably with management. The principles of management and administration are the same, but the scope of functioning for managers and administrators varies. For instance, both administrators and managers set goals, but the administrator sets goals for a department, whereas a staff nurse sets personal goals when managing his or her workload responsibilities.

**Leadership** is "shaping and sharing a vision which gives point to the work of others" (Handy, 1990, p. 134). In addition, leadership needs to be "endemic in organizations, the rule not the exception" (p. 133). For an organization to compete successfully to provide quality care, that vision must "reconceptualize the obvious, and connect the previously unconnected dream" (Handy, 1990, p. 133). At the same time that vision must make sense; it must be understandable to others. Leaders live the vision and believe in it completely. Finally, a leader realizes that unless others follow, there is no leadership.

# MANAGEMENT FUNCTIONS OF THE COMMUNITY HEALTH NURSE

The management process has both interpersonal and technical aspects that use human, physical, and technological resources to achieve well-defined goals. The process is cyclical and the functions overlap and do not always follow a sequential pattern.

Nurses, depending on their place in the organizational structure and their interests, skills, and educational backgrounds, do managing on many levels. The director of nursing and nursing supervisors will probably spend more time implementing management activities than the staff nurse will. However, staff nurses must use management functions to effectively deliver nursing services. Staff nurses also can influence how nursing administration carries out management functions.

The management functions carried out by the community health nurse are *planning, organizing, directing, coordinating, and performance management.* These functions help link the entire organizational system together and assist the nurse in effectively managing workload responsibilities.

## Planning

Planning assists an organization in establishing a vision for the future. It means deciding in advance what must be done and what the organization wants to achieve. Without planning, no set goals will be accomplished.

Planning gives purpose and direction to the decision-making process and helps the organization remain dynamic. It increases the likelihood that activities will be orderly, predictable, and less costly. Most important, planning improves the quality and effectiveness of nursing care. Although planning does not guarantee the quality of outcomes, the evaluation aspects of this process help a manager identify strengths and needs within the organization. Planning is often neglected because of the emphasis placed on carrying out day-to-day activities, the attitude that planning takes too much time, and the tendency for individuals to resist change.

Health care planning should include both the provider and the consumer. If emergencies necessitate individual decision making and planning, it is important to explain to others involved in the process the circumstances and reasons for the emergency decision.

Planning uses past, present, and future information to project what services should be provided. Currently the impact of political, social, economic, and technical forces is directly influencing the types of services provided by community health agencies and the type of personnel needed to implement these services. For instance, local health departments (LHDs) rely heavily on local tax dollars for support. When this tax base is inadequate, valuable health department services may be cut and new services may not be added.

An example of a staff nurse putting the planning process into action is a nurse working with the nursing supervisor to establish a nurse-run clinic for the homeless in the staff nurse's district. Together they would develop a written plan that might include the following elements:

1. Specific, measurable objectives related to establishment of the clinic
2. Time schedule for achieving objectives
3. Exploration of possible funding mechanisms including development of community support
4. A process for carrying out the objectives with the necessary resources
5. Evaluation methods with a timetable for periodic evaluation

These activities are discussed in further detail in Chapter 15.

A community health nurse also implements the planning function when structuring the workday and when implementing caseload management activities. During planning, many needs and goals may be identified, and priorities for them must be set. The following points should be considered when setting priorities.

ECONOMIC IMPACT. The cost-benefit aspect is always important to consider. When doing cost-benefit analysis the nurse must consider the cost and outcomes if something is not done. For example, although an immunization campaign against rubella may be initially costly, it is much less expensive socially and economically than paying for the care of children who have congenital deformities resulting from in utero rubella or who have complications from the disease. In looking at cost-benefit analysis, one LHD discontinued a screening clinic for the geriatric population because it was not cost effective. It cost the health department $40 per client to do the screening, and 90% of those screened had recently received the same screening from their private physicians and planned to do so again in the future. This was a duplication of services at a high cost to the health department. Methods other than a screening clinic could be used to reach the 10% of the population not receiving the screening privately. The money saved from this program was used for other health programs in the community.

PRACTICALITY. Is the program necessary? What is being done currently? Will enough people benefit from it to make it worthwhile? Are sufficient resources available, such as workforce and money, to accomplish the stated goals? Is there enough organizational and community support to carry out the program? Does it meet the needs of the community? All of these are questions to be answered in relation to the practicality of the program.

FEASIBILITY. Does the program fit the organization's policies and priorities? Are the resources available to carry out the program?

LEGAL REQUIREMENTS. The organization must follow its legal mandates. For example, the LHD has a legal mandate to control communicable disease. Home health agencies have regulations imposed by funding agencies such as Medicare.

URGENCY OF THE SITUATION. An emergency situation is usually given top priority. In one urban community, for instance, when a large number of people in an LHD's area developed botulism, an epidemiological investigation immediately became a top priority. Many other health department activities were stopped or modified so that this serious problem could be addressed. It was found that a large Mexican restaurant used home-canned chili peppers that were improperly prepared. The source of the outbreak was found and the epidemic was stopped. Currently community health nurses would be on the front lines of any emergency response effort to deal with biological, chemical, or nuclear casualty events. An emergency preparedness plan for the agency must be in place and all personnel must be educated on the execution of the plan.

Increasingly there are competing priorities and demands for resources of health care organizations. Nurses need to be able to defend their requests for new or enlarged programs. They also need to be able to see the "larger picture" for the total organization and perhaps defer to another colleague or discipline when requests or priorities conflict.

## Organizing

Organizing determines how activities are implemented to achieve stated goals. The organizational structure, as previously discussed, facilitates decision making and assigning of tasks. Any organizational structure has three principal components: people, work, and relationships. The interrelationship of these three variables helps determine the best way to organize activities. Well-organized activities are usually more efficient and less time consuming.

A manager's major concerns when organizing include the following:

1. *Analysis of the system,* or identifying strengths and needs of the present system to make it more effective and efficient in the future. Comparing present staff capabilities to the determined needs of clients is one example of how a system is analyzed.
2. *Analysis of functions,* which includes defining all the tasks involved in a particular job and determining the relationships among various jobs. A nurse and supervisor analyzing a staff nurse's responsibilities when she or he has a caseload of eight bedside care clients, 40 families needing health supervision, and work in six schools and two clinics weekly is an example of this principle.
3. *Assigning job responsibilities,* or grouping tasks to minimize duplication of effort and assigning responsibilities to individuals who have the knowledge and competence to carry out the job. Responsibility and authority limits should be clearly defined. Work with clients who need bedside care illustrates this principle. Assistive personnel should be assigned only basic physical care, and the com-

munity health nurse should assess and supervise the care given by the home health aide. If the health care organization has a union, labor agreements may dictate the extent to which managers can change job responsibilities.

4. *Implementation,* which involves developing an atmosphere that allows for successful completion of the work to be done by identifying the structure of authority and support mechanisms in the system and carrying out organizing activities. Team meetings that provide support, case consultation, and identification of needs illustrate this concept.

Organizing requires a cooperative effort by a health care team working together to achieve the goals of the organization. This nursing and managerial function is familiar to community health nurses because they must organize the care of a family around the family's expressed needs and the resources of the community.

## Directing

Effective programs and organizations include all levels of staff in the planning process so that information is disseminated by peers, at least in part, and "top-down" directing is minimized. The purpose of directing is to convey to workers what has occurred during the planning and organizing phases of management. The activities of directing include order giving, direction, leadership, motivating, and communicating.

*Order giving* involves helping an employee identify what needs to be done in a way that fosters understanding and acceptance. A community health nurse who clearly and completely tells assistive personnel the details of the physical care needed by a client with a cerebrovascular accident and provides opportunity for the assistant to ask questions illustrates how effective order giving can be accomplished.

*Direction* refers to the effort made in an organization to ensure that all the work is done. Professional guidance is basic to the concept of direction. Supervisors need to assist staff in developing career plans and focus on staff growth and development. They also need to explain to employees what is expected of them. Employees are more likely to effectively carry out directions if they understand them. When there is no doubt regarding what is expected of them, employees are able to work without constant supervision.

*Motivating* focuses on analyzing the needs of individual workers. Maslow's hierarchy of needs can provide a theoretical framework for examining worker needs. Maslow has developed a priority schema based on a continuum of needs beginning with those that are physiological and ending with self-actualization. He believed that a worker must satisfy lower-level needs (physiological) before the higher-level ones (self-actualization) become significant (Maslow, 1954). An effective manager attempts to build into the management system rewards that will help the employee meet these basic human needs.

*Communicating* with workers is crucial. The manager must be able to convey what is to be done, how it is to be done, who is to do it, and why it is to be done and to provide feedback on the activity. This feedback should emphasize the strengths, as well as the weaknesses, inherent in the employee's activity.

Communication is a two-way process. The manager uses skill to convey what needs to be done. Noticing staff members' responses, both verbal and nonverbal, is a critical part of the process. If the person does not hear what has been said, appropriate communication has not occurred. The interviewing skills that are a primary tool of community health nurses should be used in communicating with health care workers. These skills will help the manager direct, coordinate, and control activities within the organization.

## Coordinating

Coordination links people on the health care team together to function in such a way that the team's objectives are achieved. A problem arises when health care workers look at objectives in different ways. One nurse may consider nursing in the school setting as a low priority. The supervisor may think it a high priority. Thus coordinating can mean managing conflict. Conflict can promote growth, but it can also reduce productivity. Effective coordination reduces and prevents growth-restricting conflict.

## Performance Management

Performance management is the act of helping organizations achieve their goals by ensuring that employees perform their jobs effectively (carrying out the correct functions) and efficiently (quality and cost-effectiveness of the end product). In reengineered businesses, employees are trusted to use their own methods to achieve the purposes of the organization; therefore, mistakes can and will be made. However, employees are urged to learn from their mistakes: mistakes are to be used as an opportunity for learning and growth and not thought of as failures. Although not all mistakes can be forgiven (e.g., those that affect client safety), most can be. Again, in reality, this is a different way of thinking for many people in the health professions, where "perfection" is the accepted norm.

Performance management assists managers in identifying the current learning requirements of individual employees, as well as ways to improve the employee's work performance (Benjamin, Penland, 1995). The system has five steps:

1. Agreeing about what competencies are needed by employees to carry out their role. Competencies need to be clear and written in explicit detail so that they are understandable to all parties. Use of a collaborative process between the formal manager and employee to develop the competencies is the expectation.
2. The competencies are next prioritized in order of importance according to the needs of the organization.
3. The employee and supervisor then rate the employee on the ability to perform each of the competencies. Each

employee and supervisor must reach consensus on the ranking of the employee's performance.
4. The manager and employee develop goals for improving the employee's performance, and a performance improvement contract is written.
5. Both parties meet frequently on a formal and informal basis to examine the progress that is being made toward defined goals.

Performance management actively involves staff members in career development and provides direction for professional growth. It should examine worker *strengths*, as well as areas of concern. The emphasis on competencies helps an organization maintain a clear focus on staff, client, and organizational needs.

## NURSE MANAGERS AS CHANGE AGENTS

Nurses, as managers must be champions of change. The changing health care environment makes management of planned change to address needs and improve outcomes critical. Effective managed change can lead to improved client services, increased productivity, improved morale, and the meeting of client and staff needs.

Managers are the best change agents in the institution because they can act as role models and manage the flow of information and resources so critical to an effective change process. They are also prepared and in a position to handle resistance to change. All of the management functions covered in this chapter should be incorporated as appropriate to the situation. A manager's professional and mature approach to change helps staff adopt and support it. The Ellison Change Model for Managers (Ellison, 2001) is presented to illustrate the crucial role of managers as organizational change agents (Figure 24-2). The change model was developed based on the classic change theory of Lewin (1951) and Spradley's (1980) change model. The model has five steps with the manager influencing the process at each step. The model's steps are as follows:

1. *Recognize the need or opportunity for change.* Symptoms in the system provide evidence that a change is needed (Spradley, 1980). Managers also must be proactive to strategize changes that will make their institution more competitive in the health care environment and best demonstrate the value of their services. Data collection mechanisms for outcome and financial data must be organized in ways to identify concerns before they become problems. Staff must feel free to share concerns and ideas openly without threat of retaliation. Innovative ideas should be encouraged and credit given.
2. *Analyze the situation.* Managers can analyze the situation themselves or develop a team to analyze the situation and alternative solutions and select the change needed. A manager may construct a team with the combination of knowledge, skills, experience, and perspectives that allow a more holistic and complex analysis of the situation.

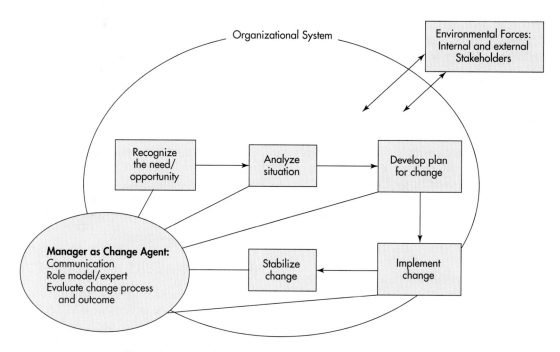

**FIGURE 24-2** Ellison change model for managers. (From Ellison KJ: *Change model for managers,* unpublished manuscript, 2001).

The risks and benefits of different changes must be analyzed in relation to resources, time, and outcomes. Lewin (1951) encourages incorporation of the driving and opposing forces for the change in the analysis process. Driving forces facilitate the change and opposing forces resist it. The stakeholders in the change, all those internal and external to the system that are affected by the change and on whom the change depends, must be identified and the effects of different decisions on those groups considered. Organizations promote hierarchical, bureaucratic structures with rules to promote stability. Both individuals and organizations need the stability that continuity in policies and procedures provide, so that recurring problems can be dealt with routinely and do not require rethinking each time they are encountered. Change creates threats to stability in various ways. Change demands investment of time and effort for relearning. Individuals may fear they do not know what is needed to make the change or they cannot learn to meet the new demands. Change also may be interpreted as a criticism—the change is occurring "because we haven't been doing it right." Many changes also threaten an organization's social system by altering how people communicate and work with each other and will be resisted because of their effects on the social customs, values, and self-esteem of members. Managers must assess the barriers to change and threats to the members' security to develop an effective plan for change.

3. *Plan the change.* A solid plan for the change is crucial to its success and ease of implementation. Plans for change should include stakeholder groups and delineate their

level of involvement in the change process. Change plans should include clear specific statements of the goals and objectives for the change and a timetable for its incorporation. Nurse managers must include plans for resource allocation including time for staff to unlearn the old ways and use the new. The manager should build in evaluation at each step in the change process. This evaluation should address both process and outcomes. A comprehensive plan also should include methods for resistance management and change stabilization. For example, a manager wanting to utilize only certified case managers might plan meetings to negotiate with current nurses regarding plans and timetables for achieving certification. A plan to stabilize a change may include featuring those successful with the change in the agency's newsletter, rewarding the champions of the new method.

4. *Implement the change.* In this step managers incorporate strategies to prepare, involve, and support those who will be affected by the change. The need for the change and ways individuals will be assisted in incorporating the change must be communicated clearly. Appropriate resources must be assigned to training and education to facilitate the change. An effective manager also will allow for flexibility and creativity so that those implementing the change can exercise their own initiative. This will help promote ownership of the change and decrease the likelihood the change will be perceived as a threat.

5. *Stabilize the change.* The manager's role in monitoring and stabilizing change is important. Managers must maintain an ongoing dialogue with those involved in the change throughout the process. Barriers to successful

integration may continue to appear as the process of change evolves. Rewards and incentives in the organization, both financial and nonfinancial, need to be directed toward the new behavior. Clear communication of incentives is important. Managers are in a position to foresee and develop strategies to prevent resistance and promote stabilization through early problem solving, conflict resolution, and negotiation. Spradley (1980) emphasized that planned change must be monitored at each step of the process to make sure the change strategies are being effective and those leading the change are being responsive to the changing system's needs.

As previously noted, the only thing that is predictable is that change will occur, and to meet the needs of our clients in the twenty-first century, nurse managers must help lead in efforts to change. Many nurses feel squeezed from unrelenting downsizing and increasing controls over their practice. They want "the good old days back." The situation cannot and will not go back to the way it was. Managers who respond to this challenge by building effective teams nurtured to expect and handle constant change will be key players in the future.

## FACILITATING EFFECTIVE TEAMWORK

Perhaps the most important outcome of good management is effective **teamwork**. No other management activity synthesizes all management functions discussed in this chapter as well. Whether working with families, community groups, or interdisciplinary groups, community health nurses need this skill. Understanding the process of teamwork and ways managers can facilitate it are important to making the best use of teams (Boxes 24-2 and 24-3). Teams can take advantage of the multiple perspectives of team members, build on each other's ideas and skills and more effectively solve problems.

Having a vision for their team is the first critical step that a manager can take in facilitating effectiveness in their team. A vision in this sense is not the kind from crystal balls or psychic predictions but one of having a clear idea of what the future should be. A leader's vision becomes the focus of the follower's activity, inspires hope, and sustains long-term motivation. A vision unites a group toward a common pur-

pose by becoming the guide for decisions and actions of the group. To create a shared vision, the leader involves members of the group empowering them to create a shared image of the future. Shared visions are particularly motivating. A vision may seem a rather nebulous concept such as "the most successful agency in the area" or "the most exciting place to work." At times a vision is hard to define usefully such as "have the highest quality." It may even be impractical such as "no client complaints." The purpose of the vision is to serve as the inspiration or motivating force driving the group's work.

A vision is translated into practicality by concrete goals. A goal must be achievable given sufficient effort and be measurable so that it is possible to tell when you have met it. Goals must also have a time limit so that strategies for meeting the goals can be organized. Managers must be astute in helping teams choose goals wisely. While a team member is working on the known and established goals, a manager needs to have the long-term view—what goals will help the team reach for the vision next week, month, year, and so on. Higher managers in the organization have to look further, accordingly. Once goals have been identified, strategies must be selected. Openness in communication, in which opinions are respected, is an important ground rule during strategy meetings. Teams lose effectiveness when there is fear of conflict, lack of trust among members, and an emphasis on blame rather than problem solving. The manager should set the example and promote consistency. An action plan will help team members know who does what by when. Teams foster accountability because group members often check on one another and group expectations are motivating.

Effective managers facilitate continued work by identifying progress of the group. Data updates related to the goals can be disseminated and displayed. A flatter organizational

**BOX 24-3**

*Ten Ways Managers Facilitate Effective Teamwork*

1. Stimulate a shared vision
2. Help members of the team become acquainted
3. Indicate the importance/value of the team and the work
4. Make individuals feel valued and their contributions/roles important
5. Make sure goals are clearly understood
6. Set ground rules for interaction: openness, respect, and trust
7. Make resources available for the group
8. Put emphasis on learning, problem solving, and improvement
9. Identify progress
10. Acknowledge achievements; give credit

**BOX 24-2**

*Teamwork Process*

- Creating shared vision—what we will look like when we are successful
- Setting goals with measurable milestones
- Choosing strategies
- Developing an action plan
- Evaluating progress and outcomes

structure where information is passed on to the worker is more motivating. An environment of openness, reflectivity, and ability to accept questions about decisions reflects a learning organization (Senge, 1990). The most effective managers build these qualities into their work environment and maximize their team member's potential. They motivate by encouraging development of members, promoting their learning and desired achievements, and coordinating those with the goals of the organization.

Managers have an initial responsibility in helping team members get to know one another. Formal and informal mechanisms can be used to facilitate members becoming knowledgeable about one another's skills and abilities and understanding the past experiences that shape their varied perspectives. Teams can flounder if they do not know each other well, resulting in a lack of trust or difficulty communicating. Even when members know each other well, they need time to talk about past experiences and what has been learned.

Team members need to be empowered to make decisions to control their work and made responsible for the outcomes. Managers provide support and encourage cooperation and learning from each other. In providing support, managers must make sure the necessary resources are allocated and coordinated, not only for today's work, but also for the work tomorrow and next week. The manager has access to information and materials as a result of their position and must use their authority wisely to help the team be more effective. Managers maintain involvement, helping workers get training as needed and encouraging and rewarding positive outcomes. Managers should be confident in their workers and help them get the knowledge and skills to be self-confident.

Managers must avoid having unreasonable high standards. A job should not be judged by just how the manager would do it, but rather by how well it meets the purpose. If certain criteria and standards must be met, these must be agreed on first. Managers then monitor the work in progress. Giving people "enough rope to hang themselves" is manager failure. A manager should always accept a decision from those they have delegated to unless it is clearly wrong and the manager's idea offers significant improvements. A good manager will not point fingers and blame, but use poor outcomes to teach, develop, and rethink their own management skills.

Managers should always praise a job well done and give credit to those involved. Managers who build and reward effective teams will most successfully navigate the swiftly changing and highly competitive health care environment.

## INFORMATION TECHNOLOGY IN COMMUNITY HEALTH NURSING

One of the key elements of reengineering discussed at the beginning of this chapter is technology. Information tech-

nology opens new possibilities for delivering more quality services, as well as for decreasing time and cost. Applying the power of modern information technology demands the ability to think deductively, recognize a powerful solution, and then seek the problems it might solve.

More and more computer applications are being nationally marketed for health care. One of the best-known management information systems (MIS) for community and home health care is one developed by the Visiting Nurse Association of Omaha, Nebraska. This system uses a classification scheme for client problems in community health nursing that adapts easily to a computerized system of record keeping. This system is addressed in Chapter 9.

The computerized system developed by the Visiting Nurse Association of Greater Philadelphia is another example of how technology is being used in community health nursing practice. The agency received a foundation grant to develop a "fully integrated computer system that would increase the cost economics that voluntary, not-for-profit home health care providers require to survive in the extremely competitive home health care market" (Visiting Nurse Association of Greater Philadelphia, 1990-1992, p. 2). During the first 3 years of the grant, the project developed and demonstrated a computerized voice messaging system for field and office staff to communicate with each other about client care and defined a comprehensive system for the development of care plans that could be computerized. During the final year the project developed a philosophy for satisfying the information needs of such an agency, produced a methodology for the identification of an agency's information management requirements, produced a methodology for the evaluation and selection of commercially available software, confirmed "open" architecture as the desired bridge between acquired software and internally developed systems, and developed several applications that track and control agency programs.

Milio (1996) has written a unique book, *The Engines of Empowerment: Using Information Technology to Create Healthy Communities and Challenge Public Policy*, that describes experiences of "ordinary people who are doing new things with computers to create healthier standards and styles of living. They are using these new tools to build social and economic renewal in their communities and to create *community*—the sense of shared responsibility that must accompany and complement viable communities" (p. 3). Milio's book is a masterful example of thinking deductively, of first finding solutions and then looking for problems.

When developing a computerized MIS, nurses must take into consideration nursing ethics. They must ensure that the rights of both client and staff are protected when information is computerized. Nurses must carefully monitor access to client and personnel data, limiting access to these types of data is essential when they are part of a computer information system.

The development and constant revamping of a MIS can create stress within an organization, especially when staff members have not previously worked much with computers. When experiencing this stress, it helps to focus on what can be achieved long range through the use of a MIS. Initially it takes additional time out of one's schedule to become knowledgeable about the functioning of this type of system. However, a new system, if used effectively, can help an agency improve the delivery of client care services and can reduce indirect service time.

Technological innovations will continue to have increasing importance in improving health care delivery and controlling costs. The health care environment is on the verge of revolutionary change in the way client information is collected, stored, transmitted, shared, and used to substantiate outcomes. Technology will make information more accessible and comparable across the continuum of care, enhancing the decision making of providers and administrators. Technology is also informing clients and improving their involvement in their own care. Information technology aids in redesigning the use of health care resources to better serve clients and in creating a knowledge-based system that continuously improves the quality of the outcomes. Telehealth is such a system.

## Telehealth

Consider the following case scenario:

**CASE Scenario**  A client with long-term diabetes uses a glucose meter to analyze his blood sugars several times a day. The glucose meter has easy-to-use screens that capture, store, and trend data. Each morning the client attaches the meter to the telephone and at a push of a button sends the previous day's results to the diabetes case manager. The case manager reviews the data and gives the client advice about care. The client did not have to see a physician, saving time and money. In this manner, health concerns can be addressed before they become problems and require hospitalization. This scenario can be replayed with many chronic conditions such as congestive heart failure, hypertension, asthma, and many others.

Telehealth is an overall term referring to use of communications networks and equipment to transfer health care information between clients and providers in different locations. Telehealth's applications include provision of long-distance health assessment and monitoring, client and provider education, and transfer of data for administrative and research purposes. The *Telemedicine Research Center* in Portland, Oregon, reported telehealth consultation has been increasing by a rate of 60% annually since 1993 (Essex, 1999). As with all technology, telehealth is a tool that can be used to break down obstacles to care (Figure 24-3). With the cost of technology decreasing and reimbursement for telehealth services increasing, telehealth is expected to

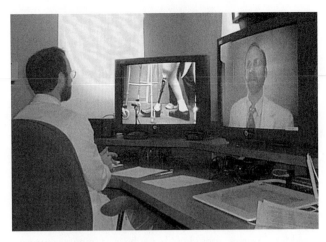

**FIGURE 24-3** Telehealth is an important part of care at the University of Tennessee Medical Center in Knoxville, Tennessee. (Courtesy UTMC Telemedicine.)

continue expansion of its role in service provision. Telehealth can increase the quality of care and improve outcomes by facilitating early diagnosis and treatment.

More timely interventions can result in improved clinical outcomes, reduced hospitalization, increased client satisfaction, and an overall improved quality of life. A study was conducted at Kaiser Permanente on the use of telecommunications with 200 chronically ill home care clients. Clients were monitored in their homes in addition to having some traditional health care visits. The study reported that the telehealth visits cost one third less than a regular visit, ambulance calls were less frequent, and client anxiety was decreased (Kincaid, 1997). Chaffee (1999) echoed these findings, reporting that the average cost of a face-to-face home visit in the late 1990s was $90, whereas the cost of a similar telehealth visit was $20 to $35. Because of the cost-saving possibilities, more emphasis is expected in developing this technology and its applications. A study by Wooten, Loane, Mair, and others (1998) suggests that as many as 45% of home visits in the United States could be done by telehealth! Kincaid (1997) concluded telehealth could be used to increase efficiency in home care by tracking client outcomes, decreasing service redundancy, and supplementing care by usual staff.

Information technology supports the focus of case management, tracking information automatically, and notifying and reminding case managers when intervention is needed. In addition, case managers can use communications systems to interact with their clients by providing monitoring, teaching, and follow-up care.

Further use of technology should also be a part of the strategic planning of an organization to improve its competitiveness in the market place. A well-designed web page is a great marketing tool. Also, using telehealth strategies can help an agency expand its market share into areas that may have been too remote or too expensive to reach before.

## *Stop and Think About It*

The administrator of the home care agency you are working for proposed the use of a new telehealth program. Discuss how this might improve the ability of the staff to give care. What client group would you like to start with and why? Describe what data you want to collect and how the data will be used. Discuss the confidentiality issues that must be addressed when using a telehealth program and how these issues will be handled.

## Outcomes Assessment and Technology

Chapter 25 discusses how measuring quality in nursing care has moved from an emphasis on structure and process to a focus on outcomes of the care provided. Health care providers, nurses included, have been somewhat uneasy with this focus because in the 1990s a major outcome was cost control. The uneasiness stems from the notion that costs should not enter into the decision to provide health care for those in need. Health care has traditionally operated on the premise that any treatment that has any chance of producing benefit, no matter how small, ought to be tried.

Providers in the future will be increasingly called on to pay attention to every aspect of their practice, including costs of their services and outcomes of their interventions. To reach the goal of maximizing quality outcomes while controlling costs, providers need information that can assist them in making sound clinical decisions.

Several factors have evoked an increasing demand for outcomes assessment (Box 24-4). Escalating health care expenditures have resulted in restructuring of health care and a demand for greater provider accountability as to the effectiveness of their services. The use of *diagnostic related groups* (DRGs) to establish prices for services and the explosive growth of various health maintenance organizations (HMO) formulations for prepaid services and other managed care initiatives have stimulated an urgency to have outcomes monitoring systems. These systems help organizations demonstrate accountability and cost effectiveness and aid in comparative evaluation of health services packages.

As Chapter 25 demonstrates, quality has become the pinnacle of the health care agenda. The changes noted in

reimbursement forced health care institutions to focus on provision of health services as a business with client care as the product. The value of that care is dependent, as in any business, on the balance of cost and quality. Evaluation of quality care must incorporate a look at the links between the processes of care and provider mix and outcomes.

The influence of business on health care also focused assessment of quality of care on how the recipients of that care defined it. As the customer of health care, clients highlighted new dimensions of quality focusing on the "service" components. Clients are not only interested in the effectiveness of treatment but also in interactions with professionals and the system as their treatment progresses. Client satisfaction with care has become an accepted benchmark for quality. Organizations with a customer service orientation that responds to client desires for increased involvement in care decisions are setting the standards for quality evaluation of many important outcomes of care.

The customer orientation in health care extends to all those paying for health care services. From individual consumers to corporate purchasers, the huge health care expenditures have resulted in a demand for quantifiable information as to the value of the dollars being spent. Comparative data on cost and outcomes are critical to making informed choices about providers and plans.

The hardware and software innovations of the past decade are fueling the demand for more and better measure of outcomes and availability of comparable data. Many for-profit companies have developed products elevating data collection, analysis, interpretation, and display to a higher plane of efficiency making more universal assessment and comparison of outcomes feasible.

Outcomes data can be used to demonstrate the value of clinical services provided. Home health has lagged behind the acute care sector in its ability to determine its impact on the health and functioning of its clients. More research like the study by Naylor, Brooten, and Campbell (1999) needs to be conducted (Box 24-5). Across the country, tremendous variation exists in the number of home-care visits conducted per client during an episode of care. Until the last 5 years, agencies used variable standards to justify extending care.

The collection of OASIS (Outcomes ASsessment and Information Set) data is now a requirement for all Medicare-certified agencies. OASIS, discussed further in Chapter 22, provides agencies with the ability to measure outcomes of care delivered in the home setting, upon admission, at follow-up points, and at discharge for 13 different areas. The 79+ items in this tool have the potential to help answer critical questions in home care such as (1) How do the number of visits impact outcomes? and (2) How can costs be decreased without hurting the quality of care? While some still question the use of OASIS for case-mix adjustments and reimbursement, most see the potential of OASIS to add to the body of evidence supporting the clinical and financial value of home care in the health care continuum.

### BOX 24-4

## *Factors Driving Outcomes Assessment*

- Restructuring of our health care system
- Growth of managed care
- Need to document quality
- Consumer demand for greater provider accountability
- Demand by purchasers for quantifiable information on the value of dollars spent
- Technological advances

**TYPES OF OUTCOMES.** To comprehensively demonstrate the value of an agency's service, a manager will want to evaluate a mix of outcomes. Several types of outcomes to consider are the following:

1. *Clinical outcomes.* Clinical measures focus on the appropriateness of clinical decision making and the processes of implementation of care. In nursing, this includes the outcomes identified for the priority diagnoses of the clients. For example, if the client is experiencing dyspnea, a nursing diagnosis of altered breathing patterns may be formulated and the outcome may be absence of dyspnea or a dyspnea rating less than 4 on a scale of 1 to 10. Once the diagnoses and outcomes for a given client population are identified, appropriate time frames for assessment and documentation need to be specified.

2. *Health status outcomes.* In its broadest sense, health status includes all manifestations of health and well-being. The content of most generic measures includes scales for physical and social functioning, role performance, and mental health. Other common measures include self-perceived health, pain, sexual functioning, and quality of life. Condition-specific instruments also exist to measure symptoms and functioning in specific disease states such as cardiac disease, asthma, arthritis, cancer, and others (Medical Outcomes Trust, 1995). Common scales currently used in practice and research include the Sickness Impact Profile, Quality of Well-being Scale, and the Short-form-36 Health Survey, developed by the Medical Outcomes Trust (1995). Normative data exist for many of these scales, especially for the SF-36, which now has comparability data across a variety of populations and languages.

3. *Satisfaction outcomes.* Measures of satisfaction are primarily centered on client perceptions of quality health care and the delivery aspects of client care for a given group. Other customer satisfaction outcomes measure satisfaction of providers and purchasers with care.

4. *Utilization outcomes.* Utilization measures are the most commonly collected and include demographics; length of stay; number of visits; readmission to the hospital; or use of emergency room, physician office, and other health services. They are often broken down by diagnostic category or case type and are a good source of service trends for the organization.

5. *Financial outcomes.* These reflect the costs of providing services. Costs may be broken down as cost of total care, cost per diagnostic category, or cost per visit or episode. An episode of care is defined as one admission to the agency for care of a particular health problem. Cost accounting systems may be used for even deeper analysis of costs and to analyze the impact of changing some aspect of care.

**NURSING OUTCOMES CLASSIFICATION SYSTEMS.** Although OASIS and other national databases have been developed to track outcomes, these databases have been criticized for being heavily focused on medical management related to the outcomes. Efforts to describe nursing sensitive outcomes began in the home health arena in the 1970s with the Omaha system, which allowed clinicians to systematically collect data on client knowledge, behavior, and health status (Martin, Scheet, Stegman, 1993). In the 1980s, a National League for Nursing (NLN) project developed outcome measures of quality care for elderly clients receiving home care, including knowledge and family support as well as clinical outcomes such as functional ability (NLN, 1994). In the last couple of decades, work at the University of Iowa has produced the *Nursing-Sensitive Outcomes Classification* (NOC), which includes client outcomes sensitive to nursing intervention (Johnson, Maas, 1997). These classification systems were discussed further in Chapters 9 and 25. Use of outcomes classifications allow practitioners to utilize technology to assess outcomes and to benchmark with other organizations.

**COLLECTING AND USING OUTCOMES DATA.** Technology used to collect the outcomes data range from written forms to higher tech palm-held and laptop computers. Once data are collected, a reporting mechanism needs to be developed. Reports and graphs aid in aggregating the individual client data or illustrating a particular point such as the number of agency clients in different age groups or the percentage of clients who have improved in different activities of daily living (ADLs). Programs such as Access and Excel allow for easy manipulation of data and can be useful in combining information such as care provider mix with clinical and financial outcomes. Statistics are also an important management tool and can document changes over time in outcomes of critical interest for quality improvement efforts

---

### BOX 24-5
### RESEARCH: *Outcomes Data*

This study demonstrates the potential of home care in promoting positive outcomes for elders at high risk for rehospitalization, while reducing the overall cost of care. The study examined the effectiveness of an advanced practice nurse (APN) in planning the hospital discharge and providing home follow-up for clients over 65 years old. The control group received the routine discharge planning at the study hospitals with no APN intervention. If control subjects were referred to home care, they received the standard of care consistent with Medicare regulations. The group who received the APN intervention had fewer inpatient readmissions and fewer hospital days per client. Authors concluded that while more studies such as this are needed, results do suggest nurses can make a positive difference with involvement in discharge planning and home visiting and can save the health care system money.

From Naylor MD, Brooten D, Campbell R, et al.: Comprehensive discharge planning and home follow-up of hospitalized elders: a randomized clinical trial, *JAMA* 281(7):613-20, 1999.

and to meet accreditation requirements. The graphics in programs such as Excel and Lotus and in presentation programs such as Powerpoint assist the manager in communicating the agency's story to others.

BENCHMARKING OUTCOMES. *Benchmarking* is a tool widely used in outcomes assessment. It involves comparing one's outcomes to others, the discovery and reporting of best practices, and meeting and exceeding the expectations of those who are monitoring one's performance. Benchmarking helps the agency or provider know how they are performing in relation to the "best in class." It can be used to identify strengths and weaknesses and in prioritizing quality improvement efforts. Benchmarking allows the standards to be set so that continuous monitoring can be done relative to those standards. For health care organizations, benchmarks are set with client outcome data. For the benchmarking process to be effective, the same data needs to be collected from all organizations using the same method.

The need for comparability of data is what is behind the mandatory reporting of data sets such as OASIS for Health Care Financing Administration (HCFA) and ORYX performance measures for the Joint Commission on Accreditation of Healthcare Organizations (JCAHO). Strategic use of outcomes and benchmarking data not only allows home care agencies to improve their service and systems for better client satisfaction but also helps the agency be more competitive in negotiations for new clients and contracts and clearly documents effectiveness to policy makers. In the current climate of change and competition, being proactive and having an edge are critical.

Benchmarking began in the business world as a way to measure and evaluate performance. In the 1990s the hospital arena began using the idea extensively as a tool for comparison and improvement. Only recently has the mandate for collecting OASIS data provided the home care industry with the opportunity to standardize definitions and outcomes and measure progress toward best practice. Most agencies begin outcome analyses with populations of high cost or utilization variation. For example, clinicians may be identified with high utilization or poor outcomes due to poor client education practices and this can be corrected. Positive extremes should be examined as well. Provider practice patterns that produce positive outcomes can be identified and duplicated. Use of the information will help the agency identify what is efficient and effective in their services. Evidence-based decisions can be made as to which programs and/or services are achieving results and which ones need to be eliminated.

## APPLYING MANAGEMENT CONCEPTS IN COMMUNITY HEALTH NURSING

In the community health nursing setting, nurses have multiple responsibilities. They may have a large number of families in their caseload, as well as a number of other nursing services to be performed. In addition, community health nurses need to develop collaborative relationships with other disciplines to coordinate family care and to establish priorities for home visits and other activities, such as school and clinic services. Community health nurses also must learn how to effectively delegate tasks to other nursing personnel.

Organizing and scheduling community health nursing activities is not an easy task for an experienced practitioner and is often overwhelming to a new staff member. These activities are easier to handle if staff apply management concepts while carrying out daily responsibilities. Nurses can more readily carry out responsibilities if the following planning activities are used.

### Scheduling Regular Conferences with the Nursing Supervisor

Scheduling regular conferences with the nursing supervisor can assist the nurse in analyzing his or her caseload responsibilities and in establishing priorities for service. With the supervisor's help, the nurse should do both a case analysis of each family who is being seen and a caseload analysis of all the work that is being done. Because turnover of clients is often rapid, this discussion becomes crucial.

### Case Analysis

Case analysis involves analyzing essential information about the family (Box 24-6). It helps nurses look at their approach to families and alter it if needed so that they can be more effective. A written summary, as well as supervisory conferences, facilitates case analyses. A written summary of work with a family, after a given number of visits in a spec-

 **BOX 24-6**

*Case Analysis*

The nurse "diagnoses" each case by answering questions such as the following:
1. What are the health problems of this family as viewed by the family and the nurse?
2. What resources does the family have for meeting these problems?
3. What movement does the family wish to make?
4. What resources are there in the community to assist families in meeting their needs?
5. What nursing activities are needed to contribute to the solution of the problems and to help bring family and community resources into proper relationship with family needs?
6. Are there some parts of the problems or needs that cannot be met at present with the resources available?
7. What has the family done to work toward solving the problem?
8. How effective have nursing interventions and family actions been in resolving current health problems?

ified time frame, helps nurses organize their care and their work. In some agencies this is part of the computerized MIS. The controlling function of management is in effect when case analysis is done as work with clients is being measured and corrections are made.

## Caseload Analysis

Caseload analysis looks at the types and numbers of cases carried, the complexity of problems in the cases visited, the age groups served, the proportion of new referrals received, and the number of emergency or crisis situations, such as individuals with sputum testing positive for tuberculosis. In addition, it examines all the other activities a nurse engages in, such as school visits, clinic services, group work, committee meetings, coordination with other community agencies, and recording and planning time. It improves the nurse's ability to schedule and plan services. A caseload analysis differs from a case analysis because it focuses more on examining the quantity of work the nurse is responsible for and the multiple activities assigned rather than on the needs of individual families.

Caseload analysis is done to determine whether a nurse has sufficient time to implement all assigned responsibilities, to ascertain whether time is being used effectively and efficiently, and to identify whether the needs present in a caseload of families reflect the needs of the population being served. When the caseload is studied, it is wise to graph or tabulate the findings so that they may be readily used and compared with caseloads in other areas or with the same area over time.

Simultaneous caseload study by several nurses may be encouraged occasionally to give a general picture of the services provided by the health agency and to allow for comparisons between nurses. When this was done in one health department, it was found that 2 of 15 census tracts had a disproportionate number of referrals. The result was that workload assignments were reallocated so that work was more evenly divided. Caseload analysis assists the nurse in examining whether there is adequate time to handle the demands of the workload.

Freeman (1949, p. 358), in her classic writings on public health nursing, emphasized that nurses should not try to develop an "average" in the caseloads they carry but should develop a caseload pattern that will provide optimum community service. Currently this continues to be a key principle to follow because of the diverse health problems in society and the dramatic changes in the population structure of the United States. When making comparisons, nurses must keep in mind that caseloads should reflect community needs and population characteristics (see Chapter 14 for the method of determining these needs and characteristics). These data are a regular part of the MIS in some agencies.

## Maintain a Tracking System

Historically, community health nurses maintained a "tickler" system wherein each family in the nurse's caseload had an identification card displaying data such as name, address, telephone number, and service classification(s). The cards were kept in a file box and when the nurse made a home visit, the date of the visit and the month and day for the next visit were indicated on the card.

Today most agencies have moved from such card systems to computer systems, and this information is part of the agency's computerized MIS. Such tracking systems assist the individual nurse in scheduling family visits and determining which families need service and when and the type of service needed. They also can be used to store other data the nurse might want to remember when visiting a client.

## Scheduling Community Health Nursing Activities

A major factor to consider when scheduling community health nursing activities is *priorities*. Once nursing activities are identified, they need to be put in order of importance or caseload priority. The competencies of the nurse, the acuity of the situation, agency policies and procedures, agency staffing, and legal mandates all need to be considered when setting priorities. The nurse makes constant decisions about priorities, with flexibility as a guiding principle. Establishing priorities helps the nurse schedule visits and activities more effectively.

Ruth Rives wrote a classic work for public health nurses on the establishment of priorities according to client needs. An update of Rives's classic article (1958), which provides a basis for determining priorities for nursing services, is provided in Appendix 24-1. Many priorities defined by Rives are still appropriate. Others have been added and some have been deleted.

When setting up a calendar for the month, the staff nurse may find that there is not enough time to carry out all the activities that she or he would like to be able to do. Community health nurses cannot meet all the health needs that are evidenced in the community setting. Money, time, and personnel are not limitless, and all three, in fact, are becoming scarcer commodities. As indicated in Chapters 11 and 13, responsibilities to aggregates in need are based on their vulnerability and their degree of risk. One way the community health nurse determines who will be seen is by setting priorities.

Several other factors need to be considered as the nurse schedules work. Ideally, at the beginning of each month the nurse will develop a calendar that identifies his or her scheduled activities for the month and allows the nurse to see how much time is available for other requests, such as new referrals. If new demands for service exceed the time available, the nurse will then have an organized calendar to share with the nursing supervisor that documents the excess demand and that helps rearrange priorities as necessary.

Nurses in a home health agency typically list all clients to be seen each day on a weekly calendar. They then inform the nurse manager of their plans for that day as priorities become apparent, such as referrals for new clients that must be seen immediately and early morning visits to check the effects of new medication orders. Factors for the community health nurse to consider when scheduling activities are given in Box 24-7.

**BOX 24-7**

*Scheduling Community Health Nursing Activities*

The community health nurse should consider the following parameters when scheduling community nursing activities for the coming week/month:

1. Schedule every case and activity requiring service during the week/month.
2. Schedule new visits around scheduled commitments.
3. Make daily visits at the same time each day, if possible.
4. Establish priorities for visits according to need and timing of visits, as illustrated by the following examples:
   A. Families with new babies: around feeding or bath time, to assess how the family handles these activities
   B. Crisis cases: as soon as possible
   C. IV medications: provide at specified times
   D. Infectious diseases: last in the day, if possible, to decrease potential for exposure to other families
5. Provide for follow-up of families with long-term and chronic diseases.
   A. Disabled or ill individuals
   B. Chronic problems
6. Set time aside for shared home visits when care is delegated to:
   A. Home health aides/assistive personnel
   B. Licensed practical nurses
7. Plan time for:
   A. Office and/or home activities
      1. Planning visits for the week; planning activities for the next week
      2. Assignment of cases
      3. Supervisory conferences
         a. Ancillary personnel
         b. Supervisor
      4. Recording and reporting
      5. Follow-up
         a. Referrals
         b. Phone calls to agencies, physicians, and families
      6. Team meetings
      7. Interdisciplinary conferences (e.g., hospice or case conference with protective service)
   B. Clinic activities
      1. Setting up
      2. Time in clinic
      3. Follow-up and evaluation
   C. School activities
   D. Agency, committee, or community coalition activities

## ORGANIZATIONAL STAFFING PATTERNS FOR COMMUNITY HEALTH NURSING

Another area of concern to nurses who are managing the care of families and groups is the staffing pattern used in a health care organization. Some agencies use a system of district nursing, whereas others use a team nursing system or a case management model. Each of these systems can work as the organizational pattern for care delivery in the agency. It is also possible to mix the patterns within an organization to fit the needs of various clients, nurse teams, and geographical areas. The method of staffing selected by an agency will determine how the nurse schedules and implements monthly and weekly activities.

### District Nursing

If the **district nursing** pattern of organization is used, the community health nurse is assigned a geographical area and is responsible for all open cases, new referrals, and sometimes schools in that district. One advantage of this method is that the same nurse follows the clients, which frequently results in better continuity of care. This method allows for independent planning and decision making, which is often less time consuming and, therefore, less expensive than group decisions. Also, the nurse serves one geographical area, which requires less travel time than traveling in several areas.

The greatest disadvantage for district nursing is the lack of flexibility of the work assignment. If an individual nurse becomes very busy with referrals or if the nurse becomes ill, coverage of the workload is difficult.

Weekly team and/or peer conferences (Figure 24-4) can assist the district nurse to manage his or her caseload. The nurse can use these conferences to increase knowledge in a specific area (e.g., available community resources) and plan for the needs of complex families.

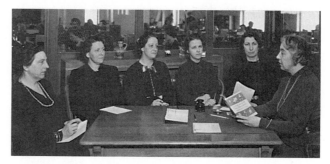

**FIGURE 24-4** The value of team conferences to deal with client, staff, and agency issues has historically been recognized in the field of community nursing. Community health nurses at all levels find it essential to maintain supportive communication with their colleagues. This communication helps them deal with workload demands, maintain an objective perspective about practice issues, and achieve cohesiveness among agency personnel. (Courtesy Metropolitan Life Insurance Company.)

## Team Nursing

Agencies can use a **team nursing** method to deliver nursing services to clients in the community. This involves assigning a team consisting of one or more community health nurses—registered nurses (RNs), licensed practical nurses (LPNs), and home health aides (HHAs) or assistive personnel—to serve a larger geographical area or larger caseload than that in a district nursing assignment. Each member of the team covers the same geographical area. Team nursing offers the advantage of lending more flexibility to work assignments because several team members can share new referrals or care of clients. Perhaps its greatest advantage is that quality of service can improve as a result of the shared planning and problem solving that occurs in regularly planned team conferences. Disadvantages are that more time is needed for planning because of the number of people involved, and travel expenses are often increased.

When the team method is used, it is important to monitor carefully the continuity of care. If cases are divided between nurses who job-share or between part-time nurses, lack of continuity of care may result. This is a major complaint from clients who "see a different nurse every time" and their physicians. When cases are shared, the number of different personnel sharing cases should be minimized, and mechanisms to maintain effective and efficient communication should be established.

## Case Management

The case management model, now used by many community agencies, has as its goal achievement of quality care outcomes while controlling costs. Standardizing resources accomplish this with clear direction for specific client interventions for like problems and with expected caregiver and system outcomes. **Case management nursing** promotes collaboration among all disciplines to provide ongoing care from preadmission to postdischarge while involving the family in the process. Although this sounds like typical community health nursing, the emphasis in case management models is on *case types*. Case managers are often allocated in home health to certain disease entities such as congestive heart failure or broader clinical specialties such as heart disease.

Chronic illnesses such as congestive heart failure, diabetes, and chronic airflow limitations often require case management services in the home after an acute exacerbation of the disease. Case managers also are commonly involved with conditions that require rehabilitation services after hospitalization such as joint replacements, strokes, and heart surgery. Services of several disciplines such as nursing, physical therapy, occupational therapy, and even speech therapy must often be coordinated and the progress of clients closely monitored to ensure positive client outcomes. Case managers are very helpful in dealing with managed care's capitated services and Medicare's prospective payment system due to strict limitations on the number of visits. In addition to monitoring the client's progress, case managers ensure that necessary services are being provided in a timely manner so the client's optimal level of wellness is being met in the time frames specified.

Some community-based case managers have a predominant focus on well populations who are at high risk for needing health care services. The goal with these populations is to maximize wellness by coordinating and integrating community services and programs (Cesta, Tahan, Fink, 1998). Community-based case managers also may manage chronically ill clients who typically have complex health needs and use a wide range of health services from multiple settings. Because of their complex pattern of health utilization, these clients are at high risk for receiving less-than-adequate, duplicative, and even delayed services.

The community-based case manager improves communication among providers across settings and provides referral and tracking services. The case manager integrates the services provided across the health care continuum so that loopholes and delays are avoided and cost-effective care is delivered in a more coordinated seamless approach. Both formal and informal mechanisms can be used to provide these services, such as community nursing clinics, home visits, and telephone and telehealth contacts. All services in this case management model are delivered on a continuous rather than episodic basis (Trella, 1996).

Illustrative of this use of case management is the focus on high-risk children at the Gloucester County Health Department in New Jersey. This health department uses the case management model to promote early identification, evaluation, diagnosis, and treatment of children with special needs and potentially disabling conditions. The case manager, a nurse who has a caseload of 300 families, is responsible for a team that counsels families, assesses the need for services, promotes and facilitates communication among the team providing services, and monitors the services received (ANA, 1988).

Case management systems often use clinical pathways designed to standardize care for common medical conditions or procedures. The plans delineate best or ideal practice specifying the timing and sequence of interventions used to achieve specific outcomes or goals for those clients. Clinical pathways are multidisciplinary in scope and reflect the standard of care at that agency. Through standardization of interventions and time lines, more efficient care is given improving quality and reducing overall costs (Cesta, Tahan, Fink, 1998). Clinical pathways thus serve as guidelines and checkpoints for the performance of the client and provider along the pathway. When a client does not meet an expected outcome on the pathway, a variance is said to have occurred. Variances may be a result of client concerns such as an infection or a learning problem, provider errors such as omitting an order, or system problems such as a break in equipment. Variances always signal the need for additional intervention.

Clinical pathways are labeled in a variety of ways in different institutions such as critical path or pathway, care maps, care steps, case management plans, anticipated recovery plans, and multidisciplinary action plans. Some of the terms (e.g., care maps) are copyrighted and others are not. Clinical pathways will not fit all clients with the diagnosis, but they are intended to fit the majority and quickly identify those clients needing different or intensive services and the further attention of the case manager. Pathways are usually most useful for client conditions that are high risk in some way such as high volume or high cost or those that have high rates of readmission, complications, customer dissatisfaction, or variability in lengths of stay. The pathways are designed to address these concerns through better communication among disciplines, delineation of responsibilities, and better allocation and coordination of resources. The goal is to provide quality of care while eliminating redundancy, fragmentation, and duplication of care activities (Cohen, Cesta, 1997). Improved outcomes are the result.

Home care pathways outline the number of visits for a particular condition and interventions for each discipline at each visit (Appendix 24-2). Expected outcomes are predetermined so that the number of client visits is appropriate to meet the expected outcomes. The allocated visits are then used to monitor the client's progress toward the outcomes (Appendix 24-3). Variances from the expected pattern can be identified early and further interventions used as necessary (see Appenidx 24-3). Visit outcome patterns can be benchmarked to provide agency and provider feedback. The termination point for the case is clearly defined related to the outcomes, and the provider no longer has to make a subjective decision as to when to close a case. Cases kept open beyond the appropriate time are very costly to the agency and signal the need for intervention. Closing cases appropriately, based on outcomes, allows resources to be allocated to those cases that truly need extended services beyond the standard.

With this model, nursing personnel are used efficiently, expected client outcomes are well delineated, timely discharge is facilitated, material resources are used appropriately, and collaborative practice is promoted. (See Chapters 10 and 24 for more discussion of case management). Continued growth of case management models and their applications in the community setting can be expected in the years to come. The disadvantage to this model is that sometimes it is applied in a strictly case-specific rather than general scope.

## USING VARIOUS LEVELS OF HEALTH PERSONNEL*

Various personnel are used in agencies to deliver community health nursing services. In nearly any community health setting, staff members who are prepared at various levels are involved in offering nursing services. In some agencies RNs (BSN-, AD-, and diploma-prepared), LPNs, and HHAs or assistive personnel are hired. In others only RNs and HHAs are available. In yet others, only BSN-prepared RNs are used. Knowledge of the educational preparation of these persons and the agency job descriptions are most helpful tools when nurses need to decide how to use personnel appropriately and determine what type of orientation and staff development is needed. Understanding a state's nurse practice act and the regulations regarding the practice of different levels of personnel is also essential.

HHAs or assistive personnel are often prepared through noncredit courses that provide 75 hours with at least 16 hours devoted to supervised practical training. Medicare regulations require that HHAs complete training and competency evaluation programs and have at least 12 hours of inservice training during each 12-month period. In the community setting HHAs can give personal care and assist with housekeeping, marketing, and preparation of meals. HHAs can give the kinds of personal care that can be taught easily to a family member if there is someone to teach.

The LPN is prepared to give physical care, to make observations about physical conditions, to carry out special rehabilitative measures after being instructed by the community health nurse, to continue the teaching of clients begun by the registered nurse, and to contribute to the nursing care plan of a client. There is a significant difference in the level of care given by LPNs and assistive personnel. The LPN has knowledge and skill that helps in making limited client assessments and contributing to the development of nursing interventions. HHAs have knowledge and skill to provide *unskilled* client care. Both the LPN and HHA, however, are prepared to function under the supervision of an RN. They both make valuable contributions on the health care team.

The RN prepared at the AD or diploma level has been prepared in institutions that have a client-centered approach to care. The RN is usually highly skilled in the care of home health service clients who are ill and who need expert care and observations in the home. Because the RN often has developed expertise in technical procedures, she or he can teach these techniques to other staff and family members. The RN has skill and knowledge to assist in the development of the nursing care plan, especially with clients who have disease conditions. Because the RN's preparation has been primarily client centered, she or he should receive orientation in relation to family-centered nursing practice, concepts related to analyzing the needs of populations, and principles relative to the coordination of care and prevention, if she or he is expected to implement all the services provided by community health nurses in a health department. This orientation is a necessity. It is un-

---

*We are indebted to Ruth Carey, former Vice President of Clinical Services, Michigan Home Health Care, Traverse City, Michigan, for the use of this material.

fair to expect the RN, prepared at the AD or diploma level, to provide comprehensive community health nursing services. She or he has not been prepared to do so. If only these RNs are available, an agency has the responsibility to provide them with orientation and staff development opportunities that adequately prepare them to carry out the demands of the job.

The baccalaureate-prepared nurse has received education in community health with an emphasis on wellness and prevention and experience in the community health setting. She or he is expected to have a family-centered focus and to function in a comprehensive fashion. This entails identifying client strengths and needs and all variables that affect health and illness (physical, social, and emotional), facilitating identification of family health goals, and assisting families to reach their goals. The community health nurse initiates, plans, and evaluates care. In addition, she or he participates in planning for the health needs of the community and works in schools, clinics, and community groups, giving service and functioning as a planning participant to see that needed services are provided.

Another caregiver seen in the community setting is the Community/Public Health Advanced Practice Nurse, who is a clinical nurse specialist or nurse practitioner in community/public health. This nurse is prepared with a master's degree in nursing and the public health sciences and functions in clinical and administrative roles. The practice of this person is focused on a community and/or population and defines and implements the nursing leadership aspects of the core public health functions of assessment, policy development, and assurance.

After orientation, which assists neophytes to the independence of the community as well as how to travel about safely and efficiently, nurses begin to develop familiarity with an organization's policies, procedures, and expectations. For the contemporary professional in the community setting, learning continues. The rapidly changing health care system and resulting complexities of care requirements make it important to have a sound staff development program in an organization.

## Delegation as a Management Function in Community Health Nursing

To carry out the diverse responsibilities of the position, the community health nurse frequently assigns tasks to other health care personnel. Delegation is the process of designating tasks and bestowing on others the authority needed to accomplish these assigned tasks. When delegating responsibilities to others, the community health nurse should follow the process outlined in Box 24-8.

A synonym for delegation is *empowerment*. Thus when nurses assign a task for which they are responsible to another person, they are empowering that person to do that

---

**● BOX 24-8**

*Process of Delegation*

1. Analyze the nature of the task to be delegated, considering the complexity and the time involved to complete it
2. Determine the capability of the individual staff member to handle the assigned responsibility, especially noting the staff member's education and experience background and other workload responsibilities
3. Identify the willingness of the staff member to accept responsibility for the assigned activity
4. Determine how much time will be needed to supervise tasks that are delegated to others
5. Prepare the person and explain the task clearly
6. Keep in touch for support and monitoring progress
7. Praise and acknowledge a job well done; use poor outcomes to teach

---

task. Carried out correctly, delegation requires instruction about what needs to be done, as well as attention to issues of employee motivation (McConnell, 1995). The key to appropriate delegation is to give the person assigned the task the equivalent authority and responsibility.

Although delegation does not negate the personal responsibility that the nurse has for the care given, appropriate delegation does mean that the person being made responsible must be given sufficient authority to complete the task. And, as discussed earlier, people need to be given the freedom to fail: mistakes need to be treated as a growth experience. The nurse provides instruction, support, resources, explains the results expected, and gives overall direction. Knowledgeable staff are empowered staff.

For nurses educated and experienced in the primary care model, the use of assistive personnel is often a challenge for which they are not prepared. A change in mindset, from "doing it all myself" to trusting one's responsibilities for care to others requires not only the ability to judge what can be delegated but also the ability to empower that person to carry out the work and to trust them in the process.

Care given by assistive personnel or LPNs should never be increased so rapidly that it is impossible for the community health nurse to adequately supervise the care delegated to them. The community health nurse must have sufficient time available to apply the principles of the five management functions when carrying out supervisory activities with HHAs and LPNs. Examples of these supervisory activities are displayed in Box 24-9. Research shows that supervision is a critical component of quality assurance (Moore, 1990; Spiegel, 1987) and personnel retention (Donovan, 1989; Feldman, 1990).

### BOX 24-9
*Example Supervisory Activities with Assistive Personnel*

1. Shared home visits with the licensed practical nurse (LPN) or home health assistant (HHA) on the initial visit to a family (planning, organizing)
2. Development of nursing care plans for each family in the caseload, based on assessment data and input from the LPN or HHA (planning, organizing)
3. Regular conferences with the LPN or HHA to determine guidance and assistance needed in specific situations (directing, organizing, coordinating)
4. Periodic shared visits with the LPN or HHA for supervision and reevaluation of the status of the family (directing, coordinating, controlling)
5. Periodic review of family records to evaluate the status of the family and the level of nursing service (controlling)
6. Inservice education related to the needs of the staff and the families in the nurse's caseload (directing)

## INTERDISCIPLINARY COLLABORATION

One of the expectations for effective health professionals repeatedly identified in the literature is the need for interdisciplinary collaboration. It is also a focus of reengineering, discussed earlier in this chapter. The emerging health care system will require all health care professionals to "work effectively as a team member in organized settings that emphasize the integration of care" (Pew Health Professions Commission, 1995, p. 5). As integrated managed care systems become the dominant source of health care, nurses will be a part of teams and will relate to other social and academic organizations. Community health nurses have had a long history of collaboration with other disciplines, and we can continue to build on this strength. Box 24-10 lists some barriers to working in collaborative teams along with strategies for successful teams. Notice the themes that have been repeated in this chapter: (1) all levels of workers are managers and leaders, (2) an emphasis on process, (3) mistakes are made and learning must occur from mistakes, and (4) trust is an important consideration.

## A DIVERSE WORKFORCE

The American population and workforce are becoming increasingly diverse. The racial and ethnic composition of the United States is changing at a dramatic rate. Estimates are that the 18% of the population that is nonwhite today will reach 40% by the year 2030.

Briggance, the Associate Director of the California Workforce Initiative, argues that "the effect of America's growing multiculturalism will outstrip all other social, economic, and technological trends both in its scope and fe-

### BOX 24-10
*Collaborative Interdisciplinary Teamwork*

*Types of Barriers to Collaborative Teamwork, With Examples*

1. *Organizational barriers:* lack of knowledge and appreciation for the roles of other professionals; legal issues related to scope of practice and liability
2. *Barriers at a team level:* role and leadership ambiguity; team too large or too small; lack of a clearly stated purpose
3. *Barriers faced by individual team members:* multiple responsibilities and job titles; competition, naiveté; gender, race, and class issues

*Strategies for Effective Interdisciplinary Teams*

1. Agree on a unifying philosophy centered around the primary care of the client and the community: define a vision of collaborative team care
2. Develop a commitment to the common goal of collaboration: simply believe in the power of the team
3. Learn about the contributions other disciplines bring to the team
4. Respect others' skills and knowledge: clients and their families and communities bring strengths to the interdisciplinary team
5. Establish positive attitudes about your own profession: when you are comfortable with yourself you will be able to value others
6. Develop trust between members
7. Be willing to share responsibility for client care: trust others' abilities
8. Establish mechanisms for negotiation and renegotiation of goals and roles over time: time and knowledge bring change to the team structure
9. Establish methods for resolving the conflicts that are inevitable among team members
10. Be willing to work continuously to overcome barriers: do not give up when the going gets rough

From Grant R: *Interdisciplinary collaborative teams in primary care: a model curriculum and resource guide*, San Francisco, 1995, Pew Health Professions Commissions.

cundity" (2001, p.1). Not only is the health care system not immune to the effects of these changes but also it is currently not prepared to handle them (Briggance, 2001). The composition of the RN workforce, as in other health-related professions, does not reflect the heterogeneity of the population it serves. In 1984 only 10.5% of the RNs employed in nursing were nonwhite (USDHHS, 1996). This has only risen to 12.3% in 2000 and has not increased to match population trends (USDHHS, 2001).

Briggance (2001) offers two proactive suggestions for the health care workforce: (1) increase the cultural awareness and sensitivity of those currently in practice, and (2) increase the diversity of the health care workforce. The pres-

### BOX 24-11

*Seven Cross-Cultural Skills*

1. *Show respect.* How can you demonstrate that you respect the people with whom you are working? Does your demonstration of respect mean the same thing to you that it does to the people with whom you are working?
2. *Tolerate uncertainty.* The ability to react to new, different, and unpredictable situations with little visible discomfort or irritation.
3. *Relate to people.* Are you concerned with the task side of the job rather than the people side? Do people feel a part of the work situation or do they feel used?
4. *Be nonjudgmental.* Do you withhold judgment and remain objective until you have enough information to understand another point of view?
5. *Personalize your observations.* Different people explain the world about them in different terms. Your knowledge and perceptions are valid only for you and not the rest of the world. What is right or true in one culture may not be right or true in another.
6. *Be empathetic.* Attempt to see things from another person's point of view.
7. *Be patient.* You may not be successful the first time and may not be able to get things done immediately, but be patient and persevere.

ence of cultural and linguistic barriers impedes the ability of nurses to provide the holistic and individualized care they desire to give. Improving cultural sensitivity of the nursing workforce will facilitate better understanding and communication between nurses and their clients. Increasing minority recruitment into nursing is just as important.

Briggance (2001) makes the point that this is far more than just increasing the cultural understanding that having providers of the same ethnic origin might provide. He stated the real goal in increasing the diversity of the workforce is to make sure that the needs of all clients are recognized in the policies, practices, and attitudes of the health care industry.

Effective leaders and managers must have and model cross-cultural skills (Box 24-11) to promote the health care environment needed for the future. They must encourage cultural sensitivity training for their workforce to provide the skills nurses need to work with people who do things differently than they do. Effective leaders and managers understand that although all people are ethnocentric to some degree (thinking that their own ways of doing things are the "right ways"), it is important to lessen the degree of ethnocentrism and promote acceptance of people for who they are.

Cultural sensitivity involves making the effort to learn how others like to do things. For example, in Germany the common form of greeting is to shake hands, extended to women before men, and one is addressed formally (Mrs. and

Mr.) even after years of working together. In Japan the group is the most important part of society and is emphasized for motivation in the workplace. In Korea, to accomplish something while causing unhappiness or discomfort for someone else is to accomplish nothing at all.

Culturally competent managers and leaders know that conflict is a natural part of working with people who do things differently. However, they have the skills to deal with that conflict and will help their colleagues to learn those skills. Leaders and managers acknowledge that diversity in a workplace can bring strength and that many ways of looking at a situation are ideal for solving problems. Overall, better use of cross-cultural skills will result in workforces that are more productive, personally and professionally.

In addition, effective leaders and managers will recognize the critical importance of increasing the diversity of their staff. If nursing is to be a leader in health care reform, we must lead in being a profession representative of those we serve. Efforts to improve recruitment and retention of a culturally diverse nursing workforce will demonstrate this resolve and help nursing improve its response to the critical needs of our society.

## SUMMARY

Community health nurses have multiple and diverse responsibilities in the practice setting, and they understand that they are both managers and leaders in carrying out these responsibilities. They have found that by applying the principles of management, they are more effective in dealing with the complex demands in the work environment. Knowledge of the five functions of management and their use in managing change and working with teams is especially helpful. The use of a management information system supports these management functions and can promote organizational effectiveness.

The development of management thought has changed over time. Reviewing the historical evolution of management helps nurses understand why it is useful to implement the five functions of management in the work setting. Analysis of the evolution of management is also beneficial because it provides a basis for defining a personal philosophy of management and leadership.

The use of management concepts in the community health nursing setting is essential. Management principles help the community health nurse organize and schedule activities, establish priorities for nursing service, effectively and efficiently utilize time, work collaboratively with others, and appropriately delegate responsibilities. All these tasks must be accomplished for the community health nurse to deliver quality care to clients in the community.

A changing health care climate and a diverse workforce contribute to a work setting that is stimulating and in flux. Principles of reengineering assist organizations with these changes in a productive manner.

## CRITICAL THINKING
*exercise*

Lieutenant General William G. Pagonis led 40,000 men and women who ran the theater logistics during the Persian Gulf War. Following are his remarks about leadership: "To lead successfully, a person must demonstrate two active, essential, and interrelated traits: expertise and empathy. In my experience, both of these traits can be deliberately and systematically cultivated; this personal development is the first important building block of leadership... The good news is that leaders are made, not born. I'm convinced that anyone who wants to work hard enough and develop these traits can lead" (Pagonis, 1992, p. 118).

Describe the type of expertise you look for in a leader and share your perceptions of the concept of *empathy* as it relates to leadership. Identify your strengths and needs in terms of these two leadership traits, expertise and empathy, and discuss how you would cultivate your leadership abilities.

## REFERENCES

American Nurses Association (ANA): *Nursing case management*, Kansas City, Mo, 1988, ANA.

American Nurses Association (ANA): *Standards for organized nursing services and responsibilities of nurse administrators across all settings*, Washington, DC, 1991, ANA.

Anderson R: Future organizational leadership, *J Professional Nurs* 13(6):334, 1997.

Benjamin S, Penland T: How developmental supervision and performance management improve effectiveness, *Health Care Superv* 14(4):12-19, 1995.

Boston Consulting Group: *Reengineering and beyond*, Boston, 1993, The Group.

Briggance MA: Impact of global immigration on health care, *February 2001 Exploring*, The Center for the Health Professions Website. Retrieved from the internet March 24, 2001. *http://www.futurehealth.ucsf.edu/ftd_archive.html*

Cesta TG, Tahan HA, Fink LF: *The case manager's survival guide: winning strategies for clinical practice*, St Louis, 1998, Mosby.

Chaffee M: A telephone odyssey, *Am J Nurs* 99(7):27-32, 1999.

Cohen EL, Cesta TG: *Nursing case management: from concept to evaluation*, ed 2, St Louis, 1997, Mosby.

Dittbrenner H: Employment outlook: put on your sunglasses, *Caring* 15(5):10-12, 1996.

Donovan R: Worker stress and job satisfaction: a study of home care workers in New York City, *Home Health Care Serv Q* 16:97-114, 1989.

Ellison KJ: *Change model for managers*, unpublished manuscript, 2001.

Essex D: Telemedicine, *Healthcare Informatics* February:100-101, 1999.

Feldman P: *Who cares for them? Workers in the home care industry*, New York, 1990, Greenwood.

Freedman DH: Is management a science? *Harvard Business Rev* 70(6):26-38, 1992.

Freeman RB: *Techniques of supervision in public health nursing*, ed 2, Philadelphia, 1949, WB Saunders.

Gleick J: *Chaos: making a new science*, New York, 1987, Viking.

Grant R: *Interdisciplinary collaborative teams in primary care: a model curriculum and resource guide*, San Francisco, 1995, Pew Health Professions Commission.

Hammer M, Champy J: *Reengineering the corporation: a manifesto for business revolution*, New York, 1993, Harper.

Handy C: *The age of unreason*, Boston, 1990, Harvard University Press.

Hersey P: *Situational selling*, Escondido, Calif, 1985, Center for Leadership Studies.

Hersey P, Blanchard KH, Johnson DE: *Management of organizational behavior: leading human resources*, ed 8, Upper Saddle River, NJ, 2001, Prentice Hall.

Johnson M, Maas M, editors: *Nursing outcomes classification (NOC)*, St Louis, 1997, Mosby.

Kincaid K: Growing home-care business benefits from telemedicine TLC, *Telemedicine and Telehealth Networks* October:23-26, 1997.

Lewin K: *Field theory in social science: selected theoretical papers*, New York, 1951, Harper and Row.

Martin KS, Scheet NJ: *The Omaha system: applications for community health nursing*, Philadelphia, 1992, WB Saunders.

Martin KS, Scheet, NJ, Stegman MR: Home health clients: characteristics, outcomes of care, and nursing interventions, *Am J Nurs* 83:1730-1734, 1993.

Maslow AH: *Motivation and personality*, New York, 1954, Harper & Row.

Medical Outcomes Trust: *Medical Outcomes Trust Bull* 3(5):1-4, 1995.

McConnell CR: Delegation versus empowerment: what, how, and is there a difference? *Health Care Superv* 14(1):66-79, 1995.

Milio N: *The engines of empowerment: using information technology to create healthy communities and challenge public policy*, Chicago, 1996, Health Administration Press.

Moore F: What about the quality of care, *Caring* 9:16-26, 1990.

National League for Nursing (NLN): *Summary of findings: In search of excellence in home care*, New York, 1994, NLN.

Naylor MD, Brooten D, Campbell R, et al.: Comprehensive discharge planning and home follow-up of hospitalized elders: a randomized clinical trial, *JAMA* 281(7):613-620, 1999.

Pagonis WG: The work of the leader, *Harvard Bus Rev* 70(6):118-126, 1992.

Pew Health Professions Commission: *Critical challenges: revitalizing the health professions for the twenty-first century. The third report of the Pew Health Professions Commission*, San Francisco, November 1995, UCSF Center for the Health Professions.

Rives R: Priorities according to needs. In Stewart DM, Vincent PA, editors: *Public health nursing*, Dubuque, Iowa, 1958, Brown.

Senge PM: *The fifth discipline: the art and practice of the learning organization*, New York, 1990, Doubleday.

Spiegel A: *Home health care*, ed 2, Owing Mills, Md, 1987, National Health Publishing.

Spradley BW: Managing change creatively, *J Nurs Adm*, May:32-37, 1980.

Timmreck TC: Use of the classical functions of management by health services midmanagers, *Health Care Manager* 19(2):50-67, 2000.

Trella B: Integrating services across the continuum: The challenge of chronic care. In Cohen E, editor: *Nursing case management in the 21st century*, St Louis, 1996, Mosby.

US Department of Health and Human Services (USDHHS), Division of Nursing: *National sample survey of registered nurses*, March, 1996. Also prior surveys.

US Department of Health and Human Services (USDHHS), Division of Nursing: *Preliminary data from the National sample survey of registered nurses*, February, 2001.

Visiting Nurse Association of Greater Philadelphia: *Software requirements, evaluation and selection for the voluntary home health agency*, Philadelphia, 1990-1992, The Association.

VNA First: *Home care steps pathways to health*, LaGrange, Ill, 2001, VNA First.

Wagner C: World trends and forecasts: demography: minority health, *Futurist* 35(3):12-13, 2001.

Wooten R, Loane M, Mair F, et al.: A joint U.S.-U.K. study of home telenursing, *J Telemedicine and Telecare* 4(1):83-85, 1998.

## SELECTED BIBLIOGRAPHY

Beckhard R, Pritchard W: *Changing the essence: the art of creating and leading fundamental change in organizations,* San Francisco, 1992, Jossey-Bass.

Budzek L, Cober S: 10 tips for success as a nurse manager, *Am J Nurs* 96(6):48-49, 1996.

Crane J, Crane N: A multilevel performance appraisal tool: transition from the traditional to a CQI approach, *Health Care Manage Rev* 25(1):64-73, 2000.

Cumbey D, Alexander J: The relationship of job satisfaction with organizational variables in public health nursing, *J Nurs Adm* 28(5):39-46, 1998.

Everson-Bates S: First line managers in the expanded role: an ethnographic study, *J Nurs Adm* 22(3):32-37, 1992.

Glen P: *It's not my department: how America can return to excellence-giving and receiving quality service,* New York, 1992, Berkley.

Hein E. *Nursing issues in the 21ˢᵗ century: perspectives from the literature,* Philadelphia, 2001, JB Lippincott.

Katzemback J: The myth of the top management team, *Harvard Business Review* 75(6):83-91, 1997.

Kiernan MJ: *The eleven commandments of 21ˢᵗ century management,* Englewood Cliffs, NJ, 1996, Prentice Hall.

Nieuenhaus SS: Legal considerations for the hiring process, *Caring* 5:20-23, 1996.

Sheerer J: Lessons in leadership: keys to success from some of corporate America's best-known leaders, *Healthcare Executive* 13(2):12-17, 1997.

Timmreck T: Developing successful performance appraisal through choosing appropriate words to effectively describe work, *Health Care Manage Rev* 23(3):48-57, 1998.

# Priorities in Community Health Nursing

## Purposes

1. To identify target population groups requiring community health nursing service
2. To identify realistic spacing of nurse service contacts according to identified target population group
3. To use levels of prevention and health promotion in planning nursing service to a community

## Code

- *Classification I: intensive visiting* is defined as visits spaced daily to 3 times a week
- *Classification II: periodic visiting* is defined as visits spaced every 1 to 2 weeks
- *Classification III: widely spaced visiting* is defined as visits spaced every 2 to 3 months

| | I. INTENSIVE VISITING | II. PERIODIC VISITING | III. WIDELY SPACED VISITING |
|---|---|---|---|
| **Communicable Disease** | | | |
| A. Tuberculosis (by law a priority) | To families who 1. Have young adults and unexamined contacts living in crowded home conditions with a client who has positive sputum 2. Have a recently diagnosed client with positive sputum 3. Have a diagnosed client with positive suptum, who is recalcitrant 4. Have a recently diagnosed client without positive sputum 5. Have a client who is immunosuppressed (AIDS, chronic illness, receiving chemotherapy) | To families who 1. Have the client with positive sputum hospitalized; have no young adults in the family; have good living standards but have some unexamined contacts 2. Need preparation for the hospital admission of the client 3. Need preparation for the discharge of the client | To families who 1. Have an arrested client returned to good home conditions 2. Have had all contacts examined and the client hospitalized under adequate medical supervision 3. Are under adequate medical supervision, with the source of infection located |
| B. Acute reportable dangerous communicable diseases | To families who 1. Have been contacts to reportable dangerous communicable disease 2. Have a diagnosed client needing home care 3. Have food handlers as a case/contact to *Salmonella* | To families who 1. Are unimmunized 2. Have a client under medical care but complications develop 3. Need follow-up for defects after recovery from acute stage | To families who 1. Are known to have immunization against communicable disease 2. Are receiving adequate medical care 3. Have a typhoid carrier in the home |
| C. Sexually transmissible diseases | To clients who 1. Need treatments and education on the prevention and spread of disease | To clients who 1. Need follow-up clinical examinations (e.g., spinal taps) | |

Modified from Rives R: Priorities according to needs, *Nurs Outlook* 6:404-408, 1958. Updated for the 3rd edition by F. Armignacco, Director of Patient Services and Community Nursing, Monroe Co. Department of Health, Rochester, NY; updated for the 4th edition by L. Randar, RN, MPH, Director, Division of Nursing, Philadelphia Department of Health, Philadelphia. Updated for the 5th edition by Joyce Kachelries, RN, BSN, Clinical Nursing Supervisor, Family Home Care, Hamilton, Ohio.

# Priorities in Community
# Health Nursing (cont'd)

| | I. INTENSIVE VISITING | II. PERIODIC VISITING | III. WIDELY SPACED VISITING |
|---|---|---|---|
| C. Sexually transmissible diseases—cont'd | 2. Have known contacts they will name<br>3. Need examination, advice on treatment, and education on how to arrest and prevent the transfer of infection<br>4. Need posttreatment observation<br>5. Need to be convinced of the necessity of the treatment ordered by the doctor<br>6. Need to be taught how to prevent further manifestations of the disease<br>7. Have babies born of mothers with active STD<br>8. To families who need instruction and assistance to care for a person with AIDS | | |

## Home Care of the Sick

| | I. INTENSIVE VISITING | II. PERIODIC VISITING | III. WIDELY SPACED VISITING |
|---|---|---|---|
| A. Cardiovascular disease | To clients who<br>1. Have cardiac failure or have had an acute cardiac episode from any cause<br>2. Have a chronic cardiac disability requiring active treatment: medical, nursing, dietetic<br>3. Have had a CVA and require active treatment: medical, nursing, occupational, and physical therapy<br>4. Have cardiac surgery | To clients who<br>1. Have a congenital heart disease: nonoperable, postoperative<br>2. Have a murmur of undetermined origin with a history of rheumatic fever<br>3. Have congenital heart disease (to be followed until a thorough medical evaluation is completed)<br>4. Have diagnosed, untreated, uncontrolled hypertension | To clients who<br>1. Have a history of rheumatic fever but no clinical heart disease<br>2. Are under medical care, stabilized for cardiovascular diagnoses |
| B. Diabetes | To clients who<br>1. Are newly diagnosed, not stabilized by diet or insulin<br>2. Cannot take own insulin (blind, aged, low mentality, and so forth)<br>3. Have difficulty understanding diet or administering their own insulin<br>4. Have uncontrolled diabetes<br>5. Have diabetes with gangrene | To clients who<br>1. Are newly diagnosed, administering own insulin but still needing supervision<br>2. Are suspected of having diabetes | To clients who<br>1. Are under medical care, stabilized as to diet or insulin, or both |

*Continued*

# Priorities in Community Health Nursing (cont'd)

| | I. INTENSIVE VISITING | II. PERIODIC VISITING | III. WIDELY SPACED VISITING |
|---|---|---|---|
| B. Diabetes—cont'd | 6. Have diabetes complicated by an infection<br>To caregivers who<br>1. Will be the persons maintaining the regimen of medications, diet, foot care, and daily assessments | | |
| C. Kidney disease | To clients who<br>1. Are on dialysis<br>2. Have comorbidities such as wound care<br>3. Need help with medications and diet and understanding disease | To clients who<br>1. Understand medications and diet but are not stabilized<br>2. Have other medical problems | To clients who<br>1. Are under medical care and are stabilized |
| D. Cancer | To clients who<br>1. Are discharged from a hospital and need active nursing care, instruction for themselves, and interpretation of their physical and emotional needs to the family<br>2. Have symptoms suspicious of cancer; need medical supervision, completion of all tests and examinations, and, if required, treatment on the earliest possible date<br>3. Are diagnosed but who, without consulting the physicians, have interrupted their treatment or discontinued having medical checkups<br>4. Are under observation for malignancy but delinquent from regular medical supervision (the urgency of a client's problem can be determined only by the attending physician)<br>5. Have hospice/terminal care needs<br>6. Need complex, high-technology interventions such as TPN intravenous feedings, dobutamine IV, or pain control | To clients who<br>1. Have precancerous lesions and are delinquent for periodic checkups (cervical erosions, leukoplakias, keratoses, mastitis, and others)<br>2. Have cancer apparently treated successfully but are not reporting for medical reexamination (cancer of the skin with no apparent recurrence)<br>3. Have advanced disease and need care (some of these clients may need to be in intensive visiting classification)<br>4. Have families that have been taught to carry out medical orders but need support in continuing medical supervision | To clients about whom<br>1. Information is needed for statistical purposes (cured, deceased, or other) |

# Priorities in Community
# Health Nursing (cont'd)

| I. INTENSIVE VISITING | II. PERIODIC VISITING | III. WIDELY SPACED VISITING |
|---|---|---|
| E. Other noncommunicable diseases, acute or chronic | To clients who<br>1. Are acutely ill and need nursing care<br>2. Are helpless or bedridden and need nursing service<br>3. Are senile and do not receive adequate home care<br>4. Are acutely ill or helpless but have families who can be taught how to give the necessary care<br>5. Are receiving terminal care | To clients who<br>1. Are acutely ill or helpless but whose families can provide care under nursing supervision<br>2. Need encouragement to continue medical care<br>3. Need emotional support to carry out health instructions | To clients who<br>1. Are under adequate medical supervision and are given good home care (by the family, a registered nurse, or a practical nurse) |

## *Health Teaching and Supervision*

| | | | |
|---|---|---|---|
| A. Maternity-antepartum | To women who<br>1. Are primiparas<br>2. Are under 17 or over 40 years of age<br>3. Are single parents<br>4. Are of low socioeconomic status<br>5. Are hypertensive<br>6. Have poor nutrition<br>7. Are not under medical care<br>8. Have had six or more pregnancies<br>9. Have had conditions associated with pregnancy resulting in infant deaths<br>10. Have had complications in past pregnancies or have signs of complications in the present pregnancy, including psychosomatic disturbances<br>11. Have a chronic disease, such as tuberculosis, diabetes, syphilis, anemia, nephritis, cardiac disease, or rheumatic fever<br>12. Have previously had premature deliveries<br>13. Are HIV-positive and/or drug abusers | To women who<br>1. Have adequate medical supervision for apparently normal pregnancies<br>2. Are in good physical and mental condition<br>3. Are able to follow advice<br>4. Have questions and desire help | (No antepartum clients in this category) |

*Continued*

# Priorities in Community
# Health Nursing (cont'd)

| | I. INTENSIVE VISITING | II. PERIODIC VISITING | III. WIDELY SPACED VISITING |
|---|---|---|---|
| B. Maternity-postpartum | To women who<br>1. Have nursing problems or breast complications, such as engorgement or abscess<br>2. Are not receiving adequate medical supervision or competent nursing care<br>3. Had complications or accidents of labor: stillbirths, abortions, or other difficulties resulting in a mishap to the mother or baby<br>4. Delivered prematurely<br>5. Had multiple births<br>6. Delivered a baby with a congenital defect<br>7. Had a baby that died during the first month of life<br>8. Evidence of poor maternal-infant bonding<br>9. Have no or few support systems<br>10. Are economically stressed (low socioeconomic status) | To women who<br>1. Had problems but are making normal progress 7 days after delivery<br>2. Have adequate medical supervision<br>3. Are coping but need guidance and support related to care of the baby, the family's adjustment, and socioeconomic variables | To women who<br>1. Are receiving good care and supervision<br>2. Are stabilizing in parenting skills and family adjustment |
| C. Infancy (higher priority is given to infants, regardless of whether they are firstborn, when they live in low economic districts where the mortality rate is highest) | To infants who<br>1. Are premature<br>2. Are newborn, especially if firstborn<br>3. Have difficulty in breastfeeding<br>4. Have consistently lost weight<br>5. Are being weaned<br>6. Have inadequate medical care<br>7. Have a reportable dangerous communicable disease<br>8. Have a physical disability resulting from a birth injury or a congenital defect—"high tech" babies such as those on respirators and who have been hospitalized at length<br>9. Need immunization<br>10. Are from substandard, poorly managed homes, or homes where there are problems of inadequate parenting<br>11. Are considered difficult babies by parents | To infants who<br>1. Are past the first month and are gaining weight slowly<br>2. Are not being fed properly<br>3. Have questionable physical and emotional delays | To infants who<br>1. Are receiving adequate medical supervision<br>2. Are receiving good home care |

# Priorities in Community
# Health Nursing (cont'd)

| | I. INTENSIVE VISITING | II. PERIODIC VISITING | III. WIDELY SPACED VISITING |
|---|---|---|---|
| C. Infancy—cont'd | 12. Are born to drug abusers<br>13. Are born to mothers who are HIV-positive<br>14. Fail to thrive<br>15. Are low birth weight | | |
| D. Preschool period | To children who<br>1. Have a reportable dangerous communicable disease<br>2. Have a physical defect<br>3. Need immunization<br>4. Need dental care<br>5. Have nutritional deficiencies<br>6. Are inconsistently disciplined<br>7. Are from homes where there is inadequate parenting<br>8. Are reported for suspected child abuse and neglect | To children who<br>1. Are insecure<br>2. Have lost weight<br>3. Lack medical supervision<br>4. Have poor health habits<br>5. Deviate from normal physical and emotional behavior | To children who<br>1. Have adequate medical supervision<br>2. Have good home care |
| E. School health | To children who<br>1. Have acute health problems<br>  a. Communicable diseases: immunization reactions or complications developing from acute communicable diseases<br>  b. Skin conditions: scabies, impetigo, ringworm, pediculosis<br>  c. Other: pregnancy, unexpected loss or gain of weight, abuse, neglect, diabetes, epilepsy<br>2. Have had an accident in school requiring hospitalization<br>3. Need immediate attention for defects discovered on physical examination: vision, hearing, cardiac, kidney, scoliosis, or other serious defects<br>4. Need follow-up of incidents indicating intense or serious emotional disturbance<br>5. Need follow-up as a contact of a diagnosed dangerous communicable disease<br>6. Have growth and other developmental delays | To children who<br>1. Need follow-up of allergies: hives, eczema, asthma<br>2. Have inadequate medical care<br>3. Have not had diagnosed defects corrected within a reasonable period of time<br>4. Are on medication for more than 3 weeks' duration during the school year<br>5. Need to be observed in relation to their growth pattern (those with structural scoliosis, those wearing braces, and so forth)<br>6. Need follow-up of minor defects: poor eating and health habits, poor dental and personal hygiene, foot and posture problems | To children who<br>1. Have a chronic health condition that is stabilized and under medical care<br>2. Have a congenital defect that does not require remedial work at the time |

*Continued*

# Priorities in Community Health Nursing (cont'd)

| | I. INTENSIVE VISITING | II. PERIODIC VISITING | III. WIDELY SPACED VISITING |
|---|---|---|---|
| F. Adult health | To clients who<br>1. Are in normative or nonnormative crisis<br>2. Are disorganized as a family and at risk for abuse and neglect of self, children, or spouse<br>3. Are homeless, in need of health and welfare services, but have not yet established contact with community resources<br>4. Have suspected dangerous communicable or chronic disease symptoms<br>5. Have no medical supervision for diagnosed physical, emotional, psychosocial problems<br>6. Are needing help adapting to chronic illness: heart disease, arthritis, multiple sclerosis, depression, etc. | To clients who<br>1. Are in crisis but have support systems<br>2. Recognize their disorganization and are working on ordering their lives<br>3. Are recently established in a home environment and are working with community resources<br>4. Have diagnosed disease and are receiving medical treatment; need help with referral to resources<br>5. Are needing help dealing with developmental tasks of parenting: sexuality and death education tasks of their children | To clients who<br>1. Have needed nursing care, are currently coping well, but are at risk for physical, emotional, and psychosocial problems |
| G. Health of older people | To clients who<br>1. Have no medical supervision<br>2. Have symptoms of a dangerous communicable, nutritional, or chronic disease<br>3. Have a diagnosed disease and need help following the treatment plan<br>4. Have no support systems<br>5. Have evidence of normative or nonnormative maturational crisis especially in relation to: loss of income, loss of spouse, loss of friends<br>6. Have evidence of intentional or unintentional alcohol or drug abuse<br>7. Are unable to maintain an environmentally safe housing situation | To clients who<br>1. Have a diagnosed medical problem<br>2. Have a complex treatment regimen and are following it<br>3. Are able to live independently but need referral sources and support | To clients who<br>1. Are under medical supervision<br>2. Have readily available support systems |

# Congestive Heart Failure *Home Care Steps*®

Patient Name: _____

Diagnosis _____       ID#: _____

Date *Home Care Steps*® protocols Opened: _____ Closed: _____ Start of Care: _____

**ASSESS/OBSERVE:** (Choose items that are currently or potentially a problem)        OTHER CoSteps or Flowsheets:
Fill in normal parameters, if applicable:                                                                      _____

_____ Vital signs _____       _____
_____ Blood pressure _____       _____
_____ Cardiovascular status _____       _____ Fatigue _____
_____ Respiratory status _____       _____ ADL _____
_____ Nutrition/Hydration (prescribed diet) _____       _____ IADL _____
_____ Weight _____       _____ Skin color/integrity _____
_____ Elimination, Bowel _____       _____ Pain control _____
_____ Elimination, Bladder _____       _____ Labs _____
_____ Edema _____       _____ Equipment _____
_____ Mobility/exercise/tolerance _____       _____ Other _____

**NURSING DIAGNOSES:** (Choose appropriate diagnoses)
_____   1.  Knowledge deficit related to disease process and home care management.
_____   2.  Knowledge deficit related to medication use.
_____   3.  Knowledge deficit related to dietary restrictions.
_____   4.  Self-care deficit, bathing/hygiene.
_____   5.  Self-care deficit, grooming/dressing.
_____   6.  Alteration in activity tolerance.
_____   7.  Alteration in lifestyle secondary to disease.
_____   8.  Ineffective coping related to diagnosis and prognosis.
_____   9.  Alteration in cardiac output related to mechanical factors.
_____  10.  Potential alteration in skin integrity related to edema.
_____  Other: _____

**GOALS:** (Check appropriate goals and/or write in date goal achieved.)
_____   1.  Patient/caregiver will demonstrate knowledge of disease process, treatment goals, and self-care management.
_____   2.  Patient will maintain stable physiological status and S/S of improved cardiac output (vitals, labs, weight, edema, cardiovascular status) within normal limits for patient.
_____   3.  Patient will achieve adequate symptom control through use of medications or other therapies/treatments.
_____   4.  Patient will demonstrate compliance with treatment plan (diet, meds, exercise, other).
_____   5.  Patient/caregiver will verbalize S/S to report to RN or physician.
_____   6.  Patient will remain safe in home environment.
_____   7.  Patient/caregiver will demonstrate effective disease management practices.
_____   8.  Patient/caregiver will verbalize appropriate measures for managing changes in body image/lifestyle.
_____   9.  Patient/caregiver will verbalize community services available and how to contact them.
_____  10.  Patient will demonstrate and maintain intact skin in edematous areas.
_____  Other: _____

**TEACHING TOOLS:**                         Care Plan Focus
_____       Safety:                 Visits 1-3 (when outcomes are met on these visit protocols)
_____       Disease control:        Visits 4-7 (when outcomes are met on these visit protocols)
_____       Health Promotion:       Visits 8-10 (when outcomes are met on these visit protocols)

**SN VISIT FREQUENCY:**
Recommended: 3 wk × 1, 2 wk × 3, 1 wk × 1       Ordered: _____
                    (10 visits total)

Other Disciplines: _____       _____ Signature and Title

*Home Care Steps*® protocols are guidelines designed to address the patient's acute episode of illness. Because each patient presents unique circumstances that must be assessed and evaluated during the provision of home care services, visit intensity and frequency may also be influenced by such factors that include, but are not limited to the home environment, resources, the presence of life-supporting therapies, and the presence of chronic illnesses or limiting handicaps.

# CHF *Home Care Steps*—Visit 2

Patient Name: _____ ID#: _____

Date: _____

☐ See CoStep: _____ ☐ See Flowsheets/Other Forms: _____

Homebound Status: ☐ Ambulation ☐ Endurance ☐ Vision ☐ Infection ☐ Respiratory ☐ Mental ☐ Other

| CARE ELEMENTS | INTERVENTIONS: USE "√" FOR COMPLETE; VARIANCE CODE FOR NOT DONE | COMMENTS |
|---|---|---|
| Disease Process | Perform physical assessment. ____ Assess weight (on patient's own scale if available). ____ Evaluate knowledge of disease process. ____ Instruct on definition, ____ S/S of exacerbation of disease process, ____ actions to take, ____ and basic treatment goals. ____ Assess for shortness of breath. ____ Assess edema. ____ | T ____ AP ____ RP ____ R ____ Wt: ____ BP R/L Sit ____, Stand ____, Lying ____ Lungs: _____ Dyspnea, cough: _____ Heart: _____ Circulation: _____ Skin color/integrity/turgor: _____ Pain: _____ |
| Medication | Instruct on medication schedule. ____ Evaluate effectiveness of medications/symptom control. ____ Instruct on purpose, action, and side effects of following medication(s): _____ Instruct on medication changes. ____ Demonstrate use of medi-planner and set up if necessary. ____ | |
| Nutrition/Hydration Elimination | Assess fluid and dietary intake. ____ Evaluate knowledge of diet restrictions/fluid requirements. ____ Instruct on diet/fluid requirements as appropriate. ____ Provide asisstance with meal planning until next scheduled visit. ____ Assess bowel and urinary function. ____ Instruct to avoid straining with bowel movements. ____ | Appetite: good ____ fair ____ poor ____ Diet intake: _____ Fluid intake: _____ Abdomen: _____ Bowel: _____ Bladder: _____ |
| Activity | Assess current activity and tolerance levels. ____ Instruct to avoid overexertion. ____ Instruct on importance of frequent rest periods and pacing activities. ____ Assess functional status and ability to perform ADLs/IADLs. ____ Evaluate need for assistive devices. ____ | ADLs: _____ IADLs: _____ Ambulation/Transfers/Endurance: _____ |
| Safety | Evaluate knowledge of how and when to call for help. ____ Provide emergency numbers. ____ Instruct on basic home safety precautions. ____ Assess environment for risk factors. ____ Instruct on modification as appropriate. ____ Instruct on safe use of oxygen (if appropriate). ____ | |
| Treatments | Administer as ordered. _____ | |
| Tests | Perform as ordered. _____ | |
| Psycho/Social | Assess family/social support systems. ____ Evaluate caregiver functioning/coping status. ____ Evaluate knowledge of Rights and Responsibilities. ____ | Level of Consciousness/Orientation: _____ Emotional: _____ |
| Interteam Services/ Community Referrals | Assess ability to purchase necessary supplies, food, etc., for treatment. ____ Initiate referrals for agency/community services as needed. ____ Evaluate knowledge of plan, ____ and barriers of care to home care services. ____ Initiate case conference: ____ SN, ____ MSS, ____ PT, ____ OT, ____ SLP, ____ HCA, ____ Physician, Other. ____ Assess for next physician appointment (Date). _____ | |

_____
Signature and Title

# CHF *Home Care Steps*—Visit 2 (cont'd)

Patient Name: _____    ID#: _____
Date: _____

**Home Care Aide Supervisory Note:** HCA Present? ☐ Yes ☐ No   Following plan of care?   ☐ Yes ☐ No
Care Plan Adequate?   ☐ Yes ☐ No   Need for continued service?   ☐ Yes ☐ No   ☐ Pt. Unable   ☐ Family Unable
Assessment of Patient/Family relationship with HCA: _____
_____

Changes in plan/goal/update: _____
☐ To HCA Supervisor                                              Date: _____   Initials _____
☐ If Applicable, HCA Name _____   HCA Signature _____   Date: _____

| PATIENT/CAREGIVER OUTCOMES | MET | NOT MET | IF NECESSARY, EXPLAIN VARIANCE CODE. |
|---|---|---|---|
| 1. Demonstrates no new or worsening symptoms. | | | |
| 2. Demonstrates ability to maintain medical condition in home without hospitalization, ER visit, or unplanned physician visit since last RN visit. | | | |
| 3. Verbalizes purpose, action, and side effects of each medication instructed (as listed above). | | | |
| 4. Verbalizes general dietary restrictions. | | | |
| 5. Verbalizes fluid restrictions if ordered. | | | |
| 6. Demonstrates optimal GI function (i.e., no S/S of N/V, diarrhea, or constipation). | | | |
| 7. Verbalizes plan to meet basic ADL/IADL needs. | | | |
| 8. Verbalizes importance of frequent rest periods and pacing activities. | | | |
| 9. Verbalizes how and when to call for help. | | | |
| 10. Verbalizes members of support system. | | | |
| 11. Verbalizes knowledge of plan/barriers to care. | | | |
| 12. Verbalizes three (3) safety issues regarding use of oxygen. | | | |
| 13. Other: | | | |

☐ If unmet outcomes from previous visits have now been met, write visit and outcome numbers: _____

**PLAN** (Include next *Home Care Step*® Visit # to be completed): _____
_____
_____

_____          _____    _____
Signature and Title                               Time In          Time Out

*Home Care Steps*® protocols are guidelines designed to address the patient's acute episode of illness. Because each patient presents unique circumstances that must be assessed and evaluated during the provision of home care services, visit intensity and frequency may also be influenced by such factors that include, but are not limited to the home environment, resources, the presence of life-supporting therapies, and the presence of chronic illnesses or limiting handicaps.

# 25

# Quality Processes in Community Health Nursing Practice

*Susan Clemen-Stone*

## OBJECTIVES

*Upon completion of this chapter, the reader should be able to:*

1. Identify dimensions of quality in health care.
2. Discuss the philosophical orientation of total quality management or continuous quality improvement efforts.
3. Describe the components of a continuous quality improvement program.
4. Discuss the concepts *structure, process,* and *outcome* as they relate to quality processes in community health nursing practice.

5. Discuss how standards and criteria guide measurement processes.
6. Discuss measurement issues in quality management.
7. Identify tools for collecting and displaying quality measurement data.

## KEY TERMS

Action strategies
Benchmarking
Continuous quality improvement (CQI)
Criteria
Customer
Health care safety net providers
Indicator
Infection control
Integrated quality management program

Joint Commission on Accreditation of Healthcare Organizations (JCAHO)
National Committee for Quality Assurance (NCQA)
Nursing-sensitive outcomes
Philosophy
Quality assessment and quality improvement (QA/QI)
Quality assurance (QA)
Quality circles

Quality of care
Risk and safety management
Standards
Structure-process-outcome conceptual framework
Threshold for evaluation
Utilization review

---

*One characteristic of a profession is the presence of a professional association that is cohesive, self-governing, and a source of professional self-discipline, standards, and ethics.*

JEROME P. LYSAUGHT, 1970, P. 41

---

"Self-review and self-regulation remain the hallmark of the healing professions" (Lohr, 1990, p. 11). Nurses share with all health care professionals the need to examine carefully the delivery of their services in light of changing societal demands. Nursing must assume the responsibility for developing, implementing, and evaluating standards of quality to validate itself as a profession and maintain the right to govern its practice. The challenge for the future will be to use an interdisciplinary approach to continuous quality improvement while containing costs in a managed care environment. Professionals across the nation are being encouraged to implement quality strategies for improving the processes, outcomes, and cost-effectiveness of health care delivery for individuals and populations (O'Neil, Pew Health Professions Commission, 1998).

# EVOLUTION OF QUALITY PROCESSES IN NURSING

Nursing's concern for quality improvement in health care delivery is not a recent phenomenon. Historical literature clearly identifies that quality improvement has always been a primary focus in the health care arena (Lummis, 1996, p. 159). Throughout history nursing and other health professionals have worked to discover ways to decrease morbidity and premature mortality and to improve their practice. Dating back to the pre-Christian era, evidence supports the idea that public health surveillance and control measures have been instrumental in achieving desired infectious disease outcomes (Lummis, 1996). Such measures laid the foundation for developing effective quality improvement strategies.

Florence Nightingale established the foundation for quality in nursing practice during the latter half of the nineteenth century. Nightingale advocated for standards in practice that would guide all nurses in the delivery of quality professional interventions (Reed, Zurakowski, 1996). Her scientific investigations demonstrated that improvements in practice (e.g., increasing the size of the nursing staff) significantly reduced mortality during the Crimean War and led to Great Britain adopting the Audit Department Act of 1866. This act established procedures for evaluating quality on an ongoing basis (Lummis, 1996).

During the early 1900s professional organizations campaigned for quality improvement in nursing practice. The initial objectives for the American Nurses Association (ANA) focused on improving standardization in nurses' training and the passage of licensure laws to protect the public from poorly trained nurses (Christy, 1971). Keeping with ANA's focus, the National Organization for Public Health Nursing (NOPHN) grew out of a concern for the right of clients to receive care from qualified persons in 1912 and emphasized the importance of accepted standards for nursing education and care in the community (Gardner, 1975).

The ANA assumed a significant leadership role in setting standards for the profession throughout the twentieth century. All divisions of nursing practice under the ANA have developed and distributed standards of practice that are revised on a regular basis. The most recent ANA standards for public health nursing practice are delineated in Box 25-1. These standards explicitly address the nurse's responsibility for ensuring quality in professional practice. Dramatic changes in health care delivery urgently necessitate a continuous focus on quality of care by the ANA in the twenty-first century.

Up until the 1960s major quality improvement efforts were primarily initiated by the health care professions. Societal influences during the 1960s, including concern for consumer protection, human rights, and health care as a right, altered this trend (Bull, 1996, p. 146). As the federal government became more actively involved in financially supporting health care for underserved populations under the Medicare and Medicaid programs, legislation was enacted to ensure accountability for quality care.

The Professional Standard Review Organizations (PSROs), established by the 1972 amendments to the Social Security Act, were developed to ensure that federal monies spent for Medicaid, Medicare, and other federal health programs would be used effectively, efficiently, and economically. Peer Review Organizations (PROs) replaced PSROs by federal legislative action under the 1982 Tax Equity and Fiscal Responsibility Act (TEFRA). PROs' structures are charged to review medical records for appropriateness, quality of care, and compliance with practice standards (Cross, 1996). In 1992, the Health Care Financing Administration (HCFA) and PROs initiated a new program for quality improvement. The *Health Care Quality Improvement Program* (HCQIP) involves analyzing and taking action to change widespread ineffective patterns of care. The national clinical priorities addressed by this program are displayed in Box 25-2. These priorities were selected based on their public health importance and available treatment methods to address the problems (HCFA, 2000).

Quality in health care service delivery from a population-focused perspective became a national priority under the *National Health Planning and Resources Development Act of 1974*. This act called for the development of national health planning goals and standards. National health goals and standards were first published in the 1979 Healthy People document. The U.S.' Healthy People (USDHHS, 2000a) initiative continues to examine ways to improve quality of life among all at-risk populations. Major tracking systems have been developed to assist local communities in assessing progress in meeting the Healthy People 2010 goals and objectives (USDHHS, 2000b).

Societal forces continue to significantly influence the emphasis on quality in health care delivery. The *President's Advisory Commission on Consumer Protection and Quality in the Health Care Industry* made health care quality visible on the national public policy agenda in 1998. At the same time, the Institute of Medicine (IOM) established the *Committee on Health Care Quality in America* for the purpose of developing a strategy for improving the threshold of quality over the subsequent ten years (Council on Graduate Medical Education, National Advisory Council on Nurse Education and Practice, 2000). Two recent IOM reports have addressed the need for a major overhaul in the U.S. health care system to improve quality and safety (IOM, 2001; Kohn, Corrigan, Donaldson, 2000).

## BOX 25-1
### Standards of Public Health Nursing Practice

### Standards of Care

**STANDARD I. ASSESSMENT**

The public health nurse assesses the health status of populations using data, community resources identification, input from the population, and professional judgment.

**STANDARD II. DIAGNOSIS**

The public health nurse analyzes collected assessment data and partners with the people to attach meaning to those data and determine opportunities and needs.

**STANDARD III. OUTCOMES IDENTIFICATION**

The public health nurse participates with other community partners to identify expected outcomes in the populations and their health status.

**STANDARD IV. PLANNING**

The public health nurse promotes and supports the development of programs, policies, and services that provide interventions that improve the health status of populations.

**STANDARD V. ASSURANCE: ACTION COMPONENT OF THE NURSING PROCESS FOR PUBLIC HEALTH NURSING**

The public health nurse assures access and availability of programs, policies, resources, and services to the population.

**STANDARD VI. EVALUATION**

The public health nurse evaluates the health status of the population.

### Standards of Professional Performance

**STANDARD I. QUALITY OF CARE**

The public health nurse systematically evaluates the availability, accessibility, acceptability, quality, and effectiveness of nursing practice for the population.

**STANDARD II. PERFORMANCE APPRAISAL**

The public health nurse evaluates his or her own nursing practice in relation to professional practice standards and relevant statutes and regulations.

**STANDARD III. EDUCATION**

The public health nurse acquires and maintains current knowledge and competency in public health nursing practice.

**STANDARD IV. COLLEGIALITY**

The public health nurse establishes collegial partnerships while interacting with health care practitioners and others and contributes to the professional development of peers, colleagues, and others.

**STANDARD V. ETHICS**

The public health nurse applies ethical standards in advocating for health and social policy, and delivery of public health programs to promote and preserve the health of the population.

**STANDARD VI. COLLABORATION**

The public health nurse collaborates with the representatives of the population and other health and human service professionals and organizations in providing for and promoting the health of the population.

**STANDARD VII. RESEARCH**

The public health nurse uses research findings in practice.

**STANDARD VIII. RESOURCE UTILIZATION**

The public health nurse considers safety, effectiveness, and cost in the planning and delivery of public health services when using available resources to ensure the maximum possible health benefit to the population.

From Quad Council of Public Health Nursing Organizations: *Scope and standards of public health nursing practice,* Washington, DC, 1999, ANA, pp. 12-21. Reprinted with permission.

## BOX 25-2
### Medicare's Health Care Quality Improvement Program: National Clinical Priority Areas

1. Acute myocardial infarction
2. Breast cancer
3. Diabetes
4. Heart failure
5. Pneumonia
6. Stroke
7. Reducing health care disparities

From Health Care Financing Administration (HCFA): *Health care quality improvement program: medicare priorities,* Washington, DC, 2000, HCFA.

## QUALITY CHALLENGES IN A MANAGED CARE ENVIRONMENT

As they strive to maintain quality in health care delivery, health care providers will face several critical challenges during the twenty-first century. They will need to expand access to care, become more accountable to those who purchase and use health services, be able to use fewer resources more effectively and efficiently, and use outcomes data to guide appropriate practice. These challenges will occur within the context of a radically changing health care system that will serve an increasingly diverse population (O'Neil, Pew Health Professions Commission, 1998) and under legislative mandates focused on improving patient care outcomes nationwide (HCFA, 2000).

A major challenge for health care providers during the twenty-first century will be to maintain a focus on quality while containing costs in a managed care environment. *Managed care* has been envisioned by the Pew Health Professions Commission "to be those processes that work to rationalize the use of health resources at the lowest possible cost and the highest possible quality" (O'Neil, Pew Health Professions Commission, 1998, p. 6). The Commission believes that managed care has the potential to improve quality, expand access, and enhance population health. However, "there is a strong need for safeguards to ensure that cost savings are not achieved by denying needed services…Managed care plans should be designed carefully so that the pursuit of least costly does not jeopardize quality of care or access to necessary services" (Managed care's conflicts of interest, 1995, p. 4). The **National Committee for Quality Assurance (NCQA),** a private, not-for-profit organization, is dedicated to establishing safeguards to ensure the delivery of quality care among managed care organizations. The Committee's survey measures examine access issues as well as clinical performance (NCQA, 2000).

A critical access issue that needs addressing throughout the coming decade is health care access for vulnerable populations (Beltran, 2000). Currently, a significant number of persons, including the 44 million Americans who are uninsured, the low-income underinsured individuals, Medicaid beneficiaries, and persons with special health care needs, have little or no access to stable health care coverage (IOM, 2000). These Americans rely on **health care safety net providers** or "those providers that organize and deliver a significant level of health care and other related services to uninsured, Medicaid, and other vulnerable patients" (IOM, 2000, p. 3). Safety net providers are not always available to address the need.

Beery, Greenwald, and Nudelman (1996) proposed that a national managed care and public health network be established to develop strategies for improving the quality of health care services for economically disadvantaged groups. These authors believe that "managed care and public health have great potential for providing mutual assistance with significant benefit to society at large" (Beery, Greenwald, Nudelman, 1996, p. 306). Their proposed network would help advance the development of coalitions between managed care and public health organizations and would encourage these coalitions to develop initiatives to safeguard the public good. These initiatives have the potential to advance quality in health care delivery for disadvantaged populations. Leviss and Hurtig (1998), Novick (1998), and Roper and Mays (2001) discuss the relationship between public health agencies and managed care organizations and the advantages of partnering to advance preventive health care for uninsured groups.

## Stop and Think About It

What providers in your local community make up the health care safety net? How well is the safety net in your community meeting the needs of vulnerable populations?

## DEFINING QUALITY IN HEALTH CARE

As the emphasis on quality increased in the health care industry, numerous definitions of the term *quality of care* have emerged. Most of these definitions imply a specified degree of excellence that is consistent with current professional standards and that results in positive client outcomes. An IOM study committee, established to design a strategy for quality review and assurance in Medicare, examined over 100 definitions of quality of care. From knowledge gained from this process, the IOM study committee developed the following definition of quality. This definition continues to guide clinical and research quality endeavors (Lohr, 1990):

"Quality of care is the degree to which health services for individuals and populations increase the likelihood of desired health outcomes and are consistent with current professional knowledge" (p. 21).

Inherent in the IOM definition of quality of care are several key concepts. This definition implies that gradations or degrees of quality can be distinguished through measurement and that health care encompasses a broad set of services. It also implies that populations as well as individuals are proper targets for quality improvement efforts. Its goal orientation links the process of health care with outcomes and reflects the belief that the outcomes of care should have a net benefit or desired health results. Additionally, it highlights the constraints placed on professional performance by the current state of professional knowledge but underscores the importance of adhering to current professional standards (Lohr, 1990, p. 129). The IOM study committee on quality believes that net benefit should "reflect considerations of patient satisfaction and well-being, broad health status or quality-of-life measures, and the processes of patient-provider interaction and decision making" (Lohr, 1990, p. 129).

A significant challenge confronting health care providers when examining quality of care is to identify dimensions of quality that can be measured and improved. The **Joint Commission on Accreditation of Healthcare Organizations (JCAHO),** a private accreditation organization dedicated to improving quality in client care, has identified nine dimensions of performance for quality monitoring. These dimensions are identified and defined in Box 25-3. They examine whether an organization is *"doing the right thing"* (appropriateness, availability, and efficacy) and whether the organization is *"doing the right thing well"* (continuity, effectiveness, efficiency, respect and caring, safety, and timeliness) (JCAHO, 1993, p. 68).

All of JCAHO's dimensions of performance for quality monitoring can be defined, measured, and improved. For example, if an organization wanted to determine whether client care was coordinated (continuity) among health care providers, it could examine such things as how often appropriate follow-up care was offered to clients, whether an adequate referral network was available, and whether referrals were successfully implemented.

The most recent Institute of Medicine Committee on Quality (IOM, 2001), designed to examine health care

**BOX 25-3**

*Definitions of the Dimensions of Performance*

**Appropriateness:**
The degree to which the care/intervention provided is relevant to the client's clinical needs, given the current state of knowledge

**Availability:**
The degree to which the appropriate care/intervention is available to meet the needs of the client served

**Continuity:**
The degree to which the care/intervention for the client is coordinated among practitioners, between organizations, and across time

**Effectiveness:**
The degree to which the care/intervention is provided in the correct manner, given the current state of knowledge, in order to achieve the desired/projected outcome(s) for the client

**Efficacy:**
The degree to which the care/intervention used for the client has been shown to accomplish the desired/projected outcome(s)

**Efficiency:**
The ratio of the outcomes (results of care/intervention) for a client to the resources used to deliver the care

**Respect and caring:**
The degree to which a client, or designee, is involved in his or her own care decisions, and that those providing the services do so with sensitivity and respect for his or her needs and expectations and individual differences

**Safety:**
The degree to which the risk of an intervention and the risk in the care environment are reduced for the client and others, including the health care provider

**Timeliness:**
The degree to which the care/intervention is provided to the client at the time it is most beneficial or necessary

From Joint Commission on Accreditation of Healthcare Organizations (JCAHO): *The measurement mandate: on the road to performance improvement in health care,* Oakbrook Terrace, Ill, 1993, JCAHO, p. 69.

quality across America, confirmed the importance of the JCAHO dimensions of performance for quality monitoring. This committee proposed that in order to improve quality in today's health care system, attention must be given to make health care safe, effective, patient-centered, timely, efficient, and equitable (IOM, 2001). Quality is a multidimensional concept influenced by many factors in the health care system.

*Stop and Think About It*

Using JCAHO's dimensions of performance for quality monitoring, evaluate how well your clinical agency is meeting the needs of clients they serve. What type of outcomes would you use to assess quality performance?

An in-depth analysis of the concept of quality in health care and quality measurement is beyond the scope of this book. Lohr (1990) and Schmele (1996) present a thoughtful discussion of both of these concepts. JCAHO (1993, 1994) and NCQA (2000) devote considerable attention to analyzing quality measurement, and the IOM (IOM, 2001; Kohn, Corrigan, Donaldson, 2000) has extensively examined strategies for improving the quality of health care.

## EVOLUTION OF TOTAL QUALITY MANAGEMENT

The focus of quality efforts from the 1960s through the mid-1980s was on **quality assurance (QA).** This process was viewed as a dynamic one through which health care professionals assumed accountability for the quality of care they provided. It was considered a commitment to excellence with an emphasis on ensuring that all health care professionals provided safe clinical care *equal to* or *better than* the standard of care designated appropriate for clients who had like characteristics.

During the 1980s the concept of quality assessment emerged. Some (O'Leary, 1991) believed that the term *quality assurance* was an "unfortunate semantic selection" because quality cannot be ensured but only improved. In contrast, a U.S. General Accounting Office report (GAO, 1990) argued that quality assessment was a prerequisite to QA and involved the use of measures of quality to assess structure, process, and outcomes of care. The GAO report viewed QA from a broader perspective, seeing it as a process that goes beyond simple assessment of quality to include quality improvement processes. In this text when the concept of QA is addressed, it is seen as a process that involves both quality assessment and quality improvement activities. QA has evolved as a significant component of the core public health function of assurance (Rowitz, 2001). Both quality assessment and QA are addressed within a total quality management framework.

The concept of total quality management (TQM), or **continuous quality improvement (CQI),** has recently come to the forefront and represents a significant philosophical shift in terms of the concept of quality. TQM moves away from the premise that problems are the result of errors by individual clinicians or other health care personnel to the belief that the majority of problems arise from defects in the design of systems and organizational processes (IOM, 2001; Pate, Stajer, 2001). In keeping with this idea, total quality management is viewed as a strategic mission that needs to focus on system issues that affect quality (IOM, 2001). A major assumption underlying this belief is that client outcomes are significantly influenced by all activities of an organization. The IOM (Kohn, Corrigan, Donaldson, 2000) asserts that "errors are usually induced by faulty systems that set people up to fail" (p. 169).

Organization-wide employee involvement is a predominant theme under TQM. TQM puts responsibility for quality control in the province of frontline managers and em-

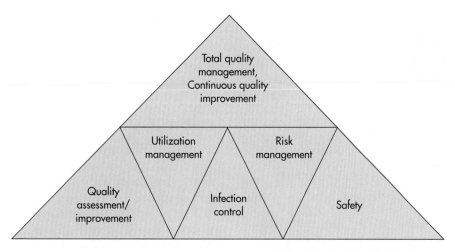

**FIGURE 25-1** Integrated quality management. (From Koch MW, Fairly TM: *Integrated quality management: the key to improving nursing care quality,* St Louis, 1993, Mosby, p. 5.)

ployees through the use of quality circles and employee education and training in the methods of quality monitoring (Baker, Gelmon, 1996; Donabedian, 1996). ***Quality circles*** are small, structured problem-solving groups of employees from the same area who work on improving productivity, efficiency, and quality using a sound database (Baker, Gelmon, 1996). Quality circles are often comprised of individuals from different disciplines. An interdisciplinary approach to quality assessment and quality improvement is a major thrust in the continuous quality improvement model (Kohn, Corrigan, Donaldson, 2000; Wakefield, O'Grady, 2000).

In addition to creating a style of management that facilitates organization-wide involvement in quality improvement, TQM challenges the prevailing concept of customer. TQM focuses on the needs and expectations of primary and secondary customers, not the values of the providers (Applebaum, 2000; Baker, Gelmon, 1996). "A **customer** is anyone who receives and benefits from the product of someone else's labor" (Melum, Sinioris, 1993, p. 60), and can be either internal or external to the organization. Within this context the recipient of clinical services, the primary customer or client, is not the only focus when implementing quality improvement activities. Attention is also placed on meeting the needs of secondary customers, such as personnel from other divisions within an organization, physicians and nurses in private practice, referral agencies, and third-party payers. In line with this philosophy, *evaluation of customer satisfaction* is seen as a significant component of the quality assessment process (ANA, 2000a; Woodward, Ostbye, Craighead, et al., 2000).

## AN INTEGRATED QUALITY MANAGEMENT PROGRAM

Total quality management (TQM) is a customer-focused process that promotes active employee participation in quality improvement efforts. It is a synergistic approach be-

tween all components of a TQM program in an organization that uses teams to promote quality service delivery. It requires an integrated program (Figure 25-1) that includes but is not limited to the following components of quality management (Koch, Fairly, 1993, p. 4):

• Quality assessment and improvement or QA
• Infection control
• Utilization management
• Risk management/safety

An **integrated quality management program** is a broad and encompassing endeavor that addresses organization-wide performance improvement according to specified standards (Katz, Green, 1997). As previously mentioned, the performance improvement framework examines *what is done* and *how well it is done* (JCAHO, 1994). JCAHO believes that an organization's level of performance is reflected in client outcomes, in the cost (or efficiency) of its services, and in clients' and others' satisfaction.

A well-established, integrated TQM program helps agencies monitor strengths and problems over time, review organizational processes and services, protect the consumer from adverse outcomes, and guard the agency from loss. It also assists agencies in maximizing resource management and educating the consumer and agency staff about reasonable and acceptable health care services at affordable prices (Koch, Fairly, 1993). An organization that cultivates an environment facilitating the achievement of these goals will maintain a competitive edge in the health care market.

## QUALITY ASSESSMENT AND IMPROVEMENT

"Quality assessment and quality improvement (QA/QI) is the systematic monitoring process that identifies opportunities for improvement in patient (client) care delivery, designs ways to improve the service, and continues to evaluate follow-up actions to make certain that improvement occurs"

**BOX 25-4**

*Desirable Attributes of a Quality Assurance Program*

- Addresses overuse, underuse, and poor technical and interpersonal quality
- Intrudes minimally into the client-provider relationship
- Is acceptable to professionals and providers
- Fosters improvement throughout the health care organization and system
- Deals with outlier practice and performance
- Uses both positive and negative incentives for change and improvement in performance
- Provides practitioners and providers with timely information to improve performance
- Has face validity for the public and for professionals (i.e., is understandable and relevant to client and clinical decision making)
- Is scientifically rigorous
- Positive impact on patient outcomes can be demonstrated or inferred
- Can address both individual and population-based outcomes
- Documents improvement in quality and progress toward excellence
- Is easily implemented and administered
- Is affordable and cost-effective
- Includes clients and the public

From Lohr KN, editor: *Medicare: a strategy for quality assurance,* vol 1, Washington, DC, 1990, National Academy Press, p. 49.

(Koch, Fairly, 1993, p. 17). Quality assessment and improvement is a complex process designed to evaluate the clinical dimensions of client care and related governance, administrative, and support services that influence health outcomes (JCAHO, 1994). It also helps agencies determine if they are meeting standards established by accreditation bodies and professional organizations and if risk management issues are being addressed (Harris, 1997). All aspects of community health nursing practice, including services to individuals, populations, and the community as a whole, are monitored through a quality assessment and improvement process.

Quality assessment and improvement activities are an important part of a sound QA program. A successful QA program provides practitioners with timely assessment data for addressing a full range of quality care issues including overuse and underuse of services, the relevancy of interventions to clients' clinical needs, the caring and respect dimensions of performance, and system forces that influence health care delivery. A successful QA program is designed to foster active client and provider participation and focuses on improving client outcomes (Box 25-4). In a QA program, emphasis is on evaluating client outcomes against standards consistent with current professional knowledge, taking action to improve unacceptable practice, and

continuously assessing and improving performance (Lohr, 1990). The ANA Quality Assurance Model has guided health care professionals in establishing appropriate standards and processes for assessing quality of care and developing strategies for improving care.

## THE ANA QUALITY ASSURANCE MODEL

In the mid-1970s the ANA adopted a QA model, developed by Dr. Norma Lang, to depict the multiple components of evaluating client care (Figure 25-2). This model illustrates that QA is a dynamic process, influenced by values and guided by standards of practice. "One strength of the model is that it suggests ongoing evaluation. The arrows around the circle indicate that the process is continuous, with subsequent evaluations incorporating previous findings as well as changes in values." This model "has stood the test of time and remains viable today" (Bull, 1996, p. 149).

There has been significant debate in the literature about the strengths and shortcomings of the QA model and the value of the industrial model of quality (TQM/CQI). Tilbury (1992, p. 12) suggests that the ANA generic model of QA can be applied to CQI with the addition of activities to monitor the new, higher level of quality achieved after action has been taken. She contends that the "differences in how the model is applied lie more in how the quality assessment and improvement processes are implemented than in the particular steps undertaken" (Tilbury, 1992, p. 12). For example, a concurrent and terminal monitoring of performance process, involving staff at *all* levels in the organization, is the norm under the CQI system. Under the traditional QA structure, retrospective chart reviews by QA personnel were emphasized (Tilbury, 1992). However, current QA processes highlight the value of concurrent and continuous quality improvement procedures (Rowitz, 2001).

JCAHO supports the integration of QA and CQI concepts. This organization's framework for improving performance incorporates the strengths of QA while broadening its scope to reflect the complexity of external and internal environmental influences on the quality of health care. During its accreditation process, JCAHO examines how well health care systems understand and align their mission with the needs of external environments. Organizations are asked to identify how the organization's departments work together for the benefit of clients (Centering the survey process, 2001).

Donabedian (1996), a world-renowned authority on health care QA, provided a thought-provoking analysis of the similarities and differences between the health care model of quality (QA) and the industrial model of quality (TQM/CQI). He concluded that despite differences in vocabulary, "the industrial model has many affinities to ours [health care model]: in its emphasis on service to the consumer; in its recognition of the worthiness, dignity, devo-

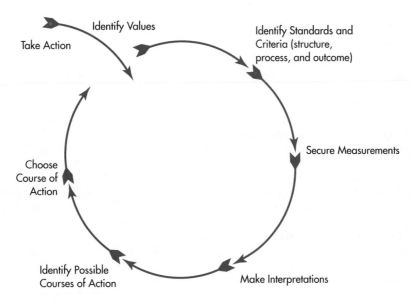

**FIGURE 25-2** A quality assurance model. (Modified from American Nurses Association: *A plan for implementation of the standards of nursing practice,* Kansas City, Mo, 1975, ANA, p. 15.)

tion, and skill of all workers; in its refusal to blame individuals for inherent deficiencies of systems and processes; in its reliance on education rather than punishment; in its reliance on leadership rather than dictation; and in its emphasis on internal self-amelioration rather than external regulation" (Donabedian, 1996, pp. 102-103). Donabedian believed that both health care professionals and industrial personnel have learned from each other. However, he cautions health care professionals not to deflect attention from clinical effectiveness to the efficiency of supportive activities as they embrace the concepts of CQI. The reader is encouraged to review in depth Donabedian's analysis of QA models.

## KEY COMPONENTS OF QUALITY ASSURANCE/ASSESSMENT

Regardless of the terminology used, all quality assurance/assessment (QA) programs have several key elements. Organizations with well-established QA programs have articulated their values about quality health care and have linked these values with their mission, vision, and philosophy statements. Additionally, these organizations have developed performance standards and established ongoing evaluation processes designed to assess and continuously improve quality outcomes.

### Mission, Philosophy, and Values

Fundamental to sound QA efforts are well-defined statements that describe an organization's mission, philosophy, vision for responding to anticipated changes in the environment, and quality of care values. These statements pro-

vide direction for all organizational activities and a blueprint for action (Katz, Green, 1997).

An organization's *mission statement* identifies the overall business of the organization (Katz, Green, 1997). In other words, it describes the purpose of the organization by delineating the nature of services to be provided, the recipients of services, and the expected level of excellence to be achieved. For example, some organizations work toward being premier centers of excellence that provide a full range of acute and community-based services to all clients within the community served. Other organizations propose to provide quality, competent home care to all clients in the community who need skilled home health services. Or they may propose to provide high-quality health promotion and disease prevention services to all vulnerable populations within the community. Mission statements in the community health setting usually reflect the value that the community is the unit of service and focus organizational efforts on designing and delivering preventive health care services to promote the health of the community and the health of vulnerable populations.

An organization's *philosophy* statement builds upon its mission statement. It describes beliefs about how things should be done to successfully carry out the business of the organization. A philosophy is "a written statement of an organization's beliefs about customer service, staff practice, and governance" (Katz, Green, 1997, p. 305). Box 25-5 presents an example of a philosophy statement that addresses these three domains. A well-written philosophy statement reflects professional and managerial values.

Beliefs and values influence how we think, how we act, and how we evaluate events and actions. In terms of QA and

## BOX 25-5

*Philosophy Written in Three Domains*

### Excellence in Service

We believe . . .

- That each of our patients, regardless of circumstances, possesses intrinsic value from God and should be treated with dignity and respect.
- That each encounter with patients and families should portray compassion and concern.
- That each patient should receive quality care that is cost-effective, competitive, and based on the latest technology.
- That patient confidentiality and privacy should be preserved.
- That meeting the needs of patients and other customers should always be our number one priority.

### Excellence in Practice

We believe . . .

- That the primary duty of health care professionals is to restore and maintain the health of patients in a spirit of compassion and concern.
- That the scientific process is an integral part of practice as health care professionals.
- That collaboration within the health care team is essential to meet the holistic needs of patients, which include physical, psychosocial, and spiritual aspects of care.
- That we should aggressively promote patient and family education to allow each individual the opportunity to prevent illness and/or achieve optimal health.
- That we are accountable to patients, patients' families, and to each other for our professional practice.
- That monitoring and evaluating health care services is our responsibility and is necessary to continuously improve care.
- That we should pursue professional growth and development through education, participation in professional organizations, and support of research.

### Excellence in Leadership

We believe . . .

- That we should provide a progressive environment, utilizing current technology, guided by responsible stewardship to promote the highest quality patient care and employee satisfaction.
- That we should encourage and support collaborative decision making by those who are closest to the situation, even at the risk of failure.
- That compassion should be characterized in our day-to-day personal interactions as well as being a motivating factor in management decisions.
- That we should be sensitive to individual needs and give support, praise, and recognition to encourage professional and personal development.
- That we should possess an energy level and personal style that empowers and inspires enthusiasm in others.
- That we should consider suggestions and criticisms as challenges for improvement and innovation.
- That justice should be applied equitably in all employment practices and personnel policies.

From Katz JM, Green E: *Managing quality: a guide to system-wide performance management in health care,* ed 2, St Louis, 1997, Mosby, p. 93.

improvement, they affect commitment to the concept of quality and how quality is defined. Identifying values in relation to quality is difficult because many forces influence the delivery of health care services. Available resources, consumer needs and wants, and professional philosophies all determine the scope of practice in the community. For example, it is unrealistic to assume that an organization can plan clinical services without taking into consideration the restrictions of limited resources. Organizations must develop realistic mission and philosophy statements consistent with the resources available or potentially available to them. Being "all things to all people" is an impossible goal that can lead to frustration and quality performance problems.

### *Stop and Think About It*

What are the values and beliefs identified in your agency's mission and philosophy statements? How do these values and beliefs guide client service?

### Standards and Criteria Guide Quality Measurement

Organizational mission and philosophy statements reflect the values and beliefs of an agency and guide the activities of all personnel. They do not provide measurable elements by which a practitioner can judge the quality of care given by health care providers. Standards and criteria must be developed so that the measurement of quality is possible. *Standards* are "broad statements of agreed-upon quality for a given element of care" (Schmele, 1996, p. 591). "Standards define a set of rules, actions or outcomes. Rules constitute the structure of the service, actions are the process of how the service is carried out, and outcomes define the results of the service" (Katz, Green, 1997, p. 9). For example, in the ANA public health nursing standards, one identified outcome is "to promote and support the development of programs, policies, and services that provide interventions that improve the health status of populations" (Standard IV: Planning) (see Box 25-1).

**Criteria** are used to measure the achievement of a standard. "Criteria are measurable statements that address the *intent* of a standard and reflect the level of accomplishment of that standard (Schmele, 1996, p. 589). An objective, measurable criterion showing the degree to which a standard has been met is labeled an **indicator**" (Schmele, 1996, pp. 589-590). Community health agencies would examine such things as immunization rates, the incidence and prevalence of disease, quality of life, and level of functioning indicators to determine how well their staff were performing in relation to the ANA standard previously discussed (Standard IV). A specific outcome or performance indicator might be "improve the immunization completion rates for 2-year-olds served by the agency's well-child clinics from 72% to at least 90% by 2003." This performance indicator is directed toward decreasing vaccine-preventable diseases and is consistent with national standards (USDHHS, 2000a). If it is not achieved, undesirable outcomes (e.g., an increase in vaccine-preventable diseases) may result.

## Structure-Process-Outcome Measurement Approach

Donabedian's (1966) classic **structure-process-outcome conceptual framework** has guided quality measurement efforts for decades and is widely used today (ANA, 2000a; Katz, Green, 1997; Lee, Mills, 2000; Schmele, Donabedian, 1996). This framework proposes that an effective quality management system evaluates quality from three perspectives: structure, process, and outcome. It provides a framework for examining both system-level and client-level outcomes against specified standards. It is based on the belief that *"good structure increases the likelihood of good process, and good process increases the likelihood of good outcome"* (Schmele, Donabedian, 1996, p. 378).

*Structural standards* assist organizations in appraising the environment in which health care is provided (Donabedian, 1969). The structure of an organization "comprises the relatively stable characteristics of the providers of care, the tools and resources they have at their disposal, and the physical and organizational settings where they work" (Schmele, Donabedian, 1996, p. 378). Structural criteria essentially measure an agency's capability to provide quality health care. Structural measures examine such variables as resource availability, the qualifications of staff, staff-client ratios, and adherence to legal standards. Licensure, certification, accreditation, and model professional standards provide guidelines for agencies by which to evaluate their structural characteristics. One such standard requires that agencies have adequate resources to achieve their stated outcomes. Criteria used to measure this standard include variables like staff qualifications, level of funding, and space and equipment needs.

*Process standards* describe how care should be delivered (Donabedian, 1969). Process criteria focus on measuring activities carried out by health care providers to assist clients in achieving desired health outcomes. They are designed to evaluate how the *clinical process* is used in the delivery of health services to clients. Process standards and criteria determine whether clinical interventions were appropriate to the needs of the family or a specified at-risk aggregate. For example, the working group on homeless health outcomes (Bureau of Primary Health Care, 1996) believes that the Health Care for the Homeless (HCH) Program plays a critical role in *reengaging* homeless people in the health and social service systems and that this dimension of service needs to be evaluated during quality assessment efforts. Specifically, a QA team would examine whether the HCH program provides access for homeless people to a wide range of comprehensive services (standard). A process indicator (criterion) to measure this standard might be "homeless clients received care for acute illness within 24 hours." Another might be "outreach activities facilitate client access to domestic violence services."

*Outcome standards* focus attention on the end results of care (Donabedian, 1969). Clinical outcome measures examine change in a client's current or future health status that can be attributed to antecedent health care (Schmele, Donabedian, 1996, p. 378). An example of a population-focused outcome standard is "reduce infant mortality by the year 2010." An outcome indicator (criterion) established to measure this standard might read "reduce the infant mortality rate to no more than 4.5 per 1000 live births-baseline: 7.2 per 1,000 live births in 1998" (USDHHS, 2000a, p. 368). Expected outcomes of care can be compared with the picture on a puzzle box: "the picture on the box of the jigsaw puzzle depicts what the end point of the process will look like when the puzzle (process) is complete, or from a patient's perspective, what the patient will look like when care is complete" (Peters, McKeon, 1998, p. 113).

Outcome measures are used to monitor the *process of care* (success, failure, or complication of an intervention), the *client's health status* (short-term or long-term functional level of the client), and *organizational outcomes* including the cost of quality care (Bureau of Primary Health Care, 1996; Harris, Dugan, 1997; Johnson, Maas, Moorhead, 2000; Peters, McKeon, 1998). Selected reasons for focusing attention on outcomes of health care delivery are displayed in Box 25-6. Accreditation bodies, those who fund services, and consumers are increasingly demanding that health care organizations measure the quality of their outcomes. "Health care organizations of all types, including providers and [managed care organizations (MCOs)] are moving toward utilizing outcomes and related analysis as a way to justify and quantify patient care and resources" (Marrelli, 1997, p. 13-1).

## Nursing-Sensitive Outcomes

Nursing is increasingly being challenged to demonstrate the impact of nursing practice on patient outcomes (ANA, 2000a; Holzemer, Henry, 1999; Johnson, Maas, Moorhead,

### BOX 25-6

*Selected Reasons for Measuring
Outcomes of Care*

- To demonstrate improvements in clients' health status, level of functioning, and quality of life.
- To know what works and what does not, and to be able to make appropriate interventions more effective.
- To build support for specific interventions that are effective with specific vulnerable populations.
- To assist with and assess internal quality improvement efforts.
- To demonstrate positive impact on public health and social issues.
- To assess cost-effectiveness.
- To assist in resource allocation.
- To exchange successful strategies.
- To increase client satisfaction.

Modified from Bureau of Primary Health Care: *The working group on homeless health outcomes: meeting proceedings,* Rockville, Md, June 1996, The Division, pp. 3-4.

### BOX 25-7

*ANA's Approved Nursing-Sensitive
Outcome Indicators for Community-Based
Settings*

- Pain management (symptom severity)
- Consistency of communication (strength of therapeutic alliance)
- Staff mix (utilization of services)
- Prevention of tobacco use (risk reduction)
- Cardiovascular prevention (risk reduction)
- Caregiver activity (protective factors)
- Identification of primary caregiver (protective factors)
- ADL/IADL (level of function)
- Psychosocial interaction (level of function)

From American Nurses Association (ANA): *Nursing quality indicators beyond acute care: literature review,* Washington, DC, 2000a, American Nurses Publishing, p. viii.

2000). Although outcome development in nursing dates back to the mid-1960s, a greater emphasis was placed on outcomes evaluation during the 1990s and into the twenty-first century. The American Nurses Association's Safety and Quality Initiative began in the 1990s (ANA, 2000a). A major component of this initiative was the development of acute care nursing quality indicators (ANA, 1995) and the community-based nonacute outcome care indicators (ANA, 2000a). Nursing-sensitive indicators for community-based settings were approved in 1999 (Box 25-7). Instruments for measuring the achievement of these outcomes can be found in *Nursing Quality Indicators Beyond Acute Care: Measurement Instruments* (ANA, 2000b). **Nursing-sensitive outcomes** address the influence of nursing practice rather than the individual nurse's contribution to client care (ANA, 2000a).

In addition to the nursing-sensitive outcomes developed under the ANA quality program, three other outcome classification systems relevant to community-based practice are the Omaha System (Martin, Norris, Leak, 1999), the Outcome and Assessment Information Set (OASIS) (Shaughnessy, Crisler, 1995), and the Nursing Outcomes Classification (NOC) (Johnson, Maas, Moorhead, 2000). These classification systems are discussed in Chapter 9.

In addition to the outcomes research being conducted by professional nursing organizations and nurse researchers, several other governmental and private sector institutes are focusing on improving quality of health care outcomes. The Agency for Healthcare Research and Quality (AHRQ) (formerly the Agency for Health Care Policy and Research) has focused on patient outcomes and effectiveness research for over a decade and is a valuable source of science-based information on clinical practice guidelines (McCormick,

Cummings, Kovner, 1997). Examples of other organizations developing outcomes initiatives are the Joint Commission on Accreditation of Healthcare Organizations, the National Committee on Quality Assurance, the Community Health Accreditation Program, the Health Care Financing Administration, and the National Cancer Institute. Websites for these organizations can be found in Table 25-1.

### Priorities for Quality Measurement

General consensus is that all-inclusive quality monitoring efforts can seldom be achieved, are costly, and tend to cause frustration and anxiety among staff. Quality monitoring efforts need to be focused on measuring the *critical* desired outcomes that the health care provider can influence and on the *key organizational functions and related processes* that have the greatest impact on client outcomes. Examples of desired outcomes that health care providers can influence are improved health status, improved level of functioning, and improved quality of life. A key function that can significantly influence these client outcomes is the care, treatment, and service function, which encompasses the care or service planning process (JCAHO, 2000). "A *function* is a goal-directed, interrelated series of processes...A *process* is a goal-directed, interrelated series of actions, events, mechanisms, or steps" (JCAHO, 1993, pp. 253, 263). For example, the care or service planning process is an interdisciplinary process that encompasses the same steps as the nursing process. Other examples of key processes that significantly affect client outcomes are the hiring processes of an organization that are designed to recruit qualified providers and an organization's infection control and safety surveillance processes.

**TABLE 25-1**

*Websites for Select Agencies Focusing on Quality Outcomes*

| AGENCIES | WEBSITES |
|---|---|
| Agency for Healthcare Research and Quality | *http://www.ahrq.gov* |
| American Nurses Association | *http://www.ana.org* |
| Community Health Accreditation Program | *http://www.chapinc.org* |
| Health Care Financing Administration | *http://www.hcfa.gov* |
| Joint Commission on Accreditation of Healthcare Organizations | *http://www.jcaho.org* |
| National Association of Home Care | *http://www.nahc.org* |
| National Cancer Institute | *http://www.nci.nih.gov* |
| National Committee for Quality Assurance | *http://www.ncqa.org* |

Four criteria commonly are used to determine which processes to review during quality monitoring efforts. "The predetermined criteria against which to measure and/or prioritize processes include deciding which are high-volume, high-risk, problem-prone, and high-cost" (Katz, Green, 1997, p. 78). These criteria are defined as follows (JCAHO, 1990b, p. 29; Katz, Green, 1997, pp. 78-80):

1. *High-volume* processes are those that occur frequently or involve a large number of clients, employees, or organizational systems (e.g., care planning for high-risk mothers and infants).

2. *High-risk* processes include those in which harm or lack of significant benefit may occur if the activity is either performed or not performed (e.g., giving a wrong medication or not giving a medication).

3. *Problem-prone* processes are those that have tended in the past to produce problems for staff or clients (e.g., wound infections after surgery or falls among elderly clients in a cluttered home environment).

4. *High-cost* processes are those that result in large expenditures for the organization or that can significantly deplete client or organizational resources immediately or over time (e.g., processes not covered by insurance or daily travel by the client to an ambulatory care center).

Structure, process, and outcome standards flow from the key organizational functions and related processes. Indicators are then selected to measure whether these standards are achieved. Refer again to the care, treatment, and service function. If a community health agency places high priority on addressing the care needs of high-risk pregnant women, this agency may use "the number of mothers served by the agency who received prenatal care during the first trimester" as an indicator of quality performance. This indicator uses the rationale that pregnant women who receive prenatal care during their first trimester are more likely to have positive pregnancy outcomes than women who do not, and that if this rate is significantly lower than the norm, opportunities for improving client service delivery exists. Oermann, Dillon, Templin (2000) found, when researching indicators of quality from the clients' perspective, that the most important indicators of health care quality to the clients in clinics were getting better, getting care and service when needed, and having diagnosis and treatment options explained.

**Thresholds for Evaluation**

Indicators focus an organization's attention on important processes and outcomes to monitor during quality improvement efforts. *Thresholds* help an organization *evaluate* data and determine when an intensive evaluation is needed to identify why a variance from the norm is occurring. When outcome, process, and structure indicators are developed, thresholds for evaluation and a time frame for goal achievement also are established.

A **"threshold for evaluation** is a level or point at which the results of data collection in monitoring and evaluation trigger intensive evaluation of a particular important aspect of care to determine whether an actual problem or opportunity for improvement exists" (JCAHO, 1990a, p. 141). In other words, a threshold or a performance target identifies how often or the percentage of time the organization adhered to agency standards (Katz, Green, 1997). Thresholds for evaluation can range from 100% of the time to 0% of the time. It is generally believed that it is neither effective nor productive to set most thresholds for evaluation at 100%. This is based on the belief that thresholds of evaluation should be designed to take into consideration the multiple factors that affect health care delivery, such as the socioeconomic and educational status of clients and caregivers, severity of a client's illness, and professional experience of staff. For example, taking into consideration the varying characteristics of family caregivers, it is not realistic to expect that instruction to caregivers on appropriate infant feeding practices be completed by the first home visit 100% of the time.

"The setting of threshold parameters for clinical indicators is guided by past performance of the organization, experts in the field, or empirical findings reported in the literature" (Wagner, 1996, p. 414). For example, based on experience, the Baltimore County Public Health Nursing division set thresholds for assessment, family evaluation, and planning at 90%; for follow-up at 85%; and for client outcomes at 75% (Zlotnick, 1992, p. 134). Although quality management efforts are aimed at improving threshold parameters, these parameters must be realistic, based on available resources and the characteristics of the clients being served. It is, for example, difficult for community health nurses to achieve desired outcomes 100% of the time when they are working with vulnerable families who are experiencing multiple physical and psychosocial problems.

## Benchmarking

Organizations that strive toward excellence in health care service delivery use the benchmarking process to identify appropriate standards and indicators for quality monitoring and thresholds for evaluation. "Benchmarking means to study someone else's processes in order to learn how to improve one's own. *Internal benchmarking* occurs within an organization. *External benchmarking* occurs between organizations that produce the same product or provide the same service" (JCAHO, 1993, p. 28). Organizations use the benchmarking process to identify what is possible and how others have achieved higher levels of performance (Czarnecki, 1996; Kaufman, 1997; Peters, McKeon, 1998).

To successfully benchmark, organizations need to identify what benchmarking issues to address, develop an internal database for comparing performance, establish partnerships with other organizations or units within their organization that are willing to benchmark, and collect and evaluate *comparative* measures of performance (Czarnecki, 1996; Wagner, 1996). Benchmarking requires a commitment to excellence and continuous performance improvement as well as resources for carrying out benchmarking activities. Benchmarking can assist organizations in establishing realistic standards of excellence and in remaining competitive in the health care environment. Health care organizations are being challenged by consumers and purchasers of health care services to document how their outcomes compare with health care industry outcomes. Competitive benchmarking helps an organization identify best practices that can be marketed.

## Secure and Use Performance Measures

TQM is a factual problem-solving process designed to monitor and evaluate organizational performance. After key functions, processes, standards, and indicators are specified, tools and methods for measuring performance must be selected. The quality improvement team answers several questions before securing methods for measuring organizational performance. These questions are displayed in Box 25-8. "Both process and outcome must drive all data collection" (Katz, Green, 1997, p. 163). Usually multiple goals are established for the data collection process (Box 25-9). An organization that has a sound management information system is more likely to accomplish multiple data collection goals than organizations that rely on traditional data recording procedures. Saba and McCormick (1996) have compiled an excellent overview of the development of computer applications in community health as well as a description of the major types of community health computer systems.

A performance management team uses multiple methods to collect data from a variety of sources (e.g., users and purchasers of health care services, staff, managers, and organizational records). Some of the methods used for collecting performance data are record audits, utilization review procedures, interviews, customer surveys, observation of clients in their environment, focus groups, and staff self-reviews. The goals established for data collection drive the selection of data collection methods. Data management efforts should be specific and support the clinical and business values, goals, and stan-

### BOX 25-8
### *Questions Asked to Guide the Data Collection Process*

- What are the goals for collecting the data?
- Who should collect the data?
- In which domain should the data be collected?
- For what purpose should the data be collected?
- What are the data sources?
- How much data should be collected?
- What tools should be used?
- What bias exists?

From Katz JM, Green E: *Managing quality: a guide to system-wide performance management in health care,* ed 2, St Louis, 1997, Mosby, p. 163.

### BOX 25-9
### *Goals for Data Collection*

- Set up a system to ensure accuracy of information on which to base future decisions.
- Avoid all punitive measures associated with the results of collected data.
- Pinpoint the exact areas of the organization that contain the performance improvement opportunities.
- Establish the degree to which improvement has occurred after the implementation of an improvement action plan.
- Collect data at regular intervals on all critical processes to demonstrate sustained improvement.
- Collect both subjective and objective data.

From Katz JM, Green E: *Managing quality: a guide to system-wide performance management in health care,* ed 2, St Louis, 1997, Mosby, p. 163.

dards of the organization (Peters, McKeon, 1998). For example, if the goal is to evaluate the care planning process and the standard specifies that this process should be individualized to address client needs, the record audit tool used to measure achievement of this standard should reflect the concept of individualization in its criteria measures. One such measure might be "the health care provider has documented the problems and needs of the client." Another might be "the health care provider has documented that the client has received information about his or her medical condition."

## Record Audit

A commonly used method for collecting performance data in community health is the record audit. Both concurrent and retrospective record auditing are carried out in community health agencies. As previously discussed, organizations subscribing to TQM or CQI emphasize concurrent review to learn about the process of care and services rather than the performance of individuals. In other words, emphasis is placed on learning how the system is currently performing, with a focus on identifying how it can be improved. The concept underlying this emphasis is that there is always opportunity for improvement and that improvement is more likely to occur if punitive measures toward individuals are avoided (Peters, McKeon, 1998).

A record audit encompasses a systematic review of a specified number of service records in a given period for the purpose of evaluating the care planning process and client outcomes. Katz and Green (1997) have established guidelines for determining sample size for record audit reviews and other measurement procedures (Table 25-2). As would be expected, the purpose of the review influences the sample size. A *routine review* is done to track trends over time. A *query review* occurs when data demonstrate that threshold parameters have not been achieved and the reasons for this can't be explained. An *intensive review* is conducted when negative client outcomes have been identified. A *sentinel event review* is done when a serious event (e.g., a medication error that compromises a client's quality of life) occurs (Katz, Green, 1997, p. 165).

**TABLE 25-2**

*Katz-Green Guidelines for Data Collection*

| TYPE OF STUDY | SAMPLE SIZE |
| --- | --- |
| Routine review | 5% or 30 (whichever is greater) |
| Query review | 10% or 60 (whichever is greater) |
| Intensive review | 15% or 90 (whichever is greater) |
| Sentinel event | 100% (every event) |

From Katz JM, Green E: *Managing quality: a guide to system-wide performance management in health care,* ed 2, St Louis, 1997, Mosby, p. 165.

Record audits are structured to ensure consistency of interpretation by all reviewers. This structure is obtained through the use of an audit tool that has a set of care standards, indicator measurements for each care standard, and a quality rating scale. Indicators are predetermined, measurable characteristics of a variable (care standard) that are used to evaluate clinical performance from both a process and an outcome perspective. One process indicator used to determine how well nurses complete assessments might read, "community health nurses collect and record data in relation to a client's family history." An outcome indicator used to assess continuity of care could be "all clients will be visited within 24 hours of referral to agency."

Each agency should have its own set of standards and indicators for its quality improvement program. These standards should address requirements of regulatory bodies. An agency functioning under a TQM philosophy empowers staff to select appropriate performance indicators and measures, based on a review of the professional literature. As previously discussed, multiple measures are used to evaluate quality performance.

## Staff Performance Appraisals

One of the most exciting aspects of a CQI program is the opportunity for staff to expand their competencies and to grow in a supportive environment. Organizations guided by the CQI model of quality encourage staff and managers to work together in the development of performance management and career advancement plans. These plans are designed to increase job satisfaction and job performance and assist human resource departments in implementing competency-based orientation and staff development programs (Benjamin, Penland, 1995).

Ongoing appraisal of one's professional performance is absolutely critical in today's rapidly changing health care environment. This appraisal can provide a safeguard for quality client care, promote professional development, and facilitate the identification of professional strengths and opportunities for professional improvement. Staff performance appraisal processes also aid organizations in identifying system barriers that impede the effective and efficient delivery of clinical services.

The performance appraisal process is based on specified standards of performance and specific indicators (criteria) for measuring these standards. "Performance standards are derived from job analysis, job descriptions, job evaluation, and other documents detailing the qualitative and quantitative aspects of jobs. They are established by authority, which may be the agency in which they are used or a professional association such as the American Nurses Association" (e.g., public health nursing standards identified earlier in this chapter) (Swansburg, 1996, p. 630).

Managers and staff focus on identifying the critical components of service delivery when developing performance standards and personnel specifications. Standards established

**TABLE 25-3**

## Milwaukee Visiting Nurse Association's Job and Personnel Specifications for a Public Health Nurse II

*Section A—job description and specifications*

*Job Summary:* Under supervision, has responsibility for case management of patients and families with a wide variety of complex health and social problems, including multiproblem families. Is expected to be able to function independently in most situations. Identifies need for consultation or supervisory help. May be assigned additional responsibilities that require leadership ability.

| DUTIES AND RESPONSIBILITIES | BASIC REQUIREMENTS |
|---|---|
| 1. Functions independently in case management of complex situations, using supervision appropriately. | Interviewing skills. Physical assessment skills. |
| 2. Admits patients and family members and gives service utilizing the nursing process. | Knowledge of health problems and illnesses. |
| a. Assessment—collects physiological, psychosocial, and financial data. Can identify the need for further data and pursues sources of data independently. | Knowledge of normal growth and development. Ability to make nursing judgments based on scientific nursing principles. |
| b. Assesses family members' health status and coping ability. Able to evaluate the family as a unit. | Knowledge of data sources within the community. |
| c. Identifies covert and overt nursing health and social problems of patients and families based on data collection. | Knowledge of family dynamics. Ability to see and interpret relationships in data and to arrive at a nursing care plan. |
| d. Implements nursing care plan as outlined. Adapts nursing procedures to the home setting. | Ability to identify objective parameters for evaluation of nursing care plan. |
| e. Evaluates results of care plan in terms of expected outcomes and takes appropriate action. | |
| 3. Recognizes and interprets behavior patterns as influenced by basic physical and emotional needs, cultural and socioeconomic differences. Sensitive and accepting of these needs and differences and adapts plan of care accordingly. | Knowledge of cultural and socioeconomic factors. Knowledge of behavioral principles. Knowledge of self. Sensitivity and ability to listen. Knowledge of dependent and independent nursing functions. |
| 4. Contacts physician to report alterations in patient's health status, to secure and share information, or to obtain medical orders. | Ability to collaborate with other disciplines regarding health care. |
| 5. Independently identifies need for consultation and initiates referral. | Knowledge of consultants available and their role in the agency. |

Reproduced by permission of the Milwaukee Visiting Nurse Association, Milwaukee, Wis, undated.

to appraise the performance of professional health care workers focus attention on how well the professional uses the care planning process. For example, the job description (Table 25-3) for a community health nurse would carefully address the role of nurse in using the nursing process to provide competent, quality care. Job descriptions are structure standards that outline "the requisite knowledge, skills, attitudes, responsibilities, and scope of authority of a specific position within an organization for the organization to function at maximum performance" (Katz, Green, 1997, p. 95).

A variety of tools and methods are used to appraise staff performance against specified standards. Some examples of these methods are peer, manager, and self-ratings; direct observation of staff in the clinical setting; and performance interview appraisals (Swansburg, 1996). Nurses who actively

participate in the development of tools and methods for measuring staff performance will be more satisfied with the results. Take the initiative to become involved. It will be a learning experience that will have long-lasting effects on the delivery of your nursing care.

## Client Reporting Measures

"Today, more than ever, the voice of the patient (client) is crucial for the continuous improvement of health care processes and clinical outcomes. As the medical care system shifts services to ambulatory and home care settings, patients' (clients') active participation in treatment and their compliance with instructions become even greater determining factors in successful clinical outcomes" (Barkley, Furse, 1996, p. 427). Most health care organizations use some type of client reporting measure to seek input from

**TABLE 25-3**

*Milwaukee Visiting Nurse Association's Job and Personnel Specifications*
*for a Public Health Nurse II—cont'd*

| DUTIES AND RESPONSIBILITIES | BASIC REQUIREMENTS |
|---|---|
| 6. Independently refers patients and families to other VNA or community services. | |
| 7. Communicates with other disciplines and services interagency and intraagency to promote continuity and coordination of services. | Knowledge of community resources. Knowledge of agency procedures. Ability to write clear, concise, informative reports. |
| 8. Teaches patients and families nursing procedures and good health practices. Interprets to patient and family the implications of the diagnosis—includes the patient and family in goal setting and plan of care according to their ability. | Knows teaching/learning principles. Ability to adapt to patient and family level of understanding and ability. |
| 9. Plans for the use of ancillary agency personnel and supervises their performance. | Knowledge of the legal functions of the RN, LPN, H-HHA. Knowledge of the legal functions of the RN, LPN, H-HHA in the agency. |
| 10. Organizes and manages caseload efficiently. a. Plans travel routes for optimum economy and efficiency. b. Establishes priorities within own caseload. c. Plans frequency of visits. d. Completes necessary records and reports as required within set time limits. | Good organizational skills. Knowledge of area and travel routes. Ability to use maps. |
| 11. May be assigned additional responsibilities (committees, research, etc.). | |
| Professional Conduct: 1. Accepts agency philosophy, purpose, and objectives. 2. Follows agency policies and procedures. 3. Demonstrates good interpersonal relationships. 4. Uses proper resources to deal with stress. | Knowledge of philosophy, purpose, and objectives. Knowledge of policies and procedures. Recognizes how behavior affects others. |
| Professional Growth: 1. Participates in performance evaluation. 2. Takes responsibility for own professional growth. | Motivated towards self-improvement. |
| *Section B—personnel specifications* 1. Wisconsin professional nurse registration. 2. Graduate of baccalaureate program accredited by the National League of Nursing and American Public Health Association. 3. Two years current experience in community health nursing. | |

clients about their level of satisfaction with the health care delivery process and its outcomes and to rate the quality of care they received. Organizations accredited by JCAHO must document that they have sought client input and have used this input to improve organizational performance as needed.

Organizations are using various methods to obtain input from clients about their perceptions of the quality of care they received and their level of satisfaction with this care. Examples of these methods are telephone or face-to-face interviews, client satisfaction and quality rating surveys, focus groups, and client representation on advisory boards.

Client reporting measures can provide information about a variety of clinical care concerns and outcomes and client satisfaction issues. A major challenge for a quality management team is to identify the type of client data needed to assess desired system-level and client-level outcomes. Client reporting measures that are sensitive to *specific* aspects of care are important because it has been documented that clients in different care settings view quality of health care differently (Edgman-Levitan, Cleary, 1996; Ketefian, Redman, Nash, Bogue, 1997; Oermann, Dillon, Templin, 2000). Client reporting measures must be valid and reliable and address differing client characteristics. Bushy (1995) firmly believes that ethnocultural factors can no longer be ignored when seeking client input. These factors significantly influence if services are acceptable and appropriate for target populations.

The increasing diversity of the American population challenges health care providers to examine carefully their continuous quality monitoring efforts to determine if they address quality improvement from a cultural perspective.

Chapters 7 and 9 identify cultural parameters to consider when developing performance standards and measurements that evaluate the cultural dimensions of care. The *Healthy People 2010* National Health Objectives (USDHHS, 2000a) assist health care providers in targeting appropriate performance outcomes for populations belonging to different ethnic groups.

## Analyze Data/Make Interpretations

Data from all clinical assessment procedures should be examined to make interpretations about clinical performance. One tool alone, such as the record audit, cannot provide a sufficient database to determine performance strengths or opportunities for improvement. Additionally, data from

multiple sources are often needed to identify the underlying reasons for inadequate care.

The purpose of QA activities is to identify discrepancies, or *variance*, between established standards and criteria and actual clinical practice. Evaluation assessments should be specific enough to identify both strengths and areas needing improvement in clinical care. If either is found lacking when analyzing evaluation data, measurement tools and processes should be reevaluated to determine if evaluation measurements discriminate between safe and unsafe care. It is also possible that staff may not be using the tools appropriately.

To identify variance between standards and actual practice, measurement data must be organized and grouped so that a composite picture is clearly presented. Summary reports should be developed so that the combined results of multiple efforts can be examined and patterns of care identified. Interpretations about overall agency performance must be based on *patterns* occurring over time, rather than on selected record reviews at a given time. There are several ways to display and summarize data such as the use of tables, histograms, graphs, and charts (see Chapter 14). Box 25-10 presents brief descriptions of some common tools used to help understand the underlying causes of assessment results. A case study analysis using the "fishbone" cause-and-effect diagram is presented later in this chapter.

## Identify, Choose, and Implement Action Strategies

Once strengths and opportunities for improvements have been delineated, **action strategies** for improvement are identified. One such strategy might be to share feedback about organizational strengths. This type of feedback provides an incentive for active participation in performance improvement efforts.

To identify action strategies for improvement, health care providers must first analyze why variance between established standards and actual performance is occurring. For example, record documentation may demonstrate limited follow-up and evaluation of provider interventions. This may be occurring for a variety of reasons, including lack of knowledge, inadequate caseload management skills, insufficient time allocated for documentation, and poor staff morale. Discourse among providers to identify the reasons for performance concerns helps providers select appropriate action strategies. If the documentation problem previously noted, for example, was a result of unrealistic time allocations for recording, an action strategy designed to improve staff's understanding of follow-up and evaluation processes would not be appropriate for improving the identified documentation problem. Rather, staff should be provided more time for recording.

Once staff choose an appropriate action strategy, it is important to develop a plan for implementing and evaluating the outcomes of this strategy that takes into consideration agency resources and identifies who is responsible for mon-

### BOX 25-10
## *Data Display Tools*

### *Flow Charts*
A flow chart graphically represents the sequence of events or steps that are required in a particular process or to produce a specific output.

### *Cause-and-Effect Diagram*
The cause-and-effect diagram looks like a fishbone with the effect being the desired outcome and the causes represented by the "spines." The causes are usually divided into four categories: materials, methods, manpower, and machines. This tool is referred to as a fishbone diagram or Ishikawa, named after a leading quality improvement authority in Japan.

### *Run Chart*
The run chart displays events or observations over time.

### *Pareto Chart*
The pareto chart displays data in a ranking order comparing factors used to determine priorities, a way to sort out the "vital few" from the "trivial many."

### *Histogram*
The histogram displays a graphic summary of how frequently something occurs.

### *Control Chart*
The control chart distinguishes common cause and special cause variation. It appears as a run chart with statistically determined upper and lower limits above and below the average.

### *Scatter Diagram*
The scatter diagram demonstrates the relationship between two variables.

From Koch MW, Fairly TM: *Integrated quality management: the key to improving nursing care quality,* St Louis, 1993, Mosby, p. 65.

itoring progress. Taking action to improve performance is one of the most significant components of a QA/QI program. It demonstrates that the organization assumes accountability for the care provided to clients by its employees. The quality assessment and monitoring cycle should continue even when expected performance is achieved. Ongoing monitoring is an important aspect of a total quality management program.

## Monitor Quality Improvement Actions

Ongoing monitoring is essential to maintain quality performance over time. A sound QA program sets in place strategies to identify whether improvement is sustained or whether new or additional improvement actions are needed. Such a program also maintains a focus on the future and continuously examines the need for new performance strategies and measurements.

The CQI process encourages staff to actively participate in identifying potential and actual opportunities for improvement and to examine how environmental factors make an impact on service delivery. Environmental factors such as the evolutionary nature of the treatment of disease and changing technology, demographic characteristics of the population, and socioeconomic conditions in society continuously influence the health care delivery process (Cesta, 1993). This in turn requires a continuous focus on how the system can improve to address these changes.

Continuous quality monitoring is in the best interest of an organization. Poor quality control can affect an organization's public image and its financial outlays directly or indirectly. Improving performance helps an organization to reduce both visible (direct) and hidden (indirect) costs, such as cost related to malpractice suits, excessive overtime, and poor client satisfaction.

## INTEGRATED QUALITY MANAGEMENT PROCESSES

Escalating health care costs and complex changes in health care delivery have resulted in increased concern over cost containment and legal issues affecting community-based health care agencies. This has led to an emphasis on utilization review, risk and safety management, and infection control activities.

**Utilization review,** or *management,* is an assessment and review process designed to evaluate the appropriateness of client care (Al-Assaf, 1996). This process focuses on the delivery of services in a cost-effective and efficient manner. It uses a client record review to identify whether the amount and type of services provided were appropriate to the needs of the clients and appropriate for the agency to provide. This review examines the care provided to determine if there was over-or-under utilization of services and whether the timing of services was appropriate. Judgments about the appropriateness of care are based on na-

tional standards or norms (Al-Assaf, 1996). Client classification systems and intensity rating instruments assist agencies in predicting the kind and amount of service needed by client groups with specific characteristics. Although client classification systems and rating instruments have been more widely used in acute care settings, several community-oriented ones are available (Ballard, McNamara, 1983; Daubert, 1997; Hardy, 1984; Hays, 1992; Hays, Kroeger, Tachenko-Achord, Peters, 1995; Martin, Scheet, 1992; Saba, 1997; Shaughnessy, Crisler, 1995).

**Risk and safety management** is a process that focuses on preventing risks or harm to clients, employees, and other individuals that come in contact with an organization. Risk management processes focus on ensuring client, employee, and visitor safety, and preventing malpractice or other legal liability (Bryant, Fields, Schaedler, 1996). Health care organizations face significant risk in relation to the delivery of client care services and employee and visitor health and safety. A recent IOM report (Kohn, Corrigan, Donaldson, 2000) estimates that health care error is a leading cause of death in the United States. A major emphasis is being placed on advancing client safety within the health care system (Levy, Lancaster, 2001; Wilson, Hatlie, 2001). A sound risk and safety management program focuses on such matters as the monitoring of staff selection, orientation, and ongoing educational processes; the development of policies to ensure client and employee safety; the evaluation of unsafe client and employee incidents; the development of educational materials to enhance caregiver/client competency; and the monitoring of laws and codes related to client care.

**Infection control** is a process focused on disease prevention, intervention, and recognition (Koch, Fairly, 1993). The concepts and principles of epidemiology form a foundation for an effective infection control program (Friedman, Chenoweth, 1996). Control actions are generally directed toward breaking the chain of transmission for infection. Examples of infection control activities are reporting and monitoring infection rates; maintaining an infection control surveillance system; orienting or providing in-service for staff about infection control issues; establishing infection control policies and procedures, including policies regarding the disposal of infectious wastes and universal precautions; and instructing clients on infection control techniques (Koch, Fairly, 1993). Nurses and clients in the community have numerous opportunities for exposure to infectious diseases. It is imperative that infection control policies and procedures be followed in all community-based settings.

## *Stop and Think About It*

You are a member of your agency's infection control committee. Conduct a "walking assessment" of the work environment and think about factors in the environment that could promote exposures to infectious diseases. How might you control these factors?

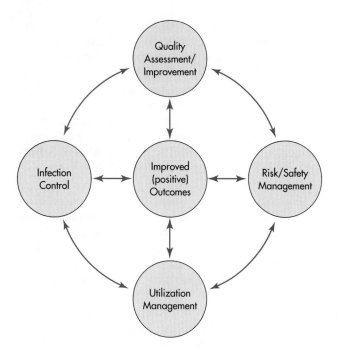

**FIGURE 25-3** Integrated quality management model: improved (positive) outcomes. (From Koch MW, Fairly TM: *Integrated quality management: the key to improving nursing care quality,* St Louis, 1993, Mosby, p. 124.)

Although utilization review, risk and safety management, infection control, and QA programs have distinctive and separate foci, they are interrelated and have a significant impact on each other. For example, selected aspects of utilization review focus on the provision of optimal or quality care. This could be reflected in the underutilization of clinical services such as referrals to other community agencies when needed. Underutilization of services can adversely influence client outcomes.

An ultimate goal of each component of CQI is improved or positive outcomes (Figure 25-3). To accomplish this goal, all CQI efforts should be integrated and coordinated to achieve a balance among the goals of the four programs. If this coordination is lacking, an agency may neglect aspects of each of these components (Harris, Yuan, 1997). Integrated quality management is the key to improving organization-wide performance, including client service delivery (Koch, Fairly, 1993).

A case scenario can best illustrate how CQI efforts are integrated and coordinated to address the important processes in an organization. The following case scenario represents a typical home care client (Koch, Fairly, 1993, pp. 235-236).

**CASE** *Scenario*  Mr. N. is a 55-year-old white male who retired early from a lucrative law practice because of a debilitating stroke (Figure 25-4). He has a

history of hypertension and workaholic behavior. He has been in a rehabilitation center and has now returned home for continued support.

He is overweight and has been unable to care for himself since the cardiovascular accident. He has several children in town, including a son who is a nurse at a local hospital. His wife employs an attendant from 10 PM to 6 AM each day to care for Mr. N. She also has a housekeeper who is available for light assistance to Mr. N. during the day. There is good family support. Mr. N.'s private insurance covers intermittent visits by a home care nurse each week.

Figure 25-4 demonstrates the proactive CQI planning process for this case, utilizing the fishbone cause-and-effect diagram described earlier in this chapter. According to Koch and Fairly (1993), this process "analyzes the possible root causes to produce a positive patient care outcome in each case" (p. 234). The possible root causes of positive outcomes for Mr. N. were defined in terms of issues related to infection control, risk/safety management, utilization management, and QA/QI. Under the QA/QI component the authors identified a need to examine the important aspects of Mr. N's care using three priority indicators defined earlier in this chapter: high-volume (HV), high-risk (HR), and problem-prone (PP). Although Mr. N. had excellent supports and was doing well, the fishbone diagram demonstrated potential risk factors. Koch and Fairly's book is an excellent resource for expanding knowledge of these concepts, as well as the concept of TQM.

## PARTNERS IN QUALITY IMPROVEMENT

Individual health care providers, professional organizations, service agencies, and clients all share responsibility for maintaining and improving quality standards for clinical practice. Input from the client is essential for determining values important to recipients of care. Client feedback is also crucial for the identification of improvements needed in practice on an ongoing basis. It is important that clients affect all components of a CQI program because client needs form a foundation from which client services emerge. Organizations that remain viable in the marketplace are ones that are customer focused in all aspects of health care delivery.

Implementing a TQM program is an exciting, challenging endeavor that promotes a client-focused system, team-building, and interdisciplinary functioning. All members of the health care team work with the client to improve health care service delivery. Through collaborative efforts all members of the health care team can help an organization maintain a competitive edge in the health care market. Such a challenge is worth working toward.

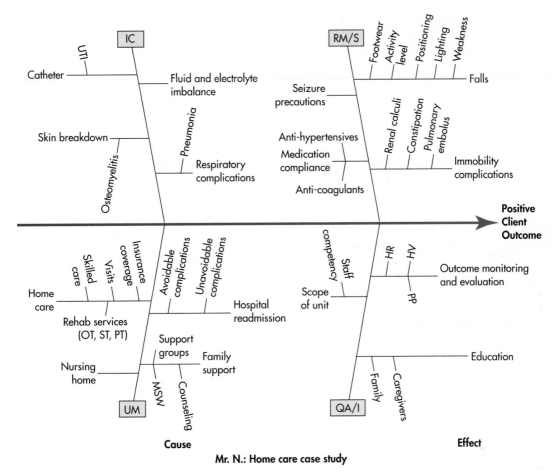

**Mr. N.: Home care case study**

**FIGURE 25-4** Integrated quality management "fishbone" diagrams: home care case study. *IC,* Infection control; *UM,* utilization management; *RM/S,* risk management/safety; *QA/I,* quality assessment/improvement; *HV,* high-volume; *HR,* high-risk; *PP,* problem-prone. (Redrawn from Koch MW, Fairly TM: *Integrated quality management: the key to improving nursing care quality,* St Louis, 1993, Mosby, p. 238.)

## SUMMARY

Daily, health care professionals are being challenged to address health care quality concerns. Nurses share with all health care professionals the need to examine carefully the delivery of their services in light of changing societal demands and unprecedented complex health care demands. An exciting approach to quality appraisal and monitoring, *total quality management,* or *continuous quality improvement,* has emerged. This concept is client oriented with a focus on achieving excellence by identifying opportunities for performance improvement. It promotes team-building and interdisciplinary functioning.

Total quality management is a dynamic process that examines how significant organizational and clinical processes facilitate or inhibit quality performance. Quality assessment, utilization review, risk and safety management, and infection control activities are systematically implemented with a focus on improving client and system outcomes. An integrated and coordinated approach is essential to achieve a balance among all quality management components. Quality management is a factual problem-solving process that uses a variety of methods for assessing and improving quality. Crucial to the successful implementation of a total quality management program is an organizational philosophy that promotes a commitment to quality improvement, a participative management leadership style, and a shared vision that places the client in the forefront.

## CRITICAL THINKING
*exercise*

Using data from a client situation in which you have been involved, complete a web-based search for national guidelines related to the care needs of this client. Using these guidelines complete a fishbone diagram (see Figure 25-4). Identify in this diagram issues related to infection control, risk/safety management, utilization management, and quality assessment and improvement that needed to be addressed. Taking into consideration the environmental conditions existing when you were caring for the identified client/family, discuss strategies that would improve service delivery performance.

## REFERENCES

Al-Assaf AF: Utilization management and the quality of health care. In Schmele J, editor: *Quality management in nursing and health care*, Albany, 1996, Delmar.

American Nurses Association (ANA): *A plan for implementation of the standards of nursing practice*, Kansas City, Mo, 1975, ANA.

American Nurses Association (ANA): *Nursing's acute care report card*, Washington, DC, 1995, American Nurses Publishing.

American Nurses Association (ANA): *Nursing quality indicators beyond acute care: literature review*, Washington, DC, 2000a, American Nurses Publishing.

American Nurses Association (ANA): *Nursing quality indicators beyond acute care: measurement instruments*, Washington, DC, 2000b, American Nurses Publishing.

Applebaum R: Assuring and improving the quality of in-home services, *Caring* 19(6):12-15, 2000.

Baker GR, Gelmon SB: Total quality management in health care. In Schmele JA, editor: *Quality management in nursing and health care*, Albany, NY, 1996, Delmar.

Ballard S, McNamara R: Quantifying nursing needs in home health care, *Nurs Res* 32(4):236-241, 1983.

Barkley WM, Furse DH: Changing priorities for improvement: the impact of low response rates in patient satisfaction, *J Qual Improvement* 22(6):427-433, 1996.

Beery WL, Greenwald HP, Nudelman PM: Managed care and public health: building a partnership, *Public Health Nurs* 13:305-310, 1996.

Beltran R: Underserved populations, the quality of their health services, *Am J Med Qual* 15(4):125, 2000 (editorial).

Benjamin S, Penland T: How developmental supervision and performance management improve effectiveness, *Health Care Superv* 14(2):19-28, 1995.

Bryant J, Fields M, Schaedler P: Risk management. In Schmele JA, editor: *Quality management in nursing and health care*, Albany, NY, 1996, Delmar.

Bull MJ: Past and present perspectives on quality of care in the United States. In Schmele JA, editor: *Quality management in nursing and health care*, Albany, NY, 1996, Delmar.

Bureau of Primary Health Care: *The working group on homeless health outcomes: meeting proceedings*, Rockville, Md, June 1996, The Division.

Bushy A: Ethnocultural sensitivity and measurement of consumer satisfaction, *J Nurs Care Qual* 9(2):16-25, 1995.

Centering the survey process, *Joint Commission Perspectives* 21(1):1,3, 2001.

Cesta TG: The link between continuous quality improvement and case management, *JONA* 23:55-61, 1993.

Christy TE: The first 50 years, *Am J Nurs* 71:1778-1784, 1971.

Council on Graduate Medical Education, National Advisory Council on Nurse Education and Practice: *Collaborative education to ensure patient safety*, Rockville, Md, 2000, Health Resources and Services Administration.

Cross LL: Legal implications of quality management. In Schmele JA, editor: *Quality management in nursing and healthcare*, Albany, NY, 1996, Delmar.

Czarnecki MT: Benchmarking: a data-oriented look at improving health care performance, *J Nurs Care Qual* 10(3):1-6, 1996.

Daubert EA: A patient classification outcome criteria system. In Harris M, editor: *Handbook of home health care administration*, ed 2, Gaithersburg, Md, 1997, Aspen.

Donabedian A: Evaluating the quality of medical care, *Milbank Q* 44:166-206, 1966.

Donabedian A: Some issues in evaluating the quality of nursing care, *Am J Public Health* 59:1833-1836, 1969.

Donabedian A: Models of quality assurance. In Schmele JA, editor: *Quality management in nursing and health care*, Albany, NY, 1996, Delmar.

Edgman-Levitan S, Cleary PD: What information do consumers want and need? *Health Affairs* 15(4):42-56, 1996.

Friedman C, Chenoweth C: Infection control. In Schmele JA, editor: *Quality management in nursing and health care*, Albany, NY, 1996, Delmar.

Gardner MS: Typewritten reminiscences, Feb. 5, 1948, NOPHN Archive Microfilm #25. In Fitzpatrick ML, editor: *The National Organization for Public Health Nursing 1912-1952: development of a practice field*, New York, 1975, National League for Nursing.

General Accounting Office (GAO): *Quality assurance: a comprehensive national strategy for health care is needed*, Gaithersburg, Md, 1990, GAO.

Hardy JA: A patient classification system for home health patients, *Caring* 3(9):26-27, 1984.

Harris M: Quality assessment/performance improvement: an administrator's viewpoint. In Harris M, editor: *Handbook of home health care administration*, ed 2, Gaithersburg, Md, 1997, Aspen.

Harris M, Dugan M: Evaluating the quality of home care services using patient outcome data. In Harris M, editor: *Handbook of home health care administration*, ed 2, Gaithersburg, Md, 1997, Aspen.

Harris M, Yuan J: Quality planning for quality patient care. In Harris M, editor: *Handbook of home health care administration*, ed 2, Gaithersburg, Md, 1997, Aspen.

Hays BJ: Nursing care requirements and resources consumption in home health care, *Nurs Res* 41(3):138-143, 1992.

Hays BJ, Kroeger RA, Tachenko-Achord SA, Peters DA: Determining intensity of need of high-risk maternal and infant clients, *J Nurs Care Qual* 9(2):67-75, 1995.

Health Care Financing Administration (HCFA): *Health care quality improvement program: medicare priorities*, Washington, DC, 2000, HCFA.

Holzemer W, Henry S: Therapeutic outcomes sensitive to nursing. In Hinshaw AS, Feethan SL, Shaver JL, editors: *Handbook of clinical nursing research*, Thousand Oaks, Calif, 1999, Sage.

Institute of Medicine: *America's health care safety net: intact but endangered*, Washington, DC, 2000, National Academy of Science.

Institute of Medicine: *Crossing the quality chasm: a new health system for the 21st century*, Washington, DC, 2001, National Academy of Science.

Johnson M, Maas M, Moorhead S, editors: *Nursing outcomes classification (NOC)*, ed 2, St Louis, 2000, Mosby.

Joint Commission on Accreditation of Healthcare Organizations (JCAHO): *Quality assurance in home care and hospice organizations*, Oakbrook Terrace, Ill, 1990a, JCAHO.

Joint Commission on Accreditation of Healthcare Organizations (JCAHO): *Primer on indicator development and application: measuring quality in health care*, Oakbrook Terrace, Ill, 1990b, JCAHO.

Joint Commission on Accreditation of Healthcare Organizations (JCAHO): *The measurement mandate: on the road to performance improvement in health care*, Oakbrook Terrace, Ill, 1993, JCAHO.

Joint Commission on Accreditation of Healthcare Organizations (JCAHO): *Framework for improving performance: from principles to practice*, Oakbrook Terrace, Ill, 1994, JCAHO.

Joint Commission on Accreditation of Healthcare Organizations (JCAHO): *CAMHC: 2001-2002 comprehensive accreditation manual for home care*, Oakbrook Terrace, Ill, 2000, JCAHO.

Katz JM, Green E: *Managing quality: a guide to system-wide performance management in health care*, ed 2, St Louis, 1997, Mosby.

Kaufman M: Home health care benchmarking. In Harris M, editor: *Handbook of home health care administration*, ed 2, Gaithersburg, Md, 1997, Aspen.

Ketefian S, Redman R, Nash MG, Bogue E: Inpatient and ambulatory patient satisfaction with nursing care, *Quality Management in Healthcare* 5(4):66-75, 1997.

Koch MW, Fairly TM: *Integrated quality management: the key to improving nursing care quality*, St Louis, 1993, Mosby.

Kohn L, Corrigan J, Donaldson M, editors: *To err is human: building a safer health system*, Washington, DC, 2000, National Academy Press.

Lee TT, Mills ME: Analysis of patient profile in predicting home care resource utilization and outcomes, *JONA* 30(2):67-75, 2000.

Leviss PS, Hurtig L: The role of local health units in a managed care environment: a case study of New York City, *J Pub Health Manag Pract* 4(1):12-20, 1998.

Levy J, Lancaster D: Collaboration to improve patient safety: the first domain of quality, *J Healthc Qual* 23(1):9-13, 2001.

Lohr KN, editor: *Medicare: a strategy for quality assurance*, vol 1, Washington, DC, 1990, National Academy Press.

Lummis M: The quality improvement movement: an epidemiologist's viewpoint. In Schmele JA, editor: *Quality management in nursing and health care*, Albany, NY, 1996, Delmar.

Lysaught JP: *An abstract for action*, New York, 1970, McGraw-Hill.

Managed care's conflicts of interest, *Caring* 14:4, 1995.

Marrelli TM: *The best of home care nurse news: manager's corner*, Tampa, 1997, Marrelli and Associates.

Martin KS, Norris J, Leak GK: Psychometric analysis of the problem rating scale for outcomes, *Outcomes Management for Nursing Practice* 3(1):20-25, 1999.

Martin KS, Scheet NJ: *The Omaha System: a pocket guide for community health nursing*, Philadelphia, 1992, WB Saunders.

McCormick KA, Cummings MA, Kovner C: The role of the Agency for Health Care Policy and Research in improving outcomes of care, *Nurs Clin North Am* 32(3):521-542, 1997.

Melum MM, Sinioris ME: Total quality management in health care: taking stock, *Quality Manage Health Care* 1(4):59-63, 1993.

National Committee for Quality Assurance (NCQA): *The state of managed care quality—2000*, Washington, DC, 2000, NCQA.

Novick LF: Managed care and public health, *J Pub Health Manag Pract* 4(1):vi, 1998.

Oermann MH, Dillon SL, Templin T: Indicators of quality of care in clinics: patients' perspectives, *J Healthc Qual* 22(6):9-11, 2000.

O'Leary DS: CQI—a step beyond QA, *Qual Rev Bull* 17(1):4-5, 1991.

O'Neil EH, Pew Health Professions Commission: *Recreating health professional practice for a new century*, San Francisco, 1998, The Center for the Health Professions.

Pate B, Stajer R: The diagnosis and treatment of blame, *J Healthc Qual* 23(1):4-7, 2001.

Peters DA, McKeon T: *Transforming home care: quality, cost, and data management*, Gaithersburg, Md, 1998, Aspen.

Quad Council of Public Health Nursing Organizations: *Scope and standards of public health nursing practice*, Washington, DC, 1999, ANA.

Reed PG, Zurakowski TL: Nightingale: foundations of nursing. In Fitzpatrick JJ, Whall AL, editors: *Conceptual models of nursing: analysis and application*, ed 3, Stamford, Conn, 1996, Appleton & Lange, pp. 27-54.

Roper W, Mays G: Managed care, public health, and the uninsured. In Novick L, Mays G, editors: *Public health administration: principles for population-based management*, Gaithersburg, Md, 2001, Aspen.

Rowitz L: *Public health leadership: putting principles into practice*, Gaithersburg, Md, 2001, Aspen.

Saba VK: The home health care classification of nursing: diagnoses and interventions. In Harris M, editor: *Handbook of home health care administration*, ed 2, Gaithersburg, Md, 1997, Aspen.

Saba VK, McCormick KA: *Essentials of computers for nurses*, ed 2, New York, 1996, McGraw-Hill.

Schmele JA: *Quality management in nursing and health care*, Albany, NY, 1996, Delmar.

Schmele JA, Donabedian A: The application of a model to measure the quality of nursing care in home health. In Schmele JA, editor: *Quality management in nursing and health care*, Albany, NY, 1996, Delmar.

Shaughnessy PW, Crisler KS: *Outcome-based quality improvement: a manual for home care agencies on how to use outcomes*, Washington, DC, 1995, National Association for Home Care.

Swansburg RC: *Management and leadership for nurse managers*, ed 2, Boston, 1996, Jones & Bartlett.

Tilbury MS: From QA to CQI: a retrospective review. In Dienemann J, editor: *CQI: continuous quality improvement in nursing*, Washington, DC, 1992, American Nurses Publishing.

US Department of Health and Human Services (USDHHS): *Healthy People 2010: volumes I and II*, Washington, DC, 2000a, US Government Printing Office.

US Department of Health and Human Services (USDHHS): *Healthy People 2010: tracking Healthy People 2010*, Washington, DC, 2000b, US Government Printing Office.

Wagner PS: Guide to identifying, collecting, and managing data. In Schmele J, editor: *Quality management in nursing and health care*, Albany, NY, 1996, Delmar.

Wakefield M, O'Grady E: Putting patients first: improving patient safety through collaborative education. In Council on Graduate Medical Education, National Advisory Council on Nurse Education and Practice: *Collaborative education to ensure patient safety*, Rockville, Md, 2000, Health Resources and Services Administration.

Wilson NJ, Hatlie MJ: Advancing patient safety: a framework for accountability and practical action, *J Healthc Qual* 23(1):30-34, 2001.

Woodward C, Ostbye T, Craighead J, et al.: Patient satisfaction as an indicator of quality care in independent health facilities: developing and assessing a tool to enhance public accountability, *Am J Med Qual* 15(3):94-106, 2000.

Zlotnick C: A public health quality assurance system, *Public Health Nurs* 9(2):133-137, 1992.

## SELECTED BIBLIOGRAPHY

Applebaum R, Mollica R, Tilly J: Assuring homecare quality: a case study of state strategies, *Generations* 21(4):57-63, 1998.

Ceglarek JE, Rife JK: Developing a public health nursing audit, *J Nurs Adm* 10:37-43, 1977.

Chassin MR, Galvin RW: The urgent need to improve health care quality—Institute of Medicine National Round Table on Health Care Quality, *JAMA* 280(11):1000-1005, 1998.

Friedman MM: Designing an infection control program to meet JCAHO standards, *Caring* 15(7):18-25, 1996.

Grube J: Learning from healthcare errors: effective reporting systems, *J Healthc Qual* 23(1):25-28, 2001.

Hays BJ, Sather L, Peters D: Quantifying client needs for care in the community: a strategy for managed care, *Public Health Nurs* 16(4):246-253, 1999.

Hill M: Outcomes measurement requires nursing to shift to outcome-based practice, *Nurs Admin Q* 21(4):57-63, 1998.

Holzemer W, Henry S: Therapeutic outcomes sensitive to nursing. In Hinshaw AS, Feethan SL, Shaver JL, editors: *Handbook of clinical nursing research*, Thousand Oaks, Calif, 1999, Sage.

Johnson M, Maas M: Nursing-sensitive patient outcomes: development and importance for use in assessing health care effectiveness. In Cohen E, De Back V, editors: *The outcomes mandate: case management in health care today*, St Louis, 1999, Mosby.

Lia-Hoagberg B, Schaffer M, Strohschein S: Public health nursing practice guidelines: an evaluation of dissemination and use, *Public Health Nurs* 16(6):397-404, 1999.

Lynn MR, McMillan BJ: Do nurses know what patients think is important in nursing care, *J Nurs Care Qual* 13(5):65-74, 1999.

Mullan F: A founder of quality assessment encounters a troubled system firsthand, *J Healthc Qual* 23(2):40-43, 2001.

Newcomer R: Community-level indicators of chronic health conditions and services, *J Healthc Qual* 22(5):29-33, 2000.

Oermann MH, Templin T: Important attributes of quality healthcare: consumer perspectives, *J Nurs Schol* 32(2):167-172, 2000.

Parris K, Place P, Orellana E, et al: Integrating nursing diagnoses, interventions, and outcomes in public health nursing practice, *Nursing Diagnosis* 10(2):49-56, 1999.

Shulkin D: Commentary: why quality improvement efforts in health care fail and what can be done about it, *Am J Med Qual* 15(2):49-53, 2000.

Upshaw V: The National Public Health Performance Standards Program: will it strengthen governance of local public health? *Health Management Practice* 6(5):88-92, 2000.

Van der Bruggen H, Groen M: Toward an unequivocal definition and classification of patient outcomes, *Nursing Diagnosis* 10(3):93-102, 1999.

Weisman C: Measuring quality in women's health care: issues and recent developments, *Quality Management in Health Care* 8(4):14-20, 2000.

# 26

# Challenges for the Future

*Susan Clemen-Stone*

## OBJECTIVES

*Upon completion of this chapter, the reader should be able to:*

1. Analyze how societal trends will influence community health nursing practice throughout the twenty-first century.
2. Articulate competencies needed by health professionals in the twenty-first century.
3. Discuss evolving ethical issues in community health nursing practice.
4. Identify the importance of nursing research in promoting the health of the nation.
5. Explain how political involvement can shape the health care delivery system.
6. Discuss the significance of the concept, "health care for all."

## KEY TERMS

Autonomy
Beneficence
Codes of ethics
Culturally appropriate services
Ethical concerns
Ethical, Legal and Social Implications (ELSI) project
Ethics

Ethnic diversification
Globalization
"Health care for all" concept
Health care safety net
Health policy
Human genome
Human Genome Project (HGP)
Justice

National Institute of Nursing Research (NINR)
Nonmaleficence
Political action
Professional competencies

---

*We are made wise not by the recollections of our past but by the responsibilities for our future.*

GEORGE BERNARD SHAW

Diversity and change will be the driving forces for the profession throughout the twenty-first century, and these will be fueled by other trends that will continue to blossom well into the new millennium. Over the next decade, the profession will be dramatically affected by changes in the U.S. health care system and the significant implication this has for health care providers and consumers (Institute for the Future, 2000; Institute of Medicine [IOM], 2001). Concurrently, the profession will be faced with unprecedented societal changes that are influencing client need and client-provider relationships. Clearly the environment is calling for innovation in service delivery and a reformulation of health care provider roles.

## SOCIETAL TRENDS

Many new things are occurring in the world today. Among these are altered demographics, increasing globalization, a knowledge explosion, a revolution in information technology, advances in biotechnology, and increasing consumer involvement in health care decision making (Brownson, Kreuter, 1997; Institute for the Future, 2000; Parks, 1997). "To be competitive in a rapidly changing environment will require an unprecedented understanding of changing health care markets, the need for developing new global competencies and capabilities, and a shift from tangible assets to an appreciation of the value of knowledge and technology" (Parks, 1997, p. 1).

### Demographics

Changing demographics will have a profound effect on community health nursing service delivery throughout the twenty-first century. Significant shifts in the age structure of the population, increasing diversity among Americans, and changing family patterns will influence both client need and service delivery strategies.

There is no debate about the graying of American society. Aging persons make up the fastest growing segment in the population. During the twentieth century, the average life expectancy increased by more than 30 years and the elderly population increased elevenfold, compared with only a threefold increase for the younger population. Population projections indicate that by 2030, one in every five Americans will be 65 years or older (American Association of Retired Persons [AARP], Administration on Aging, 2001; Institute for the Future, 2000).

The impact of the graying phenomenon has not been fully realized in the health care sector. "Although the first baby boomers won't turn 65 until 2010, the 55-year-old Americans at the leading edge of this group are beginning to suffer the chronic conditions and debilitation accompanying the aging process" (Marketing Health Services editors, 2000). The aging of our society will continue to shift the emphasis of service delivery from acute to chronic care. This shift will require the development of "new and effective interventions for promoting healthy lifestyles among the elderly to improve quality of life and reduce the complications due to disabling conditions" (Brownson, Kreuter, 1997, p. 57).

The graying of the registered nurse (RN) workforce presents significant career opportunities for younger nurses but is also a major challenge in the health care sector. A recent Robert Wood Johnson Foundation sponsored study (Buerhaus, Staiger, Ayerbach, 2000) raises serious concern about the capacity of the "aging and eventually shrinking" RN workforce to meet the health care needs of the country's expanding population (Buerhaus, 2001). The development of partnerships that include consumers, health care providers, and policy makers is needed to address the complex issues related to this concern. It is anticipated that improvements in working conditions and retention and recruitment practices, and changes in the way health care is organized will be needed. No one profession alone can address all of these changes (Buerhaus, 2001; Wilson, Mitchell, 1999).

There is also no debate about the growing ethnic diversity among the old as well as the young in America. Since the mid-1960s, higher immigration and fertility rates among racial and ethnic minority groups have dramatically altered the ethnic mix in the United States. By the year 2020, racial and ethnic minority groups will account for almost 40% of the population, up from 30% at the beginning of the twenty-first century. The increasing diversity of the population varies significantly by region and state. For example, by 2010 no one ethnic or racial group, including white non-Hispanics, will be in the majority in California (Institute for the Future, 2000).

The increasing **ethnic diversification** in the United States will provide challenges for health care providers. The practitioner of the future will need substantive transcultural knowledge to achieve favorable health outcomes (Leininger, 1997). Health care providers will also need to understand the most relevant health risks among differing ethnic populations and to develop culturally relevant interventions to address these risks (Marín, Burhansstipanov, Connell, et al., 1995). Health information will need to be targeted specifically to minority populations and presented within a cultural context that is familiar and comfortable to these populations (Harris, 2000). "The demand will become more pronounced for services that are culturally appropriate, beyond simple language competency" (Institute for the Future, 2000, p. 20).

"The concept of **culturally appropriate** services includes awareness of the complex issues related to the underdiagnosis of certain conditions and diseases among minority groups, the effects of lifestyle and cultural differences on health status, the implications of the diverse genetic endowment of the population, and the impact of patterns of assimilation on health status" (Institute for the Future, 2000, p. 20). For example, segments of ethnic minority populations continue to rely heavily on nontraditional healing alternatives. The continuing challenge for the twenty-first century will be to bridge the cultural gap between traditional and nontraditional health care.

Shifts in family patterns and continuing poverty among several segments of the American population also will present service delivery challenges in the coming century (Dalaker, Proctor, U.S. Census Bureau, 2000). With an increasing number of women entering the workforce, child and elder care arrangements are more complex, especially for families with limited income. This could provide the opportunity for community health nurses to develop specialized clinical niches, such as day care centers for ill children who cannot attend school or children from poor families, or case management services for elderly clients who want to live independently in their own homes.

Although many dual-income families may be increasingly able to purchase needed health care services, the growing income inequality between the rich and poor is likely to continue throughout the next decade. This, coupled with the fact that many places of employment are no longer providing health care benefits, will make it difficult for vulnerable populations to access essential health care services. The community health nurse will continue to play a pivotal role in linking persons to essential personal health services during the twenty-first century.

## Increasing Globalization

The globalization movement has brought both challenges and opportunities for the health care provider. Free trade agreements have enhanced our ability to exchange ideas between professionals and consumers worldwide. This allows care providers to move more quickly in solving health problems and promotes collective action for community health. The growth of the information industries is also helping to remove geographic barriers and is creating a knowledge-dependent global society. This will help people throughout the world to achieve the education needed to build productive lives and to deal with health issues (Cetron, Davies, 2001).

Preventing the spread of disease, preserving the environment, and reducing poverty will be major worldwide health challenges in the future. The globalization movement has highlighted the significant link between environmental conditions, socioeconomic developments, and other determinants of disease, mortality, and health disparities. Health disparities will continue to exist in every country because of the polarization of socioeconomic status within and between countries (Olshansky, Carnes, Rogers, Smith, 1998).

It also has become readily apparent that immigration, international travel, and free trade among nations fuel the spread of new and reemerging infectious diseases (Centers for Disease Control and Prevention [CDC], 1998). In the past 20 years at least 30 new infectious diseases have been identified internationally, and this number is projected to increase in the future (Seymour, 1997). Many of the cases of extremely rare infectious diseases in our country, such as diphtheria, have been imported from other countries (CDC, 1998). The renewed interest in strengthening the international public health surveillance system will continue throughout the century.

## An Explosion of Knowledge and Information Technology

In a world where knowledge doubles every 5 years (Society for Healthcare Planning and Marketing, 1995), it is imperative for health care professions to develop strategies for lifelong learning to prevent knowledge obsolescence. Additionally, "the successful practitioner of the next century will need to master information technologies in order to effectively manage the care of their patients. The computer allows today's generation to aggregate data about populations and understand broader patterns of health and illness" (O'Neil, Pew Health Professions Commission, 1998, p. 18).

Fortunately, the proliferation of information technologies will continue to provide exciting opportunities for self-renewal as well as for developing new approaches to health care delivery (Brownson, Kreuter, 1997). It is predicted that information technology will refine basic business processes, improve the dissemination of clinical information through electronic medical records (EMR), facilitate the analysis of health care data, and strengthen care in rural areas through telehealth and remote monitoring (Institute for the Future, 2000). Information technology can assist health care professionals to significantly improve the delivery of health care services (IOM, 2001). Box 26-1 illustrates how the use of the internet helped control an infectious disease outbreak.

● **BOX 26-1**

*Using the Internet to Help Control an Outbreak of Hantavirus Pulmonary Syndrome*

Hantavirus pulmonary syndrome (HPS), which is carried by rodents, is a lung disease that was first identified during a 1993 outbreak in the southwestern United States. People who become infected often die within days because of severe pulmonary hemorrhage. To prevent and control future outbreaks, the CDC has developed educational materials that use text, images, animation, and video to explain how the disease can be treated and how individuals can avoid infection. These materials are available on CDC's internet website on a page called "All About Hantavirus" (*http://www.cdc.gov/ncidod/diseases/hanta/hps/index.htm*).

In 1997, during an HPS outbreak in Chile, local health care workers used information from this website to mount a multimedia prevention campaign. They designed posters and radio and TV announcements that explained how people could protect themselves and their families from HPS. The announcements offered advice on how to keep rodents out of homes and workplaces and described special precautions for workers who are regularly exposed to rodents. The announcements also urged people in the affected area who experienced flulike symptoms to get immediate medical attention.

By the time an epidemiologic team from CDC arrived in the outbreak area, the campaign was already well under way. Knowing that the public had access to prevention information, the CDC team was able to concentrate its efforts on the epidemiologic investigation. Although the number of HPS cases that were avoided by preventive action cannot be counted, it is likely that many lives were saved by the rapid actions of the Chileans.

From Centers for Disease Control and Prevention (CDC): *Preventing emerging infectious diseases: a strategy for the 21st century,* Atlanta, 1998, CDC, p. 45.

Milio (1995), a nursing leader in the field of community health, has challenged public health professionals to move beyond informatics and create an electronic community infrastructure that provides worldwide linkages between international, national, and local governmental and community organizations. She proposes that such a structure would allow health care professionals to provide information and referral services to local residents and clients, promote awareness and understanding of major health problems among community citizens and policymakers, and support worldwide cooperative efforts focused on the early identification of health concerns and solutions to address these concerns. Community health professionals are increasingly developing health-related partnerships to pursue powerful goals aimed at establishing healthy, healing communities. Use of information technology will be a key component in helping these partnerships to reach their goals. Even community partnerships with limited resources can impact public policy making through the internet (Johnson, 2000) and can maintain easy communication with all members of the partnership.

## Genomics and Biotechnology Advances

In addition to information technology, numerous technological advances, such as virtual reality, robotics, telemedicine, and telenursing will continue to expand and significantly influence community health nursing service delivery in the future. Home telemedicine, telehealth, or telecare systems are currently allowing nurses in some settings to make interactive video home visits. "Telemedicine can be defined as the use of telecommunicating and information technology to provide health care services" (Finkelstein, Speedie, Lundgren, Ideker, 2000, p. 32). Telemedicine systems provide a mechanism for clients and health care providers to see and speak with each other in real time. They also allow providers to assess the client's physical health status and to monitor select blood values (Johnston, 2000).

It is projected that telecare systems will become common in many local communities. Telecare systems have the potential to save costs, improve quality, expand care to vulnerable populations, and reduce isolation for health care providers (Petersen, LaMarche, 2000). These systems make the client an active participant in the care delivery process. However, as the health care industry moves forward in its use of telehealth, professionals are being encouraged to also maintain the compassion and caring components of service delivery (Albright, Slater, 2000). The American Telemedicine Association (2001) has adopted telehomecare clinical guidelines to assist in the development of quality client care through telemedicine systems. Questions focused on client rights and liability will become paramount for ethics committees in health care organizations to consider as new service delivery options become more readily available.

Of all the advances in biotechnology affecting the health care system in the future, the greatest impact will come from the discoveries of the **Human Genome Project (HGP).** Established at the National Institutes of Health and the United States Department of Energy in 1990, this international research project is focused on mapping, sequencing, and analyzing all of the genes of the human genome (Dennis, Gallagher, Campbell, 2001). The **human genome** is the genetic makeup of all humans (Lea, 2000), or all of the chromosomes of a human. The human genome contains between 50,000 and 100,000 genes, which are located within chromosomes (CDC, Office of Genetics and Disease Prevention, 2001; Lea 2000).

The human genome project will revolutionize health care delivery. Gene mapping will promote rapid discovery of new drugs and the prevention and treatment of diseases. However, gene mapping also has the potential to lead to unprecedented ethical, legal, and social implications while bringing about sophisticated diagnostic and therapeutic developments (Heller, Oros, Durney-Crowley, 2000; National Human Genome Research Institute, 2001). The **Ethical, Legal, and Social Implications (ELSI) project,** a subproject of the HGP, is currently addressing these implications. Questions of privacy, confidentiality, genetic discrimination, the uses and misuses of genetic information, and other conceptual and philosophical issues also will become paramount in the future for consumers and ethics committees in health care organizations.

## Increasing Consumer Involvement

The twenty-first century will prove itself as the *golden era* of the consumer. Currently, sophisticated consumers are demanding more say in health care decision making and are being encouraged by health care providers to actively participate on the health care team. As information technology becomes increasingly prevalent in the home and other settings, such as public libraries, churches, and community centers, observers will witness a geometrical acceleration of this trend. Consumers will increasingly access information needed to effectively solve problems about personal health issues as well as community health concerns. Governmental officials are using the internet to seek citizen input about issues critical to the health of the nation. The internet greatly facilitates politicians' efforts to assess health needs and to make more knowledgeable judgments about critical health policy issues. The internet also can facilitate consumers' efforts to communicate effectively with health care providers and to obtain quality health information (Ford, 2000).

Community health professionals have actively promoted the position that the consumer should be the central focus in the new health care delivery system. "Public health, in a reformed health care system, will forge partnerships between communities and all levels of government. Communities and public health agencies—together—will keep the public healthy" (APHA, 1993, unnumbered foreword). Community partnerships are advancing community development efforts as well as community action for health. Provider organizations are working with communities as partners to solve health concerns and to create environments that prevent health problems. These endeavors will continue to grow (Brownson, Kreuter, 1997). It is projected that use of the partnership model will strengthen community-based public health service delivery in the future (Bruce, McKane, 2000).

As educated consumers become increasingly focused on health promotion and risk-reduction activities to improve their quality of life, community health nurses will assume a pivotal role in helping clients to promote health and prevent disease. Community health nurses are uniquely positioned to address preventive health care concerns and to facilitate self-care among various client groups. Future advances in information technology will strengthen nurses' ability to help clients readily access essential health information and develop creative approaches to health education. The challenge for all health care providers will be to effectively and efficiently use technology to benefit diverse client groups, including both the "haves" and the "have nots."

## COMPETENCIES FOR NURSING PRACTICE IN THE TWENTY-FIRST CENTURY

In response to changing societal trends, the health care delivery system has undergone dramatic change, and this change will be even more encompassing throughout the twenty-first century. The health care practitioner in the future will be functioning in a highly integrated, managed care environment focused on delivering cost-effective, high-quality, community-based services. As a new health care environment continues to evolve and the needs of consumers become increasingly complex, the health care system will rely heavily on interdisciplinary teams to effectively and efficiently manage client care in a variety of community settings (Heller, Oros, Durney-Crowley, 2000; O'Neil, Pew Health Professions Commission, 1998). It is envisioned that schools, neighborhood clinics, work sites, and other community settings will become practice sites for providing holistic family- and population-focused care. Community health nurses will be leaders in developing models of care in collaboration with clients that provide services where people live, work, and become educated.

Health care practitioners of tomorrow will need a number of skills to remain competitive in the evolving health care environment. The general consensus is that practitioners of the future need strong critical thinking skills to assist them with problem identification and problem solving (Bruce, McKane, 2000; Ibrahim, House, Levine, 1995; Misener, Alexander, Blaha, et al., 1997; O'Neil, Pew Health Professions Commission, 1998). Having these skills helps the practitioner anticipate and plan for the future. It is also generally believed that health professionals will need effective communication skills; cultural skills; political competencies; business, management, and leadership skills; and lifelong learning skills. From a community health nursing perspective, the practitioner will need a strong knowledge base from nursing, social, and public health sciences that will help them address population-and community-focused health care needs (Association of State and Territorial Directors of Nursing, 2000).

The Pew Health Professions Commission (O'Neil, Pew Health Professions Commission, 1998) argues that health care practitioners of tomorrow must have new attitudes as well as expanded competencies to meet society's evolving health care needs. The specific **professional competencies** needed by health care providers in the twenty-first century are presented in Box 26-2. These competences highlight the need for health care professionals to shift their focus from acute, disease-oriented health care delivery to a greater re-

**BOX 26-2**

*Twenty-One Competencies Needed by Health Professionals in the Twenty-First Century*

1. Embrace a personal ethic of social responsibility and service.
2. Exhibit ethical behavior in all professional activities.
3. Provide evidence-based, clinically competent care.
4. Incorporate the multiple determinants of health in clinical care.
5. Apply knowledge of the new sciences.
6. Demonstrate critical thinking, reflection, and problem-solving skills.
7. Understand the role of primary care.
8. Rigorously practice preventive health care.
9. Integrate population-based care and services into practice.
10. Improve access to health care for those with unmet health needs.
11. Practice relationship-centered care with individuals and families.
12. Provide culturally sensitive care to a diverse society.
13. Partner with communities in health care decisions.
14. Use communication and information technology effectively and appropriately.
15. Work in interdisciplinary teams.
16. Ensure care that balances individual, professional, system, and societal needs.
17. Practice leadership.
18. Take responsibility for quality of care and health outcomes at all levels.
19. Contribute to continuous improvement of the health care system.
20. Advocate for public policy that promotes and protects the health of the public.
21. Continue to learn and help others learn.

From O'Neil EH, Pew Health Professions Commission: *Recreating health professional practice for a new century,* San Francisco, 1998, Pew Health Professions Commission, p. vii.

liance on primary care, prevention, and a population-based care perspective (O'Neil, Pew Health Professions Commission, 1998). They also reflect a need to be committed to the ethical tenets of the profession while appreciating the value of knowledge and technology.

## ETHICS IN COMMUNITY HEALTH NURSING PRACTICE

Rapid changes in the health care delivery system have made life more complex and have provoked dilemmas never before faced by consumers or health care providers. It is becoming increasingly difficult for professionals in many situations to discern what should or should not be done. The ability to preserve lives that once could not be saved, advances in information technology, and governmental cutbacks in health care spending have made it increasingly difficult for community health nurses to examine the concept of human rights and choices.

Community health nurses are making decisions that impact the rights of individuals, families, and communities. They are examining how to protect client rights on the information superhighway, how to meet the needs of all client groups with shrinking resources, and how to deal with ethical issues related to new health care delivery models and biotechnology advances. They also are examining how choices about the delivery of health care services have affected various consumers and consumer groups. It is anticipated that these issues will intensify in the future and that new ethical issues will emerge. A recent survey conducted by The Electronic Privacy Information Center (Kalish, 1997), for example, reflects an urgent need to establish procedures for protecting the privacy of computer users. Issues also are being raised about the ethical implications of genetic testing (Raines, 1998) and ethical issues inherent in managed care (Newman, Dunbar, 2000). Gaining an understanding of ethics can help nurses better deal with these complex and often confusing practice issues.

## Code of Ethics

Ethics is the study of choices made by individuals and groups in their relationships with one another. The development of a code of ethics is basic to a profession because it provides a means for that profession to regulate its practice. It also helps its members make choices relative to clinical practice.

A code indicates a profession's acceptance of the responsibility and trust with which it has been invested by society. Upon entering the profession of nursing, each person inherits a measure of the responsibility and trust that has accrued to nursing over the years and the corresponding obligation to adhere to the profession's code of conduct and relationships for ethical practice. (ANA, 1985)

The American Nurses Association adopted its code of ethics in 1950 and revises it periodically. The most recent revision was published in 1985. A revised code for nurses will be discussed at the ANA national convention in 2002 (Humphrey, 2001). Professional codes of ethics are statements encompassing rules of moral responsibilities that apply to persons in professional roles and that are *voluntarily* adopted by the group themselves (Beauchamp, Childress, 2001). Many national organizations involved in promoting quality health and health-related services have developed a code of ethics for their membership. These codes are designed to preserve the basic rights of clients in an honest and ethical manner.

Implicit in codes of ethics are several fundamental principles. The general consensus is that health care professions have a responsibility to respect a client's right of self-determination in decision making (autonomy), to do

good (beneficence), to avoid harm (nonmaleficence), and to act fairly (justice) when allocating health care resources (Beauchamp, Childress, 2001). Hayne, Moore, and Osborne (1990) argued at the beginning of the 1990s that nursing ethics is at a turning point and that the profession needs to understand the ethic of caring as well as the ethic of justice.

The care-based approach to ethical inquiry focuses on the professional-client relationship and the moral obligation of the professional to protect and promote the well-being of clients in a compassionate and empathic manner (Lowdermilk, Perry, Bobak, 1997; Beauchamp, Childress, 2001). The value of caring in the nurse-client relationship is central to this approach. Throughout the next decade, increased emphasis will be placed on developing a theory of nursing ethics that delineates the uniqueness of ethics in the nurse-client relationship. Nursing has not fully reached the goals proposed by nurse ethicists in the 1990s.

## Ethical Concerns

Friedman, an ethics analyst, believes that ethical concerns in the health care system fall under four major categories (Brown, 1999, p. 259):

- *Access to care issues*, which encompasses insurance practices, provider practices, managed care practices, and access to technology and therapy;
- *Conflict of interest concerns* surrounding such things as the roles of nurse case managers and risk managers, inappropriate financial incentives for health care providers, and the loyalties of investor-owned organizations.
- *Professionalism issues* dealing with professional malpractice, client abuse, confidentiality, clinical experimentation, and other client rights and professional practice concerns; and
- *Ethics of public policy in health care*, which examines issues related to how public policy may influence inequalities in access to care, deny clients service, promote providers turning away uninsured clients, and other policy mandates.

Issues such as these are presenting ethical concerns for professionals in all health care settings. However, the American public has faith that nurses will address these concerns. In recent Gallup Surveys (Humphrey, 2001; Moore, 2001), Americans gave high ratings to nursing on honesty and ethics.

### *Stop and Think About It*

You are interested in becoming a case manager for clients with work disabilities. What type of conflict of interest concerns might you experience in this position? How might you address these concerns?

Nurses in the community setting are addressing ethical dilemmas or multiple-option situations, such as how to deal with conflicting needs of clients and caregivers; when to hospitalize a terminally ill client; resolving conflicts between what is ordered and what is needed; allowing "death with dignity"; maintaining agency standards of productivity while competently meeting increasingly complex care needs of clients; restoring access to care; and providing service, based on payer regulations (Drane, 1997; Elsner, Quinn, Fanning, et al., 1999; Michigan Home Health Association [MHHA], 1990; Newman, Dunbar, 2000). Community health nurses also are addressing how to balance the needs of populations, individuals, and families. "The care of individuals is at the center of health care delivery, but must be viewed and practiced within the overall context to continuing to generate the greatest possible health gains for groups and populations" (Tavistock Group, 1999, p. 2). During the next decade, community-based health care practitioners will increasingly need to address ethical challenges such as the rightness of shifting health care costs to informal care providers, the appropriate role of the family in medical decision making, and the fair distribution of the care burden in a family setting (Fleck, 1997).

What to do *when* (not if) an ethical crisis occurs is the key question the health care practitioner will be asking in the future (Clemen-Stone, 1997). Currently community health professionals are experiencing unprecedented demands and client care complexities on a daily basis. With the revolutionary changes occurring in the health care delivery system, there is no question that these demands and complexities will increase in the future and that most professionals will experience many ethical dilemmas throughout their career.

"Practitioners of the future must be able to frame their work in ethically sensitive ways and provide education and counseling for patients, families, and communities in situations where ethical issues arise" (Pew Health Professions Commission, 1995, p. 6). Community health organizations are increasingly establishing ethics committees to help practitioners carry out this responsibility. Ethics committees play a key role in promoting an understanding of ethical practice through education, consultation, and the development of standards for ethical practice. "Regardless of the setting, the primary purpose of ethics committees is to provide a structural format for individuals within an organization to increase their awareness of ethics and its application to clinical practice" (Haddad, 1992, pp. 8, 10). Ethics committees play a vital role in helping practitioners resolve ethical dilemmas. This role will become more paramount throughout the next decade (Maier, 2000).

The critical ethical concern for community health nurses in the future will be to ensure that cost-effective, quality health care is available to people in need. To achieve this goal, practitioners of the future must analyze social and health care situations from an ethical perspective that addresses community as well as individual needs. Practitioners also will need to shape health policy through research and political action. Health care reform will not evolve from interventions focused on individuals. Strong,

collective community action for health, supported by sound research and health policy, is needed to resolve the nation's current health crises.

## NURSING RESEARCH

Better health through nursing research was the theme of the 1996 International Nurses' Day (Holzemer, Tierney, 1996). The focus on this day was to highlight the fact that nursing care can make significant, cost-effective contributions that improve the quality of people's lives. This will be the continuing challenge for practitioners throughout the coming decade. To remain competitive in the evolving health care system, health professionals will need to conduct outcomes research to demonstrate that they can provide quality, cost-effective services that can be measured (Hadley, 1996). Demonstrating the outcomes of health promotion interventions will be particularly challenging for community health nurses in the future.

The nursing profession has actively promoted the position that nurses must engage in research to enhance the health of the nation. The **National Institute of Nursing Research (NINR)** (2000) "supports clinical and basic research to establish a scientific basis for the care of individuals across the life span" (p. 1), and families within a community context. The NINR also supports research that focuses on the special needs of subsets of the population, such as at-risk and underserved groups, with an emphasis on health disparities (NINR, 2000). This focus is consistent with the nation's national health agenda, which emphasizes eliminating health disparities by 2010 (USDHHS, 2000).

The mandates for the NINR are displayed in Box 26-3. Nursing research related to these mandates makes a significant difference. NINR-supported researchers have contributed to health care delivery and the scientific knowledge base that lays a foundation for effective nursing interventions. An example of a NINR initiative that has made a difference is the research funded by NINR to examine the impact of home visits by nurses to disadvantaged

**BOX 26-3**

*Mandates for the National Institute of Nursing Research*

- Understand and ease the symptoms of acute and chronic illness.
- Prevent or delay the onset of disease or disability or slow its progression.
- Find effective approaches to achieving and sustaining good health.
- Improve the clinical settings in which care is provided.

From National Institute of Nursing Research (NINR): *Mission statement*, Bethesda, Md, 2000, NINR. Retrieved from the internet March 12, 2001. *http://www.nih.gov/ninr/research/diversity/mission.html*

young mothers and their children. This research demonstrated that these home visits "can improve physical and mental health, reduce child injuries and abuse, and lower the numbers of arrests of mothers and of families that are dependent on welfare" (NINR, 2000, p. 4).

Community health nursing, by definition, deals with vulnerable populations that have special health problems and needs. Nurses in this practice area are uniquely positioned to identify significant, researchable questions related to NINR's research priorities. Nurses at all levels of practice are needed to identify relevant research issues and to document outcomes of nursing practice. Informing health policy through nursing research or the utilization of nursing research is an evolving tradition for the discipline in the future (Hinshaw, 1999).

## POLITICAL INVOLVEMENT

The most powerful approach that nurses can take to shape the future is the political approach. It is vital that nurses understand, actively participate in, and provide leadership in politics and the political process. Nurses make up the largest

group of health care providers in the country, and numbers alone give them a powerful majority. Today's nurses are becoming more politically active, visible, and powerful and are providing leadership in health care delivery. Practitioners in the future will need to expand their political involvement to ensure that people in need have consumer-accessible care.

**Political action** usually involves activities directed toward influencing the behavior of governmental officials and other individuals. Health care professionals focus on influencing **health policy** or "authoritative decisions made within government that pertain to health and to the pursuit of health" (Longest, 1998, p. 1). State and federal health policies and regulations significantly influence the practice of nursing and health care delivery. Politics and nursing are inseparable and, in fact, politics is an integral part of nursing. The political arena is where health care decisions are made, decisions that will bear on the profession and health care for all.

"The nursing profession has a long history of political activism that has been heightened in recent years through the politics of health care reform" (Cohen, Mason, Kouner, et al., 1996, p. 259). Nursing's political involvement in health ac-

**TABLE 26-1**

*The Progress of Nursing Through Four Stages of Political Development*

| | STAGE 1 (BUY-IN) | STAGE 2 (SELF-INTEREST) | STAGE 3 (POLITICAL SOPHISTICATION) | STAGE 4 (LEADING THE WAY) |
|---|---|---|---|---|
| Nature of action | Reactive, with a focus on nursing issues | Reactive to nursing issues (e.g., funding for nursing education) and broader issues (e.g., long-term care and immunizations) | Proactive on nursing and other health issues (e.g., Nursing's Agenda for Health Care Reform) | Proactive on leadership and agenda-setting for a broad range of health and social policy issues |
| Language | Learning political language | Using nurse jargon (e.g., caring, nursing diagnosis) | Using parlance and rhetoric common to health policy deliberations | Introducing terms that re-order the debate |
| Coalition building | Political awareness; occasional participation in coalitions | Coalition forming among nursing organizations | Coalition forming among nursing groups; active and significant participation in broader health care groups (e.g., Clinton Task Force on Health Care Reform) | Initiating coalitions beyond nursing for broad health policy concerns |
| Nurses as policy shapers | Isolated cases of nurses being appointed to policy positions, primarily because of individual accomplishments | Professional associations get nurses into nursing-related positions | Professional organizations get nurses appointed to health-related policy positions (e.g., nurse position on ProPAC) | Many nurses sought to fill nursing and health policy positions because of value of nursing expertise and knowledge |

From Cohen SS, Mason DJ, Kouner C, et al.: Stages of nursing's political development: where we've been and where we ought to go, *Nurs Outlook* 44:259-266, 1996, p. 260.

tion has evolved through several stages (Table 26-1) and reflects a movement from a reactive stance to a proactive stance. It has progressed from the "buy in," or stage of awareness where the profession recognized the importance of political activism, to the stage of political sophistication where nursing has gone beyond self-interest and is proactively campaigning on behalf of the public. The challenge for the future will be to "lead the way" in health care policy. At this stage, "nurses become the initiators of crucial health policy ideas and innovations as instigators, leaders, or formulators of health policy" (Cohen, Mason, Kouner, et al., p. 263).

There are several different ways to achieve one's goals in the legislative arena (deVries, Vanderbilt, 1992). Nurses are actively involved in writing letters, sending telegrams, making phone calls, arranging meetings with officials and legislators, making political contributions, and attending political meetings. They also are involved in political campaign efforts aimed at helping a candidate get elected, in taking an active role in the political aspects of professional organizations, in lobbying, and in running for political office (Cohen, Mason, Kouner, et al., 1996).

Individual and collective political action by nurses has significantly strengthened the political power of nursing. At last count 97 nurses have held elected positions in state legislatures (Farmer, Henderson, Ladenbeim, 2001), and many more were members of legislative staff. These nurse politicians will be focusing on such issues as the costs and coverage of prescription drugs; the parity, delivery, and funding of mental health services; health care costs; the allocation of tobacco settlement funds; women's health; and elderly abuse and neglect (Duncan, Kenny, 2001). These are issues central to the practice of nursing and to achieving health care for all.

## *Stop and Think About It*

Identify a vulnerable population (e.g., homeless, uninsured or low-income underinsured individuals, or domestic violence victims) in your local community. What type of health policy change at the local, state, or federal level could improve service delivery to this population? How and with whom might you partner to promote legislative action to assist your identified population?

## HEALTH FOR ALL: A MAJOR CHALLENGE FOR THE FUTURE

The American Public Health Association (APHA) has openly and aggressively championed the right of health for all in the United States. This is a significant goal but one that will take time and effort to achieve. In 1963 President Lyndon Johnson shared with the American public that "Yesterday is not ours to recover but tomorrow is ours to win or lose." The battle to win in the twenty-first century is the health care system's ability to extend access to health care services to all and ultimately to improve the quality of life

among Americans (USDHHS, 2000). Although data suggest that significant difficulties in our health care system presently prevent the nation from providing health for all, these obstacles can be overcome. The United States has had a long list of accomplishments in health care delivery and has a strong potential for achieving major public health goals.

The twenty-first century has brought many health care challenges. **"Health care for all"** in a managed care environment is a major one. This challenge will involve providing culturally competent health care, maintaining a "safety net" where the growing population of uninsured can obtain basic care, and addressing emerging threats to the health of public while containing costs (IOM, 2000).

A recent IOM (2000) report has found that America's health care safety net is intact but endangered. The **health care safety net** is "those providers that organize and deliver a significant level of health care and other related services to uninsured, Medicaid, and other vulnerable patients" [populations] (IOM, 2000, p. 3). Currently, safety net providers are serving a disproportionate share of low-income and uninsured clients, and the number of uninsured persons is growing significantly. There are 44 million people who lack health care coverage, an increase of 11 million since 1990 (IOM, 2000). Lack of health care coverage presents access challenges.

The "health for all" challenge emphasizes access to health care that will enable all people to lead productive and satisfying lives. This challenge involves addressing the inequities in society and within the health care system that prevent people from achieving health, and it focuses on the shared responsibility of people for their own health. This battle requires implementing strategies that promote broad-based planning for health and development rather than for health services only. It demands a strong emphasis on political action, policy formulation, multidisciplinary practice, sound managerial functioning, and constituency building (IOM, 1988; Maglacas, 1988). Constituency building is a "must." Current and future threats to our nation's public health will require collective action if they are to be resolved.

It has been well over 100 years since public health/community health nursing was started in the United States. This is a time to reflect on the rich heritage that Florence Nightingale, Lillian Wald, and many others provided for us. The health problems of today are much like the ones these women faced: communicable diseases, high infant mortality, and poverty. Wald and Nightingale viewed these problems as political ones and emphasized that the public's health had to improve to change these problems. That fact is as true today as it was during Wald and Nightingale's time. Let us take on the mantle of developing a scientific basis for the nursing care of aggregates. Let us also use the stories of our sisters of the past to guide us in our future while recognizing that because our circumstances are new, we must develop innovative

*A view
from the field*

## PUBLIC HEALTH STANDS AS A PROVEN MODEL FOR FUTURE DELIVERY SYSTEMS

When Karen Wilson became the first nurse ever appointed director of a county health district in Texas, a headline in an area newspaper read "Nursing the Public Health."

The headline captures the essence of what many nurses feel is part of the solution to America's health care crisis—the utilization of public health nurses in existing public health structures.

"Public health nurses are experts at immunization, prenatal care, well child care, screening programs, outreach into the community, education—all that is critical in a health care reform package," said Wilson, MPH, MN, RN, who now directs a staff of 43 at the Williamson County and Cities Health District in Georgetown, Texas. "The emphasis must be reshifted to preventive care and early identification of problems, and that's been the business of public health for decades."

Mike Nilsson, RN, a public health nurse from Clearwater, Fla., firmly believes that the Administration's task force on health care reform must take into account a proven model of delivery.

"We don't need a new model. We know what works. We may fine tune it. We may upgrade it. We may computerize it. But the basis is there," he said. "I want Hillary's task force to come out and say that prevention is needed from the very beginning, and in order to make that work we're going to put 'x' amount of dollars, whether it's millions or billions or whatever, into rebuilding the public health system in this country."

Wilson believes that public health nurses should have a greater voice in health care reform discussions because of their expertise. She says that not only does the public health structure emphasize wellness and prevention, but it addresses issues of access and how to provide care to underserved populations. Ensuring access is a key tenet of *Nursing's Agenda for Health Care Reform* and continues to be one of the greatest challenges facing the President's Task Force on National Health Care Reform.

"Public health nurses just laugh when they hear that the new buzzwords are case management and care coordination because that's what public health nurses have done since day one. It's helping clients get into the health programs they need," Wilson said.

In Wilson's district, a case management team of nurses, social workers, nutrition staff, and clerical staff meet often to solve problems jointly. Wilson notes that the "the more people who can form that safety net, the less likely that someone will fall through the cracks in the system."

Yet, often the groups who need health care the most will not seek it out in the present medical model of delivery, said Nilsson. "Before it was vogue, we were out in the minority communities, the communities with inadequate transportation, in the schools. We went into the homes to speak to teenagers and young women about prenatal and postnatal care or well-baby services. We discussed the whole spectrum of care."

Nilsson said, however, he has witnessed a "deterioration" of the public health system in his state and elsewhere due to a number of factors such as inadequate funding. "If the legislators and decision-makers don't value or understand prevention—if they don't see the value of public health nurses—they eliminate them." He said that legislators may not understand the "whole theory behind upfront prevention dollars—that it may take five years and cost in the short-term, but it will save you from spending thousands of dollars on the other end to take care of crack babies or a child who develops a chronic problem because of a measles outbreak."

Wilson said that current systems make it difficult for some populations to receive all the services they need—where clients must apply for Medicare and Medicaid in one office, health screenings in another office, and housing subsidies in still another location. She advocates a system where clients can "come in and tell their story one time to determine eligibility for a multiplicity of programs at once." A strength of public health nurses, she adds, is that they recognize the "needs of the whole person" and that some health care needs must wait until a family deals with more urgent social or survival needs.

Nilsson said that he hopes the administration recognizes the untapped resources of public health because "the potential is so great and we've got so much to offer."

"Our country has a lot of strong programs and a lot of experts" already available to address issues related to reform, Wilson added. "This doesn't have to be reinvented."

From Mikulencak M: Public health stands as a proven model for future delivery systems, *Am Nurse* 25(6):18, 1993.

population-focused interventions (Association of State and Territorial Directors of Nursing, 2000).

## SUMMARY

Community health professionals face many challenges. They are being asked to assume responsibility for care of unprecedented complexity and to plan services for multiple, diverse population groups. They must make some difficult decisions about the best means of allocating scarce resources, which often presents ethical dilemmas not easily solved. Competition has increased the number of selected types of community-based services but has not necessarily strengthened services for those most in need.

Sophisticated technology, spiraling health care costs, demographic changes, and increasing consumer involvement in health care decision making are dramatically influencing future directions in the health care delivery system. There is an increasing reliance on primary care, disease prevention, self-care, and cost-containment strategies. These trends present both challenges and opportunities for health care providers and consumers alike. To shape the future, health professionals must be risk takers. They must handle ethical dilemmas and engage in research activities to document the need for and the effectiveness of preventive health services, and they must be politically *active*. They also must develop new global competencies and capabilities and become technologically literate.

Let us as community health nurses think about the future so that we have the very best one possible. Let us follow Lillian Wald's ways and lead the way. Lillian Wald demonstrated the value of creating new practice roles and innovative service delivery strategies. That is our challenge for the twenty-first century.

## CRITICAL THINKING
*exercise*

The accompanying A View from the Field is a news release about a nurse who was "the first nurse ever appointed director of a county health district in Texas . . ." (Mikulencak, 1993, p. 18). The title of the article is "Public health stands as a proven model for future delivery systems." Do you believe this is feasible? Can community health nurses make a significant impact on the health care systems of this country? Justify your answers.

## REFERENCES

Albright K, Slater S: Medical devices in the home: present and future applications, *Caring* 19(7):36-38, 40, 2000.

American Association of Retired Persons (AARP), Administration on Aging: A *profile of older Americans 2000*, Washington, DC, 2001, AOA.

American Nurses Association (ANA): *Code for nurses with interpretive statements*, ANA, Pub Code No. G-58, Kansas City, Mo, 1985, ANA.

American Public Health Association (APHA): *Public health in a reformed health care system: a vision for the future*, Washington, DC, 1993, APHA.

American Telemedicine Association: *ATA adopts telehomecare clinical guidelines*, March, 2001, ATA. Retrieved from the internet June, 2001. *http://www.atmeda.org/news/guidelines.html*

Association of State and Territorial Directors of Nursing: *Public health nursing: a partner for healthy populations*, Washington, DC, 2000, American Nurses Publishing.

Beauchamp T, Childress J: *Principles of biomedical ethics*, ed 5, New York, 2001, Oxford University Press.

Brown C: Ethics, policy, and practice: interview with Emily Friedman, *Image J Nurs Sch* 31(3):259-262, 1999.

Brownson RC, Kreuter MW: Future trends affecting public health: challenges and opportunities, *J Public Health Management Practice* 3(2):49-60, 1997.

Bruce T, McKane S: *Community-based public health: a partnership model*, Washington, DC, 2000, American Public Health Association.

Buerhaus P: Aging nurses in an aging society: long-term implications, *Reflections on Nursing Leadership* 27(1):35-37, 46, 2001.

Buerhaus P, Staiger D, Ayerbach D: Implications of a rapidly aging registered nurse workforce, *JAMA* 283(22):2948-2954, 2000.

Centers for Disease Control and Prevention (CDC): *Preventing emerging infectious diseases: a strategy for the 21ˢᵗ century*, Atlanta, 1998, CDC.

Centers for Disease Control and Prevention (CDC), Office of Genetics and Disease Prevention: *Public health genetics: glossary of genetic terms*, Atlanta, 2001, CDC. Retrieved from the internet March 12, 2001. *http://www.medinfo.cam.ac.uk/phgu/info_database/glossary.asp*

Cetron M, Davies O: Trends now changing the world: economics and society, values, and concerns, energy and environment, *The Futurist* 35(1):30-43, 2001.

Clemen-Stone S: What to do when (not if) an ethical crisis occurs, *Michigan Home Health Association News* 6:1-2, 1997.

Cohen SS, Mason DJ, Kouner C, et al.: Stages of nursing's political development: where we've been and where we ought to go, *Nurs Outlook* 44:259-266, 1996.

Dalaker J, Proctor B, US Census Bureau: *Poverty in the United States: 1999*, Washington, DC, 2000, US Government Printing Office.

Dennis C, Gallagher R, Campbell P: The human genome: everyone's genome, *Nature* 409:813, 2001.

deVries CM, Vanderbilt MC: *The grass roots lobbying handbook*, Washington, DC, 1992, ANA.

Drane J: *Caring to the end*, Erie, Penn, 1997, Lake Area Health Education Center.

Duncan D, Kenny H: Survey of state health priorities for 2001: preliminary findings, *State Health Notes: special report* 22:1-3, 2001.

Elsner R, Quinn M, Fanning S, et al.: Ethical and policy considerations for centenarians—the oldest old, *Image J Nurs Sch* 31(3):263-268, 1999.

Farmer C, Henderson T, Ladenheim K: Nurses in state legislatures: gaining an edge on vital health policy issues, *State Health Notes* 22(341):1,5-6, 2001.

Finkelstein S, Speedie S, Lundgren J, Ideker M: Telehome care: connecting the home and the home care agency, *Caring* 19(7):32-35, 2000.

Fleck LM: Just caring: ethical issues in high-tech home care, *Michigan Home Health Association News* 6(2):1, 3, 7-10, 12, 1997.

Ford P: Is the internet changing the relationship between consumers and practitioners? *J Healthc Qual* 22(5):41-43, 2000.

Haddad AM: Developing an organizational ethos, *Caring* 11:4, 7-8, 10-11, 1992.

Hadley EH: Nursing in the political and economic marketplace: challenges for the 21st century, *Nurs Outlook* 44:6-10, 1996.

Harris M: Marketing health care to minorities: tapping an energy market, *Marketing Health Services* 20(2):5-9, 2000.

Hayne Y, Moore S, Osborne M: Nursing ethics: a turning point, *Nurs Forum* 25:10-12, 30, 1990.

Heller B, Oros M, Durney-Crowley J: The future of education: 10 trends to watch, *Nursing and Health Care Perspectives* 21:9-13, 2000.

Hinshaw A: Evolving nursing research traditions: influencing factors. In Hinshaw A, Feetham S, Shaver J, editors: *Handbook of Clinical Nursing Research,* Thousand Oaks, Calif, 1999, Sage Publications.

Holzemer W, Tierney A: How nursing research makes a difference, *Int Nurs Rev* 43:49-52, 1996.

Humphrey C: Nursing rated most ethical profession, *Home Healthc Nurse* 19(2):63, 2001.

Ibrahim MA, House RM, Levine RH: Educating the public health workforce for the 21st century, *Fam Community Health* 18:17-25, 1995.

Institute of Medicine (IOM): *The future of public health,* Washington, DC, 1988, National Academy Press.

Institute for the Future: *Health and health care 2010: the forecast, the challenge,* San Francisco, 2000, Jossey-Bass Publishers.

Institute of Medicine (IOM): *America's health care safety net: intact but endangered,* Washington, DC, 2000, National Academy Press.

Institute of Medicine (IOM): *Crossing the quality chasm: a new health system for the 21st century,* Washington, DC, 2001, National Academy Press.

Johnson D: The internet alters politics, *The Futurist* 34(1):11, 2000.

Johnston B: Exploring the new frontier: home care gets wired, *Caring* 19(7):6-11, 2000.

Kalish DE: Cyberspies often haunt web sites, survey says, *Ann Arbor News,* June 9, 1997, pp. A-1, A-12.

Lea D: A clinician's primer in human genetics: what nurses need to know, *Nurs Clin North Am* 35:583-614, 2000.

Leininger M: Future directions in transcultural nursing in the 21st century, *Int Nurs Rev* 44:19-23, 1997.

Longest B: *Health policy making in the United States,* ed 2, Chicago, 1998, Health Administration Press.

Lowdermilk DL, Perry SE, Bobak IM: *Maternity and women's health care,* ed 6, St Louis, 1997, Mosby.

Maglacas AM: Health for all: nursing's role, *Nurs Outlook* 36:66-71, 1988.

Maier F: Ethics in home care agencies, *Caring* 19(8):6-13, 2000.

Marín G, Burhansstipanov L, Connell CM, et al.: A research agenda for health education among underserved populations, *Health Educ Q* 22:346-363, 1995.

Marketing Health Services editors: Forecasting U.S. health care's future, *Marketing Health Services* 20(4):5-13, 2000.

Michigan Home Health Association (MHHA), Ethics Committee: *Ethical dilemmas experienced by professionals in home health care,* unpublished research project, East Lansing, Mich, 1990, MHHA.

Mikulencak M: Public health stands as a proven model for future delivery systems, *Am Nurse* 25(6):18, 1993.

Milio N: Beyond informatics: an electronic community infrastructure for public health, *J Public Health Management Practice* 1(4):84-94, 1995.

Misener TR, Alexander JW, Blaha AJ, et al.: National delphi study to determine competencies for nursing leadership in public health, *Image J Nurs Sch* 29:47-51, 1997.

Moore D: *Firefighters top Gallup's "honesty and ethics" list: nurses and members of military close behind,* 2001, Gallup Organization. Retrieved from the internet December, 2001. *http://www.gallup.com/poll/releases/pr011205.asp*

National Human Genome Research Institute: *Ethical, legal and social implications (ELSI) program areas,* March, 2001, NIH. Retrieved from the internet March 12, 2001. *http://www.nhgri.nih.gov/about-NHGRI/Der/Elsi/high-priority.html*

National Institute of Nursing Research (NINR): *Mission statement,* Bethesda, Md, 2000, NINR. Retrieved from the internet March 12, 2001. *http://www.nih.gov/ninr/research/diversity/mission.html*

Newman J, Dunbar P: Managed care and ethical conflicts, *Managed Care Quarterly* 8(4):20-32, 2000.

Olshansky S, Carnes B, Rogers R, Smith L: The challenge of prediction: the fifth stage of epidemiologic transition, *World Health Stat Q* 51(2/3/4): 99-119, 1998.

O'Neil EH, Pew Health Professions Commission: *Recreating health professional practice for a new century,* San Francisco, 1998, Pew Health Professions Commission.

Parks S: The future in dietetics. In Winterfeldt E, Ebro L, Bogle M, editors: *The profession of dietetics: present practices, future trends,* Gaithersburg, Md, 1997, Aspen.

Petersen M, LaMarche D: Telemedicine: evolving technology in an e-health care world, *Managed Care Quarterly* 8(3):15-21, 2000.

Pew Health Professions Commission: *Critical challenges: revitalizing the health professions for the 21st century,* San Francisco, 1995, UCSF Center for the Health Professions.

Raines D: Ethical implications of genetic testing, *Nurs Clin North Am* 33(2):275-286, 1998.

Seymour J: Old diseases, new danger, *Nurs Times* 93:22-24, 1997.

Society for Healthcare Planning and Marketing: *Environmental assessment, 1995-1996: renaissance for health care,* Chicago, 1995, American Hospital Association.

Tavistock Group: Journal priorities, ethical principles, *Image: J Nurs Sch* 31(1):2-3, 1999.

US Department of Health and Human Services (USDHHS): *Healthy people 2010, conference edition,* vols 1 and 2, Washington, DC, 2000, US Government Printing Office.

Wilson C, Mitchell B: Nursing 2000: collaboration to promote careers in registered nursing, *Nurs Outlook* 47:56-61, 1999.

## SELECTED BIBLIOGRAPHY

Eliss JR, Hartley CL: *Nursing in the 21st century: challenges, issues and trends,* Philadelphia, 2000, JB Lippincott.

Fos P, Fine D: *Designing health care for populations: applied epidemiology in health care administration,* San Francisco, 2000, Jossey-Bass.

Fry S: Toward a theory of nursing ethics, *Adv Nurs Sci* 11(4):9-22, 1989.

Gold R: Genetic counseling. In Association of Women's Health, Obstetric and Neonatal Nurses (AWHONN), editor: *Every woman: the essential guide for healthy living,* New York, 2000, Profile Pursuit, pp. 260-265.

Haddad A: The future of ethical decision making in health care, *Nurs Clin North Am* 33(2):373-384, 1998.

Hein EC: *Nursing issues in the 21st century,* Philadelphia, 2001, JB Lippincott.

Kramarow E, Lentzner H, Rooks R, et al.: *Health and aging chartbook. Health, United States, 1999,* Hyattsville, Md, 1999, National Center for Health Statistics.

Magilvy J, Brown N, Moritz P: Community-focused interventions and outcomes strategies. In Hinshaw A, Feetham S, Shaver J, editors: *Handbook of clinical nursing research,* Thousand Oaks, Calif, 1999, Sage.

Mason D, Leavitt J: *Policy and politics in nursing and health care,* ed 3, Philadelphia, 1998, WB Saunders.

Nicoll L: *Computers in nursing: nurses' guide to the internet,* ed 3, Philadelphia, 2000, Lippincott, Williams and Wilkins.

Ozar D, Berg J, Werhane P, et al.: *Organizational ethics in health care: toward a model for ethical decision making by provider organizations,* Chicago, 1999, American Medical Association.

Pulcini J, Mason D, Solomon C, et al.: Health policy and the private sector: new vistas for nursing, *Nursing and Health Care Perspectives* 21(1):22-28, 2000.

Rowitz L: *Public health leadership: putting principles into practice*, Gaithersburg, Md, 2001, Aspen.

White G: What we may expect from ethics and the law, *Am J Nurs* 100(10):114-116, 118, 2000.

Willard S, Dean L: AIDs in the elderly: aging raised unique treatment concerns, *Advance for Nurse Practitioners* 8(7):54, 56-58, 2000.

# Index

Page references followed by "f" indicate figures, "t" indicate tables, and "b" indicate boxes.

# Guide to Selected Key Topics*

## AIDS/HIV AND STDS

Sexually Transmitted Diseases as Contemporary Health
  Issues, *420*
Health Risks Related to STDs and HIV/AIDS, *422*
AIDS Cases in the United States at Time of Diagnosis, *422*
Risk Behaviors for STDs and HIV/AIDS, *423*
Opportunistic Conditions Related to AIDS, *423*
Levels of Prevention for STDs and HIV/AIDS, *425*
Commonly Acquired Sexually Transmitted Diseases, *443*
Sexually Transmitted Disease During Childhood, *538*
AIDS in the Workplace, *730*

## CATASTROPHIC EVENTS

Disaster Nursing, *161*
Disaster Nursing Legislation, *161*
Defining Emergency and Major Disaster, *162*
The Nursing Role in Disasters, *163*
Community Disaster Strategies for Nurses, *164*
Phases of Disaster Management, *164*
Disaster Management Responsibilities: Preparedness,
  Response, and Recovery, *165*
Phases of Emotional Reaction During a Disaster, *168*
Biological/Chemical Warfare: An Epidemiological
  Challenge, *366*
Clinical Characteristics of Critical Biological Agents, *367*
Epidemiological Clues that May Signal a Biological or
  Chemical Terrorist Attack, *369*

## CHRONIC ILLNESS

Utilizing the Epidemiological Process with Chronic
  Disease, *363*
Childhood Chronic Conditions, *534*
Adults with Chronic Illness, *590*
Chronic, Disabling, and Handicapping Conditions, *601*
Common Risk Factors for Chronic Conditions, *601*
Chronic Pain, *609*

## COMMUNICABLE DISEASE

Factors Influencing Infectious Disease Transmission and
  Progression, *345*
Stages of Infection, *347*
Infectious Diseases Designated as Notifiable at the National
  Level—United States, 2000, *357*
Infectious Disease: A Neglected Public Health
  Mandate, *360*

What Are Emerging Infectious Diseases and Why Are
  They Emerging?, *361*
Emerging Infectious Disease Issues, *361*
Tuberculosis, *362*
Common Communicable Disease, *375*
Hepatitis B and Other Bloodborne Pathogens in the
  Workplace, *731*
Tuberculosis in the Workplace, *731*

## CULTURE

Clinical Practice: The Nurse, Religious Beliefs,
  and Health, *57*
A Town in Brazil, *76*
Select Alternative Family Structures in the
  United States, *172*
Examples of Rituals and Symbols in Family Systems, *188*
Cultural Values and Attitude, *188*
Religious Beliefs, *190*
Cultural Characteristics Related to Health Care
  of Children and Families, *200*
Bloch's Ethnic/Cultural Assessment Guide, *208*
Religious Beliefs that Affect Nursing Care, *213*
Effects of Culture on Perceptions of Stress and Crisis, *232*
Giger and Davidhizar's Transcultural Assessment
  Model, *258, 293*
Cultural Factors Influence Practice, *258*
Cultural Phenomena to Be Considered Throughout the
  Nursing Process, *259*
Cross-Cultural Examples of Cultural Phenomena Affecting
  Nursing Care, *260*
Examples of Disparity in Health Beliefs, *262*
Guidelines for Relating to Clients from Different Cultures,
  *263*
Select Cultural and Biopsychosocial Characteristics of an
  Individual, *266*
Cultural Barriers to the Referral Process, *326*
Guidelines for Reporting Federal Data on Race and
  Hispanic Origin, *402*
Minority Populations and Health Disparities, *403*
Nurses and Cultural Competence, *405*
Providing Culturally Competent Care to a Target Minority
  Population, *405*
Transcultural Resources, *406*
Providing Culturally Appropriate Community Educational
  Messages, *496*
Madres a Madres: A Community Partnership
  for Health, *503*

*See table of contents and index for a comprehensive list of topics covered.